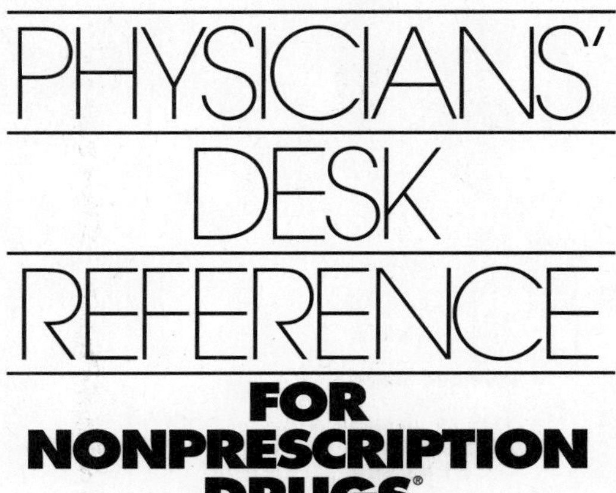

FOR NONPRESCRIPTION DRUGS®

ISBN: 1-56363-203-9

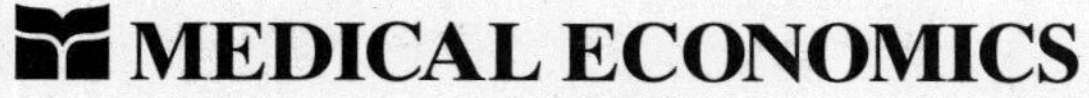
MEDICAL ECONOMICS

FOREWORD

Welcome to the eighteenth edition of *Physicians' Desk Reference For Nonprescription Drugs*, the handy companion to *PDR* that provides you with detailed information on 700 over-the-counter remedies, nutritional supplements, home diagnostic tests, and other self-care aids.

An exciting new feature in this year's edition is *PDR*'s unique Companion Drug Index—a convenient guide to over-the-counter products that may be used, in conjunction with prescription drug therapy, to reverse drug-induced side effects, relieve symptoms of the illness itself, or alleviate conditions resulting from the primary disease. For each problem, this new index lists associated categories of prescription drugs, then enumerates the various over-the-counter preparations that can be expected to provide symptomatic relief.

All the medications described in *PDR for Nonprescription Drugs* are also indexed in the popular *PDR Guide;* and you'll find an important new feature in this volume as well. The 1997 edition includes, for the first time, a comprehensive contraindications index, providing you with a handy list of drugs to avoid in any given situation. With this addition, the guide now becomes the *PDR Guide to Drug Interactions, Side Effects, Indications, Contraindications*—a truly unique database of the major prescribing considerations that concern every physician the most.

This year, you also might want to pay a visit to *PDRnet.com* on the World Wide Web. This exciting new on-line service offers registered users free MEDLINE service, as well as instant access to all the prescribing information found in *PDR* and its companion volumes.

The new *PDRnet.com* service is the latest member of the growing *PDR* family of medical references available in both traditional and electronic form. The list of printed references from *PDR* now includes:

- *Physicians' Desk Reference®*
- *PDR Guide to Drug Interactions, Side Effects, Indications, Contraindications™*
- *PDR For Nonprescription Drugs®*
- *PDR For Ophthalmology®*
- *PDR® Generics™*
- *PDR® Medical Dictionary™*
- *PDR® Nurse's Handbook™*
- *PDR® Nurse's Dictionary™*
- *PDR Supplements*

PDR and its major companion volumes are also found in the *PDR® Electronic Library™* on CD-ROM, now used in over 40,000 practices. This Windows-compatible disc provides users with a complete database of *PDR* prescribing information, electronically searchable for instant retrieval. A standard subscription includes *PDR*'s sophisticated prescription-screening program and an exhaustive file of chemical structures, illustrations, and full-color product photographs. Optional enhancements include the complete contents of *The Merck Manual* and *Stedman's Medical Dictionary*, as well as a handy file of patient handouts drawn from *PDR*'s consumer handbook, *The PDR® Family Guide to Prescription Drugs®*. The disc is available for use on individual PCs and PC networks.

For personal use—on rounds or on the go—there's also *Pocket PDR®*, a unique handheld electronic database of prescribing information that literally fits in your pocket. For facilities with large, mainframe-based information systems, *PDR* information is also available as a preformatted text file on magnetic tape. And for anyone who wants to run a fast double-check on any proposed prescription, there's the *PDR® Drug Interactions, Side Effects, Indications, Contraindications System™* — an electronic version of the *PDR Guide* capable of automatically screening a 20-drug regimen for conflicts, then proposing alternatives for any problematic medication. For more information on these or any other members of the growing family of *PDR* products, please call, toll-free, 1-800-232-7379 or fax 201-573-4956.

Physicians' Desk Reference For Nonprescription Drugs is published annually by Medical Economics Company in cooperation with participating manufacturers. The function of the publisher is the compilation, organization, and distribution of product information obtained from manufacturers. Each product description has been prepared by the manufacturer, and edited and approved by the manufacturer's medical department, medical director, and/or medical consultant. During compilation of this information, the publisher has emphasized the necessity of describing products comprehensively, in order to provide all the facts necessary for sound and intelligent decision making. The descriptions seen here include all information made available by the manufacturer.

In organizing and presenting this material in *Physicians' Desk Reference For Nonprescription Drugs,* the publisher does not warrant or guarantee any of the products described, or perform any independent analysis in connection with any of the product information contained herein. *Physicians' Desk Reference For Nonprescription Drugs* does not assume, and expressly disclaims, any obligation to obtain and include any information other than that provided to it by the manufacturer. It should be understood that by making this material available the publisher is not advocating the use of any product described herein, nor is the publisher responsible for misuse of a product due to typographical error. Additional information on any product may be obtained from the manufacturer.

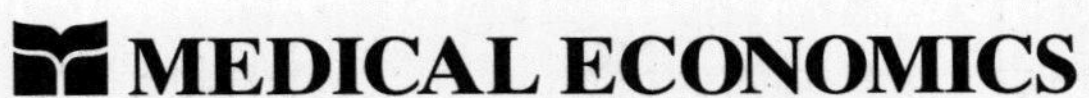
MEDICAL ECONOMICS

CONTENTS

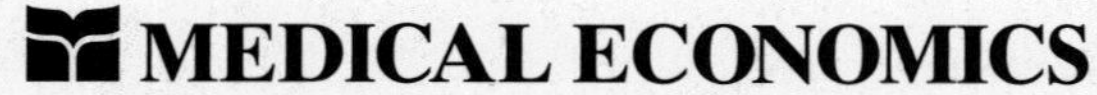
MEDICAL ECONOMICS

SECTION 1

MANUFACTURERS' INDEX

Listed in this index are all manufacturers that have supplied information in this edition. Each company's entry includes the address, phone, and fax number of its headquarters and regional offices, as well as contacts for inquiries, orders, and emergency information. A list of the company's major over-the-counter products is also included.

The ◆ symbol marks drugs shown in the "Product Identification Guide." If a company has two page numbers, the first refers to its photographs in the "Product Identification Guide," the second to its product information.

AGRO-DYNAMICS INTERNATIONAL 602
International-Bio Tech-USA
1145 Linda Vista Drive, Suite 109
San Marcos, CA 92069
Direct Inquiries to:
Jerry Stagner
(619) 471-1182
FAX: (619) 471-1878

OTC Products Available:
Latero-Flora Capsules

AK PHARMA 503, 602
P.O. Box 111
Pleasantville, NJ 08232-0111
Direct Inquiries to:
Elizabeth Wexler
(609) 645-5100
FAX: (609) 645-0767
For Medical Emergencies Contact:
Leonard P. Smith
(609) 645-5100
FAX: (609) 645-0767

OTC Products Available:
◆ Beano Liquid
◆ Beano Tablets
◆ Prelief Tablets and Granulate

AMERICAN LIFELINE, INC......... 603
103 S. Second Street
Madison, WI 53704
Direct Inquiries to:
Dave Sullivan
(800) 257-5433
(608) 836-3477

OTC Products Available:
FLORAjen Acidophilus Capsules

AML LABORATORIES 603
A Division of The Winning Combination, Inc.
1753 Cloverfield Boulevard
Santa Monica, CA 90404
Direct Inquiries to:
(800) 800-1200

OTC Products Available:
Breath + Plus
Complete for Men
Complete for Women
Fat Burning Factors
Fruit and Vegetable Safety Rinse
Natural M.D. Basic Life Prescription for Men
Natural M.D. Basic Life Prescription for Women
Natural M.D. Complete Life Prescription
Natural M.D. Essential Life Prescription
Natural M.D. Standard Life Prescription for Men
Natural M.D. Standard Life Prescription for Women
Natural M.D. Ultimate Life Prescription
Stress Gum

ASTRA USA, INC............ 503, 608
50 Otis Street
Westborough, MA 01581-4500
Direct Inquiries to:
Professional Information Department
(508) 366-1100
FAX: (508) 366-7406
For Medical Emergencies Contact:
Medical Information Services
(800) 262-0460

OTC Products Available:
◆ Xylocaine 2.5% Ointment

BAUSCH & LOMB INCORPORATED 503, 608
1400 North Goodman Street
P.O. Box 450
Rochester, NY 14692-0450
Direct Inquiries to:
Consumer Affairs
(800) 572-2931
FAX: (716) 338-0184
For Medical Emergencies Contact:
Consumer Affairs
(800) 572-2931

OTC Products Available:
◆ Curel Lotion and Cream

BAYER CORPORATION CONSUMER CARE DIVISION 503, 609
P.O. Box 1910
36 Columbia Road
Morristown, NJ 07962-1910
Direct Inquiries to:
Consumer Affairs
(800) 331-4536
For Medical Emergencies Contact:
Bayer Corporation
Consumer Care Division
(800) 331-4536

OTC Products Available:
◆ Actron Caplets and Tablets
◆ Aleve Tablets and Caplets
◆ Alka-Mints Chewable Antacid
◆ Alka-Seltzer Antacid Liquid Gelcaps
◆ Alka-Seltzer Anti-Gas Liquid Gelcaps
◆ Alka-Seltzer Original Effervescent Antacid and Pain Reliever
◆ Alka-Seltzer Cherry Effervescent Antacid and Pain Reliever

(◆) Shown in Product Identification Guide

BAYER CORPORATION CONSUMER CARE DIVISION—*cont.*
- ◆ Alka-Seltzer Extra Strength Effervescent Antacid and Pain Reliever
- ◆ Alka-Seltzer Gold Effervescent Antacid
- ◆ Alka-Seltzer Lemon Lime Effervescent Antacid and Pain Reliever
- ◆ Alka-Seltzer Plus Cold & Cough Medicine
- ◆ Alka-Seltzer Plus Cold & Cough Medicine Liqui-Gels
- ◆ Alka-Seltzer Plus Cold Medicine
- ◆ Alka-Seltzer Plus Cold Medicine Liqui-Gels
- ◆ Alka-Seltzer Plus Flu & Body Aches Effervescent Tablets
- ◆ Alka-Seltzer Plus Flu & Body Aches Liqui-Gels Non-Drowsy Formula
- ◆ Alka-Seltzer Plus Night-Time Cold Medicine
- ◆ Alka-Seltzer Plus Night-Time Cold Medicine Liqui-Gels
- ◆ Alka-Seltzer Plus Sinus Medicine
- ◆ Bactine Antiseptic/Anesthetic First Aid Liquid and Spray
- Bactine First Aid Antibiotic Plus Anesthetic Ointment
- Bactine Hydrocortisone Anti-Itch Cream
- ◆ Extra Strength Bayer Arthritis Pain Regimen Formula
- ◆ Genuine Bayer Aspirin Tablets & Caplets
- ◆ Extended-Release Bayer 8-Hour Aspirin
- ◆ Extra Strength Bayer Aspirin Caplets & Tablets
- ◆ Aspirin Regimen Bayer Regular Strength 325 mg Caplets
- ◆ Aspirin Regimen Bayer Adult Low Strength 81 mg Tablets
- ◆ Aspirin Regimen Bayer Children's Chewable Aspirin
- ◆ Aspirin Regimen Bayer 81 mg Tablets with Calcium
- Bayer Aspirin Professional Labeling (Aspirin Regimen Bayer and Genuine Bayer Aspirin)
- ◆ Extra Strength Bayer Plus Aspirin Caplets
- ◆ Extra Strength Bayer PM Aspirin Plus Sleep Aid
- Bronkaid Caplets
- Bronkaid Mist
- Bronkaid Mist Suspension
- ◆ Bugs Bunny Complete Children's Chewable Vitamins + Minerals with Iron and Calcium (Sugar Free)
- Bugs Bunny Plus Iron Children's Chewable Vitamins (Sugar Free)
- ◆ Bugs Bunny With Extra C Children's Chewable Vitamins (Sugar Free)
- Campho-Phenique Antiseptic Gel
- Campho-Phenique Cold Sore Gel
- Campho-Phenique Maximum Strength First Aid Antibiotic Plus Pain Reliever Ointment
- Campho-Phenique Liquid
- ◆ Domeboro Astringent Solution Effervescent Tablets
- ◆ Domeboro Astringent Solution Powder Packets
- ◆ Femstat 3
- ◆ Fergon Iron Supplement Tablets
- ◆ Flintstones Children's Chewable Vitamins
- ◆ Flintstones Children's Chewable Vitamins Plus Extra C
- ◆ Flintstones Children's Chewable Vitamins Plus Iron
- ◆ Flintstones Complete With Calcium, Iron & Minerals Children's Chewable Vitamins
- ◆ Flintstones Plus Calcium Children's Chewable Vitamins
- Haley's M-O, Regular & Flavored
- ◆ Maximum Strength Multi-Symptom Formula Midol
- Night Time Formula Midol PM
- ◆ PMS Multi-Symptom Formula Midol
- ◆ Maximum Strength Midol Teen Multi-Symptom Formula
- Miles Nervine Nighttime Sleep-Aid
- Mycelex OTC Cream Antifungal
- Mycelex OTC Solution Antifungal
- ◆ Mycelex-7 Combination-Pack Vaginal Inserts & External Vulvar Cream
- ◆ Mycelex-7 Vaginal Antifungal Cream with 7 Disposable Applicators
- ◆ Mycelex-7 Vaginal Cream Antifungal
- Mycelex-7 Vaginal Inserts Antifungal
- ◆ NāSal Saline Moisturizer Drops
- ◆ NāSal Saline Moisturizer Spray
- ◆ Neo-Synephrine Maximum Strength 12 Hour Nasal Spray
- Neo-Synephrine Maximum Strength 12 Hour Extra Moisturizing Nasal Spray
- ◆ Neo-Synephrine Nasal Drops, Regular and Extra Strength
- ◆ Neo-Synephrine Nasal Sprays, Regular and Extra Strength
- NTZ Long Acting Nasal Spray & Drops 0.05%
- ◆ One-A-Day Antioxidant Plus
- ◆ One-A-Day Calcium Plus
- ◆ One-A-Day Essential Vitamins
- ◆ One-A-Day 50 Plus
- ◆ One-A-Day Garlic Softgels
- ◆ One-A-Day Maximum
- ◆ One-A-Day Men's
- ◆ One-A-Day Women's
- ◆ Phillips' Gelcaps
- ◆ Phillips' Milk of Magnesia Liquid
- ◆ Vanquish Analgesic Caplets

BEACH PHARMACEUTICALS...... 627
Division of Beach Products, Inc.
EXECUTIVE OFFICE:
5220 South Manhattan Avenue
Tampa, FL 33611
(813) 839-6565
Direct Inquiries to:
Victor De Oreo, R Ph, V.P., Sales:
(803) 277-7282
Richard Stephen Jenkins, Exec. V.P.:
(813) 839-6565
Manufacturing and Distribution:
Main Street at Perimeter Road
Conestee, SC 29605
(800) 845-8210

OTC Products Available:
Beelith Tablets

BEECH-NUT NUTRITION CORPORATION 506, 627
800 Market Street
St. Louis, MO 63101
Direct Inquiries to:
Beech-Nut Nutrition Helpline
(800) 523-6633
For Medical Emergencies Contact:
Richard C. Theuer, Ph.D.
(314) 877-7146
FAX: (314) 877-7762

OTC Products Available:
- ◆ Beech-Nut Pediatric Electrolyte Solution

BEIERSDORF INC. 506, 629
360 Dr. Martin Luther King Dr.
Norwalk, CT 06856-5529
Direct Inquiries to:
Medical Division
(203) 853-8008
FAX: (203) 854-8180

OTC Products Available:
- ◆ Aquaphor Healing Ointment
- ◆ Aquaphor Healing Ointment, Original Formula
- Basis Facial Cleanser (Normal to Dry Skin)
- Basis Soap-Combination Skin
- Basis Soap-Extra Dry Skin
- Basis Soap-Normal to Dry Skin
- Basis Soap-Sensitive Skin
- Eucerin Cleansing Bar
- ◆ Eucerin Facial Moisturizing Lotion SPF 25
- ◆ Eucerin Light Moisture-Restorative Creme
- ◆ Eucerin Light Moisture-Restorative Lotion
- ◆ Eucerin Original Moisturizing Creme
- ◆ Eucerin Original Moisturizing Lotion
- ◆ Eucerin Plus Alphahydroxy Moisturizing Creme
- ◆ Eucerin Plus Alphahydroxy Moisturizing Lotion
- ◆ Eucerin Shower Therapy
- Nivea Bath and Body Oil
- Nivea Creamy Conditioning Oil
- Nivea Moisturizing Body Wash
- Nivea Moisturizing Lotion (Extra Enriched)
- Nivea Moisturizing Lotion (Original Formula)
- Nivea Moisturizing Shower Gels
- Nivea Skin Oil
- Nivea Visage Facial Nourishing Creme
- Nivea Visage No Oil, All Moisture Hydrogel
- Nivea Visage Shine Control Matifying Fluid
- Nivea Visage UV Care Daily Moisture Lotion

BEUTLICH LP PHARMACEUTICALS 631
1541 Shields Drive
Waukegan, IL 60085-8304
Direct Inquiries to:
(847) 473-1100
(800) 238-8542
FAX: (847) 473-1122
E-mail: hurricaine@aol.com
World Wide Web: www.beutlich.com

OTC Products Available:
- Ceo-Two Evacuant Suppositories
- Hurricaine Topical Anesthetic Aerosol Spray, 2 oz. (Wild Cherry Flavor)
- Hurricaine Topical Anesthetic Gel, 1 oz. Wild Cherry, Pina Colada, Watermelon, 1/8 oz. Wild Cherry, Watermelon
- Hurricaine Topical Anesthetic Liquid, .25 gm, 1 oz. Wild Cherry and Pina Colada .25 ml Dry Handle Swab Wild Cherry, 1/8 oz. Wild Cherry
- Hurricaine Topical Anesthetic Spray Extension Tubes (200)
- Hurricaine Topical Anesthetic Spray Kit
- Peridin-C Tablets

BIOZONE LABORATORIES, INC. 632
580 Garcia Avenue
Pittsburg, CA 94565
Direct Inquiries to:
(510) 473-1000, Ext. 17

OTC Products Available:
- LipoSpray Nutritional Delivery System and Products

BLAINE COMPANY, INC. 632
1465 Jamike Lane
Erlanger, KY 41018
Direct Inquiries to:
Mr. Alex M. Blaine
(800) 633-9353
FAX: (606) 283-9460

OTC Products Available:
- Mag-Ox 400
- Uro-Mag

BLAIREX LABORATORIES, INC. ... 632
3240 North Indianapolis Road
P.O. Box 2127
Columbus, IN 47202-2127
Direct Inquiries to:
Customer Service
(800) 252-4739
FAX: (812) 378-1033

For Medical Emergencies Contact:
David S. Wilson, M.D.
(800) 252-4739
FAX: (812) 378-1033

OTC Products Available:
Broncho Saline
Nasal Moist Gel
Nasal Moist Solution
Pertussin CS Children's Strength
Pertussin DM Extra Strength

BLOCK DRUG COMPANY, INC. 506, 633
257 Cornelison Avenue
Jersey City, NJ 07302
Direct Inquiries to:
Lori Hunt
(201) 434-3000, Ext. 1308
For Medical Emergencies Contact:
Consumer Service/Block
(201) 434-3000, Ext. 1308

OTC Products Available:
Balmex Ointment
BC Powder
BC Allergy Sinus Cold Powder
Arthritis Strength BC Powder
BC Sinus Cold Powder
Goody's Extra Strength Headache Powder
Goody's Extra Strength Pain Relief Tablets
◆ Nature's Remedy Tablets
Nytol QuickCaps Caplets
Maximum Strength Nytol Quickgels Softgels
◆ Phazyme Infant Drops
◆ Phazyme-95 Tablets
◆ Phazyme-125 Chewable Tablets Maximum Strength
◆ Phazyme-125 Liquid Maximum Strength
◆ Phazyme-125 Softgel Capsules Maximum Strength
Promise Sensitive Toothpaste
Original Flavor Sensodyne
Cool Gel Sensodyne
Fresh Mint Sensodyne
Sensodyne Tarter Control
Sensodyne with Baking Soda
Tegrin Dandruff Shampoo
Tegrin for Psoriasis Skin Cream & Tegrin Medicated Soap

BOIRON, THE WORLD LEADER IN HOMEOPATHY ... 638
HEADQUARTERS:
6 Campus Blvd., Building A
Newtown Square, PA 19073
Direct Inquiries to:
Gina Casey
Public Relations Manager
(610) 325-8320
For Medical Emergencies Contact:
Steven Boorstein, Pharm. D.
Branch Manager
(610) 325-7464

WEST COAST BRANCH:
98C West Cochran Street
Simi Valley, CA 93065
Direct Inquiries to:
Christophe Merville, Pharmacist
Branch Manager
(805) 582-9091

OTC Products Available:
Arnica & Calendula Gel
Arnicalm, for Bumps and Bruises
Camilia, for Baby Teething
Chestal Cough Syrup
Chestal For Children Cough Syrup
Cocyntal, for Baby Colic
Coldcalm, for Cold Symptoms
Cyclease, for Menstrual Cramps
Ginsenique, for Fatigue
Hayfever, for Pollen-Allergies
Homeodent toothpaste
Natural Phases, for PMS
Nervousness, for Stress and Tension
Optique 1 Eye Drops
Oscillococcinum, for Symptoms of Flu
Quiétude, for Sleeplessness
Sinusitis, for Sinus Inflammation
Sportenine, for Cramps and Muscle Fatigue
Yeastaway, for Vaginal Yeast Infections

BRISTOL-MYERS PRODUCTS 506, 638
A Bristol-Myers Squibb Company
345 Park Avenue
New York, NY 10154
Direct Inquiries to:
Bristol-Myers Products Division
Consumer Affairs Department
1350 Liberty Avenue
Hillside, NJ 07207
For Medical Emergencies Contact:
(800) 468-7746

OTC Products Available:
Alpha Keri Moisture Rich Body Oil
Alpha Keri Moisture Rich Cleansing Bar
Ammens Medicated Powder
Backache Caplets
BAN Antiperspirant Deodorant Cream
BAN Basic Non-Aerosol Antiperspirant Spray
BAN Clear Antiperspirant
BAN Clear Roll-On
BAN for Men Clear Antiperspirant
BAN for Men Clear Deodorant
BAN Roll-On Antiperspirant Deodorant
BAN Sensitive Touch Roll-On Antiperspirant Deodorant
BAN Sensitive Touch Solid Antiperspirant Deodorant
BAN Solid Antiperspirant Deodorant
◆ Bufferin Analgesic Tablets
◆ Arthritis Strength Bufferin Analgesic Caplets
◆ Extra Strength Bufferin Analgesic Tablets
Comtrex Deep Chest Cold and Cough Congestion Relief Non-Drowsy Liquigels
Comtrex Maximum Strength Multi-Symptom Allergy-Sinus Treatment Day/Night Tablets and Caplets
◆ Comtrex Maximum Strength Multi-Symptom Allergy-Sinus Treatment Tablets and Caplets
◆ Comtrex Maximum Strength Multi-Symptom Cold + Flu Reliever Liqui-Gels
Comtrex Maximum Strength Multi-Symptom Cold + Flu Reliever Liquid
◆ Comtrex Maximum Strength Multi-Symptom Cold + Flu Reliever Tablets and Caplets
Comtrex Maximum Strength Multi-Symptom Day/Night Tablets and Caplets
◆ Comtrex Maximum Strength Multi-Symptom Non-Drowsy Caplets
Comtrex Maximum Strength Multi-Symptom Non-Drowsy Liqui-gels
◆ Aspirin Free Excedrin Analgesic Caplets and Geltabs
◆ Excedrin Extra-Strength Analgesic Tablets, Caplets, and Geltabs
◆ Excedrin P.M. Analgesic/Sleeping Aid Tablets, Caplets, and Geltabs
Sinus Excedrin Tablets & Caplets
Fisherman's Friend Lozenges
Fostex 10% Benzoyl Peroxide Bar
Fostex 10% Benzoyl Peroxide (Vanish) Gel
Fostex 10% Benzoyl Peroxide Wash
Fostex Medicated Cleansing Bar
Fostex Medicated Cleansing Cream
◆ 4-Way Fast Acting Nasal Spray (regular and mentholated)
◆ 4-Way 12 Hour Nasal Spray
KeriCort-10 Cream
Keri Cream
◆ Keri Lotion - Original Formula
◆ Keri Lotion - Sensitive Skin, Fragrance Free
◆ Keri Lotion - Silky Smooth
Minit-Rub Analgesic Ointment
Mum Antiperspirant Cream Deodorant
Chewable No Doz Tablets
No Doz Maximum Strength Caplets
◆ Nuprin Tablets and Caplets
Pazo Hemorrhoid Ointment and Suppositories
◆ Therapeutic Mineral Ice
Therapeutic Mineral Ice Exercise Formula

CARE-TECH LABORATORIES, INC. 649
Over-The-Counter Pharmaceuticals
3224 South Kingshighway Boulevard
St. Louis, MO 63139
Direct Inquiries to:
Sherry L. Brereton
(314) 772-4610
FAX: (314) 772-4613
For Medical Emergencies Contact:
Customer Service
(800) 325-9681
FAX: (314) 772-4613

OTC Products Available:
Barri-Care Antimicrobial Ointment
Care Creme Antimicrobial Cream
CC-500 Antibacterial Skin Cleanser for Dialysis Patient Care
Clinical Care Antimicrobial Wound Cleanser
Concept Antimicrobial Dermal Cleanser
Formula Magic Antimicrobial/Anti-Fungal Powder
Humatrix Microclysmic Gel
Just Lotion - Highly Absorbent Aloe Vera Glycerine Based Skin Lotion
Loving Lather II Antibacterial Skin Cleanser
Loving Lotion Antibacterial Skin & Body Lotion
Orchid Fresh II Antimicrobial Perineal/Ostomy Cleanser
Satin Antimicrobial Skin Cleanser
Skin Magic - Antimicrobial Body Rub & Emollient
Soft Skin Non-greasy Bath Oil with Rich Emollients for Severely Damaged Dermal Tissue
Swirlsoft Whirlpool Emollient for Dry Skin Conditions
Tech 2000 Antimicrobial Oral Rinse (No Alcohol, No Sodium)
Techni-Care Surgical Scrub, Prep and Wound Decontaminant
Velvet Fresh Non-irritating Cornstarch Baby Powder

CARE TECHNOLOGIES, INC. 651
55 Holly Hill Lane
Greenwich, CT 06830
Direct Inquiries to:
Mark Watkins
VP Marketing
(203) 661-3161
FAX: (203) 661-3619
E-mail: caretec1@aol.com
WWW: http://www.clearcare.com

OTC Products Available:
Clear Total Lice Elimination System (Shampoo, Egg Remover, Nit (egg) Comb)

(◆) Shown in Product Identification Guide

CARLSBAD TECHNOLOGY INC. 652
5923 Balfour Court
Carlsbad, CA 92008
For Medical and Pharmaceutical Information, Including Emergencies Contact:
(619) 431-8284
FAX: (619) 431-7505

OTC Products Available:
Enteric Coated Pellets Aspirin Capsules

J. R. CARLSON LABORATORIES, INC. 652
15 College Drive
Arlington Heights, IL 60004-1985
Direct Inquiries to:
Customer Service
(847) 255-1600
FAX: (847) 255-1605
For Medical Emergencies Contact:
Customer Service
(847) 255-1600
FAX: (847) 255-1605

OTC Products Available:
ACES Antioxidant Soft Gels
E-Gems Soft Gels

CHATTEM, INC. 652
1715 West 38th Street
Chattanooga, TN 37409
Direct Inquiries to:
Gary Galante
Vice President of Research & Development
(423) 821-4571

OTC Products Available:
Gold Bond Medicated Anti-Itch Cream
Gold Bond Medicated Baby Powder
Gold Bond Cornstarch Plus Medicated Baby Powder
Gold Bond Triple Action Medicated Body Powder
Gold Bond Extra Strength Triple Action Medicated Body Powder
Gold Bond Maximum Strength Triple Action Medicated Foot Powder
Herpecin-L Cold Sore Lip Balm

CHURCH & DWIGHT CO., INC. 654
469 North Harrison Street
Princeton, NJ 08543-5297
Direct Inquiries to:
Nancy Sevinsky
(609) 683-7015
For Medical Emergencies Contact:
Hazard Information Services
(800) 228-5635
Extension 7

OTC Products Available:
Arm & Hammer Pure Baking Soda

CIBA SELF-MEDICATION, INC.
(See NOVARTIS CONSUMER HEALTH, INC.)

COLUMBIA LABORATORIES, INC. 507, 654
2665 South Bayshore Drive
Suite PH2B
Miami, FL 33133
Direct Inquiries to:
Professional Services Department
For Medical Emergencies Contact:
(305) 860-1670

OTC Products Available:
Diasorb Liquid
Diasorb Tablets
◆ Legatrin PM Caplets
Vaporizer in a bottle Cough Suppressant

DEL PHARMACEUTICALS, INC. ... 507, 654
A Subsidiary of Del Laboratories, Inc.
163 East Bethpage Road
Plainview, NY 11803
Direct Inquiries to:
Dr. Joseph A. Kanapka, Ph.D.
Sr. VP Scientific Affairs
(516) 844-2020
FAX: (516) 293-1515
For Medical Emergencies Contact:
Edmund Mickunas,
Director of Regulatory Affairs
(800) 952-5080

OTC Products Available:
◆ ArthriCare Odor Free Rub
◆ ArthriCare Triple Medicated Rub
◆ ArthriCare Ultra Rub
Auro-Dri Ear Water-Drying Aid
Auro Ear Wax Removal Aid
Boil-Ease Pain Relieving Ointment
Dermarest DriCort Anti-Itch Creme
Dermarest Plus Gel
Detane Desensitizing Lubricant
Diaper Guard Skin Rash Ointment
Exocaine Analgesic Rubs
Off-Ezy Wart Remover
Baby Orajel Nighttime Formula
◆ Baby Orajel Teething Pain Medicine
◆ Baby Orajel Tooth & Gum Cleanser
Orajel CoverMed Tinted Cold Sore Medicine
Orajel Denture Pain Medicine
◆ Orajel Mouth-Aid for Canker and Cold Sores
◆ Orajel Perioseptic Spot Treatment Oral Cleanser
◆ Orajel Perioseptic Super Cleaning Oral Rinse
◆ Orajel Maximum Strength Toothache Medication
Orajel PM Maximum Strength Toothache Medication
◆ Pronto Lice Killing Shampoo & Conditioner in One Kit
◆ Pronto Lice Killing Spray
Propa pH Acne Medications
Skin Shield Liquid Bandage
Stye Ophthalmic Ointment
◆ Tanac Medicated Gel
◆ Tanac No Sting Liquid
Triptone for Motion Sickness

EFFCON LABORATORIES, INC. .. 508, 657
P.O. Box 7499
Marietta, GA 30065-1499
Direct Inquiries to:
Jan Sugrue
(800) 722-2428
FAX: (770) 428-6811
For Medical Emergencies Contact:
J. Kent Burklow
(800) 722-2428
FAX: (770) 428-6811

OTC Products Available:
◆ Pin-X Pinworm Treatment

ENVIRODERM PHARMACEUTICALS, INC. 658
P.O. Box 32370
Louisville, KY 40232
Direct Inquiries to:
David W. Schropfer
(502) 634-7700
FAX: (502) 634-7701
For Medical Emergencies Contact:
Anthony A. Schulz
(800) 991-3376, ext. 7531
FAX: (502) 634-7701

OTC Products Available:
Ivy Block Skin Protectant Lotion

FISONS CORPORATION PRESCRIPTION PRODUCTS
(See MEDEVA PHARMACEUTICALS, INC.)

FLEMING & COMPANY 658
1600 Fenpark Dr.
Fenton, MO 63026
Direct Inquiries to:
Tom Fleming
(314) 343-8200
FAX: (314) 343-8203

OTC Products Available:
Chlor-3 Condiment
Impregon Concentrate
Magonate Tablets and Liquid
Marblen Suspension Peach/Apricot
Marblen Tablets
Nephrox Suspension
Nicotinex Elixir
Ocean Nasal Mist
Purge Concentrate

GEBAUER COMPANY 508, 659
9410 St. Catherine Avenue
Cleveland, OH 44104
Direct Inquiries to:
(800) 321-9348
(216) 271-5252
For Medical Information Contact:
In Emergencies:
(800) 321-9348
(216) 271-5252
After Hours and Weekend Emergencies:
Chemtrac:
(800) 424-9300

OTC Products Available:
◆ Salivart Saliva Substitute

HOGIL PHARMACEUTICAL CORP. 508, 659
Two Manhattanville Road
Purchase, NY 10577
Direct Inquiries to:
Tanya Castagna
(914) 696-7600
FAX: (914) 696-4600
For Medical Emergencies Contact:
Dr. Gilbert Spector
(914) 696-7600
FAX: (914) 696-4600

OTC Products Available:
◆ A-200 Lice Control Spray
◆ A-200 Lice Killing Shampoo
◆ A-200 Lice Treatment Kit
◆ InnoGel Plus
Innomed Lice Treatment Kit
Psor-A-Set Liquid, Shampoo, & Soap
◆ Sine-Off Night Time Formula Caplets
◆ Sine-Off No Drowsiness Formula Caplets
◆ Sine-Off Sinus Medicine Caplets
◆ Teldrin 12 Hour Allergy Relief Capsules

INTER-CAL CORPORATION 662
533 Madison Avenue
Prescott, AZ 86301
Direct Inquiries to:
Dr. Jack Hegenauer
(520) 445-8063
FAX: (520) 778-7986
For Medical Emergencies Contact:
Dr. Jack Hegenauer
(520) 445-8063
FAX: (520) 778-7986

OTC Products Available:
Ester-C Tablets, Caplets, or Capsules

IYATA PHARMACEUTICAL, INC. 663
735 North Water Street

(◆) Shown in Product Identification Guide

Suite 612
Milwaukee, WI 53202
Direct Inquiries to:
Michael B. Adekunle, M.D.
(414) 272-1982
FAX: (414) 272-2919
For Medical Emergencies Contact:
Michael B. Adekunle, M.D.
(414) 272-1982
(800) 809-7918
FAX: (414) 272-2919

OTC Products Available:
Capsagel

JOHNSON & JOHNSON • 508, 663
MERCK CONSUMER PHARMACEUTICALS CO.
Camp Hill Road
Fort Washington, PA 19034
Direct Inquiries to:
Consumer Affairs Department
(215) 233-7000
For Medical Emergencies Contact:
(215) 233-7000

OTC Products Available:
◆ ALternaGEL Liquid
◆ Dialose Tablets
◆ Dialose Plus Tablets
◆ Children's Mylanta Upset Stomach Relief Liquid
◆ Children's Mylanta Upset Stomach Relief Tablets
◆ Mylanta Gas Relief Gelcaps
◆ Mylanta Gas Relief Tablets
◆ Maximum Strength Mylanta Gas Relief Tablets
◆ Mylanta Gelcaps Antacid
◆ Mylanta Liquid
◆ Mylanta Maximum Strength Liquid
◆ Mylanta Tablets
◆ Mylanta Maximum Strength Tablets
◆ Infants' Mylicon Drops
◆ Pepcid AC Acid Controller Tablets

KONSYL PHARMACEUTICALS, INC. ... 668
4200 South Hulen
Fort Worth, TX 76109
Direct Inquiries to:
Bill Steiber
(817) 763-8011, Ext. 23
FAX: (817) 731-9389

OTC Products Available:
Konsyl Fiber Tablets
Konsyl Powder Sugar Free Unflavored

KYOLIC LTD., DIVISION OF WAKUNAGA OF AMERICA CO., LTD. 522, 669
Subsidiary of Wakunaga Pharmaceutical Co., Ltd.
23501 Madero
Mission Viejo, CA 92691
Direct Inquiries to:
(800) 421-2998

OTC Products Available:
Be Sure
Ginkgo Biloba Plus
Ginkgo-Go Caplets
Kyo-Chrome
Kyo-Dophilus
Acidophilase Capsules: L. acidophilus, B. bifidum, amylase, protease, lipase
Kyo-Dophilus Capsules: L. acidophilus, B. longum, B. bifidum
Kyo-Dophilus Chewable Tablets: L. acidophilus
Kyo-Ginseng: Aged garlic extract (300 mg), panax ginseng (50 mg), thiamine (3 mg)
Kyo-Green Powder: Barley & wheat grass, chlorella, kelp, brown rice
◆ Kyolic Aged Garlic Extract Caplets
Kyolic – Super Formula 100 Tablets & Capsules: Aged garlic extract powder (300mg), whey
Kyolic – Super Formula 101 Garlic Plus: Tablets & Capsules: Aged garlic extract powder (270mg), whey, brewer's yeast, kelp, algin
Kyolic – Super Formula 102 Tablets & Capsules: Aged garlic extract powder (350mg), amylase, protease, cellulase, lipase
Kyolic – Super Formula 103 Capsules: Aged garlic extract powder (220mg), Ester C, astragalus, calcium
Kyolic – Super Formula 104 Capsules: Aged garlic extract powder (300mg), lecithin
Kyolic – Super Formula 105 Capsules: Aged garlic extract powder (200mg), beta carotene, vitamin C, vitamin E, selenium, green tea
Kyolic – Super Formula 106 Capsules: Aged garlic extract powder (300mg), hawthorne berry, vitamin E, cayenne pepper
Kyolic Aged Garlic Extract Flavor and Odor Modified Plain Liquid
Kyolic Reserve Capsules: Aged garlic extract powder (600mg)
Premium Kyolic-EPA Gel Caps: Aged garlic extract powder (120mg), fish oil [EPA (280mg), DHA (120mg)]
Pro Formula 1000 A.G.E./SGP: Aged Garlic Extract Powder (350mg)
◆ Probiata Tablets

LAVOPTIK COMPANY, INC. 669
661 Western Avenue North
St. Paul, MN 55103
Direct Inquiries to:
661 Western Avenue North
St. Paul, MN 55103-1694
(612) 489-1351
For Medical Emergencies Contact:
B. C. Brainard
(612) 489-1351
FAX: (612) 489-0760

OTC Products Available:
Lavoptik Eye Cups
Lavoptik Eye Wash

LEDERLE CONSUMER HEALTH 670
a Division of Whitehall-Robins Healthcare
Five Giralda Farms
Madison, NJ 07940
Direct Inquiries to:
Lederle Consumer Product Information
(800) 282-8805
Distribution Centers:
GARDEN GROVE
11700 Monarch Street
Garden Grove, CA 92641
(714) 891-3743
Attn: Richard A. Benvenuti
DES PLAINS
1908 S. Mount Prospect Road
Des Plains, IL 60018
(708) 299-2206
Attn: James P. Smith
DALLAS
4116 Bronze Way
Dallas, TX 75237
(214) 399-8361
Attn: Thomas G. Culp
RICHMOND
2300 Darbytown Road
Richmond, VA 23231
(804) 226-6700
Attn: J. Stuart Smith
KINNESAW
1000 Union Court
Kennesaw, GA 30144
(404) 421-0039
Attn: E. Norman Blackwell
FRAZER
31 Morehall Road
Frazer, PA 19355
(610) 644-8000
Attn: Douglas M. Holste

OTC Products Available:
Caltrate 600 Tablets
Caltrate 600 + D Tablets
Caltrate PLUS Chewables
Caltrate PLUS Tablets
Centrum Silver Tablets
Centrum Tablets
Centrum, Jr. + Extra C Children's Chewables
Centrum, Jr. + Extra Calcium Children's Chewables
Centrum, Jr. + Iron Children's Chewables
Ferro-Sequels Tablets
FiberCon Caplets
Protegra Antioxidant Vitamin & Mineral Supplement Softgels
Stresstabs Tablets
Stresstabs + Iron Tablets
Stresstabs + Zinc Tablets

3M HEALTH CARE 509, 675
Bldg. 515-3N-02
St. Paul, MN 55144-1000
Direct Inquiries to:
Customer Service
(800) 537-2191
For Medical Emergencies Contact:
(612) 733-2882 (answered 24 hrs.)
Sales and Ordering or Returns:
(800) 832-2189

OTC Products Available:
◆ 3M Titralac Antacid Tablets
◆ 3M Titralac Extra Strength Antacid Tablets
◆ 3M Titralac Plus Antacid Tablets
◆ 3M Titralac Plus Liquid Antacid

MARLYN NUTRACEUTICALS 675
14851 North Scottsdale Road
Scottsdale, AZ 85254 USA
(800) 462-7596
(602) 991-0200
Direct Inquiries to:
Joe Lehmann
(602) 991-0200
FAX: (602) 991-0551

OTC Products Available:
4-Beauty
4-Hair, Internal
4-Hair, Topical
4-Nails, Internal
4-Nails, Topical
Hep-Forte Capsules
Marlyn Formula 50 Capsules
Marlyn PMS
Osteo Fem
Pro Skin, Internal
Pro Skin, Topical

MAYOR PHARMACEUTICAL LABORATORIES – KAREMOR INTERNATIONAL 676
2401 South 24th Street
Phoenix, AZ 85034
Direct Inquiries to:
Medical Director
(602) 244-8899

(◆) Shown in Product Identification Guide

MAYOR PHARMACEUTICAL LABORATORIES – KAREMOR INTERNATIONAL—*cont.*

OTC Products Available:
Vitamist Intra-Oral Spray Dietary Supplements
Anti-Oxidant
Blue Green Sea Spray
Colloidal Minerals
Folacin
Herbal Re-leaf
Melatonin
Multiple Adult/Prenatal/Children's Formulas
PMS
Pro-Bio Mist PB/GS
Slendermist
Smoke-less
Stress
Vitamin B-12
Vitamin C + Zinc
Vitamin E + Selenium

McNEIL CONSUMER PRODUCTS COMPANY **509, 676**
Division of McNeil-PPC, Inc.
Camp Hill Road
Fort Washington, PA 19034
Direct Inquiries to:
Consumer Affairs Department
Fort Washington, PA 19034
(215) 233-7000
Manufacturing Divisions:
Fort Washington, PA 19034

Southwest Manufacturing Plant
4001 N. I-35
Round Rock, TX 78664

Road 183 KM 19.8
Barrios Montones
Las Piedras, Puerto Rico 00771

OTC Products Available:
◆ Children's Motrin Ibuprofen Drops
◆ Children's Motrin Ibuprofen Oral Suspension
◆ Children's TYLENOL acetaminophen Chewable Tablets, Elixir and Suspension Liquid
◆ Children's TYLENOL Cold Multi Symptom Chewable Tablets and Liquid
◆ Children's TYLENOL Cold Plus Cough Multi Symptom Chewable Tablets and Liquid
◆ Children's TYLENOL Flu Liquid
◆ Imodium A-D Caplets and Liquid
◆ Infants' TYLENOL acetaminophen Suspension Drops
◆ Infants' TYLENOL Cold Decongestant & Fever Reducer Drops
◆ Junior Strength Motrin Ibuprofen Caplets
◆ Junior Strength TYLENOL acetaminophen Coated Caplets, and Chewable Tablets
◆ Lactaid Original Strength Caplets
◆ Lactaid Drops
◆ Lactaid Extra Strength Caplets
◆ Lactaid Ultra Caplets
◆ Nicotrol (Nicotine Transdermal System) Patch
◆ PediaCare Cough-Cold Chewable Tablets and Liquid
◆ PediaCare Infants' Decongestant Drops
◆ PediaCare Infants' Drops Decongestant Plus Cough
◆ PediaCare NightRest Cough-Cold Liquid
◆ Sine-Aid Maximum Strength Sinus Medication Gelcaps, Caplets and Tablets
◆ TYLENOL acetaminophen Extended Relief Caplets
TYLENOL acetaminophen, Extra Strength Adult Liquid Pain Reliever
◆ TYLENOL acetaminophen, Extra Strength Gelcaps, Caplets, Tablets, Geltabs
◆ TYLENOL acetaminophen, Regular Strength, Caplets and Tablets
◆ TYLENOL Allergy Sinus Medication NightTime, Maximum Strength Caplets
◆ TYLENOL Allergy Sinus Medication, Maximum Strength Caplets, Gelcaps, and Geltabs
◆ TYLENOL Cold Medication, Multi-Symptom Caplets and Tablets
◆ TYLENOL Cold Medication, Multi-Symptom Hot Liquid Packets
◆ TYLENOL Cold Medication, No Drowsiness Formula Caplets and Gelcaps
◆ TYLENOL Cold Severe Congestion Caplets
◆ TYLENOL Cough Medication, Multi-Symptom
◆ TYLENOL Cough Medication with Decongestant, Multi-Symptom
◆ TYLENOL Flu NightTime, Maximum Strength Gelcaps
◆ TYLENOL Flu NightTime, Maximum Strength Hot Medication Packets
◆ TYLENOL Flu No Drowsiness Formula, Maximum Strength Gelcaps
◆ TYLENOL PM Pain Reliever/Sleep Aid, Extra Strength Gelcaps, Caplets, Geltabs
◆ TYLENOL Severe Allergy Medication Caplets
◆ TYLENOL Sinus, Maximum Strength Geltabs, Gelcaps, Caplets, Tablets

MEDEVA PHARMACEUTICALS, INC. **698**
14801 Sovereign Road
Fort Worth, TX 76155-2645
Direct Inquiries to:
Customer Service Department
P.O. Box 1766
Rochester, NY 14608
(716) 274-5300
(888) 9-MEDEVA
For Emergency Medical Information Contact:
(800) 932-1950 (24 hours)
(888) 9-MEDEVA (24 hours)

OTC Products Available:
Delsym Extended-Release Suspension

MENLEY & JAMES LABORATORIES, INC. **699**
Commonwealth Corporate Center
100 Tournament Drive
Horsham, PA 19044-3697
Direct Inquiries to:
Consumer Affairs Department
(800) 321-1834
FAX: (215) 441-6576

OTC Products Available:
Acnomel Acne Medication Cream
Acryline 2 Temporary Denture Reliner
Aqua Care Cream
Aqua Care Lotion
A.R.M. Allergy Relief Medicine Caplets
Asthma Nefrin Solution Bronchodilator
AsthmaHaler Mist Aerosol Bronchodilator
Benzedrex Inhaler
B.F.I. Antiseptic First-Aid Powder
Congestac Caplets
Derifil Tablets
Hold DM Cough Suppressant Lozenge
Humibid GC Caplets
Ornex Caplets
Plate-weld Temporary Denture Repair Kit
Serutan Toasted Granules
S.T. 37 Topical Antiseptic Solution
Thermotabs Buffered Salt Tablets
Yodora Cream Deodorant

THE MENTHOLATUM COMPANY, INC. **699**
1360 Niagara Street
Buffalo, NY 14213
Direct Inquiries to:
Director of Consumer Affairs
(716) 882-7660
FAX: (716) 882-6563
For Medical Emergencies Contact:
Dr. Henry Chan
(716) 882-7660
FAX: (716) 882-6563

OTC Products Available:
Fletcher's Castoria
Fletcher's Cherry Flavor
Menthacin Cream
Mentholatum Cherry Chest Rub for Kids
Mentholatum Deep Heating Rub
Mentholatum Ointment
Red Cross Toothache Medication

MILES INC. CONSUMER HEALTHCARE PRODUCTS
(See BAYER CORPORATION CONSUMER CARE DIVISION)

NATURAL M.D.
(See AML LABORATORIES)

NICHE PHARMACEUTICALS, INC. **701**
200 N. Oak Street
P.O. Box 449
Roanoke, TX 76262
Direct Inquiries to:
Steve F. Brandon
(817) 491-2770
FAX: (817) 491-3533
For Medical Emergencies Contact:
Gerald L. Beckloff, M.D.
(817) 491-2770
FAX: (817) 491-3533

OTC Products Available:
MagTab SR Caplets
Unifiber

NOVARTIS CONSUMER HEALTH, INC. **513, 702**
Mack Woodbridge II
581 Main Street
Woodbridge, NJ 07095
Direct Product Inquiries to:
Consumer and Professional Affairs
(800) 452-0051
FAX: (800) 635-2801
Or write to the above address

OTC Products Available:
◆ Acutrim 16 Hour Steady Control Appetite Suppressant
◆ Acutrim Late Day Strength Appetite Suppressant
◆ Acutrim Maximum Strength Appetite Suppressant
Allerest Eye Drops
Allerest Maximum Strength Tablets
Allerest No Drowsiness Tablets
◆ Americaine Hemorrhoidal Ointment
◆ Americaine Topical Anesthetic Spray
◆ Regular Strength Ascriptin
◆ Arthritis Pain Ascriptin
◆ Ascriptin Enteric
◆ Maximum Strength Ascriptin
Bacid Capsules
Caldecort Anti-Itch Cream
◆ Caldesene Medicated Powder
◆ Prescription Strength Cruex Cream
◆ Cruex Spray Powder
◆ Prescription Strength Cruex Spray Powder
◆ Cruex Squeeze Powder
◆ Prescription Strength Desenex Cream
Desenex Foot and Sneaker Spray

(◆) Shown in Product Identification Guide

PHARMACIA & UPJOHN—*cont.*
- ◆ Dramamine Tablets
- ◆ Dramamine II Less Drowsy Tablets
- ◆ Dramamine Chewable Tablets
- ◆ Children's Dramamine Liquid
- ◆ Emetrol Anti-Nausea Oral Solution (Lemon-mint & Cherry Flavors)
- ◆ Kao Lectrolyte Electrolyte Replenisher (Unflavored, Grape and Bubblegum Flavors)
- ◆ Kaopectate Maximum Strength Caplets
- ◆ Kaopectate Children's Liquid
- ◆ Kaopectate Concentrated Anti-Diarrheal, Peppermint Flavor
- ◆ Kaopectate Concentrated Anti-Diarrheal, Regular Flavor
- ◆ Motrin IB Caplets, Tablets, and Gelcaps
- Motrin IB Sinus Caplets and Tablets
- ◆ Mycitracin Plus Pain Reliever
- ◆ Maximum Strength Mycitracin Triple Antibiotic First Aid Ointment
- Progaine Conditioner
- Progaine Shampoo (Extra Body)
- Progaine Shampoo (Permed & Color Treated)
- Progaine Shampoo (2 in 1)
- ◆ Rogaine for Men Hair Regrowth Treatment
- ◆ Rogaine for Women Hair Regrowth Treatment
- ◆ Surfak Liqui-Gels

PHARMANEX INC. 518, 744
625 Cochran Street
Simi Valley, CA 93065
Direct Inquiries to:
Customer Service
(800) 999-6229
FAX: (805) 582-9301
For Medical Emergencies Contact:
Michael Chang, Ph.D.
(805) 582-9300
FAX: (805) 582-9301

OTC Products Available:
- Extra Strength BioGinkgo 24/6 Tablets
- ◆ BioGinkgo 27/7 Tablets
- ◆ Cholestin Capsules
- CordyMax Cs-4 Capsules
- Tegreen 97 Capsules

PHARMATON NATURAL HEALTH PRODUCTS 518, 747
A Division of Boehringer Ingelheim Pharmaceutical Inc.
900 Ridgebury Road
Ridgefield, CT 06877
Direct Inquiries to:
Customer Service
(800) 243-0127
FAX: (203) 798-5771
For Medical Emergencies Contact:
Marvin Wetter, M.D.
(203) 798-4361
FAX: (203) 798-5771

OTC Products Available:
- ◆ Ginkoba Tablets
- ◆ Ginsana Capsules
- ◆ Ginsana Chewy Squares
- ◆ Vitasana Daily Dietary Supplement

PHARMAVITE CORPORATION 749
15451 San Fernando Mission Blvd.
Mission Hills, CA 91345
Direct Inquiries to:
Nature's Resource Brand Group
(800) 423-2405
FAX: (818) 837-6129
For Medical Information Contact:
(800) 423-2405, ext. 2281

OTC Products Available:
- Bilberry Fruit Standardized Extract
- Cascara Sagrada Bark
- Cat's Claw Standardized Extract
- Cayenne Garlic Combination
- Cayenne Pepper Fruit
- Cranberry Fruit
- Dieter's Herbal Combination
- Dong Quai Root
- Echinacea-Goldenseal Combo
- Evening Primrose Oil Standardized Extract
- Eyebright Herb
- Feverfew Leaf
- Garlic Cloves
- Ginger Root
- Ginkgo Biloba Leaf Standardized Extract Capsules
- Ginseng Gotu Kola Combination
- Ginseng Root--Korean
- Ginseng Root--Siberian
- Goldenseal Root
- Gotu Kola Root
- Grape Seed Extract
- Green Tea Standardized Extract
- Hawthorne Berries
- Kava Kava Root Standardized Extract
- Licorice Root
- Milk Thistle Standardized Extract
- St. John's Wort Standardized Extract
- Saw Palmetto Standardized Extract Capsules
- Standardized Echinacea Herb Capsules
- Standardized Valerian Root Capsules
- Yucca Stalk

PLOUGH, INC.
(See SCHERING-PLOUGH HEALTHCARE PRODUCTS)

PROCTER & GAMBLE 518, 749
P.O. Box 5516
Cincinnati, OH 45201
Direct Inquiries to:
Charles Lambert
(800) 358-8707
For Medical Emergencies Contact:
Call Collect: (513) 558-4422

OTC Products Available:
- Crest Sensitivity Protection Toothpaste
- Head & Shoulders Dandruff Shampoo
- Head & Shoulders Intensive Treatment Dandruff and Seborrheic Dermatitis Shampoo
- Metamucil Powder, Original Texture Orange Flavor
- Metamucil Powder, Original Texture Regular Flavor
- ◆ Metamucil Smooth Texture Powder, Orange Flavor
- Metamucil Smooth Texture Powder, Sugar-Free, Orange Flavor
- Metamucil Smooth Texture Powder, Sugar-Free, Regular Flavor
- ◆ Metamucil Wafers, Apple Crisp & Cinnamon Spice Flavors
- Oil of Olay Daily UV Protectant SPF 15 Beauty Fluid-Original and Fragrance Free
- ◆ Pepto-Bismol Original Liquid, Original and Cherry Tablets & Easy-to-Swallow Caplets
- Pepto-Bismol Maximum Strength Liquid
- Vicks 44 Cough Relief
- Vicks 44D Cough & Head Congestion Relief
- Vicks 44E Cough & Chest Congestion Relief
- Pediatric Vicks 44e Cough & Chest Congestion Relief
- Vicks 44M Cough, Cold & Flu Relief
- Pediatric Vicks 44m Cough & Cold Relief
- Vicks Chloraseptic Cough & Throat Drops, Menthol, Cherry and Honey Lemon Flavors
- Vicks Chloraseptic Sore Throat Lozenges, Menthol and Cherry Flavors
- Vicks Chloraseptic Sore Throat Spray, Menthol and Cherry Flavors
- Vicks Cough Drops, Menthol and Cherry Flavors
- Vicks Cough Drops, Menthol and Cherry Flavors
- Children's Vicks DayQuil Allergy Relief
- Vicks DayQuil Allergy Relief 12-Hour Extended Release Tablets
- Vicks DayQuil LiquiCaps/Liquid Multi-Symptom Cold/Flu Relief
- Vicks DayQuil SINUS Pressure & PAIN Relief with IBUPROFEN
- Children's Vicks NyQuil Cold/Cough Relief
- Vicks Nyquil Hot Therapy
- Vicks NyQuil LiquiCaps/Liquid Multi-Symptom Cold/Flu Relief, Original and Cherry Flavors
- Vicks Sinex Nasal Spray and Ultra Fine Mist
- Vicks Sinex 12-Hour Nasal Spray and Ultra Fine Mist
- Vicks Vapor Inhaler
- Vicks VapoRub Cream
- Vicks VapoRub Ointment
- Vicks VapoSteam

THE PURDUE FREDERICK COMPANY 762
100 Connecticut Avenue
Norwalk, CT 6850-3590
For Medical Information Contact:
Medical Department
(203) 853-0123

OTC Products Available:
- Betadine Brand First Aid Antibiotics + Moisturizer Ointment
- Betadine First Aid Cream
- Betadine Ointment
- Betadine Skin Cleanser
- Betadine Solution
- Senokot Children's Syrup
- Senokot Granules
- Senokot Syrup
- Senokot Tablets
- Senokot-S Tablets
- SenokotXTRA Tablets

RICHARDSON-VICKS, INC.
(See PROCTER & GAMBLE)

ROBERTS PHARMACEUTICAL CORPORATION 518, 763
4 Industrial Way West
Eatontown, NJ 07724
Direct Inquiries to:
Customer Service Department
(908) 389-1182
(800) 828-2088
FAX: (908) 389-1014
For Medical Emergencies Contact:
Medical Services Department
(800) 992-9306

OTC Products Available:
- Cheracol Cough Syrup CV
- Cheracol Cough/Sore Throat Lozenges
- ◆ Cheracol D Cough Formula
- Cheracol Nasal Spray Pump
- Cheracol Plus Multisymptom Cough/Cold Formula Cough Syrup
- Cheracol Sinus 12-hour Tablets
- Cheracol Sore Throat Spray
- ◆ Colace
- ◆ Peri-Colace Capsules and Syrup
- Squibb Cod Liver Oil
- Squibb Glycerin Suppositories
- Squibb Mineral Oil

(◆) Shown in Product Identification Guide

A. H. ROBINS CONSUMER PRODUCTS
(See WHITEHALL-ROBINS HEALTHCARE)

ROSS PRODUCTS DIVISION 766
Abbott Laboratories
Columbus, OH 43215-1724
Direct Inquiries to:
(800) 227-5767

OTC Products Available:
Clear Eyes ACR Astringent/Lubricant Redness Reliever Eye Drops
Clear Eyes CLR Soothing Drops
Clear Eyes Lubricant Eye Redness Reliever Eye Drops
Ear Drops by Murine -- (See Murine Ear Wax Removal System/Murine Ear Drops)
Murine Ear Drops
Murine Ear Wax Removal System
Murine Tears Lubricant Eye Drops
Murine Tears Plus Lubricant Redness Reliever Eye Drops
Pedialyte Oral Electrolyte Maintenance Solution
PediaSure and PediaSure with Fiber Complete Liquid Nutrition
Rehydralyte Oral Electrolyte Rehydration Solution
Ross Pediatric Nutritional Products
Alimentum Protein Hydrolysate Formula With Iron
Isomil DF Soy Formula For Diarrhea
Isomil SF Sucrose-Free Soy Formula With Iron
Isomil Soy Formula With Iron
PediaSure Complete Liquid Nutrition
PediaSure With Fiber Complete Liquid Nutrition
RCF Ross Carbohydrate Free Soy Formula Base With Iron
Similac Low-Iron Infant Formula
Similac NeoCare Infant Formula With Iron
Similac PM 60/40 Low-Iron Infant Formula
Similac Special Care With Iron 24 Premature Infant Formula
Similac With Iron Infant Formula
Selsun Blue Dandruff Shampoo 2-in-1 Treatment
Selsun Blue Dandruff Shampoo Balanced Treatment
Selsun Blue Dandruff Shampoo Medicated Treatment
Selsun Blue Dandruff Shampoo Moisturizing Treatment
Tronolane Anesthetic Cream for Hemorrhoids
Tronolane Hemorrhoidal Suppositories

SANDOZ PHARMACEUTICALS CORPORATION/CONSUMER DIVISION
(See NOVARTIS CONSUMER HEALTH, INC.)

SCANDINAVIAN NATURAL .... 771 HEALTH & BEAUTY PRODUCTS, INC.
13 North Seventh Street
Perkasie, PA 18944
Direct Inquiries to:
Catherine Peklak
(215) 453-2505

OTC Products Available:
Nasaline Preservative-Free Nasal Saline
Salix SST Lozenges Saliva Stimulant

SCHERING CORPORATION
(See SCHERING-PLOUGH HEALTHCARE PRODUCTS)

SCHERING-PLOUGH .... 518, 771 HEALTHCARE PRODUCTS
110 Allen Road
Liberty Corner, NJ 07938
Direct Product Requests to:
(908) 604-1983
FAX: (908) 604-1776
For Medical Emergencies Contact:
Clinical Department
(901) 320-2998

OTC Products Available:
◆ A + D Original Ointment
◆ A + D Ointment with Zinc Oxide
◆ Afrin Nasal Spray 0.05% and Nasal Spray Pump
Afrin Cherry Scented Nasal Spray 0.05%
◆ Afrin Extra Moisturizing Nasal Spray
◆ Afrin 4 hour Extra Moisturizing Nasal Spray
Afrin Menthol Nasal Spray 0.05%
Afrin Sinus Nasal Spray 0.05%
Afrin Nose Drops 0.05%
Afrin Saline Mist
◆ Afrin Menthol Saline Mist
◆ Chlor-Trimeton Allergy Tablets
◆ Chlor-Trimeton Allergy Decongestant Tablets
Chlor-Trimeton Allergy-Sinus Headache Caplets
◆ Coricidin Cold + Flu Tablets
◆ Coricidin Cough + Cold Tablets
◆ Coricidin 'D' Decongestant Tablets
◆ Coricidin Nighttime Cold & Cough Liquid
◆ Correctol Herbal Tea Laxative
◆ Correctol Laxative Tablets & Caplets
◆ Correctol Stool Softener Laxative Tablets
Di-Gel Antacid/Anti-Gas Liquid
Di-Gel Antacid/Anti-Gas Tablets
Drixoral Allergy/Sinus Extended Release Tablets
◆ Drixoral Cold and Allergy Sustained-Action Tablets
Drixoral Cold and Flu Extended-Release Tablets
Drixoral Nasal Decongestant Long-Acting Non-Drowsy Tablets
◆ DuoFilm Liquid Wart Remover
◆ DuoFilm Patch For Kids Wart Remover
◆ DuoPlant Gel Plantar Wart Remover
Duration 12 Hour Nasal Spray
◆ Lotrimin AF Antifungal Cream, Lotion, Solution, and Jock Itch Cream
◆ Lotrimin AF Antifungal Spray Liquid, Spray Powder, Spray Deodorant Powder, Powder and Jock Itch Spray Powder
St. Joseph Adult Chewable Aspirin Caplets (81 mg.)
◆ Shade Sunblock Gel SPF 30
◆ Shade Sunblock Lotion SPF 45
◆ Shade UVAGUARD Sunscreen Lotion SPF 15

SCOT-TUSSIN PHARMACAL ...... 782 CO., INC.
P.O. Box 8217
Cranston, RI 02920-0217
Direct Inquiries to:
(401) 942-8555
(401) 942-8556
(800) 638-SCOT (7268)
FAX: (401) 942-5690
For Medical Emergencies Contact:
Dr. S. G. Scotti
(800) 638-SCOT (7268)
FAX: (401) 942-5690

OTC Products Available:
Hayfebrol Allergy Relief Formula
Romilar DM SF
Scot-Tussin Sugar-Free Allergy Relief Formula
Scot-Tussin Diabetes Cough Formula + Sugar-Free
Scot-Tussin Senior SF Maximum Strength
Scot-Tussin Sugar-Free Original
Scot-Tussin Sugar-Free Cough Chasers Lozenges
Scot-Tussin Sugar-Free DM
Scot-Tussin Sugar-Free Expectorant
Vitalize Stress Formula
Vitalize with Ginseng High Energy Drink

SIMILASAN CORPORATION 782
1321 S. Central Avenue
Kent, WA 98032
Direct Inquiries to:
Brian S. Banks
(800) 426-1644
(305) 859-9072
FAX: (305) 859-9102
For Medical Emergencies Contact:
Alfred Knaus
(800) 426-1644
(305) 859-9072
FAX: (305) 859-9102

OTC Products Available:
Similasan Cold Drops # 1, 2 + 3
Similasan Colds and Influenza
Similasan Cough Drops # 1, 2 + 3
Similasan Eye Drops # 1
Similasan Eye Drops # 2
Similasan Hayfever Drops # 1
Similasan Nasal Spray
Similasan Sore Throat Drops # 1 + 2

SMITHKLINE BEECHAM .... 520, 783 CONSUMER HEALTHCARE, L.P.
Unit of SmithKline Beecham, Inc.
P.O. Box 1467
Pittsburgh, PA 15230
For Medical Information Contact:
(800) 245-1040 (Consumer Inquiries)
(800) 378-4055 (Healthcare Professional Inquiries)
Direct Healthcare Professional Sample Requests to:
(800) BEECHAM

OTC Products Available:
◆ CĒPASTAT Cherry Flavor Sore Throat Lozenges
◆ CĒPASTAT Extra Strength Sore Throat Lozenges
◆ CITRUCEL Orange Flavor
◆ CITRUCEL Sugar Free Orange Flavor
◆ Contac Allergy 12 Hour Tablets
◆ Contac Continuous Action Nasal Decongestant/Antihistamine 12 Hour Capsules
◆ Contac Maximum Strength Continuous Action Decongestant/Antihistamine 12 Hour Caplets
◆ Contac Day & Night Allergy/Sinus Caplets
◆ Contac Day & Night Cold/Flu Caplets
◆ Contac Day & Night Cold/Flu Night Caplets
◆ Contac Severe Cold & Flu Formula Caplets
◆ Contac Severe Cold & Flu Non-Drowsy Caplets
◆ Debrox Drops
◆ Ecotrin Enteric Coated Aspirin Low Strength Tablets
◆ Ecotrin Enteric Coated Aspirin Maximum Strength Tablets and Caplets
◆ Ecotrin Enteric Coated Aspirin Regular Strength Tablets
◆ Feosol Caplets
◆ Feosol Elixir
◆ Feosol Tablets
◆ Gaviscon Antacid Tablets
◆ Gaviscon Extra Strength Antacid Tablets
◆ Gaviscon Liquid Antacid
◆ Gaviscon Extra Strength Liquid Antacid
Gaviscon-2 Antacid Tablets
◆ Gly-Oxide Liquid

SMITHKLINE BEECHAM CONSUMER HEALTHCARE, L.P.—*cont.*
Massengill Disposable Douches
Massengill Feminine Cleansing Wash
Massengill Fragrance-Free and Baby Powder Scent Soft Cloth Towelettes
Massengill Liquid Concentrate
◆ Massengill Medicated Disposable Douche
Massengill Medicated Liquid Concentrate
Massengill Medicated Soft Cloth Towelette
Massengill Powder
N'ICE Medicated Sugarless Sore Throat and Cough Lozenges
◆ Nicoderm CQ Patch
◆ Nicorette Gum
Novahistine DMX
Novahistine Elixir
◆ Children's Panadol Chewable Tablets, Liquid, Infant's Drops
◆ Panadol Tablets and Caplets
Simron Capsules
Singlet Tablets
◆ Sucrets 4-Hour Cough Suppressant
◆ Sucrets Children's Cherry Flavored Sore Throat Lozenges
◆ Sucrets Maximum Strength Wintergreen, Maximum Strength Vapor Black Cherry Sore Throat Lozenges
◆ Sucrets Regular Strength Wild Cherry, Regular Strength Original Mint, Regular Strength Vapor Lemon Sore Throat Lozenges
◆ Tagamet HB 200 Tablets
Tums 500 Calcium Supplement Tablets
◆ Tums Antacid/Calcium Supplement Tablets
Tums Antigas/Antacid Formula Tablets, Assorted Fruit
◆ Tums E-X Antacid/Calcium Supplement Tablets
◆ Tums E-X Sugar Free Antacid/Calcium Supplement Tablets
◆ Tums ULTRA Antacid/Calcium Supplement Tablets

SMITHKLINE CONSUMER PRODUCTS
(See SMITHKLINE BEECHAM CONSUMER HEALTHCARE, L.P.)

STANDARD HOMEOPATHIC COMPANY 807
210 West 131st Street
Box 61067
Los Angeles, CA 90061
Direct Inquiries to:
Jay Borneman
(800) 624-9659

OTC Products Available:
Hyland's Bedwetting Tablets
Hyland's C-Plus Cold Tablets
Hyland's Calms Forté Tablets
Hyland's Colic Tablets
Hyland's Cough Syrup with Honey
Hyland's EnurAid Tablets
Hyland's Headache Tablets
Hyland's Leg Cramps Tablets
Hyland's Motion Sickness Tablets
Hyland's Teething Tablets
Hyland's Vaginitis Tablets

STELLAR HEALTH PRODUCTS, INC. ... 809
71 College Drive
Orange Park, FL 32065
Direct Inquiries to:
(800) 635-8372

OTC Products Available:
Arthur Itis
Diarrid Caplets

THOMPSON MEDICAL COMPANY, INC. 522, 810
222 Lakeview Avenue
West Palm Beach, FL 33401
Direct Inquiries to:
Consumer Services
(407) 820-9900
FAX: (407) 832-2297

OTC Products Available:
Aqua-Ban Maximum Strength Tablets
Arthritis Hot
◆ Aspercreme Creme Analgesic Rub
◆ Aspercreme Lotion Analgesic Rub
◆ Aspergel Gel Analgesic Rub
Breathe Free
◆ Capzasin-HP Topical Analgesic Creme
◆ Capzasin-P Topical Analgesic Creme
◆ Capzasin-P Topical Analgesic Lotion
Control Caplets
Dexatrim Maximum Strength Caffeine-Free Caplets
Dexatrim Maximum Strength Extended Duration Time Tablets
◆ Dexatrim Maximum Strength Plus Vitamin C/Caffeine-Free Caplets
◆ Dexatrim Plus Vitamins Caplets
Diar Aid Tablets
Encare Vaginal Contraceptive Suppositories
End Lice
NP-27 Cream & Spray Powder
◆ Sleepinal Night-time Sleep Aid Capsules and Softgels
Sportscreme External Analgesic Rub Cream & Lotion
Tribiotic Plus

TISHCON CORPORATION 813
30 New York Avenue
Westbury, NY 11590
Direct Inquiries to:
Product Information Department
(800) 848-8442
FAX: (516) 338-0829

OTC Products Available:
Driver's Friend Coffee Wafers
Lipo-Gel (Alpha-Lipoic Acid) Softsules
Lumitene
Dual Release Melatonin
Q-Gel Softsules
Q-Gel Forte Softsules
Q-Tab (Coenzyme Q10) Tablets
Daily Soy Capsules
Daily Soy Wafers
Stimulert Wafers
Triple Release Vitamin B12

TRITON CONSUMER PRODUCTS, INC. 814
561 West Golf Road
Arlington Heights, IL 60005
Direct Inquiries to:
Karen Shrader
(800) 942-2009
For Medical Emergencies Contact:
(800) 942-2009

OTC Products Available:
MG 217 Medicated Tar Shampoo
MG 217 Medicated Tar-Free Shampoo
MG 217 Psoriasis Ointment and Lotion
MG 217 Sal-Acid Ointment
ProTech First-Aid Stik
Retre-Gel Medicated Cold Sore Gel
Skeeter Stik Insect Bite Medication

UAS LABORATORIES 814
5610 Rowland Road #110
Minnetonka, MN 55343
Direct Inquiries to:
Dr. S.K. Dash
(612) 935-1707
FAX: (612) 935-1650
For Medical Emergencies Contact:
Dr. S.K. Dash
(612) 935-1707
FAX: (612) 935-1650

OTC Products Available:
DDS-Acidophilus Capsules, Tablets, and Powder

UNIPATH DIAGNOSTICS COMPANY 522, 814
Lever House
390 Park Avenue
New York, NY 10022
Direct Inquiries to:
(212) 888-1260

OTC Products Available:
◆ Clearblue Easy
◆ Clearplan Easy

THE UPJOHN COMPANY
(See PHARMACIA & UPJOHN)

VÄXA INTERNATIONAL, INC. 815
10307 Pacific Center Court
San Diego, CA 92121-4396
Direct Inquiries to:
(619) 625-8292
FAX: (619) 625-8272
World Wide Web:
vaxa.com

OTC Products Available:
Aller-Sine -- for allergies, sinusitis, and hayfever
Anti-Oxin+ -- purges the system of toxins, free radicals and heavy metals
Arthritin Capsules
Attend -- for ADD/ADHD and over-activity in children and adults
Buffer-pH -- pH alkalizing formula
Cholesten -- for excessive circulatory fats and lipids, cholesterol and triglycerides
Circulin -- for hypertension/high blood pressure problems
Colon-Aid+ -- depurative to cleanse the lower digestive tract
Deprex -- for mild depression, unhappiness, sadness and grief
Dermatin -- for acne, pimples, spots and blemishes
Digestin -- for normal digestive processes and relief from poor digestion
Extress -- for daily stress, anxiety and tension
Immun-Aid+ -- optimizes resistance against disease and illness
Memorin+ -- for aiding in memory, retention and retrieval
Migrin -- for migraine headaches
Nite-Rest -- for sleeplessness and insomnia
Omegacin+ Omega-3 and Omega-6 Fatty Acid Formula
Optimize -- provides extra energy and alertness for general tiredness
Pain-Eze -- for general aches and pains
Parasitin -- effectively eliminates most major parasites
PMS-Ease -- for emotional and physical pain and discomfort of premenstrual syndrome
Preserve -- for menopause, hot flashes and irregular menses
Prostatin+ -- for reduction of the enlarged prostate, BPH and associated problems
Systemex Nutraceutical Liquid Meal Replacement Formula
Tricardia+ -- for oral chelation of the cardiovascular system
Ultra CitraSlim -- repairs hypothalmic function for weight loss by increasing metabolism and decreasing appetite

Virexin Capsules

WAKUNAGA OF AMERICA CO., LTD.
(See KYOLIC LTD.)

WALLACE 522, 816
LABORATORIES
Half Acre Road
Cranbury, NJ 08512
Direct Inquiries to:
Wallace Laboratories
Div. of Carter-Wallace, Inc.
P.O. Box 1001
Cranbury, NJ 08512
(609) 655-6000
For Medical Emergencies Contact:
(800) 526-3840

OTC Products Available:
◆ Maltsupex Liquid, Powder & Tablets
Ryna Liquid
◆ Ryna-C Liquid
◆ Ryna-CX Liquid

WARNER-LAMBERT 523, 818
COMPANY
Consumer Health Products Group
201 Tabor Road
Morris Plains, NJ 07950
(See also Warner-Lambert Consumer Healthcare)
Direct Inquiries to:
1-(800) 223-0182
For Consumer Product Information Call:
1-(800) 524-2854 (Celestial Seasonings Soothers only)
1-(800) 223-0182

OTC Products Available:
◆ Celestial Seasonings Soothers Herbal Throat Drops
◆ Halls Juniors Sugar Free Cough Suppressant Drops
◆ Halls Mentho-Lyptus Cough Suppressant Drops
◆ Halls Plus Maximum Strength Cough Suppressant Drops
◆ Halls Sugar Free Mentho-Lyptus Cough Suppressant Drops
◆ Halls Vitamin C Drops
◆ Rolaids Antacid Tablets

WARNER-LAMBERT 523, 820
CONSUMER HEALTHCARE
201 Tabor Road
Morris Plains, NJ 07950
For Product Information Call:
1-(800) 223-0182
1-(800) 378-1783 (e.p.t.)
1-(800) 337-7266 (e.p.t. – Spanish)

OTC Products Available:
◆ Actifed Allergy Daytime/Nighttime Caplets
◆ Actifed Cold & Allergy Tablets
◆ Actifed Cold & Sinus Caplets and Tablets
◆ Actifed Sinus Daytime/Nighttime Tablets and Caplets
Agoral Liquid
◆ Anusol HC-1 Hydrocortisone Anti-Itch Ointment
◆ Anusol Hemorrhoidal Ointment
◆ Anusol Hemorrhoidal Suppositories
◆ Benadryl Allergy Chewables
◆ Benadryl Allergy/Cold Tablets
◆ Benadryl Allergy Decongestant Liquid Medication
◆ Benadryl Allergy Decongestant Tablets
◆ Benadryl Allergy Kapseal Capsules
◆ Benadryl Allergy Liquid Medication
◆ Benadryl Allergy Sinus Headache Caplets
◆ Benadryl Allergy Ultratab Tablets
◆ Benadryl Dye-Free Allergy Liqui-gels Softgels
◆ Benadryl Dye-Free Allergy Liquid Medication
◆ Benadryl Itch Relief Stick Extra Strength
◆ Benadryl Itch Stopping Cream Original Strength
◆ Benadryl Itch Stopping Cream Extra Strength
◆ Benadryl Itch Stopping Gel Original Strength
◆ Benadryl Itch Stopping Gel Extra Strength
◆ Benadryl Itch Stopping Spray Original Strength
◆ Benadryl Itch Stopping Spray Extra Strength
◆ Benylin Adult Cough Suppressant
◆ Benylin Cough Suppressant Expectorant
◆ Benylin Multisymptom
◆ Benylin Pediatric Cough Suppressant
◆ Borofax Skin Protectant Ointment
◆ Caladryl Clear Lotion
◆ Caladryl Cream For Kids
◆ Caladryl Lotion
Corn Husker's Lotion
Empirin Aspirin Tablets
◆ e.p.t. Pregnancy Test
◆ Listerine Antiseptic Mouthrinse
◆ Cool Mint Listerine Antiseptic Mouthrinse
◆ FreshBurst Listerine Antiseptic Mouthrinse
◆ Listermint Alcohol-Free Mouthrinse
◆ Lubriderm Bath and Shower Oil
◆ Lubriderm Dry Skin Care Lotion
◆ Lubriderm GelCreme
◆ Lubriderm Moisture Recovery Alpha Hydroxy Lotion
◆ Lubriderm Seriously Sensitive Lotion
Myadec Tablets
◆ Neosporin "Neo to Go!"
◆ Neosporin Ointment
◆ Neosporin Plus Maximum Strength Cream
◆ Neosporin Plus Maximum Strength Ointment
◆ Nix Creme Rinse
◆ Polysporin Ointment
◆ Polysporin Powder
◆ Replens Vaginal Moisturizer
◆ Sinutab Non-Drying Liquid Caps
◆ Sinutab Sinus Allergy Medication, Maximum Strength Formula, Tablets and Caplets
◆ Sinutab Sinus Medication, Maximum Strength Without Drowsiness Formula, Tablets & Caplets
◆ Sudafed 12 Hour Caplets
◆ Children's Sudafed Nasal Decongestant Chewables
◆ Children's Sudafed Nasal Decongestant Liquid Medication
◆ Sudafed Cold & Allergy Tablets
◆ Sudafed Cold & Cough Liquid Caps
◆ Sudafed Cold & Sinus Liquid Caps
◆ Sudafed Nasal Decongestant Tablets, 30 mg
◆ Sudafed Non-Drying Sinus Liquid Caps
◆ Pediatric Sudafed Nasal Decongestant Liquid Oral Drops
◆ Sudafed Severe Cold Formula Caplets
◆ Sudafed Severe Cold Formula Tablets
◆ Sudafed Sinus Caplets
◆ Sudafed Sinus Tablets
◆ Tucks Clear Hemorrhoidal Gel
◆ Tucks Premoistened Hemorrhoidal/Vaginal Pads
Tucks Take-Alongs
◆ Zantac 75 Tablets

WELLNESS INTERNATIONAL 841
NETWORK, LTD.
1501 Luna Road, Bldg. 102
Carrollton, TX 75006
Direct Inquiries to:
Director of Product Development
(972) 245-1097
FAX: (972) 389-3060

OTC Products Available:
Bio-Complex 5000 Gentle Foaming Cleanser
Bio-Complex 5000 Revitalizing Conditioner
Bio-Complex 5000 Revitalizing Shampoo
BioLean
BioLean Accelerator
BioLean Free
BioLean LipoTrim
BioLean Meal
DHEA Plus
Food for Thought
Phyto-Vite
Sleep-Tite
StePHan Bio-Nutritional Daytime Hydrating Creme
StePHan Bio-Nutritional Eye-Firming Concentrate
StePHan Bio-Nutritional Nightime Moisture Creme
StePHan Bio-Nutritional Refreshing Moisture Gel
StePHan Bio-Nutritional Ultra Hydrating Fluid
StePHan Clarity
StePHan Elasticity
StePHan Elixir
StePHan Essential
StePHan Feminine
StePHan Flexibility
StePHan Lovpil
StePHan Masculine
StePHan Protector
StePHan Relief
StePHan Tranquility
Winrgy

WHITEHALL LABORATORIES INC.
(See WHITEHALL-ROBINS HEALTHCARE)

WHITEHALL-ROBINS 849
HEALTHCARE
American Home Products Corporation
Five Giralda Farms
Madison, NJ 07940-0871
Direct Inquiries to:
Whitehall Consumer Product Information:
(800) 322-3129 (9-5 E.S.T.)
Robins Consumer Product Information:
(800) 762-4672 (9-5 E.S.T.)

OTC Products Available:
Advil Ibuprofen Tablets, Caplets and Gel Caplets
Children's Advil Oral Suspension
Advil Cold and Sinus Caplets and Tablets
Anacin Caplets and Tablets
Aspirin Free Anacin Gel Caplets
Aspirin Free Anacin Maximum Strength
Anbesol Gel and Liquid
Baby Anbesol
Axid AR Tablets
Chapstick Lip Balm
Chapstick Sunblock 15 Lip Balm
Denorex Medicated Shampoo and Conditioner
Dimetapp Allergy Dye-Free Elixir
Dimetapp Allergy Sinus Caplets
Dimetapp Cold & Allergy Chewable Tablets
Dimetapp Cold & Allergy Quick Dissolve Tablets
Dimetapp Cold & Cough Liqui-Gels, Maximum Strength
Dimetapp Cold & Fever Suspension
Dimetapp Decongestant Pediatric Drops
Dimetapp Dye-Free Allergy (Children's)
Dimetapp Elixir
Dimetapp DM Elixir
Dimetapp Extentabs
Dimetapp Liqui-Gels
Dimetapp Tablets
Dristan 12-hour Nasal Spray

WHITEHALL-ROBINS HEALTHCARE —*cont.*

Dristan Maximum Strength Cold Non-Drowsiness Gel Caplets
Orudis KT
Posture 600 mg
Preparation H Hemorrhoidal Cream
Preparation H Hemorrhoidal Ointment
Preparation H Hemorrhoidal Suppositories
Preparation H Hydrocortisone 1% Cream
Primatene Mist
Primatene Tablets
Riopan Suspension
Robitussin
Robitussin-CF
Robitussin Cold & Cough Liqui-Gels
Robitussin Cold, Cough & Flu Liqui-Gels
Robitussin Cough & Congestion
Robitussin-DM
Robitussin Liquid Center Cough Drops
Robitussin Maximum Strength Cough & Cold
Robitussin Maximum Strength Cough Suppressant
Robitussin Night-Time Cold Formula
Robitussin-PE
Robitussin Pediatric Cough & Cold Formula
Robitussin Pediatric Cough Suppressant
Robitussin Pediatric Drops
Robitussin Severe Congestion Liqui-Gels
Robitussin Sugar-Free Cough Drops

J.B. WILLIAMS COMPANY, INC. 527, 863

65 Harristown Road
Glen Rock, NJ 07452
Direct Inquiries to:
Consumer Affairs
(800) 254-8656
(201) 251-8100
FAX: (201) 251-8097
For Medical Emergencies Contact:
(800) 254-8656

OTC Products Available:

◆ Cēpacol/Cēpacol Mint Antiseptic Mouthwash/Gargle
◆ Cēpacol Maximum Strength Sore Throat Lozenges, Cherry Flavor
◆ Cēpacol Maximum Strength Sore Throat Lozenges, Mint Flavor
Cēpacol Regular Strength Sore Throat Lozenges, Cherry Flavor
Cēpacol Regular Strength Sore Throat Lozenges, Original Mint Flavor
◆ Cēpacol Maximum Strength Sore Throat Spray, Cherry Flavor
◆ Cēpacol Maximum Strength Sore Throat Spray, Cool Menthol Flavor

THE WINNING COMBINATION
(See AML LABORATORIES)

WYETH-AYERST LABORATORIES 527, 864

Division of American Home Products Corporation
P.O. Box 8299
Philadelphia, PA 19101
Direct General Inquiries to:
(610) 688-4400
For Professional Services:
(For example: Sales representative information, product pamphlets, educational materials):
(800) 395-9938
For Medical Information Contact:
Medical Affairs
Day: (800) 934-5556 (8:30 AM to 4:30 PM, Eastern Standard Time, Weekdays Only)
Night: (610) 688-4400 (Emergencies Only; non-emergencies should wait until the next day)
WYETH-AYERST DISTRIBUTION CENTERS
(Do not use freight addresses for mailing orders.)
Atlanta, GA—P.O. Box 1773
Paoli, PA 19301-1773
(800) 666-7248
Freight Address:
100 Union Court
Kennesaw, GA 30144
Mail DEA order forms to:
P.O. Box 4365
Atlanta, GA 30302
Chicago, IL – P.O. Box 1773
Paoli, PA 19301-1773
(800) 666-7248
Freight Address:
284 Lies Road
Carol Stream, IL 60188
Mail DEA order forms to:
P.O. Box 140
Wheaton, IL 60189-0140
Dallas, TX—P.O. Box 1773
Paoli, PA 19301-1773
(800) 666-7248
Freight Address:
11240 Petal Street
Dallas, TX 75238
Mail DEA order forms to:
P.O. Box 650231
Dallas, TX 75265-0231
Sparks, NV—1802 Briely Way
Sparks, NV 89431
(800) 666-7248
Freight Address:
1802 Briely Way
Sparks, NV 89431
Mail DEA order forms to:
1802 Briely Way
Sparks, NV 89431
Philadelphia, PA—P.O. Box 1773
Paoli, PA 19301-1773
(800) 666-7248
Freight Address:
31 Morehall Road
Frazer, PA 19355
Mail DEA order forms to:
P.O. Box 61
Paoli, PA 19301

OTC Products Available:

◆ Amphojel Suspension (Mint Flavor)
Amphojel Suspension without Flavor
◆ Amphojel Tablets
◆ Basaljel Capsules
◆ Basaljel Suspension
◆ Basaljel Tablets
◆ Cerose DM
◆ Donnagel Liquid and Donnagel Chewable Tablets

ZILA PHARMACEUTICALS, INC. 528, 866

5227 North 7th Street
Phoenix, AZ 85014-2800
Direct Inquiries to:
Jerry Kaster
Director of Marketing
(602) 266-6700
World Wide Web:
www.zila.com

OTC Products Available:

◆ Zilactin Medicated Gel
◆ Zilactin-B Medicated Gel with Benzocaine
◆ Zilactin-L Liquid

ZP TECH INC. 528, 866

12803 Schabarum Avenue
Irwindale, CA 91706
Direct Inquiries to:
(800) 636-6289
(818) 337-4700
FAX: (818) 338-7676

OTC Products Available:

◆ Bio-Nova Ginkgo Tablets

SECTION 2

PRODUCT NAME INDEX

This index includes all entries in the "Product Information" section. Products are listed alphabetically by brand name.

If two page numbers appear, the first refers to the product's photograph, the second to its product information.

- **Bold page numbers** indicate full product information.
- *Italic page numbers* signify partial information.

B

C

D

E

F

N

O

T

U

V

W

X

Y

Z

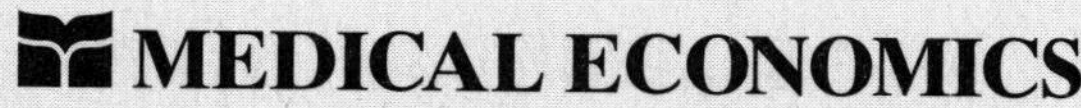
MEDICAL ECONOMICS

SECTION 3

PRODUCT CATEGORY INDEX

This index cross-references each brand by pharmaceutical category. All fully-described products in the "Product Information" section are included.

If two page numbers appear, the first refers to the product's photograph, the second to its product information.

The classification of each product is determined by the publisher in cooperation with the product's manufacturer or, when necessary, by the publisher alone.

ANTIMYCOTICS

(see SKIN & MUCOUS MEMBRANE AGENTS: ANTI-INFECTIVES, ANTIFUNGALS & COMBINATIONS; VAGINAL PREPARATIONS: ANTI-INFECTIVES, ANTIFUNGALS & COMBINATIONS)

ANTIPRURITICS

(see ANTIHISTAMINES & COMBINATIONS; SKIN & MUCOUS MEMBRANE AGENTS: ANTIPRURITICS)

ANTIPYRETICS

(see ANALGESICS: ACETAMINOPHEN & COMBINATIONS, NONSTEROIDAL ANTI-INFLAMMATORY AGENTS (NSAIDS), SALICYLATES)

RESPIRATORY AGENTS—*cont.*

ANTITUSSIVES—*cont.*

NON-NARCOTIC ANTITUSSIVES & COMBINATIONS—*cont.*

BRONCHODILATORS

SYMPATHOMIMETICS & COMBINATIONS

DECONGESTANTS & COMBINATIONS

DECONGESTANTS, EXPECTORANTS & COMBINATIONS

EXPECTORANTS & COMBINATIONS

MISCELLANEOUS COLD & COUGH PRODUCTS WITH ANALGESICS

ANESTHETICS & COMBINATIONS

ANORECTAL PREPARATIONS

ANTI-INFECTIVES

ANTIBIOTICS & COMBINATIONS

ANTIFUNGALS & COMBINATIONS

MISCELLANEOUS ANTI-INFECTIVES & COMBINATIONS

SKIN & MUCOUS MEMBRANE AGENTS —*cont.*

ANTI-INFECTIVES—*cont.*

MISCELLANEOUS ANTI-INFECTIVES & COMBINATIONS—*cont.*

SCABICIDES & PEDICULICIDES

ANTIHISTAMINES & COMBINATIONS

ANTIPRURITICS

ANTIPSORIATIC AGENTS

ANTISEBORRHEIC AGENTS

ASTRINGENTS

BATH OILS

BURN PREPARATIONS

SECTION 4

ACTIVE INGREDIENTS INDEX

This index cross-references each brand by its generic ingredients. All entries in the "Product Information" section are included. Under each generic heading, all fully described products are listed first, followed by those with only partial descriptions.

If two page numbers appear, the first refers to the product's photograph, the second to its product information.

- **Bold page numbers** indicate full product information.
- *Italic page numbers* signify partial information.

Classification of products under these headings has been determined in cooperation with the products' manufacturers or, if necessary, by the publisher alone.

Italic Page Number **Indicates Brief Listing**

Italic Page Number **Indicates Brief Listing**

SECTION 5

COMPANION DRUG INDEX

This index provides you with a quick-reference guide to over-the-counter products that may be used, in conjunction with prescription drug therapy, to reverse drug-induced side effects, relieve symptoms of the illness itself, or treat sequelae of the initial disease. All entries are derived from the product information published by *PDR.*

The products listed are generally considered effective for temporary symptomatic relief. Please bear in mind, however, that they may not be appropriate for sustained therapy, and that certain common side effects may be harbingers of more serious reactions. Remember, too, that each case must be approached on an individual basis. When making a recommendation, be sure to adjust for the patient's age, concurrent medical conditions, and complete drug regimen. Consider timing as well, since simultaneous ingestion may not be recommended in all instances.

Please note that only products fully described in *Physicians' Desk Reference* and its companion volumes are included in this index. The publisher therefore cannot guarantee that all entries are totally accurate or complete. Keep in mind, too, that although a given over-the-counter product is usually an appropriate companion for an entire class of prescription medications, certain drugs within the class may be exceptions. If you have any doubt about the suitability of a particular OTC product in a given situation, be sure to check the underlying *PDR* prescribing information and the relevant medical literature.

We hope you find this new index to be a valuable clinical tool. We are continually seeking new ways to better serve the health care community. If you have any comments or suggestions for improvement, please send us a note in care of "Companion Drug Index," *Physicians' Desk Reference,* 5 Paragon Drive, Montvale, NJ 07645.

ACUTE MOUNTAIN SICKNESS, HEADACHE SECONDARY TO

Acute mountain sickness may be treated with acetazolamide. The following products may be recommended for relief of headache:

ALCOHOLISM, HYPOCALCEMIA SECONDARY TO

Alcoholism may be treated with disulfiram or naltrexone hydrochloride. The following products may be recommended for relief of hypocalcemia:

ALCOHOLISM, HYPOMAGNESEMIA SECONDARY TO

Alcoholism may be treated with disulfiram or naltrexone hydrochloride. The following products may be recommended for relief of hypomagnesemia:

- Beelith Tablets 627
- Mag-Ox 400 632
- Magonate Tablets and Liquid 658
- MagTab SR Caplets 701
- Uro-Mag 632

ALCOHOLISM, VITAMINS AND MINERALS DEFICIENCY SECONDARY TO

Alcoholism may be treated with disulfiram or naltrexone hydrochloride. The following products may be recommended for relief of vitamins and minerals deficiency:

- Centrum Silver Tablets 673
- Centrum Tablets 670
- Complete for Men 603
- Complete for Women 604
- Natural M.D. Basic Life Prescription for Men 605
- Natural M.D. Basic Life Prescription for Women 605
- Natural M.D. Complete Life Prescription 607
- Natural M.D. Essential Life Prescription 606
- Natural M.D. Standard Life Prescription for Men 605
- Natural M.D. Standard Life Prescription for Women 606
- Natural M.D. Ultimate Life Prescription 607
- One-A-Day Essential Vitamins 624
- One-A-Day 50 Plus 624
- One-A-Day Maximum 625
- One-A-Day Men's 625
- One-A-Day Women's 626
- Stress Gum 608
- Stresstabs Tablets 674
- Stresstabs + Iron Tablets 674
- Stresstabs + Zinc Tablets 674

ANCYLOSTOMIASIS, IRON-DEFICIENCY ANEMIA SECONDARY TO

Ancylostomiasis may be treated with mebendazole or thiabendazole. The following products may be recommended for relief of iron-deficiency anemia:

- Feosol Caplets 790
- Feosol Elixir 791
- Feosol Tablets 791
- Ferro-Sequels Tablets 673
- Slow Fe Tablets 718
- Slow Fe with Folic Acid Tablets 718
- Vitron-C Tablets 727

ANEMIA, IRON-DEFICIENCY

May result from the use of chronic salicylate therapy or nonsteroidal anti-inflammatory drugs. The following products may be recommended:

- Feosol Caplets 790
- Feosol Elixir 791
- Feosol Tablets 791
- Ferro-Sequels Tablets 673
- Slow Fe Tablets 718
- Slow Fe with Folic Acid Tablets 718
- Vitron-C Tablets 727

ANGINA, UNSTABLE

May be treated with beta blockers, calcium channel blockers or nitrates. The following products may be recommended for relief of symptoms:

- Ascriptin Enteric 704
- Bayer Aspirin Professional Labeling (Aspirin Regimen Bayer and Genuine Bayer Aspirin) 615
- Bufferin Analgesic Tablets 639
- Ecotrin Enteric Coated Aspirin Low Strength Tablets 787
- Ecotrin Enteric Coated Aspirin Maximum Strength Tablets and Caplets 787
- Ecotrin Enteric Coated Aspirin Regular Strength Tablets 787
- St. Joseph Adult Chewable Aspirin Caplets (81 mg.) 781

ARTHRITIS

May be treated with corticosteroids or nonsteroidal anti-inflammatory drugs. The following products may be recommended for relief of symptoms:

- ArthriCare Odor Free Rub 654
- ArthriCare Triple Medicated Rub 654
- ArthriCare Ultra Rub 654
- Arthur Itis 809
- Aspercreme Creme Analgesic Rub 810
- Aspercreme Lotion Analgesic Rub 810
- Aspergel Gel Analgesic Rub 810
- BenGay External Analgesic Products 728
- Capsagel 663
- Capzasin-HP Topical Analgesic Creme 810
- Capzasin-P Topical Analgesic Creme 810
- Capzasin-P Topical Analgesic Lotion 810
- Eucalyptamint Arthritis Pain Relief Formula 709
- Eucalyptamint Muscle Pain Relief Formula 710
- Menthacin Cream 700
- Mentholatum Deep Heating Rub 701
- Myoflex Pain Relieving Cream 714
- Sportscreme External Analgesic Rub Cream & Lotion 813
- Therapeutic Mineral Ice 649
- Vicks VapoRub Cream 762
- Vicks VapoRub Ointment 762

BRONCHITIS, CHRONIC, ACUTE EXACERBATION OF

May be treated with quinolones, sulfamethoxazole-trimethoprim, cefixime, cefpodoxime proxetil, cefprozil, ceftibuten dihydrate, cefuroxime axetil, cilastatin sodium, clarithromycin, imipenem or loracarbef. The following products may be recommended for relief of symptoms:

- Benylin Cough Suppressant Expectorant 828
- Benylin Multisymptom 829
- Cheracol D Cough Formula 764
- Comtrex Deep Chest Cold and Cough Congestion Relief Non-Drowsy Liquigels 643
- Delsym Extended-Release Suspension 698
- PediaCare Infants' Drops Decongestant Plus Cough 684
- Primatene Tablets 857
- Robitussin 859
- Robitussin Cold & Cough Liqui-Gels 858
- Robitussin Cold, Cough & Flu Liqui-Gels 858
- Robitussin-DM 860
- Robitussin Maximum Strength Cough & Cold 861
- Robitussin-PE 860
- Robitussin Pediatric Drops 862
- Robitussin Severe Congestion Liqui-Gels 859
- Ryna-CX Liquid 817
- Sinutab Non-Drying Liquid Caps 835
- Sudafed Cold & Cough Liquid Caps 838
- Sudafed Non-Drying Sinus Liquid Caps 839
- Vicks 44E Cough & Chest Congestion Relief 754
- Pediatric Vicks 44e Cough & Chest Congestion Relief 760
- Vicks VapoRub Cream 762
- Vicks VapoRub Ointment 762
- Vicks VapoSteam 762

BURN INFECTIONS, SEVERE, NUTRIENTS DEFICIENCY SECONDARY TO

Severe burn infections may be treated with anti-infectives. The following products may be recommended for relief of nutrients deficiency:

- Bugs Bunny Complete Children's Chewable Vitamins + Minerals with Iron and Calcium (Sugar Free) 619
- Bugs Bunny Plus Iron Children's Chewable Vitamins (Sugar Free) 618
- Bugs Bunny With Extra C Children's Chewable Vitamins (Sugar Free) 620
- Centrum Silver Tablets 673
- Centrum Tablets 670
- Centrum, Jr. + Extra C Children's Chewables 671
- Centrum, Jr. + Extra Calcium Children's Chewables 671
- Centrum, Jr. + Iron Children's Chewables 672
- Complete for Men 603
- Complete for Women 604
- Ester-C Tablets, Caplets, or Capsules 662
- Flintstones Children's Chewable Vitamins 618
- Flintstones Children's Chewable Vitamins Plus Extra C 620
- Flintstones Children's Chewable Vitamins Plus Iron 618

CANCER, NUTRIENTS DEFICIENCY SECONDARY TO

Cancer may be treated with chemotherapeutic agents. The following products may be recommended for relief of nutrients deficiency:

CANDIDIASIS, VAGINAL

May be treated with antifungal agents. The following products may be recommended for relief of symptoms:

CONGESTIVE HEART FAILURE, NUTRIENTS DEFICIENCY SECONDARY TO

Congestive heart failure may be treated with ACE inhibitors, cardiac glycosides or diuretics. The following products may be recommended for relief of nutrients deficiency:

CONSTIPATION

May result from the use of ACE inhibitors, HMG-CoA reductase inhibitors, anticholinergics, anticonvulsants, antidepressants, beta blockers, bile acid sequestrants, butyrophenones, calcium and aluminum-containing antacids, calcium channel blockers, ganglionic blockers, hematinics, monoamine oxidase inhibitors, narcotic analgesics, nonsteroidal anti-inflammatory drugs or phenothiazines. The following products may be recommended:

DIABETES MELLITUS, PRURITUS SECONDARY TO
Diabetes mellitus may be treated with insulins or oral hypoglycemic agents. The following products may be recommended for relief of pruritus:

DIAPER DERMATITIS
May result from the use of cefpodoxime proxetil, cefprozil, cefuroxime axetil or varicella virus vaccine live. The following products may be recommended:

DIARRHEA
May result from the use of ACE inhibitors, beta blockers, cardiac glycosides, chemotherapeutic agents, diuretics, magnesium-containing antacids, nonsteroidal anti-inflammatory drugs, potassium supplements, acarbose, alprazolam, colchicine, divalproex sodium, ethosuximide, fluoxetine hydrochloride, guanethidine monosulfate, hydralazine hydrochloride, levodopa, lithium carbonate, lithium citrate, mesna, metformin hydrochloride, misoprostol, olsalazine sodium, pancrelipase, procainamide hydrochloride, reserpine, succimer, ticlopidine hydrochloride or valproic acid. The following products may be recommended:

DIARRHEA, ANTIBIOTIC-INDUCED
May result from the use of cephalosporins, erythromycin, erythromycin-sulfisoxazole, ampicillin or clindamycin palmitate hydrochloride. The following products may be recommended:

DIARRHEA, INFECTIOUS
May be treated with sulfamethoxazole-trimethoprim, ciprofloxacin or furazolidone. The following products may be recommended for relief of symptoms:

DRY EYE
(see under XEROPHTHALMIA)

DRY SKIN
(see under XERODERMA)

DYSPEPSIA
May result from the use of chronic systemic corticosteroid therapy, nonsteroidal anti-inflammatory drugs, ulcerogenic medications or mexiletine hydrochloride. The following products may be recommended:

DYSPEPSIA—cont.

Marblen Suspension Peach/ Apricot **658**
Marblen Tablets............................**658**
Mylanta Gelcaps Antacid **667**
Mylanta Liquid **665**
Mylanta Maximum Strength Liquid **665**
Mylanta Tablets **666**
Mylanta Maximum Strength Tablets **666**
Nephrox Suspension **658**
Phillips' Milk of Magnesia Liquid **626**
Rolaids Antacid Tablets.................**819**
3M Titralac Antacid Tablets **675**
3M Titralac Extra Strength Antacid Tablets..........................**675**
3M Titralac Plus Antacid Tablets **675**
3M Titralac Plus Liquid Antacid **675**
Tums Antacid/Calcium Supplement Tablets **806**
Tums Antigas/Antacid Formula Tablets, Assorted Fruit **807**
Tums E-X Antacid/Calcium Supplement Tablets **806**
Tums E-X Sugar Free Antacid/ Calcium Supplement Tablets **806**
Tums ULTRA Antacid/Calcium Supplement Tablets **806**

EMESIS, UNPLEASANT TASTE SECONDARY TO

Emesis may be treated with antiemetics. The following products may be recommended for relief of unpleasant taste:

Breath + Plus **603**
Cēpacol/Cēpacol Mint Antiseptic Mouthwash/Gargle **863**
Listerine Antiseptic Mouthrinse......**831**
Cool Mint Listerine Antiseptic Mouthrinse..............................**831**
FreshBurst Listerine Antiseptic Mouthrinse..............................**831**
Listermint Alcohol-Free Mouthrinse...**832**

ENTEROBIASIS, PERIANAL PRURITUS SECONDARY TO

Enterobiasis may be treated with mebendazole. The following products may be recommended for relief of perianal pruritus:

Anusol HC-1 Hydrocortisone Anti-Itch Ointment.................................**823**
Benadryl Itch Relief Stick Extra Strength.................................**827**
Caldecort Anti-Itch Cream **706**
Maximum Strength Cortaid Cream..**738**
Maximum Strength Cortaid Ointment.................................**738**
Maximum Strength Cortaid FastStick.................................**738**
Cortaid Sensitive Skin Cream with Aloe......................................**738**
Cortaid Sensitive Skin Ointment with Aloe **738**
Maximum Strength Cortaid Spray ...**738**
Cortaid Intensive Therapy Cream....**738**
Cortizone for Kids **729**
Cortizone-5 Creme and Ointment....**729**
Cortizone-10 Creme and Ointment ...**729**
Cortizone-10 External Anal Itch Relief.....................................**729**
Massengill Medicated Soft Cloth Towelette **795**
Nupercainal Hemorrhoidal and Anesthetic Ointment **715**
Nupercainal Hydrocortisone 1% Cream....................................**715**
Preparation H Hydrocortisone 1% Cream....................................**856**

FEVER

May result from the use of immunization. The following products may be recommended:

Actron Caplets and Tablets............**609**
Advil Ibuprofen Tablets, Caplets and Gel Caplets **849**
Children's Advil Oral Suspension....**850**
Aleve Tablets and Caplets **610**
Regular Strength Ascriptin **703**
Arthritis Pain Ascriptin **703**
Ascriptin Enteric...........................**704**
Maximum Strength Ascriptin **703**
Extra Strength Bayer Arthritis Pain Regimen Formula...............**616**
Genuine Bayer Aspirin Tablets & Caplets **613**
Extended-Release Bayer 8-Hour Aspirin **616**
Extra Strength Bayer Aspirin Caplets & Tablets **617**
Aspirin Regimen Bayer Regular Strength 325 mg Caplets **613**
Aspirin Regimen Bayer Adult Low Strength 81 mg Tablets............**613**
Bayer Aspirin Professional Labeling (Aspirin Regimen Bayer and Genuine Bayer Aspirin) **615**
Extra Strength Bayer Plus Aspirin Caplets **617**
Extra Strength Bayer PM Aspirin Plus Sleep Aid **617**
BC Powder **634**
BC Allergy Sinus Cold Powder **634**
Arthritis Strength BC Powder..........**634**
BC Sinus Cold Powder...................**634**
Bufferin Analgesic Tablets **639**
Arthritis Strength Bufferin Analgesic Caplets **640**
Extra Strength Bufferin Analgesic Tablets **640**
Children's Motrin Ibuprofen Drops....**676**
Children's Motrin Ibuprofen Oral Suspension **676**
Children's TYLENOL acetaminophen Chewable Tablets, Elixir and Suspension Liquid **677**
Aspirin Free Excedrin Analgesic Caplets and Geltabs **645**
Excedrin Extra-Strength Analgesic Tablets, Caplets, and Geltabs....**645**
Excedrin P.M. Analgesic/ Sleeping Aid Tablets, Caplets, and Geltabs **646**
Goody's Extra Strength Headache Powder **634**
Goody's Extra Strength Pain Relief Tablets **635**
Infants' TYLENOL acetaminophen Suspension Drops **677**
Junior Strength Motrin Ibuprofen Caplets **682**
Junior Strength TYLENOL acetaminophen Coated Caplets, and Chewable Tablets **682**
Motrin IB Caplets, Tablets, and Gelcaps **741**
Nuprin Tablets and Caplets **648**
Orudis KT **855**
Children's Panadol Chewable Tablets, Liquid, Infant's Drops ...**803**
Panadol Tablets and Caplets **803**
St. Joseph Adult Chewable Aspirin Caplets (81 mg.)............**781**
TYLENOL acetaminophen Extended Relief Caplets **687**
TYLENOL acetaminophen, Extra Strength Adult Liquid Pain Reliever **687**
TYLENOL acetaminophen, Extra Strength Gelcaps, Caplets, Tablets, Geltabs **687**
TYLENOL acetaminophen, Regular Strength, Caplets and Tablets **687**
TYLENOL PM Pain Reliever/Sleep Aid, Extra Strength Gelcaps, Caplets, Geltabs.......................**695**
Unisom With Pain Relief-Nighttime Sleep Aid and Pain Reliever **734**
Vanquish Analgesic Caplets...........**627**

FLATULENCE

May result from the use of nonsteroidal anti-inflammatory drugs, potassium supplements, acarbose, cisapride, guanadrel sulfate, mesalamine, metformin hydrochloride, methyldopa, octreotide acetate or ursodiol. The following products may be recommended:

Beano Liquid **602**
Beano Tablets **602**
Gas-X Chewable Tablets **711**
Extra Strength Gas-X Chewable Tablets **711**
Extra Strength Gas-X Softgels **711**
Maalox Anti-Gas Tablets, Regular Strength.................................**712**
Maalox Anti-Gas Tablets, Extra Strength.................................**713**
Mylanta Gas Relief Gelcaps **666**
Mylanta Gas Relief Tablets **666**
Maximum Strength Mylanta Gas Relief Tablets **666**
Phazyme Infant Drops **636**
Phazyme-95 Tablets **636**
Phazyme-125 Chewable Tablets Maximum Strength....................**636**
Phazyme-125 Liquid Maximum Strength.................................**636**
Phazyme-125 Softgel Capsules Maximum Strength....................**636**

FLU-LIKE SYNDROME

May result from the use of gemcitabine hydrochloride, interferon alfa-2b, recombinant, interferon alfa-n3 (human leukocyte derived), interferon beta-1b, interferon gamma-1b or succimer. The following products may be recommended:

GASTRITIS, IRON-DEFICIENCY SECONDARY TO

Gastritis may be treated with histamine H_2 receptor antagonists, proton pump inhibitors or sucralfate. The following products may be recommended for relief of iron deficiency:

GASTROESOPHAGEAL REFLUX DISEASE

May be treated with histamine H_2 receptor antagonists, proton pump inhibitors or sucralfate. The following products may be recommended for relief of symptoms:

GINGIVAL HYPERPLASIA

May result from the use of calcium channel blockers, cyclosporine, fosphenytoin sodium or phenytoin. The following products may be recommended:

HUMAN IMMUNODEFICIENCY VIRUS (HIV) INFECTIONS, NUTRIENTS DEFICIENCY SECONDARY TO

HIV infections may be treated with non-nucleoside reverse transcriptase inhibitors, nucleoside reverse transcriptase inhibitors or protease inhibitors. The following products may be recommended for relief of nutrients deficiency:

HUMAN IMMUNODEFICIENCY VIRUS (HIV) INFECTIONS, SEBORRHEIC DERMATITIS SECONDARY TO

HIV infections may be treated with non-nucleoside reverse transcriptase inhibitors, nucleoside reverse transcriptase inhibitors or protease inhibitors. The following products may be recommended for relief of seborrheic dermatitis:

HUMAN IMMUNODEFICIENCY VIRUS (HIV) INFECTIONS, XERODERMA SECONDARY TO

HIV infections may be treated with non-nucleoside reverse transcriptase inhibitors, nucleoside reverse transcriptase inhibitors or protease inhibitors. The following products may be recommended for relief of xeroderma:

HYPERTHYROIDISM, NUTRIENTS DEFICIENCY SECONDARY TO

Hyperthyroidism may be treated with methimazole. The following products may be recommended for relief of nutrients deficiency:

HYPOKALEMIA

May be treated with thiazides, diuretics or amphotericin B. The following products may be recommended for relief of symptoms:

HYPOKALEMIA

May result from the use of thiazides, corticosteroids, diuretics, aldesleukin, amphotericin B, carboplatin, etretinate, foscarnet sodium, mycophenolate mofetil, pamidronate disodium or tacrolimus. The following products may be recommended:

HYPOMAGNESEMIA

May result from the use of aldesleukin, aminoglycosides, amphotericin B, carboplatin, cisplatin, cyclosporine, diuretics, foscarnet, pamidronate, sargramostim or tacrolimus. The following products may be recommended:

HYPOPARATHYROIDISM

May be treated with vitamin D sterols. The following products may be recommended for relief of symptoms:

HYPOTHYROIDISM, CONSTIPATION SECONDARY TO

Hypothyroidism may be treated with thyroid hormones. The following products may be recommended for relief of constipation:

HYPOTHYROIDISM, XERODERMA SECONDARY TO

Hypothyroidism may be treated with thyroid hormones. The following products may be recommended for relief of xeroderma:

INFECTIONS, BACTERIAL, UPPER RESPIRATORY TRACT

May be treated with amoxicillin-clavulanate, cephalosporins, doxycycline, erythromycin, macrolide antibiotics, penicillins, amoxicillin trihydrate or minocycline hydrochloride. The following products may be recommended for relief of symptoms:

INFECTIONS, BACTERIAL, UPPER RESPIRATORY TRACT—cont.

INFECTIONS, BACTERIAL, UPPER RESPIRATORY TRACT—cont.

INFECTIONS, SKIN AND SKIN STRUCTURE

May be treated with aminoglycosides, amoxicillin, amoxicillin-clavulanate, cephalosporins, doxycycline, erythromycin, macrolide antibiotics, penicillins or quinolones. The following products may be recommended for relief of symptoms:

IRRITABLE BOWEL SYNDROME

May be treated with anticholinergic combinations, dicyclomine hydrochloride or hyoscyamine sulfate. The following products may be recommended for relief of symptoms:

ISCHEMIC HEART DISEASE

May be treated with beta blockers, calcium channel blockers, isosorbide dinitrate, isosorbide mononitrate or nitroglycerin. The following products may be recommended for relief of symptoms:

KERATOCONJUNCTIVITIS, VERNAL

May be treated with ophthalmic mast cell stabilizers. The following products may be recommended for relief of symptoms:

MENOPAUSAL SYMPTOMS, VAGINAL DRYNESS SECONDARY TO

Menopausal symptoms may be treated with estrogens. The following products may be recommended for relief of vaginal dryness:

MYOCARDIAL INFARCTION, ACUTE
May be treated with ACE inhibitors, anticoagulants, beta blockers, thrombolytic agents or nitroglycerin. The following products may be recommended for relief of symptoms:

NASAL POLYPS, RHINORRHEA SECONDARY TO
Nasal polyps may be treated with nasal steroidal anti-inflammatory agents. The following products may be recommended for relief of rhinorrhea:

NECATORIASIS, IRON-DEFICIENCY ANEMIA SECONDARY TO
Necatoriasis may be treated with mebendazole or thiabendazole. The following products may be recommended for relief of iron-deficiency anemia:

OSTEOPOROSIS
May be treated with biphosphonates, calcitonin or estrogens. The following products may be recommended for relief of symptoms:

OSTEOPOROSIS, SECONDARY
May result from the use of chemotherapeutic agents, phenytoin, prolonged glucocorticoid therapy, thyroid hormones, carbamazepine or methotrexate sodium. The following products may be recommended:

OTITIS MEDIA, ACUTE
May be treated with amoxicillin, amoxicillin-clavulanate, cephalosporins, erythromycin-sulfisoxazole, macrolide antibiotics or sulfamethoxazole-trimethoprim. The following products may be recommended for relief of symptoms:

OTITIS MEDIA, ACUTE—cont.

PANCREATIC INSUFFICIENCY, NUTRIENTS DEFICIENCY SECONDARY TO

Pancreatic insufficiency may be treated with pancrelipase. The following products may be recommended for relief of nutrients deficiency:

PARKINSON'S DISEASE, CONSTIPATION SECONDARY TO

Parkinson's disease may be treated with centrally active anticholinergic agents, dopaminergic agents or selective inhibitor of MAO type B. The following products may be recommended for relief of constipation:

PARKINSON'S DISEASE, SEBORRHEIC DERMATITIS SECONDARY TO

Parkinson's disease may be treated with centrally active anticholinergic agents, dopaminergic agents or selective inhibitor of MAO type B. The following products may be recommended for relief of seborrheic dermatitis:

PEPTIC ULCER DISEASE

May be treated with histamine H_2 receptor antagonists, proton pump inhibitors or sucralfate. The following products may be recommended for relief of symptoms:

PEPTIC ULCER DISEASE, IRON DEFICIENCY SECONDARY TO

Peptic ulcer disease may be treated with histamine H_2 receptor antagonists, proton pump inhibitors or sucralfate. The following products may be recommended for relief of iron deficiency:

PHARYNGITIS

May result from the use of cephalosporins, macrolide antibiotics or penicillins. The following products may be recommended:

PHARYNGITIS—cont.

PHARYNGITIS

May be treated with cephalosporins, macrolide antibiotics or penicillins. The following products may be recommended for relief of symptoms:

PHARYNGITIS—cont.

Robitussin Cold & Cough Liqui-Gels ... **858**
Robitussin Cold, Cough & Flu Liqui-Gels ... **858**
Robitussin-DM ... **860**
Robitussin Maximum Strength Cough & Cold ... **861**
Robitussin Maximum Strength Cough Suppressant ... **860**
Robitussin Night-Time Cold Formula ... **861**
Robitussin Pediatric Cough & Cold Formula ... **861**
Robitussin Pediatric Cough Suppressant ... **862**
Robitussin Pediatric Drops ... **862**
Ryna-C Liquid ... **817**
Ryna-CX Liquid ... **817**
St. Joseph Adult Chewable Aspirin Caplets (81 mg.) ... **781**
Sucrets 4-Hour Cough Suppressant ... **805**
Sucrets Children's Cherry Flavored Sore Throat Lozenges ... **804**
Sucrets Maximum Strength Wintergreen, Maximum Strength Vapor Black Cherry Sore Throat Lozenges ... **804**
Sucrets Regular Strength Wild Cherry, Regular Strength Original Mint, Regular Strength Vapor Lemon Sore Throat Lozenges ... **804**
Sudafed Cold & Cough Liquid Caps ... **838**
Sudafed Severe Cold Formula Caplets ... **839**
Sudafed Severe Cold Formula Tablets ... **839**
Theraflu Maximum Strength Flu and Cold Medicine For Sore Throat ... **721**
TheraFlu Flu, Cold and Cough Medicine ... **720**
TheraFlu Maximum Strength NightTime Flu, Cold & Cough Caplets ... **721**
TheraFlu Maximum Strength NightTime Flu, Cold & Cough Hot Liquid Packets ... **721**
TheraFlu Maximum Strength Non-Drowsy Formula Flu, Cold & Cough Hot Liquid Packets ... **722**
TheraFlu Maximum Strength Non-Drowsy Formula Flu, Cold and Cough Caplets ... **722**
Triaminic AM Cough and Decongestant Formula ... **723**
Triaminic Night Time ... **725**
Triaminic Sore Throat Formula ... **725**
Triaminic-DM Syrup ... **727**
TYLENOL acetaminophen Extended Relief Caplets ... **687**
TYLENOL acetaminophen, Extra Strength Adult Liquid Pain Reliever ... **687**
TYLENOL acetaminophen, Extra Strength Gelcaps, Caplets, Tablets, Geltabs ... **687**
TYLENOL acetaminophen, Regular Strength, Caplets and Tablets ... **687**
TYLENOL Cold Medication, Multi-Symptom Caplets and Tablets ... **688**
TYLENOL Cold Medication, Multi-Symptom Hot Liquid Packets ... **688**
TYLENOL Cold Medication, No Drowsiness Formula Caplets and Gelcaps ... **688**
TYLENOL Cold Severe Congestion Caplets ... **690**
TYLENOL Cough Medication, Multi-Symptom ... **691**
TYLENOL Cough Medication with Decongestant, Multi-Symptom ... **691**
TYLENOL Flu NightTime, Maximum Strength Gelcaps ... **693**
TYLENOL PM Pain Reliever/Sleep Aid, Extra Strength Gelcaps, Caplets, Geltabs ... **695**
Unisom With Pain Relief-Nighttime Sleep Aid and Pain Reliever ... **734**
Vanquish Analgesic Caplets ... **627**
Vicks 44 Cough Relief ... **753**
Vicks 44D Cough & Head Congestion Relief ... **754**
Vicks 44E Cough & Chest Congestion Relief ... **754**
Pediatric Vicks 44e Cough & Chest Congestion Relief ... **760**
Vicks 44M Cough, Cold & Flu Relief ... **754**
Pediatric Vicks 44m Cough & Cold Relief ... **760**
Vicks Chloraseptic Cough & Throat Drops, Menthol, Cherry and Honey Lemon Flavors ... **756**
Vicks Chloraseptic Sore Throat Lozenges, Menthol and Cherry Flavors ... **756**
Vicks Chloraseptic Sore Throat Spray, Menthol and Cherry Flavors ... **756**
Vicks Cough Drops, Menthol and Cherry Flavors ... **757**
Vicks Cough Drops, Menthol and Cherry Flavors ... **757**
Vicks DayQuil LiquiCaps/Liquid Multi-Symptom Cold/Flu Relief ... **758**
Children's Vicks NyQuil Cold/Cough Relief ... **755**
Vicks Nyquil Hot Therapy ... **759**
Vicks NyQuil LiquiCaps/Liquid Multi-Symptom Cold/Flu Relief, Original and Cherry Flavors ... **759**
Vicks VapoRub Cream ... **762**
Vicks VapoRub Ointment ... **762**
Vicks VapoSteam ... **762**

PHOTOSENSITIVITY REACTIONS

May result from the use of thiazides, antidepressants, antihistamines, estrogens, nonsteroidal anti-inflammatory drugs, phenothiazines, quinolones, sulfonamides, sulfonylurea hypoglycemic agents, tetracyclines, topical retinoids, captopril, diltiazem hydrochloride, enalapril maleate, fluorouracil, griseofulvin, labetalol hydrochloride, lisinopril, methoxsalen, methyldopa, minoxidil, nalidixic acid or nifedipine. The following products may be recommended:

Eucerin Facial Moisturizing Lotion SPF 25 ... **629**
Oil of Olay Daily UV Protectant SPF 15 Beauty Fluid-Original and Fragrance Free ... **751**
Shade Sunblock Gel SPF 30 ... **780**
Shade Sunblock Lotion SPF 45 ... **780**
Shade UVAGUARD Sunscreen Lotion SPF 15 ... **781**

PRURITUS, PERIANAL

May result from the use of broad-spectrum antibiotics. The following products may be recommended:

Anusol HC-1 Hydrocortisone Anti-Itch Ointment ... **823**
Benadryl Itch Relief Stick Extra Strength ... **827**
Caldecort Anti-Itch Cream ... **706**
Maximum Strength Cortaid Cream ... **738**
Maximum Strength Cortaid Ointment ... **738**
Maximum Strength Cortaid FastStick ... **738**
Cortaid Sensitive Skin Cream with Aloe ... **738**
Cortaid Sensitive Skin Ointment with Aloe ... **738**
Maximum Strength Cortaid Spray ... **738**
Cortaid Intensive Therapy Cream ... **738**
Cortizone for Kids ... **729**
Cortizone-5 Creme and Ointment ... **729**
Cortizone-10 Creme and Ointment ... **729**
Cortizone-10 External Anal Itch Relief ... **729**
Massengill Medicated Soft Cloth Towelette ... **795**
Nupercainal Hemorrhoidal and Anesthetic Ointment ... **715**
Nupercainal Hydrocortisone 1% Cream ... **715**
Preparation H Hydrocortisone 1% Cream ... **856**

PSORALEN WITH UV-A LIGHT (PUVA) THERAPY

May be treated with methoxsalen. The following products may be recommended for relief of symptoms:

Eucerin Facial Moisturizing Lotion SPF 25 ... **629**
Oil of Olay Daily UV Protectant SPF 15 Beauty Fluid-Original and Fragrance Free ... **751**
Shade Sunblock Gel SPF 30 ... **780**
Shade Sunblock Lotion SPF 45 ... **780**
Shade UVAGUARD Sunscreen Lotion SPF 15 ... **781**

RENAL OSTEODYSTROPHY, HYPOCALCEMIA SECONDARY TO

Renal osteodystrophy may be treated with vitamin D sterols. The following products may be recommended for relief of hypocalcemia:

Caltrate 600 Tablets ... **670**
Caltrate 600 + D Tablets ... **670**

RESPIRATORY TRACT ILLNESS, INFLUENZA A VIRUS-INDUCED

May be treated with amantadine hydrochloride or rimantadine hydrochloride. The following products may be recommended for relief of symptoms:

RESPIRATORY TRACT ILLNESS, INFLUENZA A VIRUS-INDUCED—cont.

RHEUMATOID ARTHRITIS, KERATOCONJUNCTIVITIS SICCA SECONDARY TO

Rheumatoid arthritis may be treated with corticosteroids, nonsteroidal anti-inflammatory drugs or azathioprine. The following products may be recommended for relief of keratoconjunctivitis sicca:

RHINITIS, NONALLERGIC

May be treated with nasal steroids or ipratropium bromide. The following products may be recommended for relief of symptoms:

RHINITIS, NONALLERGIC VASOMOTOR

May be treated with nasal steroids or ipratropium bromide. The following products may be recommended for relief of symptoms:

SERUM-SICKNESSLIKE REACTIONS

May result from the use of amoxicillin, amoxicillin-clavulanate, penicillins, sulfamethoxazole-trimethoprim, antivenin (crotalidae) polyvalent, antivenin (micrurus fulvius), metronidazole, ofloxacin, streptomycin sulfate, sulfadoxine, sulfamethoxazole or sulfasalazine. The following products may be recommended:

SERUM-SICKNESSLIKE REACTIONS—cont.

SINUSITIS

May be treated with amoxicillin, amoxicillin-clavulanate, cefprozil, cefuroxime axetil, clarithromycin or loracarbef. The following products may be recommended for relief of symptoms:

SINUSITIS, HALITOSIS SECONDARY TO

Sinusitis may be treated with amoxicillin, amoxicillin-clavulanate, cefprozil, cefuroxime axetil, clarithromycin or loracarbef. The following products may be recommended for relief of halitosis:

SKIN IRRITATION

May result from the use of transdermal drug delivery systems. The following products may be recommended:

STOMATITIS, APHTHOUS

May result from the use of selective serotonin reuptake inhibitors, aldesleukin, clomipramine hydrochloride, didanosine, foscarnet sodium, indinavir sulfate, indomethacin, interferon alfa-2B, recombinant, methotrexate sodium, naproxen, naproxen sodium, nicotine polacrilex or stavudine. The following products may be recommended:

TASTE DISTURBANCES

May result from the use of biguanides, acetazolamide, butorphanol tartrate, captopril, cefuroxime axetil, clarithromycin, etidronate disodium, felbamate, flunisolide, gemfibrozil, griseofulvin, interferon alfa-2B, recombinant, lithium carbonate, lithium citrate, mesna, metronidazole, nedocromil sodium, penicillamine, rifampin or succimer. The following products may be recommended:

TASTE DISTURBANCES—cont.

TONSILITIS, HALITOSIS SECONDARY TO

Tonsilitis may be treated with erythromycin, macrolide antibiotics, cefaclor, cefadroxil, cefixime, cefpodoxime proxetil, cefprozil, ceftibuten dihydrate or cefuroxime axetil. The following products may be recommended for relief of halitosis:

TRAVELER'S DIARRHEA

(see under DIARRHEA, INFECTIOUS)

TUBERCULOSIS, NUTRIENTS DEFICIENCY SECONDARY TO

Tuberculosis may be treated with capreomycin sulfate, ethambutol hydrochloride, ethionamide, isoniazid, pyrazinamide, rifampin or streptomycin sulfate. The following products may be recommended for relief of nutrients deficiency:

VAGINOSIS, BACTERIAL

May be treated with sulfabenzamide/sulfacetamide/sulfathiozole or metronidazole. The following products may be recommended for relief of symptoms:

VULVOVAGINITIS, CANDIDAL

May result from the use of estrogen-containing oral contraceptives, immunosuppressants or recent broad-spectrum antibiotic therapy. The following products may be recommended:

XEROCHILIA

May result from the use of protease inhibitors, retinoids, clomipramine hydrochloride, doxepin hydrochloride or venlafaxine hydrochloride. The following products may be recommended:

XERODERMA

May result from the use of aldesleukin, protease inhibitors, retinoids, topical acne preparations, topical corticosteroids, topical retinoids, benzoyl peroxide, clofazimine, interferon alfa-2A, recombinant, interferon alfa-2B, recombinant or pentostatin. The following products may be recommended:

XEROMYCTERIA

May result from the use of anticholinergics, antihistamines, retinoids, apraclonidine hydrochloride, clonidine, etretinate, ipratropium bromide, isotretinoin or lodoxamide tromethamine. The following products may be recommended:

XEROPHTHALMIA
May result from the use of anticholinergics, antihistamines, beta blockers or tricyclic antidepressants. The following products may be recommended:

XEROSTOMIA
May result from the use of anticholinergics, antidepressants, diuretics, phenothiazines, alprazolam, bromocriptine mesylate, buspirone hydrochloride, butorphanol tartrate, clomipramine hydrochloride, clonidine, clozapine, dexfenfluramine hydrochloride, didanosine, disopyramide phosphate, etretinate, flumazenil, fluvoxamine maleate, guanfacine hydrochloride, isotretinoin, leuprolide acetate, pergolide mesylate, selegiline hydrochloride, tramadol hydrochloride or zolpidem tartrate. The following products may be recommended:

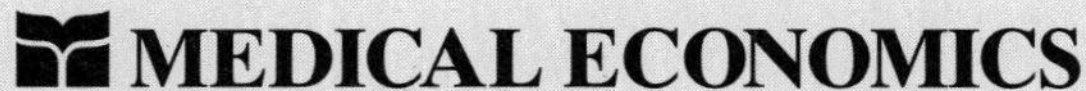

DRUG INFORMATION CENTERS

For additional information on overdosage, adverse reactions, drug interactions, and any other medication problem, specialized drug information centers are strategically located throughout the nation. Use the directory that follows to find the center nearest you. Listings are alphabetical by state and city.

ALABAMA

BIRMINGHAM

Drug Information Service
University of Alabama Hospital
619 S. 19th St.
1720 Jefferson Tower
Birmingham, AL 35233
Mon.-Fri. 8 AM-5 PM
Tel: 205-934-2162
Fax: 205-934-3501

Global Drug Information Center
Samford University
McWhorter School of Pharmacy
800 Lakeshore Dr.
Birmingham, AL 35229-7027
Mon.-Fri. 8 AM-5 PM
Tel: 205-870-2891
Fax: 205-414-4012

HUNTSVILLE

Huntsville Hospital Drug Information Center
101 Sivley Rd.
Huntsville, AL 35801
Mon.-Fri. 8 AM-5 PM
Tel: 205-517-8288
Fax: 205-517-6558

ARIZONA

TUCSON

Arizona Poison and Drug Information Center
Arizona Health Sciences Center
University Medical Center
1501 N. Campbell Ave.
Room 1156
Tucson, AZ 85724
7 days/week, 24 hours
Tel: 520-626-6016
800-362-0101 (AZ)
Fax: 520-626-2720

ARKANSAS

LITTLE ROCK

Arkansas Poison and Drug Information Center
College of Pharmacy-UAMS
4301 W. Markham St.
Little Rock, AR 72205
7 days/week, 24 hours
Tel: 800-376-4766 (AR)
Fax: 501-686-7357

CALIFORNIA

LOS ANGELES

Los Angeles Regional Drug and Poison Information Center
LAC & USC Medical Center
1200 N. State St.
Room 1107 A & B
Los Angeles, CA 90033
7 days/week, 24 hours
Tel: 213-226-2622
800-777-6476 (CA)
Fax: 213-226-4194
Poison Control Hotline:
213-222-3212

SAN DIEGO

Drug Information Analysis Service
Veterans Administration Medical Center
3350 La Jolla Village Dr.
San Diego, CA 92161
Mon.-Fri. 8 AM-4:30 PM
Tel: 619-552-8585
Fax: 619-552-7582

Drug Information Center
U.S. Naval Hospital
34800 Bob Wilson Dr.
San Diego, CA 92134-5000
Mon.-Fri. 8 AM-4 PM
Tel: 619-532-8414

Drug Information Service
University of California San Diego Medical Center
200 W. Arbor Dr.
San Diego, CA 92103-8925
Mon.-Fri. 9 AM-5 PM
Tel: 900-288-8273
Fax: 619-692-1867

STANFORD

Drug Information Center
Stanford University Hospital
Dept. of Pharmacy
H0301
300 Pasteur Dr.
Stanford, CA 94305
Mon.-Fri. 9 AM-5 PM
Tel: 415-723-6422
Fax: 415-725-5028

COLORADO

DENVER

Rocky Mountain Drug Consultation Center
8802 E. 9th Ave.
Denver, CO 80220
Mon.-Fri. 8 AM-4:30 PM
Tel: 303-893-3784
900-370-3784
(Outside Denver County, $1.99 per minute)

Drug Information Center
University of Colorado Health Science Center
4200 E. 9th Ave.
Box C239
Denver, CO 80262
Mon.-Fri. 8:30 AM-4:30 PM
Tel: 303-270-8489
Fax: 303-270-3353

CONNECTICUT

FARMINGTON

Drug Information Service
University of Connecticut
Health Center
263 Farmington Ave.
Farmington, CT 06030
Mon.-Fri. 9 AM-3 PM
Tel: 860-679-2783
Fax: 860-679-1231

HARTFORD

Drug Information Center
Hartford Hospital
P.O. Box 5037
80 Seymour St.
Hartford, CT 06102
Mon.-Fri. 8:30 AM-5 PM
Tel: 860-545-2221
860-545-2961
(main pharmacy)
after hours
Fax: 860-545-2415

NEW HAVEN

Drug Information Center
Yale-New Haven Hospital
20 York St.
New Haven, CT 06504
Mon.-Fri. 8:15 AM-4:45 PM
Tel: 203-785-2248
Fax: 203-737-4229

DISTRICT OF COLUMBIA

Drug Information Center
Washington Hospital
Center
110 Irving St., NW
Washington, DC 20010
Mon.- Fri. 7:30 AM-4 PM
Tel: 202-877-6646
Fax: 202-877-8925

Drug Information Service
Howard University
Hospital
2041 Georgia Ave. NW
Washington, DC 20060
Mon.-Fri. 9 AM-5 PM
Tel: 202-865-1325
Fax: 202-745-3731

FLORIDA

GAINESVILLE

Drug Information &
Pharmacy Resource
Center Shands Hospital at
University of Florida
P.O. Box 100316
Gainesville, FL 32610-0316
Mon.-Fri. 9 AM- 5 PM
Tel: 352-395-0408
(for health-care
professionals only)
Fax: 352-338-9860

JACKSONVILLE

Drug Information Service
University Medical Center
655 W. 8th St.
Jacksonville, FL 32209
Mon.-Fri. 8 AM-5 PM
Tel: 904-549-4095
Fax: 904-549-4272

MIAMI

Drug Information Center
(119)
Miami VA Medical Center
1201 NW 16th St.
Miami, FL 33125
Mon.-Fri. 7:30 AM-4:30
PM
Tel: 305-324-3237
Fax: 305-324-3394

NORTH MIAMI BEACH

Drug Information Service
NOVA Southeastern
University College of
Pharmacy
1750 NE 167th St.
N. Miami Beach, FL 33162
Mon.-Fri. 9 AM-5 PM
Tel: 305-948-8255

TALLAHASSEE

Drug Information
Education Center
Florida Agricultural and
Mechanical University
Tallahassee, FL 32307
Mon.-Fri. 8 AM-5 PM
Tel: 904-488-5239
Fax: 904-599-3411

GEORGIA

ATLANTA

Emory University Hospital
Dept. of Pharmaceutical
Services
1364 Clifton Rd. NE
Atlanta, GA 30322
Mon.-Fri. 8:30 AM-5 PM
Tel: 404-712-4640
Fax: 404-712-7577

Drug Information Service
Northside Hospital
1000 Johnson Ferry Rd.
Atlanta, GA 30342
Mon.-Fri. 9 AM-4 PM
Tel: 404-851-8676
Fax: 404-851-8682

Drug Information Center
Grady Memorial Hospital
and Mercer University
80 Butler St., SE
P.O. Box 26041
Atlanta, GA 30335-3801
Mon.-Fri. 8 AM-4 PM
Tel: 404-616-7725
Fax: 404-616-7727

AUGUSTA

Drug Information Center
University of Georgia
Medical College of GA
Room BIW201
1120 15th St.
Augusta, GA 30912-5600
Mon.-Fri. 8:30 AM-5 PM
Tel: 706-721-2887
Fax: 706-721-3827

IDAHO

POCATELLO

Idaho Drug Information
Service
Box 8092
Pocatello, ID 83209
Mon.-Fri. 8 AM-5 PM
Tel: 208-236-4689
Fax: 208-236-4687

ILLINOIS

BLOOMINGTON

Drug Information Center
BroMenn Life Care Center
807 N. Main St.
Bloomington, IL 61701
7 days/week, 24 hours
Tel: 309-829-0755
Fax: 309-829-0760

CHICAGO

Drug Information Center
Northwestern Memorial
Hospital
250 E. Superior St.
Wesley 153
Chicago, IL 60611
Tel: 312-908-7573
Fax: 312-908-7956

Saint Joseph Hospital
2900 N. Lake Shore Dr.
Chicago, IL 60657
Tel: 312-665-3140
Fax: 312-665-3462

Drug Information Services
University of Chicago
5841 S. Maryland Ave.
MC 0010
Chicago, IL 60637
Mon.-Fri. 8 AM-5 PM
Tel: 312-702-1388
Fax: 312-702-6631

Drug Information Center
University of Illinois
at Chicago
Room C300, MC 883
1740 W. Taylor St.
Chicago, IL 60612
Mon.-Fri. 8 AM-4 PM
Tel: 312-996-0209
Fax: 312-413-4146

HARVEY

Drug Information Center
Ingalls Memorial Hospital
1 Ingalls Dr.
Harvey, IL 60426
Mon.-Fri. 8 AM-4:30 PM
Tel: 708-333-2300
Fax: 708-210-3108

HINES

Drug Information Service
Hines Veterans
Administration Hospital
Inpatient Pharmacy (119B)
Hines, IL 60141
Mon.-Fri. 8 AM-4:30 PM
Tel: 708-343-7200

PARK RIDGE

Drug Information Center
Lutheran General Hospital
1775 Dempster St.
Park Ridge, IL 60068
Mon.-Fri. 7:30 AM-4 PM
Tel: 847-696-8128

INDIANA

INDIANAPOLIS

Drug Information Center
St. Vincent Hospital and
Health Services
2001 W. 86th St.
P.O. Box 40970
Indianapolis, IN 46260
Mon.-Fri. 8 AM-4 PM
Tel: 317-338-3200
Fax: 317-338-6547

Indiana University Medical
Center/Pharmacy
Dept. UH1410
550 N. University Blvd.
Indianapolis, IN 46202
Mon.-Fri. 8 AM-4:30 PM
Tel: 317-274-3581
Fax: 317-274-2327

IOWA

DES MOINES

Regional Drug
Information Center
Mercy Hospital
Medical Center
400 University Ave.
Des Moines, IA 50314
Mon.-Fri. 8 AM-4:30 PM
Tel: 515-247-3286
(answered
7 days/week,
24 hours)
Fax: 515-247-3966

Mid-Iowa Poison and
Drug Information Center
Iowa Methodist
Medical Center
1200 Pleasant St.
Des Moines, IA 50309
7 days/week, 24 hours
Tel: 515-241-6254
800-362-2327 (IA)
Fax: 515-241-5085

IOWA CITY

Drug Information Center
University of Iowa
Hospitals and Clinics
200 Hawkins Dr.
Iowa City, IA 52242
Mon.-Fri. 8 AM-5 PM
Tel: 319-356-2600
Fax: 319-356-4545

KANSAS

KANSAS CITY

Drug Information Center
University of Kansas
Medical Center
3901 Rainbow Blvd.
Kansas City, KS 66160
Mon.-Fri. 8 AM-5 PM
Tel: 913-588-2328
Fax: 913-588-2350

KENTUCKY

LEXINGTON

Drug Information Center
Chandler Medical Center
College of Pharmacy
University of Kentucky
800 Rose St., C-117
Lexington, KY 40536-0084
Mon.-Fri. 8 AM-5 PM
Tel: 606-323-5320
Fax: 606-323-2049

LOUISIANA

MONROE

Drug Information Center
St. Francis Medical Center
309 Jackson St.
Monroe, LA 71201
Tel: 318-327-4250
Fax: 318-327-4125

NEW ORLEANS

Xavier University Drug
Information Center
Tulane University Hospital
and Clinic
Box HC12
1415 Tulane Ave.
New Orleans, LA 70112
Mon.- Fri. 9 AM-5 PM
Tel: 504-588-5670
Fax: 504-588-5862

MARYLAND

ANDREWS AFB

Drug Information Services
89th Med Gp/SGSAP
1050 W. Perimeter Rd.
Suite B1-39
Andrews AFB, MD 20331
Mon.-Fri. 7:30 AM-6 PM
Tel: 301-981-4209
Fax: 301-981-4544

ANNAPOLIS

Drug Information Services
The Anne Arundel Medical
Center
Franklin & Cathedral Sts.
Annapolis, MD 21401
7 days/week, 24 hours
Tel: 410-267-1130
410-267-1000
Fax: 410-267-1628

BALTIMORE

Drug Information Services
Franklin Square Hospital
Center
9000 Franklin Square Dr.
Baltimore, MD 21237
7 days/week, 24 hours
Tel: 410-682-7744
Fax: 410-682-8181

Drug Information Service
Johns Hopkins Medical
Center
600 N. Wolfe St.
Halsted 503
Baltimore, MD 21287-6180
Mon.-Fri. 8:30 AM-5 PM
Tel: 410-955-6348
Fax: 410-955-8283

Drug Information Center
University of Maryland at
Baltimore School of
Pharmacy
506 W. Fayette, 3rd Floor
Baltimore, MD 21201
Mon.-Fri. 8:30 AM-5 PM
Tel: 410-706-7568
Fax: 410-706-0897

BETHESDA

Drug Information Center
Pharmacy Dept.
Warren G. Magnuson
Clinic Center
National Institutes of
Health
9000 Rockville Pike
Bldg. 10, Room IN-257
Bethesda, MD 20892-1196
Mon.-Fri. 8:30 AM-5 PM
Tel: 301-496-2407
Fax: 301-496-0210

EASTON

Drug Information Center
Memorial Hospital
219 S. Washington St.
Easton, MD 21601
7 days/week, 7 AM - Midnight
Tel: 410-822-1000
Fax: 410-820-9489

MASSACHUSETTS

BOSTON

Drug Information Services
Brigham and Women's
Hospital
75 Frances St.
Boston, MA 02115
Mon.-Fri. 7 AM-3:30 PM
Tel: 617-732-7166
Fax: 617-732-7497

Drug Information Service
New England Medical
Center Pharmacy
750 Washington St.
Box 420
Boston, MA 02111
Mon.-Fri. 8 AM-4:30 PM
Tel: 617-636-8985
Fax: 617-636-5638

WORCESTER

Drug Information Center
U.M.M.C. Hospital
55 Lake Ave. North
Worcester, MA 01655
Mon.-Fri. 8:30 AM-5 PM
Tel: 508-856-3456
508-856-2775
Fax: 508-856-1850

MICHIGAN

ANN ARBOR

Drug Information Service
University of Michigan Medical Center
1500 East Medical Center Dr.
UHB2 D301 Box 0008
Ann Arbor, MI 48109
Mon.-Fri. 8 AM-5 PM
Tel: 313-936-8200
313-936-8251
313-936-7027
(after hours)
Fax: 313-923-7027

DETROIT

Drug Information Services
Harper Hospital
3990 John R. St.
Detroit, MI 48201
Mon.-Fri. 8 AM-5 PM
Tel: 313-745-2006
313-745-8216
(after hours)
Fax: 313-745-1795

LANSING

Drug Information Center
Sparrow Hospital
1215 E. Michigan Ave.
Lansing, MI 48912
Mon.-Fri. 8 AM-4:30 PM
Tel: 517-483-2444
Fax: 517-483-2088

PONTIAC

Drug Information Center
St. Joseph Mercy Hospital
900 Woodward
Pontiac, MI 48341
Mon.-Fri. 8 AM-4:30 PM
Tel: 810-858-3055
Fax: 810-858-3010

ROYAL OAK

Drug Information Services
William Beaumont Hospital
3601 West 13 Mile Rd.
Royal Oak, MI 48073-6769
Mon.-Fri. 8 AM-4:30 PM
Tel: 810-551-4077
Fax: 810-551-4046

SOUTHFIELD

Drug Information Service
Providence Hospital
16001 West 9 Mile Rd.
P.O. Box 2043
Southfield, MI 48075
Mon.-Fri. 8 AM-4 PM
Tel: 810-424-3125
Fax: 810-424-5364

MINNESOTA

ROCHESTER

Drug Information Service
Mayo Clinic
1216 2nd St., SW
Rochester, MN 55902
Mon.-Fri. 8 AM-5 PM
Tel: 507-255-5062
507-255-5732
(after hours)
Fax: 507-255-7556

MISSISSIPPI

JACKSON

Drug Information Center
University of Mississippi Medical Center
2500 N. State St.
Jackson, MS 39216
Mon.-Fri. 8 AM-5 PM
Tel: 601-984-2060
(on call 24 hours)
Fax: 601-984-2063

MISSOURI

SPRINGFIELD

Drug Information &
Clinical Research Services
1235 E. Cherokee
Springfield, MO 65804
Mon.-Fri. 7:30 AM-4:30 PM
Tel: 417-885-3488
Fax: 417-888-7788

ST. JOSEPH

Drug Information Service
Heartland Hospital West
801 Faraon St.
St. Joseph, MO 64501
Mon.-Sat. 8 AM-8 PM
Tel: 816-271-7582
Fax: 816-271-7590

NEBRASKA

OMAHA

Drug Information Service
School of Pharmacy
Creighton University
2500 California Plaza
Omaha, NE 68178
Mon.-Fri. 8:30 AM-4:30 PM
Tel: 402-280-5101
Fax: 402-280-5149

Drug Information and Education Services
University of Nebraska Medical Center
600 S. 42nd St.
Omaha, NE 68178
Mon.-Fri. 8 AM-4:30 PM
Fax: 402-559-4907

NEW MEXICO

ALBUQUERQUE

New Mexico Poison &
Drug Information Center
University of New Mexico
Albuquerque, NM 87131
7 days/week, 24 hours
Tel: 505-843-2551
800-432-6866 (NM)
Fax: 505-277-5892

NEW YORK

BROOKLYN

International Drug Information Center
Long Island University
Arnold & Marie Schwartz College of Pharmacy
1 University Plaza
Brooklyn, NY 11201
Mon.-Fri. 9 AM-5 PM
Tel: 718-488-1064
Fax: 718-780-4056

COOPERSTOWN

Drug Information Center
The Mary Imogene Bassett Hospital
1 Atwell Rd.
Cooperstown, NY 13326
Mon.-Fri. 8:30 AM-5 PM
Tel: 607-547-3686
Fax: 607-547-3629

NEW HYDE PARK

Drug Information Center
St. John's University at Long Island Jewish Medical Center
270-05 76th Ave.
New Hyde Park, NY 11042
Mon.-Fri. 9 AM-3 PM
Tel: 718-470-DRUG
Fax: 718-470-1742

NEW YORK CITY

Drug Information Center
Memorial Sloan-Kettering Cancer Center
1275 York Ave.
New York, NY 10021
Mon.-Fri. 9 AM-5 PM
Tel: 212-639-7552
Fax: 212-639-2171

Drug Information Center
Mount Sinai Medical Center
1 Gustave Levy Place
New York, NY 10029
Mon.-Fri. 9 AM-5 PM
Tel: 212-241-6619
Fax: 212-348-7927

Drug Information Center
Bellevue Hospital Center
462 1st Ave.
New York, NY 10016
Mon.-Fri. 9 AM-5 PM
Tel: 212-562-6504
Fax: 212-562-6503

Drug Information Service
The New York Hospital
525 E. 68th St.
New York, NY 10021
Mon.-Fri. 9 AM-5 PM
Tel: 212-746-0741
Fax: 212-746-8506

ROCHESTER

Drug Information Service
Dept. of Pharmacy
University of Rochester
601 Elmwood Ave.
Rochester, NY 14642
Mon.-Fri. 8 AM-5 PM
Tel: 716-275-3718
716-275-2681
(after hours)
Fax: 716-473-9842

STONY BROOK

Suffolk Drug
Information Center
University Hospital
S.U.N.Y. - Stony Brook
Room 3-559, Z7310
Stony Brook, NY 11794
Mon.-Fri. 8 AM-4:30 PM
Tel: 516-444-2672
516-444-2680
(after hours)
Fax: 516-444-7935

NORTH CAROLINA

BUIES CREEK

Drug Information Center
School of Pharmacy
Campbell University
P.O. Box 1090
Buies Creek, NC 27506
Mon.-Fri. 8:30 AM - 4:30 PM
Tel: 910-893-1200
800-327-5467 (NC)
Fax: 910-893-1476

CHAPEL HILL

Drug Information Center
University of North
Carolina Hospitals
101 Manning Dr.
Chapel Hill, NC 27514
Mon.-Fri. 8 AM-5 PM
Tel: 919-966-2373
Fax: 919-966-1791

GREENSBORO

Triad Poison Center
Moses H. Cone
Memorial Hospital
1200 N. Elm St.
Greensboro, NC 27401
7 days/week, 24 hours
Tel: 910-574-8105
Fax: 910-574-7910

GREENVILLE

Eastern Carolina Drug
Information Center
Pitt County
Memorial Hospital
Dept. of Pharmacy Service
2100 Stantonsburg Rd.
Greenville, NC 27835
Mon.-Fri. 8 AM- 5 PM
Tel: 919-816-4257
Fax: 919-816-7425

WINSTON-SALEM

Drug Information
Service Center
NC Baptist Hospital
Bowman-Gray
Medical Center
Medical Center Blvd.
Winston-Salem, NC 27157
Mon.-Fri. 8 AM-5 PM
Tel: 910-716-2037
Fax: 910-716-2186

OHIO

ADA

Drug Information Center
Raabe College of
Pharmacy
Ohio Northern University
Ada, OH 45810
Mon.-Fri. 9 AM - 5 PM
Tel: 419-772-2307
Fax: 419-772-2289

CLEVELAND

Drug Information Center
Cleveland Clinic
Foundation
9500 Euclid Ave.
Cleveland, OH 44195
Mon.-Fri. 8 AM - 4:30 PM
Tel: 216-444-6456
Fax: 216-445-6221

COLUMBUS

Central Ohio Poison
Center
700 Children's Dr.
Columbus, OH 43205
Tel: 513-222-2227
800-682-7625 (OH)
Fax: 614-221-2672

Drug Information Center
Ohio State University
Hospital
Dept. of Pharmacy
Doan Hall 368
410 W. 10th Ave.
Columbus, OH 43210-1228
Mon.-Fri. 8 AM - 4 PM
Tel: 614-293-8679
Fax: 614-293-3264

Drug Information Center
Riverside Methodist
Hospital
3535 Olantangy River Rd.
Columbus, OH 43214
Tel: 614-566-5425
Fax: 614-566-5447

TOLEDO

Drug Information Center
The Toledo Hospital
2142 N. Cove Blvd.
Toledo, OH 43606
Mon.-Fri. 8 AM-4:30 PM
Tel: 419-471-2171
419-471-5637
(after hours)
Fax: 419-479-6926

Drug Information Services
St. Vincent Medical
Center
2213 Cherry St.
Toledo, OH 43608
Tel: 419-251-4227
Fax: 419-251-3662

OKLAHOMA

OKLAHOMA CITY

Drug Information Center
Baptist Medical Center
3300 Northwest Expressway
Oklahoma City, OK 73112
Mon.-Fri. 8 AM-4:30 PM
Tel: 405-949-3660
Fax: 405-945-5858

Drug Information Center
Presbyterian Hospital
700 NE 13th St.
Oklahoma City, OK 73104
Mon.-Fri. 7 AM-3:30 PM
Tel: 405-271-6226
Fax: 405-271-6281

Drug Information Service
University of Oklahoma
Health Sciences Center
Room LIB-380A
1000 S. L. Young Blvd.
Oklahoma City, OK 73117
Mon.-Fri. 8 AM-5 PM

TULSA

Drug Information Service
St. Francis Hospital
6161 S. Yale Ave.
Tulsa, OK 74136
Mon.-Fri. 9 AM-5:30 PM
Tel: 918-494-6339
Fax: 918-494-1893

PENNSYLVANIA

ERIE

Pharmacy and Drug
Information Services
Hamot Medical Center
201 State St.
Erie, PA 16550
7 days/week, 24 hours
Tel: 814-877-6022
Fax: 814-877-6108

PHILADELPHIA

Drug Information Center
Temple University Hospital
Dept. of Pharmacy
Broad and Ontario Sts.
Philadelphia, PA 19140
Mon.-Fri. 8 AM-4:30 PM
Tel: 215-707-4644
Fax: 215-707-3463

Drug Information Center
Thomas Jefferson
University Hospital
111 S. 11th and Walnut Sts.
Philadelphia, PA 19107
Mon.-Fri. 8 AM-5 PM
Tel: 215-955-8877

PITTSBURGH

The Center for
Drug Information
The Mercy Hospital
of Pittsburgh
1400 Locust St.
Pittsburgh, PA 15219-5166
Mon.-Fri. 8 AM-4:30 PM
Tel: 412-232-7903
412-232-7907
Fax: 412-232-8422

Drug Information and Pharmacoepidemiology Center
University of Pittsburgh Medical Center
137 Victoria Hall
Pittsburgh, PA 15261
Mon.-Fri. 8 AM-6 PM
Tel: 412-624-3784
Fax: 412-624-6350

UPLAND

Drug Information Center
Crozer-Chester Medical Center
1 Medical Center Blvd.
Upland, PA 19013
Mon.-Fri. 8 AM-4:30 PM
Tel: 610-447-2851
610-447-2862
(after hours)
Fax: 215-447-2820

WILLIAMSPORT

Drug Information Center
Susquehanna Health System
Rural Ave. Campus
Williamsport, PA 17701
Mon.-Fri. 8 AM-4 PM
Tel: 717-321-3289
Fax: 717-321-3230

PUERTO RICO

SAN JUAN

Centro Information Medicamentos
Escuela de Farmacia RCM
P.O. Box 365067
San Juan, PR 00936-5067
Mon.-Fri. 8 AM-4:30 PM
Tel. & Fax:
787-763-0196

RHODE ISLAND

PROVIDENCE

Drug Information Service
Dept. of Pharmacy
Rhode Island Hospital
593 Eddy St.
Providence, RI 02903
7 days/week, 24 hours
Tel: 401-444-5547
Fax: 401-444-8062

Drug Information Service
University of Rhode Island
Roger Williams Medical Center
825 Chalkstone Ave.
Providence, RI 02908
Mon.-Fri. 8 AM-4 PM
Tel: 401-456-2260
Fax: 401-456-2377

SOUTH CAROLINA

CHARLESTON

Drug Information Service
Medical University of South Carolina
171 Ashley Ave.
Room 515-SFX
Charleston, SC 29425-0810
Mon.-Fri. 8 AM-5:30 PM
Tel: 803-792-3896
800-922-5250
Fax: 803-792-5532

SPARTANBURG

Drug Information Center
Spartanburg Regional Medical Center
101 E. Wood St.
Spartanburg, SC 29303
Mon.-Fri. 8 AM-5 PM
Tel: 864-560-6910
Fax: 864-560-6017

SOUTH DAKOTA

BROOKINGS

South Dakota Drug Information Center
300 22nd Ave.
Brookings, SD 57006
7 days/week, 8 AM-4:30 PM
Tel: 800-456-1004 (SD)

SIOUX FALLS

Drug Information Center
McKennan Hospital
800 E. 21st St.
Sioux Falls, SD 57117-5045
7 days/week, 24 hours
Tel: 605-336-3894
800-952-0123 (SD)
800-843-0505
(IA, MN, NE, ND)
Fax: 605-322-8378

TENNESSEE

KNOXVILLE

Drug Information Center
University of Tennessee Medical Center
1924 Alcoa Highway
Knoxville, TN 37920-6999
Mon.-Fri. 8 AM-4:30 PM
Tel: 423-544-9125

MEMPHIS

South East Regional Drug Information Center
VA Medical Center
1030 Jefferson Ave.
Memphis, TN 38104
Mon.-Fri. 7:30 AM-4 PM
Tel: 901-523-8990

Drug Information Center
University of Tennessee
847 Monroe Ave.
Suite 238
Memphis, TN 38163
Mon.-Fri. 8:30 AM - 4:30 PM
Tel: 901-448-5555
Fax: 901-448-5419

TEXAS

GALVESTON

Drug Information Center
University of Texas Medical Branch
301 University Blvd. - G01
Galveston, TX 77555-0701
Mon.-Fri. 8 AM-5 PM
Tel: 409-772-2734
Fax: 409-747-9919

HOUSTON

Drug Information Center
Ben Taub General Hospital
Texas Southern University/HCHD
1504 Taub Loop
Houston, TX 77030
Mon.-Fri. 8 AM-5 PM
Tel: 713-793-2920
Fax: 713-793-2937

Drug Information Center
Methodist Hospital
6565 Fannin (DB1-09)
Houston, TX 77030
Mon.-Fri. 8 AM-5 PM
Tel: 713-790-4190
Fax: 713-793-1224

LACKLAND AFB

Drug Information Center
Dept. of Pharmacy
Wilford Hall Medical Center
2200 Berquist Dr., Suite 1
Lackland AFB, TX 78236
Mon.-Fri. 7:30 AM-5 PM
Tel: 210-670-6291
210-670-5408

LUBBOCK

Methodist Hospital
Drug Information and Consultation Service
3615 19th St.
Lubbock, TX 79410
Mon.-Fri. 8 AM-5 PM
Tel: 806-793-4012
(Attn: Pharmacy)
Fax: 806-784-5323

TEMPLE

Drug Information Center
Scott and White Memorial Hospital
2401 S. 31st St.
Temple, TX 76508
Mon.-Fri. 8 AM-6 PM
Tel: 817-724-4636
Fax: 817-724-1731

UTAH

SALT LAKE CITY

Drug Information Center
Dept. of Pharmacy Services
Room A-050
University of Utah Hospital
50 N. Medical Dr.
Salt Lake City, UT 84132
Mon.-Fri. 8:30 AM-4:30 PM
Tel: 801-581-2073
Fax: 801-585-6688

VIRGINIA

RICHMOND

Drug Information Center
St. Mary's Hospital
5801 Bremo Rd.
Richmond, VA 23226
7 days/week, 24 hours
Tel: 804-281-8058
Fax: 804-281-4411

WEST VIRGINIA

MORGANTOWN

West Virginia Drug Information Center
WV University-Robert C. Byrd Health Sciences Center
1124 HSN, P.O. Box 9520
Morgantown, WV 26506
Tel: 304-293-6640
800-352-2501 (WV)
Fax: 304-293-5483

WISCONSIN

MADISON

University of Wisconsin Hospital & Clinics
600 Highland Ave.
Madison, WI 53792
Voice mail/24 hours a day, responses in 3 days
Tel: 608-262-1315
Fax: 608-263-9424

WYOMING

LARAMIE

Drug Information Center
University of Wyoming
P.O. Box 3375
Laramie, WY 82071
Mon.-Fri. 8 AM-5 PM
Tel: 307-766-2953
Fax: 307-766-6128

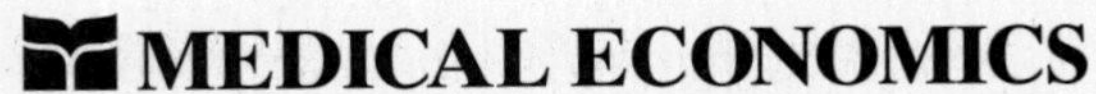
MEDICAL ECONOMICS

SECTION 6

PRODUCT IDENTIFICATION GUIDE

To aid in quick identification, this section provides full-color, actual-size photographs of tablets and capsules. A variety of other dosage forms and packages are shown at less than actual size. In all, the section contains a total of nearly 1,000 photos.

Products in this section are arranged alphabetically by manufacturer. In some instances, not all dosage forms and sizes are pictured. Letters or numbers representing the manufacturer's identification code are preceded by an asterisk.

For more information on any of the products in this section, please turn to the "Product Information" section, or check directly with the manufacturer. For easy reference, the page number of each product's text entry appears with its photographs.

While every effort has been made to guarantee faithful reproduction of the photos in this section, changes in size, color, and design are always a possibility. Be sure to confirm a product's identity with the manufacturer or your pharmacist.

MANUFACTURER'S INDEX

AKPHARMA INC.

AkPharma Inc.
P. 602

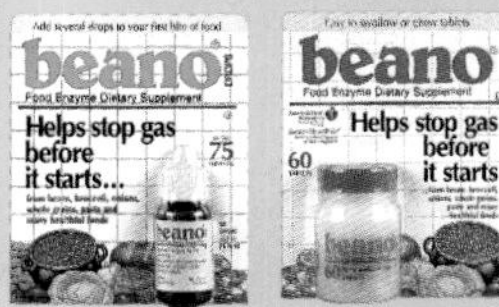

Food Enzyme Dietary Supplement Drops and Tablets.

Beano®

AkPharma Inc.
P. 602

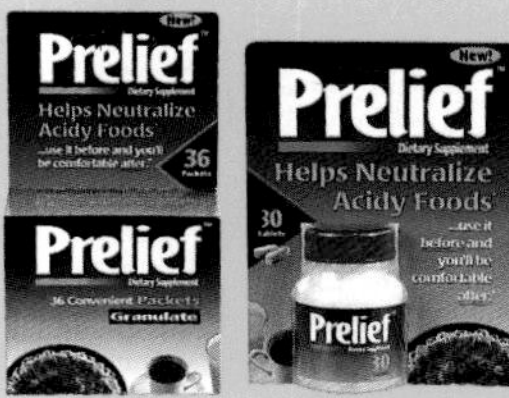

Dietary Supplement Granulate and Tablets

Prelief™

ASTRA USA

Astra USA, Inc.
P. 608

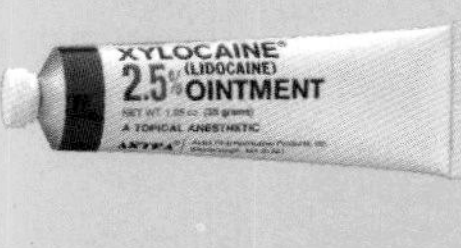

2.5% Ointment
Available in 35 gram Tube

Xylocaine®
(lidocaine)

BAUSCH & LOMB

Bausch & Lomb
P. 608

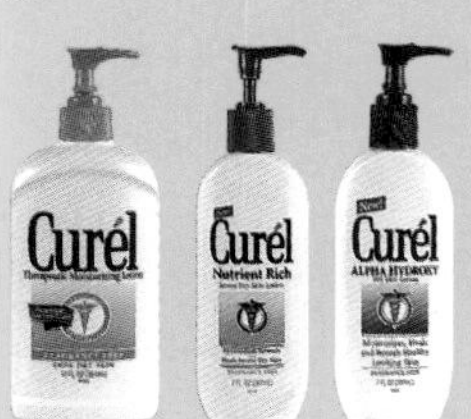

Therapeutic Moisturizing Lotion in original and fragrance free (shown) formulas, Nutrient Rich formula, and AlphaHydroxy formula.

Curél®

BAYER CORPORATION

Bayer Corporation
Consumer Care Division
P. 609

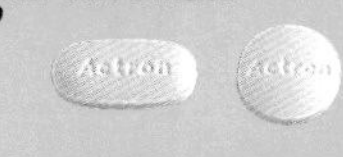

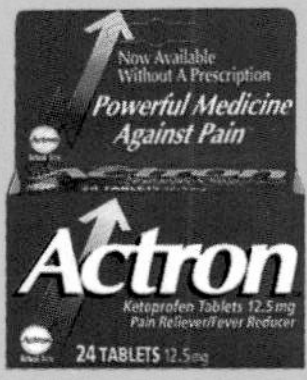

Ketoprofen Tablets and Caplets 12.5 mg

Actron™

Bayer Corporation
Consumer Care Division
P. 610

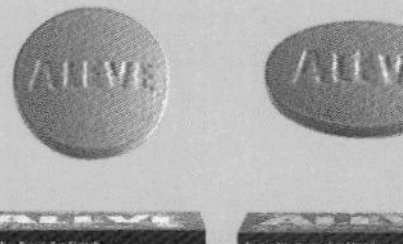

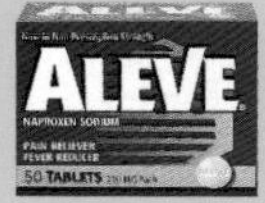

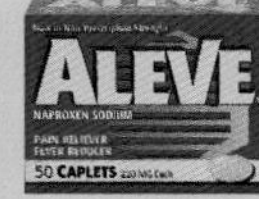

Tablets and Caplets available in 24, 50, 100 and 150 count. Caplets also available in 200 count.

Aleve®

Bayer Corporation
Consumer Care Division
P. 609

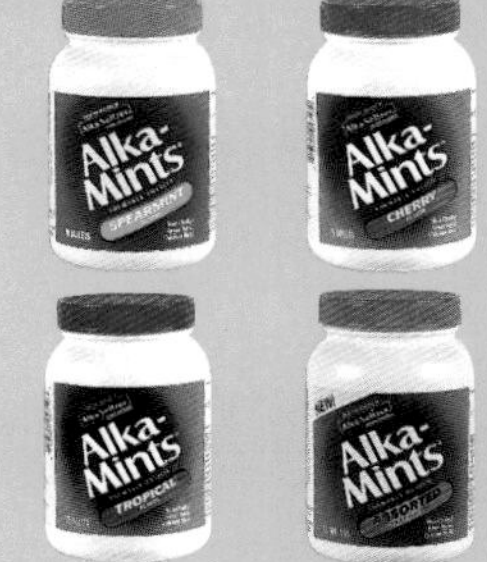

Spearmint, Cherry, Tropical and Assorted Chewable Antacid

Alka-Mints®

Bayer Corporation
Consumer Care Division
P. 611

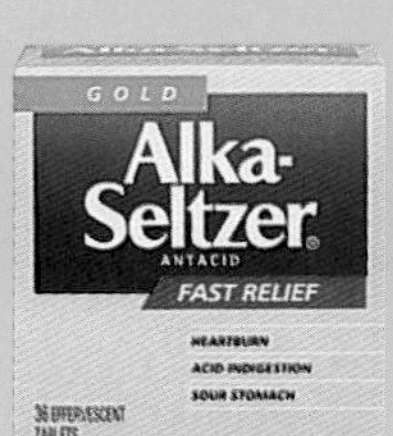

Effervescent Antacid

Alka-Seltzer® Gold

Bayer Corporation
Consumer Care Division
P. 610

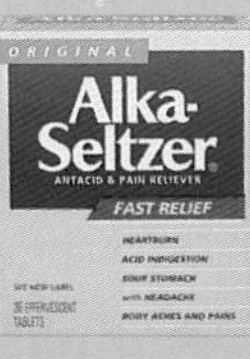

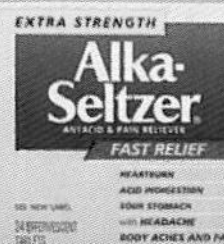

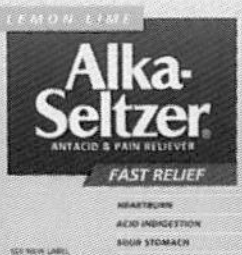

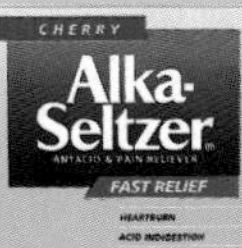

Original, Extra Strength, Lemon Lime and Cherry Effervescent Antacid and Pain Reliever

Alka-Seltzer®

Bayer Corporation
Consumer Care Division

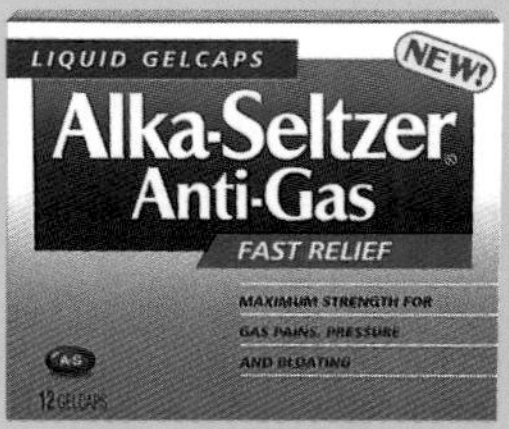

Maximum Strength Liquid Gelcaps

Alka-Seltzer® Anti-Gas

Bayer Corporation
Consumer Care Division

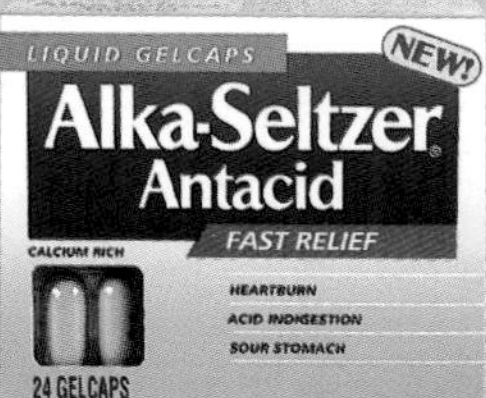

Alka-Seltzer® Antacid Liquid Gelcaps

Bayer Corporation
Consumer Care Division
P. 611

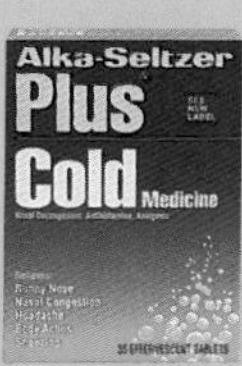

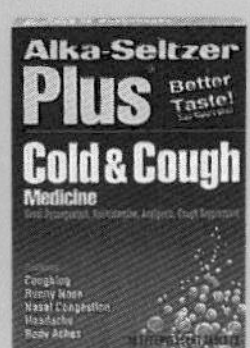

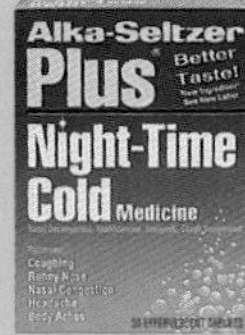

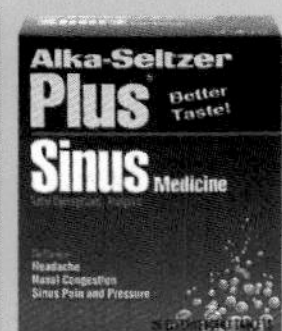

Cold, Cold & Cough, Night-Time and Sinus Effervescent Tablets

Alka-Seltzer Plus® Cold Medicine

Bayer Corporation
Consumer Care Division
P. 612

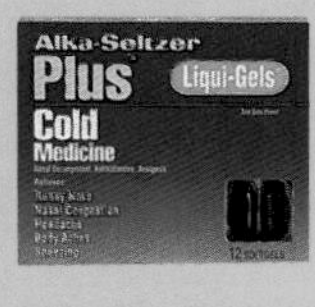

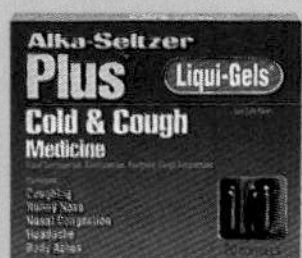

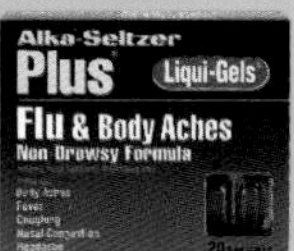

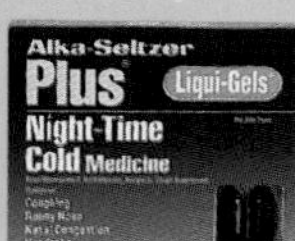

Cold, Cold & Cough, Flu & Body Aches and Night-Time.

Alka-Seltzer Plus® Cold Medicine Liqui-Gels®

Bayer Corporation
Consumer Care Division
P. 611

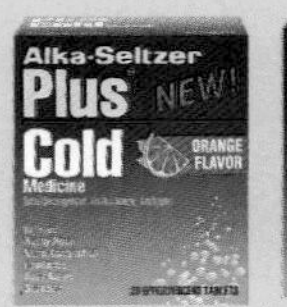

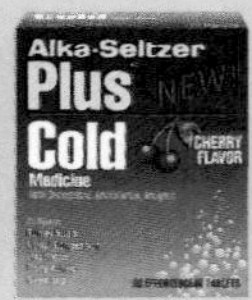

Orange and Cherry Flavors

Alka-Seltzer Plus® Cold Medicine

Bayer Corporation
Consumer Care Division
P. 612

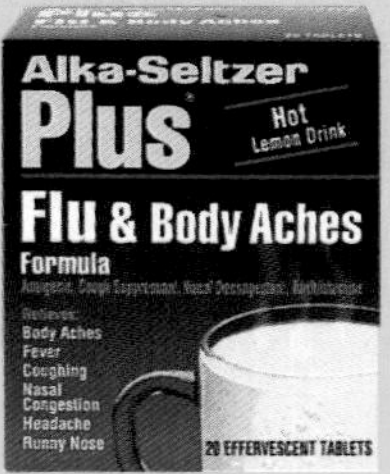

Effervescent Tablets

Alka-Seltzer Plus® Flu and Body Aches

Bayer Corporation
Consumer Care Division

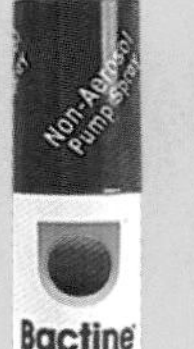

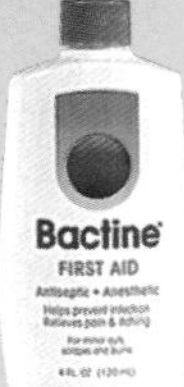

Antiseptic/Anesthetic
First Aid Spray and Liquid

Bactine®

While every effort has been made to reproduce products faithfully, this section is to be considered a Quick-Reference Identification aid.

Bayer Corporation
Consumer Care Division
P. 613

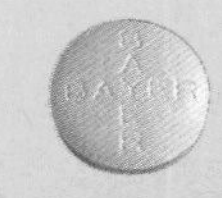

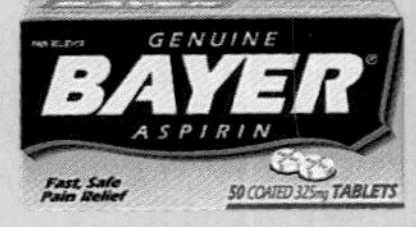

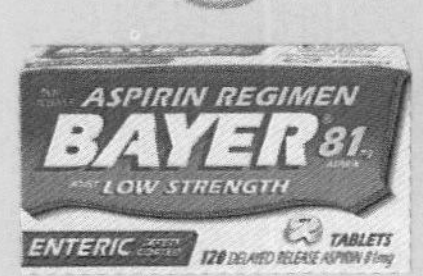

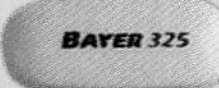

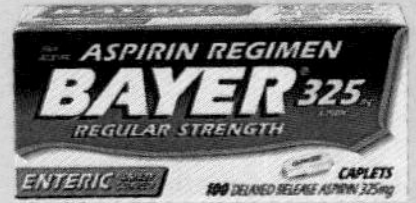

Genuine Bayer, Aspirin Regimen 81 mg,
Aspirin Regimen 325 mg

BAYER® Aspirin

Bayer Corporation
Consumer Care Division
P. 614

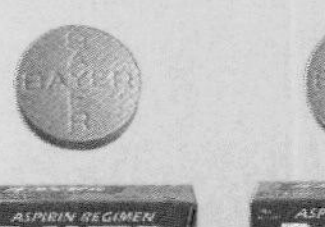

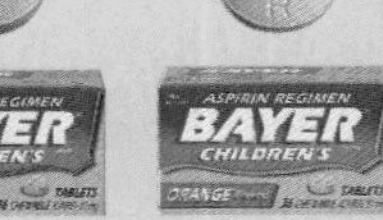

Low Strength, Chewable Aspirin
Orange and Cherry Flavors

Aspirin Regimen BAYER® Children's

Bayer Corporation
Consumer Care Division
P. 614

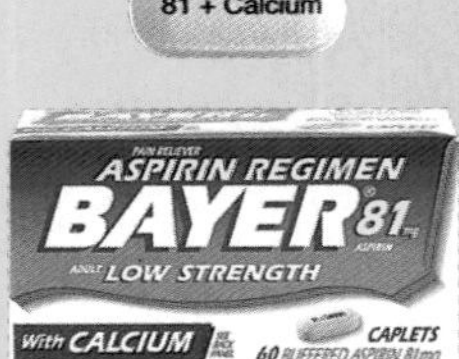

Aspirin Regimen BAYER® 81 mg with Calcium

Bayer Corporation
Consumer Care Division
P. 616

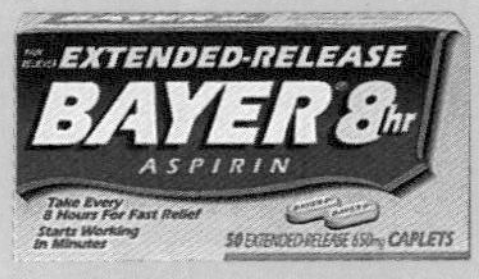

Only Extended-Release Aspirin

Extended-Release BAYER® 8 Hour

Bayer Corporation
Consumer Care Division
P. 616

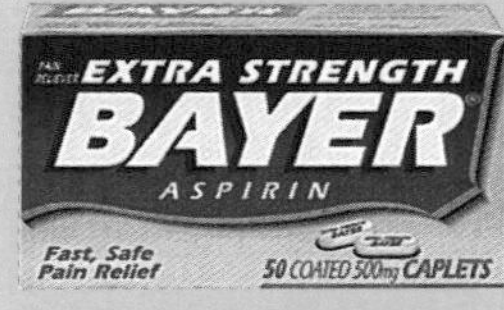

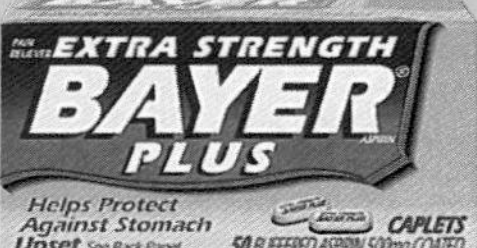

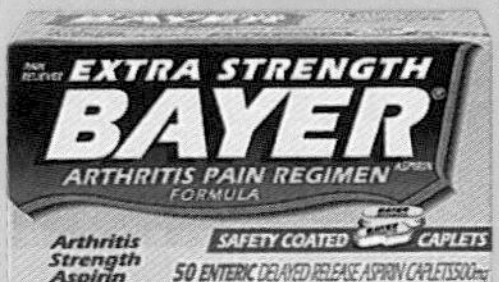

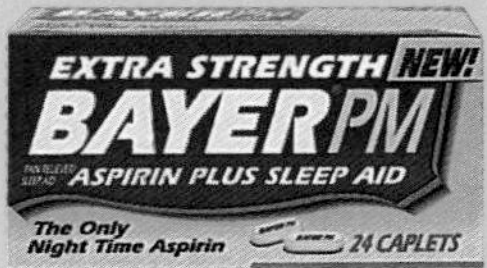

Extra Strength, Plus,
Arthritis Pain Regimen and PM

Extra Strength BAYER® Aspirin

Bayer Corporation
Consumer Care Division
P. 618

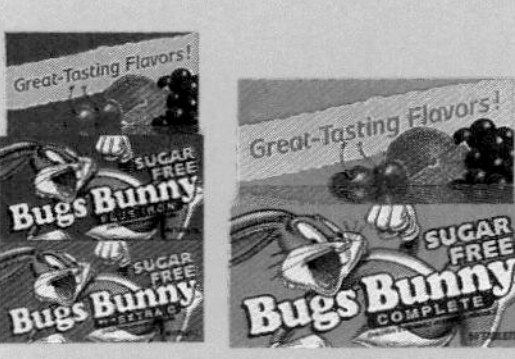

Sugar Free Children's Chewable
Complete, with Extra C and Plus Iron

Bugs Bunny™ Vitamins

Bayer Corporation
Consumer Care Division
P. 618

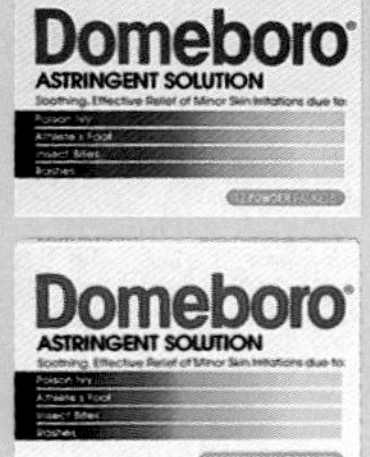

Astringent Solution
Effervescent Tablets and
Powder Packets

Domeboro®

Bayer Corporation
Consumer Care Division
P. 619

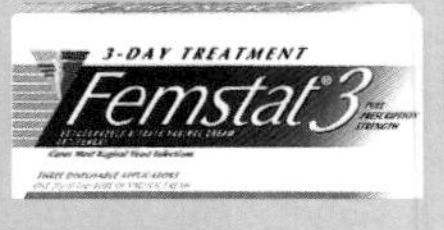

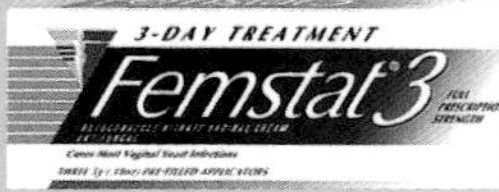

3 - Day Treatment
Full Prescription Strength

Femstat® 3

Bayer Corporation
Consumer Care Division

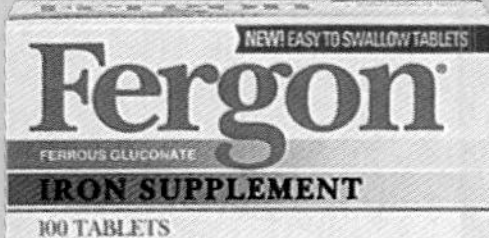

Ferrous Gluconate
Iron Supplement

Fergon®

Bayer Corporation
Consumer Care Division
P. 619

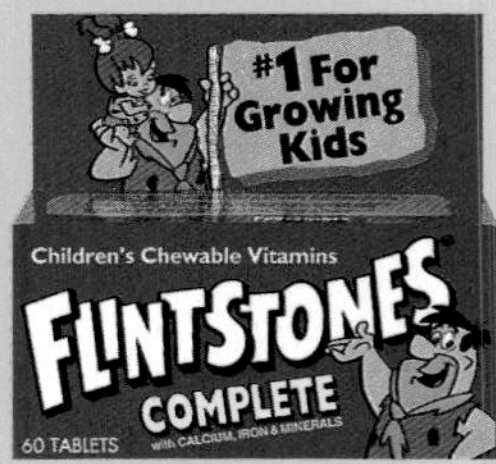

Children's Chewable Vitamins with
Iron, Calcium & Minerals

Flintstones® Complete

Bayer Corporation
Consumer Care Division
P. 618

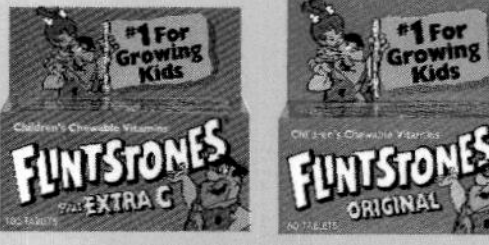

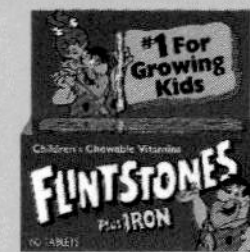

Children's Chewable Vitamins with Extra C, Original and Plus Iron

Flintstones®

Bayer Corporation
Consumer Care Division
P. 620

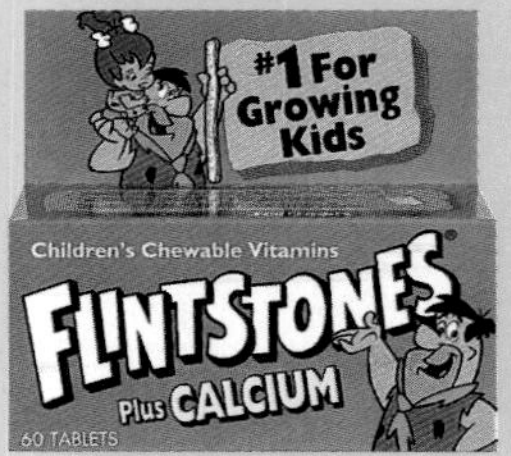

Children's Chewable Vitamins with Calcium

Flintstones® Plus Calcium

Bayer Corporation
Consumer Care Division
P. 621

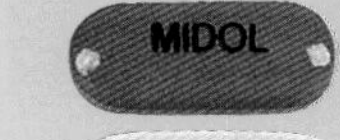

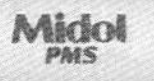

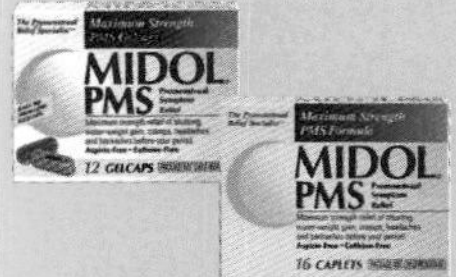

Maximum Strength Gelcaps and Caplets

Midol® PMS

Bayer Corporation
Consumer Care Division
P. 621

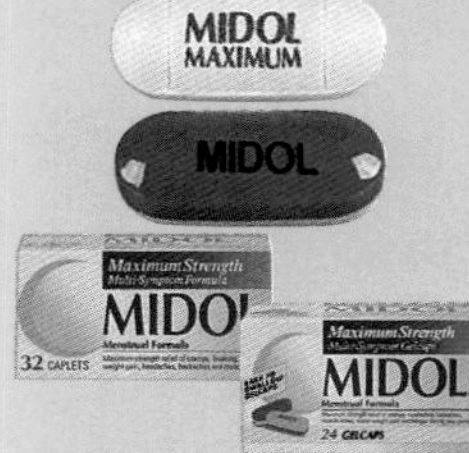

Maximum Strength Caplets and Gelcaps

Midol® Menstrual

Bayer Corporation
Consumer Care Division
P. 621

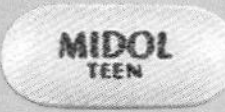

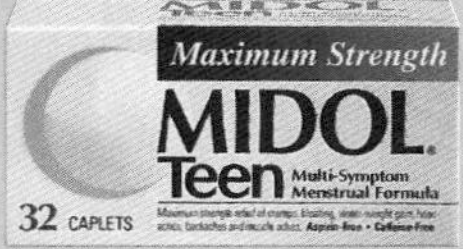

Maximum Strength Caplets

Midol® Teen

Bayer Corporation
Consumer Care Division
P. 621

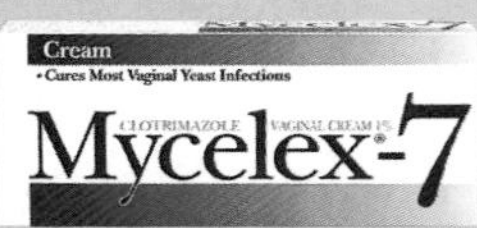

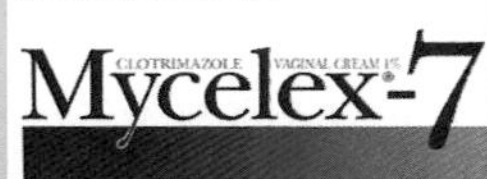

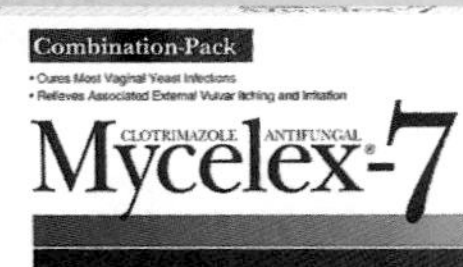

Vaginal Cream 1%
Vaginal Cream with 7 disposable applicators
Vaginal Inserts and external vulvar cream

Mycelex®-7

Bayer Corporation
Consumer Care Division

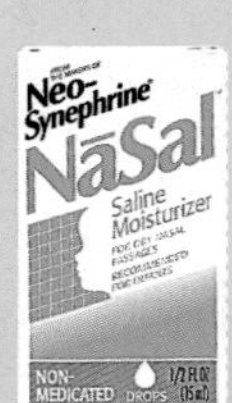

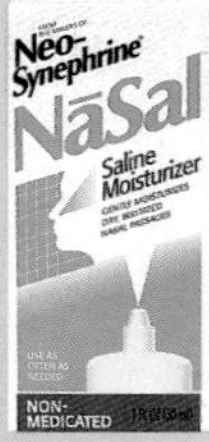

Nasal Moisturizer Spray and Drops

NaSal®

Bayer Corporation
Consumer Care Division
P. 623

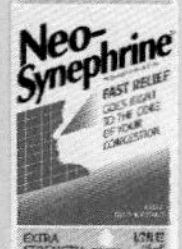

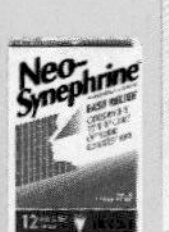

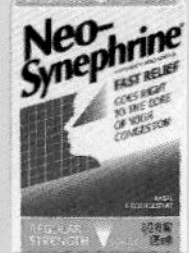

Nasal Decongestant Spray and Drops
Available in Mild, Regular, Extra Strength and Max 12-Hour Formula

Neo-Synephrine®

Bayer Corporation
Consumer Care Division
P. 624

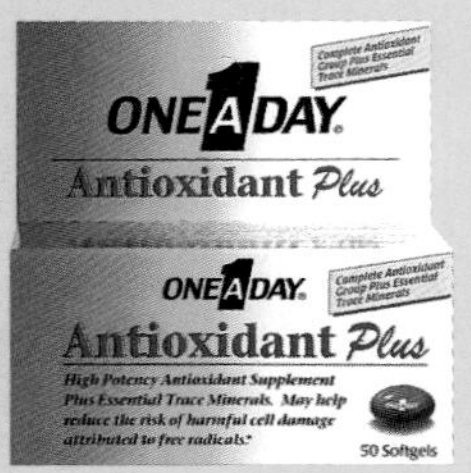

One-A-Day® Antioxidant Plus

Bayer Corporation
Consumer Care Division
P. 625

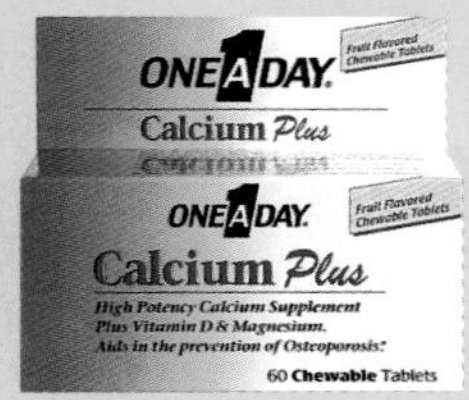

500 mg Calcium Carbonate Plus Vitamin D and Magnesium

One-A-Day® Calcium Plus

Bayer Corporation
Consumer Care Division
P. 625

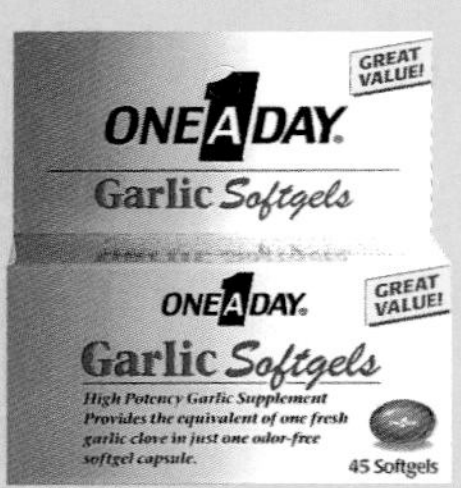

One-A-Day® Garlic Softgels

Bayer Corporation
Consumer Care Division
P. 624

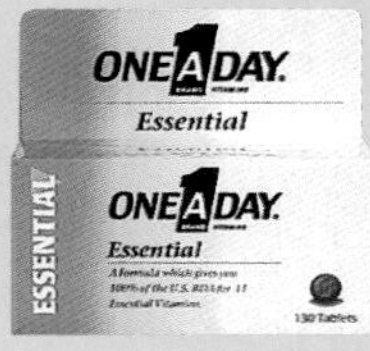

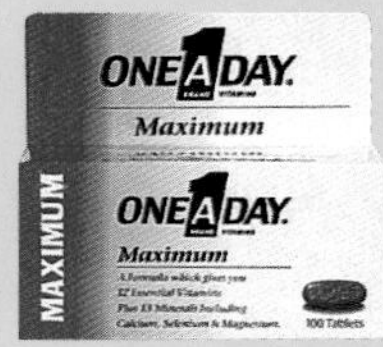

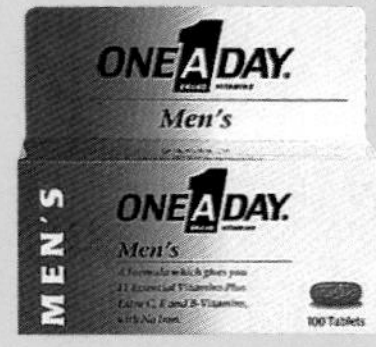

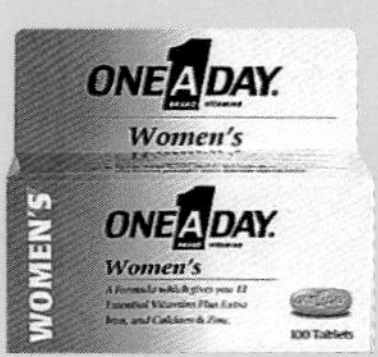

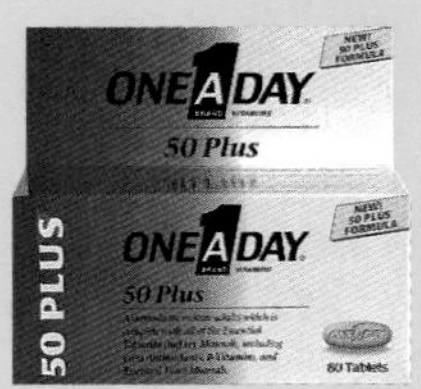

Essential, Maximum, Men's, Women's and 50 Plus.

One-A-Day® Vitamins

Bayer Corporation
Consumer Care Division
P. 626

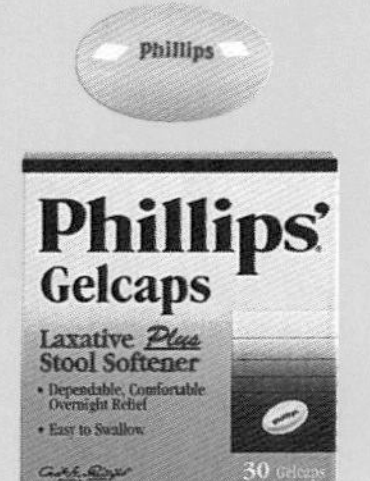

Laxative Plus Stool Softener
Avail. in 10, 30 and 60 count Gelcaps.

Phillips'® Gelcaps

Bayer Corporation
Consumer Care Division
P. 626

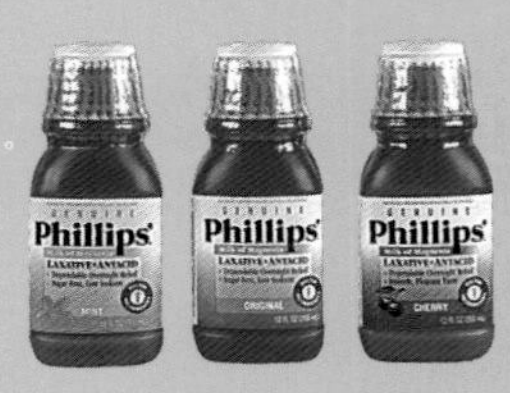

Available in Mint, Original, and Cherry Flavors
4 oz, 12 oz and 26 oz Bottles

Phillips'® Milk of Magnesia

Bayer Corporation
Consumer Care Division
P. 627

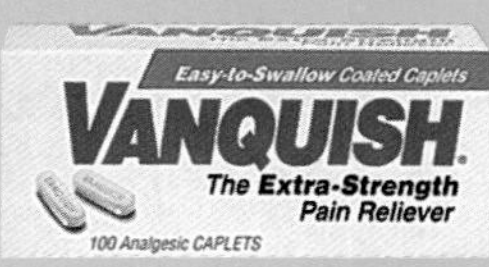

Extra-Strength Pain Formula

Vanquish®

BEECH-NUT

Beech-Nut
P. 627

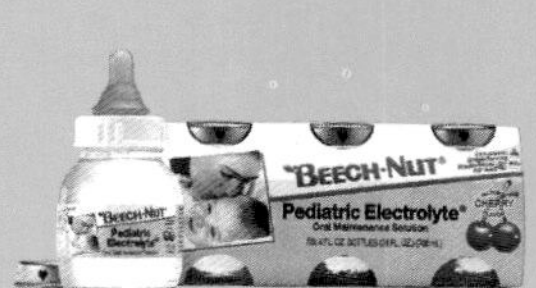

6 - 4 Fl Oz. bottles

Pediatric Electrolyte
Oral Maintenance Solution

BEIERSDORF

Beiersdorf Inc.
P. 629

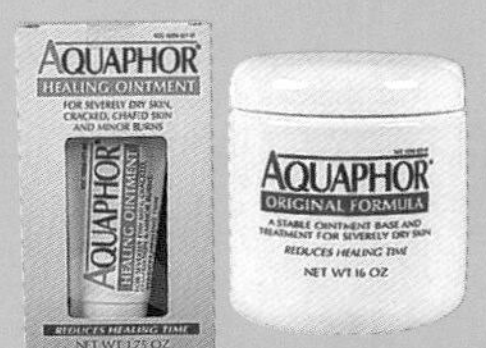

Original and Healing Ointments For Dry Skin, Minor Cuts and Burns

Aquaphor®

Beiersdorf Inc.
P. 630

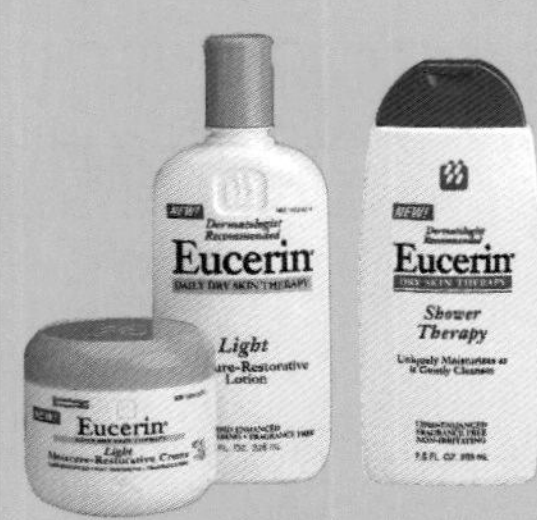

Light Moisture-Restorative Creme and Lotion, Shower Therapy

Eucerin® Daily Dry Skin Therapy

Beiersdorf Inc.
P. 629

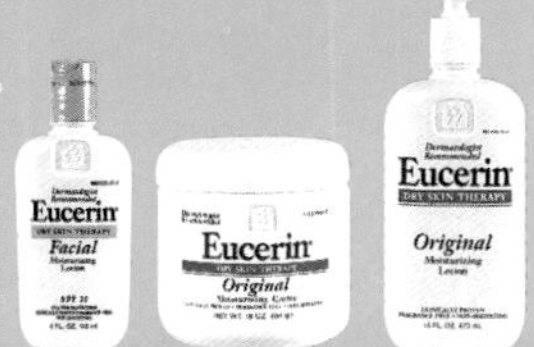

Facial Moisturizing Lotion SPF 25, Original Moisturizing Creme and Lotion

Eucerin® Dry Skin Therapy

Beiersdorf Inc.
P. 630

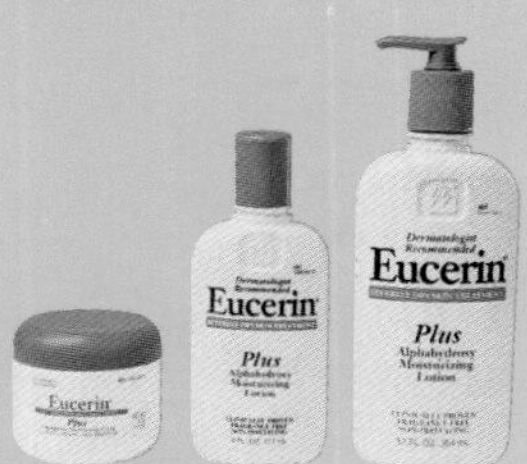

Alphahydroxy Moisturizing Creme and Lotion

Eucerin® Plus Severely Dry Skin Treatment

BLOCK DRUG

Block Drug
P. 635

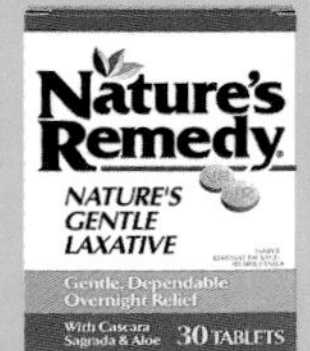

Available in boxes of 15, 30 and 60 tablets.
A stimulant laxative with natural active ingredients.

Nature's Remedy® Nature's Gentle Laxative

Block Drug
P. 636

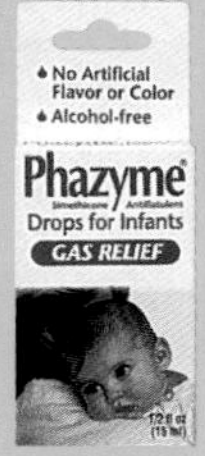

Available in 1 oz. and 1/2 oz. bottles
A liquid anti-gas that contains no alcohol, and no artificial colors, flavors or sweeteners

Phazyme® Drops for Infants

Block Drug
P. 636

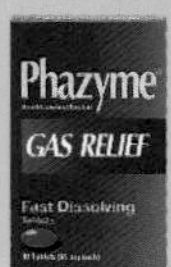

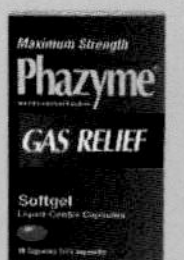

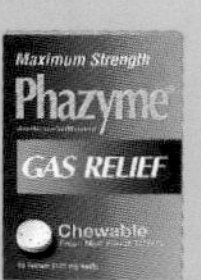

Fast dissolving tablets available in boxes of 10, 30, 50 and 100.
Maximum strength softgels and maximum strength chewable tablets available in boxes of 10, 30 and 50.

Phazyme® Gas Relief

Block Drug
P. 636

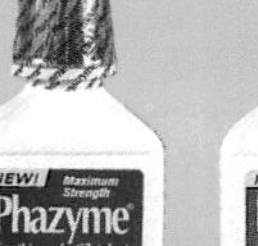

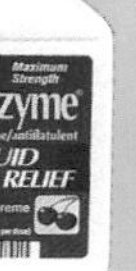

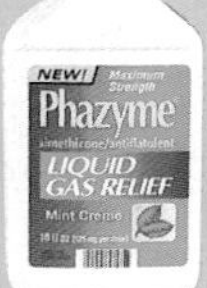

Available in 10 oz. bottles, with dosage cup, in Cherry Creme and Mint Creme

Phazyme® Liquid Gas Relief

BRISTOL-MYERS PRODUCTS

Bristol-Myers Products
P. 647

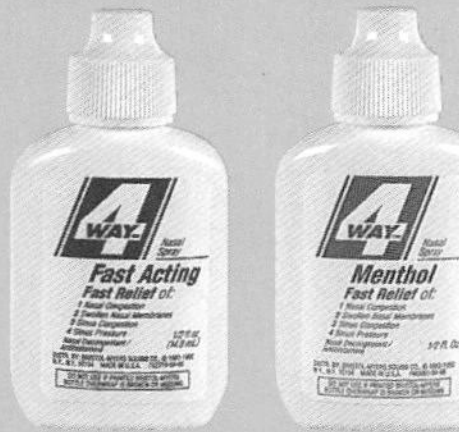

Regular available in:
1/2 oz. and 1 oz. Atomizers
Mentholated also available

4-Way® Nasal Spray

Bristol-Myers Products
P. 648

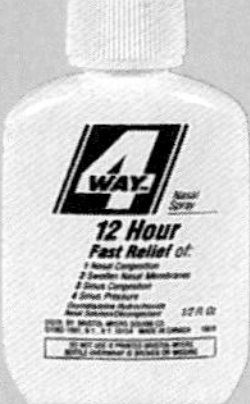

1/2 oz. Atomizers

4-Way® Nasal Spray

Bristol-Myers Products
P. 640

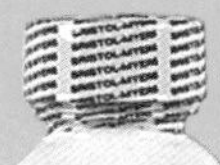

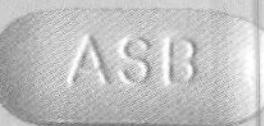

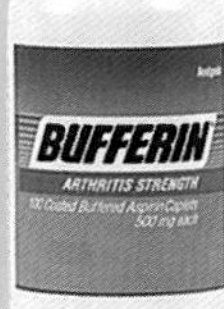

Bottles of 130 coated caplets

Bufferin® Arthritis Strength

Bristol-Myers Products
P. 639

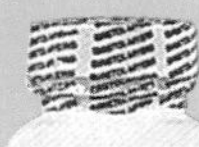

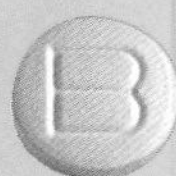

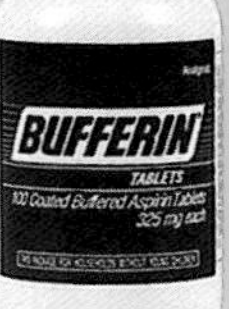

Bottles of 39, 65, 130 and 275 tablets

Bufferin® Coated Analgesic

Bristol-Myers Products
P. 640

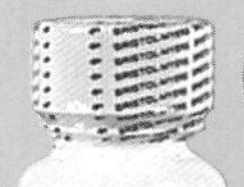

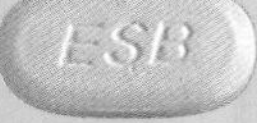

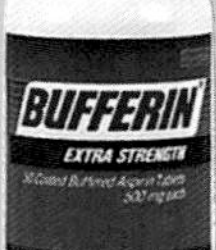

Bottles of 39, 65 and 130 coated tablets

Bufferin® Extra Strength

Bristol-Myers Products
P. 641

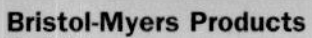
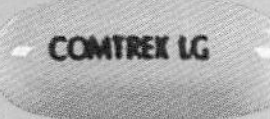
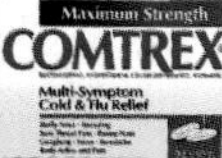
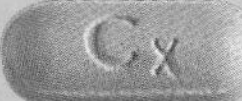
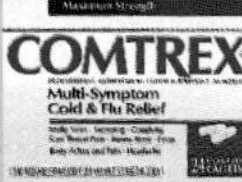
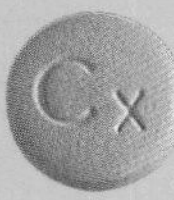
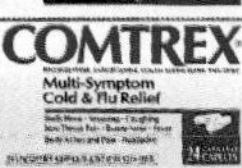

Liqui-Gels in blister packs of 24 and 50
Coated caplets in blister packs of 24 and bottles of 50
Coated tablets in blister packs of 24 and bottles of 50

Comtrex® Multi-Symptom Cold & Flu Relief

Bristol-Myers Products
P. 642

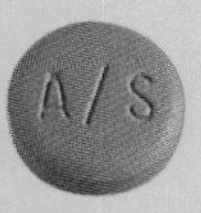
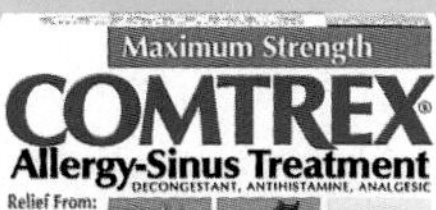
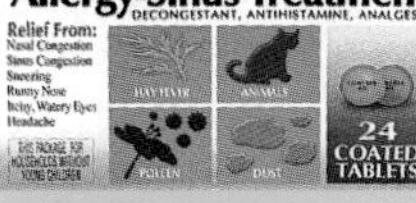

Available in blister packs of 24 and bottles of 50

Comtrex® Allergy-Sinus

Bristol-Myers Products
P. 644

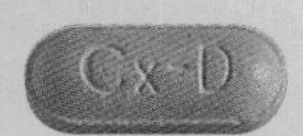
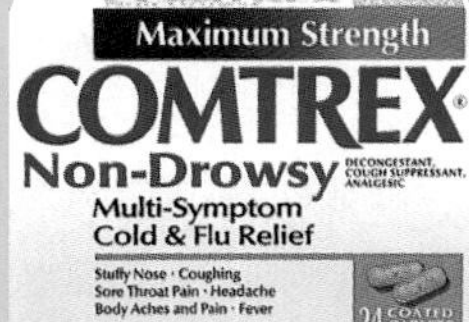

Multi-Symptom Cold Reliever Caplets
Blister packs of 24 and bottles of 50

Comtrex® Non-Drowsy Multi-Symptom Cold & Flu Relief

Bristol-Myers Products
P. 646

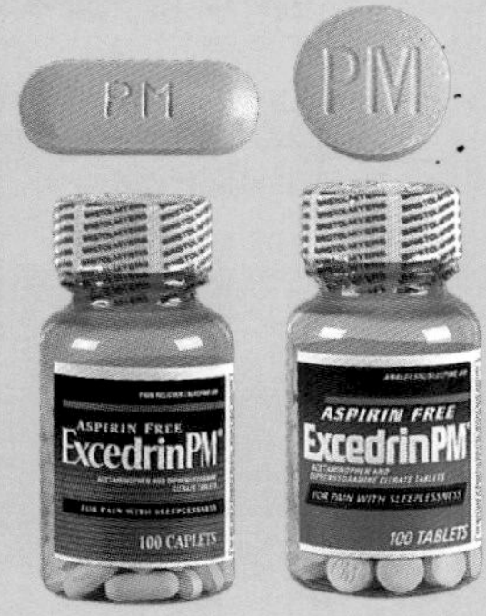
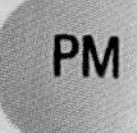
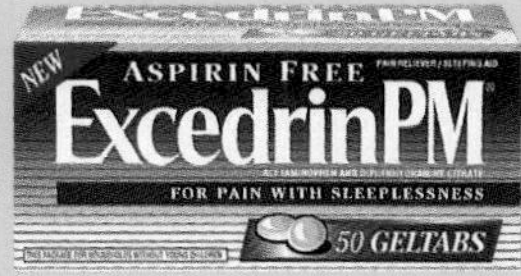

Tablets and Caplets in Bottles of 10, 24, 50 and 100
Geltabs in bottles of 24 and 50

Excedrin PM®

Bristol-Myers Products
P. 645

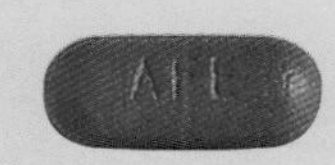
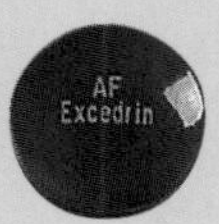

Bottles of 24, 50 and 100 caplets

Aspirin Free Excedrin®

Bristol-Myers Products
P. 645

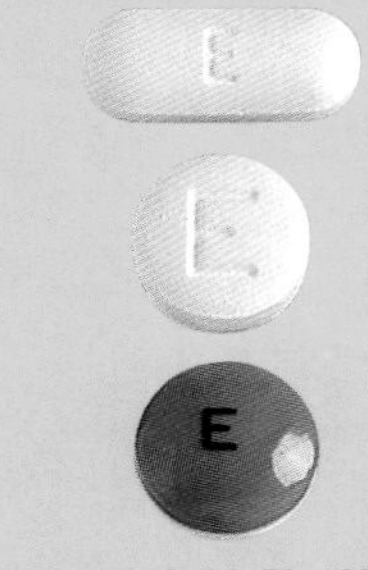

Bottles of 12, 24, 50, 100, 175 and 275, metal tins of 12 tablets

Extra Strength Excedrin®

Bristol-Myers Products
P. 648

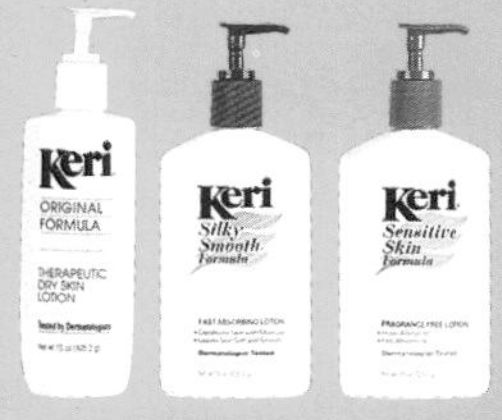

For Dry Skin Care
6.5, 11 and 15 oz. 20 oz. size for Original Formula
Silky Smooth and Fragrance Free

Keri® Lotion

Bristol-Myers Products
P. 648

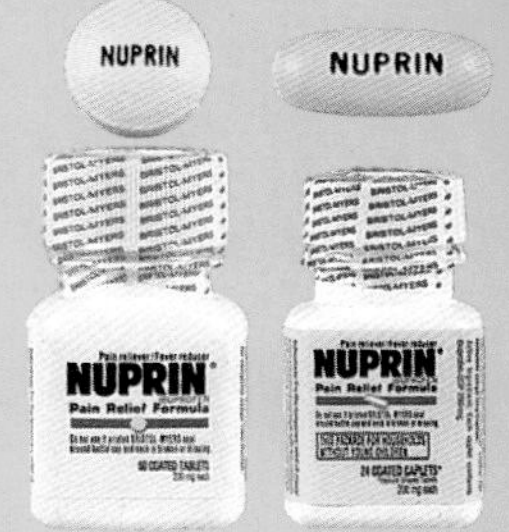

Bottles of 36, 75 and 150 tablets

Nuprin®

Bristol-Myers Products
P. 649

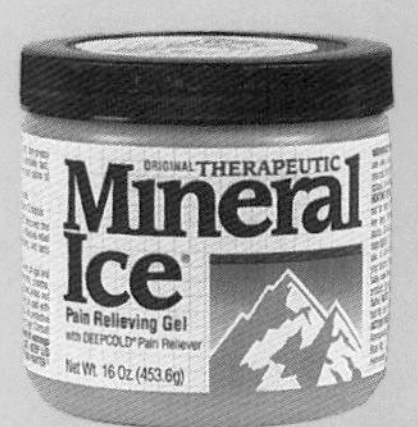

Available in: 3.5 oz., 8 oz. and 16 oz. Pain Relieving Gel

Therapeutic Mineral Ice®

For more detailed information on the products illustrated in this section, consult the Product Information Section or manufacturers may be contacted directly.

CIBA SELF-MEDICATION, INC.

IMPORTANT NOTICE:

This product line is now listed under Novartis Consumer Health, Inc.

Please see pages 513 - 516 for product identification.

COLUMBIA

Columbia
P. 654

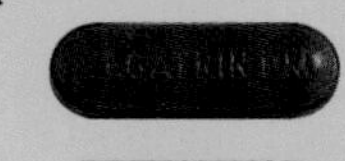
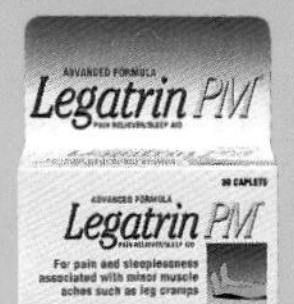

Pain Releiver / Sleep Aid
Available in packages of 30 and 50 caplets.

Advanced Formula Legatrin PM®

DEL

Del Pharmaceuticals
P. 654

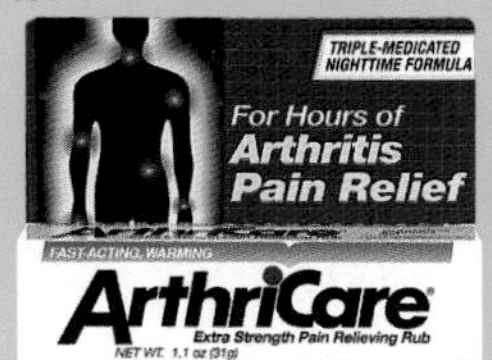
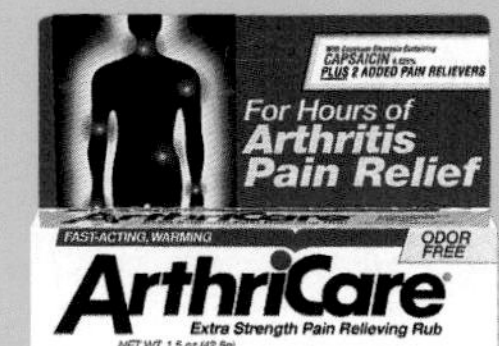
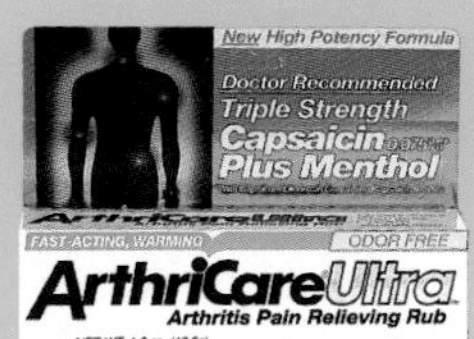

Pain Relieving Rubs

ArthriCare®

Del Pharmaceuticals
P. 655

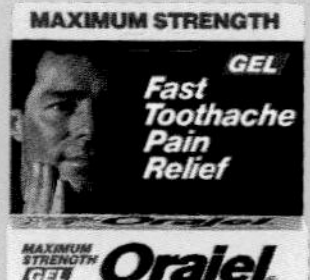

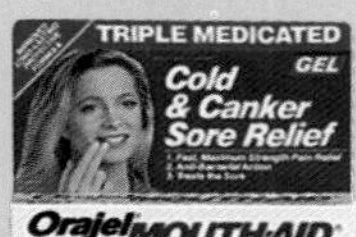

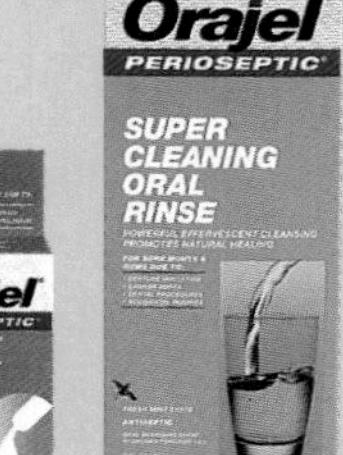

Sore Gums, Toothache Pain, and Cold & Canker Sore Relief

Orajel®

Del Pharmaceuticals
P. 655

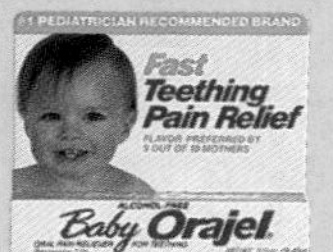

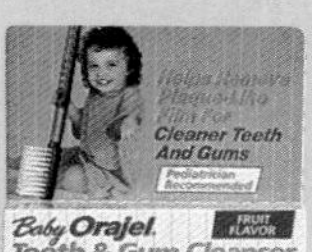

Teething Pain Medicine
Tooth & Gum Cleanser

Baby Orajel®

Del Pharmaceuticals
P. 656

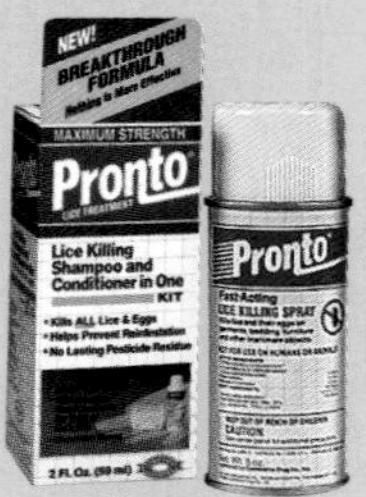

Maximum Strength
Lice Killing Shampoo
Household Spray

Pronto®

Del Pharmaceuticals
P. 657

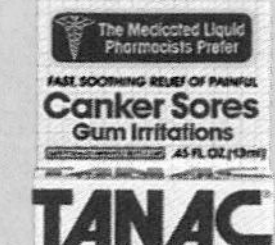

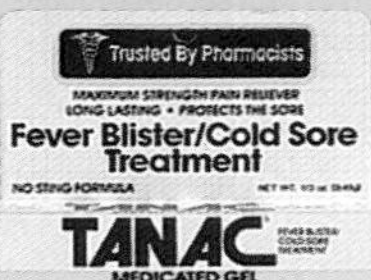

No Sting Liquid & Medicated Gel

Tanac®

EFFCON

Effcon Laboratories
P. 657

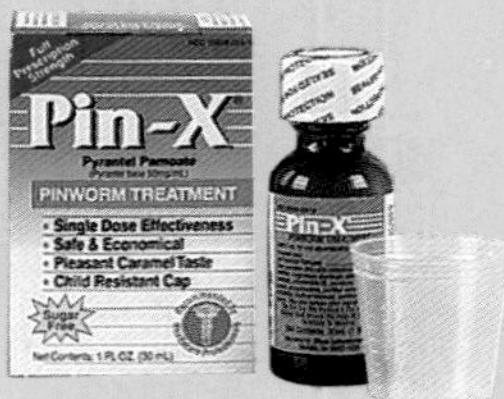

Oral Suspension 50 mg/mL
For the treatment of pinworm infections.

Pin-X®
(pyrantel pamoate)

GEBAUER

Gebauer
P. 659

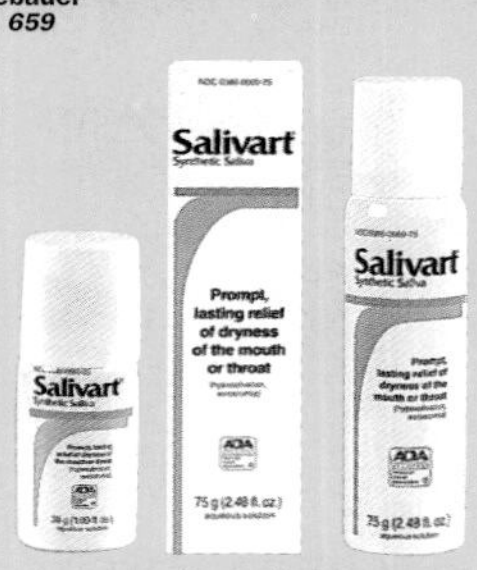

Synthetic Salivia
Available in 30 g and 75 g

Salivart®

While every effort has been made to reproduce products faithfully, this section is to be considered a Quick-Reference Identification aid.

HOGIL PHARMACEUTICAL

Hogil Pharmaceutical Corp.
P. 659

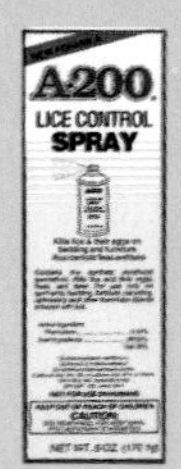

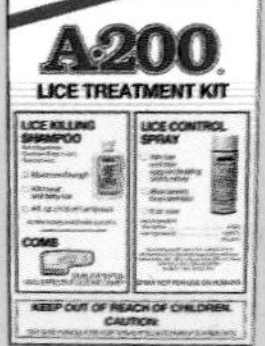

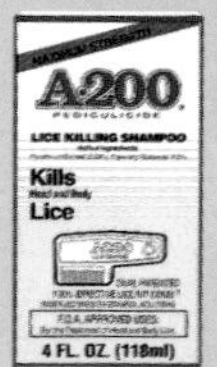

Lice Control Spray 6 oz.
Lice Treatment Kit (Kit includes shampoo, spray, and comb)
Lice Killing Shampoo 2 & 4 oz. sizes
(Special comb included)

A 200®

Hogil Pharmaceutical Corp.
P. 660

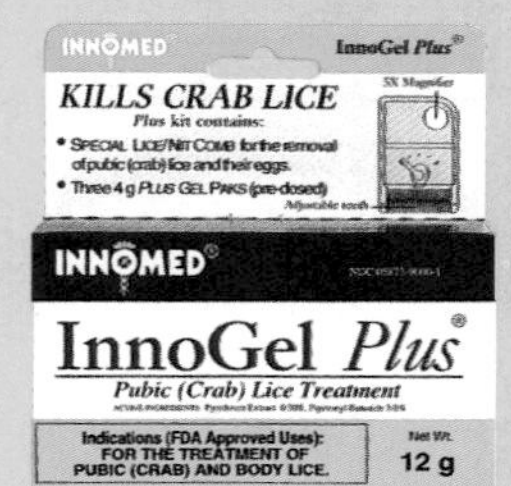

Pubic (Crab) Lice
Treatment Kit

InnoGel Plus™

Hogil Pharmaceutical Corp.
P. 661

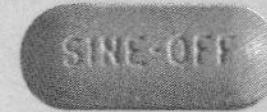

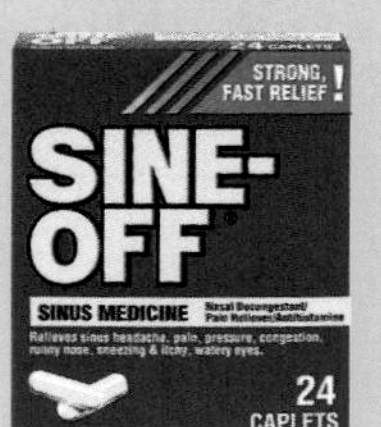

Packages of 24 and 100 caplets

Sine®-Off

Hogil Pharmaceutical Corp.
P. 660

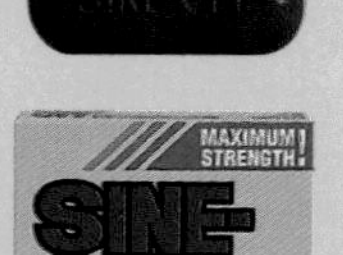

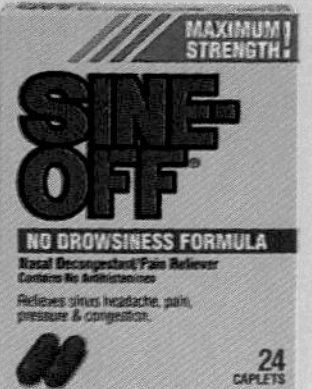

Maximum Strength
No Drowsiness Formula Caplets

Sine®-Off

Hogil Pharmaceutical Corp.
P. 661

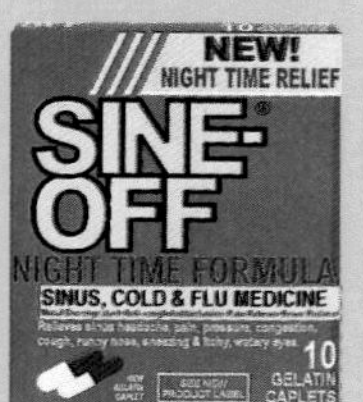

Night Time Formula Caplets

Sine®-Off

Hogil Pharmaceutical Corp.
P. 662

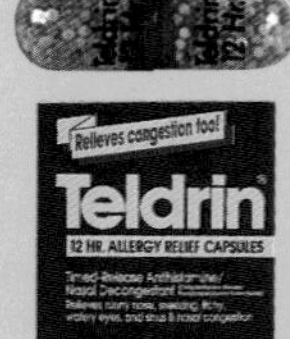

Timed-Release Capsules
Packages of 12, 24 and 48 capsules

Teldrin®

J&J-MERCK CONSUMER

J&J-Merck Consumer
P. 663

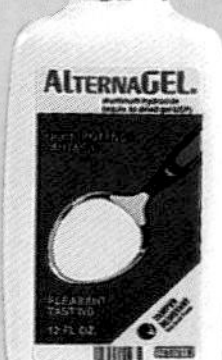

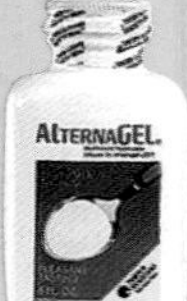

12 fl oz 5 fl oz

AlternaGel®
High potency aluminum hydroxide antacid

J&J-Merck Consumer
P. 664

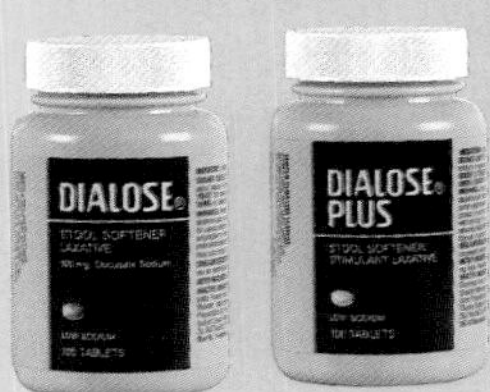

100 mg 100 mg / 65 mg
Bottles of 100 tablets

Dialose® Dialose® Plus

J&J-Merck Consumer
P. 665

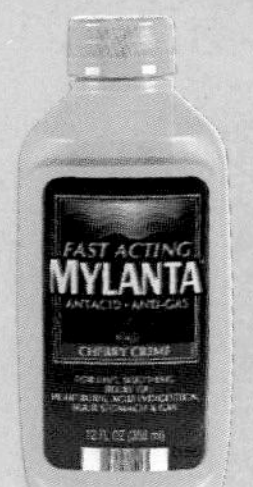

Bottles of 5, 12, 24 oz.

Fast-Acting Mylanta®

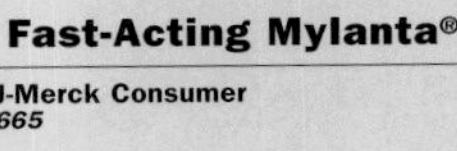

J&J-Merck Consumer
P. 665

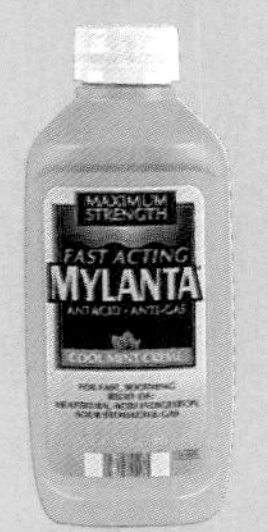

5, 12 & 24 oz. liquid

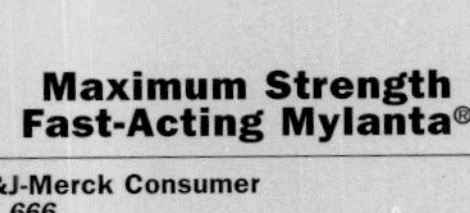

Maximum Strength Fast-Acting Mylanta®

J&J-Merck Consumer
P. 666

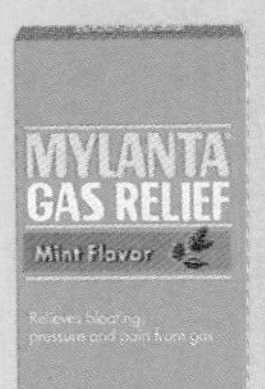

80 mg
12 & 30 tablet convenience packs, bottles of 60 and 100

Mylanta® Gas

J&J-Merck Consumer
P. 666

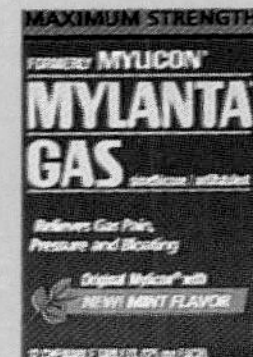

125 mg
12 & 24 tablet convenience packs

Maximum Strength Mylanta® Gas

J&J-Merck Consumer
P. 666

Boxes of 24 and 60 gelcaps

Mylanta® Gas Relief Gelcaps

J&J-Merck Consumer
P. 667

Mylanta® Gelcaps Antacid

J&J-Merck Consumer

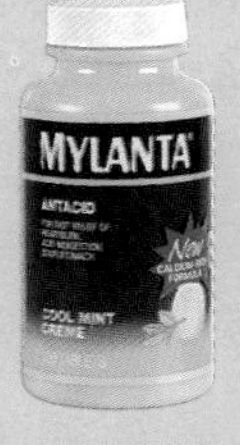

Available in Cool Mint Creme and Cherry Creme in bottles of 50 and 100 and rollpacks of 12

Mylanta® Tablets

J&J-Merck Consumer

Tablets in bottles of 35, 70 and rollpacks of 8

Mylanta® Double Strength Tablets

J&J-Merck Consumer
P. 664

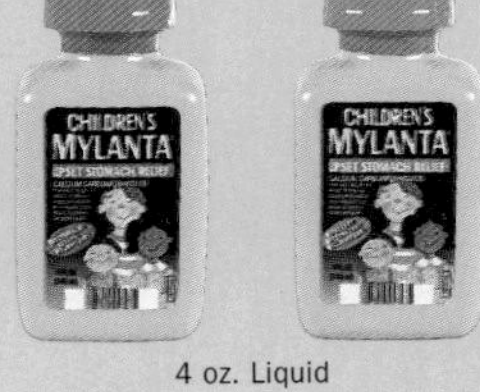

4 oz. Liquid

Children's Mylanta® Upset Stomach Relief Liquid

J&J-Merck Consumer
P. 664

Boxes of 24 tablets.

Children's Mylanta® Upset Stomach Relief Tablets

J&J-Merck Consumer
P. 664

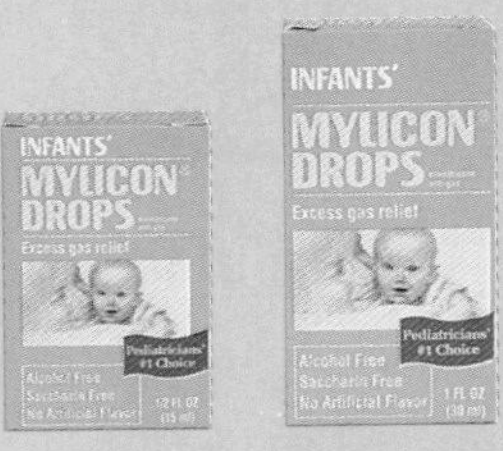

Available in 0.5 oz and 1.0 oz bottles

Infants Mylicon® Drops

J&J-Merck Consumer
P. 667

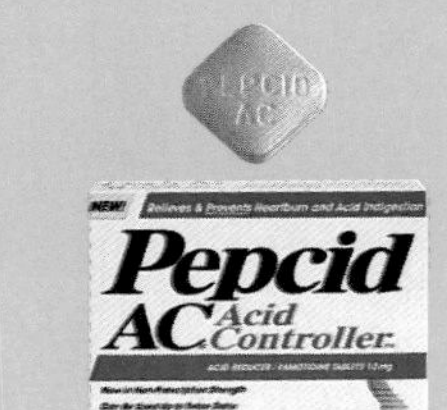

Available in 6's, 12's, 18's, 30's, 50's and 80's

Pepcid AC®

3M

3M
P. 675

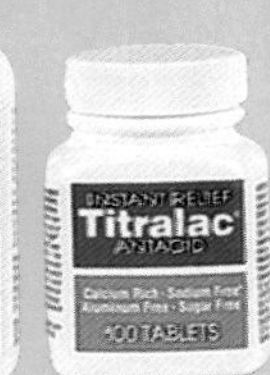

Available in: Regular Strength 40, 100, 1000 Tablets and Extra Strength 100 Tablets only

3M™ Titralac™ Antacid

3M
P. 675

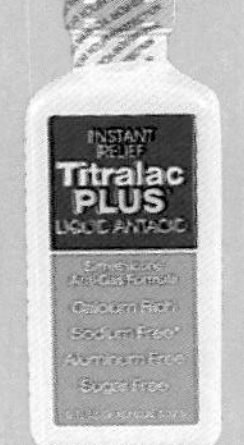

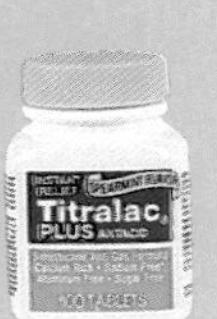

Antacid with Simethicone
Available in:
100 Tablets and 12 Fl. oz. liquid

3M™ Titralac™ Plus Antacid

MCNEIL

McNeil Consumer Products
P. 681

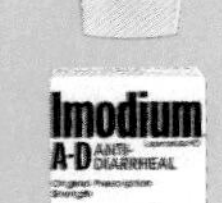

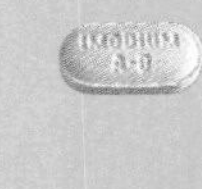

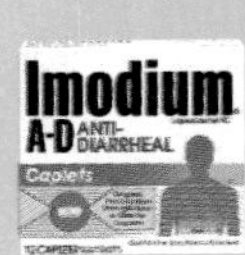

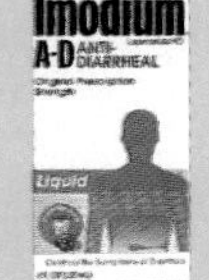

Available in 2 and 4 fl. oz. bottles with a convenient dosage cup, and caplets in 6's, 12's, 18's and 24's

Imodium® A-D

Lactaid Inc. Marked By
McNeil Consumer Products
P. 683

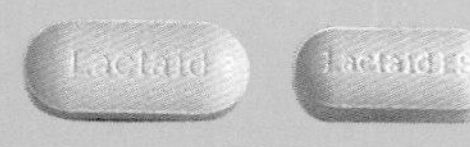

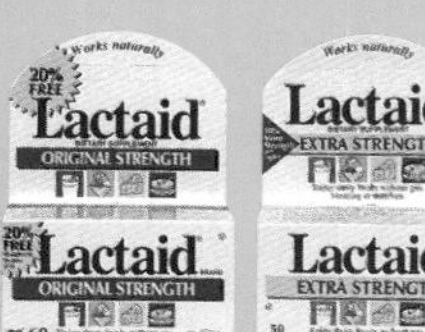

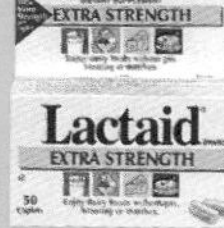

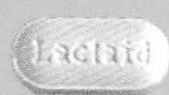

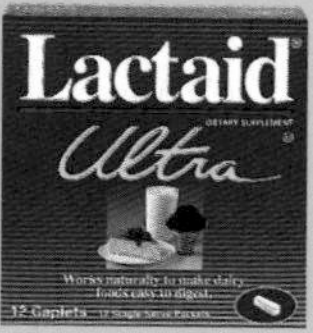

Original strength available in bottles of 60

Extra strength available in bottles of 24 and 50

Ultra available in single serve packets of 12 and 32 counts

Lactaid® Caplets

Lactaid Inc. Marked By
McNeil Consumer Products
P. 683

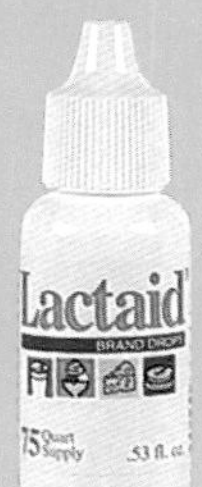

Available in 30 qt. supply

Lactaid® Drops

McNeil Consumer Products
P. 676

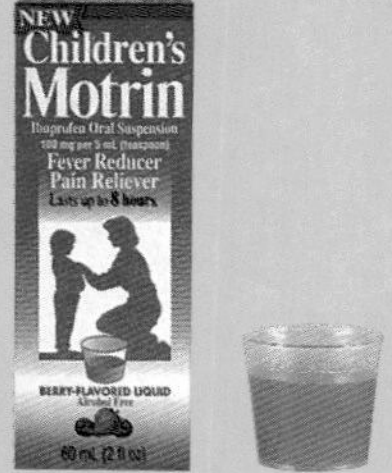

100 mg/5 mL

Children's Motrin® Ibuprofen Oral Suspension

McNeil Consumer Products
P. 676

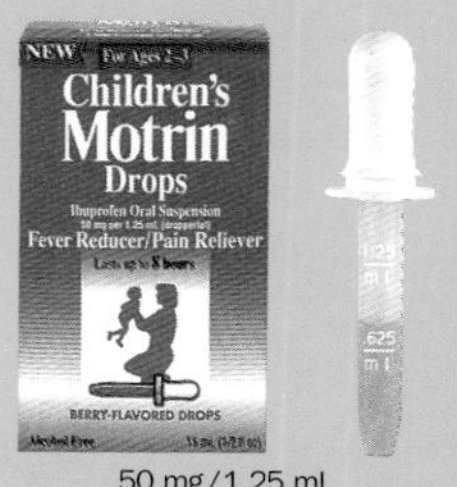

50 mg/1.25 mL
Available in 1/2 fl. oz. bottle

Children's Motrin® Drops

McNeil Consumer Products
P. 682

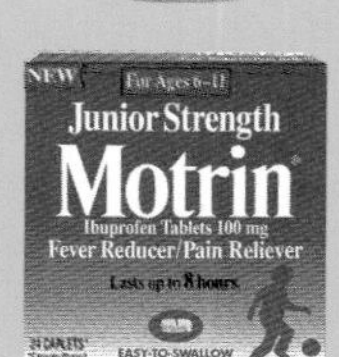

Available in blister packs of 24

Junior Strength Motrin® Ibuprofen Caplets

McNeil Consumer Products
P. 684

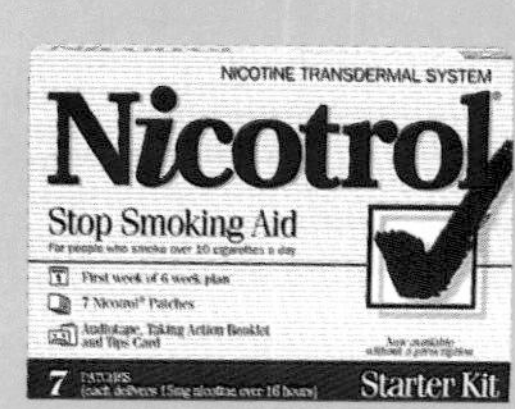

Available as Starter Kit - 7patches, Refill Kit - 7 and 14 patches

Nicotrol® Patch

McNeil Consumer Products
P. 684

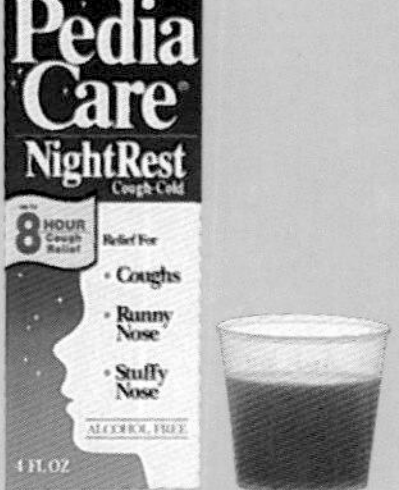

Available in 4 fl. oz. bottle with child-resistant safety cap and convenient dosage cup

PediaCare® NightRest Cough-Cold Liquid

McNeil Consumer Products
P. 684

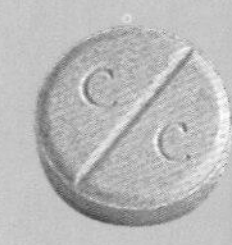

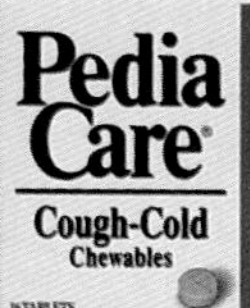

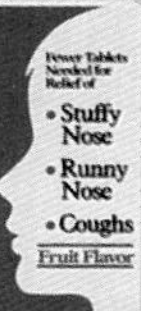

Blister Packs of 16 Chewable Tablets

Liquid available in 4 fl. oz. bottle with child-resistant safety cap and convenient dosage cup

PediaCare® Cough-Cold

McNeil Consumer Products
P. 684

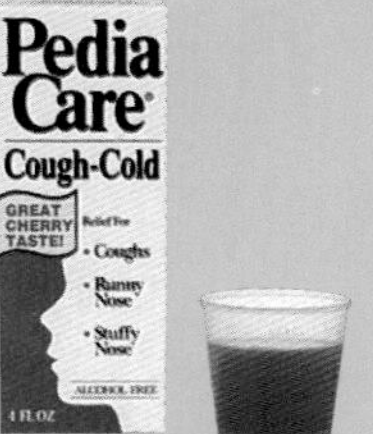

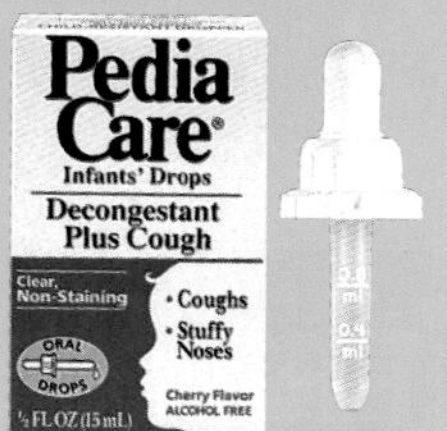

Available in $^1/_2$ fl oz. bottle with child-resistant safety cap and calibrated dropper

PediaCare® Infants' Drops Decongestant Plus Cough

McNeil Consumer Products
P. 684

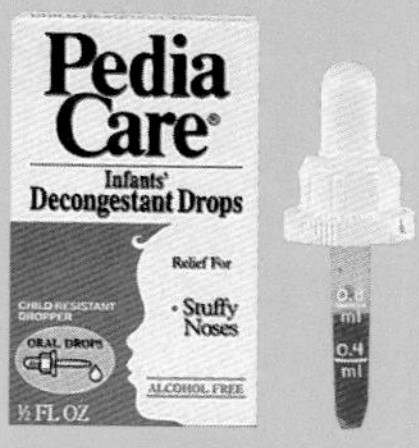

Available in 1/2 fl. oz. bottle with child-resistant safety cap and calibrated dropper

PediaCare® Infants' Decongestant Drops

McNeil Consumer Products
P. 686

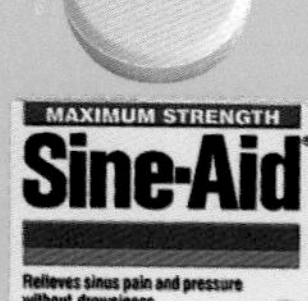

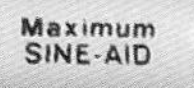

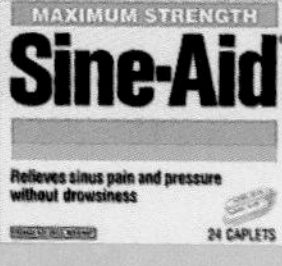

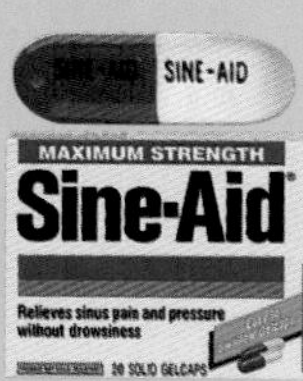

Tablets and Caplets in blister packs of 24 & bottles of 50

Gelcaps in blister packs of 20 & bottles of 40

Maximum Strength Sine-Aid®

McNeil Consumer Products
P. 677

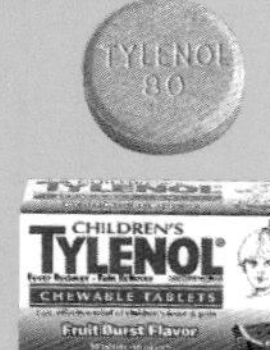

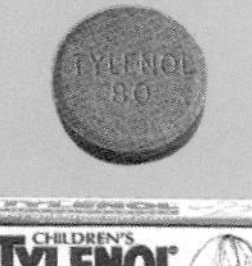

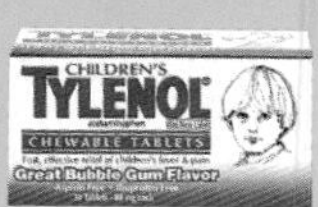

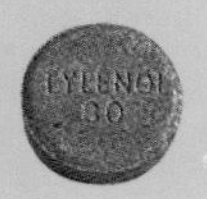

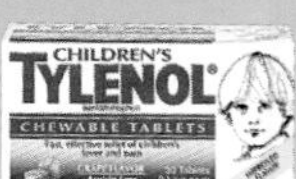

Fruit Burst Flavor: bottles of 30 with child-resistant safety cap and blister-packs of 60

Bubble Gum and Grape Flavor Bottles of 30 with child-resistant safety cap

Children's TYLENOL® 80 mg Chewable Tablets

McNeil Consumer Products
P. 677

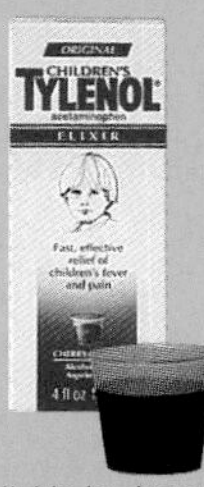

Available in cherry flavor in 2 and 4 fl. oz. bottles with child-resistant safety cap and convenient dosage cup. Alcohol Free, 80 mg. per 1/2 teaspoon

Children's TYLENOL® Elixir

McNeil Consumer Products
P. 680

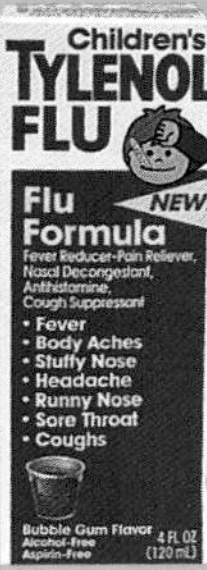

Children's TYLENOL® Flu Liquid

McNeil Consumer Products
P. 677

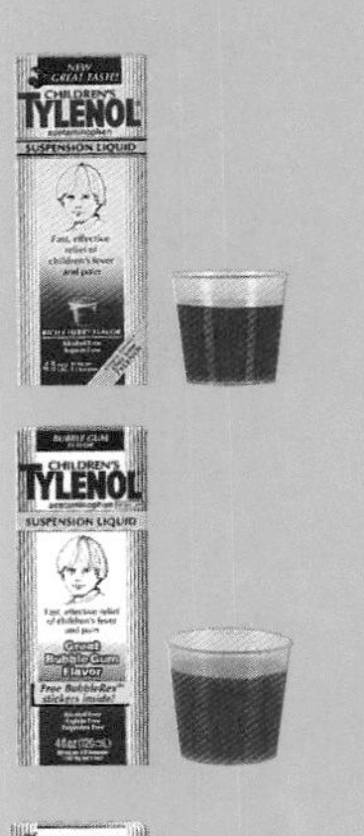

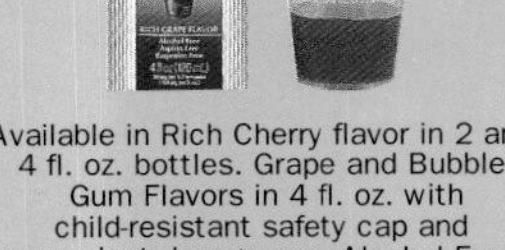

Available in Rich Cherry flavor in 2 and 4 fl. oz. bottles. Grape and Bubble Gum Flavors in 4 fl. oz. with child-resistant safety cap and convenient dosage cup. Alcohol Free, 80 mg per 1/2 teaspoon

Children's TYLENOL® Suspension Liquid

McNeil Consumer Products
P. 681

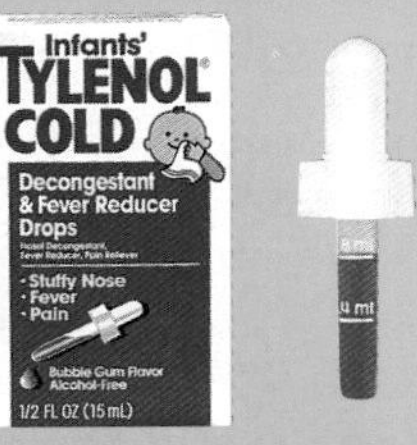

Available in 1/2 fl. oz. bottle with child-resistant safety cap and calibrated dropper. Bubble Gum Flavor, Alcohol-free.

Infant's TYLENOL® Cold Decongestant and Fever Reducer Drops

McNeil Consumer Products
P. 677

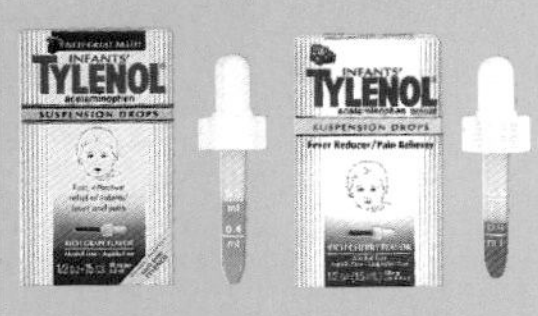

Available in rich cherry flavor and rich grape flavor 1/2 oz. bottle with child resistant safety cap and calibrated dropper. Rich Grape Flavor, Alcohol Free, 80 mg per 0.8 mL

Infants' TYLENOL® Suspension Drops

McNeil Consumer Products
P. 682

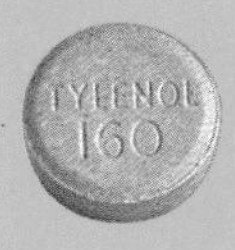

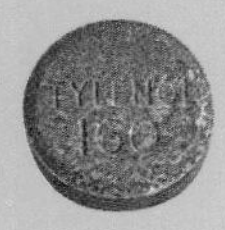

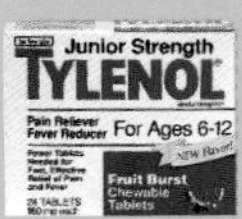

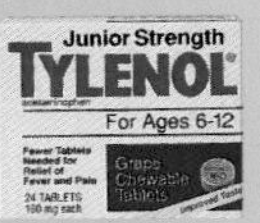

Available in Fruit Burst and Grape Flavored Chewable tablets of 160 mg available in blister pack of 24

Junior Strength TYLENOL®

McNeil Consumer Products
P. 682

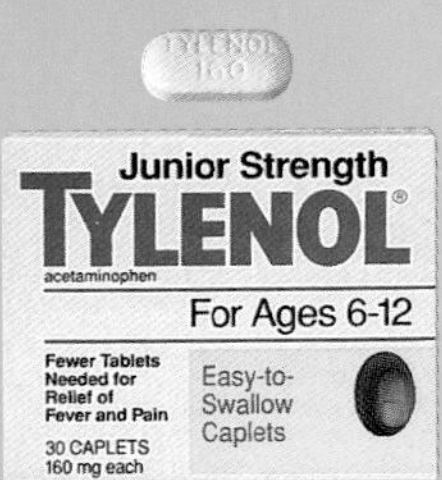

Swallowable Caplets: 160 mg blister packs of 30

Junior Strength TYLENOL®

McNeil Consumer Products
P. 678

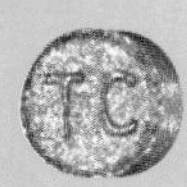

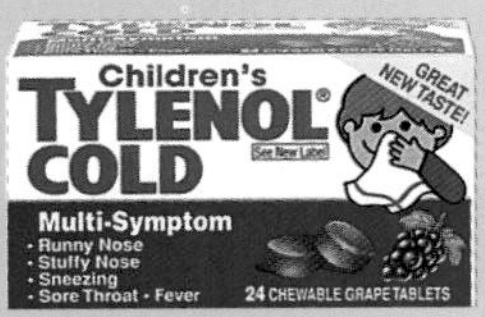

Available in bottles of 24 chewable tablets with child-resistant safety cap

Children's TYLENOL® Cold

McNeil Consumer Products
P. 678

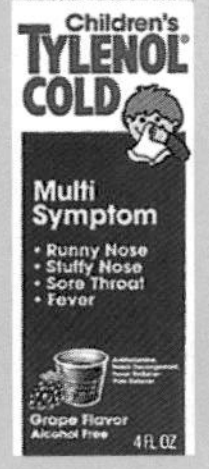

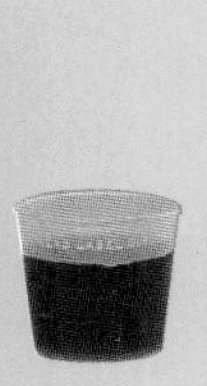

Multi-Symptom Formula

Available in 4 fl. oz. bottle with child-resistant safety cap and convenient dosage cup

Children's TYLENOL® Cold Liquid

McNeil Consumer Products
P. 679

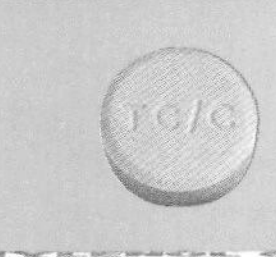

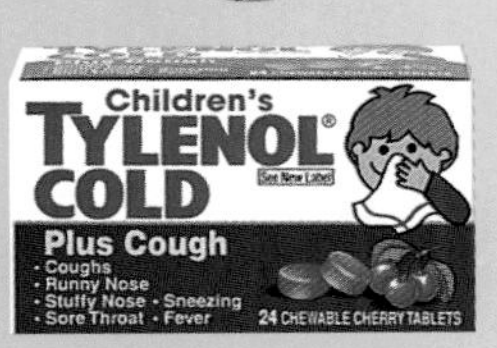

Available in bottles of 24 chewable tablets with child-resistant safety cap

Children's TYLENOL® Cold Plus Cough Chewable

McNeil Consumer Products
P. 679

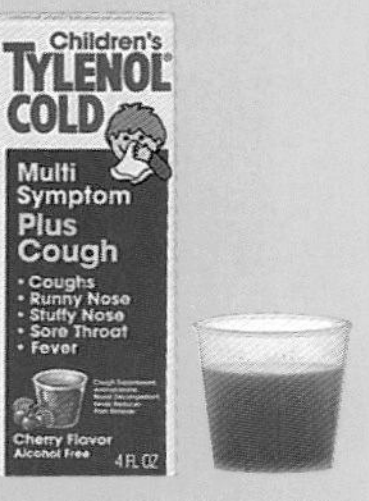

Multi-Symptom Plus Cough Formula

Available in 4 fl. oz. bottle with child-resistant safety cap and convenient dosage cup.

Children's TYLENOL® Cold Plus Cough Liquid

McNeil Consumer Products
P. 696

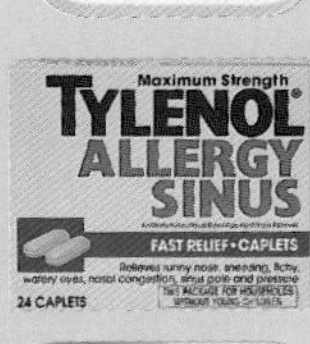

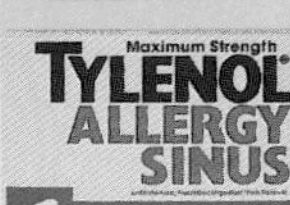

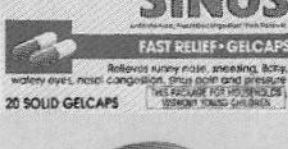

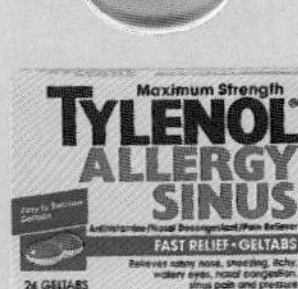

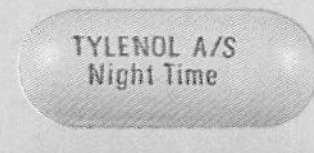

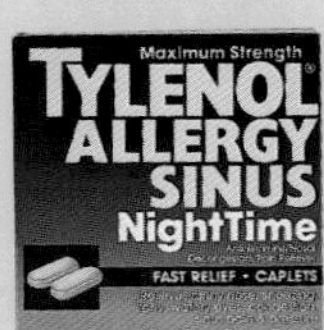

Caplets in blister packs of 24 & 48
Gelcaps in blister packs of 24 & 48
Geltabs in blister packs of 24 & 48

Maximum Strength TYLENOL® Allergy Sinus

McNeil Consumer Products
P. 696

Caplets available in blister packs of 24's

Maximum Strength TYLENOL® Allergy Sinus NightTime

McNeil Consumer Products
P. 696

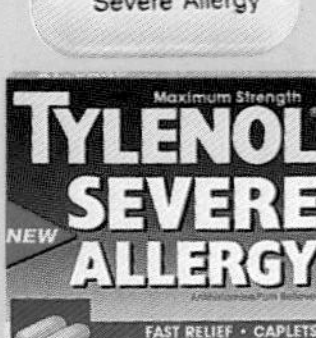

Caplets available in blister packs of 12's and 24's

Maximum Strength TYLENOL® Severe Allergy

McNeil Consumer Products
P. 688

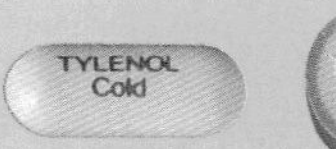

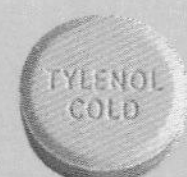

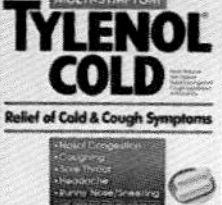

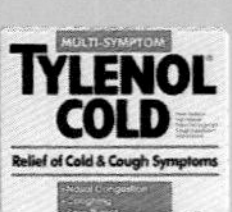

Caplets and Tablets available in blister-packs of 24 and bottles of 50

TYLENOL® Cold Medication

McNeil Consumer Products
P. 688

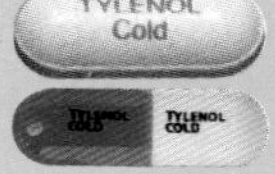

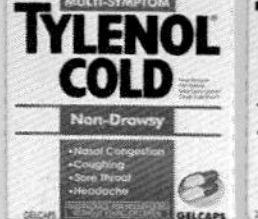

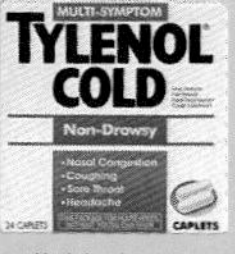

Gelcaps available in blister-packs of 24 and bottles of 40
Caplets available in blister-packs of 24 and bottles of 50
No Drowsiness Formula

TYLENOL® Cold Medication

McNeil Consumer Products
P. 688

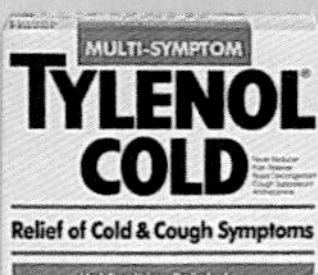

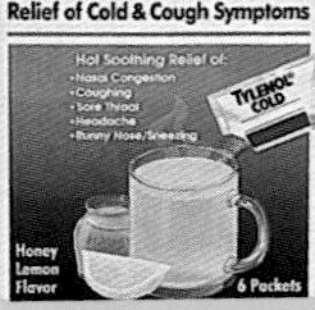

Available in cartons of 6 individual packets. Hot Liquid Medication

Multi-Symptom TYLENOL® COLD

McNeil Consumer Products
P. 690

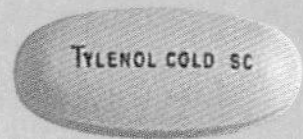

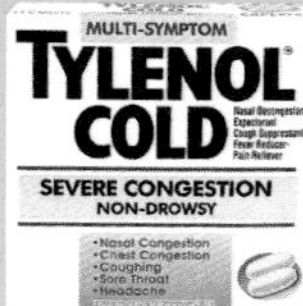

Available in blister packs of 12 and 24

TYLENOL® Cold Severe Congestion

McNeil Consumer Products
P. 691

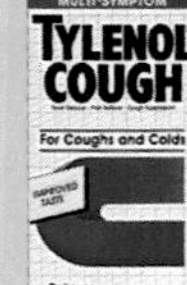

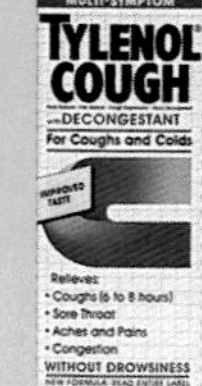

Available in 4 fl. oz. bottles

Multi-Symptom TYLENOL® Cough

McNeil Consumer Products
P. 687

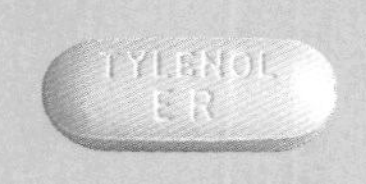

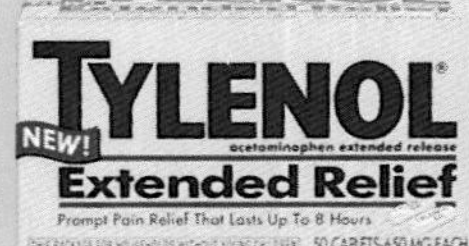

Caplets available in 24's, 50's and 100's

TYLENOL® Extended Relief

McNeil Consumer Products
P. 693

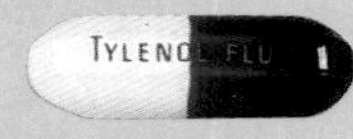

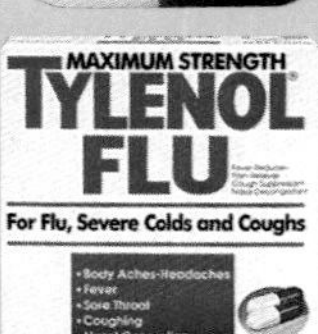

Gelcaps available in blister-packs of 10's, and 20's
No Drowsiness Formula

Maximum Strength TYLENOL® Flu

McNeil Consumer Products
P. 693

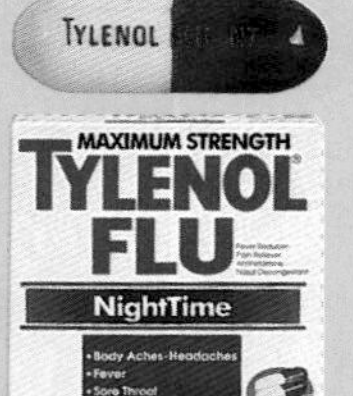

Gelcaps Available in Blister Packs of 10's and 20's

Maximum Strength TYLENOL® Flu NightTime

McNeil Consumer Products
P. 693

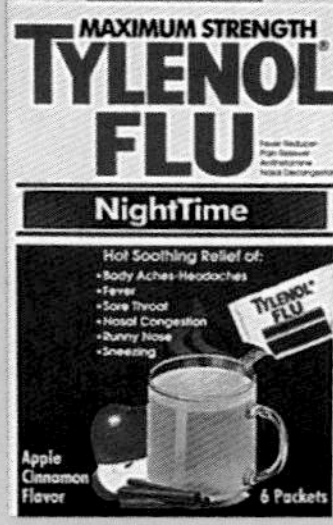

Available in cartons of 6 individual packets. Hot Liquid Medication

Maximum Strength TYLENOL® Flu NightTime

McNeil Consumer Products
P. 687

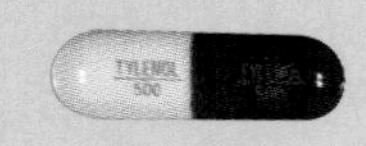

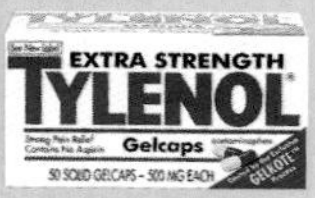

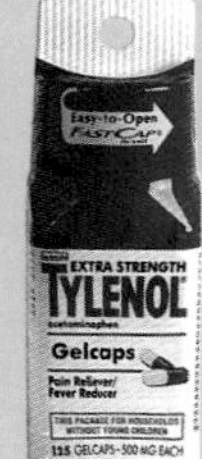

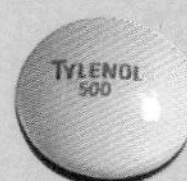

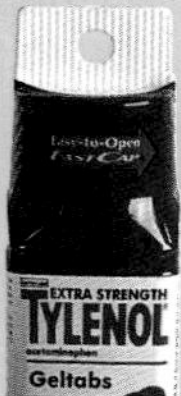

Geltabs available in tamper-resistant bottles of 24's, 50's and 100's and FastCap™ bottle of 125's "for house-holds without children"
Gelcaps available in tamper-resistant bottles of 24's, 50's, 100's, 150's and 225's and FastCap™ bottle of 125's "for households without children"

Extra Strength TYLENOL®

McNeil Consumer Products
P. 687

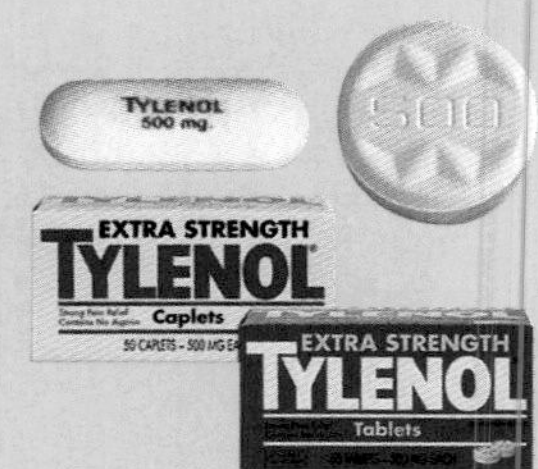

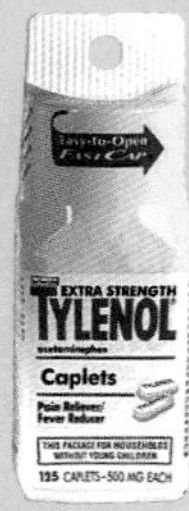

Caplets: tamper-resistant vials of 10 and bottles of 24's, 50's, 100's, 175's and 250's and FastCap™ bottle of 125's "for households with out children"
Tablets: tamper-resistant vials of 10 and bottles of 30's, 60's, 100's and 200's
Liquid: tamper-resistant bottles of 8 fl. oz.

Extra Strength TYLENOL®

McNeil Consumer Products
P. 695

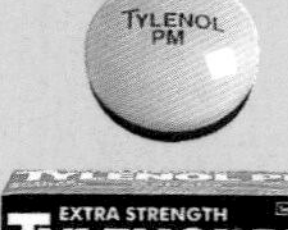

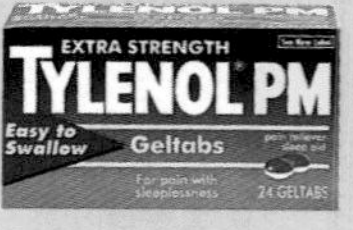

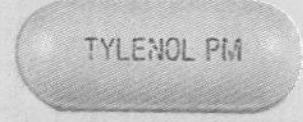

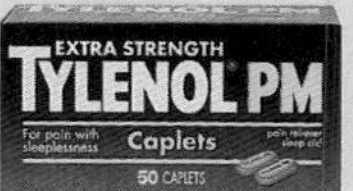

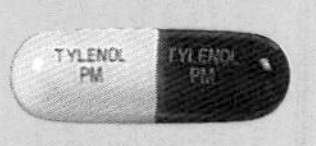

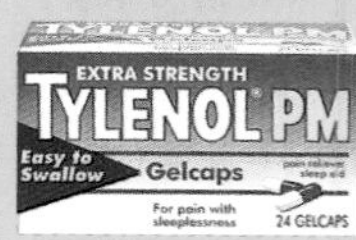

Geltabs and Gelcaps available in tamper-resistant bottles of 24's and 50's. Caplets available in tamper-resistant bottles of 24's, 50's, 100's and 150's

TYLENOL® PM

McNeil Consumer Products
P. 687

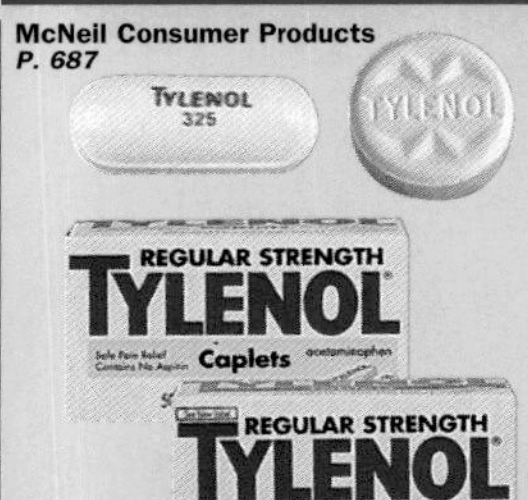

Tablets and Caplets available in:
24's, 50's, 100's and 200's and
Tins of 12's

Regular Strength
TYLENOL®

McNeil Consumer Products
P. 697

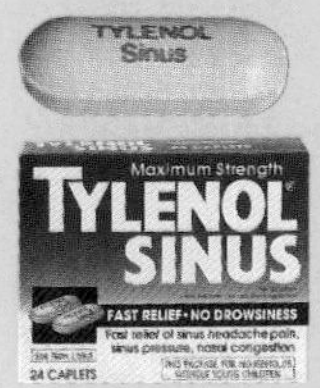

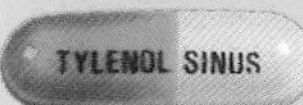

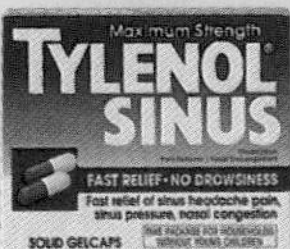

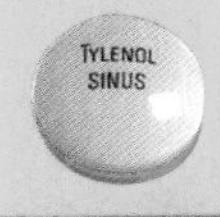

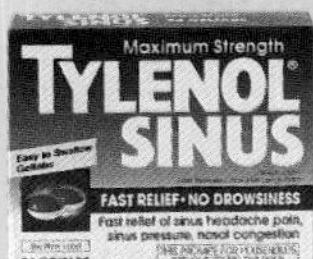

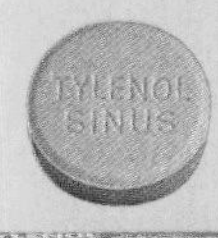

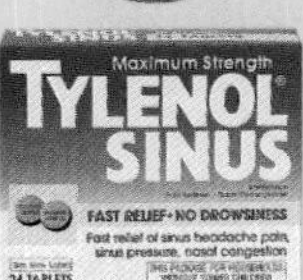

Caplets, Gelcaps, Geltabs and
Tablets in blister packs of 24 & 48

Maximum Strength
TYLENOL® Sinus

NOVARTIS CONSUMER HEALTH

Novartis Consumer Health, Inc.
P. 702

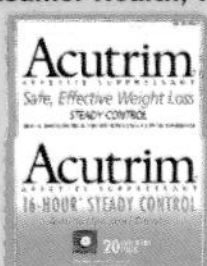

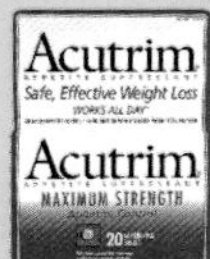

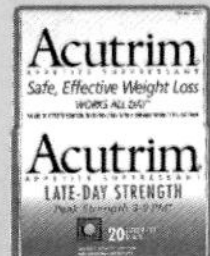

Appetite Suppressants
Caffeine Free/Works all Day

Acutrim®

Novartis Consumer Health, Inc.
P. 703

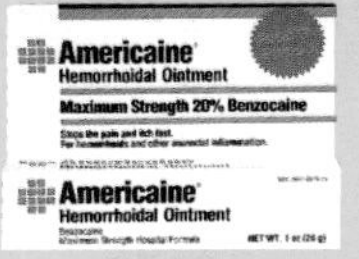

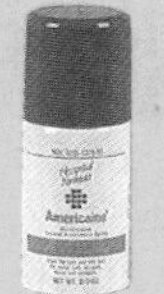

Hemorrhoidal Ointment 1 oz.
and Spray 2 oz.

Americaine®

Novartis Consumer Health, Inc.
P. 703

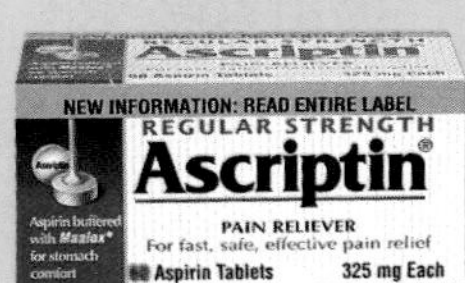

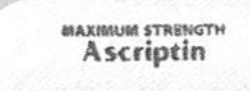

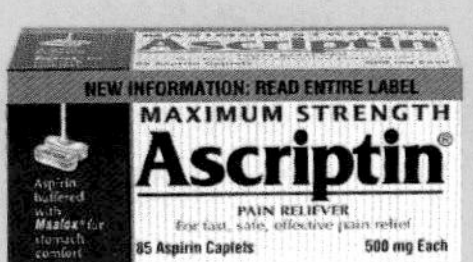

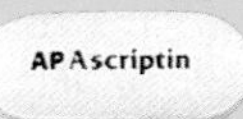

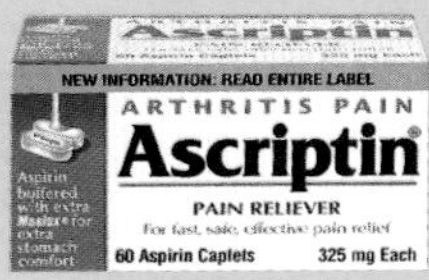

Regular Strength,
Maximum Strength and
Arthritis Pain

Ascriptin®

Novartis Consumer Health, Inc.
P. 704

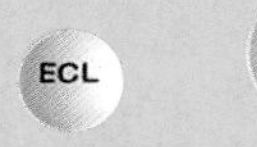

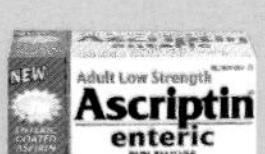

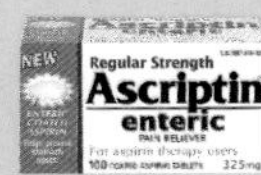

Adult Low Strength and
Regular Strength

Ascriptin® enteric

Novartis Consumer Health, Inc.
P. 706

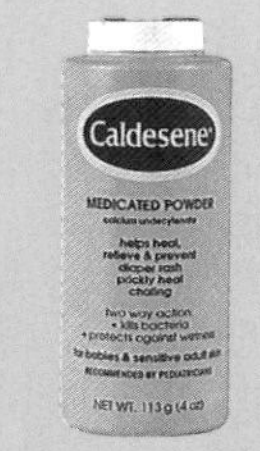

Medicated Powder
Available in 2 oz. and 4 oz.
shaker containers

Caldesene®

Novartis Consumer Health, Inc.
P. 707

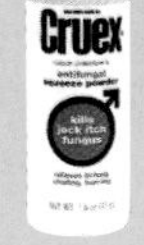

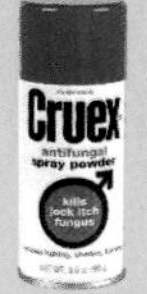

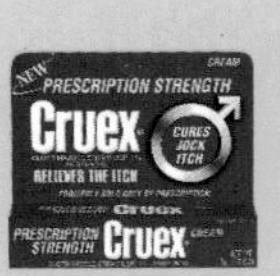

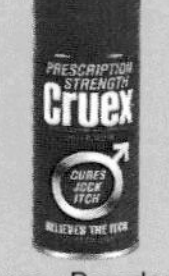

Squeeze Powder, Spray Powder,
Prescription Strength Cream and
Prescription Strength Spray Powder

Cruex®

Novartis Consumer Health, Inc.
P. 707

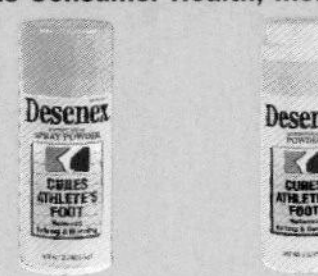

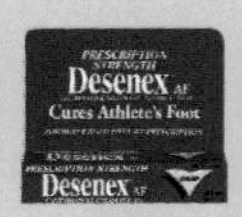

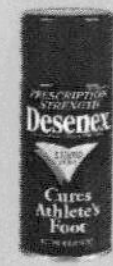

Spray Powder, Shake Powder,
Prescription Strength Cream and
Prescription Strength Spray Liquid
Also available: Ointment and
Prescription Strength Spray Powder

Desenex®

Novartis Consumer Health, Inc.
P. 709

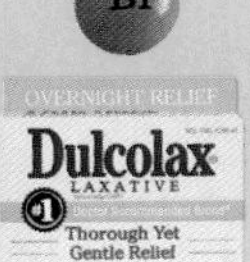

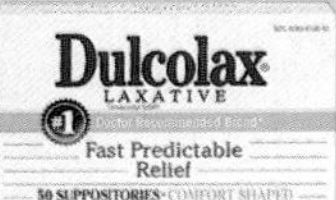

Tablets & Suppositories

Dulcolax® Laxative

Novartis Consumer Health, Inc.
P. 710

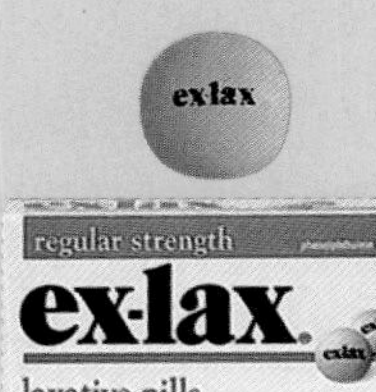

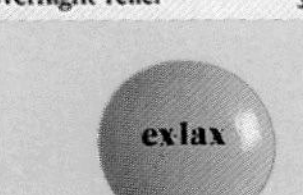

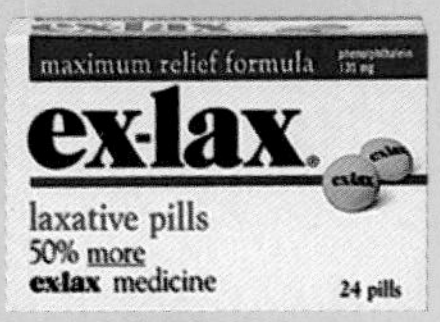

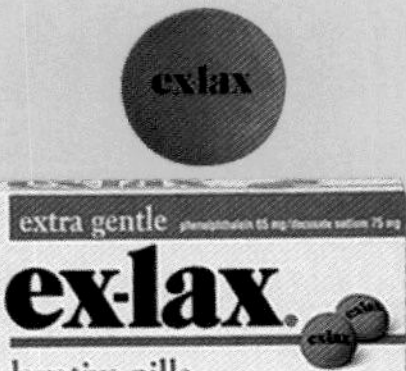

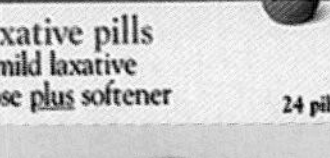

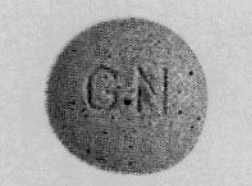

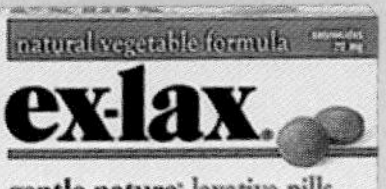

Regular Strength 8's, 30's, 60's
Maximum Relief Formula 24's, 48's
Extra Gentle 24's
Gentle Nature™ 16's

Ex-lax®

Novartis Consumer Health, Inc.
P. 710

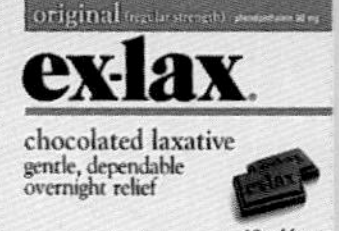

Chocolated Laxative
Tablets 6's, 18's, 48's and 72's

Ex-lax®

Novartis Consumer Health, Inc.
P. 710

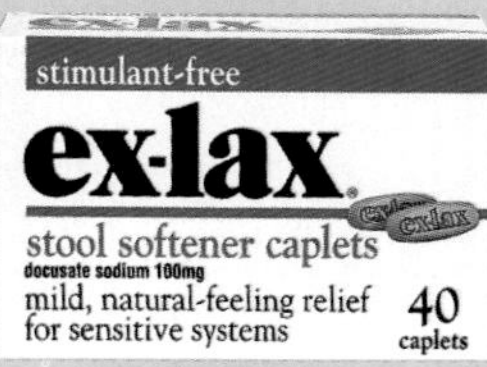

Stimulant-Free Stool
Softener Caplets

Ex-Lax®

Novartis Consumer Health, Inc.
P. 711

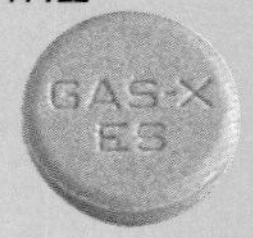

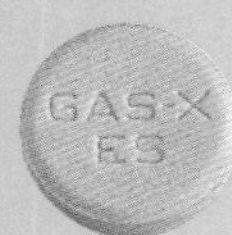

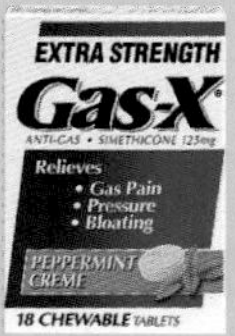

Extra-Strength Cherry 18's, 48's
Extra-Strength Peppermint 18's, 48's
(125 mg simethicone)

Gas-X®

Novartis Consumer Health, Inc.
P. 711

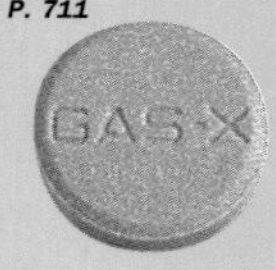

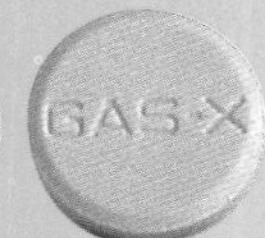

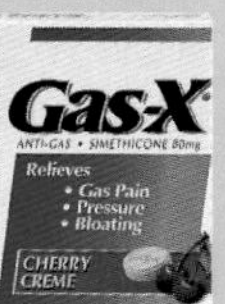

Cherry 12's, 36's
Peppermint 12's, 36's
(80 mg simethicone)

Gas-X®

Novartis Consumer Health, Inc.
P. 711

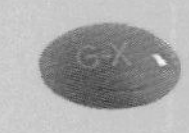
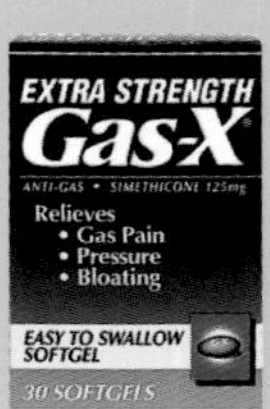

Extra Strength Softgels
in packs of 10's and 30's

Gas-X®

Novartis Consumer Health, Inc.
P. 711

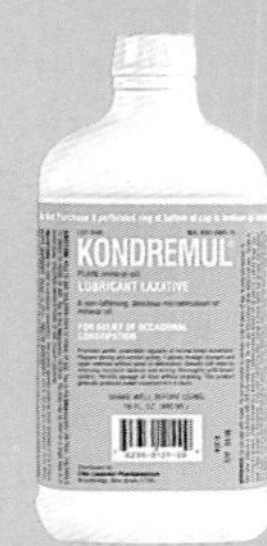

Plain (Mineral Oil)
Lubricant Laxative

Kondremul®

Novartis Consumer Health, Inc.
P. 713

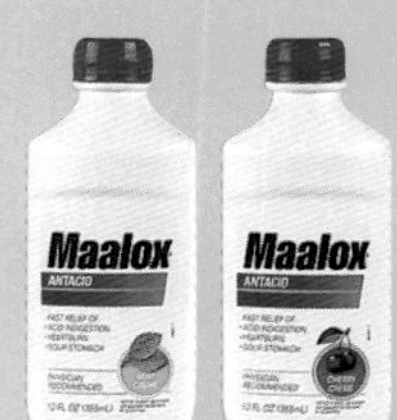

Cooling Mint and Smooth Cherry
Also available in Refreshing Lemon
Bottles of 5 (Mint Only), 12 & 26 oz.

Maalox® Antacid

Novartis Consumer Health, Inc.
P. 711

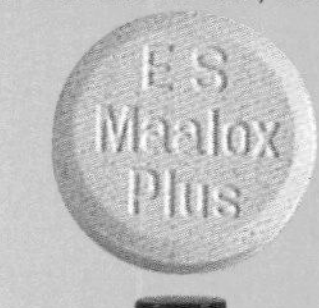

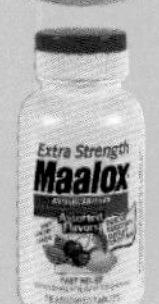

Assorted Flavors (Mint, Cherry, Lemon)
Also available in Cooling Mint
Bottles of 38 and 75

Extra Strength Maalox®
Antacid/Anti-Gas

Novartis Consumer Health, Inc.
P. 711

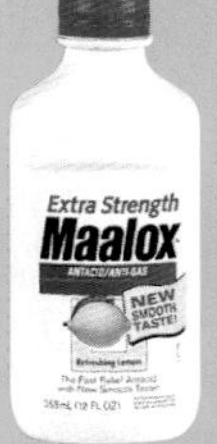

Refreshing Lemon
Also available in Cooling Mint
and Smooth Cherry
Bottles of 5 (Lemon only),
12 & 26 oz.

Extra Strength Maalox®
Antacid/Anti-Gas

Novartis Consumer Health, Inc.
P. 714

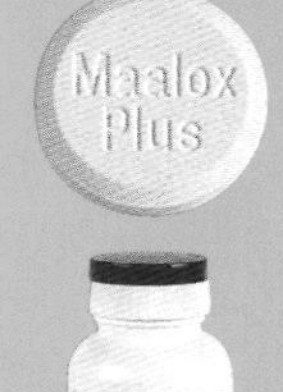

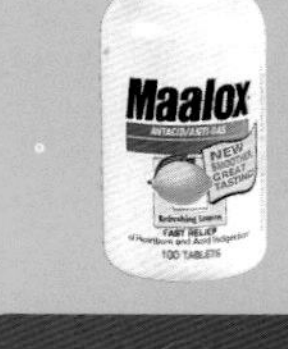

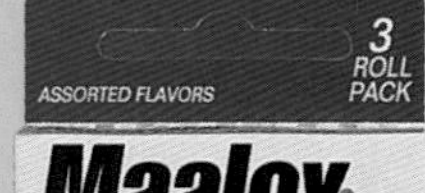

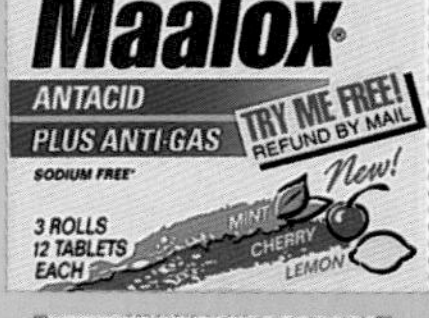

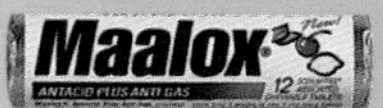

Refreshing Lemon, as well as
Assorted & Smooth Cherry Flavors
in Bottles of 50 & 100 Tablets
Rollpacks in Assorted
and Refreshing Lemon Flavors

Maalox®
Antacid/Anti-Gas

Novartis Consumer Health, Inc.
P. 712

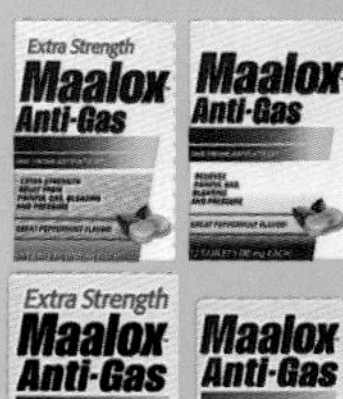

Peppermint and Sweet Lemon Flavor
Regular Strength 12's
Extra Strength 10's

Maalox® Anti-Gas

Novartis Consumer Health, Inc.
P. 714

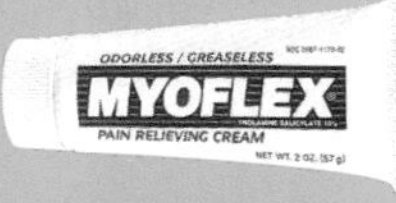

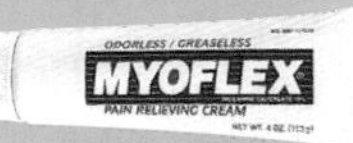

Pain Relieving Cream
Available in 2 oz. and 4 oz. tubes,
8 oz. and 16 oz. jars

Myoflex®

Novartis Consumer Health, Inc.
P. 715

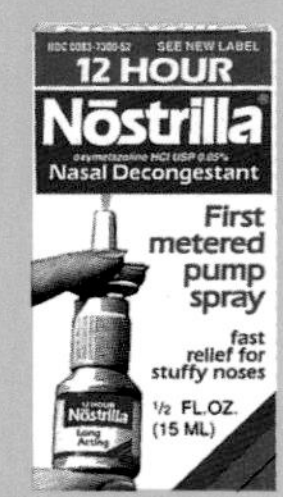

12 Hour Metered Pump Spray

Nostrilla®

Novartis Consumer Health, Inc.
P. 715

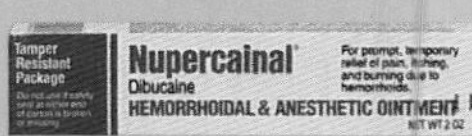

Hemorrhoidal & Anesthetic
Available in: Ointment 2 oz. & 1 oz.
Suppositories: box of 12

Nupercainal®

Novartis Consumer Health, Inc.
P. 716

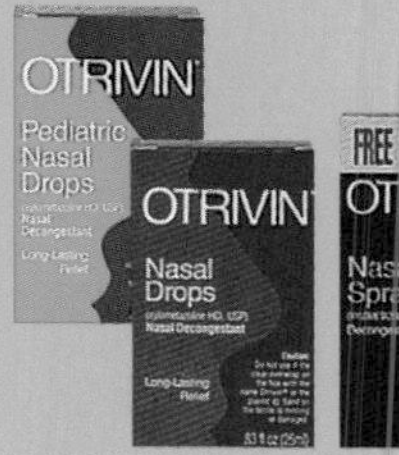

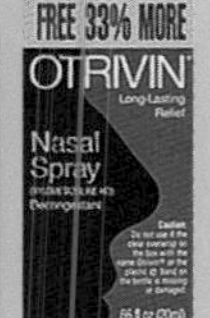

Nasal Decongestant Drops
Pediatric Drops and Nasal Spray

Otrivin®

Novartis Consumer Health, Inc.
P. 716

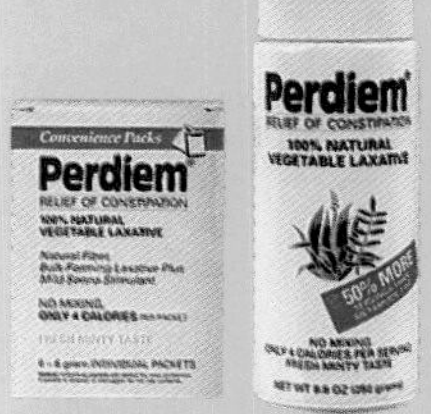

100% Natural Vegetable Laxative
250 gm and 6-6gm packets
Also available: 400 gm canisters

Perdiem®

Novartis Consumer Health, Inc.
P. 717

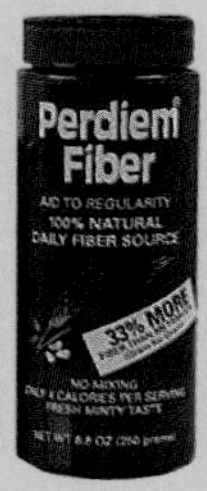

100% Natural
Daily Fiber Source
available in 250 gm

Perdiem® Fiber

Novartis Consumer Health, Inc.
P. 718

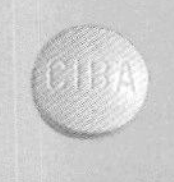
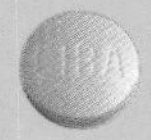
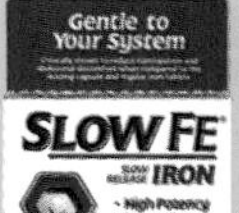
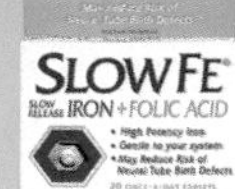

Slow Release Iron and Slow Release Iron & Folic Acid

Slow Fe®

Novartis Consumer Health, Inc.
P. 718

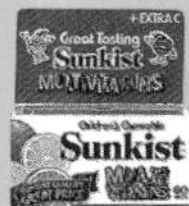
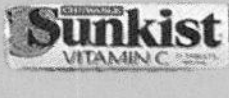
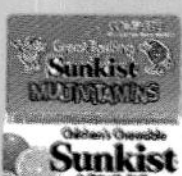
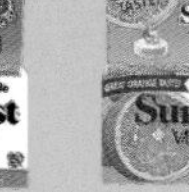

Children's Multivitamins
Extra C and Complete
Vitamin C Citrus Complex
60 mg Chewable Tablets
(11 Tablet Roll)
250 and 500 mg Chewable Tablets

Sunkist®

Novartis Consumer Health, Inc.
P. 719

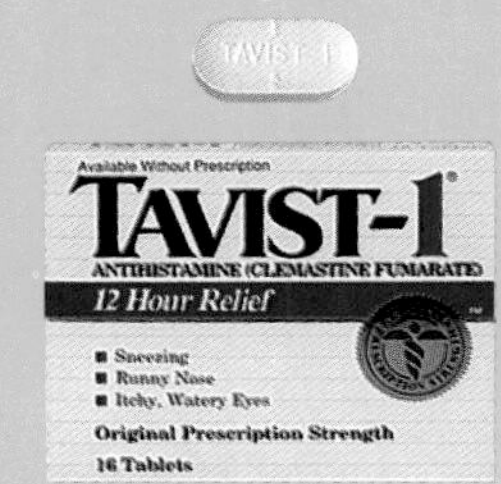

8's, 16's, 32's

Tavist-1®

Novartis Consumer Health, Inc.
P. 720

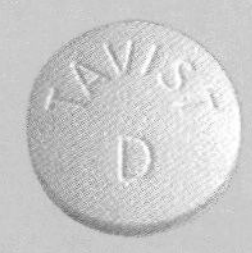
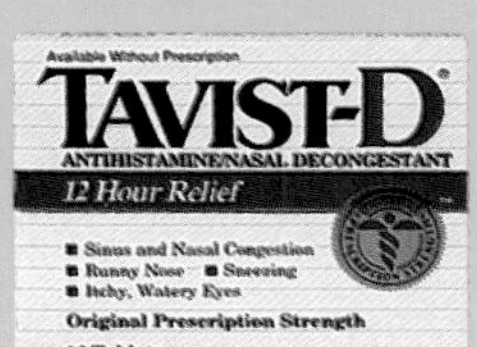

8's, 16's, 32's, 50's

Tavist-D®

Novartis Consumer Health, Inc.
P. 720

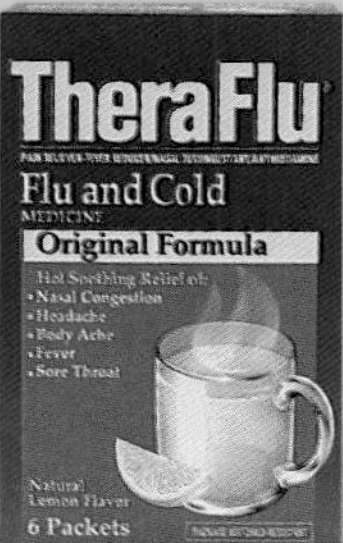
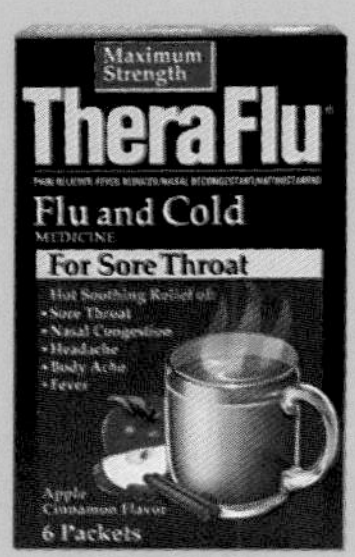

Flu and Cold Medicine
In packs of 6 and 12 ct.

Maximum Strength Flu and Cold Medicine for Sore Throat
In packs of 6.

TheraFlu®

Sandoz Consumer Division
P. 720

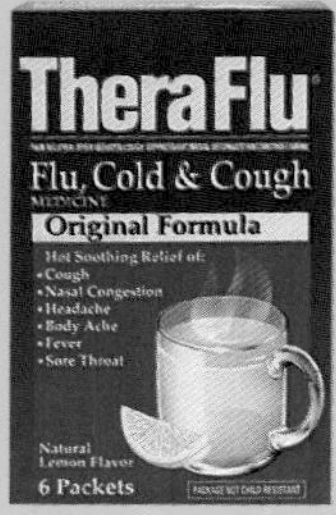
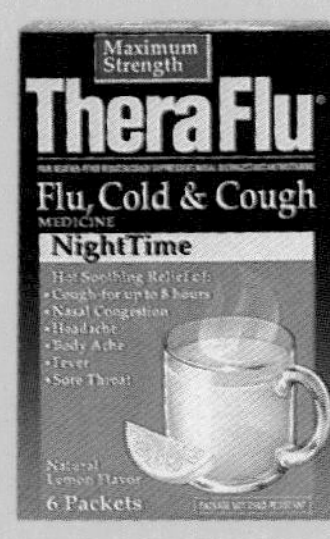
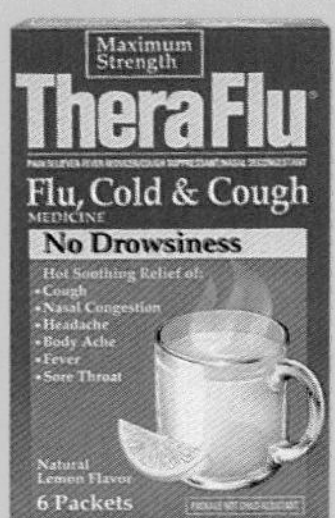

Flu, Cold & Cough Medicine
Maximum Strength Nighttime Flu, Cold & Cough Medicine
Maximum Strength, No Drowsiness Flu, Cold & Cough Medicine
In packs of 6 and 12 ct.

TheraFlu®

Novartis Consumer Health, Inc.
P. 722

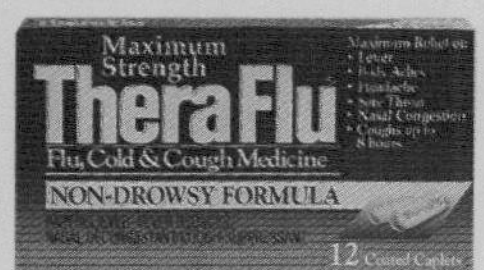

12's, 24's
Non-drowsy Flu, Cold and Cough Caplets

TheraFlu® Maximum Strength

Novartis Consumer Health, Inc.
P. 721

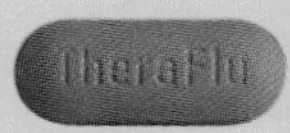
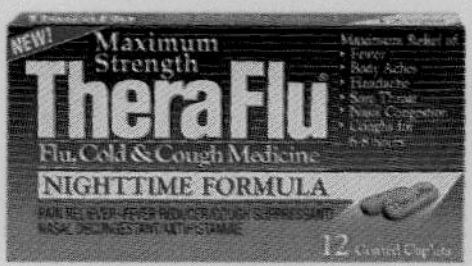

12's, 24's
Flu, Cold & Cough Medicine
Nighttime Formula

TheraFlu® Maximum Strength

Novartis Consumer Health, Inc.
P. 722

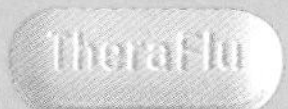
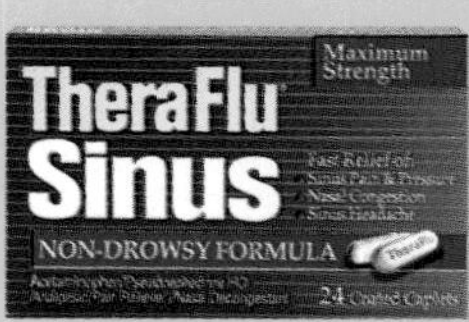

Maximum Strength Sinus Non-Drowsy Formula in packs of 24 caplets

TheraFlu® Sinus

Novartis Consumer Health, Inc.
P. 723

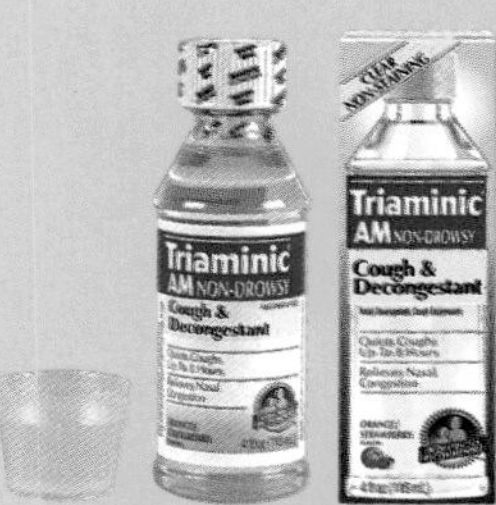

4 oz., 8 oz.

Triaminic® AM Cough & Decongestant Formula

Novartis Consumer Health, Inc.
P. 724

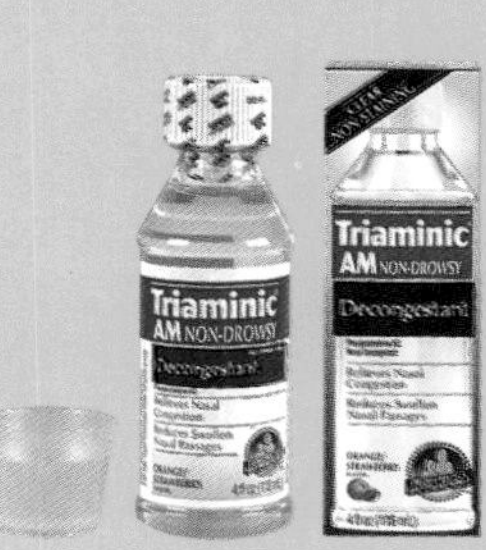

4 oz., 8 oz.

Triaminic® AM Decongestant Formula

Novartis Consumer Health, Inc.
P. 727

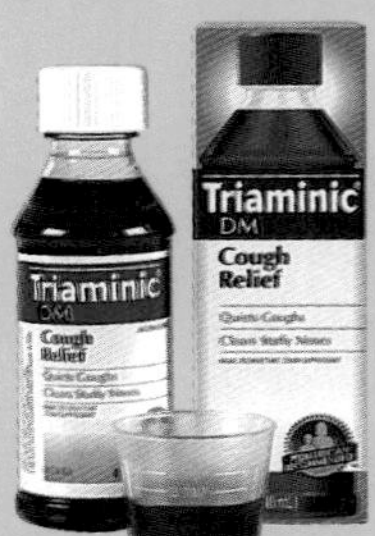

4 oz., 8 oz.

Triaminic® DM

Novartis Consumer Health, Inc.
P. 724

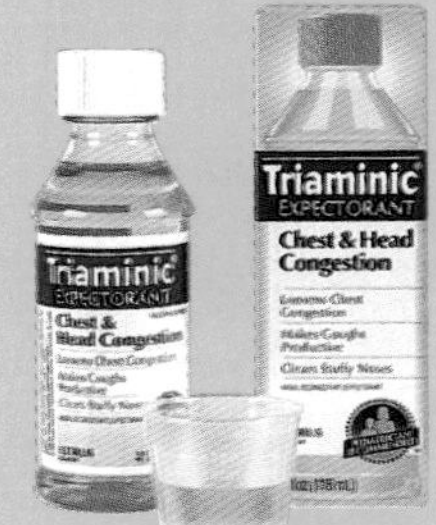

4 oz., 8 oz.

Triaminic® Expectorant

Novartis Consumer Health, Inc.
P. 725

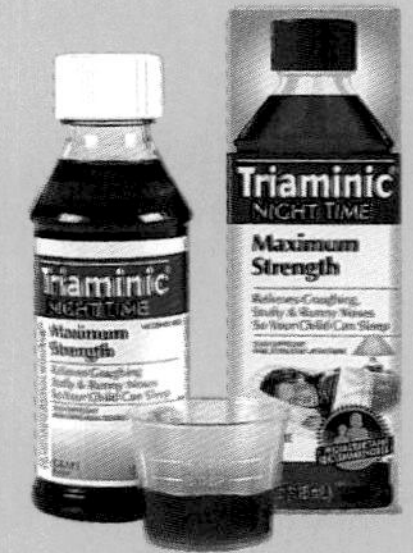

4 oz., 8 oz.

Triaminic® Night Time®

Novartis Consumer Health, Inc.
P. 725

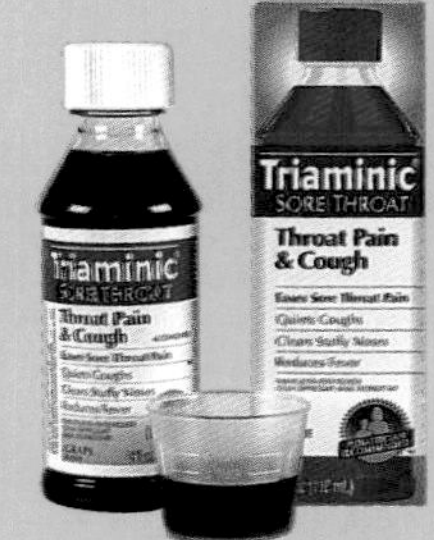

4 oz., 8 oz.

Triaminic® Sore Throat

Novartis Consumer Health, Inc.
P. 726

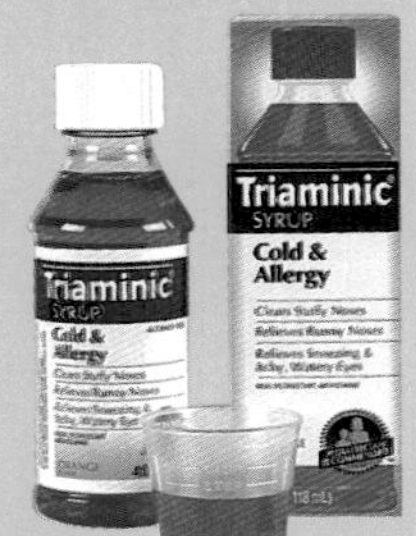

4 oz., 8 oz.

Triaminic® Syrup

Novartis Consumer Health, Inc.
P. 726

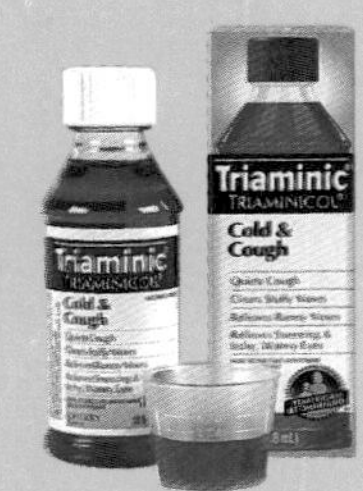

4 oz., 8 oz.

Triaminic® Triaminicol®

Novartis Consumer Health, Inc.
P. 727

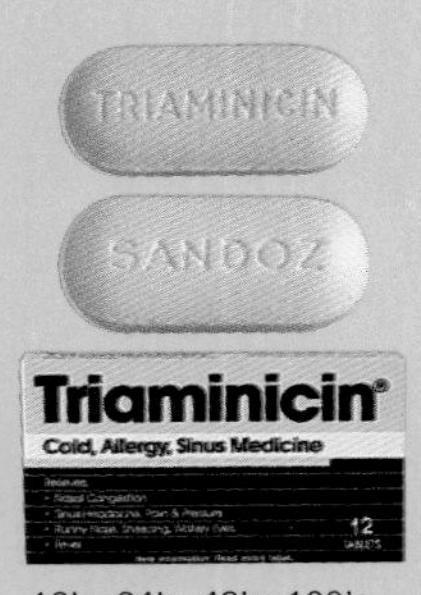

12's, 24's, 48's, 100's

Triaminicin®

For more detailed information on the products illustrated in this section, consult the Product Information Section or manufacturers may be contacted directly.

PFIZER

Pfizer Consumer Health Care
P. 728

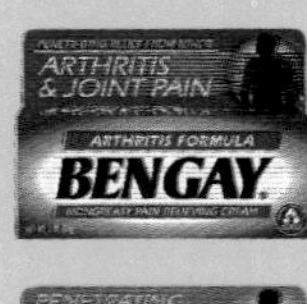

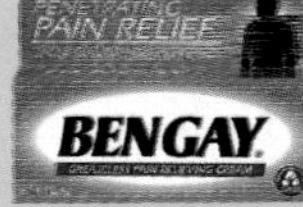

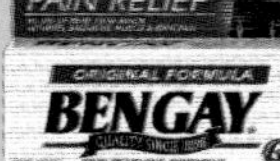

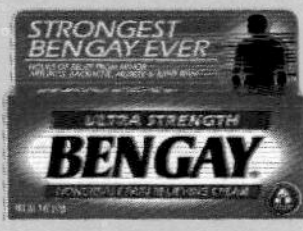

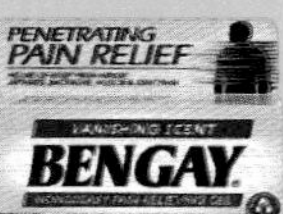

Arthritis Formula, Greaseless, Original Formula, Ultra Strength and Vanishing Scent.

BENGAY®

Pfizer Consumer Health Care
P. 729

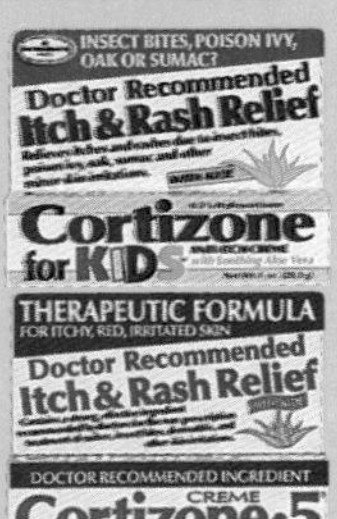

Available in 1 oz. and 2 oz. Creme and 1 oz. Ointment
Kids available in 1/2 oz. and 1 oz. Creme

Cortizone-5®

Pfizer Consumer Health Care
P. 729

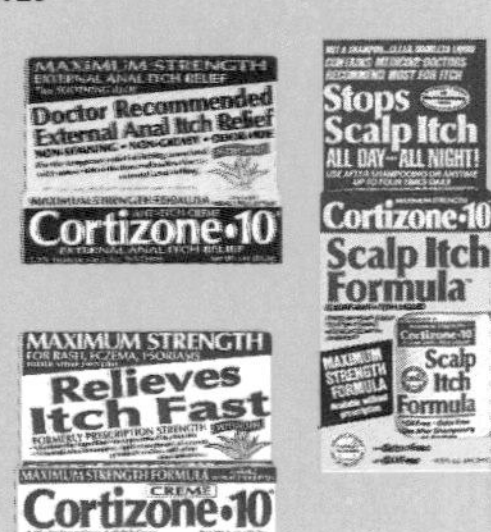

Available in 1 oz. and 2 oz. Creme and Ointment; 1.5 fl. oz. Liquid.

Cortizone-10™

Pfizer Consumer Health Care
P. 730

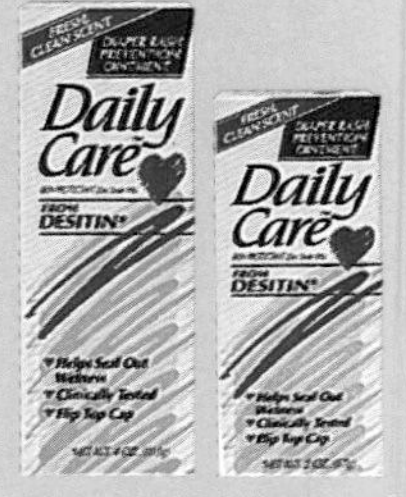

Diaper Rash Prevention Ointment

**Daily Care®
from DESITIN®**

Pfizer Consumer Health Care
P. 730

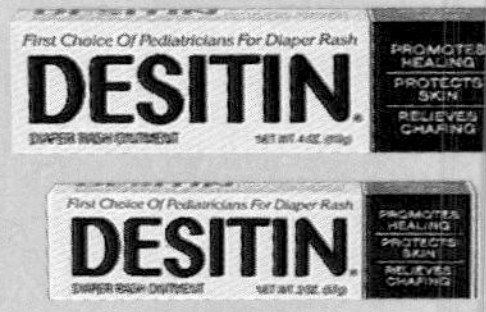

Diaper Rash Ointment

DESITIN®

Pfizer Consumer Health Care
P. 729

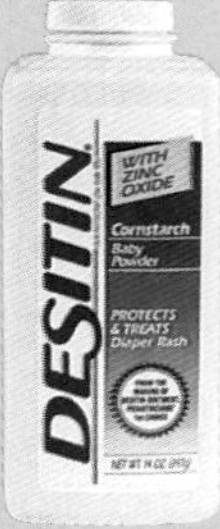

DESITIN® Cornstarch Baby Powder

Pfizer Consumer Health Care
P. 730

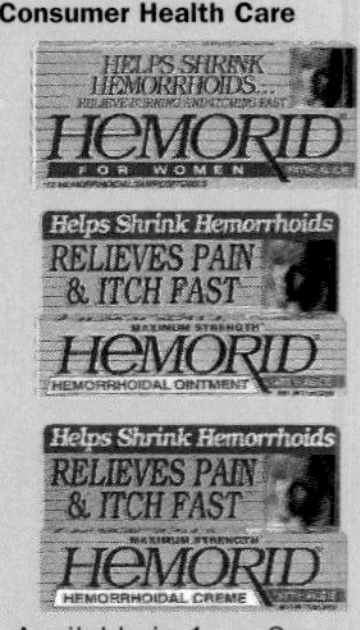

Available in 1 oz. Creme, 1 oz. Ointment, and 12 ct. Suppositories.

Hemorid®

Pfizer Consumer Health Care
P. 731

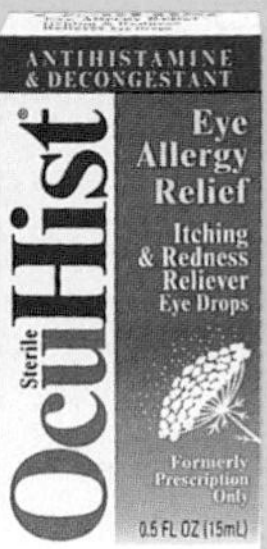

Itching and Redness Reliever Eye Drops

OcuHist®

Pfizer Consumer Health Care
P. 734

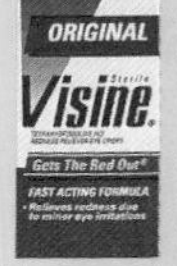

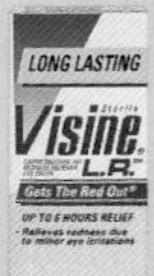

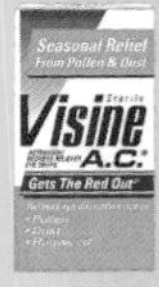

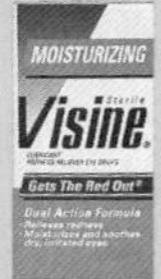

Original, Long Lasting, A.C. Seasonal Relief and Moisturizing

Visine®

PHARMABOTANIXX

PharmaBotanixx
P. 737

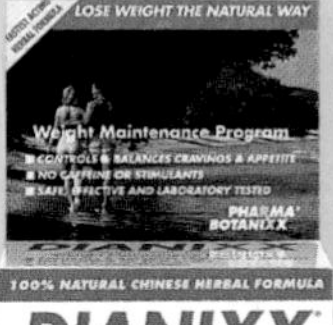

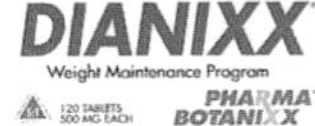

Weight Maintenance Program
Standardized Chinese Herbal Formula

Dianixx®

PharmaBotanixx
P. 737

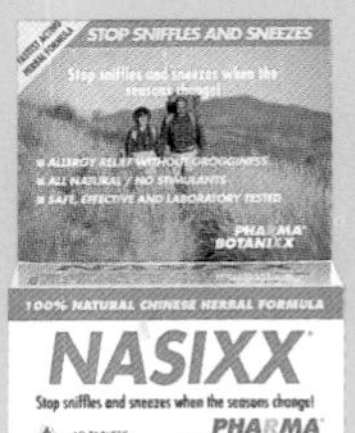

Stops Sniffles and Sneezes
Standardized Chinese Herbal Formula

Nasixx®

PharmaBotanixx
P. 738

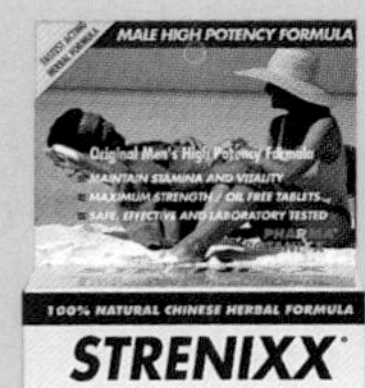

Original Men's High Potency Formula
Standardized Chinese Herbal Formula

Strenixx®

PHARMACIA & UPJOHN

Pharmacia & Upjohn
P. 738

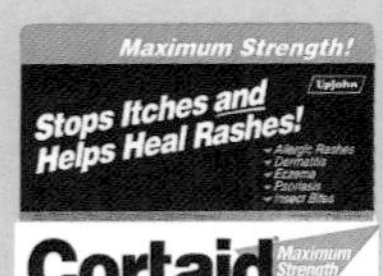

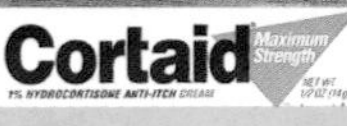

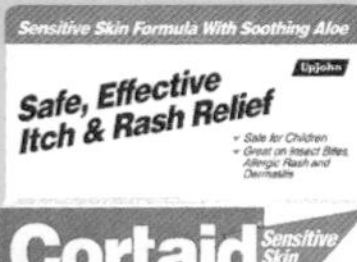

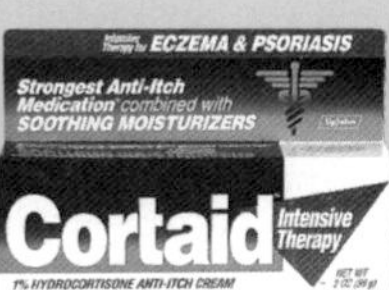

Maximum Strength (1% hydrocortisone) is available in cream, ointment, and spray.

Sensitive Skin ($^1/_2$% hydrocortisone) is available in cream and ointment.

Intensive Therapy (1% hydrocortisone) is available in cream

Cortaid®

Pharmacia & Upjohn
P. 738

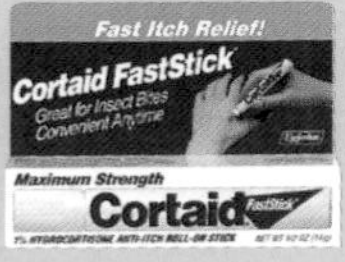

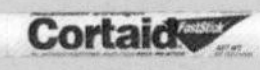

Roll-on relief for insect bites, itches and rashes

Maximum Strength

Cortaid® FastStick™
(1% hydrocortisone)

Pharmacia & Upjohn
P. 739

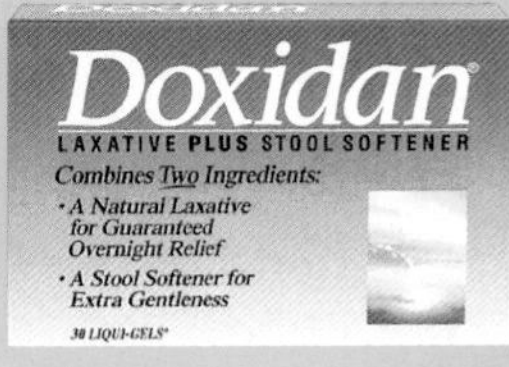

Stimulant/Stool Softener Laxative Packages of 10, 30, 100, 1,000, and 100 unit dose

Doxidan® Liqui-Gels®
(casanthranol 30 mg and docusate sodium 100 mg)

Pharmacia & Upjohn
P. 739

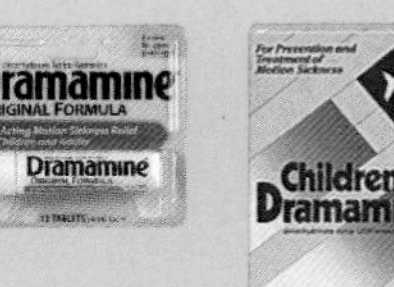

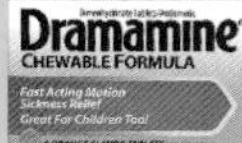

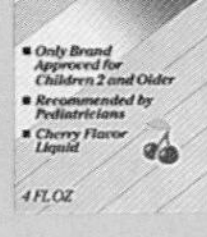

Tablets, Chewables and Children's Liquid

Dramamine®
(dimenhydrinate)

Pharmacia & Upjohn
P. 740

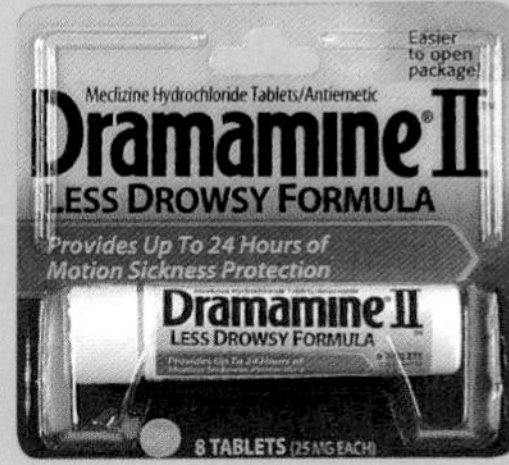

Tablets

Dramamine II™
(meclizine hydrochloride)

Pharmacia & Upjohn
P. 740

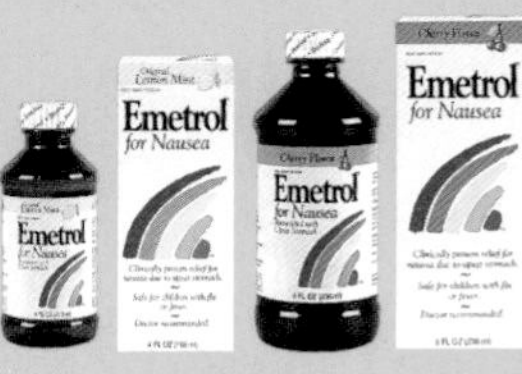

Lemon-Mint and Cherry Flavors. Available in 4oz, 8oz and 16 oz sizes

Emetrol®

Pharmacia & Upjohn
P. 741

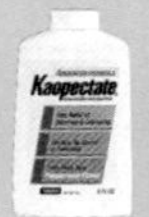

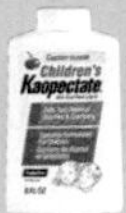

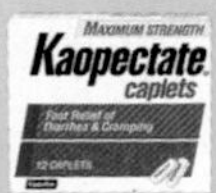

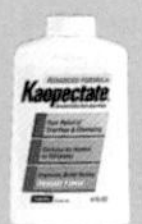

Regular, Peppermint, Children's Cherry Flavored Liquid and Maximum Strength Caplets

Kaopectate®
Anti-Diarrheal

Pharmacia & Upjohn
P. 741

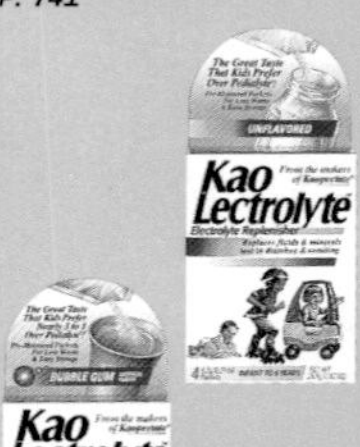

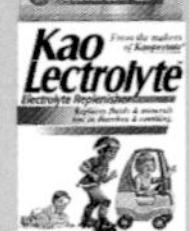

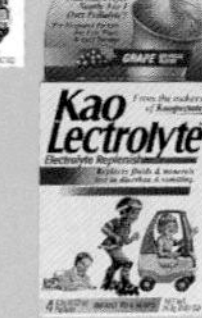

Available in Unflavored, Bubble Gum and Grape Flavors

Kao Lectrolyte™

Pharmacia & Upjohn
P. 741

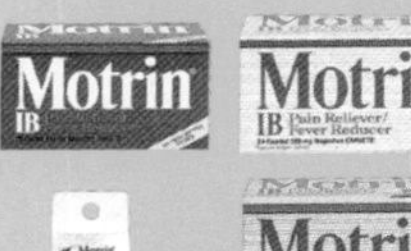

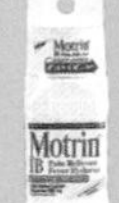

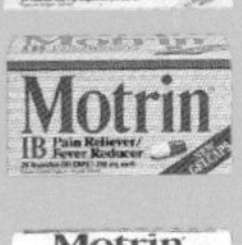

Tablets and Caplets: 24's, 50's, 100's, 130's and 165's; Gelcaps: 24's and 50's, Convenience Pack (vial) of 8 caplets

Motrin® IB
(ibuprofen, USP)

Pharmacia & Upjohn
P. 742

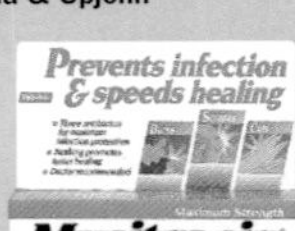

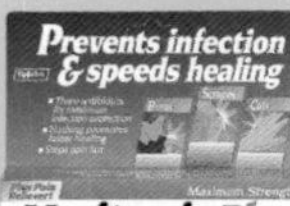

Maximum Strength Triple Antibiotic Ointment and Mycitracin Plus Pain Reliever Ointment

$^1/_2$ oz. and 1 oz. tubes

Mycitracin®

Pharmacia & Upjohn
P. 742

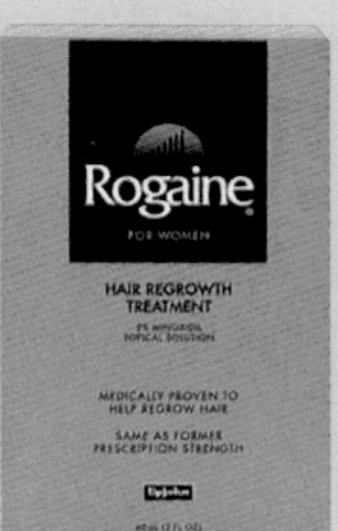

For Women

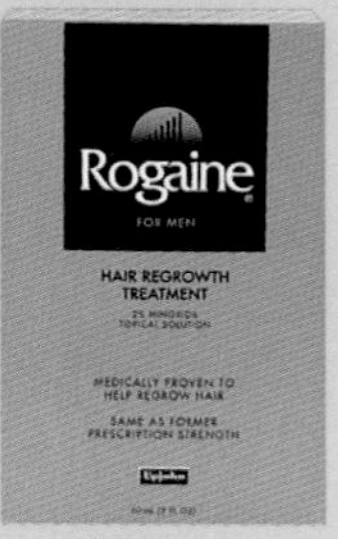

For Men

Hair Regrowth Treatment

Rogaine®
(2% minoxidil)

Pharmacia & Upjohn
P. 744

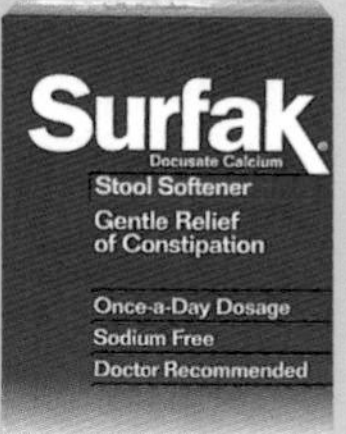

Packages of 10, 30, 100, 500 and 100 unit dose

Surfak® Liqui-Gels® Stool Softener
(docusate calcium 240 mg)

PHARMANEX, INC.

Pharmanex, Inc.
P. 744

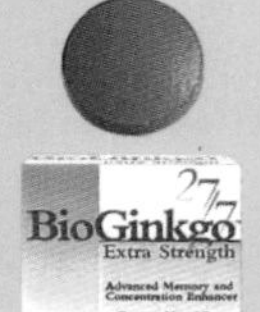

60 mg
Available in 40 ct.

BioGinkgo 27/7™

Pharmanex, Inc.
P. 745

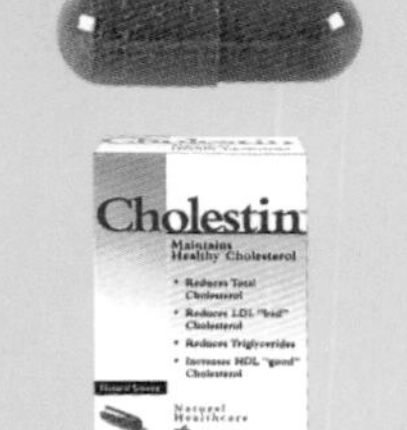

600 mg
Available in 48's and 80's.

Cholestin™

PHARMATON

Pharmaton
P. 747

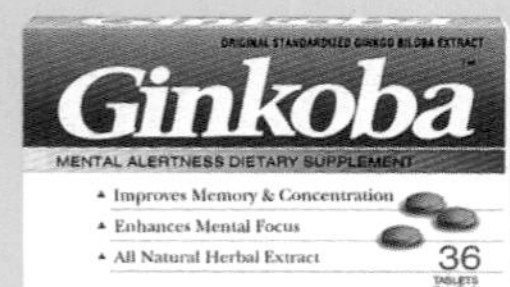

40 mg

Ginkoba™

Pharmaton
P. 748

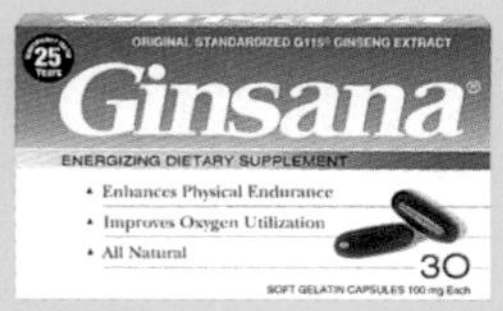

100 mg
Capsules

Ginsana®

Pharmaton
P. 748

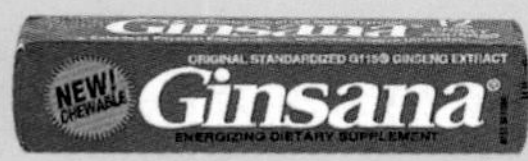

50 mg
Chewy Squares

Ginsana®

Pharmaton
P. 748

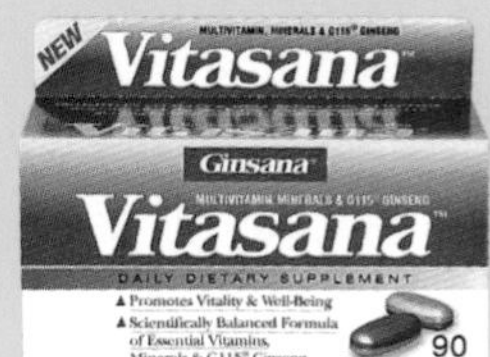

Daily Dietary Supplement

Vitasana™

PROCTER & GAMBLE

Procter & Gamble
P. 750

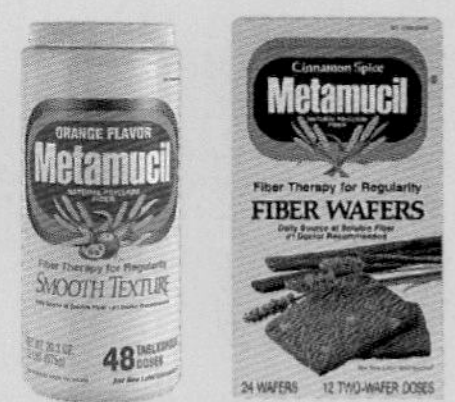

Available in 48, 72 and 114 dose canisters and 30 one-dose packets. Also available in sugar free.

Metamucil®

Procter & Gamble
P. 752

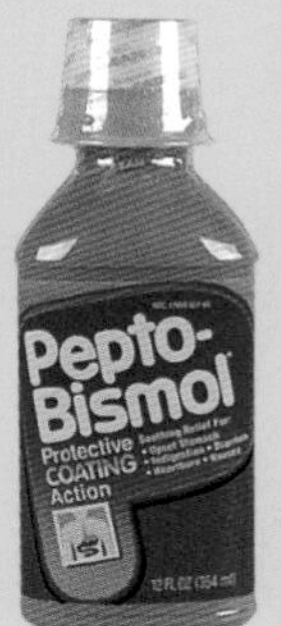

Pepto-Bismol®

ROBERTS

Roberts Pharmaceutical Corp.
P. 764

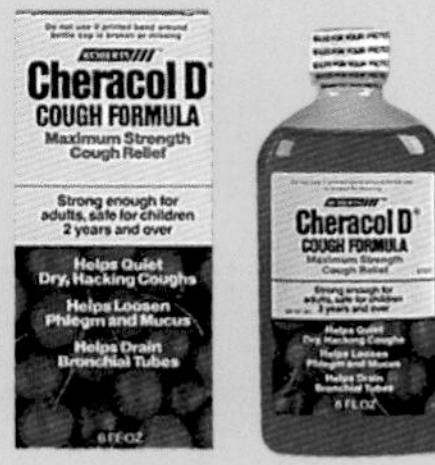

4 oz., 6 oz. Cough Formula
Also available Cheracol Plus Head Cold/Cough Formula 4 oz., 6 oz.

Cheracol D®

Roberts Pharmaceutical Corp.
P. 764

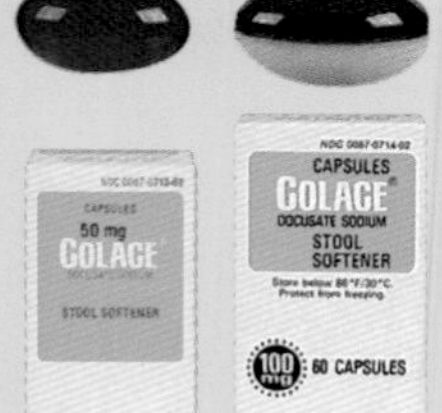

Stool softener – 50mg/100mg
100 mg available:
Two tone color 30, 60, 100, 250, 1000
50 mg available: 30, 60, 100
Available in Liquid and Syrup

Colace®

Roberts Pharmaceutical Corp.
P. 765

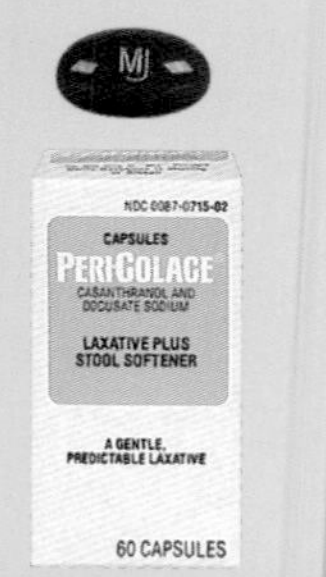

Bottles of 30, 60, 100, 250, 1000
Laxative and Stool Softener
Available in Syrup

Peri-Colace®

SANDOZ CONSUMER DIVISION

IMPORTANT NOTICE:

This product line is now listed under Novartis Consumer Health, Inc.

Please see pages 513 - 516 for product identification.

SCHERING-PLOUGH

Schering-Plough HealthCare Products
P. 771

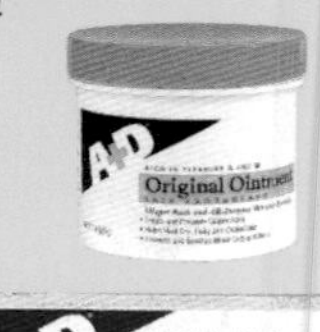

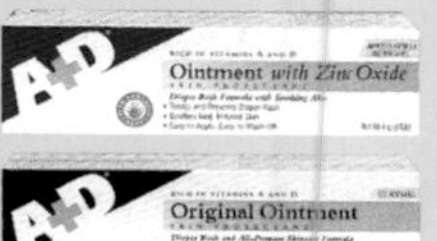

Original and with Zinc Oxide

A and D® Ointment

Schering-Plough HealthCare Products
P. 771

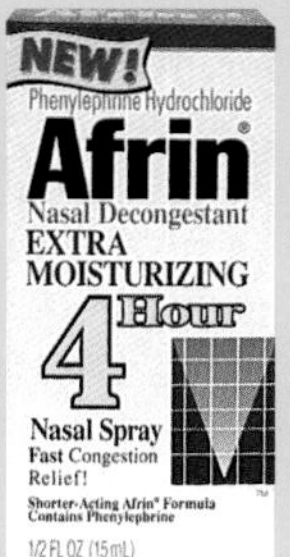

Extra-Moisturizing 4 Hour

Afrin® Extra Moisturizing Nasal Spray

Schering-Plough HealthCare Products
P. 772

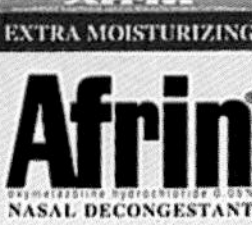

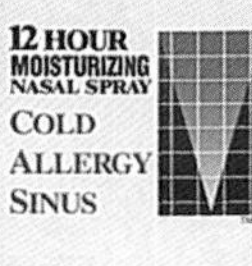

Extra-Moisturizing 12 Hour

Afrin® Extra Moisturizing Nasal Spray

Schering-Plough HealthCare Products
P. 772

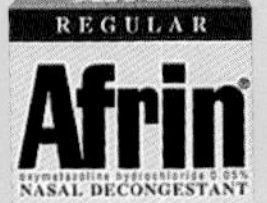

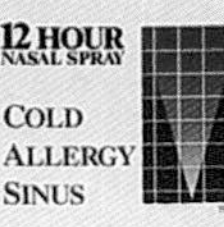

Regular 12 Hour
Safety Sealed

Afrin® Nasal Spray

Schering-Plough HealthCare Products
P. 772

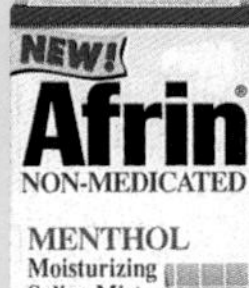

Menthol Moisturizing
Saline Mist

Afrin® Non-Medicated Saline Mist

Schering-Plough HealthCare Products
P. 772

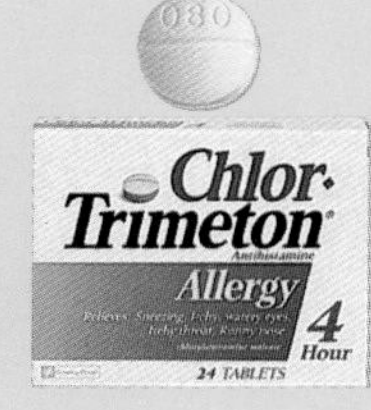

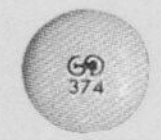

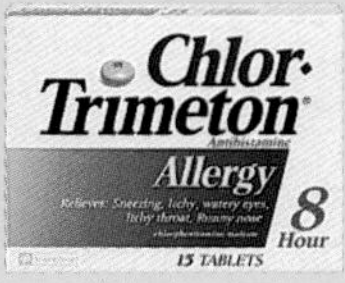

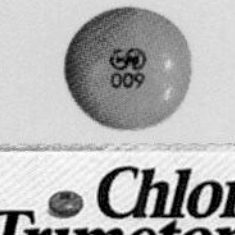

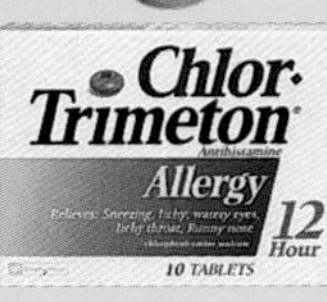

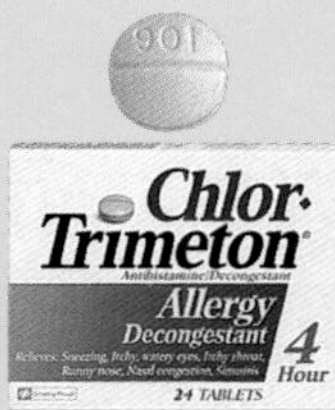

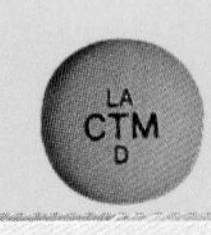

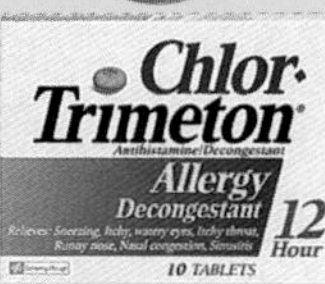

4 Hour Allergy Tablets
8 Hour Allergy Tablets
12 Hour Allergy Tablets
4 Hour Allergy Decongestant Tablets
12 Hour Allergy Decongestant Tablets

Chlor-Trimeton®

Schering-Plough HealthCare Products
P. 774

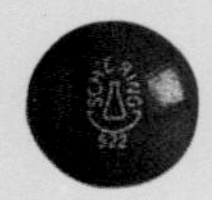

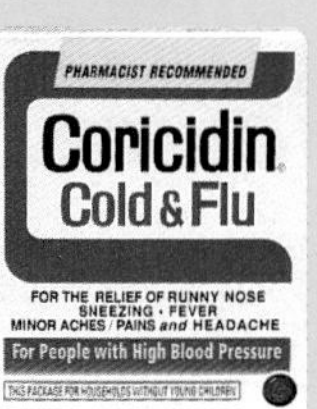

For Relief Of Cold & Flu Symptoms

Coricidin®

Schering-Plough HealthCare Products
P. 774

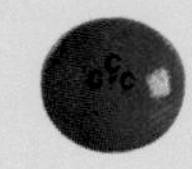

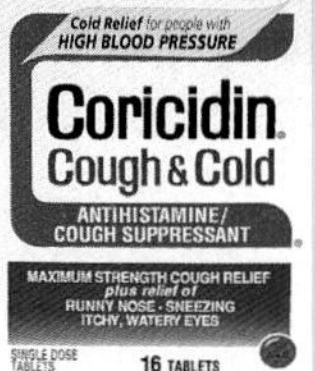

For Relief Of Cold
& Cough Symptoms

Coricidin®

Schering-Plough HealthCare Products
P. 774

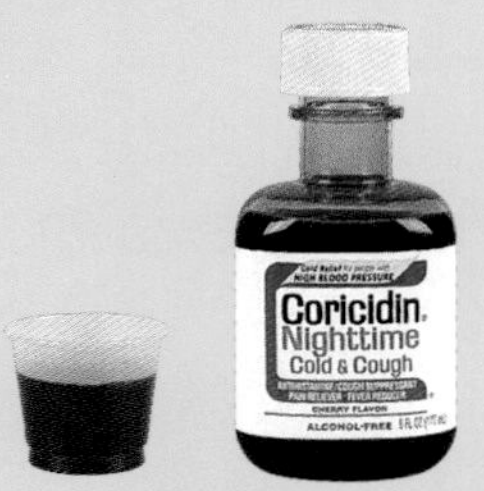

For Relief Of Cold and
Cough Symptoms.

Coricidin®

Schering-Plough HealthCare Products
P. 774

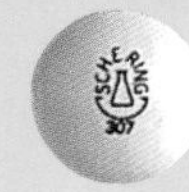

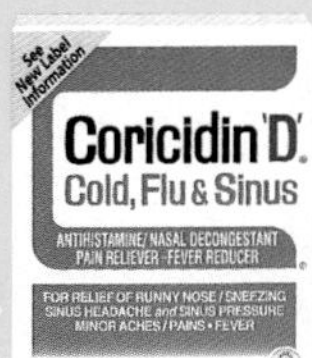

For Relief Of Cold,
Flu & Sinus Symptoms

Coricidin-D®

Schering-Plough HealthCare Products
P. 775

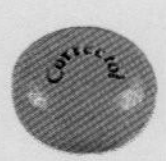

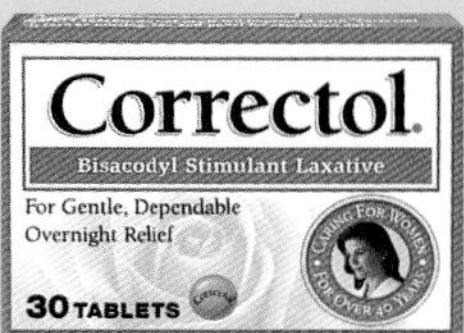

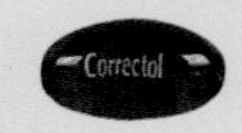

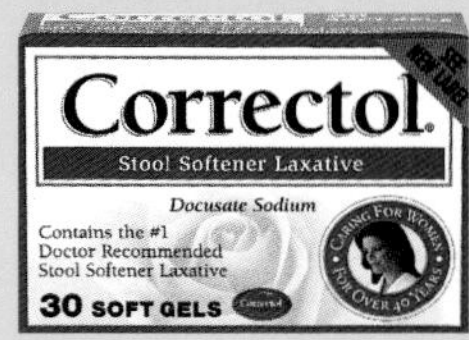

Laxative Tablets and Caplets
and Stool Softener Soft Gels

Correctol®

Schering-Plough HealthCare Products
P. 775

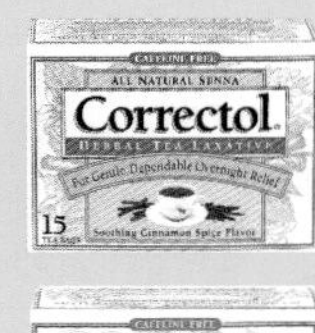

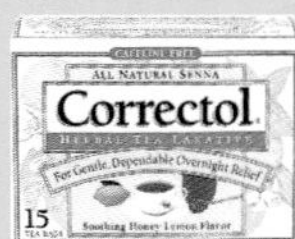

Cinnamon Spice and
Honey Lemon Flavors

Correctol® Herbal Tea Laxative

Schering-Plough HealthCare Products
P. 776

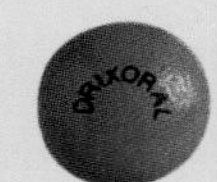

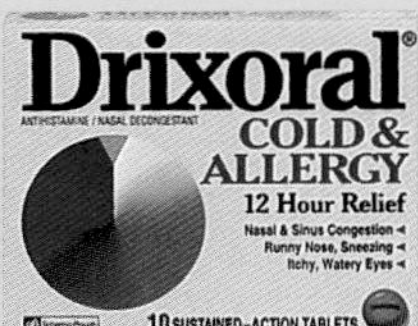

12 Hour Sustained-Action Tablets

Drixoral® Cold & Allergy

Schering-Plough HealthCare Products
P. 778

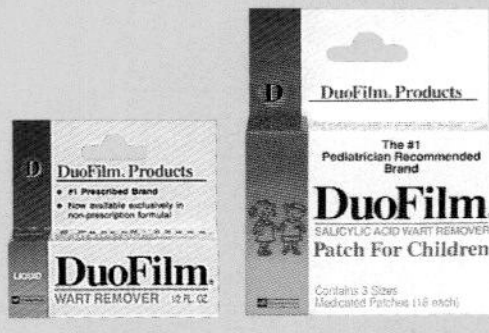

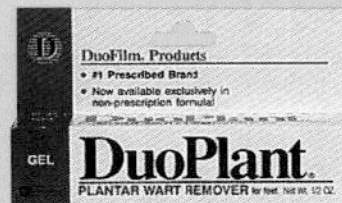

Wart Remover
and Plantar Wart Remover

DuoFilm®/DuoPlant®

Schering-Plough HealthCare Products
P. 779

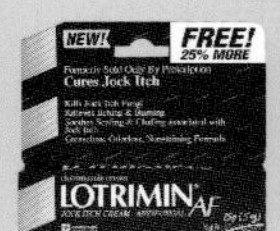

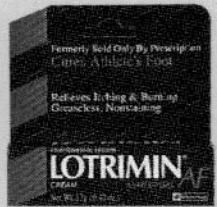

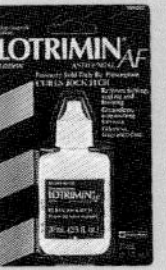

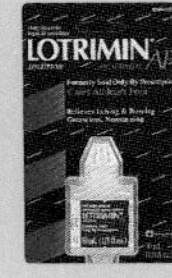

Antifungal for Athlete's Foot
and Jock Itch

Lotrimin® AF

Schering-Plough HealthCare Products
P. 779

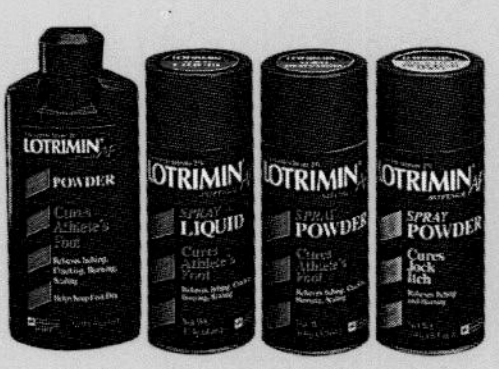

Shaker Powder, Spray Liquid, Spray
Powder and Jock Itch Spray Powder

Lotrimin® AF
(2% miconazole nitrate)

Schering-Plough HealthCare Products
P. 780

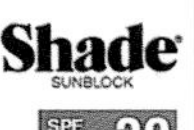

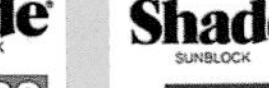

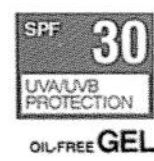

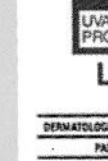

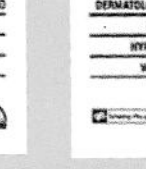

Also available:
SPF 30 Stick

Shade® Sunblock

Schering-Plough HealthCare Products
P. 781

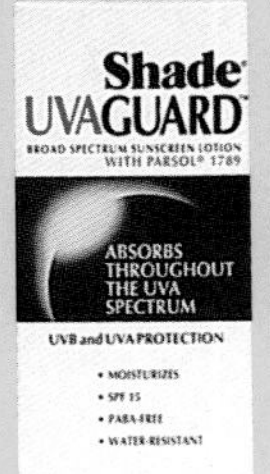

Broad Spectrum Sunscreen Lotion with
Parsol® 1789

Shade® UVAGUARD™

SMITHKLINE BEECHAM

SmithKline Beecham
Consumer Healthcare, L.P.
P. 783

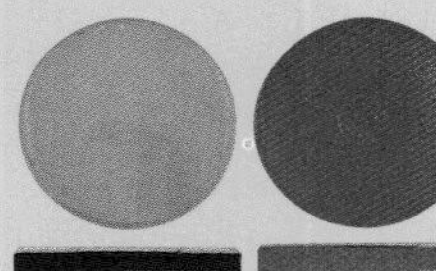
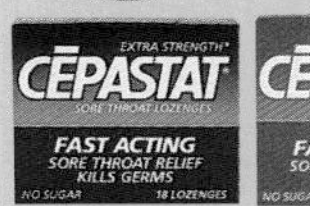

Sore Throat Lozenges
Extra Strength and Cherry
18 lozenges per package

Cepastat®

SmithKline Beecham
Consumer Healthcare, L.P.
P. 783

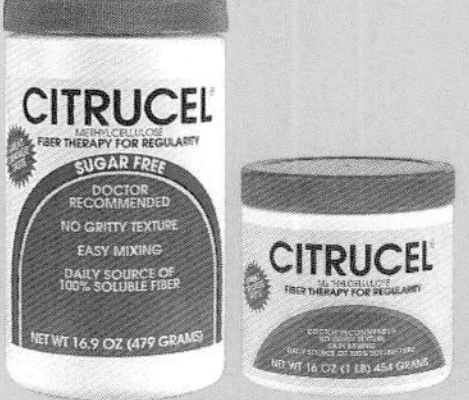

Fiber Therapy for Regularity
Sugar Free Orange available in:
8.6 oz. and 16.9 oz.
Regular Orange available in:
16 oz. and 30 oz. containers

Citrucel®

SmithKline Beecham
Consumer Healthcare, L.P.
P. 785

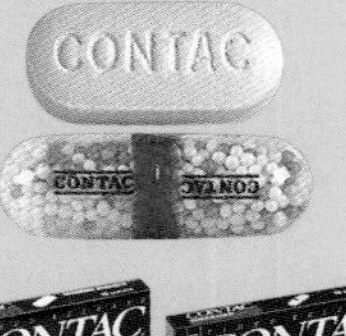

Continuous Action
Nasal Decongestant Antihistamine
Packages of 10 and 20
capsules and caplets

Contac® 12 Hour

SmithKline Beecham
Consumer Healthcare, L.P.

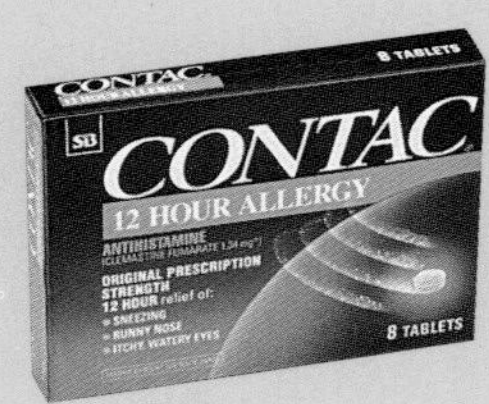

Contac® 12 Hour Allergy

SmithKline Beecham
Consumer Healthcare, L.P.
P. 784

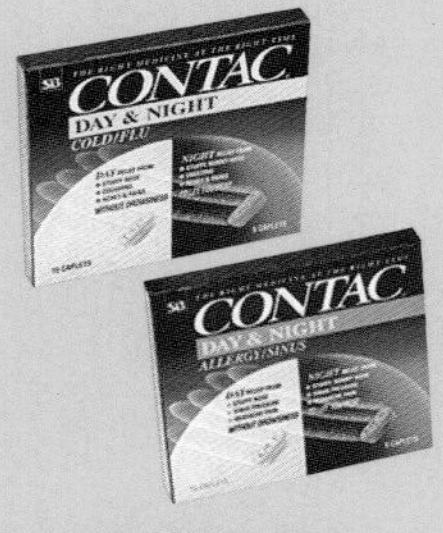

**Contac® Day & Night
Cold & Flu and
Allergy/Sinus**

SmithKline Beecham
Consumer Healthcare, L.P.
P. 786

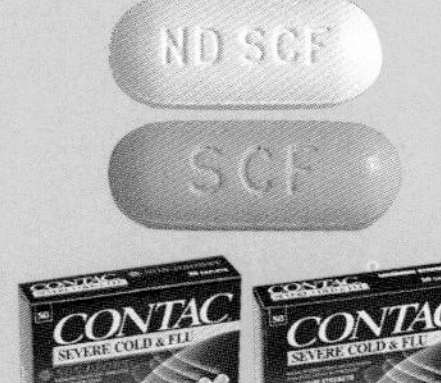

Non-Drowsy Formula
Packages of 16 caplets

**Contac® Severe
Cold & Flu**

SmithKline Beecham
Consumer Healthcare, L.P.
P. 787

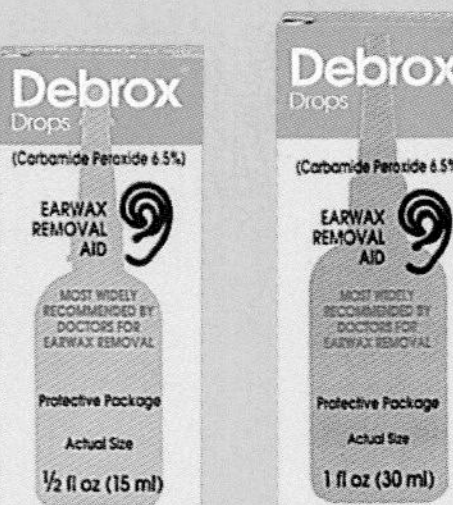

Drops
1/2 Fl. oz. 1 Fl. oz.

Debrox®

SmithKline Beecham
Consumer Healthcare, L.P.
P. 787

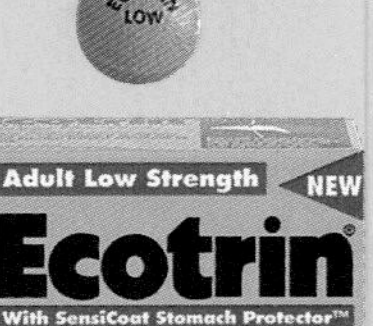

Adult Low Strength Tablets in Bottles
of 36

Ecotrin®

SmithKline Beecham
Consumer Healthcare, L.P.
P. 787

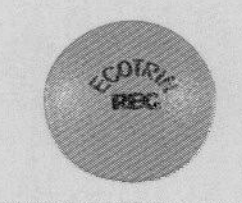
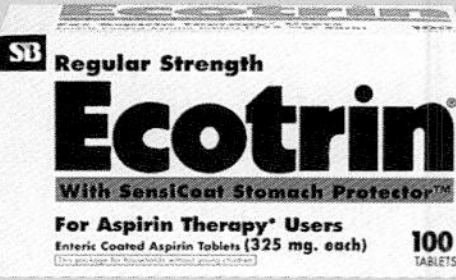

Regular Strength Tablets
in bottles of 100, 250

Ecotrin®

SmithKline Beecham
Consumer Healthcare, L.P.
P. 787

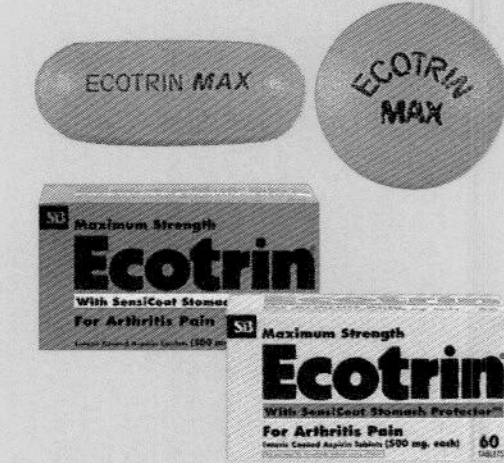

Maximum Strength Tablets
in bottles of 60, 150 and
Caplets in bottles of 60

Ecotrin®

SmithKline Beecham
Consumer Healthcare, L.P.
P. 790

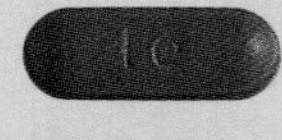
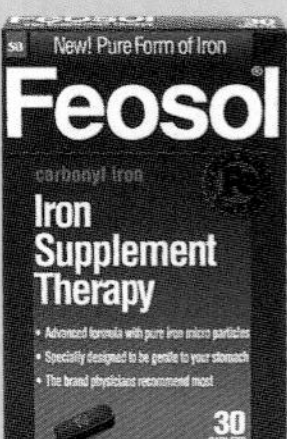

Packages of 30 caplets

Feosol®

SmithKline Beecham Consumer Healthcare, L.P.
P. 791

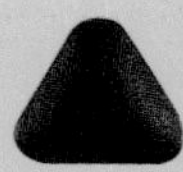

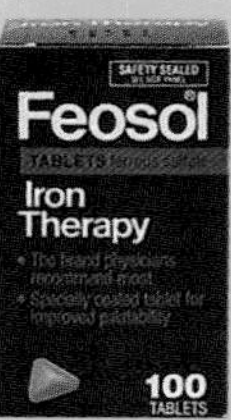

Bottles of 100 tablets

Feosol®

SmithKline Beecham Consumer Healthcare, L.P.
P. 791

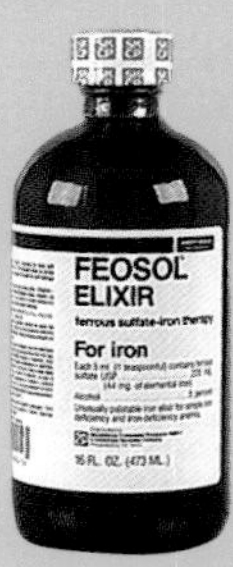

16 oz. bottle

Feosol® Elixir

SmithKline Beecham Consumer Healthcare, L.P.
P. 791

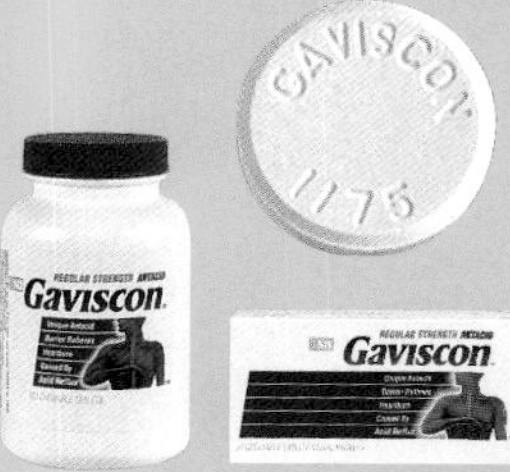

100-Tablet bottles
30-Tablet box (foil-wrapped 2s)

Gaviscon® Antacid

SmithKline Beecham Consumer Healthcare, L.P.
P. 792

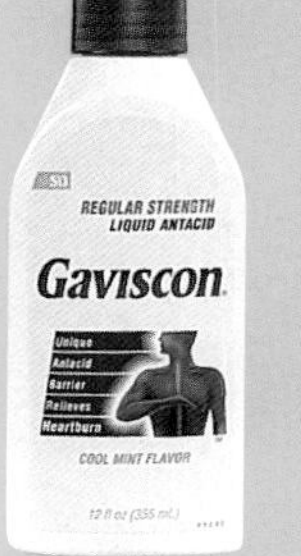

12 Fl. oz.

Gaviscon® Liquid Antacid

SmithKline Beecham Consumer Healthcare, L.P.
P. 792

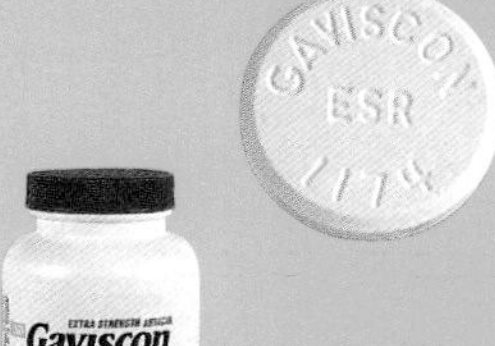

Extra Strength Relief Formula
100-Tablet bottles

Gaviscon® Extra Strength Antacid

SmithKline Beecham Consumer Healthcare, L.P.
P. 792

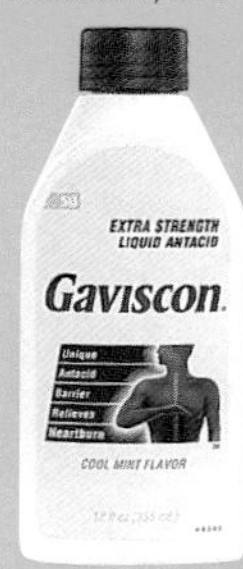

Extra Strength Relief Formula

Gaviscon® Extra Strength Liquid Antacid

SmithKline Beecham Consumer Healthcare, L.P.
P. 793

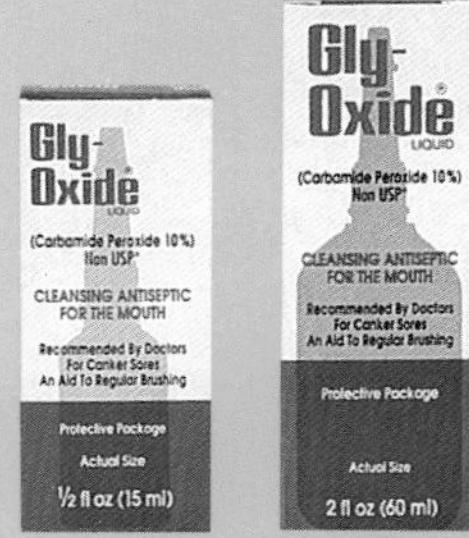

1/2 Fl. oz. 2 Fl. oz.

Gly-Oxide® Liquid

SmithKline Beecham Consumer Healthcare, L.P.
P. 794

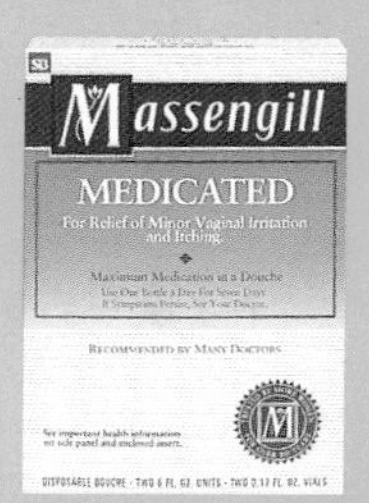

Medicated Disposable Douche
With Povidone-iodine

Available in single or twin packs

Massengill®

SmithKline Beecham Consumer Healthcare, L.P.
P. 795

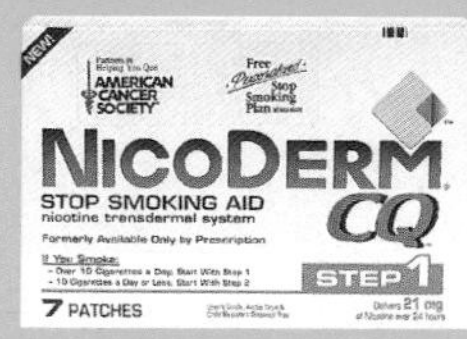

Step 1
Also available in 2 week kit

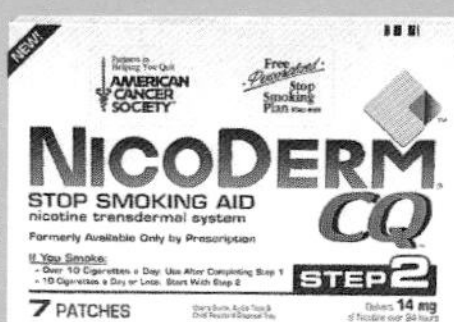

Step 2

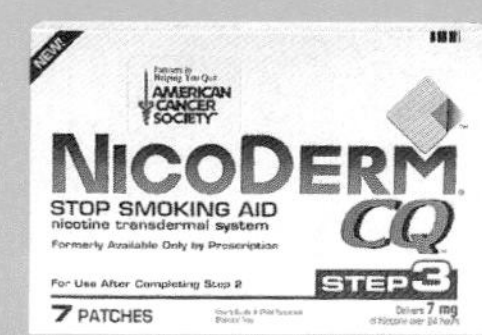

Step 3

Includes User's Guide, Audio Tape and Child Resistant Disposal Tray

Stop Smoking Aid

Nicotine Transdermal System

Nicoderm® CQ™

SmithKline Beecham Consumer Healthcare, L.P.
P. 799

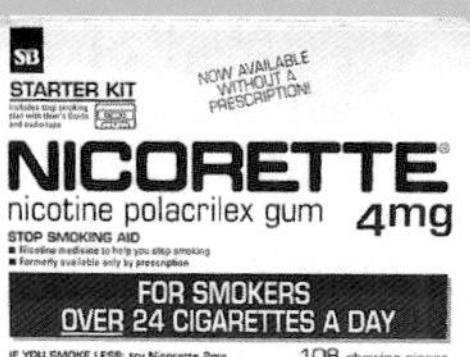

4 mg
For Smokers over 24 Cigarettes a day

Refill pack available

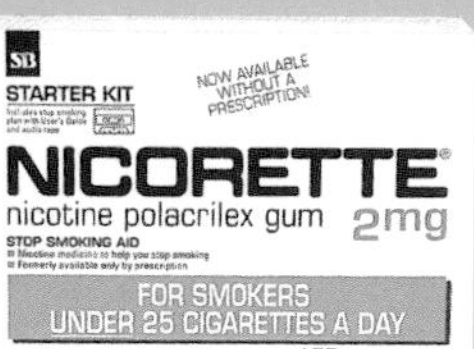

2 mg
For Smokers under 25 Cigarettes a day
Refill pack available

Stop Smoking Aid

Nicotine Polacrilex Gum

Nicorette®

SmithKline Beecham Consumer Healthcare, L.P.
P. 803

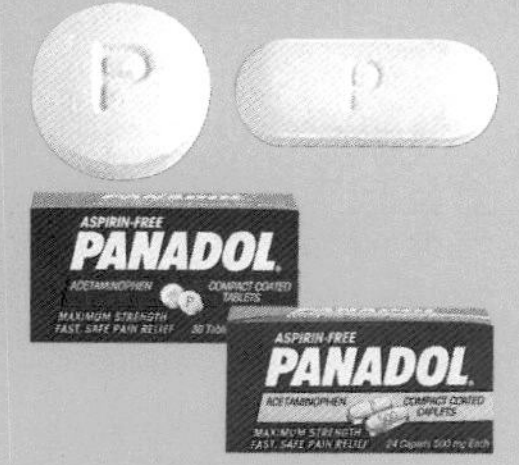

Asprin-Free Tablets and Caplets

Panadol®

SmithKline Beecham Consumer Healthcare, L.P.
P. 803

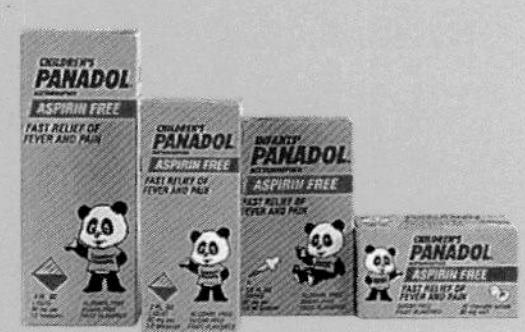

Chewable Tablets, Caplets, Liquid and Drops

Children's Panadol®

SmithKline Beecham Consumer Healthcare, L.P.
P. 804

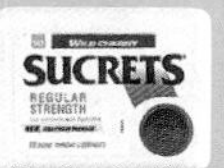

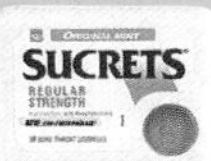

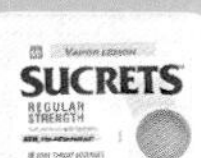

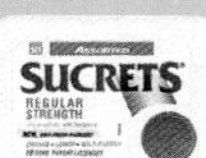

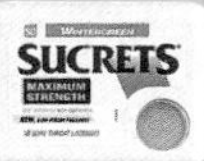

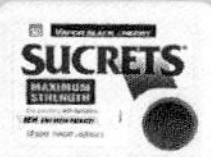

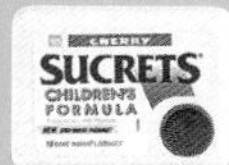

Sore Throat Lozenges
Available in: Regular Strength (Wild Cherry, Original Mint, Vapor Lemon and Assorted)
Maximum Strength (Wintergreen, Vapor Black Cherry) and Childrens Cherry

Sucrets®

SmithKline Beecham Consumer Healthcare, L.P.
P. 805

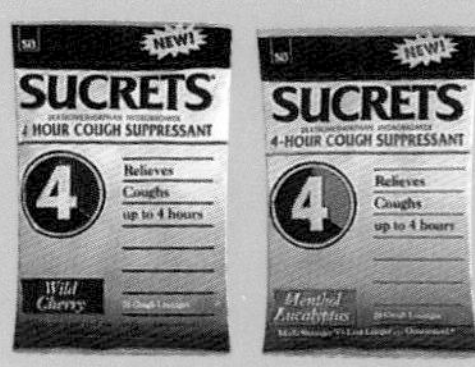

Available in Wild Cherry and Menthol-Eucalyptus

Sucrets® 4-Hour Cough Suppressant

SmithKline Beecham Consumer Healthcare, L.P.
P. 805

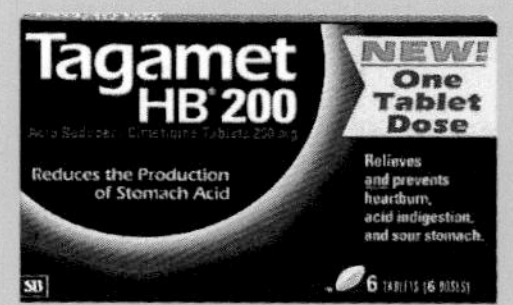

Acid Reducer
Packages of 16, 32, 48 and 64

Tagamet HB® 200

SmithKline Beecham Consumer Healthcare, L.P.
P. 806

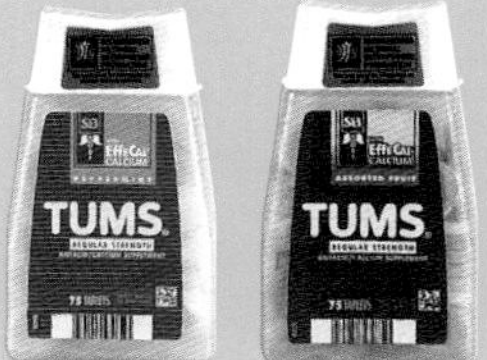

Peppermint and Assorted Flavors

Tums®

SmithKline Beecham Consumer Healthcare, L.P.
P. 806

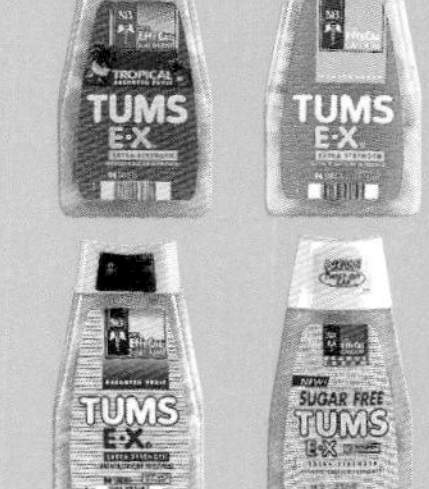

Tropical Fruit, Wintergreen, Assorted Flavors and SugarFree Orange Cream

Tums E-X®

SmithKline Beecham Consumer Healthcare, L.P.
P. 806

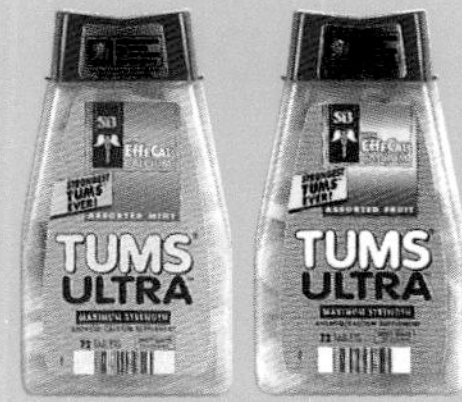

Assorted Mint and Fruit Flavors

Tums® Ultra™

THOMPSON

Thompson Medical Co., Inc.
P. 810

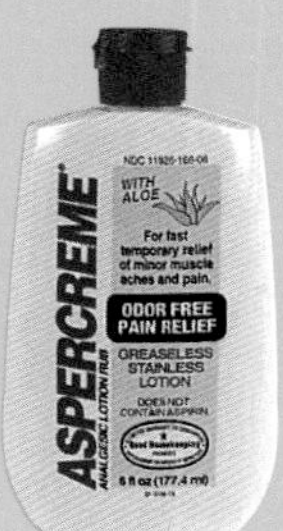

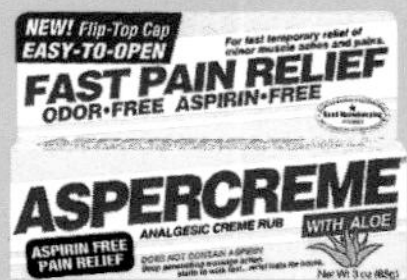

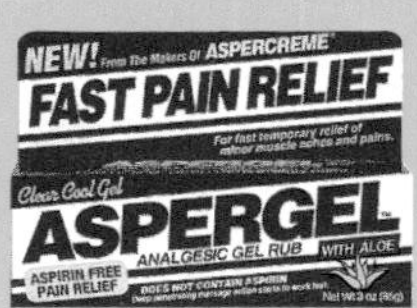

Available in 1 1/4 oz., 3 oz. and 5 oz. Creme, 6 oz. Lotion, and 3 oz. Gel

Aspercreme® with Aloe

Thompson Medical Co., Inc.
P. 810

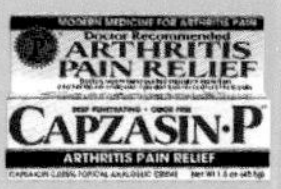

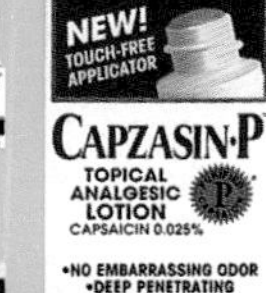

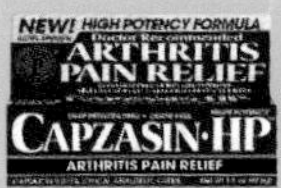

Capzasin•P available in 1.5 oz. Creme and 2 oz. Lotion, Capzasin•HP available in 1.5 oz. Creme.

Capzasin•P™

Thompson Medical Co., Inc.
P. 811

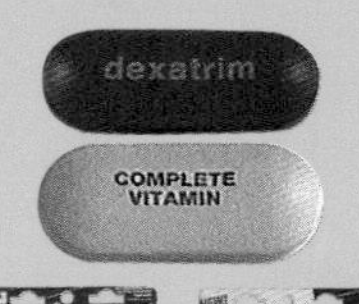

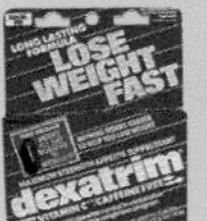

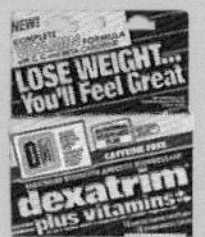

Available in 20 and 40 count package. Dexatrim Plus Vitamins available in 14 count

Maximum Strength Dexatrim®

Thompson Medical Co., Inc.
P. 812

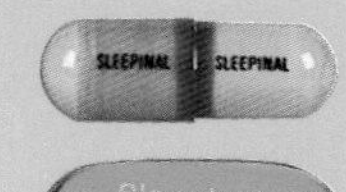

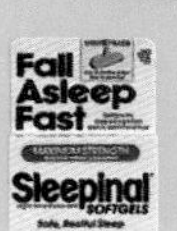

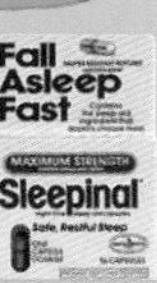

Available in 16 and 32 Capsule sizes and 8 & 16 Softgel sizes

Sleepinal®

UNIPATH

Unipath Diagnostics Company
P. 814

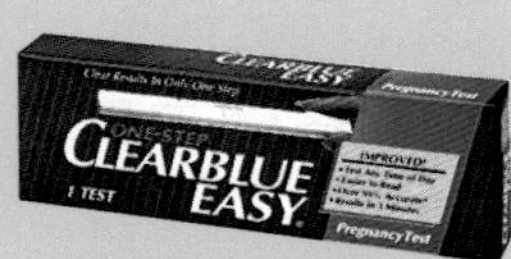

One-Step Pregnancy Test

CLEARBLUE EASY®

Unipath Diagnostics Company
P. 815

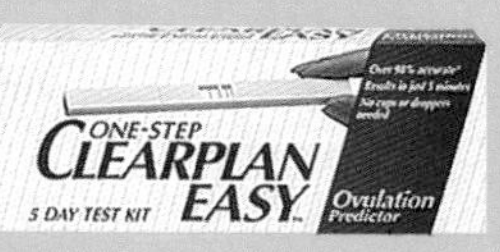

One-Step Ovulation Predictor

CLEARPLAN EASY™

WAKUNAGA

Wakunaga
P. 669

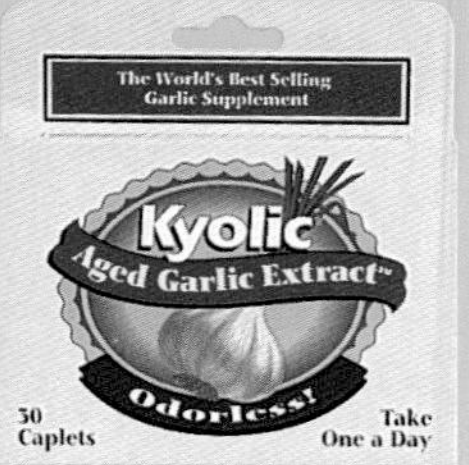

Aged Garlic Extract™

Kyolic®

Wakunaga
P. 669

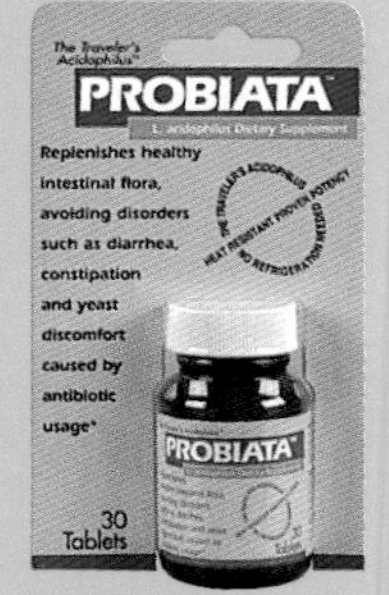

L. acidophilus

PROBIATA™

WALLACE

Wallace Laboratories
P. 816

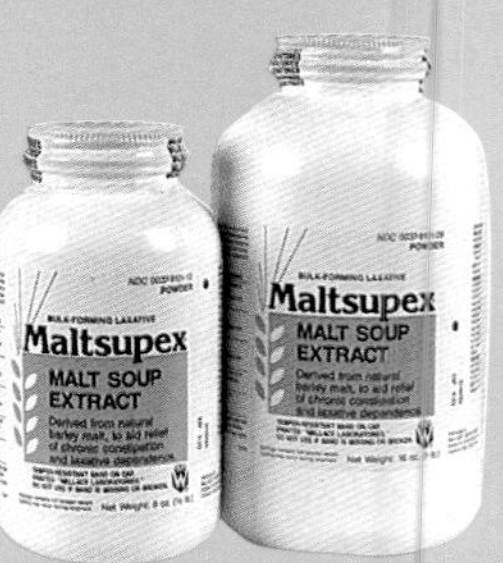

8 fl. oz. (1/2 pt) and 16 fl. oz. (1 pt)

Maltsupex® Liquid
(malt soup extract)

Wallace Laboratories
P. 816

8 oz. (1/2 lb) and 16 oz. (1 lb)

Maltsupex® Powder
(malt soup extract)

Wallace Laboratories
P. 816

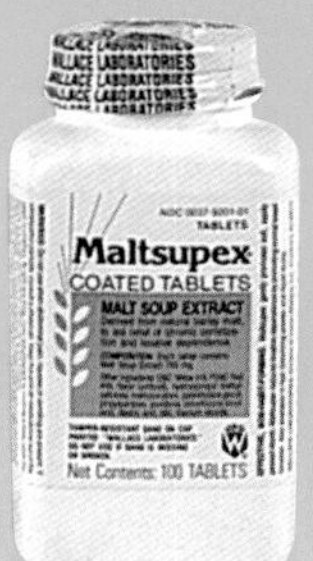

100 Tablets

Maltsupex® Tablets
(malt soup extract)

Wallace Laboratories
P. 817

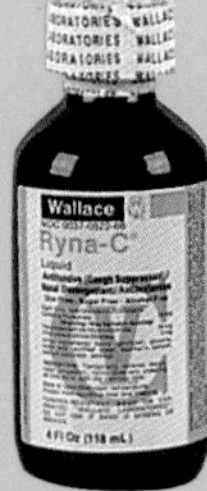

1 Pint (473 mL)
Also available: 4 fl. oz. (118 mL)

Ryna-C® Liquid
(antitussive/antihistamine/ decongestant)

Wallace Laboratories
P. 817

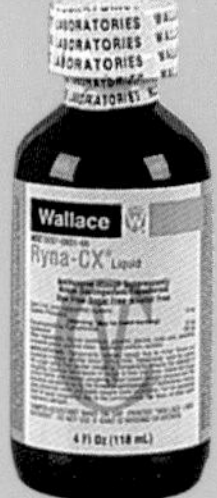

1 Pint (473 mL)
Also available: 4 fl. oz. (118 mL)

Ryna-CX® Liquid
(antitussive/decongestant/ expectorant)

WARNER-LAMBERT

Warner-Lambert Co.
P. 818

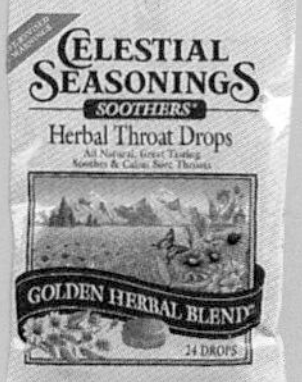

Herbal Throat Drops
New Flavor: Golden Herbal Blend
Also available in Honey-Lemon Chamomile, Harvest Cherry and Herbal Orange Spice

Celestial Seasonings® Soothers™

Warner-Lambert Co.
P. 818

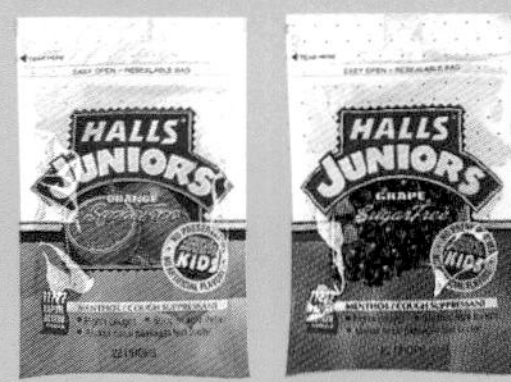

Sugar Free
Cough Suppressant Drops
Orange and Grape

Halls® Juniors Sugar Free

Warner-Lambert Co.
P. 818

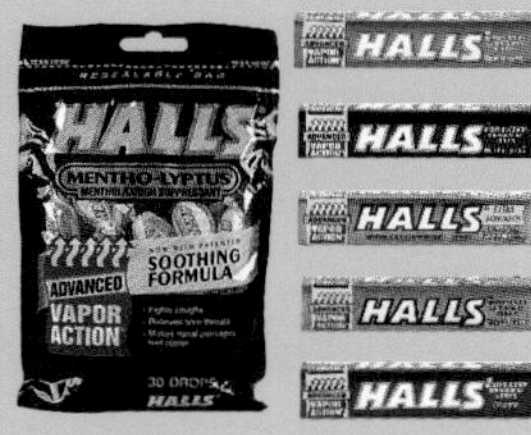

Cough Suppressant Drops
Spearmint, Mentho-Lyptus, Ice Blue, Honey-Lemon and Cherry Flavors

Halls® Mentho-Lyptus®

Warner-Lambert Co.
P. 819

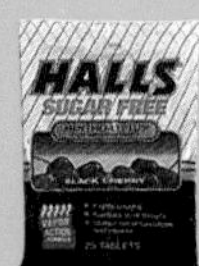

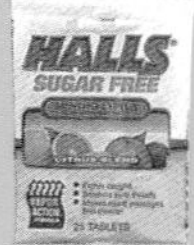

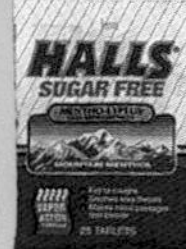

Black Cherry, Citrus Blend and Mountain Menthol

Halls® Sugar Free Mentho-Lyptus®

Warner-Lambert Co.
P. 819

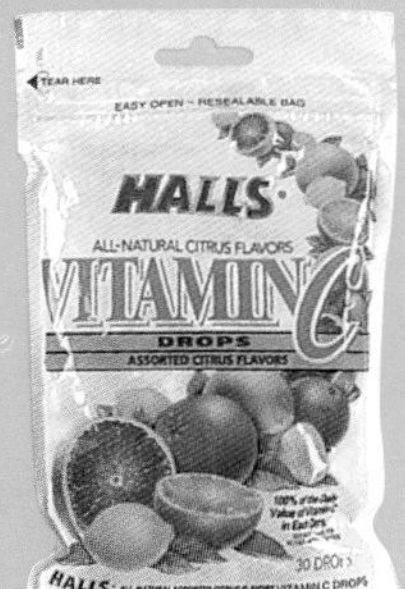

Assorted Citrus

Halls® Vitamin C Drops

Warner-Lambert Co.
P. 819

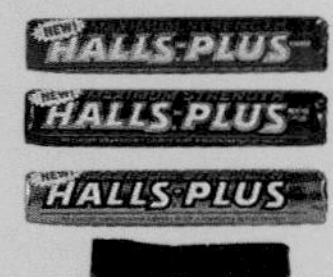

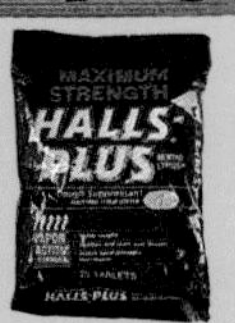

Cough Suppressant Drops with Soothing Syrup Centers
Honey-Lemon, Mentho-Lyptus and Cherry

Maximum Strength Halls® Plus

Warner-Lambert Co.
P. 819

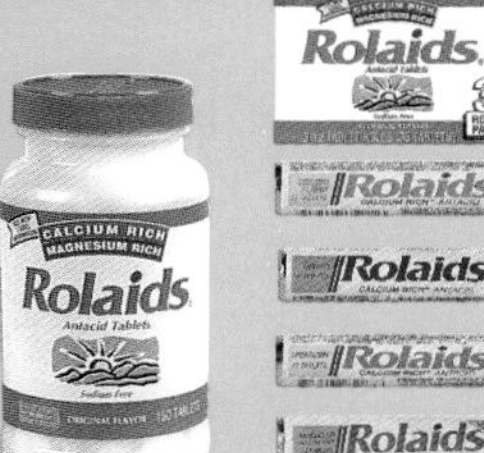

Fast, Effective Relief from Heartburn, Acid Indigestion or Sour Stomach

Original Peppermint, Spearmint, Cherry and Assorted Fruit Flavors

Rolaids®

WARNER-LAMBERT

Warner-Lambert Consumer Healthcare
P. 820

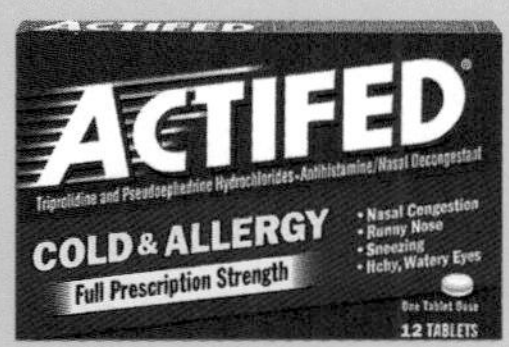

Available in 12, 24, 48 tablets and bottles of 100

Actifed® Cold & Allergy

Warner-Lambert Consumer Healthcare
P. 820

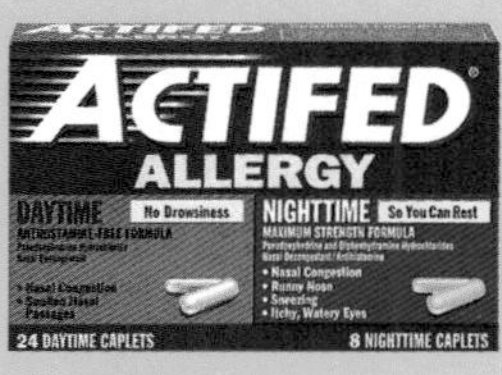

Available in 24 Daytime Caplets and 8 Nighttime Caplets

Actifed® Allergy Daytime/Nighttime

Warner-Lambert Consumer Healthcare
P. 821

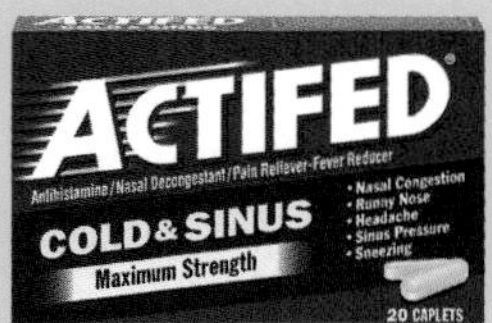

Available in 20 Tablets and Caplets

Actifed® Cold & Sinus

Warner-Lambert Consumer Healthcare
P. 821

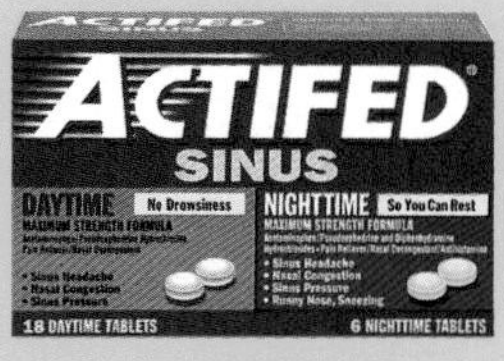

Available in 18 Daytime and 6 Nighttime Tablets or Caplets

Actifed® Sinus Daytime/Nighttime

Warner-Lambert Consumer Healthcare
P. 822

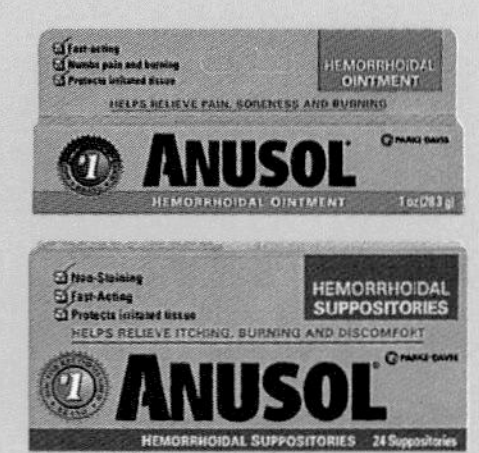

Suppositories available in boxes of 12 and 24

Ointment available in 1 oz. tubes

Anusol®

Warner-Lambert Consumer Healthcare
P. 823

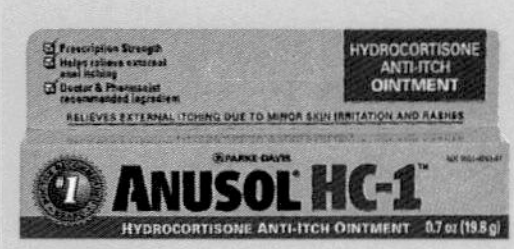

Anti-Itch Hydrocortisone Ointment
Available in 0.7 oz. tube

Anusol HC-1™

Warner-Lambert Consumer Healthcare
P. 823

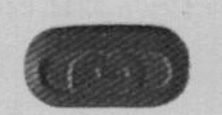
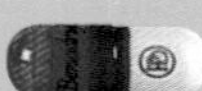
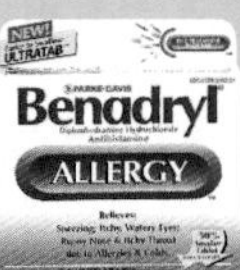

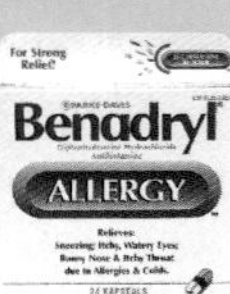

Capsules and Tablets
Available in boxes of 24 and 48
Tablets also available in
bottles of 100

Benadryl® Allergy

Warner-Lambert Consumer Healthcare
P. 825

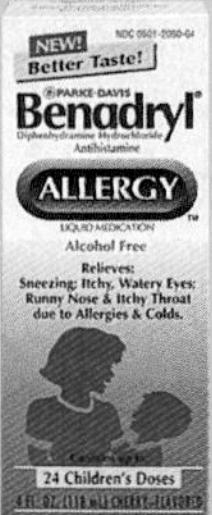

Available in 4 oz. and 8 oz. bottles

Benadryl® Allergy Liquid Medication

Warner-Lambert Consumer Healthcare
P. 824

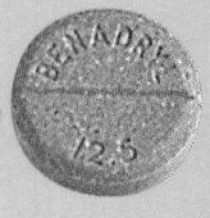

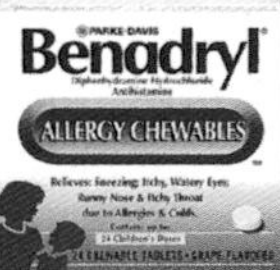

Available in boxes of 24
chewable Tablets

Benadryl® Allergy Chewables

Warner-Lambert Consumer Healthcare
P. 823

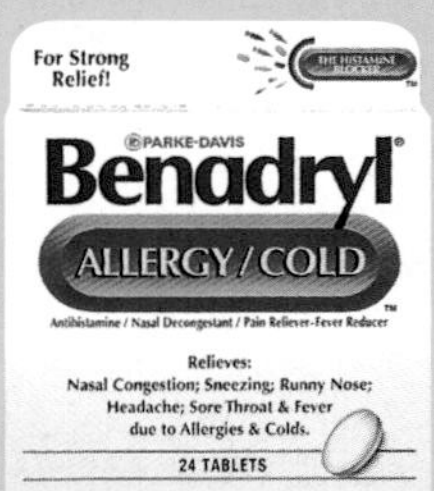

Available in boxes of 24 Tablets

Benadryl® Allergy/Cold

Warner-Lambert Consumer Healthcare
P. 824

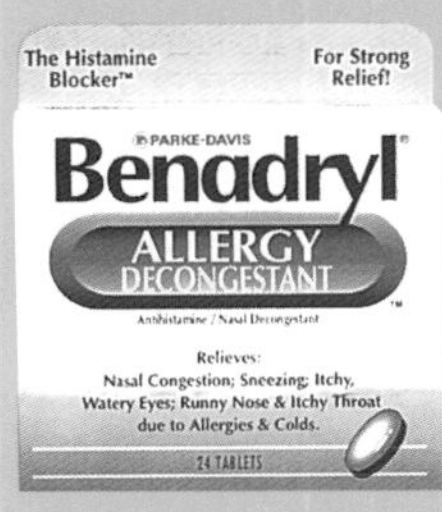

Available in boxes of 24 Tablets

Benadryl® Allergy Decongestant

Warner-Lambert Consumer Healthcare
P. 824

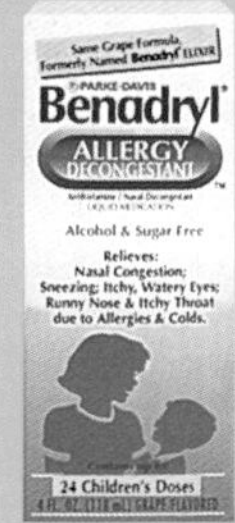

Available in 4 oz. bottles

Benadryl® Allergy Decongestant Liquid Medication

Warner-Lambert Consumer Healthcare
P. 826

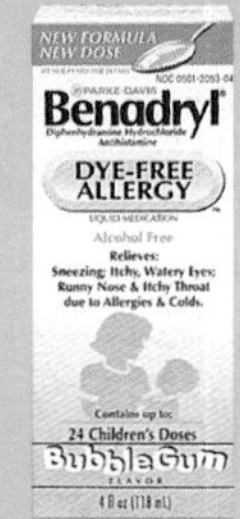

Available in 4 fl. oz. bottles

Benadryl® Dye-Free Allergy Liquid Medication

Warner-Lambert Consumer Healthcare
P. 826

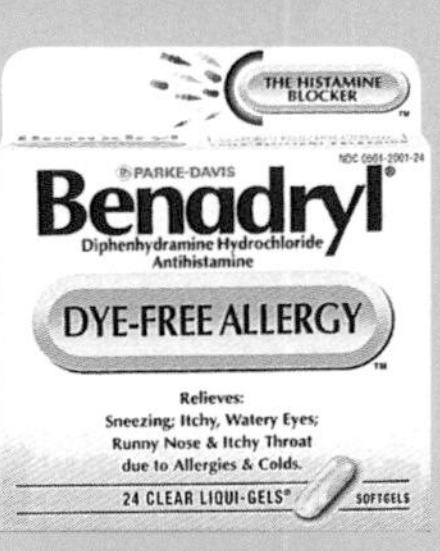

Available in Boxes of 24

Benadryl® Dye-Free Allergy Liqui-Gels® Softgels

Warner-Lambert Consumer Healthcare
P. 825

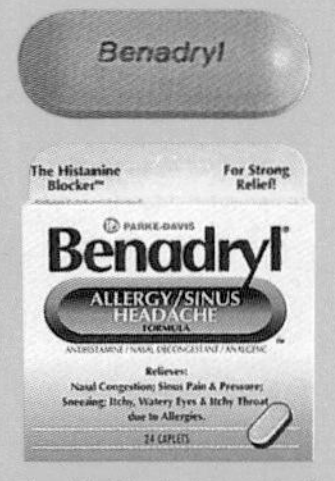

Available in boxes of
24 and 48 Caplets

Benadryl® Allergy Sinus Headache

Warner-Lambert Consumer Healthcare
P. 827

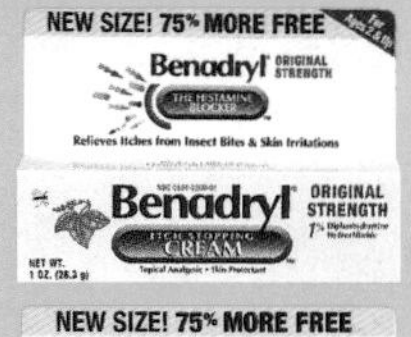

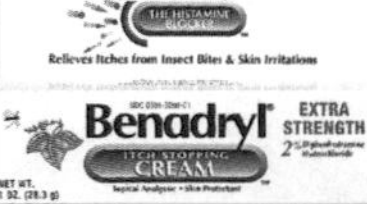

Original and Extra Strength

Benadryl® Itch Stopping Cream

Warner-Lambert Consumer Healthcare
P. 827

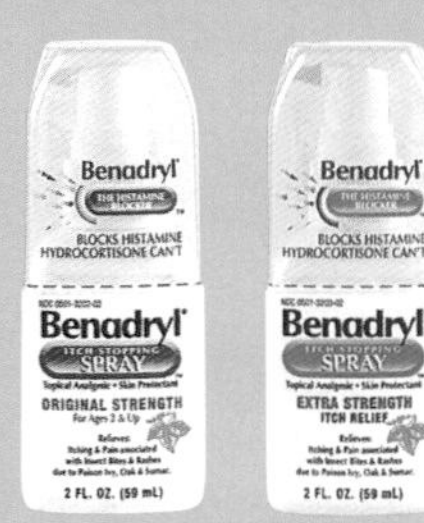

Original and Extra Strength

Benadryl® Itch Stopping Spray

Warner-Lambert Consumer Healthcare
P. 827

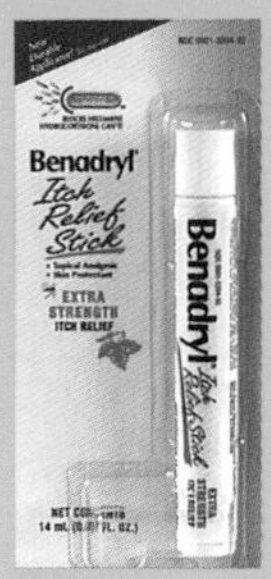

Extra Strength

Benadryl® Itch Relief Stick

Warner-Lambert Consumer Healthcare
P. 828

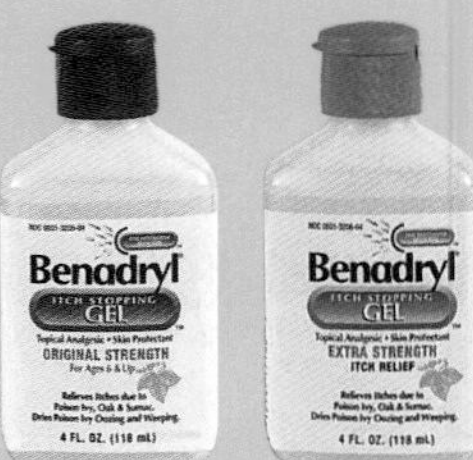

Original and Extra Strength

Benadryl® Itch Stopping Gel

Warner-Lambert Consumer Healthcare
P. 828

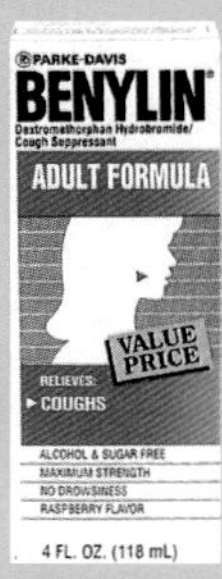

Available in 4 oz. bottles

Benylin® Adult Cough Suppressant

Warner-Lambert Consumer Healthcare
P. 828

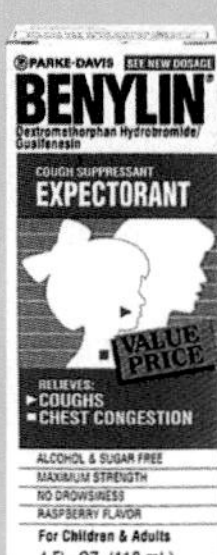

Available in 4 oz. bottles

Benylin® Cough Suppressant Expectorant

Warner-Lambert Consumer Healthcare
P. 829

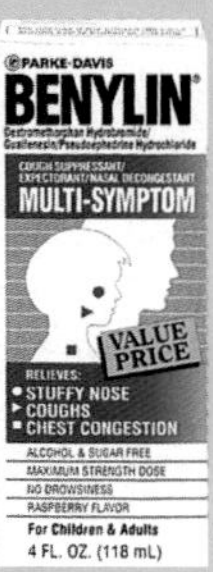

Available in 4 oz. bottles

Benylin® Multi-Symptom

Warner-Lambert Consumer Healthcare
P. 829

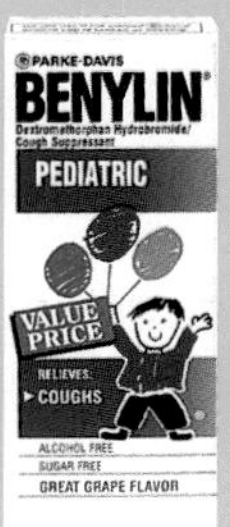

Available in 4 oz. bottles

Benylin® Pediatric Cough Suppressant

Warner-Lambert Consumer Healthcare
P. 831

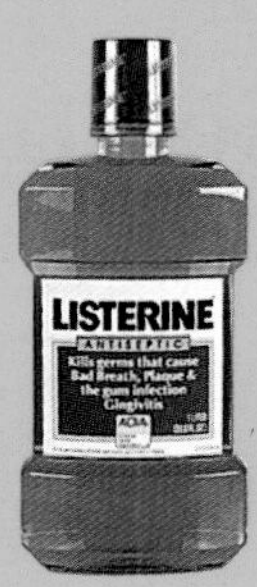

Listerine® Antiseptic

Warner-Lambert Consumer Healthcare
P. 832

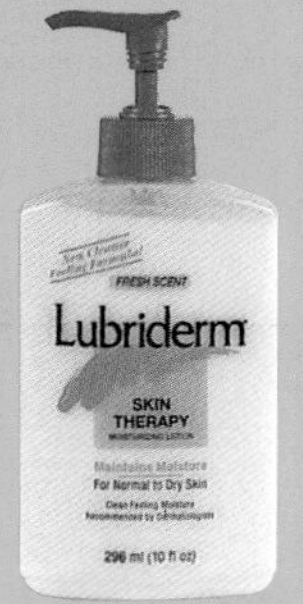

Available in Scented and Fragrance Free

Lubriderm® Lotion

Warner-Lambert Consumer Healthcare
P. 832

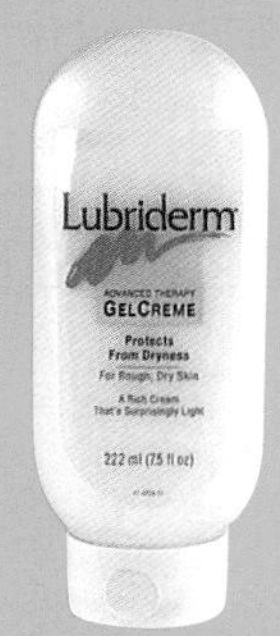

Lubriderm® GelCreme

Warner-Lambert Consumer Healthcare
P. 830

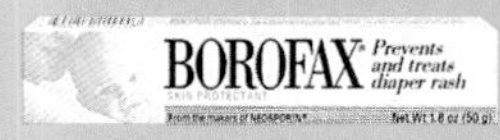

Skin Protectant Ointment
Available in 1.8 oz (50g) tube

Borofax®

Warner-Lambert Consumer Healthcare
P. 831

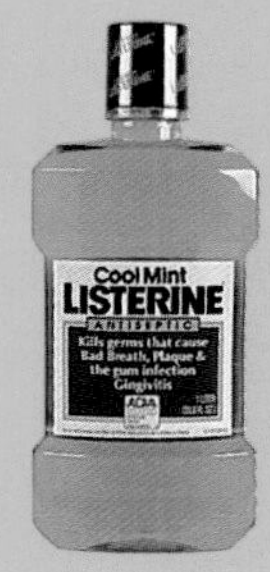

Cool Mint Listerine® Antiseptic

Warner-Lambert Consumer Healthcare
P. 832

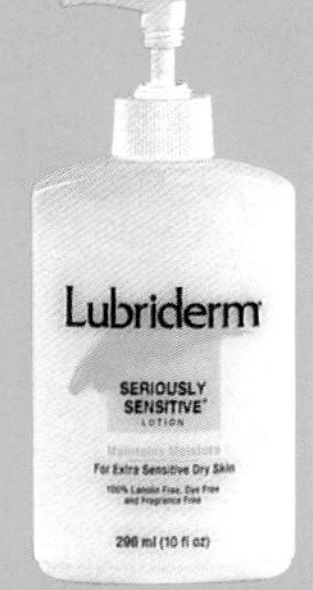

Lubriderm® Seriously Sensitive® Lotion

Warner-Lambert Consumer Healthcare
P. 833

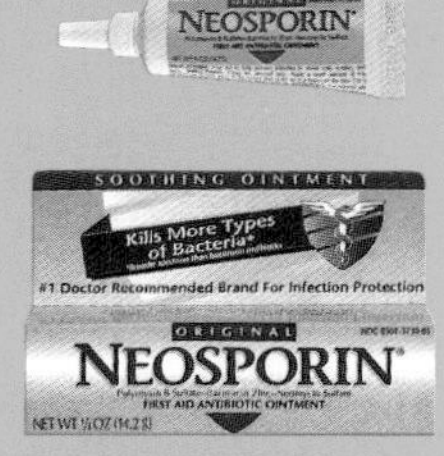

First Aid Antibiotic Ointment
Available in 1/2 oz. (14.2g) or 1 oz. (28.3g) tubes; 1/31 oz. (0.9 g)

Neosporin®

Warner-Lambert Consumer Healthcare
P. 830

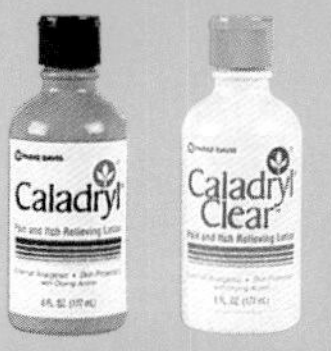

Itch Relief Plus Drying Action. Available in Lotion, Clear Lotion and Cream for Kids

Caladryl®

Warner-Lambert Consumer Healthcare
P. 831

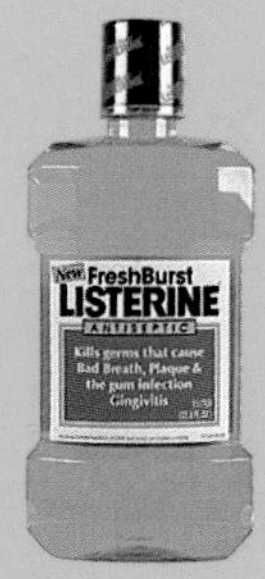

FreshBurst Listerine®

Warner-Lambert Consumer Healthcare
P. 832

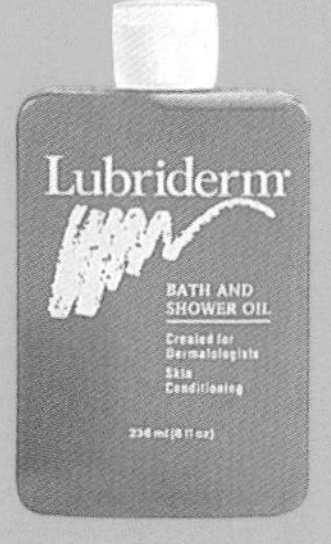

Lubriderm® Bath & Shower Oil

Warner-Lambert Consumer Healthcare
P. 833

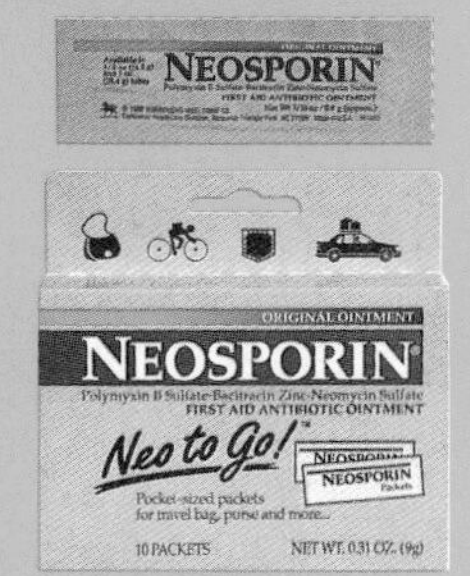

First Aid Antibiotic Ointment.
Available in Individual Foil Packets. 0.31 oz. (9g)

Neosporin® Neo to Go!™

Warner-Lambert Consumer Healthcare
P. 830

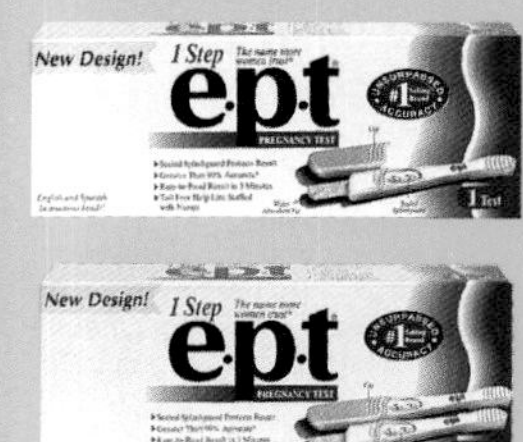

1 and 2 Pregnancy Test Kits Available
One Step. Easy to read.
Lab Accurate results.

e.p.t®

Warner-Lambert Consumer Healthcare
P. 832

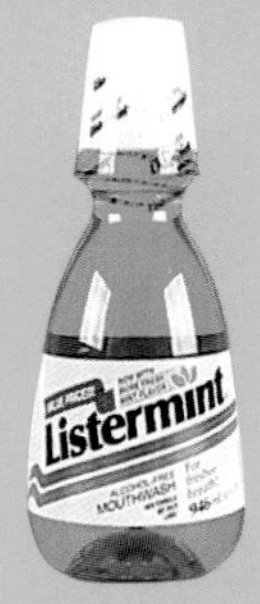

Listermint® Alcohol-Free Mouthwash

Warner-Lambert Consumer Healthcare
P. 832

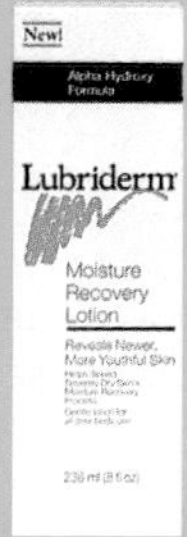

Lubriderm® Moisture Recovery Alpha Hydroxy Lotion

Warner-Lambert Consumer Healthcare
P. 833

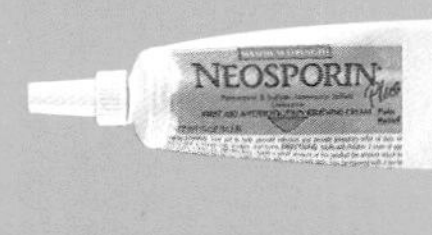

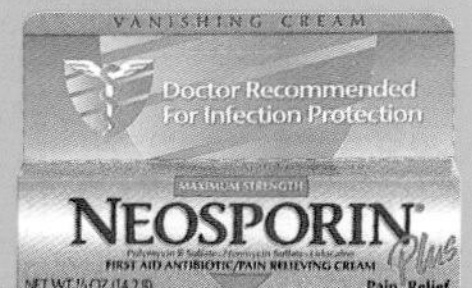

Maximum Strength Cream
Available in 1/2 oz. (14.2g) tubes

Neosporin® Plus

Warner-Lambert Consumer Healthcare
P. 833

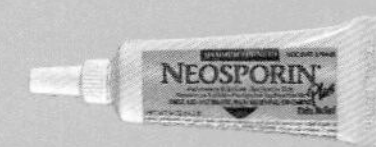

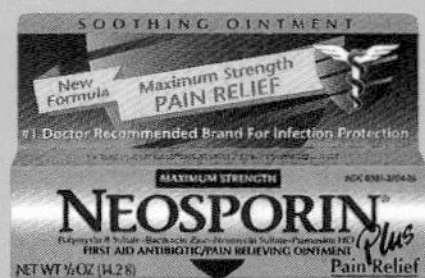

Maximum Strength Ointment
Available in 1/2 oz. (14.2g)
and 1 oz. (28.3g) tubes

Neosporin® Plus

Warner-Lambert Consumer Healthcare
P. 833

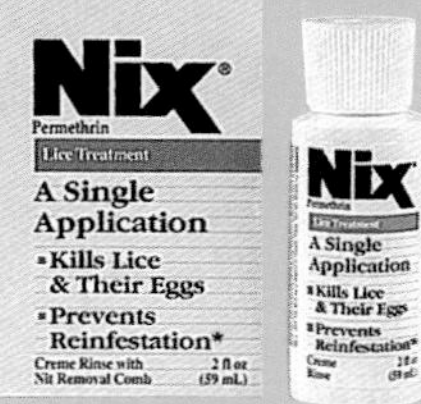

* for 14 Days

Lice Treatment Creme Rinse
2 fl. oz. (59 mL)
Also available in:
2-bottle family pack

Nix®

Warner-Lambert Consumer Healthcare
P. 834

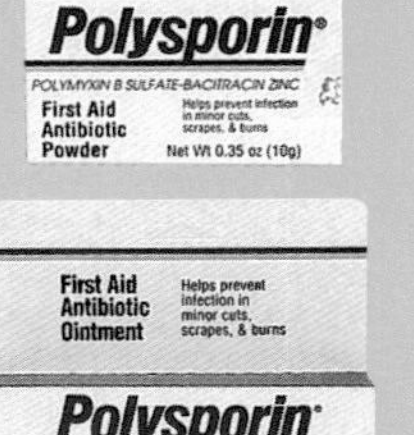

First Aid Antibiotic Powder & Ointment
Powder, 0.35 oz. (10g) Ointment,
1/2 oz. (14.2g) and 1 oz. (28.4g)

Polysporin®

Warner-Lambert Consumer Healthcare
P. 834

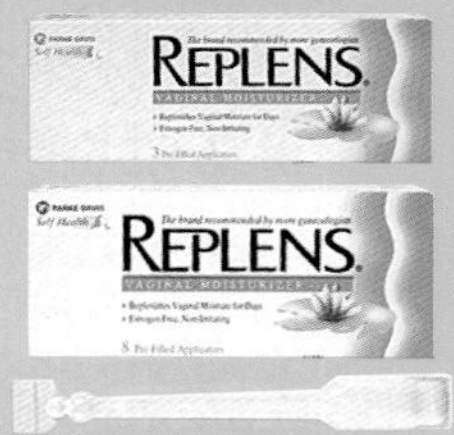

Vaginal Moisturizer
Available in boxes of 3 and 8
single-use applicators

Replens®

Warner-Lambert Consumer Healthcare
P. 835

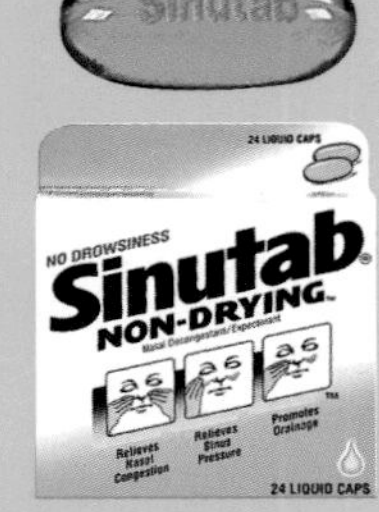

Available in Boxes of 24

Sinutab® Non-Drying Liquid Caps

Warner-Lambert Consumer Healthcare
P. 835

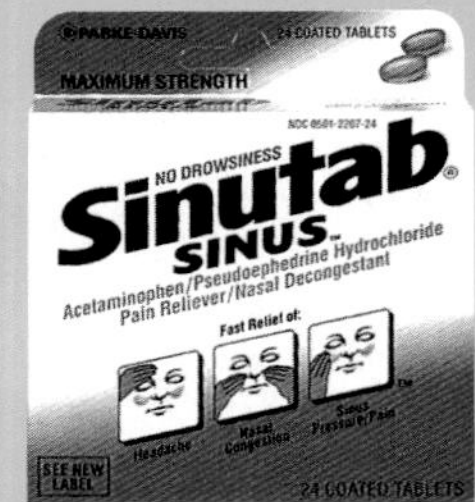

Maximum Strength
Without Drowsiness Formula
Available in 24 Caplets or Tablets

Sinutab® Sinus

Warner-Lambert Consumer Healthcare
P. 835

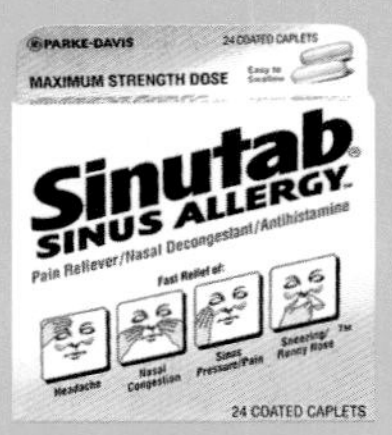

Maximum Strength Formula
Available in 24 Caplets or Tablets

Sinutab® Sinus Allergy

Warner-Lambert Consumer Healthcare
P. 838

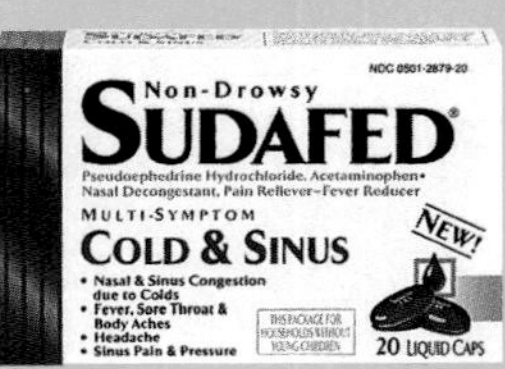

Available in boxes of
10 and 20 liquid caps

Sudafed® Cold and Sinus

Warner-Lambert Consumer Healthcare
P. 836

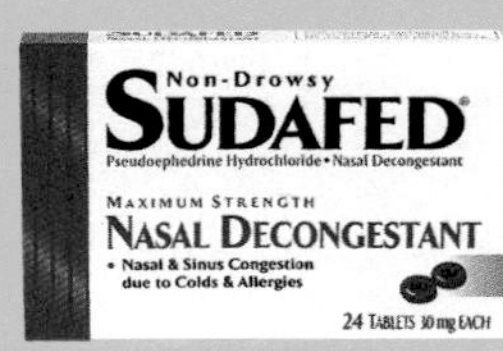

30 mg Tablets
Available in 24, 48 and 100

Sudafed® Nasal Decongestant

Warner-Lambert Consumer Healthcare
P. 836

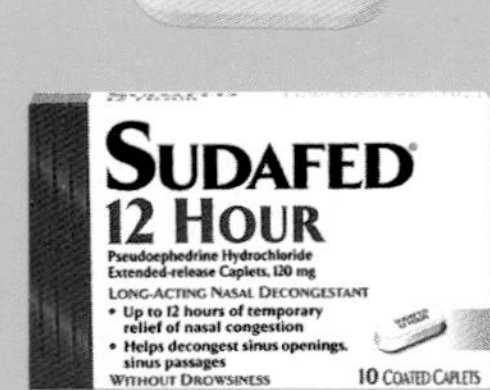

12 Hour Caplets
Available in 10 and 20 caplets

Sudafed® 12 Hour

Warner-Lambert Consumer Healthcare
P. 836

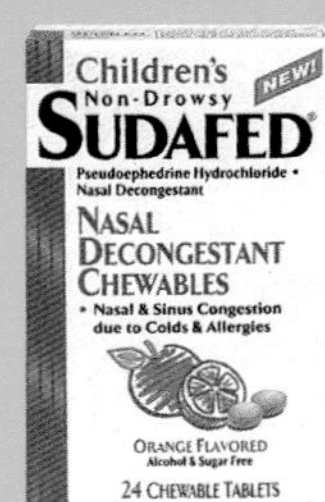

Available in boxes of
24 chewable tablets

Children's Sudafed® Nasal Decongestant

Warner-Lambert Consumer Healthcare
P. 837

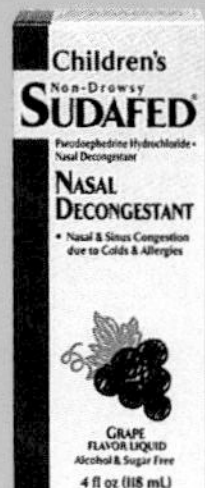

Available in 4 fl. oz. bottles

Children's Sudafed® Nasal Decongestant Liquid Medication

Warner-Lambert Consumer Healthcare
P. 838

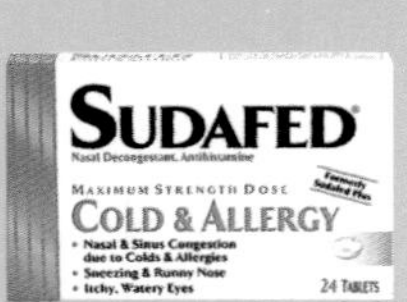

Available in boxes of 24 and
48 tablets.

Sudafed® Cold and Allergy

Warner-Lambert Consumer Healthcare
P. 838

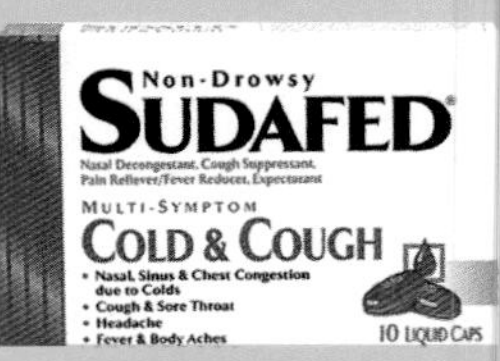

Available in 10's or 20's Liquid Caps

Sudafed® Cold & Cough

Warner-Lambert Consumer Healthcare
P. 839

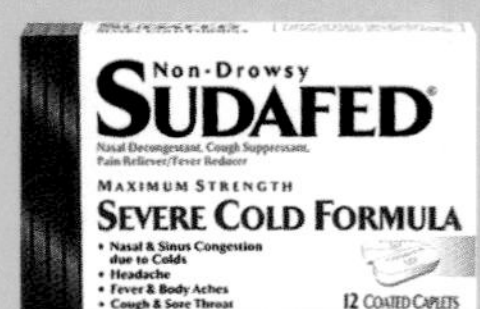

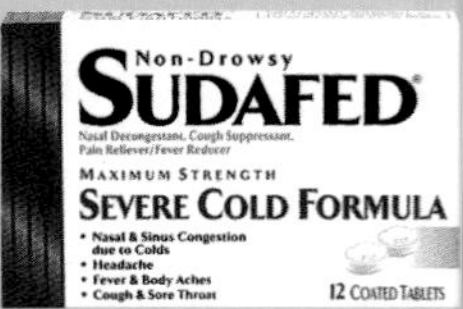

Available in 10 and 20
caplets and tablets

Sudafed® Severe Cold Formula

Warner-Lambert Consumer Healthcare
P. 839

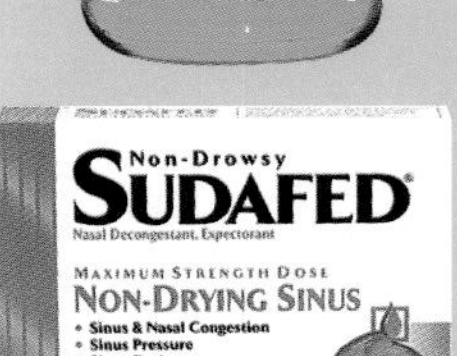

Available in 24 Liquid Caps

Sudafed® Non-Drying Sinus Liquid Caps

Warner-Lambert Consumer Healthcare
P. 840

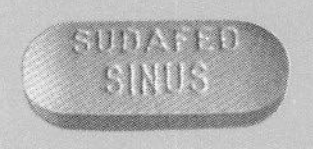

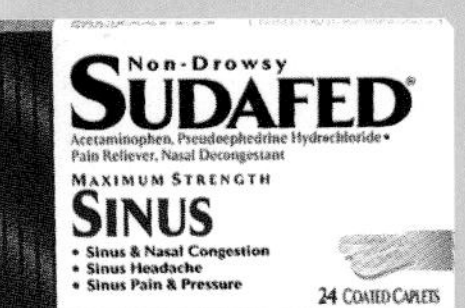

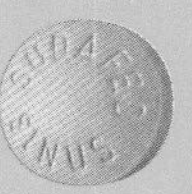

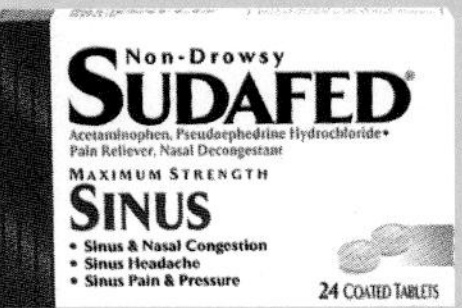

Available in 24 caplets and tablets

Sudafed® Sinus

Warner-Lambert Consumer Healthcare
P. 837

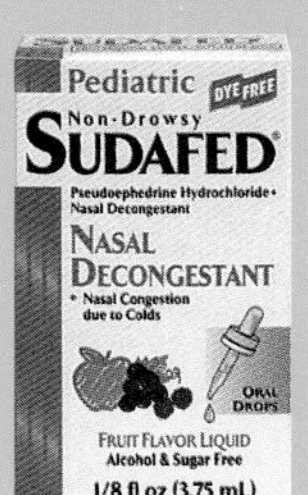

Available in 1/2 fl. oz. bottles

Pediatric Sudafed® Nasal Decongestant Liquid Oral Drops

Warner-Lambert Consumer Healthcare
P. 840

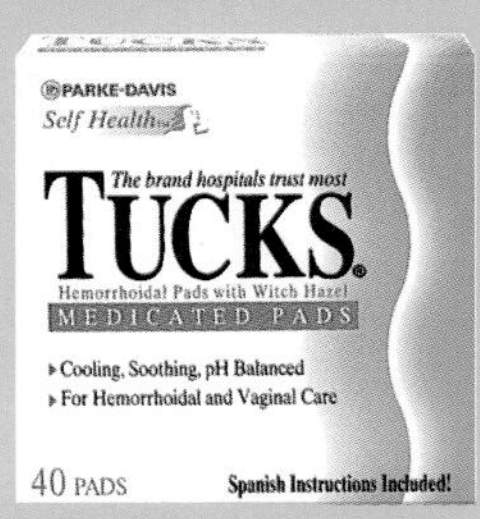

Pre-Moistened Pads
Available in 40 and 100 pad packages

Tucks®

Warner-Lambert Consumer Healthcare
P. 840

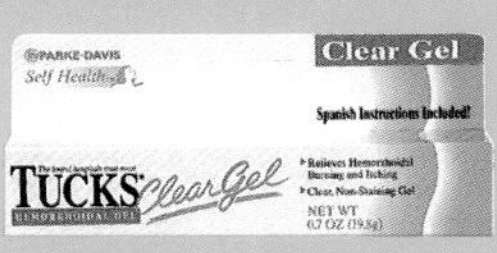

Available in 0.7 oz. (19.8 g) tubes

Tucks® Clear Gel

Warner-Lambert Consumer Healthcare
P. 841

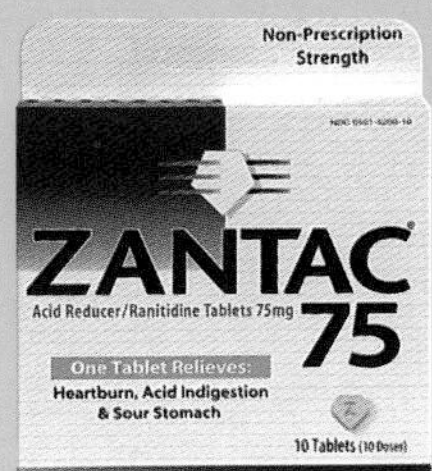

Available in boxes of
4, 10, 20 and 30 tablets

Zantac® 75

J.B. WILLIAMS CO.

J.B. Williams Co.
P. 863

Original and Mint Antiseptic Mouthwash/Gargle
Available in 4, 12, 24 and 32 Fl. oz. bottles

Cepacol®

J.B. Williams Co.
P. 863

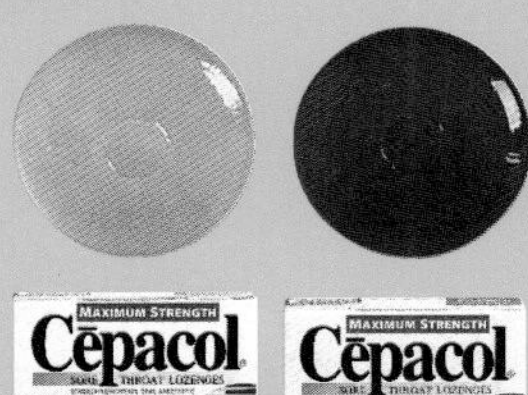

Maximum Strength Sore Throat Lozenges
Mint and Cherry Flavors
Also Available in Regular Strength.
18 lozenges per pack

Cepacol®

J.B. Williams Co.
P. 863

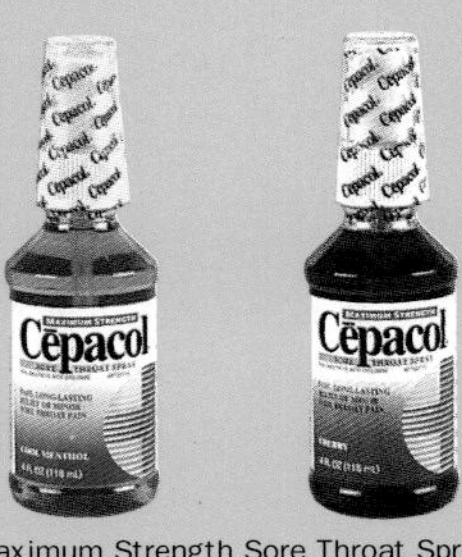

Maximum Strength Sore Throat Spray
Cool Menthol and Cherry Flavors.
4 Fl. oz. bottles

Cepacol®

WYETH-AYERST

Tamper-Resistant/ Evident Packaging

Statements alerting consumers to the specific type of Tamper-Resistant/Evident Packaging appear on the bottle labels and cartons of all over-the-counter products of Wyeth-Ayerst. This includes plastic cap seals on bottles, individually wrapped tablets or suppositories, and sealed cartons. This packaging has been developed to better protect the consumer.

Wyeth-Ayerst Laboratories
P. 864

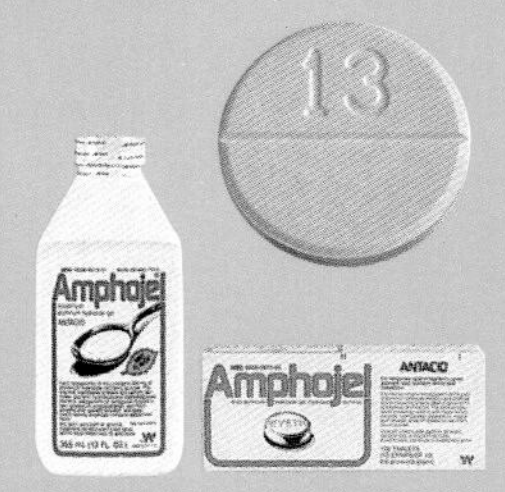

0.6 gram (10 gr.) Tablet shown above
12 Fl. oz. bottle and 100 tablets
Tablets and Suspension Antacid

Amphojel®

Wyeth-Ayerst Laboratories
P. 864

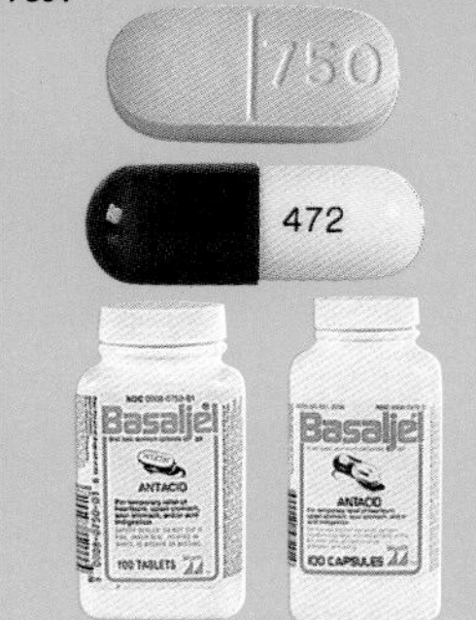

Antacid Tablets and Capsules

Basaljel®

Wyeth-Ayerst Laboratories
P. 864

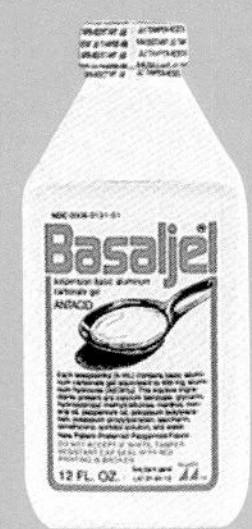

Suspension Antacid 12 Fl. oz.

Basaljel®

Wyeth-Ayerst Laboratories
P. 865

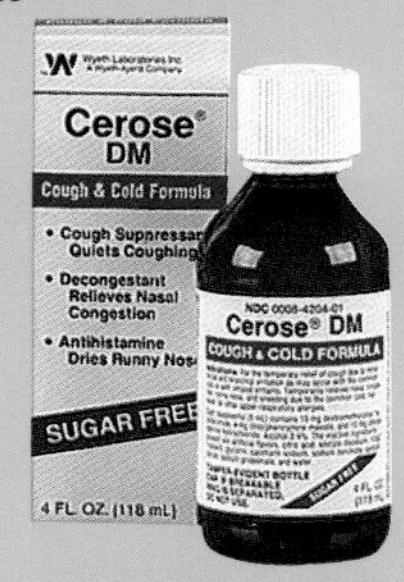

4 Fl. oz. Cough/Cold Formula
with Dextromethorphan
Also available in 1 pint bottles

Cerose® DM

Wyeth-Ayerst Laboratories
P. 865

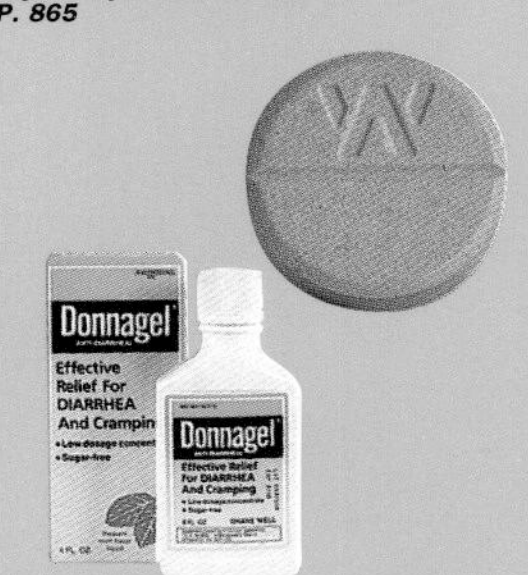

Available in bottles of 4 and 8 Fl. oz.
Chewable tablets
available in cartons of 18

Donnagel®

ZILA

Zila Pharmaceuticals, Inc.
P. 866

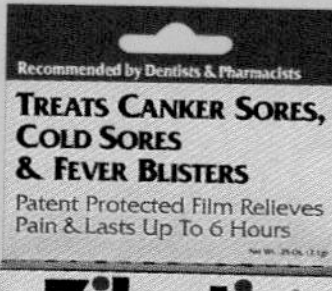

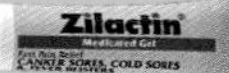

.25 oz. Medicated Gel
Unique Film Controls Pain Longer

Zilactin®

Zila Pharmaceuticals, Inc.
P. 866

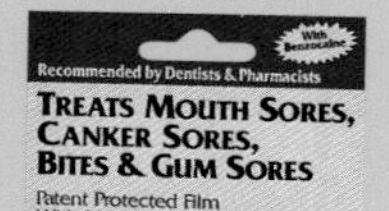

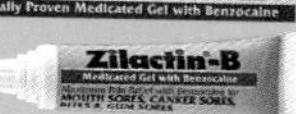

.25 oz. Medicated Gel with Benzocaine
Maximum Strength Medication

Zilactin®-B

Zila Pharmaceuticals, Inc.
P. 866

.25 Fl.oz. Medicated Liquid
Treats Cold Sores Without
Forming A Film

Zilactin®-L

ZP TECH, INC.

ZP Tech, Inc.
P. 866

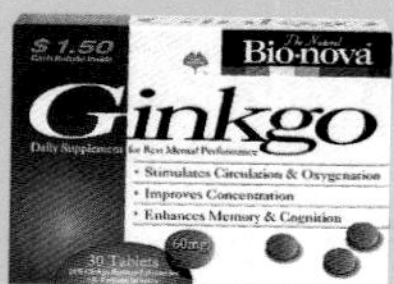

60 mg
Daily Supplement for Best
Mental Performance

Bio-nova™ Ginkgo

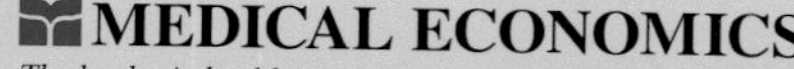

ƎECTION 7

PRODUCT INFORMATION

his section presents information on nonprescription ıedications, nutritional supplements, self-testing its, and other medical products designed for home se by consumers. It is made possible through the ourtesy of the manufacturers whose products ppear on the following pages. The information conerning each product has been prepared, edited, and pproved by the medical department, medical direcor, and/or medical counsel of the manufacturer.

he product descriptions in this section comply with abeling regulations. They are designed to provide all nformation necessary for informed use, including, vhen applicable, active ingredients, inactive ingredints, indications, actions, warnings, cautions, drug nteractions, symptoms and treatment of oral overdosage, dosage and directions for use, professional labeling, and how supplied. In some cases, additional information has been supplied to complement the standard labeling.

In compiling this section, the publisher has emphasized the necessity of describing products comprehensively. The descriptions seen here include all information made available by the manufacturer. The publisher does not warrant or guarantee any product described here, and does not perform any independent analysis of the information provided. Inclusion of a product in this book does not represent an endorsement, and the publisher does not necessarily advocate the use of any product listed.

Agro-Dynamics International
International-Bio Tech-USA
1145 LINDA VISTA DRIVE, STE. 109
SAN MARCOS, CA 92069

Direct Inquiries to:
Jerry Stagner
(619) 471–1182
FAX: (619) 471–1878

LATERO-FLORA™
(Flora Balance™)

Description: Latero-Flora™ (Flora-Balance™) Is the source of a special strain of Bacillus laterosporus (BOD Strain) a natural occurring bacteria in spore form. Each capsule contains 500,000 spores.

Indications and usage: For Candida and other yeast problems, prevention or treatment of intestinal disorders due to antibiotics and chemotherapy such as constipation, diarrhea, acne, abdominal flatulent or abdominal pain.

Administration: Adults—One or two capsules three times daily. Children —one capsule as described above.

How Supplied:
Bottle of 30 Capsules
Bottle of 60 Capsules
Storage: Store at room temperature or refrigerate.

AkPharma Inc.
P.O. BOX 111
PLEASANTVILLE, NJ 08232-0111

Direct Inquiries To:
Elizabeth Wexler: (609) 645-5100
FAX: (609) 645-0767

Medical Emergency Contact:
Leonard P. Smith: (609) 645-5100

BEANO®

PRODUCT OVERVIEW

Key Facts: Beano® alpha-galactosidase enzyme hydrolyzes raffinose, verbascose and stachyose into the digestible sugars—sucrose, fructose, glucose and galactose. Beano drops are added to food and Beano tablets are swallowed, chewed, or crumbled onto food immediately prior to eating, for *in vivo* treatment of the food during digestion.

Major Uses: Helps stop gas before it starts. Beano® enzyme has been shown to be effective in clinical studies with humans when consuming foods with high alpha-linked sugars content. Use of Beano results in substantially reduced breath hydrogen emissions and marked reduction or elimination of symptoms, compared with identical challenges with placebo.

Safety Information: Beano® enzyme should be discontinued in anyone who develops hypersensitivity to the enzyme.

PRODUCT INFORMATION

BEANO®

Description: Beano drops: each 5 drop dosage follows Food Chemical Codex (FCC) standards for activity and contains not less than 150 GalU (galactosidase units) of alpha-D-galactosidase derived from *Aspergillus niger* mold. The enzyme is in a liquid carrier of water and sorbitol. Add about 5 drops on the first bite of food serving, but remember a normal meal has 2–3 servings of the problem foods. Beano tablets: each tablet follows Food Chemical Codex (FCC) standards for activity and contains not less than 150 GalU (galactosidase units) of alpha-D-galactosidase derived from *Aspergillus niger* mold. The enzyme is in a carrier of corn starch, sorbitol, mannitol, and hydrogenated cottonseed oil. 2–3 tablets, swallowed, chewed, or crumbled onto food, should be enough for a normal meal of 2 or 3 servings of problem foods. Beano will hydrolyze complex sugars, raffinose, stachyose and verbascose, into the simple sugars—glucose, galactose and fructose, and the easily digestible disaccharide, sucrose. (Sucrose hydrolysis happens simultaneously with normal digestion.) In some cases, more enzyme than 5 drops or 3 tablets will be required, and this is a function of the quantity of food eaten, the levels of alpha-linked sugars in the food and the gas-producing propensity of the person.

Action: Hydrolysis converts raffinose, stachyose and verbascose into their monosaccharide components: glucose, galactose, fructose and sucrose. Raffinose yields sucrose + galactose; stachyose yields sucrose + galactose; verbascose yields glucose + fructose + galactose.

Indications: Flatulence and/or bloat as a result of eating a variety of grains, cereals, nuts, seeds, and vegetables containing the sugars raffinose, stachyose and/or verbascose. This includes all or most legumes and all or most cruciferous vegetables. Examples of such foods are oats, wheat, beans of all kinds, chickpeas, peas, lentils, peanuts, soy-content foods, broccoli, brussels sprouts, cabbage, carrots, corn, leeks, onions, parsnips, squash. Note: Most vegetables and beans also contain fiber, which is gas productive in some people, but usually far less so than the alpha-linked sugars. Beano® has no effect on fiber.

Usage: About 5 drops per food serving or 2–3 tablets per meal of 2 or 3 servings of problem foods; higher levels depending on symptoms.

How Supplied: Beano® is supplied in both a stable liquid form (12, 30, and 75-serving sizes, at 5 drops per serving), and a stable tablet form (12, 30, 60, 100 and 250 tablet sizes and 24 tablets in packets of 2).

Toxicity: None known

Adverse Reactions: None known; enzyme is derived from *Aspergillus niger*, a mold, and it is conceivable that mold-sensitive persons could react.

Drug Interactions: None known but because Beano is derived from a fermentation, it is advisable to avoid use with an MAO inhibitor. Beano® is classified as a dietary supplement, not a drug.

Precautions: Diabetics should be aware that the sugars in these vegetables will now be metabolically available and must be taken into account. No reports received of any diabetics' reactions. Galactosemics should not use without physician's advice, since one of the breakdown sugars is galactose.
For more information and samples, please write or call toll-free 1-800-257-8650.

Shown in Product Identification Guide, page 503

PRELIEF™

PRODUCT OVERVIEW

Key Facts: Prelief is a dietary supplement for use with acidic foods and beverages for more comfortable eating. Prelief tablets are swallowed with the first bite or sip of acidic food. Prelief granulate is added to each serving of acidic food or beverage.
Major Uses: Helps neutralize acidic foods such as spaghetti and pizza sauce, citrus and other fruit drinks, coffee, wine, and colas.
Safety Information: Prelief is made from an FDA Generally Recognized as Safe (GRAS) dietary supplement ingredient and is also listed as a food ingredient in the US Government's Food Chemicals Codex (FCC).

PRODUCT INFORMATION

PRELIEF™

Description: Prelief Tablets: each tablet contains 333 mg of calcium glycerophosphate. The tablets also contain magnesium stearate as a processing aid. One or 2 tablets should be swallowed with the first bit of food or sip of drink. Prelief Granulate: each packet contains 333 mg of calcium glycerophosphate. Add 1 or 2 packets of granulate to each serving of acidic food or beverage. Except for alcoholic beverages, the granulate dissolves rapidly in the acidic food or beverage. An additional 1–2 tablets or packets may be needed on foods that may be particularly high in acid.
One tablet or granulate packet of Prelief supplies 6% (65 mg) of the US Recommended Daily Allowance (RDA) for calcium and 5% (50 mg) of the RDA for phosphorus.
Kosher: Prelief is Kosher and Pareve.

Indications: Prelief is a dietary supplement for use with acidic foods and beverages to reduce their acid for more comfortable eating.

Action: Prelief neutralizes the acid found in many foods which many people find cause them discomfort.

Usage: 1–2 tablets or 1–2 granulate packets per serving of acidic food or beverage.

How Supplied: Prelief is supplied in both a tablet form (30 and 60-tablet bottle sizes and 24 tablets in 12-2 tablet packets), and a granulate form (36 packets).

Use Limitations: None known

Toxicity: None known

Adverse Reactions: None known

Interactions with Drugs: Calcium may interact with some medications. If you are taking a medication, check with your physician, pharmacist or other health professional about the possible interactions of calcium with that medication.

Prelief is classified as a dietary supplement, not a drug.

Precautions: People who have been advised by their physician not to take calcium, phosphorus or glycerin/glycerol should consult with their physician before using Prelief.

For more information and samples, please write or call toll-free 1-888-773-5433.

Shown in Product Identification Guide, page 503

American Lifeline, Inc.

103 S. SECOND STREET
MADISON, WI 53704

Direct Inquiries to:
Dave Sullivan
1-800-257-5433

FLORA*jen*® *Acidophilus*
Extra Strength
Non-Dairy Capsule form Refrigerated

Ingredients: Active—Over ten (10) billion viable freeze dried *Lactobacillus acidophilus* cells per capsule. Equal to the *L. acidophilus* in six (6) cups of fresh yogurt. Potency guaranteed through expiration date on label.

Inactive—Rice maltodextrin, gelatin capsule.

Directions: One capsule daily on an empty stomach with non-chlorinated water, fruit juice or preferably milk if not lactose intolerant. If taking antibiotics take FLORAjen 1–2 hours after antibiotic. While traveling, OK at room temperature for two weeks, otherwise must refrigerate.

How Supplied: 30 capsule bottle
60 capsule bottle

AML Laboratories

A Winning Combination Company
1753 CLOVERFIELD BOULEVARD
SANTA MONICA, CA 90404

TELEPHONE INFO:
For Customer Service or For Additional Product Information Call Toll Free 1 (800) 800-1200

BREATH + PLUS™
Natural Breath Freshener

Description: Each small softgel capsule contains a concentrated, balanced blend of three powerful natural breath fresheners and antioxidant vitamins.

Actions: Bad breath (halitosis) is a condition generally treated by intensive oral hygiene; however, bad breath will not respond to oral hygiene treatment when the source of bad breath is the stomach or digestive system. BREATH+PLUS™ is designed to work in the digestive system where oral hygiene has no impact. BREATH+PLUS™ is not a temporary "cover-up" like mouthwash and mints. It is a longlasting breath treatment that goes beyond brushing and flossing to neutralize unpleasant breath odors at their source—in the stomach. BREATH+PLUS™ is most effective against odors caused by spicy or pungent foods, such as garlic, onions and peppers. BREATH+PLUS™ has also been reported to be effective against tobacco, alcohol, morning breath and other odors stemming from the stomach and digestive tract. In addition to its natural breath freshening agents, BREATH+PLUS™ also contains the antioxidant nutrients Beta Carotene and Vitamin E.

Indications: For use with bad breath (halitosis) stemming from the stomach or digestive system. Effective against odors from spicy foods and can also be used immediately before bed or upon awakening for morning breath. Also reported to be effective against tobacco and alcohol odors emanating from the gastrointestinal tract.

Active Ingredients: Sunflower Oil, Parsley Seed Oil, Peppermint Oil, Chlorophyll, Vitamin E and Beta Carotene in a soft gelatin capsule.

CONTAINS NO ADDED INGREDIENTS.

Three capsules of **BREATH+PLUS™** contain the following vitamins:

	Quantity	US RDA
Vitamin A		
Beta Carotene	1,500 IU	30%
Vitamin E	15 IU	50%

Suggested Use: For odors stemming from food or beverages, SWALLOW (do not chew) 2 or 3 capsules with liquid immediately after eating. For morning breath, SWALLOW (do not chew) 2 or 3 capsules with liquid immediately before bed or upon awakening.

How Supplied: HDPE bottles of 200 softgels, or small 40-softgel dispensers, or single use 3-softgel packets.

COMPLETE FAMILY
High Antioxidant Stress Multi-Vitamin-Mineral Formulas

Description: The COMPLETE™ Multi-Vitamin-Mineral formulas are two distinct gender specific multi-vitamin multi-mineral formulas delivering over twenty essential vitamins and minerals with particular focus on providing high potencies of the antioxidant nutrients (Beta Carotene, Vitamin C and Vitamin E), as well as the B-Complex vitamins. The COMPLETE™ family of products conveniently and economically provides high levels of antioxidant protection previously only available by combining numerous separate supplement formulas.

Actions: The COMPLETE™ multi-vitamin multi-mineral product line is specially formulated to meet the widest range of requirements for a high potency anti-oxidant supplement while also providing a full complement of other essential vitamins and minerals. Antioxidants have become important because scientists and researchers now believe that antioxidant nutrients like Vitamin E, Vitamin C and Beta Carotene may neutralize the cellular damaging effects of free radicals (oxidizers). It is this potential ability of antioxidants to prevent cellular damage caused by free radicals that scientists and researchers believe may be associated with antioxidants' possible role in reducing the risk of certain degenerative diseases.

COMPLETE FOR MEN™
High Antioxidant Stress Multi-Vitamin-Mineral Formula

Description: COMPLETE FOR MEN™ is a high potency complete multi-vitamin multi-mineral formula specifically designed to meet the needs of active men and to insure optimum intake of twenty-five essential nutrients, particularly all of the antioxidant nutrients and the B-Complex vitamins. These key nutrients are provided at potencies far higher than conventional multi-vitamins in order to be consistent with the current research and therefore offer the possibility of delivering their potential health benefits.

Ingredients: Calcium ascorbate, calcium aspartate, d-alpha tocopheryl succinate, magnesium oxide, calcium carbonate, beta carotene, ascorbyl palmitate, zinc aspartate, zinc histidine, inositol hexaniacinate, zinc glycinate, iron glycinate, calcium pantothenate, riboflavin, copper glycinate, thiamine, selenomethionine, pyridoxine, chromium polynicotinate, manganese glycinate,

Continued on next page

AML Laboratories—Cont.

molybdenum glycinate, boron aspartate, cyanocobalamin, vanadium glycinate, cholecalciferol, folic acid, potassium iodide, phytonadione, biotin.

CONTAINS NO ADDED INGREDIENTS

Three capsules of **COMPLETE FOR MEN™** provide the following:

Vitamins	Quantity	US RDA
Vitamin A		
Beta Carotene	20,000 IU	400%
Vitamin D	400 IU	100%
Vitamin E	300 IU	1,000%
Vitamin K-1	80 mcg	*
Vitamin C	750 mg	1,250%
Vitamin B1	13.5 mg	900%
Vitamin B2	15.3 mg	900%
Vitamin B3	37 mg	185%
Vitamin B5	14 mg	140%
Vitamin B6	12 mg	600%
Vitain B12	19.5 mcg	325%
Folic Acid	400 mcg	100%
Biotin	60 mcg	20%

Minerals	Quantity	US RDA
Calcium	200 mg	20%
Magnesium	100 mg	25%
Iron	5 mg	27%
Zinc	30 mg	200%
Iodine	150 mcg	100%
Selenium	140 mcg	*
Chromium	100 mcg	*
Copper	1.5 mg	75%
Manganese	2 mg	*
Molybdenum	75 mcg	*
Vanadium	10 mcg	*
Boron	200 mcg	*

* No US RDA established

Suggested Use: As a dietary supplement, consume the contents of one packet with your first substantial meal of the day. SEE OWNERS MANUAL FOR MORE DETAILED INSTRUCTIONS.

How Supplied: HDPE bottle of 90 Perma-Fresh foil-mylar packets containing 3 capsules each for a total supply of 270 capsules. Also available as a 30-day supply.

COMPLETE FOR WOMEN™
High Anitoxidant Stress Multi-Vitamin-Mineral Formula

Description: COMPLETE FOR WOMEN™ is a high potency complete multi-vitamin multi-mineral formula specifically designed to meet the needs of active women and to insure optimum intake of twenty-five essential nutrients, particularly all of the antioxidant nutrients and the B-Complex vitamins. These key nutrients are provided at potencies far higher than conventional multi-vitamins in order to be consistent with the current research and therefore offer the possibility of delivering their potential health benefits. COMPLETE FOR WOMEN™ also supplies significantly higher levels of Calcium than ordinary mass market multi-vitamins, including those designed specifically for women.

Ingredients: Calcium aspartate, calcium ascorbate, calcium carbonate, magnesium oxide, d-alpha tocopheryl succinate, beta carotene, ascorbyl palmitate, zinc aspartate, zinc histidine, inositol hexaniacinate, zinc glycinate, iron glycinate, calcium pantothenate, pyridoxine, riboflavin, boron aspartate, copper glycinate, thiamine, selenomethionine, chromium polynicotinate, manganese glycinate, molybdenum glycinate, cyanocobalamin, vanadium glycinate, cholecalciferol, folic acid, potassium iodide, phytonadione, biotin.

CONTAINS NO ADDED INGREDIENTS.

Five capsules of **COMPLETE FOR WOMEN™** provide the following:

Vitamins	Quantity	US RDA
Vitamin A		
Beta Carotene	20,000 IU	400%
Vitamin D	400 IU	100%
Vitamin E	300 IU	1,000%
Vitamin K-1	80 mcg	*
Vitamin C	750 mg	1,250%
Vitamin B1	13.5 mg	900%
Vitamin B2	15.3 mg	900%
Vitamin B3	37 mg	185%
Vitamin B5	20 mg	200%
Vitamin B6	14 mg	700%
Vitamin B12	19.5 mcg	325%
Folic Acid	400 mcg	100%
Biotin	60 mcg	20%

Minerals	Quantity	US RDA
Calcium	600 mg	60%
Magnesium	200 mg	50%
Iron	10 mg	55%
Zinc	30 mg	200%
Iodine	150 mcg	100%
Selenium	140 mcg	*
Chromium	100 mcg	*
Copper	1.5 mg	75%
Manganese	2 mg	*
Molybdenum	75 mcg	*
Vanadium	10 mcg	*
Boron	800 mcg	*

*No US RDA establishd

Suggested Use: As a dietary supplement, consume the contents of one packet with your first substantial meal of the day. SEE OWNERS MANUAL FOR MORE DETAILED INSTRUCTIONS.

How Supplied: HDPE bottle of 90 Perma-Fresh foil-mylar packets containing 5 capsules each for a total supply of 450 capsules. Also available as a 30-day supply.

FAT BURNING FACTORS™
Lipotropic and Fat Metabolizing Formula

Description: FAT BURNING FACTORS™ is a dietary supplement containing lipotropics and other nutrients essential for and/or related to fat metabolism and weight loss which is offered as part of the Fat Burning Factors Lean Lifestyle Program.

Actions: FAT BURNING FACTORS™ is specifically designed for those individuals engaging in a program of physical activity designed to achieve fat loss. FAT BURNING FACTORS™ is not a stand alone weight loss product, but a dietary supplement containing all the nutrients and co-factors established by research to be essential and/or related to fat metabolism which is a necessary condition for weight loss.

Ingredients: L-carnitine tartrate, calcium ascorbate, choline bitartrate, lysine, arginine, leucine, inositol, valine, isoleucince, pyridoxine, calcium pantothenate, inositol hexaniacinate, riboflavin, thiamine, cyanocobalamin, chromium polynicotinate, folic acid, biotin.

CONTAINS NO ADDED INGREDIENTS.

Two capsules of **FAT BURNING FACTORS™** provide the following:

Vitamins	Quantity	US RDA
L-Carnitine	200 mg	*
Vitamin C	200 mg	333%
Lysine	200 mg	*
Arginine	100 mg	*
Leucine	100 mg	*
Isoleucine	25 mg	*
Valine	50 mg	*
Chromium	200 mcg	*
Vitamin B1	7.5 mg	500%
Vitamin B2	8.5 mg	500%
Vitamin B3	19 mg	95%
Vitamin B5	20 mg	200%
Vitamin B6	20 mg	1,000%
Vitamin B12	40 mcg	666%
Folic Acid	200 mcg	50%
Biotin	30 mcg	10%
Choline Bitartrate	100 mg	*
Inositol	100 mg	*

*No US RDA established

Suggested Use: As a dietary supplement to be used in conjunction with a program of regular physical activity targeted for fat loss, consume a total of two capsules daily, preferably one each with the morning and evening meal. As many as six capsules daily can be consumed divided equally over the day's meals.

How Supplied: HDPE bottle containing 180 capsules, or 90 capsules.

Natural M.D.
LIFE PRESCRIPTION FAMILY
High Antioxidant Stress Multi-Vitamin-Mineral Phytonutrient Formulas

Description: There are seven different LIFE PRESCRIPTION™ Multi-Vitamin-Mineral formulas of varying potency and/or gender specificity. Each is a comprehensive multi-vitamin multi-mineral formula delivering over twenty essential vitamins and minerals with particular focus on providing high potencies of the antioxidant nutrients (Natural

Carotenoid Complex, Vitamin C and Vitamin E), as well as the B-Complex vitamins. Several of the LIFE PRESCRIPTION™ formulas also offer high potencies of many nutritional co-factors, along with phytonutrient containing botanicals. The LIFE PRESCRIPTION™ product line conveniently and economically provides high levels of antioxidant protection previously only available by combining numerous separate supplement formulas.

Actions: The LIFE PRESCRIPTION™ multi-vitamin multi-mineral phytonutrient product line is specially formulated to meet the widest range of requirements for a high potency anti-oxidant supplement while also providing a full complement of other essential vitamins, minerals and co-factors. Antioxidants have become important because scientists and researchers now believe that antioxidant nutrients like Vitamin E, Vitamin C, Beta Carotene and other Carotenoids may neutralize the cellular damaging effects of free radicals (oxidizers). It is this potential ability of antioxidants to prevent cellular damage caused by free radicals that scientists and researchers believe may be associated with antioxidants' possible role in reducing the risk of certain degenerative diseases. The LIFE PRESCRIPTION™ formulas also contain numerous co-factors and phytonutrients because of the recent recognition of the role of these substances in achieving optimum formula efficacy and optimum health.

Natural M.D.
BASIC LIFE PRESCRIPTION FOR MEN™
High Antioxidant Stress Multi-Vitamin-Mineral Formula

Description: BASIC LIFE PRESCRIPTION FOR MEN™ is a high potency complete multi-vitamin multi-mineral formula specifically designed to meet the needs of active men and to insure optimum intake of twenty-five essential nutrients, particularly all of the antioxidant nutrients and the B-Complex vitamins. These key nutrients are provided at potencies far higher than conventional mutli-vitamins in order to be consistent with the current research and therefore offer the possibility of delivering their potential health benefits.

Ingredients: Calcium ascorbate, calcium carbonate, magnesium oxide, d-alpha tocopheryl succinate, zinc citrate, beta carotene, inositol hexaniacinate, iron glycinate, calcium pantothenate, selenomethionine, boron glycinate, molybdenum glycinate, riboflavin, thiamine, pyridoxine, manganese glycinate, ascorbyl palmitate, copper citrate, vanadium glycinate, cyanocobalamin, chromium polynicotinate, cholecalciferol, folic acid, potassium iodide, phytonadione, biotin.

CONTAINS NO ADDED INGREDIENTS.

Two capsules of **BASIC LIFE PRESCRIPTION FOR MEN™** provide the following:

Vitamins	Quantity	RDI
Vitamin A		
Beta Carotene	10,000 IU	200%
Vitamin D	400 IU	100%
Vitamin E	150 IU	500%
Vitamin K-1	80 mcg	100%
Vitamin C	300 mg	500%
Vitamin B1	13.5 mg	900%
Vitamin B2	15 mg	882%
Vitamin B3	38 mg	190%
Vitamin B5	20 mg	200%
Vitamin B6	12 mg	600%
Vitamin B12	18 mcg	300%
Folic Acid	400 mcg	100%
Biotin	300 mcg	100%
Minerals	**Quantity**	**RDI**
Calcium	160 mg	16%
Magnesium	100 mg	25%
Iron	5 mg	28%
Zinc	22.5 mg	150%
Iodine	150 mg	100%
Selenium	105 mg	150%
Chromium	100 mcg	83%
Copper	1.5 mg	75%
Manganese	2 mg	100%
Molybdenum	75 mcg	100%
Vanadium	10 mcg	*
Boron	200 mcg	*

*No RDI established

Suggested Use: As a dietary supplement, consume two capsules with your first substantial meal of the day. SEE OWNERS MANUAL FOR MORE DETAILED INSTRUCTIONS.

How Supplied: HDPE bottle containing 120 easy to swallow capsules.

Natural M.D.
BASIC LIFE PRESCRIPTION FOR WOMEN™
High Antioxidant Stress Multi-Vitamin-Mineral Formula

Description: BASIC LIFE PRESCRIPTION FOR WOMEN™ is a high potency complete multi-vitamin multi-mineral formula specifically designed to meet the needs of active women and to insure optimum intake of twenty-five essential nutrients, particularly all of the antioxidant nutrients and the B-Complex vitamins with special attention to a womans increased requirements for calcium and related nutrients. These key nutrients are provided at potencies far higher than conventional multi-vitamins in order to be consistent with the current research and therefore offer the possibility of delivering their potential health benefits.

Ingredients: Calcium carbonate, calcium ascorbate, magnesium oxide, d-alpha tocopheryl succinate, zinc citrate, beta carotene, inositol hexaniacinate, calcium pantothenate, iron glycinate, selenomethionine, boron glycinate, pyridoxine, riboflavin, molybdenum glycinate, thiamine, manganese glycincate, ascorbyl palmitate, copper citrate, cyanocobalamin, vanadium glycinate, chrominum polynicotinate, cholecalciferol, folic acid, potassium iodide, phytonadione, biotin.

CONTAINS NO ADDED INGREDIENTS.

Four capsules of **BASIC LIFE PRESCRIPTION FOR WOMEN™** provide the following:

Vitamins	Quantity	RDI
Vitamin A		
Beta Carotene	10,000 IU	200%
Vitamin D	400 IU	100%
Vitamin E	150 IU	500%
Vitamin K-1	100 mcg	125%
Vitamin C	300 mg	500%
Vitamin B1	14.5 mg	967%
Vitamin B2	16.5 mg	971%
Vitamin B3	47 mg	235%
Vitamin B5	30 mg	300%
Vitamin B6	18 mg	900%
Vitamin B12	19.5 mcg	325%
Folic Acid	400 mcg	100%
Biotin	300 mcg	100%
Minerals	**Quantity**	**RDI**
Calcium	600 mg	60%
Magnesium	200 mg	50%
Iron	5 mg	28%
Zinc	25 mg	167%
Iodine	150 mcg	100%
Selenium	105 mcg	150%
Chromium	150 mcg	125%
Copper	1.5 mg	75%
Manganese	2 mg	100%
Molybdenum	75 mcg	100%
Vanadium	10 mcg	*
Boron	1 mg	*

*No RDI established

Suggested Use: As a dietary supplement, consume four capsules with your first substantial meal of the day. SEE OWNERS MANUAL FOR MORE DETAILED INSTRUCTIONS.

How Supplied: HDPE bottle containing 240 easy to swallow capsules.

Natural M.D.
STANDARD LIFE PRESCRIPTION FOR MEN™
High Antioxidant Stress Multi-Vitamin-Mineral Formula

Description: STANDARD LIFE PRESCRIPTION FOR MEN™ is a high potency complete multi-vitamin multi-mineral formula specifically designed to deliver the precise amounts of antioxidants demanded by individuals choosing high antioxidant supplements. Specifically, it contains 400 I.U. of Vitamin E, 20,000 I.U. of natural Beta Carotene and 1,000 milligrams of Vitamin C, along with proportionately higher potencies of twenty other essential nutrients. STANDARD LIFE PRESCRIPTION FOR MEN™ does not contain Iron since many individuals choosing a high antioxidant regimen avoid supplementing additional Iron.

Continued on next page

AML Laboratories—Cont.

Ingredients: Calcium ascorbate, calcium carbonate, d-alpha tocopheryl succinate, ascorbyl palmitate, magnesium oxide, beta carotene, zinc citrate, inositol hexaniacinate, selenomethionine, pyridoxine, riboflavin, calcium pantothenate, thiamine, molybdenum glycinate, manganese glycinate, copper citrate, boron aspartate, cyanocobalamin, vanadium glycinate, chromium polynicotinate, cholecalciferol, folic acid, potassium iodide, biotin.

CONTAINS NO ADDED INGREDIENTS.

Four Capsules of **STANDARD LIFE PRESCRIPTION FOR MEN™** provide the following:

Vitamins	Quantity	RDI
Vitamin A		
Beta Carotene	20,000 IU	400%
Vitamin D	400 IU	100%
Vitamin E	400 IU	1,333%
Vitamin C	1,000 mg	1,667%
Vitamin B1	15 mg	1,000%
Vitamin B2	17 mg	1,000%
Vitamin B3	38 mg	190%
Vitamin B5	16 mg	160%
Vitamin B6	16 mg	800%
Vitamin B12	20 mcg	333%
Folic Acid	400 mcg	100%
Biotin	300 mcg	100%

Minerals	Quantity	RDI
Calcium	350 mg	35%
Magnesium	100 mg	25%
Zinc	30 mg	200%
Iodine	150 mcg	100%
Selenium	150 mcg	214%
Chromium	150 mcg	125%
Copper	1.5 mg	75%
Manganese	2 mg	100%
Molybdenum	75 mcg	100%
Vanadium	10 mcg	*
Boron	200 mcg	*

*No RDI established

Suggested Use: As a dietary supplement, consume the contents of one packet with your first substantial meal of the day. SEE OWNERS MANUAL FOR MORE DETAILED INSTRUCTIONS.

How Supplied: HDPE bottle of 60 perma-fresh, foil-mylar packets each containing four easy to swallow capsules, for a total supply of 240 capsules.

Natural M.D.
STANDARD LIFE PRESCRIPTION FOR WOMEN™
High Antioxidant Stress Multi-Vitamin-Mineral Formula

Description: Identical to STANDARD LIFE PRESCRIPTION FOR MEN™ above, except for the addition of extra Calcium (600 milligrams), Boron (800 micrograms), and Iron (10 milligrams) to address a woman's increased requirement for these nutrients.

Ingredients: Calcium carbonate, calcium ascorbate, d-alpha tocopheryl succinate, ascorbyl palmitate, magnesium oxide, beta carotene, iron glycinate, zinc citrate, inositol hexaniacinate, selenomethionine, pyridoxine, riboflavin, calcium pantothenate, thiamine, molybdenum glycinate, manganese glycinate, copper citrate, boron aspartate, cyanocobalamin, vanadium glycinate, chromium polynicotinate, cholecalciferol, folic acid, potassium iodide, biotin.

CONTAINS NO ADDED INGREDIENTS.

Five capsules of **STANDARD LIFE PRESCRIPTION FOR WOMEN™** provide the following:

Vitamins	Quantity	RDI
Vitamin A		
Beta Carotene	20,000 IU	400%
Vitamin D	400 IU	100%
Vitamin E	400 IU	1,333%
Vitamin C	1,000 mg	1,667%
Vitamin B1	15 mg	1,000%
Vitamin B2	17 mg	1,000%
Vitamin B3	38 mg	190%
Vitamin B5	16 mg	160%
Vitamin B6	16 mg	800%
Vitamin B12	20 mcg	333%
Folic Acid	400 mcg	100%
Biotin	300 mcg	100%

Minerals	Quantity	RDI
Calcium	700 mg	70%
Magnesium	200 mg	50%
Iron	10 mg	55%
Zinc	30 mg	200%
Iodine	150 mcg	100%
Selenium	150 mcg	214%
Chromium	150 mcg	125%
Copper	1.5 mg	75%
Manganese	2 mg	100%
Molybdenum	75 mcg	100%
Vanadium	10 mcg	*
Boron	1 mg	*

* No RDI established

Suggested Use: As a dietary supplement, consume the contents of one packet with your first substantial meal of the day. SEE OWNERS MANUAL FOR MORE DETAILED INSTRUCTIONS.

How Supplied: HDPE bottle of 60 perma-fresh, foil-mylar packets each containing five easy to swallow capsules, for a total supply of 300 capsules.

Natural M.D.
ESSENTIAL LIFE PRESCRIPTION™
High Potency Antioxidant Stress Multi-Vitamin-Mineral
Phytonutrient Formula

Description: ESSENTIAL LIFE PRESCRIPTION™ is an ultra-high potency complete multi-vitamin multi-mineral formula designed to meet the needs of those individuals seeking to achieve optimum moderate intake levels of antioxidant nutrients, B-Complex vitamins, along with several important nutritional cofactors and phytonutrient-containing botanicals. Its contents are selected from those nutrients and ingredients cited by the scientific literature as potentially possessing a role in the possible reduction of certain degenerative diseases.

Ingredients: Calcium ascorbate, magnesium ascorbate, garlic concentrate, d-alpha tocopheryl succinate, magnesium oxide, citrus bioflavonoid complex, green tea extract, calcium carbonate, mixed carotenoids, pyridoxine, zinc citrate, red wine proanthocyanidins, thiamine, calcium pantothenate, riboflavin, inositol hexaniacinate, selenomethionine, cranberry extract, cyanocobalamin, magnesium niacinate, pyridoxal-5'-phosphate, manganese glycinate, riboflavin-5'-phosphate, copper citrate, boron aspartate, lycopene, chromium nicotinate, folic acid, cholecalciferol, biotin.

CONTAINS NO ADDED INGREDIENTS.

Four capsules of **ESSENTIAL LIFE PRESCRIPTION™** provide the following:

Vitamins	Quantity	RDI
Vitamin A		
Total Carotenoids	20,000 IU	400%
Vitamin D	100 IU	25%
Vitamin E	400 IU	1,333%
Vitamin C	1,000 mg	1,667%
Vitamin B1	30 mg	2,000%
Vitamin B2	30 mg	1,764%
Vitamin B3	30 mg	150%
Vitamin B5	30 mg	300%
Vitamin B6	50 mg	2,500%
Vitamin B12	125 mcg	2,083%
Folic Acid	400 mcg	100%
Biotin	300 mcg	100%

Minerals	Quantity	RDI
Magnesium	68.7 mg	17%
Calcium	100 mg	10%
Copper	1 mg	50%
Zinc	15 mg	100%
Manganese	1 mg	50%
Selenium	100 mcg	143%
Chromium	100 mcg	83%
Boron	100 mcg	*

Co-Factors and Botanicals	Quantity
Lycopene	1,000 mg
Garlic Concentrate	400 mg
Citrus Bioflavonoids	100 mg
Green Tea Extract	100 mg
Red Wine Concentrate	40 mg
Cranberry Extract	20 mg

*No RDI established

Suggested Use: As a dietary supplement consume four capsules daily as needed or as directed by a physician. For best results, always consume with a substantial meal. SEE OWNERS MANUAL FOR MORE DETAILED INSTRUCTIONS.

How Supplied: HDPE bottle of 60 perma-fresh, foil-mylar packets each containing four easy to swallow capsules, for a total supply of 240 capsules.

Natural M.D.
COMPLETE LIFE PRESCRIPTION™
Ultra-High Potency Antioxidant Stress Multi-Vitamin-Mineral Phytonutrient Formula

Description: COMPLETE LIFE PRESCRIPTION™ is an ultra-high potency complete multi-vitamin multi-mineral formula designed to meet the needs of those individuals seeking the maximum potencies of antioxidant nutrients, B-Complex vitamins, along with several important nutritional co-factors and phytonutrient-containing botanicals. Its contents are selected from those nutrients and ingredients cited by the scientific literature as potentially possessing a role in the possible reduction of certain degenerative diseases.

Ingredients: Magnesium ascorbate, calcium ascorbate, d-alpha tocopheryl succinate, garlic concentrate, ascorbyl palmitate, magnesium oxide, mixed carotenoids, N acetyl cysteine, citrus bioflavonoid complex, green tea extract, pyridoxine, L-taurine, zinc citrate, co-enzyme Q-10, thiamine, L-carnitine, lipoic acid, calcium pantothenate, red wine proanthocyanidins, riboflavin, inositol hexaniacinate, selenomethionine, cyanocobalamin, shark cartilage, chondroitin sulfate, glucosamine sulfate, cranberry extract, millk thistle, magnesium niacinate, grape seed extract, pyridoxal-5'-phosphate, octacosonol, quercetin, riboflavin-5'-phosphate, manganese glycinate, bilberry extract, copper citrate, pine bark extract, boron aspartate, lycopene, chromium nicotinate, folic acid, cholecalciferol, biotin.

CONTAINS NO ADDED INGREDIENTS.

Seven capsules of **COMPLETE LIFE PRESCRIPTION™** provide the following:

Vitamins	Quantity	RDI
Vitamin A		
Total Carotenoids	25,000 IU	500%
Vitamin D	100 IU	25%
Vitamin E	600 IU	2,000%
Vitamin C	2,000 mg	3,333%
Vitamin B1	40 mg	2,667%
Vitamin B2	40 mg	2,353%
Vitamin B3	40 mg	200%
Vitamin B5	40 mg	400%
Vitamin B6	75 mg	3,750%
Vitamin B12	250 mcg	4,167%
Folic Acid	600 mcg	150%
Biotin	300 mcg	100%

Minerals	Quantity	RDI
Calcium	100 mg	10%
Magnesium	137 mg	34%
Copper	1.5 mg	75%
Zinc	22.5 mg	150%
Manganese	1 mg	50%
Selenium	150 mcg	214%
Chromium	150 mcg	125%
Boron	100 mcg	*

Co-Factors and Botanicals	Quantity
Lycopene	1,500 mcg
Co-Enzyme Q-10	60 mg
L-Carnitine	50 mg
N-Acetylcysteine	100 mg
Garlic Concentrate	400 mg
Citrus Bioflavonoids	100 mg
Green Tea Extract	100 mg
Red Wine Concentrate	40 mg
Cranberry Extract	20 mg
Grape Seed Extract	12.5 mg
Pine Bark Extract	2.5 mg
Octacosanol	0.25 mg
L-Taurine	75 mg
Lipoic Acid	50 mg
Quercetin	10 mg
Bilberry Extract	5 mg
Milk Thistle Extract	16 mg
Shark Cartilage	25 mg
Chondroitin Sulfate	25 mg
Glucosamine Sulfate	25 mg

*No RDI established

Suggested Use: As a dietary supplement consume seven capsules daily as needed or as directed by a physician. For best results, always consume with a substantial meal. SEE OWNERS MANUAL FOR MORE DETAILED INSTRUCTIONS.

How Supplied: HDPE bottle of 60 perma-fresh, foil mylar packets each containing seven easy to swallow capsules, for a total supply of 420 capsules.

Natural M.D.
ULTIMATE LIFE PRESCRIPTION™
Ultra-High Potency Antioxidant Stress Multi-Vitamin-Mineral Phytonutrient Formula

Description: ULTIMATE LIFE PRESCRIPTION™ is an ultra-high potency complete multi-mineral formula designed to meet the needs of those individuals seeking the highest available potencies of antioxidant nutrients, B-Complex vitamins, along with several important nutritional co-factors and phytonutrient-containing botanicals. Its contents are selected from those nutrients and ingredients cited by the scientific literature as potentially possessing a role in the possible reduction of certain degenerative diseases.

Ingredients: Magnesium ascorbate, calcium ascorbate, d-alpha tocopheryl succinate, garlic concentrate, ascorbyl palmitate, N-acetyl cysteine, mixed carotenoids, L-taurine, magnesium oxide, co-enzyme Q-10, pyridoxine, L-carnitine, lipoic acid, citrus bioflavonoid complex, green tea extract, zinc citrate, thiamine, calcium pantothenate, shark cartilage, chondroitin sulfate, glucosamine sulfate, riboflavin, inositol hexaniacinate, cyanocobalamin, selenomethionine, red wine proanthocyanidins, milk thistle, grape seed extract, quercetin, octacosonol, cranberry extract, pyridoxal-5'-phosphate, magnesium niacinate, bilberry extract, riboflavin-5'-phosphate, copper citrate, manganese glycinate, pine bark extract, lycopene, chromium nicotinate, boron aspartate, folic acid, cholecalciferol, biotin.

CONTAINS NO ADDED INGREDIENTS

Nine capsules of **ULTIMATE LIFE PRESCRIPTION™** provide the following:

Vitamins	Quantity	RDI
Vitamin A		
Total Carotenoids	30,000 IU	600%
Vitamin D	100 IU	25%
Vitamin E	800 IU	2,667%
Vitamin C	2,500 mg	4,167%
Vitamin B1	50 mg	3,333%
Vitamin B2	50 mg	2,941%
Vitamin B3	50 mg	250%
Vitamin B5	50 mg	500%
Vitamin B6	100 mg	5,000%
Vitamin B12	400 mcg	6,667%
Folic Acid	800 mcg	200%
Biotin	300 mcg	100%

Minerals	Quantity	RDI
Calcium	100 mg	10%
Magnesium	194 mg	49%
Copper	2 mg	100%
Zinc	30 mg	200%
Manganese	1 mg	50%
Selenium	200 mcg	286%
Chromium	200 mcg	167%
Boron	100 mcg	*

Co-Factors and Botanicals	Quantity
Lycopene	2,000 mcg
Co-Enzyme Q-10	120 mg
L-Carnitine	100 mg
N-Acetylcysteine	200 mg
Garlic Concentrate	400 mg
Citrus Bioflavonoids	100 mg
Green Tea Extract	100 mg
Red Wine Concentrate	40 mg
Cranberry Extract	20 mg
Grape Seed Extract	25 mg
Pine Bark Extract	5 mg
Octacosanol	0.5 mg
L-Taurine	150 mg
Lipoic Acid	100 mg
Quercetin	20 mg
Bilberry Extract	10 mg
Milk Thistle Extract	32 mg
Shark Cartilage	50 mg
Chondroitin Sulfate	50 mg
Glucosamine Sulfate	50 mg

*No RDI established

Suggested Use: As a dietary supplement consume nine capsules daily as needed or as directed by a physician. For best results, always consume with a substantial meal. SEE OWNERS MANUAL FOR MORE DETAILED INSTRUCTIONS.

How Supplied: HDPE bottle of 60 perma-fresh, foil-mylar packets each containing nine easy to swallow capsules, for a total supply of 540 capsules.

Fruit and Vegetable
SAFETY RINSE™
Fruit and Vegetable Cleansing Product

Description: Fruit And Vegetable SAFETY RINSE™ is a cleansing solution containing a natural blend of food grade surfactants, and emulsifiers to assist in the removal of water soluble and water insoluble topical residues such as

Continued on next page

AML Laboratories—Cont.

pesticides, fungicides, herbicides, waxes and other substances from fruits, vegetables and edible produce.

Indications: Fruit And Vegetable SAFETY RINSE™ is specifically designed for those individuals who seek to remove topical residues such as pesticides, fungicides, herbicides, waxes and other substances from fruits, vegetables and edible produce. It can be used by those individuals who possess sensitivities to many of the chemicals employed in the agricultural industry, several of which can evoke mild to severe allergic reactions. It is also intended for those individuals who are concerned about the potential long-term health risks posed by exposure to these agricultural chemicals in our food supply.

Actions: The surface active agents (surfactants) and emulsifiers present in Fruit And Vegetable SAFETY RINSE™ help remove topical residues, particularly the more persistent water insoluble pesticide, fungicide and waxy residues that do not respond to ordinary rinsing or cleansing from the surface of fruits, vegetables and edible produce.

Ingredients: Purified water and a blend of non-toxic, biodegradeable, 100% natural food grade surface active (surfactants), emulsifying and chelating agents.

Suggested Use: Soak and/or generously spray on the surface of fruits, vegetables, and edible produce. Scrub with brush or massage by hand and then rinse thoroughly with water. SEE OWNERS MANUAL FOR MORE DETAILED INSTRUCTIONS.

Warning: Individuals with severe sensitivities to topical agricultural residues should seek the approval of their physician before using this product.

How Supplied: Sixteen ounce HDPE sprayer bottle. Thirty-two ounce HDPE concentrate for refilling sprayer bottle and/or for use with produce bath.

STRESS GUM™
Complete Multivitamin Chewing Gum

Description: STRESS GUM™ is a natural mint-flavored chewing gum that freshens breath while also providing a healthy, nutrient-rich alternative to ordinary chewing gum. It is a convenient complete source of additional vitamins, particularly for those individuals who have difficulty swallowing ordinary vitamin pills or for those who do not consume a conventional multi-vitamin supplement. It contains all thirteen essential vitamins, plus two essential minerals. It supplies higher potencies of the antioxidant nutrients (Beta Carotene, Vitamin C and Vitamin E).

Actions: STRESS GUM™ is specially formulated to provide complete balanced multi-vitamin supplementation in a mint-flavored breath freshening gum. STRESS GUM™ contains higher levels of antioxidants because scientists and researchers now believe that antioxidant nutrients like Vitamin E, Vitamin C and Beta Carotene may neutralize the cellular damaging effects of free radicals (oxidizers). It is this potential ability of antioxidants to prevent cellular damage caused by free radicals that scientists believe may be associated with antioxidants' possible role in reducing the risk of certain degenerative diseases.

Ingredients: Pure natural gum base, natural spearmint flavor, natural sugars; fructose, sorbitol, and mannitol, calcium ascorbate, d-alpha tocopheryl acetate, beta carotene, niacinamide, calcium pantothenate, pyridoxine, riboflavin, thiamine, cyanocobalamin, cholecalciferol, chromium niacinate, folic acid, sodium selenate, biotin, phytonadione, **Does not contain the preservative BHT.**

CONTAINS NO ADDED INGREDIENTS.

Two pieces of **STRESS GUM™** supply the following:

	Quantity	US RDA
Vitamin A		
Beta Carotene	1,667 IU	33%
Vitamin D	20 IU	5%
Vitamin E	30 IU	100%
Vitamin C	60 mg	100%
Vitamin B1	500 mcg	33%
Vitamin B2	566 mcg	33%
Vitamin B3	6.6 mg	33%
Vitamin B5	1.3 mg	13%
Vitamin B6	666 mcg	33%
Vitamin B12	2 mcg	33%
Folic Acid	40 mcg	10%
Biotin	10 mcg	3%
Selenium	5 mcg	*
Chromium	5 mcg	*

*No US RDA established

Suggested Use: Chew STRESS GUM™ anytime throughout the day, particularly following meals. Do not exceed 20 pieces per day.

How Supplied: HDPE bottle containing 150 pieces of gum.

Astra USA, Inc.
50 OTIS ST.
WESTBOROUGH, MA
01581-4500

Direct Inquiries to:
Professional Information Department:
(508) 366-1100
FAX: (508) 366-7406

For Medical Emergencies Contact:
Medical Information Services
(800) 262-0460

XYLOCAINE® 2.5% Ointment
(lidocaine)

For temporary relief of pain and itching due to minor burns, sunburn, minor cuts, abrasions, insect bites and minor skin irritations.

Xylocaine® 2.5% Ointment should be applied liberally over the affected areas. Use enough to provide temporary relief and reapply Xylocaine 2.5% Ointment as needed for continued relief.

Warning: Use only as directed by a physician in persistent, severe or extensive skin disorders. In case of accidental ingestion, seek professional assistance or contact a poison control center immediately.

KEEP OUT OF REACH OF CHILDREN.

FOR EXTERNAL USE ONLY.

Xylocaine 2.5% Ointment is non-staining and is easily removed with water from skin or clothing.

Xylocaine 2.5% Ointment belongs in your home medicine chest and first aid kit.

Caution: Do not use in the eyes. Not for prolonged use. If the condition for which this preparation is used persists, or if a rash or irritation develops, discontinue use and consult a physician.

How Supplied: 1.25 ounce tubes containing 2.5% lidocaine base in water soluble carbowaxes.

ASTRA®
Astra USA, Inc. 021658R01
Westborough, MA 01581 11/93

Shown in Product Identification Guide, page 503

Bausch & Lomb Incorporated
ROCHESTER, NY 14692-0450

Direct Inquiries to:
Consumer Affairs (800) 572-2931

For Medical Emergency Contact:
Consumer Affairs: (800) 572-2931

CURÉL® Therapeutic Moisturizing Lotion and Cream

Indications: For control of dry skin symptoms, Curél delivers extra effective moisturization that with regular use, ends dry skin for most people.

Actions: Curél's unique cationic emulsion base enables it to be faster absorbing and more substantive to dry skin, all without a greasy after-feel. Curél is rich in humectant and occlusive ingredients, which help skin retain natural moisture and help heal dry skin problems like chapping, soreness, cracking, and erythema. Clinical skin hydration studies have shown that Curél moisturizes better than other leading therapeutic lotions, giving extra effective moisturization for softer, healthier skin. Curél Nutrient Rich Severe Dry Skin Lotion moisturizes and heals severe dry skin with extra healing moisturizers in a formula that is clinically proven to work for 12 hours, and prevents severe dry skin from returning with continued use.

Dermatologist tested and recommended, Curél contains no mineral oil or lanolin and all ingredients are non-comedogenic. Available in lightly fragranced original lotion, fragrance free lotion, fragrance free cream, alpha hydroxy fragrance free lotion, and fragrance free nutrient rich severe dry skin lotion.

Contents: Original Formula: Deionized Water, Glycerin, Distearyldimonium Chloride, Petrolatum, Isopropyl Palmitate, 1-Hexadecanol, Dimethicone, Sodium Chloride, Fragrance, Methyl Paraben, Propyl Paraben.

Fragrance Free: Deionized Water, Glycerin, Distearyldimonium Chloride, Petrolatum, Isopropyl Palmitate, 1-Hexadecanol, Dimethicone, Sodium Chloride, Methyl Paraben, Propyl Paraben.

Alpha Hydroxy: Deionized Water, Glycerin, Distearyldimonium Chloride, Petrolatum, Lactic Acid, Isopropyl Palmitate, 1-Hexadecanol, Glycolic Acid, Dimethicone, Ammonium Hydroxide, Methyl Paraben, Propyl Paraben. All products except Alpha Hydroxy lotion:

Nutrient Rich: Deionized Water, Glycerin, Petrolatum, Quaternium-5, Isopropyl Palmitate, 1-Hexadecanol, Dimethicone, Nylon 12, Methyl Paraben, Tocopheryl, Acetate, Propyl Paraben, DL-Panthenol, Ascorbyl Palmitate.

Directions for Use: Apply as often as needed. Especially effective when applied after bathing while skin is still damp. For external use only.

Alpha Hydroxy lotion: For best results, apply to skin twice a day. For external use only.

Nutrient Rich Lotion: Apply as needed to dry skin. Re-apply often to especially rough, chapped areas. For external use only.

How Supplied: Original Formula:

Lotion— 2.5 oz., 6 oz. and 10 oz. fliptop bottles
13 oz. pump bottle

Fragrance Free:

Cream— 4 oz. tube:
Lotion— 2.5 oz., 6 oz. and 10 oz. fliptop bottle
13 oz. pump bottle

Alpha Hydroxy—3.5 oz. bottle
7 oz. pump bottle

Nutrient Rich—3.5 oz. bottle
7 oz. pump bottle

For Toll-Free Product Information: Call 1-800-572-2931

Shown in Product Identification Guide, page 503

Bayer Corporation Consumer Care Division

36 Columbia Road
P.O. Box 1910
Morristown, NJ 07962-1910

Direct Inquiries to:
Consumer Affairs
(800) 331-4536

For Medical Emergency Contact:
Bayer Corporation
Consumer Care Division
(800) 331-4536

ACTRON™
Ketoprofen Tablets and Caplets, 12.5 mg

Active Ingredient: Each tablet or caplet contains 12.5 mg Ketoprofen.

Inactive Ingredients: Corn Starch, Croscarmellose Sodium, Hydroxypropyl Methylcellulose, Lactose, Magnesium Stearate, Microcrystalline Cellulose, Polyethylene Gylcol, Titanium Dioxide.

Directions: Take with a full glass of water or other fluid. ADULTS: Take 1 tablet or caplet every 4–6 hours. If pain or fever does not get better in 1 hour, you may take 1 more tablet or caplet. With experience, some people may find they need 2 tablets or caplets for the first dose. The smallest effective dose should be used.

Do not take more than: 2 tablets or caplets in any 4–6 hour period.
6 tablets or caplets in any 24 hour period.

Children: Do not give to children under age 16 unless directed by a doctor.

Indications: For the temporary relief of minor aches and pains associated with: common cold, headache, toothache, muscular aches, backache, minor arthritis, menstrual cramps. For the temporary reduction of fever.

WARNINGS: Do not take this product if you have asthma, hives or any other allergic reaction after taking any pain reliever/fever reducer. Ketoprofen could cause similar reactions. As with any drug, if you are pregnant or nursing a baby, seek the advice of a health professional before using this product. **IT IS ESPECIALLY IMPORTANT NOT TO USE KETOPROFEN DURING THE LAST 3 MONTHS OF PREGNANCY UNLESS SPECIFICALLY DIRECTED TO DO SO BY A DOCTOR BECAUSE IT MAY CAUSE PROBLEMS IN THE UNBORN CHILD OR COMPLICATIONS DURING DELIVERY.** If you generally consume 3 or more alcohol-containing drinks per day you should talk to your doctor for advice on when and how you should take Actron or other pain relievers.

DO NOT USE: With any other pain reliever/fever reducer, with any other product containing ketoprofen, for more than 3 days for fever, for more than 10 days for pain.

ASK A DOCTOR BEFORE USE IF: The painful area is red or swollen, you take other drugs on a regular basis, you are under a doctor's care for any continuing medical condition, you have had problems or side effects with any pain reliever/fever reducer.

ASK A DOCTOR AFTER USE IF: Symptoms continue or worsen, new or unexpected symptoms occur, stomach pain occurs with use of this product.

Keep this and all drugs out of the reach of children. In case of accidental overdose, seek professional assistance or contact a Poison Control Center immediately.

How Supplied: Tablets and caplets in bottles of 24's, 50's and 100's.

Shown in Product Identification Guide, page 503

ALKA-MINTS® Chewable Antacid Rich in Calcium

Active Ingredient: Each ALKA-MINTS Chewable Antacid tablet contains calcium carbonate 850 mg (340 mg of elemental calcium). Each tablet contains less than 0.5 mg sodium per tablet, and is dietarily sodium free.

Inactive Ingredients: Artificial colors, Dioctyl sodium sulfosuccinate, flavor, hydrolyzed cereal solids, magnesium stearate, polyethylene glycol, sorbitol, sugar (compressible).

Indications: For the relief of acid indigestion, heartburn and sour stomach.

Actions: Measured by the in-vitro standard established by the Food and Drug Administration, one ALKA-MINTS tablet neutralizes 15.9 mEq of acid.

Warnings: Do not take more than 9 tablets in a 24 hour period, or use the maximum dosage of this product for more than 2 weeks, except under the advice and supervision of a physician. May cause constipation. As with any drug, if you are pregnant or nursing a baby, seek the advice of a health professional before using this product. Keep this and all drugs out of the reach of children.

Drug Interaction Precaution: Antacids may interact with certain prescription drugs. If you are presently taking a prescription drug, do not take this product without checking with your doctor or other health professional.

Directions: Chew 1 or 2 tablets every 2 hours or as directed by a physician.

How Supplied: Spearmint, Cherry, Tropical and Assorted bottles of 75's.

Product Identification Mark: ALKA-MINTS embossed on each tablet.

Shown in Product Identification Guide, page 503

Continued on next page

Bayer—Cont.

ALEVE®
Naproxen Sodium Tablets, USP
Pain Reliever/Fever Reducer

Allergy Warning: Do not take this product if you have had either hives or a severe allergic reaction after taking any pain reliever. Even though this product may not contain the same ingredient, ALEVE could cause similar reactions in patients allergic to other pain relieving drugs.

Alcohol Warning: If you generally consume 3 or more alcohol-containing drinks per day, you should consult your doctor for advice on when and how you should take ALEVE and other pain relievers.

Active Ingredient: Each [tablet] [caplet] contains naproxen sodium 220 mg (naproxen 200 mg and sodium 20 mg).

Inactive Ingredients: Magnesium Stearate, Microcrystalline Cellulose, Povidone, Talc, Opadry YS-1-4215.

Indications: For the temporary relief of minor aches and pains associated with the common cold, headache, toothache, muscular aches, backache, for the minor pain of arthritis, for the pain of menstrual cramps and for the reduction of fever.

Dosage and Administration:
Adults: Take 1 [tablet] [caplet] every 8 to 12 hours while symptoms persist. With experience, some people may find that an initial dose of 2 [tablets] [caplets] followed by 1 [tablet] [caplet] 12 hours later, if necessary, will give better relief. *Do not exceed 3 [tablets] [caplets] in 24 hours unless directed to do so by a doctor.* The smallest effective dose should be used. A full glass of water or other liquid is recommended with each dose.
Adults over age 65: Do not take more than 1 [tablet] [caplet] every 12 hours, unless directed to do so by a doctor.
Children under age 12: Do not give this product to children under 12, except under the advice and supervision of a doctor.

General Warnings: Do not take ALEVE for more than 10 days for pain, or for more than 3 days for fever, unless directed by a doctor.
Consult a doctor if:
*your pain or fever persists or gets worse
*the painful area is red or swollen
*you take any other drugs on a regular basis
*you have had serious side effects from any pain reliever
*you have any new or unusual symptoms
*more than mild heartburn, upset stomach, or stomach pain occurs with use of this product or if even mild symptoms persist

Although naproxen sodium is indicated for the same conditions as aspirin, ibuprofen and acetaminophen, it should not be taken with them or other naproxen-containing products except under a doctor's direction. As with any drug, if you are pregnant or nursing a baby, seek the advice of a health professional before using this product. IT IS ESPECIALLY IMPORTANT NOT TO USE NAPROXEN SODIUM DURING THE LAST 3 MONTHS OF PREGNANCY UNLESS SPECIFICALLY DIRECTED TO DO SO BY A DOCTOR BECAUSE IT MAY CAUSE PROBLEMS IN THE UNBORN CHILD OR COMPLICATIONS DURING DELIVERY.
Keep this and all drugs out of the reach of children. In case of accidental overdose, seek professional assistance or contact a poison control center immediately. If you have questions, comments or problems, call 1-800-395-0689 to report them.

How Supplied: Light blue round tablets or oval-shaped caplets debossed with "ALEVE". Child-resistant "Safety SquEASE" bottles of 24, 50, 100, and 150 (200 available in caplets) tablets or caplets, with fold-out back label containing important information on the 24 and 50 count bottles.
Storage: Store at room temperature. Avoid excessive heat (104°F or 40°C).

Shown in Product Identification Guide, page 503

ALKA-SELTZER® Original
ALKA-SELTZER® Extra Strength
ALKA-SELTZER® Lemon Lime
ALKA-SELTZER® Cherry
Effervescent Antacid Pain Reliever

Active ingredients:
ALKA-SELTZER® Original:
Aspirin 325 mg, Heat Treated Sodium Bicarbonate 1916 mg, Citric acid 1000 mg.
ALKA-SELTZER® Extra Strength:
Aspirin 500 mg, Heat Treated Sodium Bicarbonate 1985 mg, Citric acid 1000 mg.
ALKA-SELTZER® Lemon Lime and Cherry:
Aspirin 325 mg, Heat Treated Sodium Bicarbonate 1700 mg, Citric acid 1000 mg.

Inactive Ingredients:
ALKA-SELTZER® Original:
none.
ALKA-SELTZER® Extra Strength:
Flavors.
ALKA-SELTZER® Lemon Lime:
Aspartame, Flavor Tableting Aids.
ALKA-SELTZER Cherry:
Aspartame, Flavor Tableting Aids.
Phenylketonurics:
Each tablet contain 9 mg (Lemon Lime) or 12.3 mg (Cherry) of Phenylalanine.
Sodium Content per tablet:
Alka-Seltzer® Original: 567 mg
Alka-Seltzer® Extra Strength: 588 mg
Alka-Seltzer® Lemon Lime and Cherry: 503 mg.

Indications: For fast relief of heartburn, acid indigestion, sour stomach with headache, or body aches and pain. Also for fast relief of upset stomach with headache from overindulgence in food and drink—especially recommended for taking before bed and again on arising.
Effective for pain relief alone: headache, or body and muscular aches and pains.

Directions:
Alka-Seltzer® Original, Cherry and Lemon Lime.
Adults: Dissolve 2 tablets in 4 oz. of water every 4 hours not to exceed 8 tablets in 24 hours. (60 years or older, 4 tablets in a 24-hour period).
Alka-Seltzer® Extra Strength.
Adults: Dissolve 2 tablets in 4 oz. of water every 6 hours not to exceed 7 tablets in 24 hours. (60 years or older, 4 tablets in a 24-hour period).
Caution: If symptoms persist or recur frequently, or if you are under treatment for ulcer, consult your doctor.

Warnings: Children and teenagers should not use this medicine for chicken pox or flu symptoms before a doctor is consulted about Reye syndrome, a rare but serious illness reported to be associated with aspirin. As with any drug, if you are pregnant or nursing a baby, seek the advice of a health professional before using this product. IT IS ESPECIALLY IMPORTANT NOT TO USE ASPIRIN DURING THE LAST 3 MONTHS OF PREGNANCY UNLESS SPECIFICALLY DIRECTED TO DO SO BY A DOCTOR BECAUSE IT MAY CAUSE PROBLEMS IN THE UNBORN CHILD OR COMPLICATIONS DURING DELIVERY.
Except under the advice and supervision of a doctor. Do not take more than, ADULTS: 8 tablets (Extra Strength 7 tablets) in a 24-hour period, (60 years of age or older: 4 tablets in a 24-hour period), or use the daily maximum dosage for more than 10 days. Do not take this product if you are allergic to aspirin or have asthma, if you have bleeding problems, or if you are on a sodium restricted diet.
If ringing in the ears or a loss of hearing occurs, consult a doctor before taking any more of this product.
Do not take this product for pain for more than 10 days unless directed by a doctor. If pain persists or gets worse, if new symptoms occur, or if redness or swelling is present, consult a doctor because these could be signs of a serious condition.
Keep this and all drugs out of the reach of children.

Drug Interaction Precaution: Do not take this product if you are taking a prescription drug for anticoagulation (thinning the blood), diabetes, gout, or arthritis unless directed by a doctor. Antacids may interact with certain prescription drugs. If you are presently taking a prescription drug, do not take this product without checking with your doctor or other health professional.

How Supplied: Foil sealed effervescent tablets in cartons of 12's in 6 foil twin packs; 24's in 12 foil twin packs; 36's in 18 foil twin packs.

Shown in Product Identification Guide, page 503

ALKA-SELTZER® GOLD
Effervescent Antacid
Does not contain aspirin.

Active Ingredients:
Each tablet contains heat treated sodium bicarbonate 958 mg, citric acid 832 mg, potassium bicarbonate 312 mg.

Inative Ingredient: Tableting aid.

Indications:
For relief of acid indigestion, sour stomach or heartburn.
For the symptomatic relief of hyperacidity associated with the diagnosis of peptic ulcer, gastritis, peptic esophagitis, gastric hyperacidity and hiatal hernia.

Actions: The ALKA-SELTZER® Effervescent Antacid solution provides quick and effective neutralization of gastric acid.

Warnings: Except under the advice and supervision of a physician, do not take more than: Adults: 8 tablets in a 24-hour period (60 years of age or older: 7 tablets in a 24-hour period), Children: 4 tablets in a 24-hour period; or use the maximum dosage of this product for more than 2 weeks.
Do not use this product if you are on a sodium restricted diet. Each tablet contains 311 mg of sodium.
Keep this and all drugs out of the reach of children. As with any drug, if you are pregnant or nursing a baby, seek the advice of a health professional before using this product.

Drug Interaction Precaution: Antacids may interact with certain prescription drugs. If you are presently taking a prescription drug, do not take this product without checking with your doctor or other health professional.

Directions: Adults: Take 2 tablets fully dissolved in water every 4 hours. Children: $^1/_2$ the adult dosage or as directed by a doctor.

How Supplied: Boxes of 20 tablets in 10 foil twin packs; 36 tablets in 18 foil twin packs.

Shown in Product Identification Guide, page 503

ALKA-SELTZER PLUS®
Cold & Cough Medicine,
ALKA-SELTZER PLUS®
Night-Time Cold Medicine,
ALKA-SELTZER PLUS®
Cold Medicine,
ALKA-SELTZER PLUS®
Sinus Medicine

Active Ingredients:
ALKA-SELTZER PLUS® Cold & Cough Medicine: Aspirin 325 mg*, Chlorpheniramine Maleate 2 mg, Phenylpropanolamine Bitartrate 20 mg, Dextromethorpan Hydrobromine 10 mg.
ALKA-SELTZER PLUS® Night-Time Cold Medicine: Aspirin 500 mg* Doxylamine Succinate 6.25 mg, Phenylpropanolamine Bitartrate 20 mg, Dextromethorpan Hydrochloride 15 mg.
ALKA-SELTZER PLUS® Cold Medicine: Aspirin 325 mg*, Phenylpropanolamine Bitartrate 24.08 mg, Chlorpheniramine Maleate 2 mg.
ALKA-SELTZER PLUS® Sinus Medicine: Aspirin 325 mg*, Phenylpropanolamine Bitartrate 20 mg.
*In water the aspirin is converted into its soluble ionic form, sodium acetylsalicylate.

Inactive Ingredients:
ALKA-SELTZER PLUS® Cold & Cough Medicine: Aspartame, Citric Acid, Flavor, Sodium Bicarbonate, Tableting aids.

Phenylketonurics: Contains Phenylalanine 11.2 mg per tablet.
ALKA-SELTZER PLUS® Night-Time Cold Medicine:
Aspartame, Citric Acid, Flavors, Sodium Bicarbonate, Tableting aids.

Phenylketonurics: Contains Phenylalanine 16.2 mg per tablet.
ALKA-SELTZER PLUS® Cold Medicine:
Citric Acid, Flavors, Sodium Bicarbonate. (Orange & Cherry Flavors also contain Aspartame and Tableting aids)

****Phenylketonurics:** Cherry contains Phenylalanine 10.08 mg per tablet, Orange contains Phenylalanine 14.03 mg per tablet.
ALKA-SELTZER® Sinus Medicine: Aspartame, Citric Acid, Flavors, Heat-treated Sodium Bicarbonate, Tableting aids.
PHENYLKETONURICS: Contains Phenylalanine 12.32 mg per tablet.
Sodium Content per tablet
Alka-Seltzer Plus Sinus 504 mg
Alka-Seltzer Plus Cold (Orange) 503 mg
Alka-Seltzer Plus Cold, Cherry flavor & Night-Time 506 mg
Alka-Seltzer Plus Cold & Cough 507 mg

Indications: For the temporary relief of these major cold and flu symptoms: **coughing, nasal and sinus congestion, body aches and pains, runny nose, headaches, sneezing, fever, *scratchy sore throat, so you can get the rest you need.

Directions: Adults: Dissolve 2 tablets in approximately 4 oz. of water every 4 hours. Do not exceed 8 tablets in any 24-hour period or as directed by a doctor. Children 12 yrs of age: consult a doctor.

Warning: Children and teenagers should not use this medicine for chicken pox or flu symptoms before a doctor is consulted about Reye syndrome, a rare but serious illness reported to be associated with aspirin. (If sore throat is severe, persists for more than 2 days, is accompanied by high fever, headache, nausea or vomiting, consult a physician promptly.)* As with any drug, if you are pregnant or nursing a baby, seek the advice of a health professional before using this product. **IT IS ESPECIALLY IMPORTANT NOT TO USE ASPIRIN DURING THE LAST 3 MONTHS OF PREGNANCY UNLESS SPECIFICALLY DIRECTED TO DO SO BY A DOCTOR BECAUSE IT MAY CAUSE PROBLEMS IN THE UNBORN CHILD OR COMPLICATIONS DURING DELIVERY.**
Do not exceed recommended dosage. If nervousness, dizziness or sleeplessness occur, discontinue use and consult a doctor. May cause excitability, especially in children. Do not take this product unless directed by a doctor if you are allergic to aspirin, have a breathing problem such as emphysema or chronic bronchitis, asthma, glaucoma, difficulty in urination due to enlargement of the prostate gland, heart disease, high blood pressure, diabetes, thyroid disease, bleeding problems or on a sodium restricted diet.
May cause marked drowsiness; alcohol, sedatives and tranquilizers may increase drowsiness effect. Avoid alcoholic beverages while taking this product. Do not take this product if you are taking sedatives or tranquilizers without first consulting your doctor. Use caution when driving a motor vehicle or operating machinery. [Do not take this product for persistent or chronic cough such as occurs with smoking, asthma, emphysema, or if cough is accompanied by excessive phlegm (muscus), unless directed by a doctor. A persistent cough may be a sign of a serious condition. If cough persists for more than 1 week, tends to recur or is accompanied by fever, rash, or persistent headache, consult a doctor.**] Do not take this product for more than 7 days. If symptoms do not improve or are accompanied by fever or if fever persists for more than 3 days, consult a doctor. Keep this and all drugs out of the reach of children.

Drug Interaction Precaution: Do not take this product if you are presently taking a prescription drug for anticoagulation (thinning the bood), diabetes, gout, arthritis, or are presently taking a monoamine oxidase inhibitor (MAOI) (certain drugs for depression, psychiatric or emotional conditions, or Parkinson's disease), or for 2 weeks after stopping the MAOI drug. If you are uncertain whether your prescription drug contains an MAOI, consult a health professional before taking this product.
*Does not apply to ALKA-SELTZER PLUS Sinus Medicine.
**Applies only to ALKA-SELTZER PLUS Cold & Cough Medicine and Night-Time Cold Medicine.

How Supplied: ALKA-SELTZERPLUS Cold & Cough Medicine, and Night-Time Cold Medicine: Carton of 36 tablets in 18 foil twin packs; carton of 20 tablets in 10 foil twin packs; carton of 12 tablets in 6 foil packs.

Continued on next page

Bayer—Cont.

ALKA-SELTZER PLUS Cold Medicine: Also available in the above sizes, plus carton of 48 in 24 foil twin packs.
ALKA-SELTZER PLUS Sinus: Carton of 20 tablets in 10 foil twin packs
Product Identification Mark:
Shown in Product Identification Guide, page 503

ALKA-SELTZER PLUS® NIGHT-TIME COLD MEDICINE LIQUI-GELS,

ALKA-SELTZER PLUS® COLD & COUGH MEDICINE LIQUI-GELS,

ALKA-SELTZER PLUS® COLD MEDICINE: LIQUI-GELS

Active Ingredients:
ALKA-SELTZER PLUS® NIGHT-TIME COLD MEDICINE:
Dextromethorphan Hydrobromide 10 mg, Doxylamine Succinate 6.25 mg, Pseudoephedrine HCl 30 mg, Acetaminophen 325 mg.
ALKA-SELTZER PLUS® COLD & COUGH MEDICINE:
Dextromethorphan Hydrobromide 10 mg, Chlorpheniramine Maleate 2 mg, Pseudoephedrine HCl 30 mg, Acetaminophen 325 mg.
ALKA-SELTZER PLUS® COLD MEDICINE:
Chlorpheniramine Maleate 2 mg, Pseudoephedrine HCl 30 mg, Acetominophen 325 mg.

Inactive Ingredients: Artificial Colors, Gelatin, Glycerin, Polyethylene Glycol, Potassium Acetate, Povidone, Purified Water, Sorbitol, Titanium Dioxide.

Indications: Provides temporary relief of these major symptoms of cold and flu: *coughing, runny nose, nasal and sinus congestion, headache, body aches and pains, sneezing, fever and sore throat.

Direction for Use: ALKA-SELTZER PLUS® COLD MEDICINE, and COLD & COUGH MEDICINE:
ADULTS: Swallow 2 softgels with water. CHILDREN (6–12 YEARS): Swallow 1 softgel with water. Repeat every 4 hours, not to exceed 4 doses per day, or as directed by a doctor.
CHILDREN (under 6 years): Consult a doctor:
ALKA-SELTZER PLUS® NIGHT-TIME COLD MEDICINE:
Adults: Swallow 2 softgels with water, once daily, at bedtime. Not recommended for children under 12 years.

Warnings: Do not exceed recommended dosage. If nervousness, dizziness or sleeplessness occur, discontinue use and call a doctor. If symptoms do not improve within 7 days or are accompanied by fever, consult a doctor.
If sore throat is severe, persists for more than 2 days, is accompanied by or followed by fever, rash,* headache, nausea or vomiting, consult a doctor promptly. May cause excitability especially in children. Do not take this product, unless directed by a doctor, if you have a breathing problem such as emphysema or chronic bronchitis, or glaucoma, difficulty in urination due to enlargement of the prostate gland or heart disease, high blood pressure, diabetes, or thyroid disease. May cause drowsiness; alcohol, sedatives and tranquilizers may increase drowsiness effect. Avoid alcoholic beverages while taking this product. Do not take this product if you are taking sedatives or tranquilizers without first consulting your doctor. Use caution when driving a motor vehicle or operating machinery. As with any drug, if you are pregnant or nursing a baby seek the advice of a health professional before using this product. Keep this and all medication out of the reach of children. In case of accidental overdose, contact a physician or Poison Control Center immediately. Prompt medical attention is critical for adults as well as children even if you do not notice any signs or symptoms.
(A persistent cough may be a sign of a serious condition. If cough persists for more than 1 week, tends to recur or is accompanied by fever, rash or persistent headache, consult a doctor. Do not take this product for persistent or chronic cough such as occurs with smoking, asthma, emphysema or if cough is accompanied by excessive phlegm (mucus) unless directed by a doctor.)*

Drug Interaction Precaution: Do not take this product if you are now taking a prescription monoamine oxidase inhibitor (MAOI) (certain drugs for depression, psychiatric or emotional conditions, or Parkinson's disease), or for 2 weeks after stopping the MAOI drug. If you are uncertain whether your prescription drug contains an MAOI, consult a health professional before taking this product.
*Does not apply to Alka-Seltzer Plus Cold Medicine.

How Supplied: Carton of 12 and 20 softgels.
Shown in Product Identification Guide, page 503

ALKA-SELTZER® PLUS Flu and Body Aches Formula

Active Ingredients: Acetaminophen 325 mg, Dextromethorphan Hydrobromide 10 mg, Phenylpropanolamine Bitartrate 20 mg, Chlorpheniramine, Maleate 2 mg.

Inactive Ingredients: Aspartame, Calcium Carbonate, Citric Acid, Croscarmellose Sodium, D&C Yellow #10, Flavor, Maltodextrin, Mannitol, Polyvinylpyrrolidone, Sodium Bicarbonate, Sodium Saccharin, Sorbitol, Starch, Stearic Acid, Tableting Aids.

Indications: Provides temporary relief of these symptoms associated with flu and common cold: headache, body aches, fever, coughing, minor sore throat pain, nasal and sinus congestion, runny nose and sneezing.

Directions: ADULTS: Dissolve 2 tablets in 4 oz. of hot (not boiling) water. Sip while hot. Repeat every 4 hours, but not to exceed 4 doses per day, or as directed by a doctor. Children under 12 years of age: consult a doctor.

Warnings: Not recommended for children under 12. **Do not exceed recommended dosage.** If nervousness, dizziness or sleeplessness occur, discontinue use and consult a doctor. If symptoms do not improve within 7 days or are accompanied by fever, consult a doctor. A persistent cough may be a sign of a serious condition. If cough persists for more than 1 week, tends to recur or is accompanied by fever, rash or persistent headache, consult a doctor. Do not take this product for persistent or chronic cough such as occurs with smoking, asthma, emphysema, or if cough is accompanied by excessive phlegm (mucus) unless directed by a doctor. If sore throat is severe, persists for more than 2 days, is accompanied by or followed by fever, headache, rash, nausea, or vomiting, consult a doctor promptly. May cause excitability, especially in children. Do not take this product unless directed by a doctor, if you have a breathing problem such as emphysema or chronic bronchitis, have glaucoma, heart disease, high blood pressure, thyroid disease, diabetes, or difficulty in urination due to enlargement of the prostate gland.
May cause marked drowsiness; alcohol, sedatives and tranquilizers may increase drowsiness effect. Avoid alcoholic beverage while taking this product. Do not take this product if you are taking sedatives or tranquilizers without first consulting your doctor. Use caution when driving a motor vehicle or operating machinery. As with any drug, if you are pregnant or nursing a baby, seek the advice of a health professional before using this product. Keep this and all medication out of the reach of children. In case of accidental overdose, seek professional assistance or Poison Control Center immediately. Prompt medical attention is critical for adults as well as children even if you do not notice any signs or symptoms.
Each tablet contains 111 mg sodium.

Phenylketonurics: Contains Phenylalanine 11.2 mg per tablet.

Drug Interaction Precaution: Do not use this product if you are now taking a prescription monoamine oxidase inhibitor (MAOI) (certain drugs for depression, psychiatric or emotional conditions, or Parkinson's disease) or for 2 weeks after stopping the MAOI drug. If you are uncertain whether your prescription drug contains an MAOI, consult a health professional before taking this product.

How Supplied: Carton of 20 tablets in 10 foil twin packs; carton of 36 tablets in 18 foil twin packs.
Shown in Product Identification Guide, page 504

ALKA-SELTZER® PLUS Flu & Body Aches Liqui-Gels®
Non-Drowsy Formula

Indications: Provides temporary relief of these symptoms associated with flu and common cold including: headache, body aches, fever, coughing, minor sore throat pain, nasal and sinus congestion.

Directions: ADULTS: Swallow 2 softgels with water. CHILDREN (6–12 years): Swallow 1 softgel with water. CHILDREN (under 6 years): Consult a doctor. Repeat every 4 hours, but not to exceed 4 doses per day, or as directed by a doctor.

Active Ingredients: Acetaminophen 325 mg, Pseudoephedrine Hydrochloride 30 mg, Dextromethorphan, Hydrobromide 10 mg.

Inactive Ingredients: FD&C Red #40, Gelatin, Glycerin, Polyethylene Glycol, Potassium Acetate Povidone, Purified Water, Sorbitol, Titanium Dioxide.

Warnings: Do not exceed recommended dosage. If nervousness, dizziness or sleeplessness occur, discontinue use and consult a doctor. If symptoms do not improve within 7 days or are accompanied by fever, consult a doctor. A persistent cough may be a sign of a serious condition. If cough persists for more than 1 week, tends to recur or is accompanied by fever, rash, or persistent headache, consult a doctor. Do not take this product for persistent or chronic cough such as occurs with smoking, asthma, emphysema, or if cough is accompanied by excessive phlegm (mucus) unless directed by a doctor. If sore throat is severe, persists for more than 2 days, is accompanied by or followed by fever, headache, rash, nausea, or vomiting, consult a doctor promptly. Do not take this product if you have heart disease, high blood pressure, thyroid disease, diabetes or difficulty in urination due to enlargement of the prostate gland unless directed by a doctor. As with any drug, if you are pregnant or nursing a baby, seek the advise of a health professional before using this product. Keep this and all medication out of the reach of children. In case of accidental overdose, seek professional assistance or Poison Control Center immediately. Prompt medical attention is critical for adults as well as children even if you do not notice any signs or symptoms.

Drug Interaction Precaution: Do not use this product if you are now taking a prescription monoamine oxidase inhibitor (MAOI) (certain drugs for depression, psychiatric or emotional conditions, or Parkinson's disease), or for 2 weeks after stopping the MAOI drug. If you are uncertain whether your prescription drug contains an MAOI, consult a health professional before taking this product.

How Supplied: ALKA-SELTZER® PLUS Flu and Body Aches Liqui-Gels® are available in blisters of 12 and 20 count.

Shown in Product Identification Guide, page 503

Genuine BAYER® Aspirin
Aspirin (Acetylsalicylic Acid)
Tablets and Caplets

Active Ingredients: 325 mg per tablet or caplet, coated for easy swallowing.

Inactive Ingredients: Hydroxypropyl Methylcellulose Starch and Triacetin.

Indications: For the temporary relief of: headache, pain and fever of colds, muscle aches and pains, menstrual pain, toothache pain, minor aches, and pain of arthritis.

Directions: Adults and Children 12 years and over: One or two tablets/caplets with water every 4 hours, as needed, up to a maximum of 12 tablets/caplets per 24 hours or as directed by a doctor. Do not give to children under 12 unless directed by a doctor.

Warnings: Children and teenagers should not use this medicine for chicken pox or flu symptoms before a doctor is consulted about Reye syndrome, a rare but serious illness reported to be associated with aspirin. Do not take this product for pain for more than 10 days or for fever for more than 3 days unless directed by a doctor. If pain or fever persists or gets worse, if new symptoms occur, or if redness or swelling is present consult a doctor because these could be signs of a serious condition. Do not take this product if you are allergic to aspirin, have asthma, stomach problems that persist or recur, gastric ulcers or bleeding problems unless directed by a doctor. If ringing in the ears or loss of hearing occurs, consult a doctor before taking any more of this product. Keep this and all drugs out of the reach of children. In case of accidental overdose, seek professional assistance or contact a poison control center immediately. As with any drug, if you are pregnant or nursing a baby, seek the advice of a health professional before using this product. **IT IS ESPECIALLY IMPORTANT NOT TO USE ASPIRIN DURING THE LAST 3 MONTHS OF PREGNANCY UNLESS SPECIFICALLY DIRECTED TO DO SO BY A DOCTOR BECAUSE IT MAY CAUSE PROBLEMS IN THE UNBORN CHILD OR COMPLICATIONS DURING DELIVERY.**

Drug Interaction Precaution: Do not take this product if you are taking a prescription drug for anticoagulation (thinning the blood), diabetes, gout, or arthritis unless directed by doctor.

See "Professional Labeling" listing on page 615.

How Supplied:
Genuine Bayer Aspirin 325 mg (5 grains) is supplied in packs of 12 tablets, bottles of 24, 50, 100, 200, 300, and 365 tablets, and bottles of 50 and 100 caplets. Child-resistant safety closures on 12s, 24s, 50s, 200s, 300s, 365s tablets and 50s caplets. Bottles of 100s tablets and caplets available without safety closure for households without small children.

Shown in Product Identification Guide, page 504

ASPIRIN REGIMEN BAYER® 81 mg
ASPIRIN REGIMEN BAYER® 325 mg
Delayed Release Enteric Aspirin
Adult Low Strength 81 mg Tablets and Regular Strength 325 mg Caplets

Composition: Active Ingredient: ASPIRIN REGIMEN BAYER® is an enteric-coated aspirin available in 81 mg tablet and 325 mg caplet forms. The enteric coating prevents disintegration in the stomach and promotes dissolution in the duodenum, where there is a more neutral to alkaline environment. This action aids in protecting the stomach against injuries that may occur as a result of ingesting non-enteric coated aspirin.

Safety: The safety of enteric-coated aspirin has been demonstrated in a number of endoscopic studies comparing enteric-coated aspirin and plain aspirin, as well as buffered aspirin and "arthritis strength" preparations. In these studies, endoscopies were performed in healthy volunteers before and after either 2-day or 14-day administration of aspirin doses of 3,900 or 4,000 mg per day. Compared to all the other preparations, the enteric-coated aspirin produced signficantly less damage to the gastric mucosa. There was also statistically less duodenal damage when compared with the plain, i.e., non-enteric-coated aspirin.

Bioavailability: The bioavailability of aspirin from **ASPIRIN REGIMEN BAYER®** has been confirmed. In single-dose studies[10] in which plasma acetylsalicylic acid and salicylic acid levels were measured, maximum concentrations were achieved at approximately 5 hours postdosing. **ASPIRIN REGIMEN BAYER®**, when compared with plain aspirin, achieves maximum plasma salicylate levels not significantly different from plain, i.e., non-enteric-coated, aspirin. Dissolution of the enteric coating occurs at a neutral to basic pH and is therefore dependent on gastric emptying into the duodenum. With continued dosing, appropriate therapeutic plasma levels are maintained.

Regular Strength 325mg—D&C Yellow #10, FD&C Yellow #6, Hydroxypropyl Methylcellulose, Methacrylic Acid Copolymer, Starch, Titanium Dioxide, Triacetin.

Adult Low Strength 81mg—Croscarmellose Sodium, D&C Yellow #10, FD&C Yellow #6, Hydroxypropyl Methylcellulose, Iron Oxides, Lactose, Methacrylic Acid, Microcrystalline Cellulose,

Continued on next page

Bayer—Cont.

Polysorbate 80, Sodium Lauryl Sulfate, Starch, Titanium Dioxide, Triacetin.

Indications: ASPIRIN REGIMEN BAYER® is an anti-inflammatory, analgesic, and antiplatelet agent indicated for the relief of painful discomfort and muscular aches and pains associated with conditions requiring long-term aspirin therapy, e.g., arthritis or rheumatism, and for situations where compliance with aspirin usage may be hindered by gastrointestinal side effects of non-enteric-coated or buffered aspirin. For additional **Anti-inflammatory, Antiarthritic,** and **Antiplatelet** indications, see the **PROFESSIONAL LABELING** section.

Directions: For nonprescription analgesic indications: Adults & children 12 years and older: Take two 325 mg caplets or eight 81 mg tablets every 4 hours or three 325 mg caplet or twelve 81 mg tablet every 6 hours with water.
Do not exceed 4000 mg in 24 hours. Dosage may modified as directed by a doctor.

Warnings: Children and teenagers should not use this medicine for chicken pox or flu symptoms before a doctor is consulted about Reye Syndrome, a rare but serious illness reported to be associated with aspirin. Do not take for pain for more than 10 days or for fever for more than 3 days unless directed by a doctor. If pain or fever persists or gets worse, if new symptoms occur, or if redness or swelling is present, consult a doctor because these could be signs of a serious condition. Do not take this product if you are allergic to aspirin, have asthma, have stomach problems (such as heartburn, upset stomach or stomach pain) that persist or recur, or have gastric ulcers or bleeding problems unless directed by a doctor. If ringing in the ears or loss of hearing occurs, consult a doctor before taking any more of this product. Keep this and all drugs out of the reach of children. In case of accidental overdose, seek professional assistance or contact a poison control center immediately. As with any drug, if you are pregnant or nursing a baby, seek the advice of a health professional before using this product. **IT IS ESPECIALLY IMPORTANT NOT TO USE ASPIRIN DURING THE LAST 3 MONTHS OF PREGNANCY UNLESS SPECIFICALLY DIRECTED TO DO SO BY A DOCTOR BECAUSE IT MAY CAUSE PROBLEMS IN THE UNBORN CHILD OR COMPLICATIONS DURING DELIVERY.**

Drug Interaction Precaution: Do not take this product if you are taking a prescription drug for anticoagulation (thinning the blood), diabetes, gout, or arthritis unless directed by a doctor.
See "Professional Labeling" listing on page 615.

How Supplied: ASPIRIN REGIMEN BAYER 325 mg—Regular strength 325 mg caplets in bottles of 100 with child-resistant safety closure.
ASPIRIN REGIMEN BAYER 81 mg—Adult Low Strenth 81 mg tablets in bottles of 120 with child-resistant safety closure.

REV. 11/94

Shown in Product Identification Guide, page 504

ASPIRIN REGIMEN BAYER® 81 mg WITH CALCIUM

Each caplet provides 81 mg of aspirin and 10% (100 mg) of the Daily Value of Calcium as part of the buffered base of Calcium Carbonate.

Indications. For the temporary relief of minor aches and pains or as recommended by your doctor.

Directions: Adults and Children 12 years and over, take 4 to 8 caplets with water every 4 hours, as needed, up to a maximum of 32 caplets per 24 hours or as directed by a doctor.

Warnings: Children and teenagers should not use this medicine for chicken pox or flu symptoms before a doctor is consulted about Reye Syndrome, a rare but serious illness reported to be associated with aspirin. Do not take for pain for more than 10 days or for fever for more than 3 days unless directed by a doctor. If pain or fever persists or gets worse, if new symptoms occur or if redness or swelling is present, consult a doctor because these could be signs of a serious condition. Do not take this product if you are allergic to aspirin, have asthma, have stomach problems (such as heartburn, upset stomach or stomach pain) that persist or recur, gastric ulcers or bleeding problems unless directed by a doctor. If ringing in the ears or loss of hearing occurs, consult a doctor before taking any more of this product. Keep this and all drugs out of the reach of children. In case of accidental overdose, seek professional assistance or contact a poison control center immediately. As with any drug, if you are pregnant or nursing a baby, seek the advice of a health professional before using this product. IT IS ESPECIALLY IMPORTANT NOT TO USE ASPIRIN DURING THE LAST 3 MONTHS OF PREGNANCY UNLESS DIRECTED TO DO SO BY A DOCTOR BECAUSE IT MAY CAUSE PROBLEMS IN THE UNBORN CHILD OR COMPLICATIONS DURING DELIVERY.

Drug Interaction Precaution: Do not take this product if you are taking any prescription drug including those for anticoagulation (thinning the blood), diabetes, gout or arthritis unless directed by a doctor.

Active Ingredients: 81 mg Aspirin per caplet in a buffered base of Calcium Carbonate (250 mg = 100 mg of elemental calcium).

Inactive Ingredients: Colloidal Silicon Dioxide, FD&C Blue #2 Lake, Hydroxypropyl Methylcellulose, Microcrystalline Cellulose, Propylene Glycol, Sodium Starch Glycolate, Starch, Titanium Dioxide, Zinc Stearate.
See "Professional Labeling" listing on page 615.

How Supplied: Bottles of 60 count.

Shown in Product Identification Guide, page 504

Aspirin Regimen BAYER® Children's Chewable 81 mg Aspirin Orange & Cherry Flavored

Active Ingredients: 81 mg Aspirin per tablet

Inactive Ingredients: Orange Flavored: Dextrose Excipient, FD&C Yellow #6, Flavor, Saccharin Sodium, Starch. Cherry Flavored: D&C Red #27, Dextrose Excipient, FD&C Red #40, Flavor, Saccharin Sodium, Starch.

Indications: For the temporary relief of minor aches, pains and headaches, and to reduce fever associated with colds, sore throats and teething.

Directions:
Children's Dose: To be administered only under adult supervision.

Age (Years)	Weight (lb)	Dosage
2 to under 4	32 to 35	2 tablets
4 to under 6	36 to 45	3 tablets
6 to under 9	46 to 65	4 tablets
9 to under 11	66 to 76	4–5 tablets
11 to under 12	77 to 83	4–6 tablets
Adults and Children		
12 yrs and over		5–8 tablets

Dosage may be repeated every four hours, while symptoms persist, up to a maximum of five doses per 24 hours or as directed by a doctor. For larger or more frequent doses or for children under 2, consult your doctor before taking.
Ways to Administer: Tablets may be chewed, swallowed or dissolved on tongue followed with a half a glass of liquid. Tablets may also be crushed in a teaspoonful of water followed with a half a glass of liquid.

Warnings: Children and teenagers should not use this medicine for chicken pox or flu symptoms before a doctor is consulted about Reye syndrome, a rare but serious illness reported to be associated with aspirin. Do not take this product for pain for more than 10 days (for adults) or 5 days (for children), and do not take for fever for more than 3 days unless directed by a doctor. If pain or fever persists or gets worse, if new symptoms occur, or if redness or swelling is present, consult a doctor because these could be signs of a serious condition. Do not give this product to children for the pain of arthritis unless directed by a doctor. If sore throat is severe, persists for more than 2 days, is accompanied or followed by fever, head-

ache, rash, nausea, or vomiting, consult a doctor promptly. Do not take this product for at least 7 days after tonsillectomy or oral surgery unless directed by a doctor. Do not take this product if you are allergic to aspirin, have asthma, have stomach problems (such as heartburn, upset stomach or stomach pain) that persist or recur or have gastric ulcers or bleeding problems unless directed by a doctor. If ringing in the ears or loss of hearing occurs, consult a doctor before taking any more of this product.
KEEP THIS AND ALL DRUGS OUT OF THE REACH OF CHILDREN. IN CASE OF ACCIDENTAL OVERDOSE, SEEK PROFESSIONAL ASSISTANCE OR CONTACT A POISON CONTROL CENTER IMMEDIATELY. AS WITH ANY DRUG, IF YOU ARE PREGNANT OR NURSING A BABY, SEEK THE ADVICE OF A HEALTH PROFESSIONAL BEFORE USING THIS PRODUCT. **IT IS ESPECIALLY IMPORTANT NOT TO USE ASPIRIN DURING THE LAST 3 MONTHS OF PREGNANCY UNLESS SPECIFICALLY DIRECTED TO DO SO BY A DOCTOR BECAUSE IT MAY CAUSE PROBLEMS IN THE UNBORN CHILD OR COMPLICATIONS DURING DELIVERY.**

Drug Interaction Precaution: Do not take this product if taking a prescription drug for anticoagulation (thinning the blood), diabetes, gout or arthritis unless directed by a doctor.
See "Professional labeling" listing on page 615.

How Supplied: Bottles of 36 tablets with child-resistant safety closure.
Store at room temperature.

Shown in Product Identification Guide, page 504

PROFESSIONAL LABELING

Genuine Bayer Aspirin
Aspirin Regimen Bayer 325 mg
Aspirin Regimen Bayer 81 mg
Aspirin Regimen Bayer 81 mg with Calcium
Aspirin Regimen Bayer Childrens Chewable 81 mg

Professional Labeling: ANTIARTHRITIC EFFECT

Indication: Conditions requiring chronic or long-aspirin therapy for pain and/or inflammation, e.g., rheumatoid arthritis, juvenile rheumatoid arthritis, systemic lupus erythematosus, osteoarthritis (degenerative joint disease), ankylosing spondylitis, psortatic arthritis, Reiter's syndrome, and fibrositis.

ANTIPLATELET EFFECT
In MI Prophylaxis:

Indication: Aspirin is indicated to reduce the risk of death and/or nonfatal myocardial infarction in patients with a previous infarction or unstable angina pectoris.

Clinical Trials: The indication is supported by the results of six large randomized, multicenter, placebo-controlled studies[1–7] involving 10,816 predominantly male post-myocardial infarction (MI) patients and one randomized placebo-controlled study of 1,266 men with unstable angina.
Aspirin therapy in MI patients was associated with about a 20% reduction in the risk of subsequent death and/or nonfatal reinfarction, a median absolute decrease of 3% from the 12% to 22% event rates in the placebo groups. In the aspirin-treated unstable angina patients, the reduction in risk was about 50%, a reduction in the event rate of 5% from the 10% rate in the placebo group over the 12 weeks of study.
Daily dosage of aspirin in the post-myocardial infarction studies was 300 mg in one study and 900–1,500 mg in five studies. A dose of 325 mg was used in the study of unstable angina.

Adverse Reactions: Gastrointestinal reactions: Doses of 1,000 mg per day of aspirin caused gastrointestinal symptoms and bleeding that, in some cases, were clinically significant. In the largest postinfarction study (the Aspirin Myocardial Infarction Study [AMIS] with 4,500 people), the percentage of incidences of gastrointestinal symptoms for the aspirin (1,000 mg of a standard, solid-tablet formulation), and placebo-treated subjects, respectively, were stomach pain (14.5%, 4.4%), heartburn (11.9%, 4.8%), nausea and/or vomiting (7.6%, 2.1%), hospitalization for GI disorder (4.9%, 3.5%). In the AMIS and other trials, aspirin-treated patients had increased rates of gross gastrointestinal bleeding. Symptoms and signs of gastrointestinal irritation were not significantly increased in subjects treated for unstable angina with buffered aspirin in solution.
Cardiovascular and Biochemical: In the AMIS trial, the dosage of 1,000 mg per day of aspirin was associated with small increases in systolic blood pressure (BP) average 1.5 to 2.1 mm) and diastolic BP (0.5 to 0.6 mm), depending upon whether maximal or last available readings were used. Blood urea nitrogen and uric acid levels were also increased but by less than 1.0 mg percent.
Subjects with marked hypertension or renal insufficiency had been excluded from the trial so that the clinical importance of these observations for such subjects or for any subjects treated over more prolonged periods is not known. It is recommended that patients placed on long-term aspirin treatment, even at doses of 300 mg per day, be seen at regular intervals to assess changes in these measurements.

Dosage and Administration: Although most of the studies used dosages exceeding 300 mg, two trials used only 300 mg daily and pharmacologic data indicate that this dose inhibits platelet function fully. Therefore, 300 mg or a conventional 325 mg aspirin dose daily is a reasonable routine dose that would minimize gastrointestinal adverse reactions. This use of aspirin applies to both solid oral dosage forms (buffered and plain aspirin) and buffered aspirin in solution.

In Transient Ischemic Attacks:

Indication: Aspirin is indicated for reducing the risk of recurrent transient ischemic attacks (TIAs) or stroke in men who have transient ischemia of the brain due to fibrin emboli. There is no evidence that aspirin is effective in reducing TIAs in women, or is of benefit in the treatment of completed strokes in men or women.

Clinical Trials: The indication is supported by the results of a Canadian study[8] in which 585 patients with threatened stroke were followed in a randomized clinical trial for an average of 28 months to determine whether aspirin or sulfinpyrazone, singly or in combination, was superior to placebo in preventing transient ischemic attacks, stroke, or death. The study showed that, although sulfinpyrazone had no statistically significant effect, aspirin reduced the risk of continuing transient ischemic attacks, stroke, or death by 19 percent and reduced the risk of stroke or death by 31 percent. Another aspirin study carried out in the United States with 178 patients showed a statistically significant number of "favorable outcomes," including reduced transient ischemic attacks, stroke, and death.[9]

Precautions: Patients presenting with signs and/or symptoms of TIAs should have a complete medical and neurologic evaluation. Consideration should be given to other disorders which may resemble TIAs. It is important to evaluate and treat, if appropriate, diseases associated with TIAs and stroke, such as hypertension and diabetes.
Concurrent administration of absorbable antacids at therapeutic doses may increase the clearance of salicylates in some individuals. The concurrent administration of nonabsorbable antacids may alter the rate of absorption of aspirin, thereby resulting in a decreased acetylsalicylic acid/salicylate ratio in plasma. The clinical significance of these decreases in available aspirin is unknown.
Aspirin at dosages of 1,000 milligrams per day has been associated with small increases in blood pressure, blood urea nitrogen, and serum uric acid levels. It is recommended that patients placed on long-term aspirin treatment be seen at regular intervals to assess changes in these measurements.

Adverse Reactions: At dosages of 1,000 milligrams or higher of aspirin per day, gastrointestinal side effects include stomach pain, heartburn, nausea and/or vomiting, as well as increased rates of gross gastrointestinal bleeding.

Dosage and Administration: Adult oral dosage for men is 1,300 milligrams a day, in divided doses of 650 milligrams twice a day or 325 milligrams four times a day.

Continued on next page

Bayer—Cont.

Occasional reports have documented individuals with impaired gastric emptying in whom there may be retention of one or more enteric-coated tablets over time. This phenomenon may occur as a result of outlet obstruction from ulcer disease alone or combined with hypotonic gastric peristalsis. Because of the integrity of the enteric coating in an acidic environment, these tablets may accumulate and form a bezoar in the stomach. Individuals with this condition may present with complaints of early satiety or of vague upper abdominal distress.
Diagnosis may be made by endoscopy or by abdominal films, which show opacities suggestive of a mass of small tablets.[11] Management may vary according to the condition of the patient. Options include gastrotomy and alternating slightly basic and neutral lavage.[12] While there have been no clinical reports, it has been suggested that such individuals may also be treated with parenteral cimetidine to reduce acid secretion and then given sips of slightly basic liquids to effect gradual dissolution of the enteric coating. Progress may be followed with plasma salicylate levels or via recognition of tinnitus by the patient. **It should be kept in mind that individuals with a history of partial or complete gastrectomy may produce reduced amounts of acid and therefore have less acidic gastric pH. Under these circumstances, the benefits offered by the acid-resistant enteric coating may not exist.**

References: 1. Elwood PC, et al: A randomized controlled trial of acetylsalicylic acid in the secondary prevention of mortality from myocardial infarction. *Br Med J* 1974;1:436–440. 2. The Coronary Drug Project Research Group: Aspirin in coronary heart disease. *J Chronic Dis* 1976;29:625–642. 3. Breddin K, et al: Secondary prevention of myocardial infarction: A comparison of acetylsalicylic acid, phenprocoumon or placebo. *Homeostasis* 1979;470:263–268. 4. Aspirin Myocardial Infarction Study Research Group: A randomized, controlled trial of aspirin in persons recovered from myocardial infarction. *JAMA* 1980;245:661–669. 5. Elwood PC, Sweetnam PM: Aspirin and secondary mortality after myocardial infarction. *Lancet.* December 22–29, 1979, pp 1313–1315. 6. The Persantine-Aspirin Reinfarction Study Research Group: Persantine and aspirin in coronary heart disease. *Circulation* 1980; 62:449–460. 7. Lewis, IID, et al: Protective effects of aspirin against acute myocardial infarction and death in men with unstable angina: Results of a Veterans Administration Cooperative Study. *N Engl J Med* 1983;309:396–403. 8. The Canadian Cooperative Study Group: A randomized trial of aspirin and sulfinpyrazone in threatened stroke. *N Engl J Med* 1978;299:53–59. 9. Fields WS, et al: Controlled trial of aspirin in cerebral ischemia. *Stroke* 1977;8:301–316. 10. Data on file (Bayer Corporation). 11. Bogacz K. Caldron P: Enteric-coated aspirin bezoar: Evaluation of serum salicylate level by barium study. *Am J Med* 1987; 83:783–786. 12. Baum J, Enteric-coated aspirin and the problem of gastric retention. *J Rheumatol* 1984;11:250–251.

Extra Strength BAYER® Aspirin Arthritis Pain Regimen Formula [aspirin, 500 mg]

Enteric Coated Caplets

The enteric coating on BAYER® Aspirin Arthritis Pain Regimen Formula is designed to allow the caplet to pass through the stomach to the intestine before it dissolves, providing protection against stomach upset.

Indications: For the temporary relief of minor aches and pains of arthritis, rheumatoid arthritis, juvenile rheumatoid arthritis, systemic lupus erythematosus, osteoarthritis, ankylosing spondylitis, psoriatic arthritis, Reiter's syndrome, and fibrositis or as recommended by your doctor.
Because of its delayed action, BAYER® Aspirin Arthritis Pain Regimen Formula will not provide fast relief of headaches, fever or other symptoms needing immediate relief.

Direction: Adults and Children 12 years and over, take 2 caplets with water every 6 hours, as needed, up to a maximum of 8 caplets per 24 hours. Ask your doctor about recommended dosages for other indications.

Warnings: Children and teenagers should not use this medicine for chicken pox or flu symptoms before a doctor is consulted about Reye Syndrome, a rare but serious illness reported to be associated with aspirin. Do not take for pain for more than 10 days or for fever for more than 3 days unless directed by a doctor. If pain or fever persists or gets worse, if new symptoms occur or if redness or swelling is present, consult a doctor because these could be signs of a serious condition. Do not take this product if you are allergic to aspirin, have asthma, have stomach problems (such as heartburn, upset stomach or stomach pain) that persist or recur, gastric ulcers or bleeding problems unless directed by a doctor. If ringing in the ears or loss of hearing occurs, consult a doctor before taking any more of this product. Keep this and all drugs out of the reach of children. In case of accidental overdose, seek professional assistance or contact a poison control center immediately. As with any drug, if you are pregnant or nursing a baby, seek the advice of a health professional before using this product. IT IS ESPECIALLY IMPORTANT NOT TO USE ASPIRIN DURING THE LAST 3 MONTHS OF PREGNANCY UNLESS SPECIFICALLY DIRECTED TO DO SO BY A DOCTOR BECAUSE IT MAY CAUSE PROBLEMS IN THE UNBORN CHILD OR COMPLICATIONS DURING DELIVERY.

Drug Interaction Precaution: Do not take this product if you are taking a prescription drug for anticoagulation (thinning the blood), diabetes, gout or arthritis unless directed by a doctor.

Active Ingredient: 500 mg Aspirin per caplet.

Inactive Ingredients: D&C Yellow #10 FD&C Yellow #6, Hydroxypropyl Methylcellulose, Iron Oxide, Methacrylic Acid Copolymer, Starch, Titanium Dioxide, Triacetin.
Store at room temperature.

How Supplied: Bottles of 50 caplets with a child-resistant safety closure.

Shown in Product Identification Guide, page 504

Extended-Release BAYER® 8-Hour Aspirin Aspirin (acetylsalicylic acid)

Active Ingredients: 650 mg of aspirin in microencapsulated form.

Inactive Ingredients: Guar Gum, Microcrystalline Cellulose, Starch and other ingredients.

Indications: For the temporary relief of nagging, recurring pain of backache, bursitis, minor pain and stiffness of arthritis and rheumatism, sprains, headaches, sinusitis pain, and painful discomfort and fever due to colds and flu.

Directions: Adults and children 12 yrs and over: Take 2 caplets with water every 8 hours. Children under 12 yrs. Consult a doctor. Do not exceed 6 caplets in 24 hours. Two Extended-Release BAYER 8-Hour Aspirin caplets every 8 hours provide effective long-lasting pain relief. Whenever necessary, two caplets 1300 mg or (20 grains) should be given before retiring to provide effective analgesic and anti-inflammatory action—for relief of pain throughout the night and lessening of stiffness upon arising. Do not exceed 6 caplets in 24 hours. This two-caplet 1300 mg or (20-grain) dose of extended-release aspirin promptly produces salicylate blood levels greater than those achieved by a 650 mg (10-grain) dose of regular aspirin, and in the second 4-hour period produces a salicylate blood level curve which approximates that of two successive 650 mg (10-grain) doses of regular aspirin at 4-hour intervals. The 650 mg (10-grain) scored Extended-Release BAYER 8-Hour Aspirin caplets permit administration of aspirin in multiples of 325 mg (5-grains) allowing individualization of dosage to meet the specific needs of the patient. For the convenience of patients on a regular aspirin dosage schedule, two 650 mg (10-grain).

Warnings: Children and teenagers should not use this medicine for chicken pox or flu symptoms before a doctor is consulted about Reye syndrome, a rare but serious illness reported to be associated with aspirin. Do not take for pain for more than 10 days or for fever for more than 3 days unless directed by a doctor. If pain or fever persists or gets worse, if new symptoms occur, or if redness or swelling is present consult a doctor because these could be signs of a serious condition. Do not take this product if you are allergic to aspirin, have asthma, stomach problems that persist or recur, gastric ulcers or bleeding problems unless directed by a doctor. If ringing in the ears or loss of hearing occurs, consult a doctor before taking any more of this product. Keep this and all drugs out of the reach of children. In case of accidental overdose, seek professional assistance or contact a poison control center immediately. As with any drug, if you are pregnant or nursing a baby, seek the advice of a health professional before using this product. **IT IS ESPECIALLY IMPORTANT NOT TO USE ASPIRIN DURING THE LAST 3 MONTHS OF PREGNANCY UNLESS SPECIFICALLY DIRECTED TO DO SO BY A DOCTOR BECAUSE IT MAY CAUSE PROBLEMS IN THE UNBORN CHILD OR COMPLICATIONS DURING DELIVERY.**

Drug Interaction Precaution: Do not take this product if you are taking a prescription drug for anticoagulation (thinning of the blood), diabetes, gout, or arthritis unless directed by a doctor.

How Supplied: Bottles of 50 caplets with a child-resistant safety closure. Store at room temperature.

Shown in Product Identification Guide, page 504

Extra Strength BAYER® Aspirin
Aspirin (Acetylsalicylic Acid)
Caplets and Tablets

Active Ingredients: Extra Strength Bayer Aspirin—Aspirin 500 mg (7.7 grains) contains a thin, inert, Hydroxypropyl Methylcellulose coating for easier swallowing. This is not an enteric coating and does not alter the onset of action of Bayer Aspirin.

Inactive Ingredients: Starch and Triacetin.

Indications: Analgesic, antipyretic, anti-inflammatory. For relief of headache; painful discomfort and fever of colds; muscular aches and pains; temporary relief of minor pains of arthritis; toothache, and pain following dental procedures; menstrual pain.

Directions: Adults and Children 12 years and over: Take 1 or 2 tablets/caplets with water every 4 to 6 hours, as needed up to a maximum of 8 tablets/caplets per 24 hours or as directed by a doctor. Do not give to children under 12 unless directed by a doctor.

Warnings: Children and teenagers should not use this medicine for chicken pox or flu symptoms before a doctor is consulted about Reye syndrome, a rare but serious illness reported to be associated with aspirin. Do not take this product for pain for more than 10 days or for fever for more than 3 days unless directed by a doctor. If pain or fever persists or gets worse, if new symptoms occur, or if redness or swelling is present consult a doctor because these could be signs of a serious condition. Do not take this product if you are allergic to aspirin, have asthma, stomach problems that persist or recur, gastric ulcers or bleeding problems unless directed by a doctor. If ringing in the ears or loss of hearing occurs, consult a doctor before taking any more of this product. Keep this and all drugs out of the reach of children. In case of accidental overdose, seek professional assistance or contact a poison control center immediately. As with any drug, if you are pregnant or nursing a baby, seek the advice of a health professional before using this product. **IT IS ESPECIALLY IMPORTANT NOT TO USE ASPIRIN DURING THE LAST 3 MONTHS OF PREGNANCY UNLESS SPECIFICALLY DIRECTED TO DO SO BY A DOCTOR BECAUSE IT MAY CAUSE PROBLEMS IN THE UNBORN CHILD OR COMPLICATIONS DURING DELIVERY.**

Drug Interaction Precaution: Do not take this product if you are taking a prescription drug for anticoagulation (thinning the blood), diabetes, gout, or arthritis unless directed by a doctor.

How Supplied: Extra Strength Bayer Aspirin 500 mg (7.7 grains) is available in bottles of 24, 50 and 100 caplets, and bottles of 50 tablets.

Shown in Product Identification Guide, page 504

Extra Strength BAYER® PLUS
Buffered Aspirin
Extra Strength BAYER® Aspirin
Caplets and Tablets

Active Ingredients: 500 mg Aspirin
Extra Strength BAYER Plus is buffered with Calcium Carbonate
Extra Strength BAYER aspirin is coated for easier swallowing.

Inactive Ingredients: Extra Strength BAYER Aspirin: Hydroxypropyl Methylcellulose, Starch and Triacetin.
Extra Strength BAYER PLUS: Colloidal Silicon Dioxide, D&C Red #7 Lake, FD&C Blue #2 Lake, Hydroxypropyl Methylcellulose, Microcrystalline Cellulose, Propylene Glycol, Sodium Starch Glycolate, Starch, Titanium Dioxide, Zinc Stearate.

Indications: Temporary relief of: headache, pain and fever of colds, muscle aches and pains, menstrual pain, toothache pain, minor aches and pains of arthritis.

Directions: Adults and Children 12 years and over: Take 1 or 2 tablets or caplets with water every 4 to 6 hours, as needed, up to a maximum of 8 tablets/caplets per 24 hours or as directed by a doctor. Do not give to children under 12 unless directed by a doctor.

Warnings: Children and teenagers should not use this medicine for chicken pox or flu symptoms before a doctor is consulted about Reye syndrome, a rare but serious illness reported to be associated with aspirin. Do not take this product for pain for more than 10 days or for fever for more than 3 days unless directed by a doctor. If pain or fever persists or gets worse, if new symptoms occur, or if redness or swelling is present consult a doctor because these could be signs of a serious condition. Do not take this product if you are allergic to aspirin, have asthma, stomach problems that persist or recur, gastric ulcers or bleeding problems unless directed by a doctor. If ringing in the ears or loss of hearing occurs, consult a doctor before taking any more of this product. Keep this and all drugs out of the reach of children. In case of accidental overdose, seek professional assistance or contact a poison control center immediately. As with any drug, if you are pregnant or nursing a baby, seek the advice of a health professional before using this product. **IT IS ESPECIALLY IMPORTANT NOT TO USE ASPIRIN DURING THE LAST 3 MONTHS OF PREGNANCY UNLESS SPECIFICALLY DIRECTED TO DO SO BY A DOCTOR BECAUSE IT MAY CAUSE PROBLEMS IN THE UNBORN CHILD OR COMPLICATIONS DURING DELIVERY.**

Drug Interaction Precaution: Do not take this product if you are taking a prescription drug for anticoagulation (thinning the blood), diabetes, gout or arthritis unless directed by a doctor.

How Supplied: Extra Strength Bayer Plus Aspirin (500 mg) —bottles of 50 caplets pouches of 2's.
Extra Strength Bayer Aspirin—bottles of 24's and 50's and 100's.

Shown in Product Identification Guide, page 504

Extra Strength BAYER® PM
Aspirin Plus Sleep Aid
[500 mg aspirin/diphenhydramine HCl]

Indications: For the temporary relief of occasional headaches and minor aches and pains with accompanying sleeplessness.

Directions: Adults and Children 12 years of age and over, take 2 caplets with water at bedtime, if needed, or as directed by a doctor.

Warnings: Do not give to children under 12 years of age. **Children and teenagers should not use this medicine for chicken pox or flu symptoms before a doctor is consulted about Reye Syndrome, a rare but serious illness reported to be associated with aspirin.**

Continued on next page

Bayer—Cont.

Do not take this product for pain for more than 10 days or for fever for more than 3 days unless directed by a doctor. If pain or fever persists or gets worse, if new symptoms occur, or if redness or swelling is present, consult a doctor because these could be signs of a serious condition. Do not take this product if you are allergic to aspirin or if you have asthma unless directed by a doctor. If ringing in the ears or a loss of hearing occurs, consult a doctor before taking any more of this product. Do not take this product if you have stomach problems (such as heartburn, upset stomach, or stomach pain) that persist or recur, or if you have ulcers or bleeding problems, unless directed by a doctor. If sleeplessness persists continuously for more than 2 weeks, consult your doctor. Insomnia may be a symptom of serious underlying medical illness. Do not take this product, unless directed by a doctor, if you have a breathing problem such as emphysema or chronic bronchitis, or if you have glaucoma or difficulty in urination due to enlargement of the prostate gland. Avoid alcoholic beverages while taking this product. Do not take this product if you are taking sedatives or tranquilizers, without first consulting your doctor. Keep this and all drugs out of the reach of children. In case of accidental overdose, seek professional assistance or contact a poison control center immediately. As with any drug, if you are pregnant or nursing a baby, seek the advice of a health professional before using this product. IT IS ESPECIALLY IMPORTANT NOT TO USE ASPIRIN DURING THE LAST 3 MONTHS OF PREGNANCY UNLESS SPECIFICALLY DIRECTED TO DO SO BY A DOCTOR BECAUSE IT MAY CAUSE PROBLEMS IN THE UNBORN CHILD OR COMPLICATIONS DURING DELIVERY.

Drug Interaction Precaution: Do not take this product if you are taking a prescription drug for anticoagulation (thinning the blood), diabetes, gout, or arthritis unless directed by a doctor.

Active Ingredients: 500 mg Aspirin, 25 mg Diphenhydramine Hydrochloride per caplet.

Inactive Ingredients: Colloidal Silicon Dioxide, Dibasic Calcium Phosphate, Dibutyl Sebacate, Ethylcellulose, FD&C Blue #1 Lake, FD&C Blue #2 Lake, Hydroxypropyl Methylcellulose, Microcrystalline Cellulose, Oleic Acid, Propylene Glycol, Starch, Titanium Dioxide, Zinc Stearate.
Store at room temperature.

How Supplied: Bottles of 24 caplets with a child-resistant safety closure.

Shown in Product Identification Guide, page 504

BUGS BUNNY™ Children's Chewable Vitamins Plus Iron (Sugar Free)
FLINTSTONES® Children's Chewable Vitamins
FLINTSTONES® Plus Iron Children's Chewable Vitamins

Vitamin Ingredients: Each multivitamin supplement with iron contains the ingredients listed in the chart below:

BUGS BUNNY™ Children's Chewable Vitamins Plus Iron (Sugar Free)
FLINTSTONES® Children's Chewable Vitamins Plus Iron

Vitamins	Quantity per Tablet	% Daily Value for Children 2–4 Years of Age	% Daily Value for Adults/Children 4 or More Years of Age
Vitamin A (As Acetate and Beta Carotene)	2500 I.U.	100%	50%
Vitamin C	60 mg	150%	100%
Vitamin D	400 I.U.	100%	100%
Vitamin E	15 I.U.	150%	50%
Thiamin	1.05 mg	150%	70%
Riboflavin	1.2 mg	150%	70%
Niacin	13.5 mg	150%	67%
Vitamin B_6	1.05 mg	150%	52%
Folate	300 mcg	150%	75%
Vitamin B_{12}	4.5 mcg.	150%	75%
Iron (Elemental)	15 mg	150%	83%

FLINTSTONES® Children's Chewable Vitamins provide the same quantities of vitamins, but do not provide iron.

Indication: Dietary supplementation.

Dosage and Administration: For adults and children two years and older chew one tablet daily. Tablet must be chewed.

Warning
For Bugs Bunny Only: Phenylketonurics: Contains Phenylalanine.

Precaution:
IRON SUPPLEMENTS ONLY.
Close tightly and keep out of reach of children. Contains iron, which can be harmful or fatal to children in large doses. In case of accidental overdose, seek professional assistance or contact a Poison Control Center immediately.
KEEP OUT OF REACH OF CHILDREN.

CHILD RESISTANT CAP
Do not use this product if safety seal bearing Bayer Corporation under cap is torn or missing.

How Supplied: Flintstones are supplied in bottles of 60 and 100, Bugs Bunny in bottles of 60 with child-resistant caps.

Shown in Product Identification Guide, page 504

DOMEBORO® Astringent Solution (Powder Packets)

DOMEBORO® Astringent Solution (Effervescent Tablets)

Active Ingredients: When dissolved in water, the active ingredient is aluminum acetate resulting from the reaction of calcium acetate (938 mg) and aluminum sulfate (1191 mg) for powder packets, and calcium acetate (604 mg) and aluminum sulfate (878 mg) for the effervescent tablets. The resulting astringent solution is buffered to an acid pH.

Inactive Ingredients: DOMEBORO Astringent Solution (Powder Packets) Dextrin
DOMEBORO Astringent Solution (Effervescent Tablets) Dextrin, Polyethylene Glycol, Sodium Bicarbonate

Directions: For powder packets dissolve 1 or 2 packets, or for effervescent tablets 1 or 2 tablets in water and stir the solution until fully dissolved. Do not strain or filter the solution. Can be used as a compress, wet dressing or as a soak. AS A COMPRESS OR WET DRESSING: Saturate a clean, soft, white cloth (such as a diaper or torn sheet) in the solution; gently squeeze and apply loosely to the affected area. Saturate the cloth in the solution every 15 to 30 minutes and apply to the affected area. Discard solution after each use. Repeat as often as necessary. AS A SOAK: Soak affected area in the solution for 15 to 30 minutes. Discard solution after each use. Repeat 3 times a day.

Indications: For temporary relief of minor skin irritations due to poison ivy, poison oak, poison sumac, insect bites, athlete's foot or rashes caused by soaps, detergents, cosmetics or jewelry.

Warnings: If condition worsens or symptoms persist for more than 7 days discontinue use of the product and consult a doctor. For external use only. Avoid contact with eyes. Do not cover compress or wet dressing with plastic to prevent evaporation. Keep this and all drugs out of the reach of children. In case of accidental ingestion, seek professional assistance or contact a Poison Control Center immediately.

How Supplied: Boxes of 12 or 100 effervescent tablets or powder packets.

Shown in Product Identification Guide, page 504

FEMSTAT® 3
(butoconazole nitrate)
2% vaginal cream
Antifungal

ACTIVE INGREDIENTS: Butoconazole Nitrate (2%).

INACTIVE INGREDIENTS: Cetyl Alcohol, Glyceryl Stearate (and) PEG-100 Stearate, Methylparaben and Propylparaben (preservatives), Mineral Oil, Polysorbate 60, Propylene Glycol, Sorbitan Monostearate, Stearyl Alcohol and Water (purified).

Femstat® 3 is the first 3-day medicine available without a prescription for the treatment of vaginal yeast (Candida) infections.

Femstat 3 is clinically proven to cure most yeast infections with only 3 days of treatment.

IF THIS IS THE FIRST TIME YOU HAVE HAD VAGINAL ITCH AND DISCOMFORT, CONSULT YOUR DOCTOR. IF YOU HAVE HAD A DOCTOR DIAGNOSE A VAGINAL YEAST INFECTION BEFORE AND HAVE THE SAME SYMPTOMS NOW, USE FEMSTAT 3 AS DIRECTED FOR 3 CONSECUTIVE DAYS.

Directions For Use: Disposable Cardboard Applicator

IMPORTANT: In order to help ensure proper dosage, please familiarize yourself with the disposable applicator before using the product. To do this, pull the ends of the disposable applicator apart until you see an arrow pointing to the "full" line as described in step 3. Push the disposable applicator back together.

1. Open the tube of cream.

- *Remove the cap from the tube.*
- *Turn the cap upside down.*
- *Using the point on the cap, puncture the protective seal on the tube.*

2. Attach white end *of disposable applicator over opening of tube of cream and push until secure.*

3. Slowly squeeze *the tube of cream until you see the "full" line on the disposable applicator appear.*

4. Remove *disposable applicator from tube of cream and use immediately.*

5. Insert the disposable applicator into the vagina.

- *Lie down with your knees bent to insert.*
- *Hold the applicator with your thumb and forefinger.*
- *Beginning with the white end, gently insert the applicator into the vagina.*
- *Insert as far as the applicator will go comfortably.*

6. To dispense the cream, *slowly push the blue end of the applicator in as far as it will go.*

7. Remove the cardboard applicator and throw it away.

- *Some cream may be left in the applicator, but if you pushed the blue end of the applicator until it stopped, you will be getting the proper dosage.*
- *Do not flush the disposable applicator in toilet.*

8. Repeat steps #2 through #7 for the next two days, preferably at bedtime.

DO NOT USE TAMPONS.

Pre-Filled Applicator

1. Tear open the foil wrapper and remove one Femstat 3 pre-filled applicator. The Femstat 3 applicator has a special tip on the end. Do not remove tip; do not use if tip has been removed. Do not warm applicator before using.

2. While holding the applicator firmly, pull the ring back to fully extend the plunger.

3. Hold the applicator by the outer cylinder with the thumb and forefinger. Lie down with your knees bent to insert the applicator into the vagina as far as it will go comfortably.

4. Push the plunger to release the cream. Remove the applicator and throw it away. Some cream may be left in the applicator, but if you pushed the plunger until it stopped, you are getting the proper dosage.

5. Repeat this procedure for the next two days, preferably at bedtime.

DO NOT USE TAMPONS.

WARNINGS:

- **Do not use if you have abdominal pain, fever, or foul-smelling discharge. Contact your doctor immediately.**
- **If your infection isn't gone in three days, you may have a condition other than a yeast infection or you may need to use more medication. Consult your doctor. If your symptoms return within two months or if you think you have been exposed to the human immunodeficiency virus (HIV) that causes AIDS, consult your doctor immediately. Recurring infections may be a sign of pregnancy or a serious condition, such as AIDS or diabetes.**
- **Do not use this product if you are pregnant or think you may be pregnant, have diabetes, a positive HIV test or AIDS. Consult Your Doctor.**
- Do not rely on condoms or diaphragms to prevent sexually transmitted diseases or pregnancy while using this product. This product may damage condoms and diaphragms and may cause them to fail. Use another method of birth control to prevent pregnancy while using this product.
- Do not use tampons while using this medicine.
- Do not use in girls under 12 years of age.
- **Keep this and all drugs out of the reach of children.**
- For vaginal use only. Do not use in eyes or take by mouth. In case of accidental ingestion, seek professional assistance or contact a Poison Control Center immediately.
- If your doctor has previously told you that you are sensitive or allergic to any Femstat product, do not use Femstat 3 without talking to your doctor first.

The tube opening should be sealed. Do not use if seal has a hole in it or if the seal can not be seen.

CONTENTS: Disposable Cardboard Applicator: One 20g (0.67 oz) tube of vaginal cream and 3 disposable applicators. Pre-Filled Applicator: Three disposable applicators pre-filled to deliver 5 g vaginal cream (butoconazole nitrate 2%).

Avoid excessive heat above 30°C (86°F) and avoid freezing.

Distributed by
Bayer Corporation
Consumer Care Division
Morristown, NJ 07960 USA

Shown in Product Identification Guide, page 504

FLINTSTONES® COMPLETE
With Iron, Calcium & Minerals
Children's Chewable Vitamins

BUGS BUNNY™ COMPLETE
Children's Chewable
Vitamins + Minerals
With Iron and Calcium
(Sugar Free)

Ingredients: Each supplement provides the ingredients listed in the chart below:

FLINTSTONES® COMPLETE
Children's Chewable Vitamins
BUGS BUNNY™ COMPLETE
Children's Chewable
Vitamins + Minerals
(Sugar Free)

		% Daily Value for	
Vitamins	**Quantity per Tablet**	**Children 2–4 Years of Age**	**Adults/ Children 4 or More Years of Age**
Vitamin A (As Acetate and Beta Carotene)	5000 I.U.	100%	100%
Vitamin C	60 mg	75%	100%
Vitamin D	400 I.U.	50%	100%
Vitamin E	30 I.U.	150%	100%

Continued on next page

Bayer—Cont.

Thiamin	1.5 mg	107%	100%
Riboflavin	1.7 mg	106%	100%
Niacin	20 mg	111%	100%
Vitamin B_6	2 mg	143%	100%
Folate	400 mcg	100%	100%
Vitamin B_{12}	6 mcg	100%	100%
Biotin	40 mcg	13%	13%
Pantothenic Acid	10 mg	100%	100%
Calcium	100 mg	6%	10%
Iron (Elemental)	18 mg	90%	100%
Phosphorus	100 mg	6%	10%
Iodine	150 mcg	107%	100%
Magnesium	20 mg	5%	5%
Zinc	15 mg	94%	100%
Copper	2 mg	100%	100%

Indication: Dietary Supplementation.

Dosage and Administration: 2–4 years of age: Chew one-half tablet daily. Over 4 years of age: Chew one tablet daily.

Warning for Bugs Bunny only: Phenylketonurics: Contains Phenylalanine.

Precaution: Close tightly and keep out of reach of children. Contains iron, which can be harmful or fatal to children in large doses. In case of accidental overdose, seek professional assistance or contact a Poison Control Center immediately.

KEEP OUT OF REACH OF CHILDREN.
CHILD RESISTANT CAP

Do not use this product if safety seal bearing Bayer Corporation under cap is torn or missing.

How Supplied: Bottles of 60's with child-resistant caps.

Shown in Product Identification Guide, page 504

FLINTSTONES® PLUS CALCIUM with Beta Carotene Children's Chewable Vitamins

Ingredients: Calcium Carbonate, Sorbitol, Starch, Sodium Ascorbate, Natural & Artificial Flavors (including fruit acids), Glycerides of Stearic & Palmitic Acid, Gelatin, Magnesium Stearate, Vitamin E Acetate, Niacinamide, Artificial Colors (including Yellow #6), Aspartame* (a sweetener), Pyridoxine Hydrochloride, Riboflavin, Thiamine Mononitrate, Vitamin A Acetate, Monoammonium Glycyrrhizinate, Folic Acid, Beta Carotene, Vitamin D, Vitamin B_{12}.

* Phenylketonurics: contains phenylalanine

One Tablet Daily Provides: Vitamins	Quantity Per Tablet	Percent U.S. RDA For Children 2 to 4 Years of Age	For Adults and Children Over 4 Years of Age
Vitamin A (as Acetate and Beta Carotene)	**2500 I.U.**	**100**	**50**
Vitamin D	400 I.U.	100	100
Vitamin E	15 I.U.	150	50
Vitamin C	60 mg	150	100
Folic Acid	0.3 mg	150	75
Thiamin	1.05 mg	150	70
Riboflavin	1.20 mg	150	70
Niacin	13.50 mg	150	67
Vitamin B_6	1.05 mg	150	52
Vitamin B_{12}	4.5 mcg	150	75

Minerals	Quantity	Percent U.S. RDA	
Calcium	200 mg	25	20

Indications: For dietary supplementation.

Dosage and Administration: FOR ADULTS AND CHILDREN 2 YEARS AND OLDER CHEW ONE TABLET DAILY. TABLET MUST BE CHEWED

KEEP OUT OF REACH OF CHILDREN.
CHILD RESISTANT CAP

Do not use this product if safety seal bearing Bayer Corporation under cap is torn or missing.

How Supplied: Bottle of 60 Tablets

Shown in Product Identification Guide, page 505

FLINTSTONES® Plus Extra C Children's Chewable Vitamins
BUGS BUNNY™ With Extra C Children's Chewable Vitamins (Sugar Free)

Vitamin Ingredients: Each multivitamin supplement contains the ingredients listed in the chart below:

BUGS BUNNY™ With Extra C Children's Chewable Vitamins (Sugar Free)
FLINTSTONES® Plus Extra C Children's Chewable Vitamins

Vitamins	Quantity per Tablet	% Daily Value for Children 2–4 Years of Age	Adults/Children 4 or More Years of Age
Vitamin A Acetate and Beta Carotene	2500 I.U.	100%	50%
Vitamin C	250 mg	625%	417%
Vitamin D	400 I.U.	100%	100%
Vitamin E	15 I.U.	150%	50%
Thiamin	1.05 mg	150%	70%
Riboflavin	1.2 mg	150%	70%
Niacin	13.5 mg	150%	67%
Vitamin B_6	1.05 mg	150%	52%
Folate	300 mcg	150%	75%
Vitamin B_{12}	4.5 mcg	150%	75%

Indication: Dietary supplementation.

Dosage and Administration: One tablet daily for adults and children two years and older; tablet must be chewed.

Warning
For Bugs Bunny Only: Phenylketonurics: Contains Phenylalanine.

KEEP OUT OF REACH OF CHILDREN.
CHILD RESISTANT CAP

Do not use this product if safety seal bearing Bayer Corporation under cap is torn or missing.

How Supplied: Flintstones in bottles of 60's & 100's, Bugs Bunny in bottles of 60 with child-resistant caps.

Shown in Product Identification Guide, page 505

Maximum Strength
MIDOL®Teen
Menstrual Formula
Multi-Symptom Formula
Aspirin and Caffeine Free

Active Ingredients: Each caplet contains Acetaminophen 500 mg and Pamabrom 25 mg.

Inactive Ingredients: Croscarmellose Sodium, D&C Red #7 Lake, FD&C Blue #2 Lake, Hydroxpropyl Methylcellulose, Magnesium Stearate, Microcrystaline Cellulose, Starch, Titanium Dioxide and Triacetin.

Indications: Relieves cramps, bloating, water-weight gain, headaches, backaches and muscular aches and pains.

Directions: Adults and children 12 years and over: Take 2 caplets with water. Repeat every 4 hours, as needed, up to a maximum of 8 caplets per day. Under age 12: Consult your doctor.

Warnings: Do not use for more than 10 days unless directed by a doctor. If pain persists for more than 10 days, consult a doctor immediately. Keep this and all drugs out of reach of children. In case of accidental overdose, immediate medical attention is essential for adults as well as for children even if you do not notice any signs or symptoms. As with any drug, if you are pregnant or nursing a baby, seek the advice of a health professional before using this product.

How Supplied: White capsule-shaped caplets available in packages of 2 blisters of 8 caplets each and bottles of 32 caplets. Child-resistant safety closure on bottles of 32 caplets.

Shown in Product Identification Guide, page 505

Maximum Strength
Multi-Symptom Formula
MIDOL®
Menstrual Formula
Aspirin Free

Active Ingredients: Each caplet or gelcap contains Acetaminophen 500 mg, Caffeine 60 mg and Pyrilamine Maleate 15 mg.

Inactive Ingredients: Caplets—Croscarmellose Sodium, FD&C Blue #2, Hydroxypropyl Methylcellulose, Magnesium Stearate, Microcrystalline Cellulose, Pregelatinized Starch and Triacetin.
Gelcaps—Croscarmellose Sodium, D&C Red #33 Lake, EDTA Sodium, FD&C Blue #1 Lake, Gelatin, Glycerin, Hydroxypropyl Methylcellulose, Iron Oxide, Magnesium Stearate, Microcrystalline Cellulose, Starch, Stearic Acid, Titanium Dioxide, Triacetin.

Indications: Relieves all of these physical menstrual symptoms: cramps, bloating, water-weight gain, headaches, backaches, muscular aches and fatigue.

Directions: Adults and children 12 years and over: Take 2 caplets or gelcaps with water. Repeat every 4–6 hours, as needed, up to a maximum of 8 caplets or gelcaps per day. Under age 12: Consult your doctor.

Warnings: Do not use for more than 10 days unless directed by a doctor. If pain persists for more than 10 days, consult a doctor immediately. May cause drowsiness; alcohol, sedatives and tranquilizers may increase drowsiness. Avoid alcoholic beverages while taking this product. Do not take this product if you are taking sedatives and tranquilizers without first consulting your doctor. Use caution when driving or operating machinery. May cause excitability, especially in children. The recommended dose of this product contains about as much caffeine as a cup of coffee. Limit the use of caffeine-containing medications, foods, or beverages while taking this product because too much caffeine may cause nervousness, irritability, sleeplessness, and occasionally, rapid heartbeat. Do not take this product, unless diected by a doctor, if you have a breathing problem such as emphysema or chronic bronchitis or if you have glaucoma or difficulty in urination due to enlargement of the prostate gland. Keep this and all drugs out of reach of children. In case of accidental overdose, immediate medical attention is essential for adults as well as for children even if you do not notice any signs or symptoms. As with any drug, if you are pregnant or nursing a baby, seek the advice of a health professional before using this product.

How Supplied: Caplets—White capsule-shaped caplets available in bottles of 8 and 32 caplets, and packages of 2 blisters of 8 caplets each. Child-resistant safety closures on bottles of 8 and 32 caplets.
Gelcaps—Dark/light blue capsule-shaped gelcaps available in bottles of 24 gelcaps and packages of 2 blisters of 6 gelcaps each. Child-resistant safety closure on bottle of 24 gelcaps.

Shown in Product Identification Guide, page 505

MIDOL®
PMS Formula
Premenstrual Symptom Relief
Aspirin and Caffeine Free

Active Ingredients: Each caplet or gelcap contains Acetaminophen 500 mg, Pamabrom 25 mg and Pyrilamine Maleate 15 mg.

Inactive Ingredients: Caplets—Croscarmellose Sodium, D&C Red #30, D&C Yellow #10, Hydroxypropyl Methylcellulose, Magnesium Stearate, Microcrystalline Cellulose, Pregelatinized Starch and Triacetin.
Gelcaps—Croscarmellose Sodium, D&C Red #27 Lake, EDTA Disodium, FD&C Blue #1, FD&C Red #40 Lake, Gelatin, Glycerin, Hydroxypropyl Methylcellulose, Iron Oxide, Magnesium Stearate, Microcrystalline Cellulose, Starch, Stearic Acid, Titanium Dioxide, Triacetin.

Indications: Contains maximum strength medication for all these premenstrual symptoms: bloating, water-weight gain, cramps, headaches and backaches.

Directions: Adults and children 12 years and over: Take 2 caplets or gelcaps with water. Repeat every 4 hours, as needed, up to a maximum of 8 caplets or gelcaps per day. Under age 12: Consult your doctor.

Warnings: Do not use for more than 10 days unless directed by doctor. If pain persists for more than 10 days, consult a doctor immediately. May cause drowsiness; alcohol, sedatives and tranquilizers may increase drowsiness. Avoid alcoholic beverages while taking this product. Do not take this product if you are taking sedatives or tranquilizers without first consulting your doctor. Use caution when driving or operating machinery. May cause excitability especially in children. Do not take this product, unless directed by a doctor, if you have a breathing problem such as emphysema or chronic bronchitis or if you have glaucoma or difficulty in urination due to enlargement of the prostate gland. Keep this and all drugs out of the reach of children. In case of accidental overdose, immediate medical attention is essential for adults as well as for children even if you do not notice any signs or symptoms. As with any drug, if you are pregnant or nursing a baby, seek the advice of a health professional before using this product.

How Supplied: Caplets—White capsule-shaped caplets available in packages of 2 blisters of 8 caplets each and bottles of 32 caplets. Child-resistant safety closure on bottles of 32 caplets.
Gelcaps—Dark/light pink capsule-shaped gelcaps available in bottles of 24 gelcaps and packages of 2 blisters of 6 gelcaps each. Child-resistant safety closure on bottle of 24 gelcaps.

Shown in Product Identification Guide, page 505

MYCELEX® OTC
CREAM ANTIFUNGAL

Active Ingredient: Clotrimazole 1%

Inactive Ingredients: Benzyl alcohol (1%) as a preservative, cetostearyl alcohol, cetyl esters wax, octyldodecanol, polysorbate 60, purified water, sorbitan monostearate.
Store between 2°–30°C (36°–86°F).

Indications: Cures athlete's foot (tinea pedis), jock itch (tinea cruris), and ringworm (tinea corporis). For effective relief of the itching, cracking, burning and discomfort which can accompany these conditions.

Continued on next page

Bayer—Cont.

Warnings: For external use only. Do not use on children under 2 years of age except under the advice and supervision of a doctor. If irritation occurs or if there is no improvement within 4 weeks (for athlete's foot or ringworm) or within 2 weeks (for jock itch) discontinue use and consult a doctor or pharmacist. Keep this and all drugs out of the reach of children. In case of accidental ingestion seek professional assistance or contact a Poison Control Center immediately. Use only as directed.

Directions: Cleanse skin with soap and water and dry thoroughly. Apply a thin layer and gently massage over affected area morning and evening or as directed by a doctor. For athlete's foot, pay special attention to the spaces between the toes. It is also helpful to wear well-fitting, ventilated shoes and to change shoes and socks at least once daily. Best results in athlete's foot and ringworm are usually obtained with 4 weeks' use of this product and in jock itch with 2 weeks' use. If satisfactory results have not occurred within these times, consult a doctor or pharmacist. Children under 12 years of age should be supervised in the use of this product. This product is not effective on the scalp or nails.

FOR BEST RESULTS, FOLLOW DIRECTIONS AND CONTINUE TREATMENT FOR LENGTH OF TIME INDICATED.

How Supplied: Cream Tube 15 g (½ oz.)

MYCELEX-7®
VAGINAL CREAM ANTIFUNGAL

Active Ingredient: Clotrimazole 1%

Inactive Ingredients: Benzyl alcohol, cetostearyl alcohol, cetyl esters wax, octyldodecanol, polysorbate 60, purified water, sorbitan monostearate

Indications: For treatment of vaginal yeast (Candida) infection.

Actions: Cures most vaginal yeast infections. MYCELEX®-7 Antifungal Vaginal Cream can kill the yeast that may cause vaginal infection. It is greaseless and does not stain clothes.

Precautions: IF THIS IS THE FIRST TIME YOU HAVE HAD VAGINAL ITCH AND DISCOMFORT, CONSULT YOUR DOCTOR. IF YOU HAVE HAD A DOCTOR DIAGNOSE A VAGINAL YEAST INFECTION BEFORE AND HAVE THE SAME SYMPTOMS NOW, USE THIS CREAM AS DIRECTED FOR 7 CONSECUTIVE DAYS.

WARNING: DO NOT USE IF YOU HAVE ABDOMINAL PAIN, FEVER, OR FOUL-SMELLING DISCHARGE. CONTACT YOUR DOCTOR IMMEDIATELY.

IF YOU DO NOT IMPROVE IN 3 DAYS OR IF YOU DO NOT GET WELL IN 7 DAYS, YOU MAY HAVE A CONDITION OTHER THAN A YEAST INFECTION. CONSULT YOUR DOCTOR. If your symptoms return within two months or if you have infections that do not clear up easily with proper treatment, consult your doctor. You could be pregnant or there could be a serious underlying medical cause for your infections, including diabetes or a damaged immune system (including damage from infection with HIV-the virus that causes AIDS). (PLEASE READ PATIENT PACKAGE PAMPHLET.)

Do not use during pregnancy except under the advice and supervision of a doctor. Do not use tampons while using this medication. Keep this and all drugs out of the reach of children. In case of accidental ingestion, seek professional assistance or contact a Poison Control Center immediately. NOT FOR USE IN CHILDREN LESS THAN 12 YEARS OF AGE.

Dosage and Administration: Before using, read the enclosed pamphlet. **Directions:** Fill the applicator and insert one applicatorful of cream into the vagina, preferably at bedtime. Repeat this procedure daily for 7 consecutive days.

How Supplied: 1.5 oz. (45 g) tube and applicator. (7-Day Therapy)

Shown in Product Identification Guide, page 505

MYCELEX-7 VAGINAL ANTIFUNGAL CREAM WITH 7 DISPOSABLE APPLICATORS

Description: MYCELEX®-7 Antifungal Vaginal Cream can kill the yeast that may cause vaginal infection. It is greaseless and does not stain clothes.

Indications: For treatment of vaginal yeast (Candida) infection.

IF THIS IS THE FIRST TIME YOU HAVE HAD VAGINAL ITCH AND DISCOMFORT, CONSULT YOUR DOCTOR. IF YOU HAVE HAD A DOCTOR DIAGNOSE A VAGINAL YEAST INFECTION BEFORE AND HAVE THE SAME SYMPTOMS NOW, USE THIS CREAM AS DIRECTED FOR 7 CONSECUTIVE DAYS.

WARNING: DO NOT USE IF YOU HAVE ABDOMINAL PAIN, FEVER, OR FOUL-SMELLING DISCHARGE. CONTACT YOUR DOCTOR IMMEDIATELY.

Before using, read the enclosed pamphlet.

Directions: Fill the applicator and insert one applicatorful of cream into the vagina, preferably at bedtime. Dispose of each applicator after use. Do not flush in toilet. Repeat this procedure daily with a new applicator for 7 consecutive days.

WARNING: IF YOU DO NOT IMPROVE IN 3 DAYS OR IF YOU DO NOT GET WELL IN 7 DAYS, YOU MAY HAVE A CONDITION OTHER THAN A YEAST INFECTION. CONSULT YOUR DOCTOR. If your symptoms return within two months or if you have infections that do not clear up easily with proper treatment consult your doctor. You could be pregnant or there could be a serious underlying medical cause for your infections, including diabetes or a damaged immune system (including damage from infection with HIV–the virus that causes AIDS). (PLEASE READ PATIENT PACKAGE PAMPHLET.)

Do not use during pregnancy except under the advice and supervision of a doctor. Do not use tampons while using this medication. Keep this and all drugs out of the reach of children.

In case of accidental ingestion, seek professional assistance or contact a Poison Control Center immediately. NOT FOR USE IN CHILDREN LESS THAN 12 YEARS OF AGE.

If you have any questions about MYCELEX®-7 or vaginal yeast infection, contact your physician.

Store at room temperature between 2[illegible] and 30°C (36° and 86°F).

See end panel of carton and tube crimp for lot number and expiration date.

Active Ingredient: Clotrimazole 1%.

Inactive Ingredients: Benzyl alcohol, cetostearyl alcohol, cetyl esters wax, octyldodecanol, polysorbate 60, purified water, sorbitan monostearate.

How Supplied: One 45g (1.5 oz.) tube of vaginal cream and 7 applicators (7 day therapy)

Consumer Questions or Comments
Call 1-800-800-4793
8:30–5:00 EST M–F

Shown in Product Identification Guide, page 505

MYCELEX-7®
VAGINAL INSERTS ANTIFUNGAL

Active Ingredient: Each insert contains 100 mg clotrimazole.

Inactive Ingredients: Corn starch, lactose, magnesium stearate, povidone.

Indications: For treatment of vaginal yeast (Candida) infection.

Actions: Cures most vaginal yeast infections. MYCELEX-7 Antifungal Vaginal Inserts can kill the yeast that may cause vaginal infection. They do not stain clothes.

Precautions: IF THIS IS THE FIRST TIME YOU HAVE HAD VAGINAL ITCH AND DISCOMFORT, CONSULT YOUR DOCTOR. IF YOU HAVE HAD A DOCTOR DIAGNOSE A VAGINAL YEAST INFECTION BEFORE AND HAVE THE SAME SYMPTOMS NOW, USE THESE INSERTS AS DIRECTED FOR 7 CONSECUTIVE DAYS.

WARNING: DO NOT USE IF YOU HAVE ABDOMINAL PAIN, FEVER, OR FOUL-SMELLING DISCHARGE. CONTACT YOUR DOCTOR IMMEDIATELY.
IF YOU DO NOT IMPROVE IN 3 DAYS OR IF YOU DO NOT GET WELL IN 7 DAYS, YOU MAY HAVE A CONDITION OTHER THAN A YEAST INFECTION. CONSULT YOUR DOCTOR. If your symptoms return within two months or if you have infections that do not clear up easily with proper treatment, consult your doctor. You could be pregnant or there could be a serious underlying medical cause for your infections, including diabetes or a damaged immune system (including damage from infection with HIV-the virus that causes AIDS). (PLEASE READ PATIENT PACKAGE PAMPHLET) Do not use during pregnancy except under the advice and supervision of a doctor. Do not use tampons while using this medication. Keep this and all drugs out of the reach of children. In case of accidental ingestion, seek professional assistance or contact a Poison Control Center immediately. NOT FOR USE IN CHILDREN LESS THAN 12 YEARS OF AGE.

Dosage and Administration: Before using, read the enclosed pamphlet. **Directions:** Unwrap one insert, place it in the applicator, and use the applicator to place the insert into the vagina, preferably at bedtime. Repeat this procedure daily for 7 consecutive days.

How Supplied: 7 vaginal inserts and applicator. (7-Day Therapy)

Shown in Product Identification Guide, page 505

MYCELEX-7 Combination-Pack VAGINAL INSERTS & EXTERNAL VULVAR CREAM

- **Cures Most Vaginal Yeast Infections**
- **Relieves Associated External Vulvar Itching and Irritation**

MYCELEX®-7 Antifungal Vaginal Inserts and External Vulvar Cream can kill the yeast that may cause vaginal infection. They do not stain clothes.

Indications: For treatment of vaginal yeast *(Candida)* infection and the relief of external vulvar itching and irritation associated with vaginal yeast infection.

IF THIS IS THE <u>FIRST</u> TIME YOU HAVE HAD VAGINAL OR VULVAR ITCH AND DISCOMFORT, CONSULT YOUR DOCTOR. IF YOU HAVE HAD A DOCTOR DIAGNOSE A VAGINAL YEAST INFECTION BEFORE AND HAVE THE SAME SYMPTOMS NOW, USE THESE INSERTS AND CREAM AS DIRECTED FOR 7 CONSECUTIVE DAYS.

WARNING: DO NOT USE IF YOU HAVE ABDOMINAL PAIN, FEVER, OR FOUL-SMELLING DISCHARGE. CONTACT YOUR DOCTOR IMMEDIATELY.

Before using, read the enclosed pamphlet.

Directions:

Inserts: Unwrap one insert, place it in the applicator, and use the applicator to place the insert into the vagina, preferably at bedtime. Repeat this procedure daily for 7 consecutive days to treat vaginal *(Candida)* yeast infection.

Cream: Squeeze a small amount of cream onto your finger and gently spread the cream onto the irritated area of the vulva. Use once or twice daily for up to 7 days as needed to relieve external vulvar itching.

THE CREAM SHOULD NOT BE USED FOR VULVAR ITCHING DUE TO CAUSES OTHER THAN A YEAST INFECTION.

WARNING: IF YOU DO NOT IMPROVE IN 3 DAYS OR IF YOU DO NOT GET WELL IN 7 DAYS, YOU MAY HAVE A CONDITION OTHER THAN A YEAST INFECTION. CONSULT YOUR DOCTOR. If your symptoms return within two months or if you have infections that do not clear up easily with proper treatment, consult your doctor. You could be pregnant or there could be a serious underlying medical cause for your infections, including diabetes or a damaged immune system (including damage from infection with HIV—the virus that causes AIDS). (PLEASE READ ENCLOSED PATIENT PACKAGE PAMPHLET.)

Do not use during pregnancy except under the advice and supervision of a doctor.

Do not use tampons while using this medication.

Keep this and all drugs out of the reach of children. In case of accidental ingestion, seek professional assistance or contact a Poison Control Center immediately.

NOT FOR USE IN CHILDREN LESS THAN 12 YEARS OF AGE.

If you have any questions about MYCELEX®-7 Combination-Pack or vaginal yeast infection, contact your physician.

Active Ingredient:

Inserts: Each insert contains 100 mg clotrimazole

Cream: Clotrimazole 1%

Inactive Ingredients:

Inserts: Corn starch, lactose, magnesium stearate, povidone

Cream: Benzyl alcohol, cetostearyl alcohol, cetyl esters wax, octyldodecanol, polysorbate 60, purified water, sorbitan monostearate

How Supplied: 7 vaginal inserts and applicator (7-day therapy) and one 7g. (.25 oz.) tube of external vulvar cream.

Store at room temperature between 2° and 30°C (36° and 86°F).

See end panel of carton, foil wrappers and tube crimp for lot number and expiration date.

Consumer Questions or Comments call 1-800-800-4793
8:30–5:00 EST M-F

Shown in Product Identification Guide, page 505

NEO-SYNEPHRINE®
Regular Strength, and Extra Strength.

Description: This line of nasal sprays, and drops contains Phenylephrine Hydrochloride in strengths ranging from 0.25% to 1%. Also contains: Benzalkonium Chloride and Thimerosal 0.001% as preservatives, Citric Acid, Purified Water, Sodium Chloride, Sodium Citrate.

Action: Rapid-acting nasal decongestant.

Directions: For a 0.25% solution (Mild):
Adults and children 6 to under 12 years of age (with adult supervision): 2 or 3 drops or sprays in each nostril not more often than every 4 hours. Children under 6 years of age: consult a doctor.
For a 0.5% solution (Regular):
Adults and children 12 years of age and over: 2 or 3 drops or sprays in each nostril not more often than every 4 hours. Do not give to children under 12 years of age unless directed by a doctor.
For a 1% solution (Extra):
Adults and children 12 years of age and over: 2 or 3 drops or sprays in each nostril not more often than every 4 hours. Do not give to children under 12 years of age unless directed by a doctor.

Indications: For temporary relief of nasal congestion due to common cold, hay fever, sinusitis, or other upper respiratory allergies.

Warnings: For adults:
Do not exceed recommended dosage. This product may cause temporary discomfort such as burning, stinging, sneezing, or an increase in nasal discharge. The use of this container by more than one person may spread infection. Do not use this product for more than 3 days. Use only as directed. Frequent or prolonged use may cause nasal congestion to recur or worsen. If symptoms persist, consult a doctor. Do not use this product if you have (or give this product to a child who has) heart disease, high blood pressure, thyroid disease, diabetes, or difficulty in urination due to enlargement of the prostate gland unless directed by a doctor.

How Supplied: Mild Formula (0.25%) in 15 mL spray. Regular Strength (0.5%) in 15 mL drops and spray. Extra Strength (1.0%) in 15 mL drops and spray.

Shown in Product Identification Guide, page 505

Continued on next page

Bayer—Cont.

NEO-SYNEPHRINE®
Maximum Strength 12 Hour (nasal spray)
Maximum Strength 12 Hour Extra Moisturizing (nasal spray)

Active Ingredient: Oxymetazoline Hydrochloride 0.05%.

Inactive Ingredients: Benzalkonium Chloride and Phenylmercuric Acetate 0.002% as preservatives, Glycine, Purified Water, Sorbitol.

Indications: For temporary relief, up to 12 HOURS, of nasal congestion due to a cold, hay fever, or other upper respiratory allergies or associated with sinusitis. Temporarily relieves stuffy nose. Temporarily restores freer breathing through the nose. Helps decongest sinus openings and passages; temporarily relieves sinus congestion and pressure.

Directions: Adults and children 6 to under 12 years of age (with adult supervision): 2 or 3 sprays in each nostril not more often than every 10 to 12 hours. Do not exceed 2 doses in any 24-hour period. Children under 6 years of age: consult a doctor.

Warnings: Do not exceed recommended dosage. This product may cause temporary discomfort such as burning, stinging, sneezing, or an increase in nasal discharge. The use of the container by more than one person may spread infection. Do not use this product for more than 3 days. Use only as directed. Frequent or prolonged use may cause nasal congestion to recur or worsen. If symptoms persist, consult a doctor. Do not use this product if you have (or give this product to a child who has) heart disease, high blood pressure, thyroid disease, diabetes, or difficulty in urination due to enlargement of the prostate gland unless directed by a doctor.
Keep this and all drugs out of the reach of children. In case of accidental ingestion, seek professional assistance or contact a Poison Control Center immediately. As with any drug, if you are pregnant or nursing a baby, seek the advice of a health professional before using this product.

How Supplied: *Nasal Spray Maximum Strength* — plastic squeeze bottles of 15 ml (½ fl. oz.); Maximum Strength 12 Hour Extra Moisturizing Nasal Spray — 15 ml (½ fl. oz).

Shown in Product Identification Guide, page 505

ONE-A-DAY® 50 PLUS
Multivitamin/Mineral Supplement

Description: *ONE-A-DAY 50 Plus is scientifically balanced to meet the changing nutritional needs of adults over 50. This special formula is complete with all of the essential vitamins plus more of the key nutrients important for mature adults, including extra Antioxidants, B Vitamins, and Essential Trace Minerals.*

MULTIVITAMIN/MULTIMINERAL SUPPLEMENT

Directions For Use: Adults take one tablet daily with food.

VITAMINS	QUANTITY	% U.S. RDA
Vitamin A (as Acetate) and Beta Carotene	5000 I.U.	100
Vitamin C	120 mg	200
Vitamin D	400 I.U.	100
Vitamin E	60 I.U.	200
Vitamin K	20 mcg	25
Thiamin (B_1)	4.5 mg	300
Riboflavin (B_2)	3.4 mg	200
Niacin	20 mg	100
Vitamin B_6	6 mg	300
Folic Acid	0.4 mg	100
Vitamin B_{12}	30 mcg	500
Biotin	30 mcg	10
Pantothenic Acid	15 mg	150

MINERALS	QUANTITY	% U.S. RDA
Calcium (elemental)	120 mg	12
Iodine	150 mcg	100
Magnesium	100 mg	25
Zinc	22.5 mg	150
Selenium	105 mcg	150
Copper	2 mg	100
Manganese	4 mg	200
Chromium	180 mcg	150
Molybdenum	93.75 mcg	125
Chloride	34 mg	1
Potassium	37.5 mg	*

*No U.S. RDA established.

Indication: Dietary supplementation

Ingredients: Calcium Carbonate, Magnesium Hydroxide, Niacinamide Ascorbate, Ascorbic Acid, Potassium Chloride, Vitamin E Acetate, Gelatin, Zinc Sulfate, Starch, Modified Cellulose Gum, Cellulose, Calcium Silicate, Hydroxypropyl Methylcellulose, Citric Acid, Calcium Panthothenate, Hydroxypropyl Cellulose, Manganese Sulfate, Zinc Oxide, Pyridoxine Hydrochloride, Thiamine Mononitrate, Cupric Sulfate, Riboflavin, Vitamin A Acetate, Chromium Chloride, Artificial Color (FD&C Yellow #6), Beta Carotene, Folic Acid, Sodium Selenate, Potassium Iodide, Sodium Molybdate, Vitamin B12, Vitamin K, Biotin, Vitamin D.

KEEP OUT OF REACH OF CHILDREN
CHILD RESISTANT CAP

Do not use this product if safety seal bearing Bayer Corporation under cap is torn or missing.

How Supplied: Bottles of 50's and 80's with child-resistant caps.

Shown in Product Identification Guide, page 505

ONE-A-DAY® Essential Vitamins
100% USRDA of 11 Essential Vitamins in a small easy-to-swallow tablet.

Ingredients: Calcium Carbonate, Ascorbic Acid, Gelatin, Vitamin E Acetate, Starch, Niacinamide, Calcium Pantothenate, Calcium Silicate, Hydroxypropyl Methylcellulose, Artificial Color, Hydroxypropylcellulose, Vitamin A Acetate, Pyridoxine Hydrochloride, Riboflavin, Thiamine Mononitrate, Magnesium Stearate, Folic Acid, Beta Carotene, Sodium Hexametaphosphate, Vitamin D, Vitamin B-12, Lecithin.

Vitamins	Quantity	U.S. RDA
Vitamin A (as Acetate and Beta Carotene)	5000 I. U.	100%
Vitamin C	60 mg	100%
Vitamin D	400 I.U.	100%
Vitamin E	30 I.U.	100%
Thiamin (B_1)	1.5 mg	100%
Riboflavin (B_2)	1.7 mg	100%
Niacin	20 mg	100%
Vitamin B_6	2 mg	100%
Folic Acid	0.4 mg	100%
Vitamin B_{12}	6 mcg	100%
Pantothenic Acid	10 mg	100%

Indication: Dietary supplementation.

Dosage and Administration: Adults take one tablet daily.

KEEP OUT OF REACH OF CHILDREN.
CHILD RESISTANT CAP

Do not use this product if safety seal bearing Bayer Corporation under cap is torn or missing.

How Supplied: Bottles of 75's and 130's with child-resistant caps.

Shown in Product Identification Guide, page 505

ONE-A-DAY® ANTIOXIDANT PLUS
Complete Antioxidant Group Plus Essential Trace Minerals

Ingredients: Ascorbic Acid, Vitamin E Acetate, Gelatin, Glycerin, Soybean Oil, Selenium Yeast, Lecithin, Zinc Oxide, Vegetable Oil (Partially Hydrogenated Cottonseed and Soybean Oils), Yellow Wax (Beeswax, Yellow) Manganese Sulfate, Beta Carotene, Cupric Oxide, Titanium Dioxide, Artificial Colors including FD&C Yellow #5 (Tartrazine).

Directions for Use: Adults take one softgel capsule daily alone or with your everyday ONE-A-DAY multivitamin. To preserve quality and freshness, keep bottle tightly closed and store at room temperature.

VITAMINS	QUANTITY	% US RDA
Vitamin E	200 I.U.	667
Vitamin C	250 mg	417
Vitamin A (as Beta Carotene)	5000 I.U.	100

MINERALS	QUANTITY	% US RDA
Zinc	7.5 mg	50
Copper	1.0 mg	50
Selenium	15.0 mcg	21
Manganese	1.5 mg	75

Indications: For dietary supplementation. ONE-A-DAY ANTIOXIDANT PLUS may reduce the risk of harmful cell damage attributed to free radicals. Antioxidant Vitamins (C, E, and Beta Carotene) may neutralize the effects of free radicals (oxidants) which may be a cause of harmful cell damage. One-A-Day Antioxidant Plus provides antioxidant nutrients plus the essential trace minerals necessary for antioxidant enzyme activity.

KEEP OUT OF REACH OF CHILDREN
CHILD RESISTANT CAP
Do not use this product if safety seal bearing Bayer Corporation under cap is torn or missing.

How Supplied: Bottle of 50 softgels.
Shown in Product Identification Guide, page 505

ONE-A-DAY® CALCIUM PLUS
Calcium Supplement

VITAMINS:

Each Tablet Contains	Quantity	RDA
Vitamin D	100 IU	25%

MINERALS:

Each Tablet Contains	Quantity	RDA
Calcium (elemental)	500 mg	50%
Magnesium (elemental)	50 mg	12.5%

Indication: Dietary supplementation.

Ingredients: Calcium Carbonate, Sorbitol, Magnesium Carbonate, Maltodextrin, Xylitol, Starch, Stearic Acid, Aspartame* (a sweetener), Natural and Artificial Flavors, Magnesium Stearate, Polyethylene Glycol, Gelatin, Polydextrose, Poloxamer 407, Docusate Sodium, Vitamin D3
*PHENYLKETONURICS: CONTAINS PHENYLALANINE.

Directions For Use: Adults and children 12 years of age or older take one to two chewable tablets daily (with food), or as recommended by your doctor, to supplement your normal dietary intake.
Two tablets provide 1,000 mg of elemental calcium, 100% of the Recommended Daily Value for adults and children 12 years of age or older.
Special Note for Pregnant and Lactating Women: Three tablets provide 1,500 mg of elemental calcium (125% of the Recommended Daily Value).

Actions: ONE-A-DAY Calcium Plus aids in the prevention of the bone disease osteoporosis. This high potency formula contains 500 mg of the most concentrated form of Calcium, plus Vitamin D and Magnesium, in a fruit flavored chewable tablet. Calcium is essential for building and maintaining strong and healthy bones. Vitamin D is necessary for optimal absorption and utilization of calcium by the body. Magnesium is necessary for strong teeth and bones.

KEEP OUT OF REACH OF CHILDREN
CHILD RESISTANT CAP
Do not use this product if safety seal bearing Bayer Corporation under cap is torn or missing.

How Supplied: Bottles of 60 Chewable Tablets.
Shown in Product Identification Guide, page 505

ONE-A-DAY® GARLIC SOFTGELS

Ingredients: Garlic Oil Macerate, Gelatin, Glycerin, Sorbitol, Xylose.

Indication: Dietary supplementation

Directions For Use: Adults take one softgel capsule daily with a meal, alone or with your everyday multivitamin. Do not chew. Swallow whole with liquid to ensure maximum strength and fresh breath. To preserve quality and freshness, keep bottle tightly closed and store at room temperature.

Indications: One-A-Day GARLIC SOFTGELS are specially formulated to contain 600 mg of concentrated garlic, the equivalent of one fresh garlic clove, in each odor-free softgel capsule. One-A-Day Garlic Softgels provide the benefits of garlic without the unpleasant after-odor typical of fresh garlic.

KEEP OUT OF REACH OF CHILDREN
CHILD RESISTANT CAP
Do not use this product if safety seal bearing Bayer Corporation under cap is torn or missing.

How Supplied: Bottles of 45 softgels
Shown in Product Identification Guide, page 505

ONE-A-DAY® MAXIMUM
Multivitamin/Multimineral Supplement for Adults

Ingredients: Dicalcium Phosphate, Magnesium Hydroxide, Cellulose, Potassium Chloride, Ascorbic Acid, Ferrous Fumarate, Zinc Sulfate, Modified Cellulose Gum, Gelatin, Vitamin E Acetate, Citric Acid, Hydroxypropyl Methylcellulose, Niacinamide, Magnesium Stearate, Calcium Pantothenate, Selenium Yeast, Manganese Sulfate, Artificial Color, Copper Sulfate, Chromium Yeast, Molybdenum Yeast, Pyridoxine Hydrochloride, Vitamin A Acetate, Riboflavin, Thiamine Mononitrate, Beta Carotene, Folic Acid, Biotin, Potassium Iodide, Vitamin D3, Vitamin B12.
One tablet daily of ONE-A-DAY® Maximum provides:

Vitamins	Quantity	% of U.S. RDA
Vitamin A (as Acetate and Beta Carotene)	5000 I.U.	100
Vitamin C	60 mg	100
Thiamin (B_1)	1.5 mg	100
Riboflavin (B_2)	1.7 mg	100
Niacin	20 mg	100
Vitamin D	400 I.U.	100
Vitamin E	30 I.U.	100
Vitamin B_6	2 mg	100
Folic Acid	0.4 mg	100
Vitamin B_{12}	6 mcg	100
Biotin	30 mcg	10
Pantothenic Acid	10 mg	100

Minerals	Quantity	% of U.S. RDA
Iron (Elemental)	18 mg	100
Calcium (Elemental)	130 mg	13
Phosphorus	100 mg	10
Iodine	150 mcg	100
Magnesium	100 mg	25
Copper	2 mg	100
Zinc	15 mg	100
Chromium	10 mcg	8
Selenium	10 mcg	14
Molybdenum	10 mcg	13
Manganese	2.5 mg	125
Potassium	37.5 mg	*
Chloride	34 mg	1

*No U.S. RDA established

Indication: Dietary supplementation.

Dosage and Administration: Adults take one tablet daily with food.

Warning: Contains iron, which can be harmful or fatal to children in large doses. Close tightly and keep out of reach of children. In case of overdose, seek professional assistance or contact a Poison Control Center immediately.

KEEP OUT OF REACH OF CHILDREN.
CHILD RESISTANT CAP
Do not use this product if safety seal is bearing Bayer Corporation under cap is torn or missing.

How Supplied: Bottles of 60 and 100 with child-resistant caps.
Shown in Product Identification Guide, page 505

ONE-A-DAY® MEN'S MULTIVITAMIN/MULTIMINERAL SUPPLEMENT

Description: ONE-A-DAY Men's is scientifically balanced to meet the unique nutritional needs of men. This special formula provides essential vitamins and minerals plus higher levels of the key nutrients that help keep men healthy, including extra C, E, and B Vitamins.

Ingredients: Magnesium Hydroxide, Niacinamide Ascorbate, Potassium Chloride, Zinc Sulfate, Gelatin, Vitamin E Acetate, Ascorbic Acid, Modified Cellu-

Continued on next page

Bayer—Cont.

lose Gum, Cellulose, Calcium Pantothenate, Hydroxypropyl Methylcellulose, Calcium Silicate, Manganese Sulfate, Citric Acid, Povidone, Dicalcium Phosphate, Hydroxypropyl Cellulose, Cupric Sulfate, Pyridoxine Hydrochloride, Riboflavin, Thiamine Mononitrate, Vitamin A Acetate, Chromium Chloride, Beta Carotene, Folic Acid, Artificial Color (FD&C Yellow #6), Potassium Iodide, Sodium Selenate, Sodium Molybdate, Vitamin D, Vitamin B12.

VITAMINS	QUANTITY	% U.S. RDA
Vitamin A (as Acetate and Beta Carotene	5000 I.U.	100
Vitamin C	90 mg	150
Vitamin D	400 I.U.	100
Vitamin E	45 I.U.	150
Thiamin (B_1)	2.25 mg	150
Riboflavin (B_2)	2.55 mg	150
Niacin	20 mg	100
Vitamin B_6	3 mg	150
Folic Acid	0.4 mg	100
Vitamin B_{12}	9 mcg	150
Pantothenic Acid	10 mg	100

MINERALS	QUANTITY	% U.S. RDA
Iodine	150 mcg	100
Magnesium	100 mg	25
Zinc	15 mg	100
Selenium	87.5 mcg	125
Copper	2 mg	100
Manganese	3.5 mg	175
Chromium	150 mcg	125
Molybdenum	75 mcg	100
Chloride	34 mg	1
Potassium	37.5 mg	*

* No U.S. RDA established.

Indication: Dietary Supplementation.
KEEP OUT OF REACH OF CHILDREN
CHILD RESISTANT CAP

Directions for Use: Adults take one tablet daily.
Do not use this product if safety seal bearing Bayer Corporation under cap is torn or missing.

How Supplied: Bottles of 60's & 100's with child-resistant caps.

Shown in Product Identification Guide, page 505

ONE-A-DAY® WOMEN'S
Multivitamin/Multimineral Supplement

Description: ONE-A-DAY Women's is scientifically balanced to meet the unique nutritional needs of women. This special formula provides 100% U.S. RDA of 11 essential vitamins plus extra Calcium and Iron, the two minerals women need most, and Zinc.

Ingredients: Calcium Carbonate, Starch, Ferrous Fumarate, Ascorbic Acid, Gelatin, Vitamin E Acetate, Hydroxypropyl Methylcellulose, Niacinamide, Modified Cellulose Gum, Zinc Oxide, Calcium Pantothenate, Artificial Colors [including FD&C Yellow No. 5 (Tartrazine) and FD&C Yellow No. 6], Pyridoxine Hydrochloride, Vitamin A Acetate, Riboflavin, Thiamine Mononitrate, Beta Carotene, Folic Acid, Vitamin D, Vitamin B12.

Vitamins	Quantity	% of U.S. RDA
Vitamin A (as Acetate and Beta Carotene)	5000 I.U.	100
Vitamin C	60 mg	100
Thiamine (B_1)	1.5 mg	100
Riboflavin (B_2)	1.7 mg	100
Niacin	20 mg	100
Vitamin D	400 I.U.	100
Vitamin E	30 I.U.	100
Vitamin B_6	2 mg	100
Folic Acid	0.4 mg	100
Vitamin B_{12}	6 mcg	100
Pantothenic Acid	10 mg	100

Minerals	Quantity	% of U.S. RDA
Iron (Elemental)	27 mg	150
Calcium (Elemental)	450 mg	45
Zinc	15 mg	100

Indication: Dietary supplementation.

Dosage and Administration: Adults take one tablet daily with food.

Warning: Contains iron, which can be harmful or fatal to children in large doses. Close tightly and keep out of reach of children. In case of overdose, seek professional assistance or contact a Poison Control Center immediately.
KEEP OUT REACH OF CHILDREN
CHILD RESISTANT CAP
Do not use this product if safety seal bearing Bayer Corporation under cap is torn or missing.

How Supplied: Bottles of 60 and 100 with child-resistant caps.

Shown in Product Identification Guide, page 505

PHILLIPS'® GELCAPS
Laxative plus Stool Softener

Active Ingredients: Phenolphthalein (90 mg) and docusate sodium (83 mg) per gelcap.

Inactive Ingredients: FD&C Blue # 2, gelatin, glycerin, PEG 400 and 3350, propylene glycol, sorbitol, and titanium dioxide.

Indications: For relief of occasional constipation (irregularity). This product generally produces bowel movement in 6 to 12 hours.

Action: Phenolphthalein is a stimulant laxative which increases the peristaltic activity of the intestine. Docusate sodium is a stool softener which allows easier passage of the stool.

Directions: Adults and children 12 and over take one (1) or two (2) gelcaps daily with a full glass (8 oz) of liquid, or as directed by a doctor. For children under 12, consult your doctor.

Drug Interaction Precaution: Do not take this product if you are presently taking mineral oil, unless directed by a doctor.

Warnings: Do not take any laxative if abdominal pain, nausea or vomiting are present unless directed by a doctor. If you have noticed a sudden change in bowel habits persisting for over 2 weeks, consult a doctor before using a laxative. Laxative products should not be used for a period longer than 1 week, unless directed by a doctor. Rectal bleeding or failure to have a bowel movement after use of a laxative may indicate a serious condition. Discontinue use and consult your doctor. If skin rash appears, do not use this product or any other preparation containing phenolphthalein. Keep this and all drugs out of the reach of children. In case of accidental overdose, seek professional assistance or contact a poison control center immediately. As with any drug, if you are pregnant or nursing a baby, seek the advice of a health professional before using this product.

How Supplied: Blister packs of 30 and 60 gelcaps.

Shown in Product Identification Guide, page 505

PHILLIPS' ® MILK OF MAGNESIA
Laxative/Antacid

Active Ingredients: Magnesium Hydroxide. Phillips' Milk of Magnesia contains 400 mg per teaspoon (5 mL) of magnesium hydroxide.

Inactive Ingredients: Original—Purified water. Mint—Flavor, Mineral Oil, Purified water, Saccharin Sodium.
Cherry—Carboxymethylcellulose Sodium, Citric Acid, D&C Red #28, Flavor Glycerine, Microcrystalline Cellulose Propylene Glycol, Purified water, Sorbitol, Sugar, Xantham Gum.

Indications: For relief of occasional constipation (irregularity), relief of acid indigestion, sour stomach and heartburn. The laxative dosage generally produces bowel movement in $^1/_2$ to 6 hours.

Action at Laxative Dosage: Phillips' Milk of Magnesia is a mild saline laxative which acts by drawing water into the gut, increasing intraluminal pressure and increasing intestinal motility.

Action at Antacid Dosage: Phillips Milk of Magnesia is an effective acid neutralizer.

Directions: Laxative: Adults and children 12 years and older, 2–4 tbsp followed by a full glass (8 oz) of liquid; children 6–11 years, 1–2 tbsp followed by a full glass (8 oz) of liquid; children 2–5 years, 1–3 tsp followed by a full glass (8 oz) of liquid. Children under 2, consult a doctor.
Antacid: Adults & children 12 & older 1–3 tsp with a little water, up

to four times a day, or as directed by a doctor.

Drug Interaction Precaution: Antacids may interact with certain prescription drugs. If you are presently taking a prescription drug do not take this product without checking with your doctor or other health professional.

Laxative Warnings: Do not take any laxative if abdominal pain, nausea, vomiting or kidney disease are present unless directed by a doctor. If you have noticed a sudden change in bowel habits persisting for over 2 weeks, consult a doctor before using a laxative. Laxative products should not be used for a period longer than 1 week, unless directed by a doctor. Rectal bleeding or failure to have a bowel movement after use of a laxative may indicate a serious condition. Discontinue use and consult your doctor. Phillips® Milk of Magnesia is a saline laxative.

Antacid Warnings: Do not take more than the maximum recommended daily dosage in a 24-hour period (see Directions), or use the maximum dosage of this product for more than two weeks, or use this product if you have kidney disease, except under the advice and supervision of a doctor. May have laxative effect.

General Warnings: As with any drug, if you are pregnant or nursing a baby, seek the advice of a health professional before using this product. Keep this and all drugs out of reach of children. In case of accidental overdose, seek professional assistance or contact a poison control center immediately.

How Supplied: Phillips' Milk of Magnesia is available in original, mint and cherry flavor in 4, 12 and 26 fl oz bottles. Also available in tablet form and concentrated liquid form.

Shown in Product Identification Guide, page 506

VANQUISH® Analgesic Caplets

Active Ingredients: Each caplet contains aspirin 227 mg, acetaminophen 194 mg, caffeine 33 mg, dried aluminum hydroxide gel 25 mg, magnesium hydroxide 50 mg.

Inactive Ingredients: Hydroxypropyl Methylcellulose, Microcrystalline Cellulose, Polyethylene Glycol, Polysorbate 80, Silicon Dioxide, Starch, Titanium Dioxide, Zinc Stearate.

Indications: Fast, safe, temporary relief of minor aches and pains associated with headaches, colds and flu, backaches, muscle aches, menstrual pain and minor pain of arthritis.

Directions: Adults (12 years and over), take 2 caplets with water every 4 hours, as needed, up to a maximum of 12 caplets in 24 hours or as directed by a doctor. **Children under 12 years**, consult a doctor.

Warnings: Children and teenagers should not use this medicine for chicken pox or flu symptoms before a doctor is consulted about Reye syndrome, a rare but serious illness reported to be associated with aspirin. Do not take this product for pain for more than 10 days or for fever for more than 3 days unless directed by a doctor. If pain or fever persists or gets worse, if new symptoms occur, or if redness or swelling is present consult a doctor immediately. Do not take this product if you are allergic to aspirin, have asthma, stomach problems that persist or recur, gastric ulcers or bleeding problems unless directed by a doctor. If ringing in the ears or loss of hearing occurs, consult a doctor before taking any more of this product. Keep this and all drugs out of the reach of children. In case of accidental overdose, immediate medical attention is essential for adults as well as for children even if you do not notice any sign or symptoms. As with any drug, if you are pregnant or nursing a baby, seek the advice of a health professional before using this product. **IT IS ESPECIALLY IMPORTANT NOT TO USE ASPIRIN DURING THE LAST 3 MONTHS OF PREGNANCY UNLESS SPECIFICALLY DIRECTED TO DO SO BY A DOCTOR BECAUSE IT MAY CAUSE PROBLEMS IN THE UNBORN CHILD OR COMPLICATIONS DURING DELIVERY.**

Drug Interaction Precaution: Do not take this product if you are taking a prescription drug for anticoagulation (thinning of the blood), diabetes, gout, or arthritis unless directed by a doctor.

How Supplied:
Bottles of 30, 60 and 100 caplets. Child-resistant safety closures on bottles of 30 and 60 caplets. Bottle of 100 caplets available without safety closure for households without young children.

Shown in Product Identification Guide, page 506

Beach Pharmaceuticals

Division of Beach Products, Inc.
5220 SOUTH MANHATTAN AVE.
TAMPA, FL 33611

Direct Inquiries to:
Richard Stephen Jenkins, Exec. V.P.:
(813) 839-6565

BEELITH Tablets
MAGNESIUM SUPPLEMENT WITH PYRIDOXINE HCL

Each tablet supplies 362 mg (30 mEq) of magnesium and 25 mg of pyridoxine hydrochloride.

Description: Each tablet contains magnesium oxide 600 mg and pyridoxine hydrochloride (Vitamin B_6) 25 mg equivalent to B_6 20 mg. Each tablet yields 362 mg of magnesium and supplies 90% of the Adult U.S. Recommended Daily Allowance (RDA) for magnesium and 1000% of the Adult RDA for Vitamin B_6.

Indications: As a dietary supplement for patients with magnesium and/or Vitamin B_6 deficiencies resulting from malnutrition, alcoholism, magnesium depleting drugs, chemotherapy, and inadequate nutritional intake or absorption. Also, increases urinary magnesium levels.

Dosage: One tablet daily or as directed by a physician.

Drug Interaction Precaution: Do not take this product if you are presently taking a prescription drug without consulting your physician or other health professional.

Warnings: If you have kidney disease, take only under the supervision of a physician. Excessive dosage may cause laxation. **KEEP OUT OF THE REACH OF CHILDREN.** As with any drug, if your are pregnant or nursing a baby, seek the advice of a health professional before using this product.

How Supplied: Golden yellow, film coated tablet with the name **BEACH** and the number **1132** printed on each tablet. Packaged in bottles of 100 (NDC 0486-1132-01) tablets.

Beech-Nut Nutrition Corporation

800 MARKET STREET
ST. LOUIS, MO 63101

Direct Inquiries to:
Beech-Nut Nutrition Helpline:
1-800-523-6633

For Medical Emergency Contact:
Richard C. Theuer, Ph.D.:
(314) 877-7146
FAX: (314) 877-7762

BEECH-NUT® PEDIATRIC ELECTROLYTE
Oral Maintenance Solution

Usage: Maintenance and replacement of water and electrolytes in infants and young children

- during mild to moderate diarrhea, with or without vomiting
- following parenteral treatment of severe diarrhea

1. Specifically formulated to meet the recommendations of the Committee on Nutrition, American Academy of Pediatrics, for Oral Maintenance Solutions for Treating Pediatric Patients with Gastrointestinal Fluid Losses
2. Made with glucose as the only carbohydrate. Glucose is the preferred sugar for use in oral rehydration solutions because it facilitates the transport of sodium across the bowel wall.

Continued on next page

Beech-Nut—Cont.

3. Available in delicious, natural cherry flavor; contains no artificial sweeteners (Aspartame), colors or flavors.
4. Convenient, easy-to-open and easy-to-use 4-fl. oz. single-serving jar accepts a standard nipple to facilitate feeding to infants and young children.
5. pH-buffered to improve tolerance.

Availability: 4-fl. oz. (118 mL) jars with 40 mm finish to accept standard U.S. nipple fitting. Retail multipack unit of six 4-fl. oz. jars, packed four multipacks to the case.

Dosage: To replace and maintain fluid and electrolyte losses in infants and young children with mild or moderate dehydration due to acute diarrhea, with or without vomiting.

Fluid maintenance requirements

a. Body weight general rule:

100 mL/kg/day for the first 10 kg of body weight

50 mL/kg/day for the next 10 kg of body weight

20 mL/kg/day for each kg above 20 kg

b. Adjustments:

fever—increase water requirement by 12% for each 1°C rise

excessive sweating—increase water by 10 to 25 mL/kg/day

high environmental humidity—decrease water by 0 to 15 mL/kg/day

Fluid deficit requirements

1. Determine previous healthy (recent) body weight: ___ kg (A)
2. Determine current weight of sick child ___ kg (B)
3. Calculate the difference (fluid loss) ___ kg (C=A−B)
4. Express fluid loss as a percentage ___ (C/A ×100)

Degrees of fluid deficit

[See first table above.]

Sample chart for infants and children with 5% fluid deficit

[See second table above.]

In mild dehydration, small amounts of oral rehydration solution should be given ad libitum to provide approximately 50 mL/kg over the first four hours. In moderate dehydration, the dose should be increased to 100 mL/kg over the first six hours. Intake should not exceed 150 mL/kg in a 24-hour period. If additional fluid is needed to satisfy thirst, a low-solute fluid such as breast milk or water should be offered.

When rehydration is complete, patients with mild diarrhea usually can be maintained with 100 mL/kg/24 hours until the diarrhea stops.

In severe diarrhea, the initial objective is to correct the fluid and electrolyte deficits. After fluid and electrolyte deficits have been corrected, usually parenterally, the continuing losses of significant fluid and electrolytes associated with severe diarrhea must be replaced. Oral maintenance solution should be given in amounts that equal the measured volume of stool losses. If stool volume cannot be measured, an intake of 10 to 15 mL/kg/hr is appropriate.

	Infants	Child	Correct fluid deficit
Mild dehydration	less than 5%	less than 3%	orally over 4 hours
Moderate dehydration	5% to 10%	3% to 6%	orally over 6 hours
Severe dehydration	10% or more	7% or more	with parenteral fluids

Weight of child	Number of bottles to give in the first 4–6 hours	Total number of bottles to give in first 24 hours	Number of bottles to give in later days
5 kg (11 to 12 lb.)	$2^1/_2$	6	4 to 5
6 kg (12 to 15 lb.)	3	7 to 8	5 to 6
8 kg (15 to 20 lb.)	4	9 to 11	6 to 7
10 kg (20 to 25 lb.)	5	12 to 13	8 to 9
13 kg (25 to 30 lb.)	6	14 to 15	10 to 11
15 kg (30 to 35 lb.)	7	16 to 17	12 to 13

Per liter	American Academy of Pediatrics recommendation	Beech-Nut® Pediatric Electrolyte	Pedialyte® Fruit Flavor
Sodium, mEq	40 to 60	50	45
Potassium, mEq	20	20	20
Chloride, mEq	—	50	35
Anions			
Base (citrate)	20–30%	29%	46%
Chloride	70–80%	71%	54%
Glucose grams	20 to 25	25	20
Fructose grams	only glucose is recommended	0	5

The infant or child who vomits may tolerate 5 to 10 mL (1 to 2 teaspoonfuls) given every 5 minutes until vomiting ends, when volumes of 30 to 60 mL (1 to 2 fluid ounces) may be offered.

Fever significantly increases water requirements—12% for each 1°C rise or 6% for each 1°F rise—so fever control is important.

Ingredients: Water, glucose, natural cherry flavor, sodium chloride (salt), potassium citrate and citric acid.

Composition:

[See third table above.]

Rationale: Children are more likely to experience gastrointestinal disease, especially gastroenteritis. Gastrointestinal symptoms occur with many nongastrointestinal diseases. Dehydration from fluid loss, most commonly diarrhea and vomiting, can be especially dangerous to infants because of their high turnover of water (15–20% in a 24-hour period) and because they cannot independently respond to thirst or secure access to fluids.

The goal of management of mild and moderate diarrheal dehydration in healthy well-nourished infants and young children is to provide fluid support during the two or three days of acute illness and to avoid complications related to dehydration or to inappropriate measures taken to prevent dehydration.

Oral rehydration with a solution with an appropriate ratio of sodium to glucose exploits the fact that glucose facilitates the transport of sodium across the bowel wall, even in the face of inflammation of the small intestine or the presence of enterotoxin. Home remedies, including decarbonated soda beverages, fruit juices, Jell-O®, Kool-Aid® and tea, are not suitable because they have inappropriately high osmolalities, due to too much carbohydrate, which can make the diarrhea worse; low sodium concentrations which can cause hyponatremia; and inappropriate carbohydrate to sodium ratios.

Giving rehydration solution orally is intrinsically safer than parenteral fluid administration. Thirst regulates fluid intake by the infant or child so that overrehydration is less likely. Infection and thromboembolic phenomena also are less likely with oral fluids. Oral rehydration is less painful and is less emotionally traumatic to the infant or child. The cost of oral fluids is considerably less than the cost of parenteral fluids.

Severe dehydration requires parenteral rehydration or a special oral rehydration solution. Oral maintenance solutions should be used in severe diarrhea only after correction of acute fluid deficits.

Oral maintenance solutions are designed to correct dehydration but do not stop diarrhea. Diarrhea usually stops spontaneously. After rehydration is complete, the early reintroduction of food may shorten the duration of diarrhea and reduce stool frequency. Food should be reintroduced while the oral electrolyte solution is continued to replace ongoing diarrheal fluid losses and for normal maintenance requirements.

Pedialyte® assigned to Abbott Laboratories

Jell-O® assigned to Kraft General Foods

Kool-Aid® assigned to Kraft General Foods

Contraindications: Oral rehydration therapy requires the careful attention of a qualified caregiver and patient compliance. If the child refuses to consume the ral maintenance solution or if the care-iver is judged incapable of following in-tructions, parenteral therapy is indi-ated.

)ral maintenance solution is contraindi-ated for initial therapy of severe dehy-ration. Parenteral rehydration or a spe-ial oral electrolyte solution are requir-d to correct fluid and electrolyte deficits n severely dehydrated infants and hildren.

)ral maintenance solution is contraindi-ated for patients with persistent, severe omiting. Parenteral fluid therapy is in-icated in these circumstances.

ackage Warnings for Caregivers:

onsult your doctor immediately if:

your child has fever or is lethargic (not responsive).

your child has severe vomiting for more than four to six hours.

your child has decreased urination (dry diapers for 4 to 6 hours for infants less than three months of age; dry diapers for 6 to 8 hours for infants three months to twelve months of age; or dry diapers for 12 hours for toddlers).

your child refuses to consume oral maintenance solution.

your child has blood in the stool or the diarrhea continues beyond 24 hours.

Shown in Product Identification Guide, page 506

Beiersdorf Inc.

360 Dr. Martin Luther King Dr.
NORWALK, CT 06856-5529

)irect Inquiries To:
/ledical Division: (203) 853-8008
'AX: (203) 854-8180

AQUAPHOR®—
)riginal Formula Ointment
NDC Numbers— 10356-020-01
10356-020-02

omposition: Petrolatum, mineral oil, nineral wax and wool wax alcohol.

ctions and Uses: Aquaphor is a sta-le, neutral, odorless, anhydrous oint-nent base. Miscible with water or aque-us solutions, Aquaphor will absorb sev-ral times its own weight, forming mooth, creamy water-in-oil emulsions. n its pure form, Aquaphor is recom-nended for use as a topical preparation o help heal severely dry skin. Aquaphor ontains no preservatives, fragrances or nown irritants.

dministration and Dosages: Use quaphor alone or in compounding vir-ually any ointment using aqueous solu-ions or in combination with other oil-ased substances and all common topical nedications. Apply Aquaphor liberally o affected area.

recautions: For external use only. void contact with eyes. Not to be ap-lied over third degree burns, deep or uncture wounds, infections or lacerations. If condition worsens or does not improve within 7 days, patient should consult a doctor.

How Supplied: 16 oz. jar—List No. 45585
5 lb. jar—List. No. 45586

Shown in Product Identification Guide, page 506

AQUAPHOR
Healing Ointment
NDC Number—10356-021-01

Composition: Petrolatum, Mineral Oil, Mineral Wax, Wool Wax Alcohol, Panthenol, Bisabolol, Glycerin.

Actions and Uses: Aquaphor Healing Ointment is specially formulated for faster healing of severely dry skin, cracked skin and minor burns. It is recommended for patients suffering from severe skin chapping and from skin disorders that result in severely dry skin. This formula is also indicated as a follow-up skin treatment for patients undergoing radiation therapy or other drying/burning medical therapies. It is preservative-free, fragrance-free and hypoallergenic.[1].

Administration and Dosage: Use Aquaphor Healing Ointment whenever a mild healing agent is needed. Apply liberally to affected areas two to three times a day. In the case of minor wounds, clean area prior to application.

Precautions: For external use only. Avoid contact with the eyes. Not to be applied over third degree burns, deep or puncture wounds, infections or lacerations. If condition worsens or does not improve within seven days, patient should consult a physician.

How Supplied: 1.75 oz. tube
1. Data on file, BDF Inc

Shown in Product Identification Guide, page 506

EUCERIN® BAR
[*ū 'sir-in*]
Dry Skin Therapy Cleansing Bar

Indications: Use with warm water to cleanse skin.

Contains: Disodium Lauryl Sulfosuccinate, Sodium Cocoyl Isethionate, Cetearyl Alcohol, Corn Starch, Glyceryl Stearate, Paraffin, Water, Titanium Dioxide, Octyldodecanol, Cyclopentadecanolide, Lanolin Alcohol, Bisabolol.

Actions and Uses: Eucerin® Cleansing Bar has been specially formulated for use on sensitive skin. The formulation contains Eucerite®, a special blend of ingredients that closely resemble the natural oils of the skin, thus providing excellent moisturizing properties. This formulation is fragrance-free and non-comedogenic. Additionally, the pH value of Eucerin Cleansing Bar is neutral so as not to affect the skin's normal acid mantle.

Directions: Use during shower, bath, or regular cleansing.

How Supplied: 3 oz. bar—List No. 03852

EUCERIN® Creme
[*ū 'sir-in*]
Original Moisturizing Creme
NDC Numbers—10356-090-01
10356-090-05
10356-090-04
10356-090-07

Indications: Use daily to help relieve dry and very dry skin conditions.

Composition: Water, Petrolatum, Mineral Oil, Ceresin, Lanolin Alcohol, Methylchloroisothiazolinone, Methylisothiazolinone.

Actions and Uses: A gentle, non-comedogenic, fragrance-free water-in-oil emulsion. Eucerin can be used for treating dry skin conditions associated with eczema, psoriasis, chapped or chafed skin, sunburn, windburn and itching associated with dryness.[1].

Administration and Dosages: Apply freely to affected areas of the skin as often as necessary or as directed by a physician.

Precautions: For external use only. Avoid contact with the eyes. Discontinue use if signs of irritation occur.

How Supplied:
16 oz. jar—List Number 00090
8 oz. jar—List Number 03774
4 oz. jar—List Number 03797
2 oz. tube—List Number 03868
1. Data on File.

Shown in Product Identification Guide, page 506

EUCERIN®
FACIAL MOISTURIZING LOTION SPF 25
NDC Number—10356-972-01

Indications: Use daily to help relieve dry skin and provide broad spectrum sun protection.

Composition:
Active Ingredients: Octyl Methoxycinnamate, Octyl Salicylate, Titanium Dioxide.

Other Ingredients: Water, Octyldodecyl Neopentanoate, Dioctyl Malate, Glycerin, Petrolatum, Zinc Oxide, Cetearyl Alcohol, DEA-Cetyl Phosphate, PEG-40 Castor Oil, Glyceryl Stearate, Sodium Hyaluronate, Lactic Acid, Lanolin Alcohol, Sodium Cetearyl Sulfate, Xanthan

Continued on next page

Beiersdorf—Cont.

Gum, Methicone, Dimethicone, EDTA, Sodium Hydroxide, Methylchloroisothiazolinone, Methylisothiazolinone.

Actions and Uses: Eucerin Facial Moisturizing Lotion SPF 25 is fragrance-free and non-comedogenic, with a unique sun screen (titanium dioxide) to protect skin from UVA and UVB light. It is specially formulated for dry, sensitive skin or for those undergoing therapies which irritate delicate facial skin. This light, oil-in-water formula is non-greasy and is easily absorbed into the skin.

Administration and Dosage: Apply Eucerin Facial Moisturizing Lotion SPF 25 twice a day (especially in the morning) or as directed by a physician, to nourish and moisturize skin and protect it from harmful UVA and UVB rays.

Precautions: For external use only. Avoid contact with eyes. Keep out of the reach of children. Discontinue use if signs of irritation occur.

How Supplied: 4-oz. bottle.—List No. 03972

Shown in Product Identification Guide, page 506

EUCERIN Light
Moisture-Restorative Creme
[*ū ' sir-in*]
NDC Number-10356-282-01

Indications: Use daily to help relieve dry skin

Composition: Active ingredient: Dimethicone

Other ingredients: Water, Sunflower Seed Oil (Helianthus annuus), Glycerin, Cetearyl Alcohol, Panthenol, Octyldodecanol, Caprylic/Capric Triglyceride, Stearic Acid, Tocopheryl Acetate (Vitamin E), Glycerl Stearate, Triethanolamine, Sodium Lactate, Sodium PCA, Cholesterol, Allantoin, Ceresin, Carbomer, Disodium EDTA, BHT, Methylchloroisothiazolinone, Methylisothiazolinone

Actions and Uses: Eucerin Light Moisture-Restorative Creme is a lipid enhanced, fragrance free formulation that helps reinforce the skin's own structure for extra protection against dry skin[1]. Light, fast-absorbing formulation leaves skin feeling smoother, softer and healthier.

Administration and Dosage: Apply liberally as often as necessary or directed by a physician.

Precautions: For external use only. Avoid contact with eyes and areas where skin is inflamed or cracked. Discontinue use if signs of irritation occur.

How Supplied: 4 oz. jar-List no. 03282

[1] Data on File.

Shown in Product Identification Guide, page 506

EUCERIN Light
Moisture-Restorative Lotion
[*ū ' sir-in*]
NDC Number-10356-032-01

Indications: Use daily to help relieve dry skin

Composition: Active Ingredient: Dimethicone

Other Ingredients: Water, Sunflower Seed Oil (Helianthus annuus), Petrolatum, Glycerin, Glyceryl Stearate SE, Octyldodecanol, Panthenol, Caprylic/Capric Triglyceride, Tocopheryl Acetate (Vitamin E), Stearic Acid, Cholesterol, Triethanolamine, Carbomer, Disodium EDTA, BHT, Methylchloroisothiazolinone, Methylisothiazolinone

Actions and Uses: Eucerin Light Moisture-Restorative Lotion is a lipid enhanced, fragrance free formulation that helps reinforce the skin's own structure for extra protection against dry skin[1]. Light, fast-absorbing formulation leaves skin feeling smoother, softer and healthier.

Administration and Dosage: Apply liberally as often as necessary or directed by a physician.

Precautions: For external use only. Avoid contact with eyes. Not to be applied over deep or puncture wounds, infections or lacerations. Discontinue use if signs of irritation occur.

How Supplied: 8 oz. bottle-List no. 03276

[1] Data on File.

Shown in Product Identification Guide, page 506

EUCERIN® Lotion
[*ū 'sir-in*]
Original Moisturizing Lotion
NDC Numbers—10356-793-01
10356-793-04

Indications: Use daily to help relieve dry skin.

Composition: Water, Mineral Oil, Isopropyl Myristate, PEG-40 Sorbitan Peroleate, Glyceryl Lanoleate, Sorbitol, Propylene Glycol, Cetyl Palmitate, Magnesium Sulfate, Aluminum Stearate, Lanolin Alcohol, BHT, Methylchloroisothiazolinone, Methylisothiazolinone.

Actions and Uses: Eucerin Lotion is a non-comedogenic, fragrance-free, unique water-in-oil formulation that will help to alleviate and soothe dry skin, and provide long-lasting moisturization.

Administration and Dosage: Use daily on dry skin or as directed by a physician.

Precautions: For external use only. Avoid contact with the eyes. Discontinue use if signs of irritation occur.

How Supplied: 8 oz. bottle—List Number 03793

16 oz. bottle—List number 03794

Shown in Product Identification Guide, page 506

EUCERIN PLUS CREME
Moisturizing Alphahydroxy Creme
NDC 10356-036-01

Indications: Use daily to help reliev severely dry, flaky skin.

Composition: Water, Mineral Oil Urea, Magnesium Stearate, Ceresin Polyglyceryl-3 Diisostearate, Sodiun Lactate, Isopropyl Palmitate, Benzy Alcohol, Panthenol, Bisabolol, Lanoli Alcohol, Magnesium Sulfate.

Action and Uses: Eucerin Plus Crem is a unique alphahydroxy acid moisturiz ing creme (2.5% sodium lactate, 10% urea) that is clinically proven to help re lieve severely dry, flaky skin conditions[1] Unlike other alphahydroxy acid moistur izers, Eucerin Plus Creme has low irrita tion potential, is fragrance-free and nor comedogenic.

Administration and Dosage: Us daily on severely dry, scaly skin or as di rected by a physician.

Precautions: Avoid contact with eye or areas where skin is inflamed o cracked. Discontinue use if signs of irri tation occur. For external use only. Kee out of reach of children.

How Supplied: 4 oz. jar—List No. 0361

1.Data on file.

Shown in Product Identification Guide, page 506

EUCERIN PLUS LOTION
Alphahydroxy Moisturizing Lotion
NDC 10356-967-01
10356-967-03

Indications: Use daily to help reliev severely dry, flaky skin.

Composition: Water, Mineral Oi PEG-7 Hydrogenated Castor Oil, Isohex adecane, Sodium Lactate 5%, Urea 5% Glycerin, Isopropyl Palmitate, Pan thenol, Ozokerite, Magnesium Sulfate Lanolin Alcohol, Bisabolol, Methy chloroisothiazolinone, Methylisothiazoli none.

Action and Uses: Eucerin Plus Lotio is a unique, patented alphahydroxy aci moisturizing lotion (5% Sodium Lactate 5% Urea) that is clinically proven to hel relieve severely dry, flaky skin condi tions.[1] Unlike other alphahydroxy aci moisturizing lotions, Eucerin Plus ha low irritation potential, is fragrance fre and non-comedogenic.

Administration and Dosage: Us daily on severely dry, flaky skin or as di rected by a physician.

Precautions: Avoid contact with eye or areas where skin is inflamed o cracked. Discontinue use if signs of irri tation occur. For external use only. Kee out of reach of children.

How Supplied: 6 oz bottle—List No. 03967
12 oz bottle—List No. 03321
1. Data on File.
Shown in Product Identification Guide, page 506

EUCERIN Shower Therapy
[*ū' sir-in*]

Indications: Use daily to moisturize and gently cleanse.

Composition: Soybean Oil, MIPA-Laureth Sulfate, Castor Oil, Laureth-4, Cocamide DEA, Poloxamer 101, Laureth-9, Water, Citric Acid, Diammonium Citrate, BHT, Propyl Gallate.

Actions and Uses: Eucerin Shower Therapy is a lipid enhanced, fragrance free, non-irritating formulation that restores moisture to the skin as it gently cleanses. Shower Therapy adds lipids to help reinforce the skin's natural barrier function for long-lasting protection against dryness.[1]

Administration and Dosage: Massage onto wet skin. Cleanse body then rinse off.

Precautions: Discontinue use if signs of irritation occur. Avoid contact with eyes. Guard against slipping in shower.

How Supplied: 7.5 oz. bottle-List no. 03241
1 Data on File.
Shown in Product Identification Guide, page 506

Beutlich LP Pharmaceuticals
1541 SHIELDS DRIVE
WAUKEGAN, IL 60085-8304

Direct Inquiries to:
847-473-1100
800-238-8542
FAX 847–473-1122

CEO–TWO® EVACUANT SUPPOSITORIES

NDC #0283-0763-09

Composition: Each adult rectal suppository contains sodium bicarbonate and potassium bitartrate in a water soluble polyethylene glycol base.

Actions: CEO-TWO suppositories are easy to use, effective and predictable. They will not disturb the homeostasis of the bowel. They are gentle and will not irritate the bowel which often would result in a secondary urge to defecate. CEO-TWO will not cause cramping.
CEO-TWO suppositories combine with the natural moisture in the bowel to gently release approximately 175 cc's of carbon dioxide. The slowly released CO_2 distends the rectal ampulla thus stimulating peristalsis. The emollient base allows for easy insertion and lubricates the bowel wall to facilitate passage of feces. Defecation generally occurs within 10 to 30 minutes after insertion of the suppository.

Indications: CEO-TWO is indicated for the relief of constipation in adolescents through geriatrics. It is used effectively in bowel training and maintenance programs. It will provide predictable results prior to lower endoscopic procedures as well as pre and post operative or pre and post partum bowel emptying. CEO-TWO should be used whenever the last 25 cm of the bowel must be evacuated.

Administration and Dosage: One or two suppositories can be used as needed. Moisten CEO-TWO with warm water before inserting. Patient should retain as long as possible. Dosage can be repeated in 4–6 hours if necessary.

Contraindications: As with other enemas or laxatives.

Warnings: Do not use CEO-TWO when abdominal pain, nausea or vomiting are present unless directed by a physician.

How Supplied: In packages of 10, white opaque suppositories. Keep in cool, dry place.
DO NOT REFRIGERATE

HURRICAINE® TOPICAL ANESTHETIC

Composition: HURRICAINE contains 20% benzocaine in a flavored, water soluble polyethylene glycol base.

Action and Indications: HURRICAINE is a topical anesthetic that provides rapid anesthesia on all accessible mucous membrane in 15 to 30 seconds, short duration of 15 minutes, has virtually no systemic absorption, and tastes good. Hurricaine is used as a lubricant and topical anesthetic to facilitate passage of fiberoptic gastroscopes, laryngoscopes, proctoscopes and sigmoidoscopes. In addition, Hurricaine is effective in suppressing the pharyngeal and tracheal gag reflex during the placement of nasogastric tubes. Hurricaine is used to control pain and discomfort during certain gynecological procedures such as IUD insertion, vaginal speculum placement, and as a preinjection anesthesia prior to LEEP procedures and paracervical blocks. Hurricaine is also effective for the temporary relief of pain due to sore throat, stomatitis and mucositis. It is also effective in controlling various types of pain associated with dental procedures and the temporary relief of minor mouth irritations, canker sores and irritation to the mouth and gums caused by dentures or orthodontic appliances.

Contraindications: Patients with a known hypersensitivity to benzocaine should not use HURRICAINE. True allergic reactions are rare.

Adverse Reactions: Methemoglobinemia has been reported following the use of benzocaine on extremely rare occasions. Intravenous methylene blue is the specific therapy for this condition.

Cautions: DO NOT USE IN THE EYES. NOT FOR INJECTION. KEEP THIS AND ALL DRUGS OUT OF THE REACH OF CHILDREN.

Packaging Available
Gel
1 oz. Jar Wild Cherry NDC #0283-0871-31
1 oz. Jar Pina Colada NDC #0283-0886-31
1 oz. Jar Watermelon NDC #0283-0293-31
1/8 oz. Tube Wild Cherry NDC #0283-0871-12
1/8 oz. Tube Watermelon NDC #0283-0293-12
Liquid
1 fl. oz. Jar Wild Cherry NDC #0283-0569-31
1 fl. oz. Jar Pina Colada NDC #0283-1886-31
1/8 oz. Tube Wild Cherry NDC #0283-0569-12
.25 gm. Packet Wild Cherry NDC #0283-0569-50
.25 gm. Packet Pina Colada NDC #0283-1886-50
.25 ml Dry Handle Swab Wild Cherry NDC #0283-0693-01
Spray
2 oz. Aerosol Wild Cherry NDC #0283-0679-02
Spray Kit
2 oz. Aerosol Wild Cherry NDC #0283-0183-02 with 200 Disposable Extension Tubes

---

PERIDIN-C®

Composition: Each orange colored tablet contains 2 popular antioxidants; Vitamin C and Bioflavonoids.
Ascorbic Acid 200 mg.
Hesperidin Complex 150 mg.
Hesperidin Methyl Chalcone 50 mg. F.D. & C. #6.

Dosage: 1 tablet daily or as directed.

How Supplied: In bottles of:
100 tablets NDC #0283-0597-01
500 tablets NDC #0283-0597-05

UNKNOWN DRUG?
Consult the
Product Identification Guide
(Gray Pages)
for full-color photos of
leading over-the-counter
medications

BioZone Laboratories, Inc.

580 GARCIA AVENUE
PITTSBURG, CA 94565

Direct Inquiries to:
(510) 473–1000, ext. 17

LipoSpray™ Nutritional Delivery System

Descriptions: LipoSpray™ is a patent pending liposomal delivery system designed to optimize the sublingual absorption of nutrients and pharmaceuticals.

Studies Show: LipoSpray™ vs. Tablets

- Faster onset
- Greater Bioavailability
- Longer duration of action

When compared to conventional oral dosage forms.

Recommended Use: Spray one-two full sprays under tongue, hold for 20–30 seconds, then swallow.

How Supplied: In 1 fl. Oz. (30 ml) and 2 fl. oz. (60 ml) plastic sprayer bottles.

Bioavailability Study

Plasma Levels after 10mg Dose

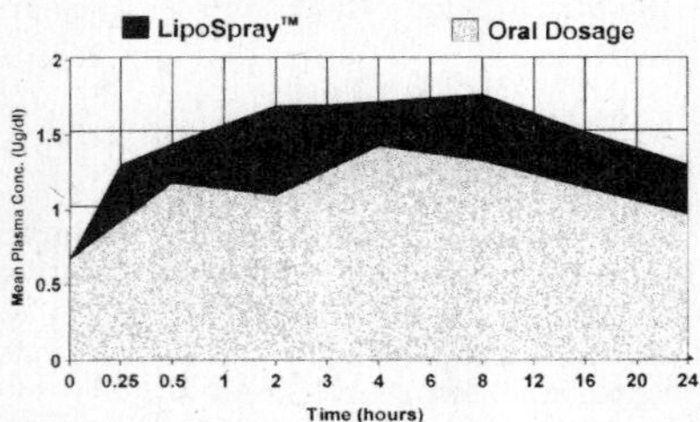

LipoSpray™ Products:

LipoSpray™ Alpha Tocopherol 40 I.U./Spray

LipoSpray™ Antioxidant Formula

LipoSpray™ Vitamin B Complex

LipoSpray™ Vitamin C 125 mg/Spray
Vitamin B_2 1 mg/Spray
Vitamin B_6 5 mg/Spray

LipoSpray™ Cat's Claw 75 mg/Spray

LipoSpray™ CoQ_{10} 10 mg, 15 mg, 25 mg, and 30 mg/Spray

LipoSpray™ DHEA 5 mg, 10 mg and 15 mg

LipoSpray™ Diet Suppressant, Citrimax 80 mg/Chromate 100 mcg/Spray

LipoSpray™ Ginkgo Biloba Extract 20 mg/Spray

LipoSpray™ Kava Kava 25 mg, 50 mg, and 75 mg/Spray

LipoSpray™ Melatonin 0.5 mg and 1.5 mg/Spray

LipoSpray™ Milk Thistle 50 mg/Spray

LipoSpray™ Panax Ginseng Extract 15 mg/Spray

LipoSpray™ Phosphotidyl Serine 25 mg/Spray

LipoSpray™ Multi Vitamin	mg/Spray	% DV/2 Sprays*
Vitamin A	1500.0 I.U.	1000%
Vitamin C	15.0 mg	100%
Vitamin D	100.0 I.U.	100%
Vitamin E	3.0 I.U.	100%
Thiamine	0.5 mg	100%
Riboflavin	0.3 mg	100%
Niacinamide	4.0 mg	100%
Vitamin B6	0.5 mg	100%
Biotin	5.0 mcg	100%
Folic Acid	100.0 mcg	100%
Pantothenic Acid	3.0 mg	100%
Vitamin B_{12}	0.5 mcg	100%

*Children's DV

LipoSpray™ Colloidal Multimineral

LipoSpray™ Echinacea 60 mg, and 125 mg

Blaine Company, Inc.

1465 JAMIKE LANE
ERLANGER, KY 41018

Direct Inquiries to:
Mr. Alex M. Blaine
(800) 633-9353
FAX: (606) 283-9460

MAG–OX 400

Description: Each tablet contains Magnesium Oxide 400 mg. U.S.P. (Heavy), or 241.3 mg. Elemental Magnesium (19.86 mEq.)

Indications and Usage: Hypomagnesemia, magnesium deficiencies and/or magnesium depletion during therapy with diuretics and/or digitalis, aminoglycosides, amphotericin B, cyclosporin, chemotherapy, and during pregnancy, PMS, menopause, diabetes, hyperoxaluria, malnutrition, weight/strength training, restricted diet, or alcoholism.

Warnings: Do not use this product except under the advice and supervision of a physician if you have a kidney disease. May have laxative effect.

Dosage: Adult dose 1 or 2 tablets daily with meals or as directed by a physician.

Professional Labeling: Serum magnesium levels do not accurately represent total body, tissue, or bone magnesium levels.

How Supplied: Bottles of 100, 1000, and hospital unit dose (U.D. 100s)

URO–MAG

Description: Each capsule contains Magnesium Oxide 140 mg. U.S.P. (Heavy), or 84.5 mg. Elemental Magnesium (6.93 mEq.)

Indications and Usage: Hypomagnesemia, magnesium deficiencies and/or magnesium depletion during therapy with diuretics and/or digitalis, aminoglycosides, amphotericin B, cyclosporin, chemotherapy, and during pregnancy, PMS, menopause, diabetes, hyperoxaluria, malnutrition, weight/strength training, restricted diet, or alcoholism.

Warnings: Do not use this product except under the advice and supervision of a physician if you have a kidney disease. May have laxative effect.

Dosage: Adult dose 3–4 capsules daily with meals or as directed by a physician.

Professional Labeling: Serum magnesium levels do not accurately represent total body, tissue, or bone magnesium levels.

How Supplied: Bottles of 100 and 1000.

EDUCATIONAL MATERIAL

Cardiovascular system charts, female reproductive system charts, samples, and literature available to physicians upon request.

Blairex Laboratories, Inc

3240 NORTH INDIANAPOLIS ROAD
P.O. BOX 2127
COLUMBUS, IN 47202-2127

Direct Inquiries to:
Customer Service
(800) 252-4739
FAX (812) 378-1033

For Medical Emergency Contact:
David S. Wilson, M.D.
(800) 252-4739
FAX (812) 378-1033

BRONCHO SALINE®

0.9% Sodium Chloride Aerosol for the dilution of bronchodilator inhalation solutions. Sterile normal saline for diluting bronchodilator solutions for oral inhalation.

Description: Broncho Saline® is for patients using bronchodilator solutions for oral inhalation that require dilution with sterile normal saline solution. Broncho Saline is a sterile liquid solution consisting of 0.9% sodium chloride for oral inhalation with a pH of 4.5 to 7.5. Not to be used for injection.

How Supplied: Broncho Saline® comes in 90cc (mL) (NDC 50486-078-22) and 240cc (mL) (NDC 50486-078-23) Pressurized Containers.

Store between 15–25°C (59–77°F). Keep out of reach of children. See WARNINGS.

NASAL MOIST®
Sodium Chloride 0.65%

Description: Isotonic saline solution buffered with sodium bicarbonate. Preserved with Benzyl alcohol.

Actions and Uses: Use for dry nasal membranes caused by chronic sinusitis, allergy, asthma, dry air, and oxygen therapy. May be used as often as needed.

Directions: Squeeze twice into each nostril as needed.

How Supplied: 45 mL (1.5 oz.) plastic squeeze bottle with drop capability, (NDC 50486-027-01) 15 mL (.5 oz.) plastic squeeze bottle with drop capability (NDC 50486-027-05) and 15 mL (.5 oz.) fine mist metered pump (NDC 50486-027-55).

NASAL MOIST® GEL

Description: Nasal Moist Gel with aloe vera is designed to relieve dryness and soreness caused by nasal cannula or BiPAP/CPAP use. Non-petroleum based, Nasal Moist Gel treats dry nasal passages caused by chronic sinusitis, allergies, asthma, common colds and dry air.

Directions: Apply in and around your nose to relieve dryness and soreness. Use as often as needed.

How Supplied: 1 oz. (28.5g) flip-top tube (NDC 50486-027-35)

PERTUSSIN® DM EXTRA STRENGTH
Cough Suppressant

Description: Each 5mL (one teaspoonful) contains:
Dextromethorphan Hydrobromide, USP 15mg

Inactive Ingredients: Carmel, Carboxymethylcellulose Sodium, Citric Acid, D&C Red No. 33, Flavor, Sorbic Acid, Sorbitol, Sugar, Purified Water. Contains 4% alcohol.

Indications: Temporarily relieves cough due to minor throat and bronchial irritation associated with the common cold.

Warnings: A persistent cough may be a sign of a serious condition. If cough persists more than 1 week, tends to recur, or is accompanied by a fever, rash, or persistent headache, consult a doctor. Do not take this product for persistent or chronic cough such as occurs with smoking, asthma, chronic bronchitis, emphysema, or if cough is accompanied by excessive phlegm (mucus) unless directed by a doctor. As with any drug, if you are pregnant or nursing a baby, seek the advise of a health professional before using this product.
KEEP THIS AND ALL DRUGS OUT OF THE REACH OF CHILDREN, IN CASE OF ACCIDENTAL OVERDOSE, SEEK PROFESSIONAL ASSISTANCE OR CONTACT A POISON CONTROL CENTER IMMEDIATELY.

Drug Interaction Precaution: Do not use this product if you are taking a prescription drug containing a monoamine oxidase inhibitor (MAOI) (certain drugs for depression or psychiatric or emotional conditions or Parkinson's disease), without first consulting your doctor. If you are uncertain whether your prescription drug contains an MAOI, consult a health professional before taking this product.

Directions: Adults and children 12 years of age and older: 2 teaspoonfuls every 6–8 hours as needed. Not to exceed 8 teaspoonfuls in 24 hours. Children 6 to under 12 years of age: One teaspoonful every 6–8 hours as needed. Not to exceed 4 teaspoonfuls in 24 hours. Do not administer to children under 6 years of age: Consult a doctor.

How Supplied: Available in shatter-resistant bottles of 4 fl. oz. (NDC 50486-048-20).

PERTUSSIN® CS CHILDREN'S STRENGTH
Cough Suppressant

Description: Each 5mL (one teaspoonful) contains:
Dextromethorphan Hydrobromide, USP 3.5mg

Inactive Ingredients: Citric Acid, Colors, Flavor, Sorbic Acid, Sorbitol, Sucrose, Purified Water. Alcohol-free.

Indications: Temporarily relieves cough due to minor throat and bronchial irritation associated with the common cold.

Warnings: A persistent cough may be a sign of a serious condition. If cough persists more than 1 week, tends to recur, or is accompanied by a fever, rash, or persistent headache, consult a doctor. Do not take this product for persistent or chronic cough such as occurs with smoking, asthma, chronic bronchitis, emphysema, or if cough is accompanied by excessive phlegm (mucus) unless directed by a doctor. As with any drug, if you are pregnant or nursing a baby, seek the advise of a health professional before using this product.
KEEP THIS AND ALL DRUGS OUT OF THE REACH OF CHILDREN, IN CASE OF ACCIDENTAL OVERDOSE, SEEK PROFESSIONAL ASSISTANCE OR CONTACT A POISON CONTROL CENTER IMMEDIATELY.

Drug Interaction Precaution: Do not give this product to a child who is taking a prescription drug containing a monoamine oxidase inhibitor (MAOI) (certain drugs for depression or psychiatric or emotional conditions or Parkinson's disease), without first consulting the child's doctor. If you are uncertain whether your child's prescription drug contains an MAOI, consult a health professional before giving this product.

Directions: Children 2 to under 6 years of age: 1 teaspoonful. Children 6 to under 12 years of age: 2 teaspoonfuls. Adults and children 12 years of age and older: 4 teaspoonfuls. Repeat every 4 hours as needed. Do not exceed 6 doses in a 24 hour period. Children under 2 years of age: Consult a doctor.

How Supplied: Available in shatter-resistant bottles of 4 fl. oz. (NDC 50486-048-40).

Block Drug Company, Inc.
257 CORNELISON AVENUE
JERSEY CITY, NJ 07302

Direct Inquiries to:
Lori Hunt
(201) 434-3000 Ext. 1308

For Medical Emergencies Contact:
Consumer Service/Block
(201) 434-3000 Ext. 1308

BALMEX® OINTMENT
for diaper rash

Description: Balmex® contains Zinc Oxide (11.3%) in a unique formulation including Peruvian Balsam suitable for topical application for the treatment and prevention of diaper rash.

Indications and Uses: Balmex helps treat and prevent diaper rash in four ways: 1. Soothes irritation. 2. Provides protection. 3. Promotes healing. 4. Reduces inflammation.
The zinc oxide based formulation provides a protective barrier on the skin against the natural causes of irritation. Balmex spreads on smooth and wipes off the baby easily, without causing irritation to the affected area. Balmex tactile properties promote compliance amongst mothers, and clinical studies have demonstrated that Balmex is effective in treating diaper rash.

Directions: At the first sign of diaper rash or redness apply Balmex three or more times daily as needed. To help prevent diaper rash, apply Balmex liberally as often as necessary, with each diaper change, especially at bedtime or anytime when exposure to wet diapers may be prolonged.

Warnings: Avoid contact with the eyes. For external use only. If condition worsens or does not improve within 7 days, contact a physician. Keep out of reach of children.

Active Ingredient: Zinc Oxide.

Inactive Ingredients: Balsam (Specially Purified Balsam Peru), Beeswax,

Continued on next page

Block Drug—Cont.

Benzoic Acid, Bismuth Subnitrate, Mineral Oil, Purified Water, Silicone, Synthetic White Wax, and other ingredients.

How Supplied: 2 oz. (57 g.) and 4 oz. (113 g.) tubes and 16 oz. (454 g.) jars.

BC® POWDER
ARTHRITIS STRENGTH BC® POWDER
BC® COLD POWDER

Description: BC® POWDER: Active Ingredients: Each powder contains Aspirin 650 mg, Salicylamide 195 mg and Caffeine 32 mg. ARTHRITIS STRENGTH BC® POWDER: Active Ingredients: Each powder contains Aspirin 742 mg, Salicylamide 222 mg and Caffeine 36 mg. BC® ALLERGY SINUS COLD POWDER
Active Ingredients: Aspirin 650 mg, Phenylpropanolamine Hydrochloride 25 mg, and Chlorpheniramine Maleate 4 mg per powder. BC® SINUS COLD POWDER. Active Ingredients: Aspirin 650 mg and Phenylpropanolamine Hydrochloride 25 mg per powder.

Indications: BC Powder is for relief of simple headache; for temporary relief of minor arthritic pain, neuralgia, neuritis and sciatica; for relief of muscular aches, discomfort and fever of colds; and for relief of normal menstrual pain and pain of tooth extraction.
Arthritis Strength BC Powder is specially formulated to fight occasional minor pain and inflammation of arthritis. Like Original Formula BC, Arthritis Strength BC provides fast temporary relief of minor arthritis pain and inflammation, neuralgia, neuritis and sciatica; relief of muscular aches, discomfort and fever of colds; and pain of tooth extraction.
BC Allergy Sinus Cold Powder is for relief of multiple symptoms such as body aches, fever, nasal congestion, sneezing, running nose, and watery itchy eyes associated with Allergy Sinus and Colds. BC Sinus Cold Powder is for relief of such symptoms as body aches, fever, and nasal congestions.

BC Powder®, Arthritis Strength BC® Powder:

Warnings: BC Powder and Arthritis Strength BC® Powder: Children and teenagers should not use this medicine for chicken pox or flu symptoms before a doctor is consulted about Reye Syndrome, a rare but serious illness reported to be associated with aspirin. Do not take this product if you are allergic to aspirin. If pain persists for more than 10 days or redness is present, discontinue use of this product and consult a physician immediately. Keep this and all medication out of children's reach. In case of accidental overdose contact a physician or poison control center immediately. As with any drug, if you are pregnant or nursing a baby, consult your physician before using this product.

Alcohol Warning: If you generally consume 3 or more alcohol-containing drinks per day, you should consult your physician for advice on when and how you should take BC and other pain relievers.
IT IS ESPECIALLY IMPORTANT NOT TO USE ASPIRIN DURING THE LAST 3 MONTHS OF PREGNANCY UNLESS SPECIFICALLY DIRECTED TO DO SO BY A DOCTOR BECAUSE IT MAY CAUSE PROBLEMS IN THE UNBORN CHILD OR COMPLICATIONS DURING DELIVERY.
BC Cold Powder Line:

Warnings: Children and teenagers should not use BC for chicken pox or flu symptoms before a doctor is consulted about Reye Syndrome, a rare but serious illness reported to be associated with aspirin. Keep BC and all medicines out of children's reach. In case of accidental overdose, contact a physician or poison control center immediately.
As with any drug, if you are pregnant or nursing a baby seek the advice of a health professional before using BC.

Alcohol Warning: If you generally consume 3 or more alcohol-containing drinks per day, you should consult your physician for advice on when and how you should take BC and other pain relievers.
IT IS ESPECIALLY IMPORTANT NOT TO USE ASPIRIN DURING THE LAST 3 MONTHS OF PREGNANCY UNLESS SPECIFICALLY DIRECTED TO DO SO BY A DOCTOR BECAUSE IT MAY CAUSE PROBLEMS IN THE UNBORN CHILD OR COMPLICATIONS DURING DELIVERY.
Nervousness, dizziness or sleeplessness may occur if recommended dosage is exceeded. If symptoms do not improve within 7 days, or are accompanied by fever that lasts more than 3 days, or if new symptoms occur, consult a physician before continuing use. Do not take BC if you are sensitive to aspirin, or have heart disease, high blood pressure, thyroid disease, diabetes, asthma, glaucoma, emphysema, chronic pulmonary disease, shortness of breath, difficulty in breathing or difficulty in urination due to enlargement of the prostrate gland, or if you are presently taking a prescription antihypertensive or antidepressant drug containing a monoamine oxidase inhibitor unless directed by a doctor. BC Allergy Sinus Cold Powder with antihistamine may cause drowsiness. Use caution when driving a motor vehicle or operating machinery. May cause excitability, especially in children.

Overdosage: In case of accidental overdosage, contact a physician or poison control center immediately.

Dosage and Administration: BC® Powder, Arthritis Strength BC® Powder, BC® Cold Powder Line:
Place one powder on tongue and follow with liquid. If you prefer, stir powder into glass of water or other liquid. May be used every three to four hours, up to 4 powders each 24 hours. For children under 12, consult a physician.

How Supplied: BC Powder: Available in tamper resistant overwrapped envelopes of 2 or 6 powders, as well as tamper resistant boxes of 24 and 50 powders.
Arthritis Strength BC Powder: Available in tamper resistant over wrapped envelopes of 6 powders, and tamper resistant overwrapped boxes of 24 and 50 powders.
BC Cold Powder Line:
Available in tamper-resistant overwrapped envelopes of 6 powders, as well as tamper-resistant boxes of 12 powders.

GOODY'S
Extra Strength Headache Powder

Indications: For Temporary Relief of Minor Aches & Pain Due to Headaches, Arthritis, Colds & Fever

Directions: Adults: Place one powder on tongue and follow with liquid or stir powder into a glass of water or other liquid. May be repeated in 4 to 6 hours. Do not take more than 4 powders in any 24-hour period. Children under 12 years of age: Consult a doctor.

Warnings: Children and teenagers should not use this medicine for chicken pox or flu symptoms before a doctor is consulted about Reye Syndrome, a rare but serious illness reported to be associated with aspirin.
As with any drug, if you are pregnant, or nursing a baby, seek the advice of a health professional before using this product.
IT IS ESPECIALLY IMPORTANT NOT TO USE ASPIRIN DURING THE LAST 3 MONTHS OF PREGNANCY UNLESS SPECIFICALLY DIRECTED TO DO SO BY A DOCTOR BECAUSE IT MAY CAUSE PROBLEMS IN THE UNBORN CHILD OR COMPLICATIONS DURING DELIVERY. Alcohol Warning: If you generally consume 3 or more alcohol-containing drinks per day, you should consult your physician for advice on when and how you should take Goody's® and other pain relievers. **Keep this and all medicines out of the reach of children. In case of accidental overdose, contact a doctor or poison control center immediately.**
This product contains aspirin and should not be taken by individuals who are sensitive to aspirin. If pain persists for more than 10 days or redness is present, consult a physician immediately.

Active Ingredients: Each Powder contains 520 mg. aspirin in combination with 260 mg. acetaminophen and 32.5 mg. caffeine.

Inactive Ingredients: Lactose and Potassium Chloride.

Dist. By: GOODY'S PHARMACEUTICALS
Memphis, TN 38113

GOODY'S®
Extra Strength Pain Relief Tablets

Indications: Goody's EXTRA STRENGTH tablets are a specially developed pain reliever that provide fast & effective temporary relief from minor aches & pain due to headaches, arthritis, colds or "flu," muscle strain, backache & menstrual discomfort. It is recommended for temporary relief of toothaches and to reduce fever.

Dosage: Adults: Two tablets with water or other liquid. May be repeated in 4 to 6 hours. Do not take more than 8 tablets in any 24-hour period. Children under 12 years of age: Consult a doctor.

Warning: Children and teenagers should not use this medicine for chicken pox or flu symptoms before a doctor is consulted about Reye Syndrome, a rare but serious illness reported to be associated with aspirin. As with any drug, if you are pregnant, or nursing a baby, seek the advice of a health professional before using this product. IT IS ESPECIALLY IMPORTANT NOT TO USE ASPIRIN DURING THE LAST 3 MONTHS OF PREGNANCY UNLESS SPECIFICALLY DIRECTED TO DO SO BY A DOCTOR BECAUSE IT MAY CAUSE PROBLEMS IN THE UNBORN CHILD OR COMPLICATIONS DURING DELIVERY. **Alcohol Warning:** If you generally consume 3 or more alcohol-containing drinks per day, you should consult your physician for advice on when and how you should take Goody's® and other pain relievers. Keep this and all medicines out of the reach of children. In case of accidental overdose, contact a doctor or poison control center immediately. This product contains aspirin and should not be taken by individuals who are sensitive to aspirin. If pain persists for more than 10 days, or redness is present, consult a physician immediately.
Active Ingredients: Each tablet contains 260 mg. aspirin in combination with 130 mg. acetaminophen and 16.25 mg. caffeine. **Inactive Ingredients:** Corn Starch, Modified Starch, Polyvinylpyrrolidone and Stearic Acid.
Dist. By: GOODY'S PHARMACEUTICALS
Memphis, TN 38113

NATURE'S REMEDY®
Nature's Gentle LAXATIVE

Description: Nature's Remedy is a stimulant laxative with natural active ingredients that work gently, overnight. It is the only laxative on the market with the natural active ingredients Cascara Sagrada and Aloe.
Active Ingredients: Each tablet contains Cascara Sagrada 150 mg and Aloe 100 mg.

Inactive Ingredients: Calcium Stearate FD&C Blue #2, FD&C Yellow #6, Hydroxypropyl Cellulose, Hydroxypropyl Methylcellulose, Lactose, Microcrystalline Cellulose, Polyethylene Glycol, Titanium Dioxide.

Actions: Nature's Remedy has two natural active ingredients, Cascara Sagrada and Aloe, that gently stimulate the body's natural function.

Indications: For relief of occasional constipation. Nature's Remedy tablets generally produce bowel movement in 6 to 12 hours.

Warnings: Keep this and all drugs out of the reach of children. Do not use laxative products when abdominal pain, nausea, or vomiting are present unless directed by a doctor. If you have noticed a sudden change in bowel habits that persists over a period of 2 weeks consult a doctor before using a laxative. Laxative products should not be used for a period longer than 1 week unless directed by a doctor. Rectal bleeding or failure to have a bowel movement after use of a laxative may indicate a serious condition. Discontinue use and consult your doctor. In case of accidental overdose, seek professional assistance or contact a poison control center immediately. As with any drug, if you are pregnant or nursing a baby, seek the advice of a health professional before using this product.
Store at room temperature, avoid excessive heat (greater than 100°F) or high humidity.

Dosage: Adults and children 15 years of age and over: Swallow 2 tablets daily along with a full glass of water; Children 8 to under 15 years of age: 1 tablet daily along with a full glass of water, or as directed by a physician; Children under 8 years of age: Consult a physician.

How Supplied: Beige, film-coated tablets with foil-backed blister packaging in boxes of 15, 30 and 60.

Shown in Product Identification Guide, page 506

Maximum Strength
NYTOL® Quickgels® Softgels

Active Ingredient: Diphenhydramine Hydrochloride 50 mg per softgel.

Inactive Ingredients: Polyethylene Glycol, Gelatin, Glycerin, Sorbitol, Purified Water, Edible Ink.

Indications: For relief of occasional sleeplessness.

Do not give to children under 12 years of age. If sleeplessness persists continuously for more than two weeks, consult your doctor. Insomnia may be a symptom of a serious underlying medical illness. **DO NOT TAKE THIS PRODUCT, UNLESS DIRECTED BY A DOCTOR, IF YOU HAVE A BREATHING PROBLEM SUCH AS EMPHYSEMA OR CHRONIC BRONCHITIS, OR IF YOU HAVE GLAUCOMA OR DIFFICULTY IN URINATION DUE TO ENLARGEMENT OF THE PROSTATE GLAND.** Avoid alcoholic beverages while taking this product. Do not take this product if you are taking sedatives or tranquilizers, without first consulting your doctor. In case of accidental overdose, seek professional assistance or contact Poison Control Center immediately. As with any drug, if you are pregnant or nursing a baby seek the advice of a health professional before using this product. Keep this and all drugs out of the reach of children.

Drug Interaction: Alcohol and other drugs which cause CNS depression will heighten the depressant effect of this product. Monoamine oxidase (MAO) inhibitors will prolong and intensify the anticholinergic effects of antihistamines.

Symptoms and Treatment of Oral Overdosage: In adults overdose may cause CNS depression resulting in hypnosis and coma. In children CNS hyperexcitability may follow sedation; the stimulant phase may bring tremor, delirium and convulsions. Gastrointestinal reactions may include dry mouth, appetite loss, nausea and vomiting. Respiratory distress and cardiovascular complications (hypotension) may be evident. Treatment includes inducing emesis, and controlling symptoms.

Dosage and Administration: Adults and children 12 years of age and over: oral dosage is one softgel (50 mg) at bedtime if needed, or as directed by a doctor.

How supplied: Available in packages of 8 and 16 softgels.

NYTOL® QUICK CAPS® CAPLETS

Active Ingredient: Diphenhydramine Hydrochloride, 25 mg per caplet.

Inactive Ingredients: Corn Starch, Lactose, Microcrystalline Cellulose, Silica, Stearic Acid.

Indications: For relief of occasional sleeplessness. Diphenhydramine Hydrochloride is an antihistamine with anticholinergic and sedative effects which induces drowsiness and helps in falling asleep.

Warnings: Do not give to children under 12 years of age. If sleeplessness persists continuously for more than 2 weeks, consult your doctor. Insomnia may be a symptom of serious underlying medical illness. Do not take this product, unless directed by a doctor, if you have a breathing problem such as emphysema or chronic bronchitis, or if you have glaucoma or difficulty in urination due to enlargement of the prostate gland. Avoid alcoholic beverages while taking this product. Do not take this product if you are taking sedatives or tranquilizers, without first consulting your doctor. In case of accidental overdose seek professional assistance or contact a poison con-

Continued on next page

Block Drug—Cont.

trol center immediately. As with any drug, if your are pregnant or nursing a baby, seek the advice of a health professional before using this product. Keep this and all drugs out of the reach of children.

Drug Interaction: Alcohol and other drugs which cause CNS depression will heighten the depressant effect of this product. Monoamine oxidase (MAO) inhibitors will prolong and intensify the anticholinergic effects of antihistamines.

Symptoms and Treatment of Oral Overdosage: In adults overdose may cause CNS depression resulting in hypnosis and coma. In children CNS hyperexcitability may follow sedation; the stimulant phase may bring tremor, delirium and convulsions. Gastrointestinal reactions may include dry mouth, appetite loss, nausea and vomiting. Respiratory distress and cardiovascular complications (hypotension) may be evident. Treatment includes inducing emesis, and controlling symptoms.

Dosage and Administration: Adults and children 12 years of age and over, take 2 NYTOL with DPH at bedtime if needed, or as directed by a physician.

How Supplied: Available in tamper resistant packages of 16, 32, and 72 caplets NYTOL with DPH.

PHAZYME®-95

[*fay-zime*]

Tablets

Description: Contains simethicone, an antiflatulent to alleviate or relieve the symptoms referred to as gas. It has no known side effects or drug interactions.

Actions: Simethicone minimizes gas formation and relieves gas entrapment in both the stomach and the lower G.I. tract. This action combats the distress due to gastrointestinal gas.
Sodium Content: 12 mg./tablet

Indication: To alleviate or relieve the symptoms referred to as gas.

Warnings: Keep this and all drugs out of the reach of children. If condition persists, consult your physician.

Store at room temperature.

Active Ingredient: Each tablet contains simethicone 95 mg.

Inactive Ingredients: Acacia, carnauba wax, compressible sugar, crosscarmellose sodium, FD&C red No. 40 aluminum lake, FD&C yellow No. 6 aluminum lake, hydroxypropyl methylcellulose, microcrystalline cellulose, polyoxyl 40 stearate, povidone, sodium benzoate, sucrose, talc, titanium dioxide, white wax.

Dosage: One tablet four times a day after meals and at bedtime. Do not exceed 5 tablets per day unless directed by a physician.

How Supplied: Red coated tablet imprinted "Phazyme 95" in 10 pack, 30 pack and bottles of 50's and 100's.

Shown in Product Identification Guide, page 506

PHAZYME® INFANT DROPS

[*fay-zime*]

Description: Contains simethicone in a natural, orange flavor, an antiflatulent to alleviate or relieve the symptoms referred to as gas. It has no known side effects or drug interactions.

Active Ingredient: Each 0.6 mL contains simethicone, 40 mg.

Inactive Ingredients: Carbomer 974P, citric acid, flavor (natural orange), hydroxypropyl methylcellulose, PEG-8 stearate, sodium benzoate, sodium citrate, water.

Actions: Simethicone minimizes gas formation and relieves gas entrapment in both the stomach and the lower G.I. tract. This action combats the distress due to gastrointestinal gas.

Indication: To alleviate or relieve the symptoms referred to as gas.

Warnings: Keep this and all drugs out of the reach of children. If condition persists, consult your physician.

Store at room temperature.

Dosage/Administration: Shake well before using.

Infants (under 2 years):
0.3 ml four times daily after meals and at bedtime or as directed by a physician. Can also be mixed with liquids for easier administration.

Children (2 to 12 years):
0.6 ml four times daily after meals and at bedtime or as directed by a physician.

Adults: 1.2 ml (take two 0.6 ml doses) four times daily after meals and at bedtime. Do not take more than six times per day unless directed by a physician.

How Supplied: Dropper bottles of 15 mL (0.5 fl oz) and 30 mL (1 fl oz).

Shown in Product Identification Guide, page 506

Maximum Strength PHAZYME®-125 Chewable Tablets

[*fayzime*]

Description: Phazyme Chewables contains simethicone in a single, fresh mint tasting chewable tablet. It has no known side effects or drug interactions.

Active Ingredient: Each tablet contains simethicone 125 mg.

Inactive Ingredients: Citric acid, D&C Yellow #10, dextrates, FD&C Blue #1, peppermint flavor, sorbitol, starch, sucrose, talc, tribasic calcium phosphate.

Actions: Simethicone minimizes gas formation and relieves gas entrapment in both the stomach and the lower G.I. tract. This action combats the distress due to gastrointestinal gas.

Indication: To alleviate or relieve the symptoms referred to as gas.

Warnings: Keep this and all drugs out of the reach of children. If condition persists, consult your physician.

Store at room temperature.

Dosage: One tablet, chewed thoroughly, four times a day after meals and at bedtime. Do not exceed 4 chewable tablets per day unless directed by a physician.

How Supplied: White, bevel-edged tablets with green speckles and imprinted with "Phazyme 125" in 10 pack, 30 pack and 50 pack.

Shown in Product Identification Guide, page 506

Maximum Strength PHAZYME—125 LIQUID

[*fay' zime*]

Description: Phazyme Liquid is the only liquid made specifically for fast gas relief. Contains simethicone, an antiflatulent to alleviate or relieve the symptoms referred to as gas, in smooth Cherry Creme and Mint Creme. It has no known side effects or drug interactions.

Active Ingredient: Each teaspoonful (5ml) contains 62.5 mg simethicone.

Inactive Ingredients: Bentonite, flavor, glycerin, hydrochloric acid, hydroxyethylcellulose, PEG 40 stearate, sodium benzoate, sodium saccharin, titanium dioxide, water.
Mint: Sodium Content: 6 mg./dose
Cherry: Sodium Content: 5 mg./dose

Actions: Simethicone minimizes gas formation and relieves gas entrapment in both the stomach and the lower G.I. tract. This action combats the distress due to gastrointestinal gas.

Indication: To alleviate or relieve the symptoms referred to as gas.

Warnings: Keep this and all drugs out of the reach of children. If condition persists, consult our physician.
Store at room temperature.

Directions: Shake well before using. Take two teaspoons four times a day after meals and at bedtime. Do not exceed 8 teaspoons per day unless directed by a physician.

How Supplied: 10 oz. bottles with dosage cup shrink wrapped to cap.

Shown in Product Identification Guide, page 506

Maximum Strength PHAZYME®-125 Softgel Capsules

[*fayzime*]

Description: A red easy to swallow softgel containing simethicone to alleviate or relieve the symptoms referred to as gas. It has no known side effects or drug interactions.

Active Ingredient: Each capsule contains simethicone, 125 mg.

Inactive Ingredients: FD&C red No. 40, gelatin, glycerin, hydrogenated soybean oil, lecithin, methylparaben, polysorbate 80, propylparaben, soybean oil, titanium dioxide, vegetable shortening, yellow wax.

Actions: Simethicone minimizes gas formation and relieves gas entrapment in both the stomach and the lower G.I. tract. This action combats the distress due to gastrointestinal gas.

Indication: To alleviate or relieve the symptoms referred to as gas.

Warnings: Keep this and all drugs out of the reach of children. If condition persists, consult your physician.

Store at room temperature.

Dosage: One softgel capsule four times a day after meals and at bedtime. Do not exceed 4 softgel capsules per day unless directed by a physician.

How Supplied: Red softgel capsule imprinted Phazyme 125 in 10 pack, 30 pack and 50 count bottle.

Shown in Product Identification Guide, page 506

PROMISE® SENSITIVE TOOTHPASTE
Anticavity Toothpaste for Sensitive Teeth

Active Ingredients: Potassium Nitrate and Sodium Monofluorophosphate in a pleasantly mint-flavored dentifrice.

Inactive Ingredients: Water, Dicalcium Phosphate Dihydrate, Glycerin, Sorbitol, Dicalcium Phosphate, Sodium Lauryl Sulfate, Hydroxyethylcellulose, Flavor, Silica, Sodium Saccharin, Methylparaben, Propylparaben, D&C Yellow #10, FD&C Blue #1.

Promise contains Potassium Nitrate for relief of dentinal hypersensitivity resulting from the exposure of tooth dentin due to periodontal surgery, cervical (gumline) erosion, abrasion or recession which causes pain on contact with hot, cold, or tactile stimuli. Promise also contains Sodium Monofluorophosphate for cavity prevention.

Indications: Promise builds increasing protection against painful sensitivity of the teeth to cold, heat, acids, sweets or contact and aids in the prevention of dental cavities.

Actions: Promise significantly reduces tooth hypersensitivity, with response to therapy evident after two weeks of use. Controlled double-blind clinical studies provide substantial evidence of the safety and effectiveness of Promise. The current theory on mechanism of action is that the potassium nitrate in Promise has an effect on neural transmission, interrupting the signal which would result in the sensation of pain. Sodium Monofluorophosphate protects the tooth surfaces to prevent cavities.

Warning: Sensitive teeth may indicate a serious problem that may need prompt care by a dentist. See your dentist if the problem persists or worsens. Do not use this product longer than 4 weeks unless recommended by a dentist or physician. **Keep this and all drugs out of the reach of children. If you accidentally swallow more than used for brushing seek professional assistance or contact a Poison Control Center immediately.**

Directions: Adults and children 12 years of age and older:
Apply at least a 1-inch strip of the product onto a soft bristle toothbrush. Brush teeth thoroughly for at least 1 minute twice a day (morning and evening) or as recommended by a dentist or doctor. Make sure to brush all sensitive areas of the teeth. Children under 12 years of age: Consult a dentist or physician.

How Supplied: Promise Sensitive is supplied in 3.0 oz. (85 g) and 4.5 oz. (128 g) tubes.

FRESH MINT SENSODYNE®
COOL GEL SENSODYNE®
SENSODYNE® WITH BAKING SODA
SENSODYNE® TARTAR CONTROL
ORIGINAL FLAVOR SENSODYNE®
Anticavity toothpaste for sensitive teeth

Active Ingredients: 5% Potassium Nitrate and Sodium Monofluorophosphate (Fresh Mint and Original Flavor) or Sodium Fluoride (Cool Gel, Baking Soda, Tartar Control) in a pleasantly mint-flavored dentifrice.

Fresh Mint Sensodyne, Cool Gel Sensodyne, Sensodyne with Baking Soda, Sensodyne Tartar Control and Original Flavor Sensodyne contain Potassium Nitrate for relief of dentinal hypersensitivity resulting from the exposure of tooth dentin due to periodontal surgery, cervical (gum line) erosion, abrasion or recession which causes pain on contact with hot, cold, or tactile stimuli and fluoride for cavity prevention. Fresh Mint Sensodyne has been given the Seal of Acceptance by the ADA Council on Dental Therapeutics as an effective desensitizing dentifrice for otherwise normal teeth.

Actions: All Sensodyne Formulas significantly reduce tooth hypersensitivity, with response to therapy evident after two weeks of use. Controlled double-blind clinical studies provide substantial evidence of the safety and effectiveness of potassium nitrate. The current theory on mechanism of action is that potassium nitrate has an effect on neural transmission, interrupting the signal which would result in the sensation of pain. Fluorides are anticariogenic, forming fluoroapatite in the outer surface of the dental enamel which is resistant to acids and caries.

Warnings: Sensitive teeth may indicate a serious problem that may need prompt care by a dentist. See your dentist if the problem persists or worsens. Do not use this product longer than 4 weeks unless recommended by a dentist or physician. Keep this and all drugs out of the reach of children. If you accidentally swallow more than used for brushing, seek professional assistance or contact a Poison Control Center immediately.

Dosage and Administration: Adults and children 12 years of age and older: Apply at least a 1-inch strip of the product onto a soft bristle toothbrush. Brush teeth thoroughly for at least 1 minute twice a day (morning and evening) or as recommended by a dentist or doctor. Make sure to brush all sensitive areas of the teeth. Children under 12 years of age: consult a dentist or physician.

How Supplied: All Sensodyne formulas are supplied in 2.1 (60 g), 4.0 (113 g) and 6.0 oz. (170 g) tubes.

TEGRIN® DANDRUFF SHAMPOO
TEGRIN® FOR PSORIASIS SKIN CREAM AND MEDICATED SOAP

Description: Tegrin® Dandruff Shampoo contains 7% coal tar solution equivalent to 1.1% coal tar, in a pleasantly scented, high-foaming, cleansing shampoo base with emollients, conditioners and other formula components.

Tegrin® for Psoriasis Skin Cream and Medicated Soap each contain 5% coal tar solution, equivalent to 0.8% coal tar. The Cream also contains alcohol (4.9% and 4.7%, respectively).

Indications: For relief of itching, flaking and irritation of the skin associated with psoriasis and seborrheic dermatitis.

Directions: CREAM Apply to affected areas one to four times daily or as directed by a doctor.

SHAMPOO SHAKE WELL. Wet hair. Lather, rinse, repeat. For best results use at least twice a week or as directed by a doctor.

SOAP: Use on affected areas in place of your regular soap.

Coal Tar is obtained in the destructive distillation of bituminous coal and is a highly effective agent for controlling the flaking and itching of the scalp associated with dandruff, seborrheic dermatitis and psoriasis. The action of coal tar is believed to be keratolytic, antiseptic, antipruritic and astringent. The coal tar solution used in Tegrin Dandruff Shampoo is prepared in such a way as to reduce the pitch and other irritant components found in crude coal tar without reduction in therapeutic potency.

Continued on next page

Block Drug—Cont.

Coal tar solution has been used clinically for many years as a remedy for dandruff and for scaling associated with scalp disorders such as seborrhea and psoriasis. Its mechanism of action has not been fully established, but it is believed to retard the rate of turnover of epidermal cells with regular use. A number of clinical studies have demonstrated the performance attributes of Tegrin Dandruff Shampoo against dandruff and seborrheic dermatitis. In addition to relieving the above symptoms, Tegrin shampoo, used regularly, maintains scalp and hair cleanliness and leaves the hair lustrous and manageable.

Warnings: For external use only. Avoid contact with eyes. If contact occurs, rinse eyes thoroughly with water. If condition worsens or does not improve after regular use of this product as directed consult a doctor. Do not use cream in or around the rectum or in the genital area or groin except on the advice of a doctor. Use caution in exposing skin to sunlight after applying this product. It may increase tendency to sunburn for up to 24 hours after application. Do not use for prolonged periods without consulting a doctor. Do not use this product with other forms of psoriasis therapy, such as ultraviolet radiation or prescription drugs unless directed by a doctor. If the condition covers a large area of the body, consult your doctor before using this product. Keep out of reach of children. In case of accidental ingestion, seek professional assistance or contact a Poison Control Center immediately.

How Supplied: Tegrin Dandruff Shampoo is supplied in 7 fl. oz. (207 ml) plastic bottles.
Tegrin Cream 2 oz. (57 g) and 4.4 oz. (124 g) tubes, Tegrin Soap 4.5 oz. (127 g) bars.

Boiron, The World Leader In Homeopathy

6 CAMPUS BLVD.
BUILDING A
NEWTOWN SQUARE, PA 19073

HEADQUARTERS
6 Campus Blvd., Building A
Newtown Square, PA 19073
(610) 325-7464

Direct Inquiries to:
Gina Casey
Public Relations Manager
(610) 325-8320

For Medical Emergencies Contact:
Steven Boorstein, Pharm. D.
Branch Manager
(610) 325-7464

WEST COAST BRANCH:
98C West Cochran Street
Simi Valley, CA 93065

Direct Inquiries to:
Christophe Merville, Pharmacist
Branch Manager
(805) 582-9091

OSCILLOCOCCINUM®

[ah-sill'o-cox-see'num']

Active Ingredient: Anas barbariae hepatis et cordis extractum HPUS 200CK

Indications: For the relief of symptoms of flu such as fever, chills, body aches and pains.

Actions: Like most homeopathic medicine, Oscillococcinum® acts gently by stimulating the patient's natural defense mechanisms.

Dosage and Administration: (Adults and Children over 2 years of age):
At the onset of symptoms, place the entire contents of one tube in the mouth and allow to dissolve under the tongue. Repeat for 2 more doses at 6 hour intervals. For maximum results, Oscillococcinum® should be taken early, at the onset of symptoms, and at least 15 minutes before or 1 hour after meals.

Warnings: If symptoms persist for more than three days or worsen, consult your physician. Keep this and all medication out of reach of children. As with any drug if you are pregnant or nursing a baby, seek professional advice before using this product. Diabetics: this product contains sugar (0.85 g sucrose, 0.15 g lactose per unit dose).

How Supplied: boxes of 3 unit doses or 6 unit doses of 0.04 oz. (1 gram) each (NDC #0220-9280-32 and NDC #0220-9288-33) Tamper resistant package.
Manufactured by Boiron, France.
Distributor: Boiron, Newtown Square, PA 19073

EDUCATIONAL MATERIAL

Boiron Product Catalogue
General description of the most popular Boiron products.

***Oscillococcinum*® Brochure**
Brochure describing clinical research on the product.

"What Is Homeopathy?"
Booklet describing the basic principles of homeopathy.

"An Introduction to Homeopathy for the Practicing Pharmacist"
An ACPE-approved continuing education booklet for pharmacists (0.2 CEUs).

Research Bibliography
A listing of current research in homeopathic medicine.

Bristol-Myers Products

(A Bristol-Myers Squibb Company)
345 PARK AVENUE
NEW YORK, NY 10154

For Medical Information Contact:
Generally:
Bristol-Myers Products Division
Consumer Affairs Department
1350 Liberty Avenue
Hillside, NJ 07207

In Emergencies:
(800) 468-7746

ALPHA KERI®
Moisture Rich Body Oil

Composition: Contains mineral oil, PEG-4 dilaurate, lanolin oil, fragrance, benzophenone-3, D&C green 6.

Indications: ALPHA KERI is a water-dispersible oil for the care of dry skin. ALPHA KERI effectively deposits a thin, uniform, emulsified film of oil over the skin. This film lubricates and softens the skin. ALPHA KERI Moisture Rich Body Oil is an all-over skin moisturizer. Only Alpha Keri contains Hydroloc™—the unique emulsifier that provides a more uniform distribution of the therapeutic oils to moisturize dry skin. ALPHA KERI is valuable as an aid for dry skin and mild skin irritations.

Directions for Use: ALPHA KERI *should always be used with water, either added to water or rubbed on to wet skin.* Because of its inherent cleansing properties it is not necessary to use soap when ALPHA KERI is being used.
For external use only.
Label directions should be followed for use in shower, bath and cleansing.

Precaution: The patient should be warned to guard against slipping in tub or shower.

How Supplied: 4 fl. oz., 8 fl. oz., and 16 fl. oz., plastic bottles.

BACKACHE CAPLETS

Composition: Each caplet contains Magnesium Salicylate Tetrahydrate 580 mg (equivalent to 467 mg of anhydrous Magnesium Salicylate)
Other Ingredients: Carnauba Wax, Hydrogenated Vegetable Oil, Hydroxypropyl Methylcellulose, Magnesium Stearate, Microcrystalline Cellulose, Polyethylene Glycol, Polysorbate 80, Titanium Dioxide

Indications: For the temporary relief of minor aches and pains associated with backache and muscular aches (e.g., sprains and strains).

Directions: Adults: 2 caplets with water every 6 hours while symptoms persist, not to exceed 8 caplets in 24 hours or as directed by a doctor. Children under 12: Consult a doctor.

Warnings: Children and teenagers should not use this medicine for chicken pox or flu symptoms before a doctor is consulted about Reye syndrome, a rate but serious illness. **KEEP THIS AND ALL OTHER MEDICATIONS OUT OF THE REACH OF CHILDREN. IN CASE OF ACCIDENTAL OVERDOSE, SEEK PROFESSIONAL ASSISTANCE OR CONTACT A POISON CONTROL CENTER IMMEDIATELY.** As with any drug, if you are pregnant or nursing a baby, seek the advice of a health professional before using this product. Do not take this product for more than 10 days unless directed by a doctor. If pain persists or gets worse, if new symptoms occur, or if redness or swelling is present, consult a doctor because these could be signs of a serious condition. Do not take this product if you are allergic to salicylates (including aspirin), have asthma, have stomach problems (such as heartburn, upset stomach or stomach pain) that persists or recur, or if you have ulcers or bleeding problems, unless directed by a doctor. If ringing in the ears or loss of hearing occurs, consult a doctor before taking any more of this product.

Drug Interaction Precaution: Do not take this product if you are taking a prescription drug for anticoagulation (thinning of blood), diabetes, gout or arthritis unless directed by a doctor.

How Supplied: BACKACHE is a white caplet with the logo "N-BACK" debossed on one side.
Supplied in blister cards of 24's.
Store at room temperature.

BUFFERIN®
[*bŭf'fĕr-ĭn*]
Analgesic

Composition:
Active Ingredient: Aspirin 325 mg in a formulation buffered with Calcium Carbonate, Magnesium Oxide and Magnesium Carbonate.
Other Ingredients: Benzoic Acid, Citric Acid, Corn Starch, FD&C Blue No. 1, Hydroxypropyl Methylcellulose, Magnesium Stearate, Mineral Oil, Polysorbate 20, Povidone, Propylene Glycol, Simethicone Emulsion, Sodium Phosphate, Sorbitan Monolaurate, Titanium Dioxide. May also contain: Carnauba Wax, Zinc Stearate.
Indications: For fast temporary relief of headaches, minor arthritis pain and inflammation, muscle aches, pain and fever of colds, menstrual pain and toothaches.

Directions: Adults and chldren 12 years of age and over: 2 tablets with water every 4 hours while symptoms persist, not to exceed 12 tablets in 24 hours, or as directed by a doctor. Children under 12 years of age: Consult a doctor.

Warnings: Children and teenagers should not use this medicine for chicken pox or flu symptoms before a doctor is consulted about Reye syndrome, a rare but serious illness reported to be associated with aspirin. Keep this and all drugs out of the reach of children. In case of accidental overdose, seek professional assistance or contact a poison control center immediately. As with any drug, if you are pregnant or nursing a baby, seek the advice of a health professional before using this product. **IT IS ESPECIALLY IMPORTANT NOT TO USE ASPIRIN DURING THE LAST 3 MONTHS OF PREGNANCY UNLESS SPECIFICALLY DIRECTED TO DO SO BY A DOCTOR BECAUSE IT MAY CAUSE PROBLEMS IN THE UNBORN CHILD OR COMPLICATIONS DURING DELIVERY.** Do not take this product for pain for more than 10 days or for fever for more than 3 days unless directed by a doctor. If pain or fever persists or gets worse, if new symptoms occur, or if redness or swelling is present, consult a doctor because these could be signs of a serious condition. Do not take this product if you are allergic to aspirin, have asthma, have stomach problems (such as heartburn, upset stomach or stomach pain) that persist or recur, or if you have ulcers or bleeding problems, unless directed by a doctor. If ringing in the ears or loss of hearing occurs, consult a doctor before taking or giving any more of this product.

Drug Interaction Precaution: Do not take this product if you are taking a prescription drug for anticoagulation (thinning of blood), diabetes, gout or arthritis unless directed by a doctor.

How Supplied: BUFFERIN is supplied as:
Coated circular white tablet with letter "B" debossed on one surface.
Supplied in bottles of 39's, 65's, 130's and 275's.
All consumer sizes have child resistant closures except 130's tablets which are sizes recommended for households without young children. Store at room temperature.

Professional Labeling

1. BUFFERIN® FOR RECURRENT TRANSIENT ISCHEMIC ATTACKS

Indication: For reducing the risk of recurrent transient ischemic attacks (TIA's) or stroke in men who have had transient ischemia of the brain due to fibrin platelet emboli. There is inadequate evidence that aspirin or buffered aspirin is effective in reducing TIA's in women at the recommended dosage. There is no evidence that aspirin or buffered aspirin is of benefit in the treatment of completed strokes in men or women.

Clinical Trials: The indication is supported by the results of a Canadian study (1) in which 585 patients with threatened stroke were followed in a randomized clinical trial for an average of 26 months to determine whether aspirin or sulfinpyrazone, singly or in combination, was superior to placebo in preventing transient ischemic attacks, stroke, or death. The study showed that, although sulfinpyrazone had no statistically significant effect, aspirin reduced the risk of continuing transient ischemic attacks, stroke, or death by 19 percent and reduced the risk of stroke or death by 31 percent. Another aspirin study carried out in the United States with 178 patients, showed a statistically significant number of "favorable outcomes," including reduced transient ischemic attacks, stroke, and death (2).

Precautions: Patients presenting with signs and symptoms of TIA's should have a complete medical and neurologic evaluation. Consideration should be given to other disorders that resemble TIA's. Attention should be given to risk factors: it is important to evaluate and treat, if appropriate, other diseases associated with TIA's and stroke, such as hypertension and diabetes.
Concurrent administration of absorbable antacids at therapeutic doses may increase the clearance of salicylates in some individuals. The concurrent administration of nonabsorbable antacids may alter the rate of absorption of aspirin, thereby resulting in a decreased acetylsalicylic acid/salicylate ratio in plasma. The clinical significance of these decreases in available aspirin is unknown.
Aspirin at dosages of 1,000 milligrams per day has been associated with small increases in blood pressure, blood urea nitrogen, and serum uric acid levels. It is recommended that patients placed on long-term aspirin treatment be seen at regular intervals to assess changes in these measurements.

Adverse Reactions: At dosages of 1,000 milligrams or higher of aspirin per day, gastrointestinal side effects include stomach pain, heartburn, nausea and/or vomiting, as well as increased rates of gross gastrointestinal bleeding.

Dosage and Administration: Adult oral dosage for men is 1,300 milligrams a day, in divided doses of 650 milligrams twice a day or 325 milligrams four times a day.

References:
(1) The Canadian Cooperative Study Group. "A Randomized Trial of Aspirin and Sulfinpyrazone in Threatened Stroke," *New England Journal of Medicine,* 299:53–59, 1978.
(2) Fields, W.S., et al., "Controlled Trial of Aspirin in Cerebral Ischemia," *Stroke* 8:301–316, 1977.

2. BUFFERIN® FOR MYOCARDIAL INFARCTION

Indication: Aspirin is indicated to reduce the risk of death and/or nonfatal myocardial infarction in patients with a previous infarction or unstable angina pectoris.

Clinical Trials: The indication is supported by the results of six, large, randomized multicenter, placebo-controlled studies[1–7] involving 10,816, predomi-

Continued on next page

Bristol-Myers—Cont.

nantly male, post-myocardial infarction (MI) patients and one randomized placebo-controlled study of 1,266 men with unstable angina. Therapy with aspirin was begun at intervals after the onset of acute MI varying from less than 3 days to more than 5 years and continued for periods of from less than one year to four years. In the unstable angina study, treatment was started within 1 month after the onset of unstable angina and continued for 12 weeks and complicating conditions such as congestive heart failure were not included in the study.

Aspirin therapy in MI patients was associated with about a 20 percent reduction in the risk of subsequent death and/or nonfatal reinfarction, a median absolute decrease of 3 percent from the 12 to 22 percent event rates in the placebo groups. In the aspirin-treated unstable angina patients the reduction in risk was about 50 percent, a reduction in the event rate of 5% from the 10% rate in the placebo group over the 12 weeks of the study.

Daily dosage of aspirin in the post-myocardial infarction studies was 300 mg. in one study and 900 and 1500 mg. in five studies. A dose of 325 mg. was used in the study of unstable angina.

Adverse Reactions: Gastrointestinal Reactions: Doses of 1000 mg. per day of aspirin caused gastrointestinal symptoms and bleeding that in some cases were clinically significant. In the largest post-infarction study (The Aspirin Myocardial Infaraction Study (AMIS) with 4,500 people), the percentage incidences of gastrointestinal symptoms for the aspirin (1000 mg. of a standard, solid-tablet formulation) and placebo-treated subjects, respectively, were: stomach pain (14.5%; 4.4%); heartburn (11.9%; 4.8%); nausea and/or vomiting (7.6%; 2.1%); hospitalization for gastrointestinal disorder (4.8%; 3.5%). In the AMIS and other trials, aspirin treated patients had increased rates of gross gastrointestinal bleeding. Symptoms and signs of gastrointestinal irritation were not significantly increased in subjects treated for unstable angina with buffered aspirin in solution.

Cardiovascular and Biochemical: In the AMIS trial, the dosage of 1000 mg. per day of aspirin was associated with small increases in systolic blood pressure (BP) (average 1.5 to 2.1 mm) and diastolic BP (0.5 to 0.6 mm), depending upon whether maximal or last available readings were used. Blood urea nitrogen and uric acid levels were also increased, but by less than 1.0 mg%.

Subjects with marked hypertension or renal insufficiency had been excluded from the trial so that the clinical importance of these observations for such subjects or for any subjects treated over more prolonged periods is not known. It is recommended that patients placed on long-term aspirin treatment, even at doses of 300 mg. per day, be seen at regular intervals to assess changes in these measurements.

Administration and Dosage: Although most of the studies used dosages exceeding 300 mg., two trials used only 300 mg. and pharmacologic data indicate that this dose inhibits platelet function fully. Therefore, 300 mg. or a conventional 325 mg. aspirin dose is a reasonable, routine dose that would minimize gastrointestinal adverse reactions.

References: 1. Elwood P.C., et al., "A Randomized Controlled Trial of Acetylsalicylic Acid in the Secondary Prevention of Mortality from Myocardial Infarction," *British Medical Journal,* 1:436–440, 1974. 2. The Coronary Drug Project Research Group, "Aspirin in Coronary Heart Disease," *Journal of Chronic Disease,* 29:625–642, 1976. 3. Breddin K, et al., "Secondary Prevention of Myocardial Infarction; Comparison of Acetylsalicylic Acid Phenprocoumon and Placebo," *Thromb. Haemost.,* 41:225–236, 1979. 4. Aspirin Myocardial Infarction Study Research Group, "A Randomized, Controlled Trial of Aspirin in Persons Recovered from Myocardial Infarction," *Journal American Medical Association,* 243:661–669, 1980. 5. Elwood P.C., and Sweetnam, P.M., "Aspirin and Secondary Mortality after Myocardial Infarction," *Lancet,* pp. 1313–1315, December 22–29, 1979. 6. The Persantine-Aspirin Reinfarction Study Research Group. "Persantine and Aspirin in Coronary Heart Disease," *Circulation* 62;449–460, 1980. 7. Lewis H.D., et al., "Protective Effects of Aspirin Against Acute Myocardial Infarction and Death in Men with Unstable Angina, Results of a Veterans Administration Cooperative Study," *New England Journal of Medicine,* 309;396–403, 1983.

Shown in Product Identification Guide, page 506

Arthritis Strength BUFFERIN®
[*bŭf'fĕr-ĭn*]
Analgesic

Composition:
Active Ingredient: Aspirin (500 mg) in a formulation buffered with Calcium Carbonate, Magnesium Oxide and Magnesium Carbonate.
Other Ingredients: Benzoic Acid, Citric Acid, Corn Starch, FD&C Blue No. 1, Hydroxypropyl Methylcellulose, Magnesium Stearate, Mineral Oil, Polysorbate 20, Povidone, Propylene Glycol, Simethicone Emulsion, Sodium Phosphate, Sorbitan Monolaurate, Titanium Dioxide. May also contain: Carnauba Wax, Zinc Stearate.

Indications: For fast temporary relief of the minor aches and pains, stiffness, swelling and inflammation of arthritis.

Directions: Adults and children 12 years of age and over: 2 caplets with water every 6 hours while symptoms persist, not to exceed 8 caplets in 24 hours or as directed by a doctor. Children under 12 years of age: consult a doctor.

Warnings: Children and teenagers should not use this medicine for chicken pox or flu symptoms before a doctor is consulted about Reye syndrome, a rare but serious illness reported to be associated with aspirin. Keep this and all drugs out of the reach of children. In case of accidental overdose, seek professional assistance or contact a poison control center immediately. As with any drug, if you are pregnant or nursing a baby, seek the advice of a health professional before using this product.
IT IS ESPECIALLY IMPORTANT NOT TO USE ASPIRIN DURING THE LAST 3 MONTHS OF PREGNANCY UNLESS SPECIFICALLY DIRECTED TO DO SO BY A DOCTOR BECAUSE IT MAY CAUSE PROBLEMS IN THE UNBORN CHILD OR COMPLICATIONS DURING DELIVERY. Do not take this product for pain for more than 10 days or for fever for more than 3 days unless directed by a doctor. If pain or fever persists or gets worse, if new symptoms occur, or if redness or swelling is present, consult a doctor because these could be signs of a serious condition. Do not take this product if you are allergic to aspirin, have asthma, have stomach problems (such as heartburn, upset stomach or stomach pain) that persist or recur, or if you have ulcers or bleeding problems, unless directed by a doctor. If ringing in the ears or loss of hearing occurs, consult a doctor before taking any more of this product.

Drug Interaction Precaution: Do not take this product if you are taking a prescription drug for anticoagulation (thinning of blood), diabetes, gout or arthritis unless directed by a doctor.

How Supplied: Arthritis Strength BUFFERIN® is supplied as:
Plain white coated caplet "ASB" debossed on one side.
Supplied in bottles of 130's
Store at room temperature.

Shown in Product Identification Guide, page 506

Extra Strength BUFFERIN®
[*bŭf'fĕr-ĭn*]
Analgesic

Composition:
Active Ingredient: Aspirin (500 mg) in a formulation buffered with Calcium Carbonate, Magnesium Oxide and Magnesium Carbonate.
Other Ingredients: Benzoic Acid, Citric Acid, Corn Starch, FD&C Blue No. 1, Hydroxypropyl Methylcellulose, Magnesium Stearate, Mineral Oil, Polysorbate 20, Povidone, Propylene Glycol, Simethicone Emulsion, Sodium Phosphate, Sorbitan Monolaurate, Titanium Dioxide. May also contain: Carnauba Wax, Zinc Stearate.

Indications: For fast temporary relief of headaches, minor arthritis pain and inflammation, muscle aches, pain and fever of colds, menstrual pain and toothaches.

Directions: Adults and children 12 years of age and over: 2 tablets with water every 6 hours while symptoms persist, not to exceed 8 tablets in 24 hours or as directed by a doctor. Children under 12 years of age: Consult a doctor.

Warnings: Children and teenagers should not use this medicine for chicken pox or flu symptoms before a doctor is consulted about Reye syndrome, a rare but serious illness reported to be associated with aspirin. Keep this and all drugs out of the reach of children. In case of accidental overdose, seek professional assistance or contact a poison control center immediately. As with any drug, if you are pregnant or nursing a baby, seek the advice of a health professional before using this product. **IT IS ESPECIALLY IMPORTANT NOT TO USE ASPIRIN DURING THE LAST 3 MONTHS OF PREGNANCY UNLESS SPECIFICALLY DIRECTED TO DO SO BY A DOCTOR BECAUSE IT MAY CAUSE PROBLEMS IN THE UNBORN CHILD OR COMPLICATIONS DURING DELIVERY.** Do not take this product for more than 10 days or for fever for more than 3 days unless directed by a doctor. If pain or fever persists or gets worse, if new symptoms occur, or if redness or swelling is present, consult a doctor because these could be signs of a serious condition. Do not take this product if you are allergic to aspirin, have asthma, have stomach problems (such as heartburn, upset stomach or stomach pain) that persist or recur, or if you have ulcers or bleeding problems, unless directed by a doctor. If ringing in the ears or loss of hearing occurs, consult a doctor before taking any more of this product.

Drug Interaction Precaution: Do not take this product if you are taking a prescription drug for anticoagulation (thinning of blood), diabetes, gout or arthritis unless directed by a doctor.

How Supplied: Extra Strength BUFFERIN® is supplied as:
White elongated coated tablet with "ESB" debossed on one side.
Supplied in bottles of 39's, 65's, 130's.
All sizes have child resistant closures except 65's which is recommended for households without young children.
Store at room temperature.

Shown in Product Identification Guide, page 506

COMTREX® Maximum Strength
[*cŏm 'trĕx*]
Multi-Symptom Cold & Flu Reliever

Composition: Each tablet, caplet, liqui-gel and fluidounce (30 ml.) contains:
[See table below.]

Indications: For the temporary relief of the following symptoms associated with the common cold and flu: minor aches, pains, headache, muscular aches, sore throat pain, and fever; cough; nasal congestion; runny nose and sneezing.

Directions:
Tablets or Caplets: Adults and children 12 years of age and over: 2 tablets or caplets every 6 hours while symptoms persist, not to exceed 8 tablets or caplets in 24 hours, or as directed by a doctor. Children under 12 years of age: Consult a doctor.

Liqui-Gel: Adults and children 12 years of age and over: 2 liqui-gels every 6 hours, while symptoms persist, not to exceed 8 liqui-gels in 24 hours, or as directed by a doctor. Children under 12 years of age: consult a doctor.

Liquid: Adults and children 12 years of age and over: One fluidounce using dosage cup provided or 2 tablespoonfuls every 6 hours while symptoms persist, not to exceed 4 doses in 24 hours or as directed by your doctor. Children under 12 years of age: consult a doctor.

Warnings: Keep this and all drugs out of the reach of children. In case of accidental overdose, seek professional assistance or contact a poison control center immediately. Prompt medical attention is critical for adults as well as children even if you do not notice any signs or symptoms. As with any drug, if you are pregnant or nursing a baby, seek the advice of a health professional before using this product. Do not take this product for more than 7 days. A persistent cough may be a sign of a serious condition. If cough persists for more than 7 days, tends to recur, or is accompanied by rash, persistent headache, fever that lasts for more than 3 days, or if new symptoms occur, consult a doctor. If sore throat is severe, persists for more than 2 days, is accompanied or followed by fever, headache, rash, nausea, or vomiting, consult a doctor promptly. Do not take this product for persistent or chronic cough such as occurs with smoking, asthma, emphysema, or if cough is accompanied by excessive phlegm (mucus) unless directed by a doctor. **Do not exceed recommended dosage.** If nervousness, dizzi-

	COMTREX Per Tablet or Caplet	COMTREX Liquid-Gel per Liqui-Gel	COMTREX Liquid* Per Fl. Ounce
Acetaminophen:	500 mg.	500 mg.	1000 mg.
Pseudoephedrine HCl:	30 mg.	—	60 mg.
Phenylpropanolamine HCl:	—	12.5 mg.	—
Chlorpheniramine Maleate:	2 mg.	2 mg.	4 mg.
Dextromethorphan HBr:	15 mg.	15 mg.	30 mg.

Tablet/Caplet	**Liqui-Gels**	**Liquid**
Benzoic Acid	D&C Yellow No. 10	Alcohol (10% by volume)
Corn Starch	FD&C Red No. 40	Benzoic acid
D&C Yellow No. 10 Lake	Gelatin	D&C Yellow No. 10
FD&C Red No. 40 Lake	Glycerin	FD&C Blue No. 1
Hydroxypropyl Methylcellulose	Polyethylene Glycol	FD&C Red No. 40
Magnesium Stearate	Povidone	Flavors
Methylparaben	Propylene Glycol	Glycerin
Mineral Oil	Silicon Dioxide	Polyethylene Glycol
Polysorbate 20	Sorbitol	Povidone
Povidone	Titanium Dioxide	Saccharin Sodium
Propylene Glycol	Water	Sodium Citrate
Propylparaben		Sucrose
Simethicone Emulsion		Water
Sorbitan Monolaurate		
Stearic Acid		
Titanium Dioxide		
May also contain:		
Carnauba wax		
D&C Yellow No. 10		
FD&C Red No. 40		

*contains 15 mg sodium per fluid ounce (30 ml)

Continued on next page

ness, or sleeplessness occur, discontinue use and consult a doctor. If symptoms do not improve within 7 days or are accompanied by fever, consult a doctor. Do not take this product unless directed by a doctor, if you have a breathing problem such as emphysema or chronic bronchitis, heart disease, high blood pressure, thyroid disease, diabetes, glaucoma, or difficulty in urination due to enlargement of the prostate gland. May cause excitability especially in children. May cause marked drowsiness; alcohol, sedatives, and tranquilizers may increase the drowsiness effect. Avoid alcoholic beverages while taking this product. Do not take this product if you are taking sedatives or tranquilizers, without first consulting your doctor. Use caution when driving a motor vehicle or operating machinery. If you generally consume 3 or more alcohol-containing drinks per day, you should consult your physician for advice on when and how you should take Comtrex and other pain relievers.

Drug Interaction Precaution: Do not use this product if you are now taking a prescription monoamine oxidase inhibitor (MAOI) (certain drugs for depression, psychiatric or emotional conditions, or Parkinson's disease), or for 2 weeks after stopping the MAOI drug. If you are uncertain whether your prescription drug contains an MAOI, consult a health professional before taking this product.

Overdose:

MUCOMYST (acetylcysteine) As An Antidote For Acetaminophen Overdose)

Acetaminophen is rapidly absorbed from the upper gastrointestinal tract with peak plasma levels occurring between 30 and 60 minutes after therapeutic doses and usually within 4 hours following an overdose. The parent compound, which is nontoxic, is extensively metabolized in the liver to form principally the sulfate and glucuronide conjugates which are also nontoxic and are rapidly excreted in the urine. A small fraction of an ingested dose is metabolized in the liver by the cytochrome P-450 mixed function oxidase enzyme system to form a reactive, potentially toxic, intermediate metabolite which preferentially conjugates with hepatic glutathione to form the nontoxic cysteine and mercapturic acid derivatives which are then excreted by the kidney. Therapeutic doses of acetaminophen do not saturate the glucuronide and sulfate conjugation pathways and do not result in the formation of sufficient reactive metabolite to deplete glutathione stores. However, following ingestion of a large overdose (150 mg/kg or greater) the glucuronide and sulfate conjugation pathways are saturated resulting in a larger fraction of the drug being metabolized via the P-450 pathway. The increased formation of reactive metabolite may deplete the hepatic stores of glutathione with subsequent binding of the metabolite to protein molecules within the hepatocyte resulting in cellular necrosis. Acetylcysteine has been shown to reduce the extent of liver injury following acetaminophen overdose. Early symptoms following a potentially hepatotoxic overdose may include: nausea, vomiting, diaphoresis and general malaise. Clinical and laboratory evidence of hepatic toxicity may not be apparent until 48 to 72 hours postingestion. In most adults and adolescents, regardless of the quantity of acetaminophen reported to have been ingested, administer MUCOMYST® acetylcysteine immediately. MUCOMYST acetylcysteine therapy should be initiated and continued for a full course of therapy. Its effectiveness depends on early administration, with benefit seen principally in patients treated within 16 hours of the overdose. If acetaminophen plasma assay capability is not available, and the estimated acetaminophen ingestion exceeds 150 mg/kg., MUCOMYST acetylcysteine therapy should be initiated and continued for a full course of therapy.

For full prescribing information, refer to the MUCOMYST package insert. Do not await the results of assays for acetaminophen level before initiating treatment with MUCOMYST acetylcysteine. The following additional procedures are recommended: The stomach should be emptied promptly by lavage or by induction of emesis with syrup of ipecac. A serum acetaminophen assay should be obtained as early as possible, but no sooner than four hours following ingestion. Liver function studies should be obtained initially and repeated at 24-hour intervals.

For additional emergency information call your regional poison center or toll-free (1-800-525-6115) to the Rocky Mountain Poison Center for assistance in diagnosis and for directions in the use of MUCOMYST acetylcysteine as an antidote.

How Supplied:

COMTREX® is supplied as:

Coated yellow tablet with letters "Cx" debossed on one surface.

Supplied in Blister packages of 24's and Bottles of 50's

Coated yellow caplet with "Cx" debossed on one side.

Supplied in Blister packages of 24's and Bottles of 50's

Yellow Liqui-Gel with "COMTREX LG" printed in red on one side.

Supplied in Blister packages of 24's and 50's

Clear Red Cherry Flavored liquid:

Supplied in 6 oz. plastic bottles.

All sizes packaged in child resistant closures except for 24's for tablets, caplets and liqui-gels which are sizes recommended for households without young children. Store caplets, tablets and liquid at room temperature.

Store liqui-gels below 86° F. (30° C.). Keep from freezing.

Shown in Product Identification Guide, page 507

COMTREX ALLERGY–SINUS TREATMENT Maximum Strength

[*cŏm ′trĕx*]

Multi-Symptom Allergy/Sinus Formula

Composition:

Active Ingredients: Each coated tablet or caplet contains 500 mg acetaminophen, 30 mg pseudoephedrine HCl, 2 mg chlorpheniramine maleate.

Other Ingredients: Benzoic acid, carnauba wax, corn starch, D&C yellow No. 10 lake, FD&C blue No. 1 lake, FD&C Red No. 40 lake, hydroxypropyl methylcellulose, mineral oil, polysorbate 20, povidone, propylene glycol, simethicone emulsion, sodium citrate, sorbitan monolaurate, stearic acid, titanium dioxide. May also contain: crospovidone, D&C yellow No. 10, erythorbic acid, FD&C blue No. 1, magnesium stearate, methylparaben, microcrystalline cellulose, polysorbate 80, propylparaben, silicon dioxide, wood cellulose.

Indications: For the temporary relief of the following symptoms associated with upper respiratory allergies, hay fever and sinusitis: runny nose, sneezing, itching of the nose or throat, itchy, watery eyes; nasal congestion, sinus pressure; and headache pain.

Directions: Adults and children 12 years of age and over: 2 tablets every 6 hours, while symptoms persist, not to exceed 8 tablets in 24 hours, or as directed by your doctor. Children under 12 years of age; consult a doctor.

Warnings: Keep this and all drugs out of the reach of children. In case of accidental overdose, seek professional assistance or contact a poison control center immediately. Prompt medical attention is critical for adults as well as for children even if you do not notice any signs or symptoms. As with any drug, if you are pregnant or nursing a baby, seek the advice of a health professional before using this product. Do not take this product for more than 7 days unless directed by a doctor. If symptoms do not improve or are accompanied by a fever that lasts for more than 3 days, or if new symptoms occur, consult a doctor. Do not exceed recommended dosage. If nervousness, dizziness or sleeplessness occur, discontinue use and consult a doctor. Do not take this product unless directed by a doctor if you have a breathing problem such as emphysema, or chronic bronchitis, heart disease, high blood pressure, thyroid disease, diabetes, glaucoma, or difficulty in urination due to enlargement of the prostate gland. May cause excitability especially in children. May cause drowsiness; alcohol, sedatives and tranquilizers may increase the drowsiness effect. Avoid alcoholic beverages, while taking this product. Do not take this product if you are taking sedatives or tranquilizers without first consulting your doctor. Use caution when driving a motor vehicle or operating machinery. If you generally consume 3 or more alcohol-containing drinks per day, you should consult your physician for advice on when and how you should take Comtrex and other pain relievers.

Drug Interaction Precaution: Do not use this product if you are now taking a prescription monoamine oxidase inhibitor (MAOI) (certain drugs for depression, psychiatric or emotional conditions, or Parkinson's disease), or for 2 weeks after stopping the MAOI drug. If you are uncertain whether your prescription drug contains an MAOI, consult a health professional before taking this product.

Overdose:
MUCOMYST (acetylcysteine) As An Antidote For Acetaminophen Overdose)
Acetaminophen is rapidly absorbed from the upper gastrointestinal tract with peak plasma levels occurring between 30 and 60 minutes after therapeutic doses and usually within 4 hours following an overdose. The parent compound, which is nontoxic, is extensively metabolized in the liver to form principally the sulfate and glucuronide conjugates which are also nontoxic and are rapidly excreted in the urine. A small fraction of an ingested dose is metabolized in the liver by the cytochrome P-450 mixed function oxidase enzyme system to form a reactive, potentially toxic, intermediate metabolite which preferentially conjugates with hepatic glutathione to form the nontoxic cysteine and mercapturic acid derivatives which are then excreted by the kidney. Therapeutic doses of acetaminophen do not saturate the glucuronide and sulfate conjugation pathways and do not result in the formation of sufficient reactive metabolite to deplete glutathione stores. However, following ingestion of a large overdose (150 mg/kg or greater) the glucuronide and sulfate conjugation pathways are saturated resulting in a larger fraction of the drug being metabolized via the P-450 pathway. The increased formation of reactive metabolite may deplete the hepatic stores of glutathione with subsequent binding of the metabolite to protein molecules within the hepatocyte resulting in cellular necrosis. Acetylcysteine has been shown to reduce the extent of liver injury following acetaminophen overdose. Early symptoms following a potentially hepatotoxic overdose may include: nausea, vomiting, diaphoresis and general malaise. Clinical and laboratory evidence of hepatic toxicity may not be apparent until 48 to 72 hours postingestion. In most adults and adolescents, regardless of the quantity of acetaminophen reported to have been ingested, administer MUCOMYST® acetylcysteine immediately. MUCOMYST acetylcysteine therapy should be initiated and continued for a full course of therapy. Its effectiveness depends on early administration, with benefit seen principally in patients treated within 16 hours of the overdose. If acetaminophen plasma assay capability is not available, and the estimated acetaminophen ingestion exceeds 150 mg/kg, MUCOMYST acetylcysteine therapy should be initiated and continued for a full course of therapy.
For full prescribing information, refer to the MUCOMYST package insert. Do not await the results of assays for acetaminophen level before initiating treatment with MUCOMYST acetylcysteine. The following additional procedures are recommended: The stomach should be emptied promptly by lavage or by induction of emesis with syrup of ipecac. A serum acetaminophen assay should be obtained as early as possible, but no sooner than four hours following ingestion. Liver function studies should be obtained initially and repeated at 24-hour intervals.
For additional emergency information call your regional poison center or toll-free (1-800-525-6115) to the Rocky Mountain Poison Center for assistance in diagnosis and for directions in the use of MUCOMYST acetylcysteine as an antidote.

How Supplied: Allergy-Sinus COMTREX® is supplied as:
Coated green tablets or caplets with "A/S" debossed on one side.
Supplied in bottles of 24's, 50's.
All sizes packaged in child resistant closures except 24's which are sizes recommended for households without young children.
Store at room temperature.

Shown in Product Identification Guide, page 507

COMTREX®
DEEP CHEST COLD
& Congestion Relief

Composition: Each liquigel contains: Acetaminophen 325 mg, Guaifenesin 200 mg, Phenylpropanolamine Hydrochloride 12.5 mg, and Dextromethorphan Hydrobromide 10 mg.
Other ingredients: FD&C Red No. 40, Gelatin, Glycerin, Polyethylene Glycol, Povidone, Propylene Glycol, Silicon Dioxide, Sorbitol, Titanium Dioxide, Water.

Indications: For the temporary relief of the following symptoms associated with the common cold and flu: minor aches, pains, headache, muscular aches, sore throat, and fever; cough; and nasal congestion. Helps loosen phlegm (mucus) and thin bronchial secretions to drain bronchial tubes and make coughs more productive.

Directions: Adults and children 12 years of age and over: 2 liquigels every 4 hours, while symptoms persist, not to exceed 12 liquigels in 24 hours, or as directed by your doctor. Children under 12 years of age: consult a doctor.

Warnings: Keep this and all drugs out of the reach of children. In case of accidental overdose, seek professional assistance or contact a poison control center immediately. Prompt medical attention is critical for adults as well as for children even if you do not notice any signs or symptoms. As with any drug, if you are pregnant or nursing a baby, seek the advice of a health professional before using this product. Do not take this product for more than 7 days or for fever for more than 3 days unless directed by a doctor. If pain or fever persists or gets worse, if new symptoms occur, consult a doctor. A persistent cough may be a sign of a serious condition. If cough persists for more than 1 week, tends to recur, or is accompanied by fever, rash, or persistent headache, consult a doctor. Do not take this product for persistent or chronic cough such as occurs with smoking, asthma, chronic bronchitis, emphysema, or where cough is accompanied by excessive phlegm (mucus) unless directed by a doctor. If sore throat is severe, persists for more than 2 days, is accompanied or followed by fever, headache, rash, nausea, or vomiting, consult a doctor promptly. **Do not exceed recommended dosage.**
If nervousness, dizziness, or sleeplessness occur, discontinue use and consult a doctor. If symptoms do not improve within 7 days or are accompanied by fever, consult a doctor. Do not take this product if you have heart disease, high blood pressure, thyroid disease, diabetes, or difficulty in urination due to enlargement of the prostate gland unless directed by a doctor. If you generally consume 3 or more alcohol-containing drinks per day, you should consult your physician for advice on when and how you should take Comtrex Deep Chest Cold and other pain relievers.

Drug Interaction Precaution: Do not use this product if you are now taking a prescription monoamine oxidase inhibitor (MAOI) (certain drugs for depression, psychiatric or emotional conditions, or Parkinson's disease), or for 2 weeks after stopping the MAOI drug. If you are uncertain whether your prescription drug contains an MAOI, consult a health professional before taking this product.

Overdose: MUCOMYST (acetylcysteine) As An Antidote For Acetaminophen Overdose)
Acetaminophen is rapidly absorbed from the upper gastrointestinal tract with peak plasma levels occurring between 30 and 60 minutes after therapeutic doses and usually within 4 hours following an overdose. The parent compound, which is nontoxic, is extensively metabolized in the liver to form principally the sulfate and glucuronide conjugates which are also nontoxic and are rapidly excreted in the urine. A small fraction of an ingested dose is metabolized in the liver by the cytochrome P-450 mixed function oxidase enzyme system to form a reactive, potentially toxic, intermediate metabolite which preferentially conjugates with hepatic glutathione to form the nontoxic cysteine and mercapturic acid derivatives which are then excreted by the kidney. Therapeutic doses of acetaminophen do not saturate the glucuronide and

Continued on next page

Bristol-Myers—Cont.

sulfate conjugation pathways and do not result in the formation of sufficient reactive metabolite to deplete glutathione stores. However, following ingestion of a large overdose (150 mg/kg or greater) the glucuronide and sulfate conjugation pathways are saturated resulting in a larger fraction of the drug being metabolized via the P-450 pathway. The increased formation of reactive metabolite may deplete the hepatic stores of glutathione with subsequent binding of the metabolite to protein molecules within the hepatocyte resulting in cellular necrosis. Acetylcysteine has been shown to reduce the extent of liver injury following acetaminophen overdose. Early symptoms following a potentially hepatotoxic overdose may include: nausea, vomiting, diaphoresis and general malaise. Clinical and laboratory evidence of hepatic toxicity may not be apparent until 48 to 72 hours postingestion. In most adults and adolescents, regardless of the quantity of acetaminophen reported to have been ingested, administer MUCOMYST® acetylcysteine immediately. MUCOMYST acetylcysteine therapy should be initiated and continued for a full course of therapy. Its effectiveness depends on early administration, with benefit seen principally in patients treated within 16 hours of the overdose.

If acetaminophen plasma assay capability is not available, and the estimated acetaminophen ingestion exceeds 150 mg/kg., MUCOMYST acetylcysteine therapy should be initiated and continued for a full course of therapy.

For full prescribing information, refer to the MUCOMYST package insert. Do not await the results of assays for acetaminophen level before initiating treatment with MUCOMYST acetylcysteine. The following additional procedures are recommended: The stomach should be emptied promptly by lavage or by induction of emesis with syrup of ipecac. A serum acetaminophen assay should be obtained as early as possible, but no sooner than four hours following ingestion. Liver function studies should be obtained initially and repeated at 24-hour intervals.

For additional emergency information call your regional poison center or toll-free (1-800-525-6115) to the Rocky Mountain Poison Center for assistance in diagnosis and for directions in the use of MUCOMYST acetylcysteine as an antidote.

How Supplied: Red Oval shaped liquigel printed with "Comtrex CC" in white supplied in bottles of 24's.

Non-Drowsy COMTREX® Maximum Strength

Each caplet or liqui-gel contains: [See table at right.]

Other Ingredients (Caplet): Benzoic acid, Corn starch, D&C Yellow No. 10 Lake, FD&C Red No. 40 Lake, Hydroxypropyl methylcellulose, Magnesium Stearate, Methylparaben, Mineral Oil, Polysorbate 20, Povidone, Propylene Glycol, Propylparaben, Simethicone Emulsion, Sorbitan Monolaurate, Stearic Acid, Titanium Dioxide.

May also contain: Carnauba Wax, D&C Yellow No. 10, FD&C Red No. 40

Other Ingredients (Liqui-gel): FD&C Yellow No. 6, Gelatin, Glycerin, Polyethylene Glycol, Povidone, Propylene Glycol, Silicon Dioxide, Sorbitol, Titanium Dioxide, Water

Indications: For the temporary relief of the following symptoms associated with the common cold and flu: minor aches, pains, headache, muscular aches, and fever; cough; and nasal congestion.

Warnings: Keep this and all drugs out of the reach of children. In case of accidental overdose, seek professional assistance or contact a poison control center immediately. Prompt medical attention is critical for adults as well as children even if you do not notice any signs or symptoms. As with any drug, if you are pregnant or nursing a baby, seek the advice of a health professional before using this product. Do not take this product for more than 7 days. A persistent cough may be a sign of a serious condition. If cough persists for more than 7 days, tends to recur, or is accompanied by rash, persistent headache, fever that lasts for more than 3 days, or if new symptoms occur, consult a doctor. Do not take this product for persistent or chronic cough such as occurs with smoking, asthma or emphysema, or if cough is accompanied by excessive phlegm (mucus) unless directed by a doctor. **Do not exceed recommended dosage.** If nervousness, dizziness, or sleeplessness occur, discontinue use and consult a doctor. If symptoms do not improve within 7 days or are accompanied by fever, consult a doctor. Do not take this product if you have heart disease, high blood pressure, thyroid disease, diabetes, or difficulty in urination due to enlargement of the prostate gland unless directed by a doctor. If you generally consume 3 or more alcohol-containing drinks per day, you should consult your physician for advice on when and how you should take Maximum Strength Comtrex Non-Drowsy and other pain relievers.

DRUG INTERACTION PRECAUTION: Do not use this product if you are now taking a prescription monoamine oxidase inhibitor (MAOI) (certain drugs for depression, psychiatric or emotional conditions, or Parkinson's disease), or for 2 weeks after stopping the MAOI drug. If you are uncertain whether your prescription drug contains an MAOI, consult a health professional before taking this product.

Directions: Adults and children 12 years of age and over: 2 caplets or liquigels every 6 hours, while symptoms persist, not to exceed 8 caplets or liquigels in 24 hours, or as directed by your doctor. Children under 12 years of age: consult a doctor.

Overdose: MUCOMYST (acetylcysteine) As An Antidote For Acetaminophen Overdose)

Acetaminophen is rapidly absorbed from the upper gastrointestinal tract with peak plasma levels occurring between 30 and 60 minutes after therapeutic doses and usually within 4 hours following an overdose. The parent compound, which is nontoxic, is extensively metabolized in the liver to form principally the sulfate and glucuronide conjugates which are also nontoxic and are rapidly excreted in the urine. A small fraction of an ingested dose is metabolized in the liver by the cytochrome P-450 mixed function oxidase enzyme system to form a reactive, potentially toxic, intermediate metabolite which preferentially conjugates with hepatic glutathione to form the nontoxic cysteine and mercapturic acid derivatives which are then excreted by the kidney. Therapeutic doses of acetaminophen do not saturate the glucuronide and sulfate conjugation pathways and do not result in the formation of sufficient reactive metabolite to deplete glutathione stores. However, following ingestion of a large overdose (150 mg/kg or greater) the glucuronide and sulfate conjugation pathways are saturated resulting in a larger fraction of the drug being metabolized via the P-450 pathway. The increased formation of reactive metabolite may deplete the hepatic stores of glutathione with subsequent binding of the metabolite to protein molecules within the hepatocyte resulting in cellular necrosis. Acetylcysteine has been shown to reduce the extent of liver injury following acetaminophen overdose. Early symptoms following a potentially hepatotoxic overdose may include: nausea, vomiting, diaphoresis and general malaise. Clinical and laboratory evidence of hepatic toxicity may not be apparent until 48 to 72 hours postingestion. In most adults and adolescents, regardless of the quantity of acetaminophen reported to have been ingested, administer MUCOMYST® acetylcysteine immediately. MUCOMYST acetylcysteine therapy should be initiated and continued for a full course of therapy. Its effectiveness depends on early administration, with benefit seen principally in patients treated within 16 hours of the overdose.

If acetaminophen plasma assay capability is not available, and the estimated

Active:	**Comtrex Non-Drowsy per caplet**	**Comtrex Non-Drowsy per liqui-gel**
Acetaminophen	500 mg	500 mg
Pseudoephedrine HCL	30 mg	—
Dextromethorphan HBr	15 mg	15 mg
Phenylpropanolamine HCL	—	12.5 mg

acetaminophen ingestion exceeds 150 mg/kg, MUCOMYST acetylcysteine therapy should be initiated and continued for a full course of therapy.

For full prescribing information, refer to the MUCOMYST package insert. Do not await the results of assays for acetaminophen level before initiating treatment with MUCOMYST acetylcysteine. The following additional procedures are recommended: The stomach should be emptied promptly by lavage or by induction of emesis with syrup of ipecac. A serum acetaminophen assay should be obtained as early as possible, but no sooner than four hours following ingestion. Liver function studies should be obtained initially and repeated at 24-hour intervals.

For additional emergency information call your regional poison center or toll-free (1-800-525-6115) to the Rocky Mountain Poison Center for assistance in diagnosis and for directions in the use of MUCOMYST acetylcysteine as an antidote.

How Supplied: Non-Drowsy Comtrex® is supplied as:

Coated orange caplet with "CX-D" debossed on one surface. Supplied in blister packages of 24's and Bottles of 50's.

Liquigel printed with "COMTREX DAY" supplied in Blister packages of 24's and of 50's.

The 24 size does not have a child resistant closure and is recommended for households without young children.

Store at room temperature.

Shown in Product Identification Guide, page 507

Aspirin Free EXCEDRIN®

Composition: Each caplet and geltab contains Acetaminophen 500 mg. and Caffeine 65 mg. Other Ingredients: (caplet) Benzoic Acid, Carnauba Wax, Corn starch, D&C Red No. 27 Lake, D&C Yellow No. 10 Lake, FD&C Blue No. 1 Lake, Hydroxypropyl methylcellulose, Magnesium stearate, Methylparaben, Microcrystalline Cellulose, Mineral Oil, Polysorbate 20, Povidone, Propylene Glycol, Propylparaben, Simethicone Emulsion, Sorbitan Monolaurate, Stearic Acid, Titanium Dioxide.

May also contain: Croscarmellose sodium, FD&C Red No. 40, Saccharin sodium, Sodium starch glycolate

Other Ingredients: (geltab) Benzoic Acid, Corn Starch, FD&C Blue No. 1, FD&C Red No. 40, FD&C Yellow No. 6, Gelatin, Glycerin, Hydroxypropyl methylcellulose, Magnesium stearate, Methylparaben, Microcrystalline cellulose, Mineral oil, Polysorbate 20, Povidone, Propylene glycol, Propylparaben, Simethicone emulsion, Sorbitan monolaurate, Stearic acid, Titanium dioxide.

May also contain: Croscarmellose sodium, Sodium starch glycolate

Indications: For temporary relief of the minor pain of headache, sinusitis, colds, muscular aches, menstrual discomfort, toothaches and arthritis pain.

Directions: Adults: 2 caplets or geltabs every 6 hours while symptoms persist, not to exceed 8 caplets or geltabs in 24 hours, or as directed by a doctor. Children under 12 years of age: Consult a doctor.

Warnings: Keep this and all drugs out of the reach of children. In case of accidental overdose, seek professional assistance or contact a poison control center immediately. Prompt medical attention is critical for adults as well as for children even if you do not notice any signs or symptoms. As with any drug, if you are pregnant or nursing a baby, seek the advice of a health professional before using this product. Do not take this product for pain for more than 10 days or for fever for more than 3 days unless directed by a doctor. If pain or fever persists or gets worse, if new symptoms occur, of if redness or swelling is present, consult a doctor because these could be signs of a serious condition. Consult a dentist promptly for toothache. If you generally consume 3 or more alcohol-containing drinks per day, you should consult your physician for advice on when and how you should take Aspirin Free Excedrin and other pain relievers.

Overdose: MUCOMYST (acetylcysteine) As An Antidote For Acetaminophen Overdose)

Acetaminophen is rapidly absorbed from the upper gastrointestinal tract with peak plasma levels occurring between 30 and 60 minutes after therapeutic doses and usually within 4 hours following an overdose. The parent compound, which is nontoxic, is extensively metabolized in the liver to form principally the sulfate and glucuronide conjugates which are also nontoxic and are rapidly excreted in the urine. A small fraction of an ingested dose is metabolized in the liver by the cytochrome P-450 mixed function oxidase enzyme system to form a reactive, potentially toxic, intermediate metabolite which preferentially conjugates with hepatic glutathione to form the nontoxic cysteine and mercapturic acid derivatives which are then excreted by the kidney. Therapeutic doses of acetaminophen do not saturate the glucuronide and sulfate conjugation pathways and do not result in the formation of sufficient reactive metabolite to deplete glutathione stores. However, following ingestion of a large overdose (150 mg/kg or greater) the glucuronide and sulfate conjugation pathways are saturated resulting in a larger fraction of the drug being metabolized via the P-450 pathway. The increased formation of reactive metabolite may deplete the hepatic stores of glutathione with subsequent binding of the metabolite to protein molecules within the hepatocyte resulting in cellular necrosis. Acetylcysteine has been shown to reduce the extent of liver injury following acetaminophen overdose. Early symptoms following a potentially hepatotoxic overdose may include: nausea, vomiting, diaphoresis and general malaise. Clinical and laboratory evidence of hepatic toxicity may not be apparent until 48 to 72 hours postingestion. In most adults and adolescents, regardless of the quantity of acetaminophen reported to have been ingested, administer MUCOMYST® acetylcysteine immediately. MUCOMYST acetylcysteine therapy should be initiated and continued for a full course of therapy. Its effectiveness depends on early administration, with benefit seen principally in patients treated within 16 hours of the overdose.

If acetaminophen plasma assay capability is not available, and the estimated acetaminophen ingestion exceeds 150 mg/kg, MUCOMYST acetylcysteine therapy should be initiated and continued for a full course of therapy.

For full prescribing information, refer to the MUCOMYST package insert. Do not await the results of assays for acetaminophen level before initiating treatment with MUCOMYST acetylcysteine. The following additional procedures are recommended: The stomach should be emptied promptly by lavage or by induction of emesis with syrup of ipecac. A serum acetaminophen assay should be obtained as early as possible, but no sooner than four hours following ingestion. Liver function studies should be obtained initially and repeated at 24-hour intervals.

For additional emergency information call your regional poison center or toll-free (1-800-525-6115) to the Rocky Mountain Poison Center for assistance in diagnosis and for directions in the use of MUCOMYST acetylcysteine as an antidote.

How Supplied: Aspirin Free EXCEDRIN® is supplied as: Coated red caplets with AFE debossed on one side supplied in bottles of 24's, 50's, 100's and bonus packages of 125's.

All sizes packaged in child resistant closures except 100's size for caplets which is recommended for households without young children.

Easy to swallow red geltabs with "AF Excedrin" printed in white on one side supplied in bottles of 20's, 40's, 80's and bonus packages of 100's.

All sizes packaged in child resistant closures except 40's which is recommended for households without young children.

Store at room temperature.

Shown in Product Identification Guide, page 507

EXCEDRIN® Extra-Strength Analgesic

[ĕx ″cĕd ′rĭn]

Composition: Each tablet, caplet, or geltab contains Acetaminophen 250 mg.; Aspirin 250 mg.; and Caffeine 65 mg.

Other Ingredients: (tablet, caplet) Benzoic acid, Hydroxypropylcellulose, Hy-

Continued on next page

Bristol-Myers—Cont.

droxypropyl methylcellulose, Microcrystalline Cellulose, Mineral Oil, Polysorbate 20, Povidone, Propylene Glycol, Simethicone Emulsion, Sorbitan Monolaurate, Stearic Acid,
Tablets and caplets may also contain: Carnauba wax, FD&C Blue No. 1, Saccharin Sodium, Titanium Dioxide
Other Ingredients: (geltab) Benzoic Acid, D&C Yellow #10 Lake, Disodium EDTA, FD&C Blue #1 Lake, FD&C Red # 40 Lake, Ferric Oxide, Gelatin, Glycerin, Hydroxypropylcellulose, Hydroxypropyl Methylcellulose, Maltitol Solution, Microcrystalline Cellulose, Mineral Oil, Pepsin, Polysorbate 20, Povidone, Propylene Glycol, Propyl Gallate, Simethicone Emulsion, Sorbitan Monolaurate, Stearic Acid, Titanium Dioxide.

Indications: For temporary relief of the pain of headache, sinusitis, colds, muscular aches, menstrual discomfort, toothache and minor arthritis pain.

Warnings: Children and teenagers should not use this medicine for chicken pox or flu symptoms before a doctor is consulted about Reye syndrome, a rare but serious illness reported to be associated with aspirin. Keep this and all drugs out of the reach of children. In case of accidental overdose, seek professional assistance or contact a physician or poison control center immediately. Prompt medical attention is critical for adults as well as for children even if you do not notice any signs or symptoms. As with any drug, if you are pregnant or nursing a baby, seek the advice of a health professional before using this product. IT IS ESPECIALLY IMPORTANT NOT TO USE ASPIRIN DURING THE LAST 3 MONTHS OF PREGNANCY UNLESS SPECIFICALLY DIRECTED TO DO SO BY A DOCTOR BECAUSE IT MAY CAUSE PROBLEMS IN THE UNBORN CHILD OR COMPLICATIONS DURING DELIVERY. Do not take this product for pain for more than 10 days or for fever for more than 3 days unless directed by a doctor. If pain or fever persists or gets worse, if new symptoms occur, or if redness or swelling is present, consult a doctor because these could be signs of a serious condition. Consult a dentist promptly for toothache. Do not take this product if you are allergic to aspirin, have asthma, have stomach problems (such as heartburn, upset stomach or stomach pain) that persist or recur, or if you have ulcers or bleeding problems, unless directed by a doctor. If ringing in the ears or loss of hearing occurs, consult a doctor before taking any more of this product. If you generally consume 3 or more alcohol-containing drinks per day, you should consult your physician for advice on when and how you should take Excedrin and other pain relievers.

Drug Interaction Precaution: Do not take this product if you are taking a prescription drug for anticoagulation (thinning of blood), diabetes, gout or arthritis unless directed by a doctor.

Directions: Adults: 2 tablets, caplets or geltabs with water every 6 hours while symptoms persist, not to exceed 8 tablets, caplets or geltabs in 24 hours, or as directed by a doctor. Children under 12 years of age: Consult a doctor.

Overdose: MUCOMYST (acetylcysteine) As An Antidote For Acetaminophen Overdose)
Acetaminophen is rapidly absorbed from the upper gastrointestinal tract with peak plasma levels occurring between 30 and 60 minutes after therapeutic doses and usually within 4 hours following an overdose. The parent compound, which is nontoxic, is extensively metabolized in the liver to form principally the sulfate and glucuronide conjugates which are also nontoxic and are rapidly excreted in the urine. A small fraction of an ingested dose is metabolized in the liver by the cytochrome P-450 mixed function oxidase enzyme system to form a reactive, potentially toxic, intermediate metabolite which preferentially conjugates with hepatic glutathione to form the nontoxic cysteine and mercapturic acid derivatives which are then excreted by the kidney. Therapeutic doses of acetaminophen do not saturate the glucuronide and sulfate conjugation pathways and do not result in the formation of sufficient reactive metabolite to deplete glutathione stores. However, following ingestion of a large overdose (150 mg/kg or greater) the glucuronide and sulfate conjugation pathways are saturated resulting in a larger fraction of the drug being metabolized via the P-450 pathway. The increased formation of reactive metabolite may deplete the hepatic stores of glutathione with subsequent binding of the metabolite to protein molecules within the hepatocyte resulting in cellular necrosis. Acetylcysteine has been shown to reduce the extent of liver injury following acetaminophen overdose. Early symptoms following a potentially hepatotoxic overdose may include: nausea, vomiting, diaphoresis and general malaise. Clinical and laboratory evidence of hepatic toxicity may not be apparent until 48 to 72 hours postingestion. In most adults and adolescents, regardless of the quantity of acetaminophen reported to have been ingested, administer MUCOMYST® acetylcysteine immediately. MUCOMYST acetylcysteine therapy should be initiated and continued for a full course of therapy. Its effectiveness depends on early administration, with benefit seen principally in patients treated within 16 hours of the overdose.
If acetaminophen plasma assay capability is not available, and the estimated acetaminophen ingestion exceeds 150 mg/kg, MUCOMYST acetylcysteine therapy should be initiated and continued for a full course of therapy.
For full prescribing information, refer to the MUCOMYST package insert. Do not await the results of assays for acetaminophen level before initiating treatment with MUCOMYST acetylcysteine. The following additional procedures are recommended: The stomach should be emptied promptly by lavage or by induction of emesis with syrup of ipecac. A serum acetaminophen assay should be obtained as early as possible, but no sooner than four hours following ingestion. Liver function studies should be obtained initially and repeated at 24-hour intervals.
For additional emergency information call your regional poison center or toll free (1-800-525-6115) to the Rocky Mountain Poison Center for assistance in diagnosis and for directions in the use of MUCOMYST acetylcysteine as an antidote.

How Supplied: Extra Strength EXCEDRIN® is supplied as:
White circular tablet with letter "E" debossed on one side. Supplied in bottles of 12's, 24's, 50's, 100's, 175's and metal tins of 12's.
Coated while caplets with "E" debossed on one side. Supplied in bottles of 24's 50's, 100's, 175's.
Coated round geltabs–green on one side white on the other, printed with black "E" on one side. Supplied in bottles of 20's, 40's, 80's and 2's.
All sizes packaged in child resistant closures except 100's for tablets, 50's for caplets which are sizes recommended for households without young children.

Shown in Product Identification Guide, page 507

EXCEDRIN P.M.®
[*ĕx "cĕd 'rĭn*]
Analgesic Sleeping Aid

Composition: Each tablet, caplet or geltab contains:

	EXCEDRIN®PM Per Tablet or Caplet
Acetaminophen	500 mg.
Diphenhydramine Citrate:	38 mg.
Other Ingredients:	—

Tablet or Caplet
- benzoic acid
- carnauba wax
- corn starch
- D&C yellow no. 10
- D&C yellow no. 10 aluminum lake
- FD&C blue no. 1
- FD&C blue no. 1 aluminum lake
- hydroxypropyl methylcellulose
- magnesium stearate
- methylparaben
- pregelatinized starch
- propylene glycol
- propylparaben
- simethicone emulsion
- stearic acid
- titanium dioxide

May also contain:
- mineral oil
- polysorbate 20
- povidone
- sodium citrate
- sorbitan monolaurate

	EXCEDRIN®PM Per Geltab
Acetaminophen	500 mg.
Diphenhydramine Citrate	38 mg.

Other Ingredients:

Benzoic Acid
Corn starch
D&C Red No. 33 Lake
D&C Yellow No. 10
D&C Yellow No. 10 Lake
Edetate Disodium
Fd&C Blue No. 1
Fd&C Blue No. 1 Lake
Gelatin
Glycerin
Hydroxypropyl Methylcellulose
Magnesium Stearate
Methylparaben
Mineral Oil
Polysorbate 20
Povidone
Pregelatinized Starch
Propylene Glycol
Propylparaben
Simethicone Emulsion
Sorbitan Monolaurate
Stearic Acid
Titanium Dioxide

Indications: For temporary relief of occasional headaches and minor aches and pains with accompanying sleeplessness.

Warnings: Keep this and all drugs out of the reach of children. In case of accidental overdose, seek professional assistance or contact a poison control center immediately. Prompt medical attention is critical for adults as well as for children even if you do not notice any signs or symptoms. As with any drug, if you are pregnant or nursing a baby, seek the advice of a health professional before using this product. Do not give to children under 12 years of age or use for more than 10 days unless directed by a doctor. If symptoms persist or get worse, if new ones occur, or if sleeplessness persists continuously for more than 2 weeks, consult your doctor. Insomnia may be a symptom of serious underlying medical illness. Do not take this product, unless directed by a doctor, if you have a breathing problem such as emphysema or chronic bronchitis, or if you have glaucoma or difficulty in urination due to enlargement of the prostate gland. Avoid alcoholic beverages while taking this product. Do not take this product if you are taking sedatives or tranquilizers, without first consulting your doctor. If you generally consume 3 or more alcohol-containing drinks per day, you should consult your physician for advice on when and how you should take Excedrin PM and other pain relievers.

Directions:
Adults and children 12 years of age and over: 2 tablets, caplets, or geltabs at bedtime if needed or as directed by a doctor.

Overdose: MUCOMYST (acetylcysteine) As An Antidote For Acetaminophen Overdose)

Acetaminophen is rapidly absorbed from the upper gastrointestinal tract with peak plasma levels occurring between 30 and 60 minutes after therapeutic doses and usually within 4 hours following an overdose. The parent compound, which is nontoxic, is extensively metabolized in the liver to form principally the sulfate and glucuronide conjugates which are also nontoxic and are rapidly excreted in the urine. A small fraction of an ingested dose is metabolized in the liver by the cytochrome P-450 mixed function oxidase enzyme system to form a reactive, potentially toxic, intermediate metabolite which preferentially conjugates with hepatic glutathione to form the nontoxic cysteine and mercapturic acid derivatives which are then excreted by the kidney. Therapeutic doses of acetaminophen do not saturate the glucuronide and sulfate conjugation pathways and do not result in the formation of sufficient reactive metabolite to deplete glutathione stores. However, following ingestion of a large overdose (150 mg/kg or greater) the glucuronide and sulfate conjugation pathways are saturated resulting in a larger fraction of the drug being metabolized via the P-450 pathway. The increased formation of reactive metabolite may deplete the hepatic stores of glutathione with subsequent binding of the metabolite to protein molecules within the hepatocyte resulting in cellular necrosis. Acetylcysteine has been shown to reduce the extent of liver injury following acetaminophen overdose. Early symptoms following a potentially hepatotoxic overdose may include: nausea, vomiting, diaphoresis and general malaise. Clinical and laboratory evidence of hepatic toxicity may not be apparent until 48 to 72 hours postingestion. In most adults and adolescents, regardless of the quantity of acetaminophen reported to have been ingested, administer MUCOMYST® acetylcysteine immediately. MUCOMYST acetylcysteine therapy should be initiated and continued for a full course of therapy. Its effectiveness depends on early administration, with benefit seen principally in patients treated within 16 hours of the overdose.
If acetaminophen plasma assay capability is not available, and the estimated acetaminophen ingestion exceeds 150 mg/kg, MUCOMYST acetylcysteine therapy should be initiated and continued for a full course of therapy.
For full prescribing information, refer to the MUCOMYST package insert. Do not await the results of assays for acetaminophen level before initiating treatment with MUCOMYST acetylcysteine. The following additional procedures are recommended: The stomach should be emptied promptly by lavage or by induction of emesis with syrup of ipecac. A serum acetaminophen assay should be obtained as early as possible, but no sooner than four hours following ingestion. Liver function studies should be obtained initially and repeated at 24-hour intervals.
For additional emergency information call your regional poison center or toll-free (1-800-525-6115) to the Rocky Mountain Poison Center for assistance in diagnosis and for directions in the use of MUCOMYST acetylcysteine as an antidote.
For overdose treatment information, consult a regional poison control center.

How Supplied: EXCEDRIN P.M.® is supplied as:
Light blue circular coated tablets with "PM" debossed on one side. Supplied in bottles of 10's, 24's, 50's, 100's, 150's.
Light blue coated caplet with "PM" debossed on one side. Supplied in bottles of 24's, 50's, 100's.
Light blue geltabs with "Excedrin PM" printed on one side. Supplied in bottles of 24's, 50's.
All sizes packaged in child resistant closures except 50's, which are recommended for households without young children.
Store at room temperature.

Shown in Product Identification Guide, page 507

4-WAY® Fast Acting Nasal Spray

Composition: Regular formula contains:
Phenylephrine hydrochloride 0.5%, naphazoline hydrochloride 0.05%, pyrilamine maleate 0.2%, in a buffered solution. Also Contains: Benzalkonium Chloride, Boric Acid, Sodium Borate, Water.
Also available in a mentholated formula containing: Phenylephrine hydrochloride 0.5%, naphazoline hydrochloride 0.05%, pyrilamine maleate 0.2%, in a buffered solution. Also Contains: Benzalkonium Chloride, Boric Acid, Camphor, Eucalyptol, Menthol, Poloxamer 188, Polysorbate 80, Sodium Borate, Water.

Indications: For prompt, temporary relief of nasal congestion due to the common cold, sinusitis, hay fever or other upper respiratory allergies.

Directions and Use Instructions:
Directions: Adults: Spray twice into each nostril not more often than every 6 hours. Do not give to children under 12 years of age unless directed by a doctor.
Use Instructions: For Metered Pump—Remove protective cap. Hold bottle with thumb at base and nozzle between first and second fingers. With head upright, insert metered pump spray nozzle into nostril. Depress pump all the way down, with a firm even stroke and sniff deeply. Repeat in other nostril. Do not tilt head backward while spraying. Wipe tip clean after each use. Note: This bottle is filled to correct level for proper pump action. Before using the first time, remove the protective cap from the tip and prime the metered pump by depressing pump firmly several times.
Use Instructions: For Atomizer—
With head in a normal upright position, put atomizer tip into nostril. Squeeze

Continued on next page

Bristol-Myers—Cont.

bottle with firm, quick pressure while inhaling.

Warnings: **KEEP THIS AND ALL OTHER MEDICATIONS OUT OF THE REACH OF CHILDREN. IN CASE OF ACCIDENTAL OVERDOSE OR INGESTION, SEEK PROFESSIONAL ASSISTANCE OR CONTACT A POISON CONTROL CENTER IMMEDIATELY.** Do not exceed recommended dosage because burning, stinging, sneezing, or increase of nasal discharge may occur. The use of this container by more than one person may spread infection. Do not use this product for more than 3 days. If symptoms persist, consult a doctor. Do not use this product in children under 12 years of age because it may cause sedation if swallowed. Do not use this product if you have heart disease, high blood pressure, thyroid disease, diabetes, or difficulty in urination due to enlargement of the prostate gland should not use this product unless directed by a doctor.

How Supplied:
Regular formula:
Supplied as Atomizer 1/2 fluid, and 1 fluid ounce size.
Mentholated formula:
Supplied as Atomizer of 1/2 fluid ounce.
Store at room temperature.

Shown in Product Identification Guide, page 506

4-WAY® 12 Hour Nasal Spray

Composition: Oxymetazoline Hydrochloride 0.05% in a buffered isotonic aqueous solution. Phenylmercuric Acetate 0.002% added as a preservative. **Also Contains:** Benzalkonium Chloride, Glycine, Sorbitol, Water.

Indications: Temporarily relieves nasal congestion due to the common cold, hay fever or other upper respiratory allergies associated with sinusitis.

Directions and Use Instructions:
Directions: Adults and children 6 to under 12 years of age (with adult supervision): 2 or 3 sprays in each nostril not more often than every 10 to 12 hours. Do not exceed 2 doses in any 24-hour period. Children under 6 years of age: Consult a doctor.
Use Instructions:
With head in a normal, upright position, put atomizer tip into nostril. Squeeze bottle with firm, quick pressure while inhaling. Wipe nozzle clean after each use.

Warnings: Keep this and all drugs out of the reach of children. In case of accidental overdose or ingestion, seek professional assistance or contact a poison control center immediately. **Do not exceed recommended dosage.** This product may cause temporary discomfort such as burning, stinging, sneezing, or an increase in nasal discharge. The use of this container by more than one person may spread infection. Do not use this product for more than 3 days. Use only as directed. Frequent or prolonged use may cause nasal congestion to recur or worsen. If symptoms persist, consult a doctor. Do not use this product if you have heart disease, high blood pressure, thyroid disease, or diabetes or difficulty in urination due to enlargement of the prostate gland unless directed by a doctor. Do not use this product in a child who has heart disease, high blood pressure, thyroid disease, or diabetes unless directed by a doctor.

How Supplied: 4-WAY 12 Hour Nasal Spray is supplied as:
Atomizer of 1/2 fluid ounce.
Store at room temperature.

Shown in Product Identification Guide, page 506

KERI LOTION
Skin Lubricant—Moisturizer

Available in three formulations:
KERI Original, Silky Smooth and Sensitive Skin

KERI Original

Composition: Water, mineral oil, propylene glycol, PEG-40 stearate, glyceryl stearate/PEG-100 stearate, PEG-4 dilaurate, laureth-4, lanolin oil, methyl paraben, carbomer, propylparaben, fragrance triethanolamine, dioctyl sodium sulfosuccinate, quaternium-15.

Direction for Use: Apply wherever skin feels dry, rough or irritated. For external use only.

KERI Silky Smooth recommended for daily use on dry skin.

Composition: Water, petrolatum, glycerin, dimethicone, steareth-2, cetyl alcohol, benzyl alcohol, laureth-23, magnesium aluminum silicate, tocopheryl acetate or tocopheryl linoleate, carbomer, fragrance, sodium hydroxide, disodium EDTA, quaternium-15.

Directions for Use: Apply liberally after bathing, before bed or whenever skin feels dry. Use daily on hands, arms, legs, or anywhere skin feels dry for softer, smoother, healthier-looking skin. For external use only.

KERI Sensitive Skin

Composition: Water, petrolatum, glycerin, dimethicone, steareth-2, cetyl alcohol, benzyl alcohol, laureth-23, magnesium aluminum silicate, tocopheryl acetate or tocopheryl linoleate, carbomer, sodium hydroxide, disodium EDTA, quaternium-15.

Directions for Use: Apply liberally after bathing, before bed or whenever skin feels dry. Use daily on hands, arms, legs, or anywhere skin feels dry for softer, smoother, healthier-looking skin. For external use only.

How Supplied: KERI Lotion Original 6 1/2 oz., 11 oz., 15 oz. and 20 oz. plastic bottles. KERI Silky Smooth 6 1/2 oz., 11 oz. and 15 oz. plastic bottles. KERI Sensitive Skin 6 1/2 oz., 11 oz. and 15 oz. plastic bottles.

Shown in Product Identification Guide, page 507

NO DOZ® Maximum Strength Caplets

Composition: Each caplet contains 200 mg. Caffeine. Other ingredients: Benzoic Acid, Corn Starch, FD&C Blue No. 1, Flavors, Hydroxypropyl Methylcellulose, Microcrystalline Cellulose, Propylene Glycol, Simethicone Emulsion, Stearic Acid, Sucrose, Titanium Dioxide. May also contain: Carnauba Wax, Mineral Oil, Polysorbate 20, Povidone, Sorbitan Monolaurate.

Indications: Helps restore mental alertness or wakefulness when experiencing fatigue or drowsiness.

Directions: Adults: one-half to one caplet not more often than every 3 to 4 hours.

Warnings: KEEP THIS AND ALL OTHER MEDICATIONS OUT OF THE REACH OF CHILDREN. IN CASE OF ACCIDENTAL OVERDOSE, SEEK PROFESSIONAL ASSISTANCE OR CONTACT A POISON CONTROL CENTER IMMEDIATELY. As with any drug, if you are pregnant or nursing a baby, seek the advice of a health professional before using this product. Do not give to children under 12 years of age. For occasional use only. Not intended for use as a substitute for sleep. If fatigue or drowsiness persists or continues to occur, consult a doctor. The recommended dose of this product contains about as much caffeine as a cup of coffee. Limit the use of caffeine-containing medications, foods, or beverages while taking this product because too much caffeine may cause nervousness, irritability, sleeplessness and, occasionally, rapid heart beat.

How Supplied: NO DOZ® Maximum Strength is supplied as: White coated caplets with "NO DOZ" debossed on one side. The opposite side is scored.
Supplied in bottles of 16's, 36's, 60's.
Store at room temperature.

NUPRIN®
(ibuprofen)
Analgesic

Warning: ASPIRIN SENSITIVE PATIENTS. Do not take this product if you have had a severe allergic reaction to aspirin, e.g.—asthma, swelling, shock or hives, because even though this product contains no aspirin or salicylates, cross-reactions may occur in patients allergic to aspirin.

Composition: Each tablet or caplet contains ibuprofen USP, 200 mg. **Other Ingredients:** Carnauba wax, cornstarch, D&C Yellow No. 10, FD&C Yellow No. 6, hydroxypropyl methylcellulose, propylene glycol, silicon dioxide, stearic acid, titanium dioxide.

Indications: For the temporary relief of minor aches and pains associated with the common cold, headache, toothache, muscular aches, backache, for the minor pain of arthritis, for the pain of menstrual cramps and for reduction of fever.

Warnings: Do not take for pain for more than 10 days or for fever for more than 3 days unless directed by a doctor. If pain or fever persists or gets worse, if new symptoms occur, or if the painful area is red or swollen, consult a doctor. These could be signs of serious illness. If you are under a doctor's care for any serious condition, consult a doctor before taking this product. As with aspirin and acetaminophen, if you have any condition which requires you to take prescription drugs or if you have had any problems or serious side effects from taking any non-prescription pain reliever, do not take NUPRIN without first discussing it with your doctor. If you experience any symptoms which are unusual or seem unrelated to the condition for which you took ibuprofen, consult a doctor before taking any more of it. Although ibuprofen is indicated for the same conditions as aspirin and acetaminophen, it should not be taken with them except under a doctor's direction. Do not combine this product with any other ibuprofen-containing product. As with any drug, if you are pregnant or nursing a baby, seek the advice of a health professional before using this product. IT IS ESPECIALLY IMPORTANT NOT TO USE IBUPROFEN DURING THE LAST 3 MONTHS OF PREGNANCY UNLESS SPECIFICALLY DIRECTED TO DO SO BY A DOCTOR BECAUSE IT MAY CAUSE PROBLEMS IN THE UNBORN CHILD OR COMPLICATIONS DURING DELIVERY. Keep this and all drugs out of the reach of children. In case of accidental overdose, seek professional assistance or contact a poison control center immediately.

Caution: Store at room temperature. Avoid excessive heat 40°C (104°F).

Directions: Adults: Take 1 tablet or caplet every 4 to 6 hours while symptoms persist. If pain or fever does not respond to 1 tablet or caplet, 2 tablets or caplets may be used but do not exceed 6 tablets or caplets in 24 hours, unless directed by a doctor. The smallest effective dose should be used. Take with food or milk if occasional and mild heartburn, upset stomach, or stomach pain occurs with use. Consult a doctor if these symptoms are more than mild or if they persist. Children: Do not give this product to children under 12 except under the advice and supervision of a doctor.

Overdose: For overdose treatment information, consult a regional poison control center.

How Supplied:
NUPRIN® is supplied as:
Golden yellow round tablets with "NUPRIN" printed in black on one side.
Golden yellow caplets with "NUPRIN" printed in black on one side.
Supplied in bottles of 36's, 75's, 150's.
All sizes packaged in child resistant closures.

Store at room temperature. Avoid excessive heat 40°C. (104°F.).
Distributed by Bristol-Myers Company

Shown in Product Identification Guide, page 507

THERAPEUTIC MINERAL ICE®

Composition:
Active Ingredient: Menthol 2%
Other Ingredients: Ammonium Hydroxide, Carbomer 934, Cupric Sulfate, FD&C Blue No. 1, Isopropyl Alcohol, Magnesium Sulfate, Sodium Hydroxide, Thymol, Water.

Indications: For the temporary relief of minor aches and pains of muscles and joints associated with arthritis, simple backache, strains, bruises, sprains and sports injuries. **USE ONLY AS DIRECTED. Read all warnings before use.**

Warnings: KEEP OUT OF THE REACH OF CHILDREN. For external use only. Not for internal use. Avoid contact with eyes and mucous membranes. Do not use with other ointments, creams, sprays, or liniments. **Do not use with Heating Pads or Heating Devices.** If condition worsens, or if symptoms persist for more than 7 days, or clear up and occur again within a few days, discontinue use of this product and consult your doctor. Do not apply to wounds or damaged skin. Do not bandage tightly. If you have sensitive skin, consult doctor **before** use. If skin irritation develops, discontinue use and consult your doctor. As with any drug, if you are pregnant or nursing a baby, seek the advice of a health professional before using this product. Keep cap tightly closed. Do not use, pour, spill or store near heat or open flame. **Note:** You can always use Mineral Ice as directed, but its use is never intended to replace your doctor's advice.

Directions: Adults and children 2 years of age and older: Clean skin of all other ointments, creams, sprays, or liniments. Apply to affected areas not more than 3 to 4 times daily. May be used with wet or dry bandages or with ice packs. No protective cover needed. Children under 2 years of age: Consult a doctor.

How Supplied:
3.5, 8 and 16 ounce.
Store at room temperature.

Shown in Product Identification Guide, page 507

Care-Tech® Laboratories, Inc.

Over-The-Counter Pharmaceuticals
3224 SOUTH KINGSHIGHWAY BOULEVARD
ST. LOUIS, MO 63139

Direct Inquiries to:
Sherry L. Brereton
(314) 772-4610
FAX: (314) 772-4613

For Medical Emergencies Contact:
Customer Service
(800) 325-9681
FAX: (314) 772-4613

BARRI-CARE®
ANTIMICROBIAL OINTMENT

Composition: Active Ingredient: Chloroxylenol
Inactive Ingredients: Petrolatum, Water, Paraffin, Propylene Glycol, Milk Protein, Cod Liver Oil, Aloe Vera Gel, Fragrance, Potassium Hydroxide, Methyl Paraben, Propyl Paraben, Vitamin A & D_3, (E) dl Alpha-Tocopheryl Acetate, (E) dl-Alpha-Tocopherol, D&C Yellow #11 and D&C Red #17.

Actions and Uses: Topical, antimicrobial for prevention and treatment of bacterial infection. Formulated for diabetic feet, topical staph infection and immune compromised patient care. For use around edges of chronic wounds to halt additional breakdown, trac sites, I.V. sites. Proven antimicrobial action against E. coli, MRSA, S. aureus and Pseudomonas aeruginosa. Protects perineal area of the incontinent patient from painful skin rashes and relieves irritation around stoma sites. Utilize on Grades I–IV pressure ulcers to halt skin breakdown. Can be used also on minor burns. Will not melt under feverish conditions. No Contra-indications. Three year shelf life.

Precautions: External Use Only. Non-Toxic. Avoid eye contact.—Ointment-base.

Directions: Cleanse affected area with Satin thoroughly. Apply ointment topically to affected area. Reapply 2–3 times daily or as directed by physician.

How Supplied: 1 ounce tubes, 4 oz. tubes, 8 oz. jar. NDC #46706-206

CARE CREME®
ANTIMICROBIAL CREAM

Composition: Active Ingredient: Chloroxylenol .8%
Inactive Ingredients: Water, Cetyl Alcohol, Lanolin Oil, Cod Liver Oil, Sodium Laureth Sulfate, Triethanolamine, Propylene Glycol, Petrolatum, Lanolin Alcohol, Methyl Gluceth 20 Distearate, Beeswax, Citric Acid, Methyl Paraben, Fra-

Continued on next page

Care-Tech—Cont.

grance, Propyl Paraben, Vitamins A, D_3 and E-dl Alpha-Tocopherol.

Actions and Uses: Vitamin enriched broad spectrum topical, antimicrobial cream for treatment of atopic dermatitis, psoriasis, severe itching, staph infections. Transdermal, antimicrobial action on gram-negative, gram-positive, yeast and fungi. Extremely effective on oncology radiation burns. Use at first sign of reddened skin or initial breakdown. Vitamin and oil enriched to promote skin integrity. Contains no metallic ions. Provides moisture and vitamin enriched wound therapy.

Precautions: Non-toxic, External Use Only. Avoid use around eye area. No Contra-indications. Three year shelf life.

Directions: Cleanse affected area with Satin and gently massage Care Creme into skin until completely absorbed or as directed by physician. Apply 3–4 times daily or as needed.

How Supplied: 1 ounce tubes, 4 oz. tubes, 9 oz. jar. NDC #46706-205

CLINICAL CARE® ANTIMICROBIAL WOUND CLEANSER

Composition: Active Ingredient: Benzethonium Chloride .1%
Inactive Ingredients: Water, Amphoteric 2, Aloe Vera Gel, DMDM Hydantoin, Citric Acid.

Actions and Uses: Clinical Care is an antimicrobial, emulsifying solution which aids in removing debris and particulate matter from open, dermal wounds. Clinical Care inhibits the growth of pathogenic organisms. Proven effective at eliminating S. aureus, P. aeruginosa, S. typhimurium, Aspergillus, E. coli, MRSA, S. pyogenes and K. pneumonia. Will not produce dermal irritation.

Precautions: External Use Only. Non-Toxic. No contra-indicators.

Directions: Spray affected area as necessary to debride. Use sterile gauze to gently remove debris and necrotic tissue at dermal surface.

How Supplied: 4 oz. spray, 12 oz. spray

CONCEPT® ANTIMICROBIAL DERMAL CLEANSER

Composition: Active Ingredient: Chloroxylenol
Inactive Ingredients: Water, Amphoteric 9, Polysorbate 20, PEG-150 Distearate, Cocamide DEA, Cocoyl Sarcosine, Fragrance, D&C Green #5.

Actions and Uses: Concept is a geriatric shampoo and body wash for patients whose skin is irritated by soaps and harsh detergents. Concept is non-eye irritating and eliminates bacteria on the skin. Excellent for replenishing moisture in dry, flaky dermal tissues and eliminating body odors. Safe for use on infants to address rashing or atopic dermatitis. Excellent for use on HIV and oncology patients to reduce topical infection.

Precautions: External Use Only. Non-Toxic. No Contra-indications.

Directions: Use in normal manner of bathing and shampooing. Rinse thoroughly.

How Supplied: 8 oz., Gallons

FORMULA MAGIC® ANTIMICROBIAL/ANTI-FUNGAL POWDER

Composition: Active Ingredient: Benzethonium Chloride .1%
Inactive Ingredients: Talc, Mineral Oil, Magnesium Carbonate, Fragrance, DMDM Hydantoin.

Actions and Uses: Broad spectrum antimicrobial/antifungal talc base powder for treatment of diabetic feet and limbs. Aids in preventing excoriation, friction chafing and eliminating odor. Antibacterial action proven effective at 99.9% inhibition where Formula Magic is applied. Excellent for use on diabetic patients, feet and under breasts to relieve redness and skin irritation caused by excessive moisture and resulting bacterial growth.

Precautions: Non-irritating to skin, non-toxic, slightly irritating to eyes.

Directions: Apply liberally to body and rub gently into skin.

How Supplied: 4 oz. and 12 oz. NDC #46706-202

HUMATRIX® MICROCLYSMIC GEL
Burn/Wound Healing Gel

Composition: Water, Propylene Glycol, Glycerine, Hydrolyzed Collagen, Citric Acid, Carbomer, Triethanolamine, Chondroitin Sulfate, Preservatives.

Actions and Uses: Provides endothermic and biomimetic properties to cool traumatized tissue and aid in the homeostasis of healing. HUMATRIX® provides the ultimate moisturization for burns, autograft procedures, radiation irritation, glycolic acid peel irritation, mechanical injuries, laser treatment, and chronic wound therapy. Humatrix is almost pure protein in content and aids in rapid cellular regeneration (New Technology).

Precautions: External use only. Non-toxic. No contra-indications.

Directions: Cleanse the area with Techni-Care® Surgical Scrub, Prep. and Wound Cleanser, Rinse thoroughly with Clinical Care® Antimicrobial Wound Cleanser. Do not pat dry. Apply a layer of HUMATRIX® Microclysmic Gel approximately 2–4mm. thick. Cover the wound with a non-occlusive dressing. Reapply at every dressing change to maintain a moist wound environment.

How Supplied: 8.5 oz. Spray Bottle. NDC# 46706-440-03

ORCHID FRESH II® ANTIMICROBIAL PERINEAL/ OSTOMY CLEANSER
Perineal/Ostomy Cleanser

Composition: Active Ingredient: Benzethonium Chloride .1%
Inactive Ingredients: Water, Amphoteric 2, DMDM Hydantoin, Fragrance, Citric Acid.

Actions and Uses: Orchid Fresh II is an amphoteric, topical antimicrobial cleansing solution which gently cleans and emulsifies feces and urine on the incontinent patient. Use also on stoma sites and ostomy bags to deodorize and eliminate odor. Broad spectrum antimicrobial action on Pseudomonas, E. coli, Staphylococcus aureus, MRSA, etc. Orchid Fresh II will aid in reducing skin breakdown or tears. Significantly reduces UTI infection in the incontinent, geriatric patient.

Precautions: External Use Only, Non-Toxic—Non-Dermal Irritating No Contra-indications.

Directions: Spray topically and remove feces and urine with warm, moist washcloth. Spray directly on peristomal skin areas, clean gently and pat dry. Utilize Care Creme on reddened skin areas.

How Supplied: 4 oz., 8 oz., 16 oz. and Gallons NDC #46706-115

SATIN® ANTIMICROBIAL SKIN CLEANSER

Composition: Active Ingredient: Chloroxylenol .8%
Inactive Ingredients: Water, Sodium Laureth Sulfate, Cocamidopropyl Betaine, PEG-8, Cocamide DEA, Glycol Stearate, Lanolin Oil, Tetrasodium EDTA, D&C Yellow #10.

Actions and Uses: Satin has been specially formulated for use on sensitive or aging dermal tissue, atopic dermatitis and psoriasis. Effective in eliminating gram-positive and gram-negative pathogens such as E. coli, S. aureus, Pseudomonas, etc. Contains emollients to replenish natural oils and proteins. Satin also eliminates skin odor and dry, itchy skin.

Precautions: No contra-indicators. External use only. Non-Toxic.

Directions: Use daily during shower, bath or regular cleansing or as directed by physician.

How Supplied: 4 oz., 8 oz., 12 oz. 16 oz., 1 Gallon NDC #46706-101

TECHNI–CARE® SURGICAL SCRUB, Prep and Wound Decontaminant

Composition: Active Ingredient: Chloroxylenol 3%
Inactive Ingredients: Water, Sodium Lauryl Sulfate, Cocamide DEA, Propylene Glycol, Cocamidopropyl Betaine, Cocamidopropyl PG-Dimonium Chloride Phosphate, Citric Acid, Tetrasodium EDTA, Aloe Vera Gel, Hydrolyzed Animal Protein, D&C Yellow #10.

Actions and Uses: Techni-Care represents entirerly new technology in a broad-spectrum, topical, antiseptic microbicide for skin degerming. 99.99% Bacterial reduction in 30 second contact usage. Techni-Care may be used for disinfection of wounds, for pre-op and post-op along with surgical scrub applications. Non-staining and non-irritating to dermal tissue. Techni-Care conditions dermal tissue and phospholipid promotes a more rapid rate of cellular regeneration. Use for treatment of acute, chronic wounds in replacement of topical, antibiotic therapy.

Precautions: Non-Toxic, Non-Irritating, External Use Only. Can be used safely around ears and eyes or as directed by a physician. No Contra-indications.

Directions: Apply, lather and rinse well. For pre-op, apply and let dry, no rinsing required.

How Supplied: 20 mL packets, 4 oz., 8 oz., 12 oz., 16 oz., 32 oz., Gallons and peel paks

---

Care Technologies, Inc.
55 HOLLY HILL LANE
GREENWICH, CT 06830

Direct Inquiries to:
Mark Watkins
VP Marketing
(203) 661-3161
FAX: (203) 661-3619
E-mail: caretec1@aol.com
http://www.clearcare.com

CLEAR™ Total Lice Elimination System
CLEAR™Lice Killing Shampoo
CLEAR® Lice Egg Remover
CLEAR™ Nit (egg) Comb

PRODUCT OVERVIEW
Key Facts: Clear™ Total Lice Elimination System offers the only combination treatment product with enzymatic lice egg remover. This lice killing shampoo kills lice and their eggs with a full strength pyrethrum extract shampoo. It is effective against head, body and pubic (crab) lice.
The active ingredients are pyrethrum extract and piperonyl butoxide, technical which work against the louse and egg nervous system. There is almost no skin absorption. The piperonyl butoxide acts as a synergist. The pyrethrum extract in Clear™ shampoo residues disappears within minutes after rinsing out. Each **Clear™** Total System package also contains a patented enzymatic lice egg remover in a tube plus an effective nit (egg) comb. Together, these combing aids make the difficult job of lice egg removal faster and easier so that children can return to school more quickly.

Major Uses: Clear™ Total System is used to treat head lice infestations as quickly as possible and allow children to return to school. Only one package is required to do the complete job.
Safety Information: Clear™ Lice Killing Shampoo should be used with caution by individuals sensitive to ragweed. This product is intended for external use only. It is harmful if swallowed. Keep this and all drugs out of the reach of children. In case of accidental lice treatment ingestion, seek professional assistance or contact a Poison Control Center immediately.
Clear® Lice Egg Remover contains no harsh chemicals and is safe for use at any time. It is not a treatment product and needs to be used in conjunction with a lice treatment product if it is used in the process of eliminating a lice infestation and returning a child to school. **Clear®** Lice Egg Remover is for external use only. If it does get into the eye, gently flush with water.

PRESCRIBING INFORMATION
Clear™ Lice Killing Shampoo
2 OZ-NDC# 62653-210-02
4 OZ-NDC# 62653-210-04

Description: Clear™ Lice Killing Shampoo contains a liquid pediculicide whose active ingredients are pyrethrum extract 0.33% and piperonyl butoxide, technical 4.00%. Inert ingredients (95.67%) are: octylphenoxypolyethoxyethanol non-ionic surfactant, benzyl alcohol, petroleum distillate, and water.

Actions: Clear™ Lice Killing Shampoo kills head lice (Pediculus humanus capitus), body lice (Pediculus humanus humanus), and pubic (crab) lice (Pthirus pubis), and their eggs. The pyrethrum extract acts as a contact poison affecting the nervous system, resulting in paralysis and death. The efficacy of the pyrethrum extract pediculicide is synergized by piperonyl butoxide. The pyrethrum extract is rinsed out after treatment leaving no appreciable residue. In addition, the pyrethrum molecules are not readily absorbed through the skin. Any minute amounts which are absorbed, are rapidly metabolized and eliminated from the body with no ill effects.

Indications: For the treatment of head, pubic (crab) and body lice.

Dosage and Administration: Apply to affected areas until hair is thoroughly saturated. Allow product to remain on area for 10 minutes but not longer. Add sufficient warm water to form a lather and shampoo as usual. Rinse thoroughly. Apply the **Clear** Lice Egg Remover directly to the affected areas, massage in and wait three minutes for it to loosen the nits (eggs). Use the **Clear ™** nit (egg) comb comb out the nits from the hair (Follow the detailed instructions in the package insert). A second treatment must be given in 7 to 10 days to kill any newly hatched lice.
Since there is no immunity to lice, daily inspections and continued personal care will help prevent reinfestation. The following additional steps are important to minimize the opportunities for environmental reinfestation. Disinfect all personal clothing, bed linen, and bath linen items by machine washing in hot water and drying, using the hot cycle of the dryer for at least 20 minutes. Personal clothing and bedding that cannot be washed may be dry-cleaned, sealed in plastic bags for a period of two weeks, or thoroughly vacuumed. Personal combs and brushes may be disinfected by soaking hot water (above 130°F) for 5 to 10 minutes. Thorough vacuuming of rooms inhabited by infected persons is recommended.

Warnings: Clear™ Lice Killing Shampoo should be used with caution by individuals sensitive to ragweed. This product is intended for external use only. It is harmful if swallowed. Do not use near the eyes or permit contact with mucous membranes, such as inside the nose, mouth, or vagina, as irritation may occur. Keep out of eyes when rinsing hair. Adults and children: Close eyes tightly and do not open eyes until product is rinsed out. Also, protect children's eyes with a washcloth, towel or other suitable material, or by a similar method. If pyrethrum product gets into eyes, immediately flush with water. If skin irritation or infection is present or develops, discontinue use and consult your doctor. Consult your doctor if infestation of eyebrows or eyelashes occurs. As with any drug, if you are pregnant or nursing a baby, seek the advice of a health professional before using this product. Keep this and all drugs out of the reach of children. In case of accidental lice treatment ingestion, seek professional assistance or contact a Poison Control Center immediately.

FACED WITH AN Rx SIDE EFFECT?
Turn to the
Companion Drug Index
(Green Pages)
for products that
provide symptomatic
relief.

Carlsbad Technology Inc.
5923 BALFOUR COURT
CARLSBAD, CA 92008

For Medical and Pharmaceutical Information Including Emergencies:
(619) 431-8284
FAX: (619) 431-7505

ENTERIC COATED PELLETS ASPIRIN
81 mg, Delayed Release Enteric Coated Pellets Aspirin
Adult Low Strength 81 mg Pellets Capsules

Active Ingredients: Each capsule contains Aspirin 81 mg. Adult Low Strength 81 mg Aspirin Capsule contains the same low strength of Aspirin as Aspirin tablet but in an Encapsulated Enteric Coated Pellets made for adults. The Enteric Coated Pellet provides protection against stomach upset and those side effects in the small intestine due to a sudden, highly localized dose of drug at one site.

Indications: For temporary relief of minor aches and pains or as recommended by your doctor.

Directions: Adults: Take 4 to 8 capsules every 4 hours while symptoms persist, not to exceed 48 capsules in 24 hours or as directed by a doctor. Drink a full glass of water with each dose.

Warnings: Keep out of reach of children and see labels and cases for detail information.

Drug Interaction Precaution: Do not take this product if you are taking a prescription drug for anticoagulation (thinning of the blood), diabetes, gout, or arthritis unless directed by a doctor.

How Supplied: One bottle contains 120 capsules.

J. R. Carlson Laboratories, Inc.
15 COLLEGE DR.
ARLINGTON HEIGHTS, IL 60004

Direct Inquiries to:
Customer Service
(847) 255-1600
FAX: (847) 255-1605

For Medical Emergency Contact:
Customer Service
(847) 255-1600
FAX: (847) 255-1605

ACES®
Vitamin, Antioxidants

Description: ACES provides four natural antioxidant nutrients.

Two Soft Gels Contain:	% U.S. RDA
Beta-Carotene (Pro-Vitamin A) 10,000 IU	200%
Vitamin C (Calcium Ascorbate) 1,000 mg	1667%
Vitamin E (d-Alpha Tocopherol) 400 IU	1333%
Selenium (L-Selenomethionine) 100 mcg	*

RDA: Recommended Daily Allowance - Adults
*U.S. RDA not determined

The nutrients in ACES are: Beta-Carotene (Pro-vitamin A) derived from tiny sea plants or algae (D. salina) grown in the fresh ocean waters off southern Australia; Vitamin C provided as the gentle, buffered calcium ascorbate; Vitamin E 100% natural-source from soy, the most biologically active form; and Selenium, organically bound with the essential nutrient methionine to promote assimilation.

Suggested Use: For dietary supplementation, take two soft gels daily, preferably at mealtime.
CORN-Free, WHEAT-Free, MILK-Free, SUGAR-Free, YEAST-Free, PRESERVATIVE-Free, Soft Gel Contents: Nutrients listed above, soybean oil, vegetable stearin, lecithin, beeswax, Soft Gel Shell: Beef gelatin, glycerin, water, carob.

How Supplied: In bottles of 50, 90, 200, and 360.
Also available as ACES (R) plus ZINC.

E-GEMS®
Vitamins, Antioxidants

Description: 100% natural-source vitamin E (d-alpha tocopheryl acetate) soft gels. Available in 8 strengths: 30IU, 100IU, 200IU, 400IU, 600IU, 800IU, 1000IU, 1200IU.

How Supplied: Supplied in a variety of bottle sizes. Also in creams, ointments, spray, and more.

Chattem, Inc.
1715 WEST 38TH STREET
CHATTANOOGA, TN 37409

Direct Inquiries to:
Gary Galante
Vice President of Research & Development
(423) 821-4571

GOLD BOND® MEDICATED ANTI-ITCH CREAM
A Pain Relieving Anti-Itch Cream With Essential Oils

Indications: For temporary relief from the pain and itching associated with minor skin irritations, minor cuts, scrapes, minor burns, sunburn, dry skin, insect bites, or rashes due to poison ivy, oak or sumac. Also helps soothe sensitive skin.

Directions: Adults and children 2 years of age and older: Apply to affected area not more than 3 to 4 times daily. Children under 2 years of age: consult a doctor.

Warning: For external use only. Avoid contact with the eyes. If condition worsens or if symptoms persist for more than 7 days or clear up and occur again within a few days, discontinue use of this product and consult a doctor. Do not use in large quantities, particularly over raw surfaces or blistered areas. Keep out of reach of children. Do not swallow. In case of accidental ingestion, seek professional assistance or contact a Poison Control center immediately
Questions or comments? Call us toll free at 1-800-745-2429 between 9 AM and 5 PM Eastern Time.

Active Ingredients: Lidocaine Hydrochloride, Menthol.
MADE IN USA
Distributed by CHATTEM, INC., Chattanooga, TN 37409

How Supplied: NET WT. 1.0 OZ. (28 g.)

GOLD BOND®
Medicated Baby Powder

GOLD BOND® Cornstarch Plus
Medicated Baby Powder

DESCRIPTION:
GOLD BOND Medicated Baby Powder Active Ingredients: Talc and Zinc Oxide. **Also Contains:** Fragrance.
Gold Bond® Medicated Baby Powder is a blend of the finest talcum powder and zinc oxide designed to help keep skin fresh and irritation free.
GOLD BOND Cornstarch Plus Medicated Baby Powder Active Ingredients: Cornstarch, Zinc Oxide, Kaolin. Also Contains: Fragrance, Silica.
Gold Bond® Cornstarch Plus Medicated Baby Powder helps relieve diaper rash with a combination of three effective skin protecting ingredients that soothes, protects and softens baby's delicate skin, absorbs moisture and forms a protective barrier to repel moisture.

Indications:
- Helps prevent and treat diaper rash
- Protects from chafed skin and minor skin irritations due to diaper rash
- Helps protect from wetness

Warning: For external use only. If condition worsens or does not improve within 7 days, consult a doctor. Do not use on broken skin. Keep powder away from child's face to avoid inhalation, which can cause breathing problems. Avoid contact with eyes. Keep this and all other drugs out of the reach of children. In case of accidental ingestion, seek professional assistance or contact a Poison Control Center immediately.

Directions For Baby: Change wet or soiled diaper promptly, cleanse the diaper area and allow to dry. Carefully shake the powder into the diaper or hand and apply to diaper area. Apply powder

close to the body, away from child's face. Apply powder as often as necessary, with each diaper change, especially at bedtime or anytime when exposure to wet or soiled diapers may be prolonged.
Directions For Adults: Use every day to feel dry and fresh and to soothe and protect skin from chafing and minor skin irritations.

How Supplied: Net weight 4 oz. (113 g.) & 10 oz. (283 g.)
Questions or comments? Call toll-free at 1-800-745-2429.
MADE IN USA
Distributed by
CHATTEM, INC.
Chattanooga, TN 37409

GOLD BOND®
Triple Action Medicated Body Powder
Skin Protectant and Pain Relieving Powder

GOLD BOND® Extra Strength
Triple Action Medicated Body Powder
Skin Protectant and Pain Relieving Powder

Description: GOLD BOND—Active Ingredients: Menthol, Zinc Oxide.
Also Contains: Acacia, Eucalyptol, Methyl Salicylate, Salicylic Acid, Talc, Thymol, Zinc Stearate.
GOLD BOND® Extra Strength—Active Ingredients: Menthol, Zinc Oxide.
Also Contains: Acacia, Eucalyptol, Methyl Salicylate, Salicylic Acid, Talc, Thymol, Zinc Stearate.
Gold Bond® Medicated Powder is a blend of 2 medically proven ingredients, combined with the finest powder and essential oils to provide relief of the pain and itching due to:

- Minor Cuts
- Scrapes
- Burns
- Sunburn
- Prickly Heat
- Rashes
- Insect Bites
- Poison Ivy
- Poison Oak
- Poison Sumac

Great for after shower, bath or exercise–for deodorant protection and a cool, refreshing feeling. Gold Bond will leave your skin feeling soft and smooth. Also use in footwear and on feet for cool, soothing comfort. Gold Bond also helps absorb excess moisture.

Indications: For temporary relief from the pain and itching associated with minor cuts, scrapes, minor burns, sunburn, insect bites or other minor skin irritations. Helps dry up poison ivy, oak or sumac. Also helps soothe sensitive skin and helps protect against rashes and prickly heat.

Warning: For external use only. Avoid contact with eyes. Keep out of reach of children. If condition worsens or does not improve within 7 days, consult a doctor. In case of accidental ingestion, seek professional assistance or contact a Poison Control Center immediately.

Directions: Adults and children 2 years of age or older: For best results, dry skin thoroughly and apply freely up to 3 or 4 times daily.
Children under 2 years of age: Consult a doctor.

How Supplied: Net weight 4 oz. (113 g.) & 10 oz. (283 g)
Questions or comments: Call toll-free at 1-800-745-2429.
MADE IN USA
Distributed by
CHATTEM, INC.
Chattanooga, TN 37409

GOLD BOND MAXIMUM STRENGTH
Triple Action Medicated Foot Powder with Menthol

Gold Bond® Medicated Foot Powder is specially formulated for foot itch. Its unique formula of medically proven ingredients:

- Provides Maximum Strength Itch Relief
- Cools, soothes and helps protect irritated skin
- Absorbs excess moisture
- Controls foot odor and odor-causing bacteria

Active Ingredient: Menthol
Also Contains: Acacia, Benzethonium Chloride, Eucalyptus Oil, Peppermint Oil, Sodium Bicarbonate, Talc.

Indications: For temporary relief of pain and itching associated with minor skin irritations on the feet. Also formulated to cool, soothe and help protect against wetness or other foot discomforts.

Directions: Thoroughly wash and dry feet, sprinkle powder liberally over feet, between toes and on bottom of feet. For best results, apply to affected areas up to 3 or 4 times daily. Children under 2 years of age: consult a doctor.

Warning: For external use only. Avoid contact with eyes. Keep this and all drugs out of the reach of children. If condition worsens or does not improve within 7 days, consult a doctor. In case of accidental ingestion, seek professional assistance or contact a Poison Control Center immediately.

How Supplied: Net weight 4 oz. (113 g.) & 10 oz. (283 g.)
Questions or comments? Call toll-free at 1-800-745-2429.
MADE IN USA
Distributed by
CHATTEM, INC.
Chattanooga, TN 37409

HERPECIN-L® Cold Sore Lip Balm
[*her "puh-sin-el"*]

PRODUCT OVERVIEW
Key Facts: HERPECIN-L Lip Balm is a convenient, easy-to-use treatment for perioral herpes simplex infections. Sunscreens provide an SPF of 15.
Major Uses: HERPECIN-L not only treats cold sores, sun and fever blisters, but with prophylactic use, its sunscreens also protect to help prevent them. Users report early use at the prodromal stages of an attack will often abort the lesions and prevent scabbing. Prescribe: "early, often and liberally."
Safety Information: For topical use only. A rare sensitivity may occur.

PRESCRIBING INFORMATION

HERPECIN-L® Cold Sore Lip Balm

Composition: A soothing, emollient, lip balm incorporating the sunscreen, Padimate O, and allantoin, in a balanced, slightly acidic lipid base that includes petrolatum and titanium dioxide at a cosmetically acceptable level. (Does not contain any caines, phenol or camphor.)

Actions and Use: HERPECIN-L relieves dryness and chapping by providing a lipid barrier to help restore normal moisture balance to the lips. Skin protectants help to soften the crusts and scabs of "cold sores." The sunscreen is effective in 2900–3200 AU range while titanium dioxide, though at low levels, helps to block, scatter and reflect the sun's rays. Applied as a lip balm, SPF is 15. Reapply often during sun exposure.

Administration: (1) *Recurrent "cold sores, sun and fever blisters":* Simply put, use **soon and often.** Frequent sufferers report that with prophylactic use (BID/PRN), attacks are fewer and less severe. Most recurrent herpes labialis patients are aware of the prodromal symptoms: tingling, itching, burning. At this stage, or if the lesion has already developed, HERPECIN-L should be applied liberally as often as convenient—at least *every hour.* (2) *Outdoor protection:* Apply before and during sun exposure, after swimming and again at bedtime. (h.s.). (3) *Dry, chapped lips:* Apply as needed.

Adverse Reactions: If sensitive to any of the ingredients, discontinue use.

Contraindications: None.

How Supplied: 2.8 gm. swivel tubes.

Church & Dwight Co., Inc.

469 N. HARRISON STREET
PRINCETON, NJ 08543-5297

Direct Inquiries to:
Nancy Sevinsky
(609) 683-7015

For Medical Emergencies Contact:
Hazard Information Services
(800) 228-5635
Extension 7

ARM & HAMMER®
Pure Baking Soda

Active Ingredient: Sodium Bicarbonate U.S.P.

Indications: For alleviation of acid indigestion, also known as heartburn or sour stomach. Not a remedy for other types of stomach complaints such as nausea, stomachache, abdominal cramps, gas pains, or stomach distention caused by overeating and/or overdrinking. In the latter case, one should not ingest solids, liquids or antacid but rather refrain from all physical activity and—if uncomfortable—call a physician.

Actions: ARM & HAMMER® Pure Baking Soda provides fast-acting, effective neutralization of stomach acids. Each level ½ teaspoon dose will neutralize 20.9 mEq of acid.

Warnings: Except under the advice and supervision of a physician: (1) do not administer to children under five years of age, (2) do not take more than eight level ½ teaspoons per person up to 60 years old or four level ½ teaspoons per person 60 years or older in a 24-hour period, (3) do not use this product if you are on a sodium restricted diet, (4) do not use the maximum dose for more than two weeks.

Stomach Warning: To avoid serious injury, do not take until powder is completely dissolved. It is very important not to take this product when overly full from food or drink. Consult a physician if severe stomach pain occurs after taking this product.

Drug Interaction Precaution: Antacids may interact with certain prescription drugs. If you are presently taking a prescription drug, do not take this product without checking with your physician or other health professional.

Dosage and Administration: Level ½ teaspoon in ½ glass (4 fl. oz.) of water every two hours up to maximum dosage or as directed by a physician. Accurately measure level ½ teaspoon. Each level ½ teaspoon contains 20.9 mEq (.476 gm) sodium.

How Supplied: Available in 8 oz., 16 oz., 32 oz., 64 oz., and 160 oz. boxes.

Ciba Self-Medication, Inc.

For product information, please see Novartis Consumer Health, Inc.

Columbia Laboratories, Inc.

2665 SOUTH BAYSHORE DRIVE
SUITE PH2B
MIAMI, FL 33133

Direct Inquiries to:
Professional Services Department

For Medical Emergencies Contact:
(305) 860-1670

Advanced Formula
LEGATRIN PM®
[leg'a-trin]
Pain Reliever/Sleep Aid

Advanced Formula Legatrin PM® a special night-time medicine which combines extra-strength pain reliever to relieve your muscle aches and pains, with an ingredient to help you fall asleep safely.

Advanced Formula Legatrin PM® caplets are specially coated and shaped for easy swallowing.

Indications: For the occasional relief of sleeplessness and minor muscle aches and pains, such as leg cramps.

Dosage: Adults and Children 12 years of age and older: One caplet at bedtime or as directed by your physician. Do not exceed recommended dosage.

Warnings: Do not give to Children under 12 years of age or use for more than 10 days unless directed by your physician. Consult your physician if symptoms persist or new ones occur, or if fever persists for more than 3 days, or if sleeplessness persists for more than 2 weeks. Insomnia may be a symptom of serious underlying medical illness. Do not take this product if you have asthma, glaucoma, emphysema, chronic pulmonary disease, shortness of breath, difficulty in breathing or difficulty in urination due to enlargement of the prostate gland unless directed by a physician. Avoid alcoholic beverages while taking this product. Do not take if you are taking sedatives or tranquilizers without first consulting your physician. Do not use with other products containing acetaminophen.

Alcohol Warning: If you generally consume 3 or more alcohol-containing drinks per day, you should consult your physician for advice on when and how you should take Legatrin PM® and other pain relievers.

Active Ingredients (per caplet): Acetaminophen 500 mg and Diphenhydramine HCl 50 mg.

Inactive Ingredients: Dicalcium phosphate, stearic acid, microcrystalline cellulose, magnesium stearate, FD&C blue No. 2 aluminum lake, FD&C red No. 40 aluminum lake, hydroxypropyl methylcellulose, polyethylene glycol, talc, titanium dioxide.

Caution: This product will cause drowsiness. Do not drive a motor vehicle or operate machinery after use.

How Supplied: Supplied in child resistant bottles of 30 and 50 count caplets. DO NOT USE IF PRINTED OVERWRAP ON NECK OF THE BOTTLE OR PRINTED FOIL INNER SEAL IS BROKEN. KEEP THIS AND ALL MEDICATIONS OUT OF THE REACH OF CHILDREN. IN CASE OF ACCIDENTAL OVERDOSE, CONTACT A PHYSICIAN OR POISON CONTROL CENTER IMMEDIATELY. AS WITH ANY DRUG, IF YOU ARE PREGNANT OR NURSING A BABY, SEEK THE ADVICE OF A HEALTH PROFESSIONAL BEFORE USING THIS PRODUCT.
Store at room temperature.
See side panel or below for expiration date.
Distributed by:
Columbia Laboratories, Inc.
Miami, FL 33133

Shown in Product Identification Guide, page 507

Del Pharmaceuticals, Inc.

A Subsidiary of Del Laboratories, Inc.
163 E. BETHPAGE ROAD
PLAINVIEW, NY 11803

Direct Inquiries to:
Dr. Joseph A. Kanapka, Ph.D.,
Sr. VP Scientific Affairs
(516) 844-2020
FAX: (516) 293-1515

For Medical Emergencies Contact:
Serap Ozelkan, Director
Edmund Mickunas, Director
of Regulatory Affairs
1-800-952-5080

ARTHRICARE®
Pain Relieving Rubs

Description: **ArthriCare Odor Free** is perfect for daytime use anywhere. Its unique greaseless and stainless formula provides the warming pain relief of medicinal rubs without the embarrassing medicinal odor. This special formula provides temporary relief of minor aches and pains of muscles and joints associated with arthritis, simple back pain, sprains and strains. This unique formulation contains Capsicum Oleoresin (containing Capsaicin 0.025%), a strong, penetrating pain blocker not commonly found in other rubs. In addition, it has

two added fast-acting pain relievers to ease stiffness of muscles and joints.
ArthriCare Triple Medicated is specially formulated with three fast acting pain relievers. It's strong medicine that penetrates deep. You don't have to rub it in; just apply gently. ArthriCare Triple-Medicated provides temporary relief of minor aches and pains of muscles and joints associated with arthritis, simple backache, sprains and strains. Perfect for nightime use to help one sleep.
ArthriCare Ultra is a triple strength capsaicin* 0.075% formulation *plus* menthol. This fast-acting arthritis rub contains the doctor recommended ingredient, capsaicin, for the relief of minor aches and pains associated with arthritis, simple backache, sprains and strains. The product should be used 3–4 times daily for maximum effectiveness.
*as capsicum oleoresin.

Active Ingredients: ArthriCare Odor Free Menthol 1.25%, Methyl Nicotinate 0.25%, Capsicum Oleoresin (containing Capsaicin 0.025%).
ArthriCare Triple Medicated Methyl Salicylate 30%, Menthol 1.25%, Methyl Nicotinate 0.25%.
ArthriCare Ultra Menthol USP 2.0%, Capsicum Oleoresin (Containing Capsaicin 0.075%).

Inactive Ingredients: ArthriCare Odor Free Aloe Vera Gel, Carbomer 940, Cetyl Alcohol, DMDM Hydantoin, Emulsifying Wax, Glyceryl Stearate SE, Isocatyl Alcohol, Myristyl Propionate, Propylparaben, Purified Water, Stearyl Alcohol, Triethanolamine.
ArthriCare Triple Medicated Carbomer 940, Dioctyl Sodium Sulfosuccinate, FD&C Blue No. 1, Glycerin, Isopropyl Alcohol, Polysorbate 60, Propylene Gycol, Purified Water.
ArthriCare Ultra Aloe Vera Gel, Carbomer, Cetyl Alcohol, DMDM Hydantoin, Emulsifying Wax, Glyceryl Stearate SE, Isocetyl Alcohol, Myristyl Propionate, Propylparaben, Purified Water, Stearyl Alcohol.

Directions: Adults and children 2 years of age and older: Apply to affected area not more than 3 to 4 times daily. Children under 2 years of age: Consult a physician. Read package insert before using.

Warnings: For external use only. Avoid contact with the eyes. If condition worsens, or if symptoms persist for more than 7 days or clear up and occur again within a few days, discontinue use of this product and consult a physician. Do not apply to wounds or damaged skin. Do not bandage tightly. Avoid contact with mucous membranes, broken or irritated skin. Do not use with a heating pad, or immediately before or after taking a shower or bath. As part of its warming action, temporary redness may occur Keep this and all drugs out of the reach of children. In case of accidental ingestion, seek professional assistance or contact a Poison Control Center immediately. Store at room temperature 15–30 C (59–86 F).

Shown in Product Identification Guide, page 507

BABY ORAJEL®
Teething Pain Medicine

Description: Baby Orajel with fast-acting benzocaine (7.5%) relieves teething pain within one minute. It's pleasant tasting and contains no alcohol.

Active Ingredient: Benzocaine 7.5%.

Inactive Ingredients: FD&C Red No. 40, Flavor, Glycerin, Polyethylene Glycols, Purified Water, Sodium Saccharin, Sorbic Acid, Sorbitol.

Indications: For the temporary relief of sore gums due to teething in infants and children 4 months of age and older. Baby Orajel is a safe, soothing, pleasantly flavored product which helps to immediately relieve teething pain by its topical anesthetic effect on the gums.

Actions: Benzocaine is a topical, local anesthetic commonly used for pain, discomfort, or pruritis associated with wounds, mucous membranes and skin irritations.

Warnings: Do not use this product for more than 7 days unless directed by a dentist or physician. If sore mouth symptoms do not improve in 7 days; if irritation, pain or redness persists or worsens; or if swelling, rash or fever develops, see your dentist or physician promptly. Do not exceed recommended dosage. Do not use this product if you have a history of allergy to local anesthetics such as procaine, butacaine, benzocaine, or other "caine" anesthetics. Fever and nasal congestion are not symptoms of teething and may indicate the presence of infection. If these symptoms persist, consult your physician. Keep this and all drugs out of the reach of children. In case of accidental overdose or allergic reaction, seek professional assistance or contact a Poison Control Center immediately. Do not use if tube tip is cut prior to opening.

Precaution: For persistent or excessive teething pain, consult your physician.

Directions: Wash hands. Cut open tip of tube on score mark. Use your fingertip or cotton applicator to apply a small pea-size amount of Baby Orajel. Apply to affected area not more than four times daily or as directed by a dentist or physician. For infants under 4 months of age, there is no recommended dosage or treatment except under the advice and supervision of a dentist or physician.

How Supplied: Baby Orajel: Gel in 1/3 oz (9.45 g) tube.

Shown in Product Identification Guide, page 508

BABY ORAJEL® TOOTH & GUM CLEANSER

Description: Baby Orajel Tooth & Gum Cleanser is specifically designed for children under four. Safe to swallow, non-foaming, fluoride- and abrasive-free, it contains Microdent®, which helps remove plaque and fight its build-up. Available in Fruit and Peaches 'n Cream flavors.

Active Ingredients: Microdent® (Poloxamer 407 2.0%, Simethicone 0.12%).

Inactive Ingredients: Carboxymethylcellulose Sodium, Citric Acid, Flavor, Glycerin, Methylparaben, Potassium Sorbate, Propylene Glycol, Propylparaben, Purified Water, Sodium Saccharin, Sorbitol.

Indications and Actions: Baby Orajel Tooth & Gum Cleanser is the first oral cleanser specially formulated to remove the plaque-like film on babies' teeth and gums. It's fluoride-free, non-abrasive and does not foam so it's safe to swallow. It's sugar-free and has a flavor babies love. Only Baby Orajel Tooth & Gum Cleanser contains patented Microdent® to help remove plaque and fight its buildup.

Warnings: Keep out of the reach of children. Do not use if tube tip is cut prior to opening.

Dosage and Administration: Wash hands. Cut open tip of tube on score mark. Apply a small amount to baby's gums and teeth with your finger, a gauze pad or a toothbrush. Gently rub or brush the gums and teeth to remove food and plaque-like film. For best results, use in the morning and at bedtime.

How Supplied: Gel in ½ oz. (14.2g) tube. Available in assorted flavors.

Shown in Product Identification Guide, page 508

Maximum Strength ORAJEL®
[ōr 'ah-jel]
Toothache Medicine

Descriptions: Maximum Strength Orajel with 20% benzocaine provides immediate, long lasting toothache pain relief.
Orajel PM is the first nighttime toothache pain relief medicine. This long-lasting paste is formulated to stay in place for extended duration of relief.

Active Ingredient: Benzocaine 20%.

Inactive Ingredients: Flavor, Polyethylene Glycols, Sodium Saccharin, Sorbic Acid.
Orajel PM Cellulose Gum, Gelatin, Menthol, Methyl Salicylate, Pectin, Plasticized Hydrocarbon Gel, Polyethylene Glycol, Sodium Saccharin.

Indications: Maximum Strength Orajel and Orajel PM are formulated to provide fast, long lasting relief from daytime and nighttime toothache pain for hours.

Continued on next page

Del—Cont.

Actions: Benzocaine is a topical, local anesthetic commonly used for pain, discomfort, or pruritis associated with wounds, mucous membranes and skin irritation.

Warning: Keep this and all drugs out of the reach of children. Do not use if tube tip is cut prior to opening. Do not use this product if you have a history of allergy to local anesthetics such as procaine, butacaine, benzocaine or other "caine" anesthetics. In case of accidental overdose or allergic reaction, seek professional assistance or contact a Poison Control Center immediately.

Precaution: This preparation is intended for use in cases of toothache only as a temporary expedient until a dentist can be consulted. Do not use continuously.

Directions: Remove cap. Cut open tip of tube on score mark. Squeeze a small quantity of Maximum Strength Orajel directly into cavity and around gum surrounding the teeth. Firmly squeeze a one inch strip of Orajel PM onto a finger or cotton swab. Apply it to affected cavity and around the gum surrounding the teeth.

How Supplied: Gel in two sizes—3/16 oz (5.3 g) and 1/3 oz (9.45 g) tubes. Paste in 1/4 oz (7.08 g) tube.

Shown in Product Identification Guide, page 508

ORAJEL® COVERMED®
Fever Blister/Cold Sore Treatment

Description: Orajel CoverMed conceals unsightly cold sores or fever blisters for hours as it protects and relieves pain.

Active Ingredients: Dyclonine Hydrochloride 1.0%, Allantoin 0.5%.

Inactive Ingredients: Beeswax, Citric Acid, Colloidal Silicone Dioxide, Flavor, Iron Oxides, Lanolin, Petrolatum, Propylene Glycol, Purified Water, PVP/Hexadecene Copolymer, Titanium Dioxide.

Warnings: For external use only. Avoid contact with the eyes. If condition worsens, or if symptoms persist for more than 7 days or clear up and occur again within a few days, discontinue use of this product and consult a physician. Keep this and all drugs out of the reach of children. In case of accidental overdose, seek professional assistance or contact a Poison Control Center immediately. Do not use if tube tip is cut prior to opening.

Dosage and Administration: Remove cap and cut open tip of tube on score mark. Adults and children 2 years of age and older: Apply to fever blisters/cold sores not more than 3 to 4 times daily. Children under 2 years of age: consult a physician.

How Supplied: Available in 3/16 oz. (5.3g) tube.

ORAJEL® Mouth-Aid®
[ōr ′ah-jel]
Cold/Canker Sore Medicine

Description: **Orajel Mouth-Aid** is a unique triple-acting medication which provides fast relief from painful minor mouth and lip sores. It has a protective formula that stays on the sore.

Active Ingredients: Benzocaine 20%, Benzalkonium Chloride 0.02%, Zinc Chloride 0.1%.

Inactive Ingredients: Allantoin, Carbomer, Edetate Disodium, Peppermint Oil, Polyethylene Glycol, Polysorbate 60, Propyl Gallate, Propylene Glycol, Purified Water, Povidone, Sodium Saccharin, Sorbic Acid, Stearyl Alcohol.

Indications: For the temporary relief of pain associated with canker sores, cold sores, fever blisters and minor irritation or injury of the mouth and gums.

Actions: Benzocaine is a topical, local anesthetic commonly used for pain, discomfort, or pruritis associated with wounds, mucous membranes and skin irritations. Benzalkonium chloride is a rapidly acting surface disinfectant and detergent. Zinc chloride provides an astringent effect.

Warnings: Do not use this product for more than 7 days unless directed by a dentist or physician. If sore mouth symptoms do not improve in 7 days; if irritation, pain, or redness persists or worsens; or if swelling, rash or fever develops, see your dentist or physician promptly. Do not exceed recommended dosage. Do not use this product if you have a history of allergy to local anesthetics such as procaine, butacaine, benzocaine or other "caine" anesthetics. Keep this and all drugs out of the reach of children. In case of accidental overdose or allergic reaction, seek professional assistance or contact a Poison Control Center immediately. Do not use if tube tip is cut prior to opening.

Precaution: If condition persists, discontinue use and consult your physician or dentist. Not for prolonged use.

Directions: Cut open tip of tube on score mark. Adults and children 2 years and older: Apply to the affected area. Use up to 4 times daily or as directed by a dentist or physician. Children under 12 years of age should be supervised in the use of the product. Children under 2 years of age: Consult a dentist or physician.

How Supplied: Gel in 2 sizes—a 1/3 oz (9.45 g) tube and a 3/16 oz (5.3 g) tube.

Shown in Product Identification Guide, page 508

ORAJEL® PERIOSEPTIC®

Description: Orajel Perioseptic Spot Treatment Oral Cleanser and Orajel Periospetic Super Cleaning Oral Rinse are oral wound cleansers that use the debriding action of peroxide to cleanse sore mouths and gums due to denture irritation, canker sores, dental procedures, accidental injuries, and gum irritation. They both have a fresh minty taste, and can supplement your regular mouthwash routine.

Active Ingredients: Spot Treatment Oral Cleanser—Carbamide peroxide 15% (maximum strength) in anhydrous glycerin. Super Cleaning Oral Rinse—Hydrogen peroxide 1.5%.

Inactive Ingredients: Spot Treatment Oral Cleanser—Citric acid, Edetate disodium, Flavor, Methylparaben, Propylene glycol, Purified water, Sodium chloride, Sodium saccharin. Super Cleaning Oral Rinse—Edetate disodium, Ethyl alcohol (4% v/v), FD&C Blue No. 1, Methyl salicylate, Methylparaben, Phosphoric acid, Poloxamer 338, Purified water, Sodium saccharin, Sorbitol.

Indications: For temporary use in cleansing minor wounds or minor gum inflammation resulting from minor dental procedures, dentures, orthodontic appliances, accidental injury, canker sores, or other irritations of the mouth or gums.

Warning: Do not use this product for more than 7 days unless directed by a dentist or doctor. If sore mouth symptoms do not improve in 7 days; if irritation, pain, or redness persists or worsens, or if swelling, rash, or fever develops, see your dentist or doctor promptly. Cap bottle tightly. Keep away from heat and direct sunlight. Do not swallow.

Dosage and Administration: Adults and children 2 years of age and older: Apply several drops of Spot Treatment Oral Cleanser directly to the affected area of the mouth with cotton swab or applicator, or swish around Super Cleaning Oral Rinse in the mouth over the affected area. Allow the medication to remain in place at least 1 minute and then spit out. Use up to 4 times daily after meals and at bedtime or as directed by a dentist or doctor. Children under 12 years of age should be supervised in the use of this product. Children under 2 years of age: Consult a dentist or doctor.

How Supplied: Spot Treatment Oral Cleanser—0.4 fl. oz (11.8 ml) bottle with applicator and stand. Super Cleaning Oral Rinse—8 fl oz (236 ml) bottle.

Shown in Product Identification Guide, page 508

PRONTO® Lice Killing Shampoo & Conditioner in One Kit

Description: **Pronto Concentrate** Lice Killing Shampoo & Conditioner in One contains the maximum strength of pyrethrum extract and piperonyl butoxide. In laboratory testing it has been shown to be effective in killing 100% of lice and their eggs. In addition, a conditioner is included in the formulation to reduce tangles, for easy, effective comb-out of lice and eggs.

Active Ingredients: Piperonyl Butoxide 4%, Pyrethrum Extract 0.33%

Inactive Ingredients: Ammonium Laureth Sulfate, Benzyl Alcohol, BHT, Decyl Alcohol, Disodium EDTA, Fragrance, Isopropyl Alcohol, Glycerin, PEG-14M, Poloxamer 183, Purified Water

Indications: For the treatment of head, pubic (crab), and body lice.

Actions: Pronto contains the maximum strength of pyrethrum extract and piperonyl butoxide. Pyrethrum extract acts directly on the nervous system of insects and piperonyl butoxide enhances the neurotoxic effect of pyrethrum extract by inhibiting the oxidative breakdown of pyrethrum extract by the insect's detoxification system. This results in a longer amount of time which the pyrethrum extract may exert its toxic effect on the insect.

Warning: Use with caution on persons allergic to ragweed. For external use only. Do not use near the eyes or permit contact with mucous membranes, such as inside the nose, mouth, or vagina, as irritation may occur. Keep out of eyes when rinsing hair. Adults and children: Close eyes tightly and do not open eyes until product is rinsed out. Also, protect children's eyes with washcloth, towel or other suitable material, or by similar method. If product gets into the eyes, immediately flush with water. If skin irritation or infection is present or develops, discontinue use and consult a doctor. Consult a doctor if infestation of eyebrows or eyelashes occurs. Wash thoroughly with soap and water after handling. Do not exceed two applications within 24 hours.

Directions: Shake well. Apply to affected area until all the hair is thoroughly wet with product. Allow product to remain on area for 10 minutes but no longer. Add sufficient warm water to form a lather and shampoo as usual. Rinse thoroughly. A fine-toothed comb or a special lice/nit-removing comb may be used to help remove dead lice or their eggs (nits) from hair. A second treatment must be done in 7 to 10 days to kill any newly hatched lice. Handy applicator gloves are provided for your convenience in applying the shampoo to avoid contact with lice.

How Supplied: 2 fl. oz. (59 ml) and 4 fl. oz. (118 ml) plastic bottles.

Shown in Product Identification Guide, page 508

TANAC® Medicated Gel
Fever Blister/Cold Sore Treatment

Description: **Tanac Medicated Gel** treats cold sores with a unique, long lasting maximum strength pain reliever, Dyclonine Hydrochloride (1.0%). It also protects lip sores while it treats them.

Active Ingredients: Dyclonine Hydrochloride 1.0%, Allantoin 0.5%.

Inactive Ingredients: Citric Acid, Flavor, Hydroxylated Lanolin, Petrolatum, Propylene Glycol, Purified Water, PVP/Hexadecene Copolymer, Yellow Wax.

Indications: For the temporary relief of pain and itching associated with fever blisters and cold sores. Relieves dryness and softens cold sores and fever blisters.

Warnings: DO NOT USE IF TIP IS CUT PRIOR TO OPENING. For external use only. Avoid contact with the eyes. If condition worsens, or if symptoms persist for more than 7 days or clear up and occur again within a few days, discontinue use of this product and consult a physician. Keep this and all other drugs out of reach of children. In case of accidental ingestion, seek professional assistance, or contact a Poison Control Center immediately.

Dosage and Administration: Cut open tip of tube on score mark. Adults and children 2 years of age and older: Apply to fever blisters/cold sores not more than 3 to 4 times daily. Children under 2 years of age: consult a physician.

How Supplied: Available in ⅓ oz. (9.45g) plastic tube.

Shown in Product Identification Guide, page 508

TANAC® No Sting Liquid
Canker Sore Medicine

Description: **Tanac Liquid** provides fast, soothing relief from painful canker sores and gum irritations because it contains an effective anesthetic plus an antiseptic. It's alcohol-free so it doesn't sting.

Active Ingredients: Benzocaine 10%, Benzalkonium Chloride 0.12%.

Inactive Ingredients: Flavor, Polyethylene Glycol 400, Propylene Glycol, Purified Water, Sodium Saccharin, Tannic Acid.

Indications: For temporary relief of pain from mouth sores, canker sores, fever blisters and gum irritations.

Warnings: If the condition for which this preparation is used persists or if a rash or irritation develops, discontinue use and consult a physician. Use as indicated but not for more than 5 consecutive days. Not for prolonged use. Avoid getting into eyes. Do not use if you have a history of allergy to local anesthetics such as procaine, butacaine, benzocaine, or other "caine" anesthetics. KEEP THIS AND ALL DRUGS OUT OF THE REACH OF CHILDREN. In case of accidental overdose or allergic reaction, seek professional assistance or contact a Poison Control Center immediately. Do not use if imprinted bottle cap safety seal is broken or missing prior to opening.

Dosage and Administration: Apply with cotton or cotton swab to affected area not more than 3 to 4 times daily.

How Supplied: Available in 0.45 fl. oz. (13 ml) glass bottle.

Shown in Product Identification Guide, page 508

Effcon Laboratories, Inc.

P.O. BOX 7499
MARIETTA, GA 30065-1499

Address inquiries to:
Jan Sugrue
(800-722-2428)
Fax: (770-428-6811)

For Medical Emergency Contact:
J. Kent Burklow,
(800-722-2428)
Fax: (770-428-6811)

PIN-X®
Pinworm Treatment

Description: Each 1 mL of liquid for oral administration contains:

Pyrantel base .... 50 mg
(as Pyrantel Pamoate)

Indication: For the treatment of pinworms.

Warnings: Keep this and all drugs out of the reach of children. In case of accidental overdose, seek professional assistance or contact a poison control center immediately.
If you are pregnant or have liver disease, do not take this product unless directed by a doctor.

Directions for Use: Adults and children 2 years to under 12 years of age: oral dosage is a single dose of 5 milligrams of pyrantel base per pound, or 11 milligrams per kilogram, of body weight not to exceed 1 gram. Dosage information is summarized on the following dosing schedule:

Weight		Dosage (taken as a single dose)
25 to 37 lbs.	=	½ tsp.
38 to 62 lbs.	=	1 tsp.
63 to 87 lbs.	=	1½ tsp.
88 to 112 lbs.	=	2 tsp.
113 to 137 lbs.	=	2½ tsp.
138 to 162 lbs.	=	3 tsp. (1 tbsp.)
163 to 187 lbs.	=	3½ tsp.
188 lbs. & over	=	4 tsp.

SHAKE WELL BEFORE USING

How Supplied: Pin-X is supplied as a tan to yellowish, caramel-flavored sus-

Continued on next page

Effcon—Cont.

pension which contains 50 mg of pyrantel base (as pyrantel pamoate) per mL, in bottles of 30 mL (1 fl oz). NDC 55806-024-10
Store at controlled room temperature 15°–30°C (59°–86°F).
Manufactured for:
Effcon Laboratories Inc.
Marietta, GA 30065-1499
Manufactured by:
MIKART, INC.
Atlanta, GA 30318
Rev. 1/89
Code 587A00

Shown in Product Identification Guide, page 508

EnviroDerm Pharmaceuticals, Inc.

P.O. BOX 32370
LOUISVILLE, KY 40232

Direct Inquiries to:
David W. Schropfer
(502) 634-7700
FAX: (502) 634-7701

Medical Emergency Contact:
Anthony A. Schulz
(800) 991-3376, ext. 7531
FAX: (502) 634-7701

IVY BLOCK™
[*ī-vē-blok*]

Ivy Block skin protectant is a lotion which helps protect against poison ivy, poison oak, and poison sumac rash when applied BEFORE contact.

Active Ingredient: Bentoquatam 5%

Inactive Ingredients: SDA 40 denatured alcohol (25% by weight), diisopropyl adipate, bentonite, benzyl alcohol, methylparaben, purified water.

Directions: For maximum protection, avoid contact with poison ivy, oak, and sumac. Shake bottle before each use. Apply at least 15 minutes before possible contact with plants. Rub enough lotion on exposed skin to leave smooth wet film. A visible coating indicates where skin is protected. Apply every four hours for continued protection or sooner if needed to maintain coating. May be removed with soap and water.

Warnings: For external use only. Do not use on children under 6 years of age, unless directed by a doctor, if you are allergic to any ingredients, or if you already have a rash from poison ivy, poison oak, or poison sumac. Avoid contact with eyes. If contact occurs, flush with water for at least 20 minutes. Keep this and all drugs out of the reach of children. In case of accidental ingestion, seek professional assistance or contact a Poison Control Center immediately.

Flammable: Ivy Block contains alcohol. Keep away from fire or flame. Ivy Block will remain flammable until it dries on the skin. Cap bottle tightly and store at room temperature (15–30°C or 59–86°F). Keep away from heat.

How Supplied: Ivy Block lotion 4 fl. oz. (120 ml) bottle

Fleming & Company

1600 FENPARK DR.
FENTON, MO 63026

Direct Inquiries to:
Tom Fleming
(314) 343-8200
FAX (314) 343-8203

CHLOR-3
Medicinal Condiment

Active Ingredients: A troika of sodium chloride (50% 24.3 mEq/half tsp. iodized); potassium chloride (30% 11.5 mEq/half tsp.); magnesium chloride (20% 5.6 mEq/half tsp.).

Indications: The first medicinal condiment to restore needed K^+ & Mg^{++} lost during diuresis, at the expense of Na^+. To restore electrolytes lost by overcooking foods, or to add to diets that lack green vegetables, bananas, etc. And to replace conventional salting of foods in culinary and gourmet arts.

Symptoms and Treatment of Oral Overdosage: Hyperkalemia and hypermagnesemia are not end-stage results of usage.

How Supplied: In 8-oz plastic shaker, tamper-evident bottles.

IMPREGON Concentrate

Active Ingredient: Tetrachlorosalicylanilide 2%

Indications: Diaper Rash Relief, 'Staph' control, Mold inhibitor.

Actions: This is a bacteriostatic/fungistatic agent for home usage and hospital usage.

Warnings: Impregon should not be exposed to direct sunlight for long periods after applications.

Precaution: Addition of bleach prior to diaper treatment negates application effects.

Dosage and Administration: One capful (5ml) per gallon of water to impregnate diapers in the diaper pail. Dilutions for many home areas accompany the full package.

Note: For disposable-type diapers, add one teaspoonful to 8 oz of water to a 'Windex-type' sprayer. Spray middle half area of diapers until damp, and allow to dry before using, to prevent rashes.

How Supplied: Four ounce amber plastic bottles.

MAGONATE TABLETS
MAGONATE LIQUID
Magnesium Gluconate (Dihydrate)

Active Ingredients: Each tablet contains magnesium gluconate (dihydrate) 500mg (27mg of Mg^{++}). Each 5cc of Magonate Liquid contains magnesium gluconate (dihydrate) 1000mg (54mg of Mg^{++}).

Indications: For all patients in negative magnesium balance.

Precaution: Excessive dosage may cause loose stools.

Dosage and Administration: Magonate is recommended during and for three weeks after a course in chemotherapy, then monitored regularly.
Adults and children over 12 yrs.—one or two tablets or ½ to 1 teaspoon of liquid t.i.d. Under 12 yrs.—one tablet or ½ teaspoon of liquid t.i.d. Dosage may be increased in severe cases.

How Supplied: Magonate Tablets are supplied in bottles of 100 and 1000 tablets. Magonate Liquid is supplied in pints and gallons.

MARBLEN Suspension and Tablet

Composition: A modified 'Sippy Powder' antacid containing magnesium and calcium carbonates.

Action and Uses: The peach/apricot (pink) antacid suspension is sugar-free and neutralizes 18 mEq acid per teaspoonful with a low sodium content of 18mg per fl. oz. Each pink tablet consumes 18.0 mEq acid.

Administration and Dosage: One teaspoonful rather than a tablespoonful or one tablet to reduce patient cost by ⅔.

How Supplied: Plastic pints and bottles of 100 and 1000.

NEPHROX SUSPENSION
(aluminum hydroxide)
Antacid Suspension

Composition: A watermelon flavored aluminum hydroxide (320mg as gel)/mineral oil (10% by volume) antacid per teaspoonful.

Action and Uses: A sugar-free/saccharin-free pink suspension containing no magnesium and low sodium (19mg/oz). Extremely palatable and especially indicated in renal patients. Each teaspoon consumes 9 mEq acid.

Administration and Dosage: Two teaspoonfuls or as directed by a physician.

Caution: To be taken only at bedtime. Do not use at any other time or administer to infants, expectant women, and nursing mothers except upon the advice of a physician as this product contains mineral oil.

How Supplied: Plastic pints and gallons.

NICOTINEX Elixir
nicotinic acid

Composition: Contains niacin 50 mg./tsp. in a sherry wine base (amber color).

Action and Uses: Produces flushing when tablets fail. To increase micro-circulation of inner-ear in Meniere's, tinnitus and labyrinthine syndromes. For 'cold hands & feet', and as a vehicle for additives.

Administration and Dosage: One or two teaspoonsful on fasting stomach.

Side Effects: Patients should be warned of dermal flush. Ulcer and gout patients may be affected by 14% alcoholic content.

Contraindications: Severe hypotension and hemorrhage.

How Supplied: Plastic pints and gallons.

OCEAN MIST
(buffered saline)

Composition: A 0.65% special saline made isotonic by a dual preservative system and buffering excipients prevent nasal irritation.

Action and Uses: Rhinitis medicamentosa, rhinitis sicca and atrophic rhinitis. For patients 'hooked on nose drops' and glaucoma patients on diuretics having dry nasal capillaries. OCEAN may also be used as a mist or drop.

Administration and Dosage: One or two squeezes in each nostril P.R.N.

Supplied: Plastic 45cc spray bottles and pints.

PURGE
(flavored castor oil)

Composition: Contains 95% castor oil (USP) in a sweetened lemon flavored base that completely masks the odor and taste of the oil.

Indications: Preparation of the bowel for x-ray, surgery and proctological procedures, IVPs, and constipation.

Dosage: Infants—1–2 teaspoonfuls. Children—adjust between infant and adult dose. Adult—2–4 tablespoonfuls.

Precaution: Not indicated when nausea, vomiting, abdominal pain or symptoms of appendicitis occur. Pregnancy, use only on advice of physician.

Supplied: Plastic 1 oz. & 2 oz. bottles.

Gebauer Company

9410 ST. CATHERINE AVE.
CLEVELAND, OH 44104

Direct Inquiries to:
(800) 321-9348
(216) 271-5252

For Medical Information Contact:
In Emergencies:
(800) 321-9348
(216) 271-5252
After Hours and Weekend Emergencies:
Chemtrac:
(800) 424-9300

SALIVART®
[sal 'ĭ-vart]
Saliva Substitute

Description: Prompt, lasting relief of dryness of the mouth or throat (hyposalivation, xerostomia).

Contains:	**% W/W**
Sodium carboxymethylcellulose	1.000
Sorbitol	3.000
Sodium chloride	0.084
Potassium chloride	0.120
Calcium chloride, dihydrate	0.015
Magnesium chloride, hexahydrate	0.005
Potassium phosphate, dibasic	0.034
Purified water	95.742
	100.000

Propellant: Nitrogen

Indications: For reduced salivary flow, caused by medications, salivary gland infection, mouth or throat inflammation, dental or oral surgery, fever, emotional factors, and radiation therapy near the mouth or throat. Also for relieving nasal crusting and bad taste.

Actions: Moistens and lubricates the oral cavity like natural saliva to allow normal eating, swallowing, and talking. Improves adherence of dentures.

Warnings: Avoid spraying in eyes. Keep out of reach of children. Contents under pressure. Do not puncture or incinerate. Protect from direct sunlight and from heat above 50°C (120°F).

Dosage and Administration: The Salivart spray should be directed carefully into the mouth or throat, for 1 to 2 seconds, using it as often as needed to maintain moistness, or as instructed by the physician. Relief of nasal crusting has been reported following Salivart application into the nostrils.
The Salivart spray can should always be held upright, with nozzle pointed into the mouth (or applied to cotton swab for nostrils—if instructed by the physician). The nozzle should be pushed down for 1 to 2 seconds. The valve opening should be cleaned if it clogs.
Salivart is safe to swallow.

How Supplied:

75 g (2.48 fl. oz.)	NDC 0386-0009-75
30 g (1.00 fl. oz.)	NDC 0386-0009-25

Shown in Product Identification Guide, page 508

Hogil Pharmaceutical Corp.

TWO MANHATTANVILLE RD.
PURCHASE, NY 10577

Direct Inquiries to:
Tanya Costagna
(914) 696-7600
FAX: (914) 696-4600

For Medical Information Contact:
Dr. Gilbert Spector
(914) 696-7600
FAX: (914) 696-4600

A•200®
Lice Control Spray

Description: A•200 Lice Control Spray contains the synthetic pyrethroid permethrin.

Active Ingredients:

*Permethrin	0.50%
Inert Ingredients	99.50%
	100.00%

*(3-phenoxyphenyl) methyl (+/−) cis/trans 3-(2,2-dichloroethenyl) 2,2- dimethylcyclopropanecarboxylate. Cis/ trans ratio: Min. 35% (+/−) cis and max. 65% (+/−) trans.

Indications: A•200 Lice control Spray is indicated for use only on garments, bedding, furniture, carpeting, upholstery and other inanimate objects infested with lice. Also for control of fleas and ticks on dogs.

Actions: Permethrin, a highly active synthetic pyrethroid, acts on nerve cell membranes to disrupt polarization creating paralysis of the insect.

Warnings: **PRECAUTIONARY STATEMENTS: HAZARDS TO HUMANS AND DOMESTIC ANIMALS-CAUTION:** Harmful if swallowed. May be absorbed through the skin. Avoid inhalation of spray mist. Avoid contact with skin, eyes or clothing. Wash thoroughly after handling and before smoking or eating. Avoid contamination of feed and food-stuffs. Remove pets and birds and cover fish aquaria before space spraying or surface applications.
THIS PRODUCTS IS NOT FOR USE ON HUMANS. ANIMALS: Do not spray directly in/on eyes, mouth or genitalia. Do not cause exposure to puppies less than four weeks old.
Environmental Hazards: This product is toxic to fish. Do not apply directly to water.
STATEMENT OF PRACTICAL TREATMENT: IF INHALED: Remove affected person to fresh air. Apply artificial respiration if indicated.
IF IN EYES: Flush with plenty of water. Contact a physician if irritation persists.
IF ON SKIN: Wash affected areas immediately with soap and water. Get medical attention if irritation persists.
Physical or Chemical Hazards: Contents under pressure. Do not use or store

Continued on next page

Hogil Pharmaceutical—Cont.

near heat or open flame. Do not puncture or incinerate container. Exposure to temperatures above 130°F may cause bursting.

Directions For Use: It is a violation of Federal law to use this product in a manner inconsistent with its labeling. Do not use in food areas of food handling establishments, restaurants or other areas where food is commercially prepared or processed. Do not use in serving areas while food is exposed or facility is in operation. Serving areas are areas where prepared foods are served such as dining rooms but excluding areas where foods may be preapred or held. In the home, all food processing surfaces and utensils should be covered during treatment or thoroughly washed before use. Exposed food should be covered or removed. Do not use this product in or on electrical equipment due to the possibility of shock hazards.

SHAKE WELL BEFORE USING. Remove protective cap, hold container upright and spray from a distance of 12 to 15 inches. Remove birds and cover fish aquariums before spraying.

To Kill Lice and Louse Eggs: Spray in an inconspicuous area to test for possible staining or discoloration. Inspect again after drying, then proceed to spray entire area to be treated. Hold container upright with nozzle away from you. Depress valve and spray from a distance of 8 to 10 inches. Spray each square foot for three seconds.

Spray only those garments and parts of bedding, including mattresses and furniture that can not be either laundered or dry cleaned. Allow all sprayed articles to dry thoroughly before use.

Storage and Disposal: Store in a cool dry area. Do not transport or store below 32°F. Storage. Wrap container in several layers of newspaper and dispose of in trash. Do not incinerate or puncture.

How Supplied: 6 Oz. aerosol can. Also available in combination with A•200 Lice Treatment Kit.

Shown in Product Identification Guide, page 508

A•200®
LICE KILLING SHAMPOO

Description: A•200 Pediculicide, a synergized pyrethrum extract contains:

Active Ingredients:
Pyrethrum Extract 0.33%
Piperonyl Butoxide 4.0%

Other Ingredients: Benzyl Alcohol, $C_{13}C_{14}$Isoparaffin, Isopropyl Alcohol, Fragrance, Octoxynol-9, Water.

Indications: A•200 is indicated for the treatment of head and body lice.

Actions: Pyrethrum Extract disrupts nervous transmission in lice resulting in paralysis and death. Piperonyl Butoxide is a synergist that potentiates the lethal actions of pyrethrum extract by blocking detoxification of the drug by the lice. Pyrethrum extract is poorly absorbed through the skin.

Warning: Should be used with caution on persons allergic to ragweed.

Precautions: For external use only. Do not use near the eyes or permit contact with mucous membranes, such as inside the nose, mouth or vagina, as irritation may occur. Keep out of eyes when rinsing hair. Adults and children: Close eyes tightly and do not open until product is rinsed out. Also protect children's eyes with washcloth, towel or other suitable material, or by a similar method. If product gets in the eyes: immediately flush with water. If skin irritation or infection is present or develops, discontinue use and consult a physician. Consult a physician if infestation of eyebrows or eye-lashes occurs. In case of accidental ingestion, seek professional assistance or call a poison control center. If pregnant or nursing a baby, seek advice from a health professional before using this product.

Storage and Disposal: Do not contaminate water, food or feed by storage or disposal. Do not reuse container. Wrap and put in trash collection. Do not transport or store below 32°F (0°C).

Directions for Use: Important—Read Warnings Before Using. Shake well before using. Apply to the affected area until all the hair is thoroughly wet with product. Allow product to remain on the area for 10 minutes but no longer. Then add sufficient warm water to form a lather and shampoo as usual. Rinse thoroughly. Use the special A•200 Lice/Nit comb supplied to help remove the dead lice and their eggs(nits) from the hair. A second treatment must be done in 7 to 10 days to kill any newly hatched lice.

How Supplied: In 2 and 4 oz. unbreakable plastic bottles. A special patented A•200 Lice/Nit Comb for lice and egg (nit) removal and a patient insert in both English and Spanish are included.

Shown in Product Identification Guide, page 508

INNOGel PLUS®
Pubic (Crab) Lice Treatment Gel

Description: Active Ingredients:
Pyrethrum Extract 0.30%
Piperonyl Butoxide 3.0%

Other Ingredients: Benzyl Alcohol, Carbomer 934, D&C Red #33, FD&C Blue #1, Isopropyl Alcohol, Octoxynol-9, Trolamine, Water.

Indications: InnoGel Plus is indicated for the treatment of pubic(crab) and body lice.

Actions: Pyrethrum extract disrupts nervous transmission in lice resulting in paralysis and death. Piperonyl Butoxide is a synergist that potentiates the lethal actions of pyrethum extract by blocking detoxification of the drug by the lice. Pyrethrum extract is poorly absorbed through the skin.

Warning: Should be used with caution on persons allergic to ragweed.

Precautions: For external use only. Do not use near the eyes or permit contact with mucous membranes, such as inside the nose, mouth or vagina, as irritation may occur. Keep out of eyes when rinsing hair. Adults and children: Close eyes tightly and do not open until product is rinsed out. Also protect children's eyes with washcloth, towel or other suitable material, or by a similar method. If product gets in the eyes: immediately flush with water. If skin irritation or infection is present or develops, discontinue use and consult a physician. Consult a physician if infestation of eyebrows or eyelashes occurs. In case of accidental ingestion, seek professional assistance or call a poison control center. If pregnant or nursing a baby, seek advice from a health professional before using this product.

Directions for Use: Apply InnoGel Plus to affected area until hair is thoroughly covered with product. Allow product to remain on the area for 10 minutes but no longer. Wash area thoroughly with warm water and soap or shampoo. Use the special InnoGel Plus Lice/Nit Comb supplied to remove dead lice and their eggs(nits) from the hair. A second treatment must be done in 7 to 10 days to kill any newly hatched lice.

How Supplied: Consumer package containing 3-4 gram pre-dosed gel packettes and a special InnoGel Lice/Nit Comb and a patient insert (English/Spanish).

Shown in Product Identification Guide, page 508

SINE-OFF®
No Drowsiness Formula
Caplets
Nasal Decongestant/Pain Reliever
Contains No Antihistamines

Relieves sinus headache, pain, pressure & congestion.

Indications: For temporary relief of sinus and headache pain and nasal congestion associated with sinusitis or due to a cold, hay fever or other upper respiratory allergies (allergic rhinitis). Temporarily restores freer breathing through the nose. Helps decongest sinus openings and passages; temporarily relieves sinus congestion and pressure.

Directions: Adults and children 12 years and older: 2 caplets every 6 hours, not to exceed 8 caplets in 24 hours, or as directed by a doctor. Children under 12 years of age: Consult a doctor.

Warnings: Do not take this product for more than 10 days. If symptoms do not improve or are accompanied by fever that lasts for more than 3 days, or if new symptoms occur, consult a doctor. Do not take this product if you have heart disease, high blood pressure, thyroid disease, diabetes, or difficulty in urination due to enlargement of the prostate gland unless directed by a doctor. **Do not exceed recommended dosage.** If nervousness, dizziness, or sleeplessness occur, discontinue use and consult a doctor. **KEEP THIS AND ALL DRUGS OUT OF THE REACH OF CHILDREN.** In case of accidental overdose, see professional assistance or contact a Poison Control Center immediately. Prompt medical attention is critical for adults as well as for children even if you do not notice any signs or symptoms. As with any drug, if you are pregnant or nursing a baby, seek the advice of a health professional before using this product.

Drug Interaction Precaution: Do not use this product if you are now taking a prescription monoamine oxidase inhibitor (MAOI) (certain drugs for depression, psychiatric or emotional conditions, or Parkinson's disease), or for 2 weeks after stopping the MAOI drug. If you are uncertain whether your prescription drug contains an MAOI, consult a health professional before taking this product.

Active Ingredients: Each caplet contains: Acetaminophen 500 mg. and Pseudoephedrine Hydrochloride 30 mg.

Inactive Ingredients: Crospovidone, FD&C Red 40, Hydroxypropyl Methylcellulose, Magnesium Stearate, Microcrystalline Cellulose, Polyethylene Glycol, Polysorbate 80, Povidone, Starch and Titanium Dioxide.

Tamper-Evident Package Features For Your Protection:

- Each caplet is encased in a clear plastic cell with a printed foil back.
- The name SINE-OFF appears on each caplet (see product illustration on front of carton).
- DO NOT USE THIS PRODUCT IF ANY OF THESE TAMPER-EVIDENT FEATURES ARE MISSING OR BROKEN.

Avoid storing at high temperature (greater than 100°F).

RETAIN OUTER CARTON FOR COMPLETE DIRECTIONS AND WARNINGS.

Distributed By: Hogil Pharmaceutical Corporation
Purchase, New York 10557-2118
Made in U.S.A.

Shown in Product Identification Guide, page 508

SINE–OFF®
SINUS MEDICINE
Nasal Decongestant/Pain Reliever/ Antihistamine

Relieves sinus headache, pain, pressure, congestion, runny nose, sneezing & itchy, watery eyes.

Each Caplet Contains These Active Ingredients:

Nasal Decongestant (Pseudoephedrine HCl 30 mg)

Analgesic/Antipyretic (Acetaminophen 500 mg)

Antihistamine (Chlorpheniramine Maleate 2 mg)

For the Temporary Relief of the Following Symptoms:
Sinus and nasal congestion
Sinus headache and pain
Runny nose and sneezing associated with the common cold and hay fever

Inactive Ingredients: Camauba Wax, Croscarmellose Sodium, D&C Yellow #10 Al. Lake, FD&C Yellow #6 Al. Lake, Hydrogenated Vegetable Oil, Hydroxypropyl Cellulose, Hydroxypropyl Methylcellulose, Magnesium Stearate, Microcrystalline Cellulose, Polyethylene Glycol, Pregelatinized Starch, Silicon Dioxide, Titanium Dioxide.

Directions: Adults and children 12 or more years of age - 2 caplets every 6 hours, not to exceed 8 caplets in any 24 hour period, or as directed by a doctor. Children under 12 years - consult a doctor.

Warnings: Do not take this product for pain for more than 10 days. If symptoms do not improve or are accompanied by fever that lasts for more than 3 days, or if new symptoms occur, consult a doctor. Do not exceed recommended dosage because at higher doses nervousness, dizziness, or sleeplessness may occur. Do not take this product if you have heart disease, high blood pressure, thyroid disease, diabetes, asthma, glaucoma, emphysema, chronic pulmonary disease, shortness of breath, difficulty in breathing, or difficulty in urination due to enlargement of the prostate gland unless directed by a doctor. May cause excitability especially in children. May cause drowsiness; alcohol, sedatives and tranquilizers may increase the drowsiness effect. Avoid alcoholic beverages while taking this product. Do not take this product if you are taking sedatives or tranquilizers, without first consulting your doctor. Use caution when driving a motor vehicle or operating machinery. As with any drug, if you are pregnant or nursing a baby, seek the advice of a health professional before using this product.

Drug Interaction Precaution: Do not use this product if you are now taking a prescription monoamine oxidase inhibitor (MAOI) (certain drugs for depression, psychiatric or emotional conditions, or Parkinson's disease), or for 2 weeks after stopping the MAOI drug. If you are uncertain whether your prescription drug contains an MAOI, consult a health professional before taking this product.

Keep this and all drugs out of the reach of children! In case of accidental overdose, seek professional assistance or contact a poison control center immediately!

KEEP IN A DRY PLACE.
DO NOT EXPOSE TO EXCESSIVE HEAT.

Distributed by:
Hogil Pharmaceutical Corporation
Purchase, New York 10557-2118
Made in U.S.A.

Shown in Product Identification Guide, page 508

SINE-OFF® Night Time Formula
SINUS, COLD & FLU MEDICINE
Nasal Decongestant • Antihistamine • Pain Reliever • Fever Reducer

Relieves sinus headache, pain, pressure, congestion, runny nose, sneezing & itchy, watery eyes.

Each Caplet Contains These Active Ingredients:
Analgesic (Acetaminophen 500 mg)
Antihistamine (Diphenhydramine HCL 25 mg)
Nasal Decongestant (Pseudoephedrine HCL 30 mg)

For The Temporary Relief Of The Following Symptoms:
Headache, sore throat, fever and muscular aches and pains
Runny nose, and sneezing associated with the common cold, flu or hay fever
Sinus and nasal congestion

Inactive Ingredients: Croscamellose Sodium. D&C Red #28, FD&C Blue #1, FD&C Yellow #6, Gellatin, Hydroxypropyl Methylcellulose, Polysorbate 80, Silicon Dioxide, Sodium Lauryl Sulfate, Stearic Acid, Titanum Dioxide.

Directions: Adults and children 12 or more years of age 2 gelatin caplets at bedtime. May repeat every 6 hours. Do not exceed 8 gelatin caplets in 24 hours, or as directed by a doctor. Children under 12 years. Consult a doctor.

Warnings: Do not take this product for pain for more than 10 days. If symptoms do not improve or are accompanied by fever that lasts for more than 3 days or if new symptoms occur, consult a doctor. If sore throat is severe, persists for more than 2 days, is accompanied or followed by fever, headache, rash, nausea, or vomiting, consult a doctor promptly. Do not exceed recommended dosage because at higher doses nervousness, dizziness, or sleeplessness may occur. Do not take this product if you have heart disease, high blood pressure, thyroid disease, diabetes, or if you have a breathing problem such as emphysema or chronic bronchitis, or if you have glaucoma, or difficulty in urination due to enlargement of the prostate gland. May cause excitability especially in children. May cause marked drowsiness; alcohol, sedatives and tranquilizers may increase the drowsiness effect. Avoid alcoholic beverages while taking this product. Do not take this product if you are taking sedatives or tranquilizers without first consulting your doctor. Use caution when driving a motor vehicle or operating machinery. As with any drug, if you are pregnant or nursing a baby, seek the advise of a

Continued on next page

Hogil Pharmaceutical—Cont.

health professional before using this product.

Drug Interaction Precaution: Do not use this product if you are now taking a prescription monoamine oxidase inhibitor (MAOI) (certain drugs for depression, psychiatric or emotional conditions, or parkinson's disease) or for 2 weeks after stopping the MAOI drug. If you are uncertain whether your prescription drug contains an MAOI, consult your health professional before taking this product.

Keep this and all drugs out of the reach of children. In case of accidental overdose, seek professional assistance or contact a poison control center immediately. Prompt medical attention is critical for adults as well as for children even if you do not notice any signs or symptoms.

KEEP IN A DRY PLACE

DO NOT EXPOSE TO EXCESSIVE HEAT

Made in U.S.A.

Distributed by:

HOGIL **PHARMACEUTICAL CORP.**

Purchase, NY 10557/Made in U.S.A.

Shown in Product Identification Guide, page 508

TELDRIN®
12 HR. ALLERGY RELIEF CAPSULES
Timed-Release Antiistamine/Nasal Decongestant
(Chlorpheniramine Maleate Phenylpropanolamine Hydrochloride)

Relieves runny nose, sneezing, itchy, watery eyes, and sinus & nasal congestion.

Product Benefits: Hay fever and allergies may be commonly caused by such things as pollen, dust, and dander. TELDRIN provides up to 12 hours of relief from hay fever and allergy symptoms, plus relieves sinus and nasal congestion. TELDRIN is formulated to release some medication initially and the rest gradually over a prolonged period.

Indications: Temporarily relieves runny nose and reduces sneezing, itching of the nose or throat, and itchy watery eyes due to hay fever or other upper respiratory allergies. Also temporarily relieves nasal congestion due to the common cold, hay fever, or associated with sinusitis.

Directions: Adults and children over 12 years of age: One capsule every 12 hours, not to exceed 2 capsules in 24 hours, or as directed by a doctor. Children under 12 years of age: Consult a doctor.

This carton is protected by a clear overwrap printed with "safety sealed"; do not use if overwrap is missing or broken.

Tamper-Evident Package Features For Your Protection:

- Each capsule is encased in a plastic cell with a foil back; do not use if cell or foil is broken.
- Each capsule is protected by a red Perma-Seal™ band which bonds the two capsule halves together; do not use if capsule or band is broken.

Warnings: Do not exceed recommended dosage. If nervousness, dizziness, or sleeplessness occur, discontinue use and consult a doctor. If symptoms do not improve within 7 days or are accompanied by fever, consult a doctor. Do not take this product, unless directed by a doctor, if you have a breathing problem such as emphysema or chronic bronchitis, or if you have heart disease, high blood pressure, thyroid diabetes, glaucoma, or difficulty in urination due to enlargement of the prostate gland. Do not take this product if you are taking another medication containing phenylpropanolamine. May cause excitability especially in children. May cause drowsiness; alcohol, sedatives, and tranquilizers may increase the drowsiness effect. Avoid alcoholic beverages while taking this product. Do not take this product if you are taking sedatives or tranquilizers, without first consulting your doctor. Use caution when driving a motor vehicle or operating machinery. **KEEP THIS AND ALL DRUGS OUT OF THE REACH OF CHILDREN.** In case of accidental overdose, seek professional assistance or contact a Poison Control Center immediately. As with any drug, if you are pregnant or nursing a baby, seek the advice of a health professional before using this product.

Drug Interaction Precaution: Do not use this product if you are now taking a prescription monoamine oxidase inhibitor (MAOI) (certain drugs for depression, psychiatric or emotional conditions, or Parkinson's disease), or for 2 weeks after stopping the MAOI drug. If you are uncertain whether your prescription drug contains an MAOI, consult a health professional before taking this product.

Store in a dry place at controlled room temperature: 15°–30°C (59°–86°F).

Each Capsule Contains: Active Ingredients: Chlorpheniramine Maleate 8 mg. and Phenylpropanolamine Hydrochloride 75 mg.

Inactive Ingredients: Benzyl Alcohol, Butylparaben, D&C Red No. 33, Edetate Calcium Disodium, FD&C Red No. 3, FD&C Yellow No. 6, Gelatin, Methylparaben, Pharmaceutical Glaze, Propylparaben, Sodium Lauryl Sulfate, Sodium Propionate, Starch, Sucrose, and other ingredients. May also contain Polysorbate 80.

RETAIN OUTER CARTON FOR COMPLETE DIRECTIONS AND WARNINGS.

Distributed by:

Hogil Pharmaceutical Corporation

Purchase, New York 10557-2118

Shown in Product Identification Guide, page 508

EDUCATIONAL MATERIAL

The Contemporary Approach to the Control of Head Lice in Schools and communities. (A comprehensive training Manual for health Professionals)

Head Lice: Differential Diagnosis Cards

Inter-Cal Corporation
533 MADISON AVENUE
PRESCOTT, AZ 86301

Direct Inquiries to:

Dr. Jack Hegenauer: (520) 445-8063

FAX: (520) 778-7986

For Medical Emergency Contact:

Dr. Jack Hegenauer: (520) 445-8063

FAX: (520) 778-7986

ESTER-C®
(Calcium Ascorbate with C Metabolites)

Description: Each Ester-C® tablet, caplet, or capsule contains 500 mg vitamin C in the form of calcium ascorbate. Tablets and caplets may also contain vegetable-derived cellulose as an excipient. Ester-C® calcium ascorbate contains no preservatives, sugars, artificial colorings, or flavorings. The primary constituent of Ester-C® is calcium ascorbate, the calcium salt of L-ascorbic acid, having an empirical formula of $CaC_{12}H_{14}O_{12}$. The water-based neutralization process used to prepare the patented Ester-C® complex yields natural C metabolites, including the calcium salt of threonic acid.

Actions: Vitamin C is essential for the prevention of scurvy. In humans, an exogenous source of the vitamin is required for collagen formation and tissue repair. The C metabolites (e.g., threonic acid) aid in the transport of vitamin C by the cells. Biochemically, vitamin C serves as a reducing agent in many important hydroxylation reactions in the body. The vitamin participates in collagen cross-linking and synthesis; synthesis of adrenal hormones and vasoactive amines; microsomal drug metabolism; carnitine synthesis; iron metabolism; folate metabolism; leukocyte activity and resistance to infection; and wound healing.

Indications and Usage: Vitamin C and its salts, such as calcium ascorbate, are recommended as nutritional supplements in the prevention of scurvy. Ascorbate deficiency results in impaired collagen formation, leading to defective bone formation, poor wound healing, and rupture of capillaries. Symptoms of mild deficiency may include faulty development of bones, bleeding gums, gingivitis, and loose teeth. An increased need for the vitamin exists in inflammatory or febrile states, diabetes, chronic illness, and infection. An increased daily intake of ascorbate is indicated in trauma, burns, physical stress, delayed healing of bone fractures and wounds, hemovascular disorders, and capillary fragility. Vitamin C requirements are increased for smokers.

Contraindications: Because of its calcium content, Ester-C® is contraindicated in hypercalcemic states, e.g., from dosing with parathyroid hormone, overdosage of vitamin D, or dysfunctional calcium metabolism. High-dose supplementation with vitamin C is contraindicated in individuals predisposed to form urinary calcium oxalate stones.

Adverse Reactions: No adverse reactions following ingestion of Ester-C® are known. Gastric disturbances characteristic of large doses of ascorbic acid are absent or greatly diminished when the nonacidic form of calcium ascorbate present in Ester-C® is utilized as the source of vitamin C supplementation.

Dosage and Administration: The U.S. Recommended Dietary Allowance (RDA) for vitamin C to prevent scurvy is 60 mg per day. The RDA for smokers is 100 mg per day. Optimum daily allowances for the maintenance of cellular and body reserves are significantly greater. For adults, doses in excess of 200 mg per day are required to saturate blood cells and plasma. Supplementation with doses of 1-10 grams of vitamin C (e.g., 2-20 Ester-C® tablets, caplets, or capsules) is common in the U.S. and is considered to be a safe practice.

How Supplied: Tablets, caplets, or capsules of Ester-C® (equal to 500 mg of vitamin C) in 100 or 250 count bottles. The Inter-Cal Corporation manufactures Ester-C® ascorbates as powdered raw materials. Many distributors supply Ester-C® in varying potencies, formulations, and packages. Also available as magnesium, potassium, sodium and zinc salts. Store at room temperature.

U.S. Patent No. 4,822,816, granted April 18, 1989.

Literature revised: 2 October 1996.
Mfd. by Inter-Cal Corp.
Prescott, AZ 86301

IYATA Pharmaceutical, Inc.

735 NORTH WATER STREET
SUITE 612
MILWAUKEE, WI 53202

Direct Inquiries to:
Michael B. Adekunle, M.D.:
(414) 272-1982
FAX: (414) 272-2919

For Medical Emergency Contact:
(414) 272-1982
(800) 809-7918
FAX: (414) 272-2919

CAPSAGEL®

Product Information: Capsagel® contains natural purified capsaicin in a patented gel formulation developed by doctors.

Indications: For the temporary relief of minor aches and pains associated with Arthritis, Joint aches, Backaches, Sprains, Strains, Bruises, Bursitis, Tendinitis, Athralgias and Neuralgia.

Warnings: For external use only. Keep this and all medicines out of the reach of children. Avoid contact with eyes and mucous membranes. Do not apply to open or damaged skin. Do not bandage tightly. If condition worsens or if symptoms persist for more than seven days, or clear up and occur again within a few days, discontinue use and consult a doctor. If pregnant, consult your physician before using this product.

Directions: For adults and children over the age of two years. Apply a 1/8 inch dab (about the size of a pea) to the affected area and massage until the gel is completely absorbed into the skin. Wash hands thoroughly with soap and water after each application. Capsagel® may be applied three to four times daily, as needed.

Inactive Ingredients: Carbopol 1382, Neutrol TE, Polysorbate 20, Uvinol MS 40, Germall II, Disodium EDTA USP, Ethyl alcohol SDA 40, Ion exchanged or Distilled water q. ed.

How Supplied: Capsagel is available in 3 strengths: .025%, .05% and .075% natural purified capsaicin in a unique patented gel formula.
U.S. patents: 6,178,879; 5,296,225 and 5,431,914
Distributed by IYATA Pharmaceutical Inc. Capsagel® is a registered trademark of IYATA Pharmaceutical Inc., Milwaukee, WI 53202 Made in U.S.A.

Johnson & Johnson • MERCK

Consumer Pharmaceuticals Co.
CAMP HILL ROAD
FORT WASHINGTON, PA 19034

Direct Inquiries to:
Consumer Affairs Department
Fort Washington, PA 19034
(215) 233-7000
For Medical Information Contact:
In Emergencies:
(215) 233-7000

ALternaGEL™
[al-tern 'a-jel]
Liquid
High-Potency Aluminum Hydroxide Antacid

Description: ALternaGEL is available as a white, pleasant-tasting, high-potency aluminum hydroxide liquid antacid.

Ingredients: Each 5 mL teaspoonful contains: Active: 600 mg aluminum hydroxide (equivalent to dried gel, USP) providing 16 milliequivalents (mEq) of acid-neutralizing capacity (ANC), and less than 2.5 mg (0.109 mEq) of sodium and no sugar. Inactive: butylparaben, flavors, propylparaben, purified water, simethicone, and other ingredients.

Indications: ALternaGEL is indicated for the symptomatic relief of hyperacidity associated with peptic ulcer, gastritis, peptic esophagitis, gastric hyperacidity, hiatal hernia, and heartburn.
ALternaGEL will be of special value to those patients for whom magnesium-containing antacids are undesirable, such as patients with renal insufficiency, patients requiring control of attendant GI complications resulting from steroid or other drug therapy, and patients experiencing the laxation which may result from magnesium or combination antacid regimens.

Directions: One to two teaspoonfuls, as needed, between meals and at bedtime, or as directed by a physician: May be followed by a sip of water if desired. Concentrated product. Shake well before using. Keep tightly closed.

Warnings: Keep this and all drugs out of the reach of children. ALternaGEL may cause constipation.
Except under the advice and supervision of a physician: do not take more than 18 teaspoonfuls in a 24-hour period, or use the maximum dose of ALternaGEL for more than two weeks. ALternaGEL may cause constipation.
Prolonged use of aluminum-containing antacids in patients with renal failure may result in or worsen dialysis osteomalacia. Elevated tissue aluminum levels contribute to the development of the dialysis encephalopathy and osteomalacia syndromes. Small amounts of aluminum are absorbed from the gastrointestinal tract and renal excretion of aluminum is impaired in renal failure. Aluminum is not well removed by dialysis because it is bound to albumin and transferrin, which do not cross dialysis membranes. As a result, aluminum is deposited in bone, and dialysis osteomalacia may develop when large amounts of aluminum are ingested orally by patients with impaired renal function.
Aluminum forms insoluble complexes with phosphate in the gastrointestinal tract, thus decreasing phosphate absorption. Prolonged use of aluminum-containing antacids by normophosphatemic patients may result in hypophosphatemia if phosphate intake is not adequate. In its more severe forms, hypophosphatemia can lead to anorexia, malaise, muscle weakness, and osteomalacia.

Drug Interaction Precaution: Antacids may interact with certain prescription drugs. If you are presently taking a prescription drug, do not take this product without checking with your physician or other health professional.

How Supplied: ALternaGEL is available in bottles of 12 fluid ounces and 1 fluid ounce hospital unit doses. NDC 16837-860.

Shown in Product Identification Guide, page 508

Continued on next page

J&J • Merck—Cont.

DIALOSE® Tablets
[di 'a-lose]
Stool Softener Laxative

Description: DIALOSE is a very low sodium, nonhabit forming, stool softener containing 100 mg docusate sodium per tablet.
The docusate in DIALOSE is a highly efficient surfactant which facilitates absorption of water by the stool to form a soft, easily evacuated mass. Unlike stimulant laxatives, DIALOSE does not interfere with normal peristalsis, neither does it cause griping nor sensations of urgency.

Ingredients: Active: Docusate Sodium, 100 mg per tablet
Inactive: Colloidal Silicone Dioxide, Dextrates, Flavors, Hydroxypropyl Methylcellulose, Magnesium Stearate, Microcrystalline Cellulose, Polyethylene Glycol, Polysorbate 80, Pregelatinized Starch, Propylene Glycol, Sodium Starch Glycolate, Titanium Dioxide, D&C Red No. 28, D&C Red No. 27 Aluminum Lake, FD&C Blue No. 1, FD&C Blue No. 1 Aluminum Lake, FD&C Red No. 40.

Indications: DIALOSE is indicated for the relief of occasional constipation (irregularity).
DIALOSE is an effective aid to soften or prevent formation of hard stools in a wide range of conditions that may lead to constipation. DIALOSE helps to eliminate straining associated with obstetric, geriatric, cardiac, surgical, anorectal, or proctologic conditions. In cases of mild constipation, the fecal softening action of DIALOSE can prevent constipation from progressing and relieve painful defecation.

Directions: *Adults:* One tablet, one to three times daily; adjust dosage as needed.
Children 6 to under 12 years: One tablet daily as needed.
Children under 6 years: As directed by physician.
It is helpful to increase the daily intake of fluids by taking a glass of water with each dose.

Warnings: Unless directed by a physician: Do not use when abdominal pain, nausea, or vomiting are present. Do not use for a period longer than one week. Do not take this product if you are presently taking a prescription drug or mineral oil. As with any drug, if you are pregnant or nursing a baby, seek the advice of a health professional before using this product. Keep out of the reach of children.

How Supplied: Bottles of 100 pink tablets. Also available in 100 tablet unit dose boxes (10 strips of 10 tablets each). NDC-16837-870.

Shown in Product Identification Guide, page 509

DIALOSE® PLUS Tablets
[di 'a-lose Plus]
Stool Softener/Stimulant Laxative

Description: DIALOSE PLUS provides a very low sodium tablet formulation of 100 mg docusate sodium and 65 mg yellow phenolphthalein.

Ingredients: Each tablet contains: Actives: Docusate Sodium, 100 mg., yellow phenolphthalein, 65 mg.
Inactive: Dextrates, Dibasic Calcium Phosphate Dihydrate, Flavors, Hydroxypropyl Methylcellulose, Magnesium Stearate, Microcrystalline Cellulose, Polydextrose, Polythylene Glycol, Polysorbate 80, Propylene Glycol, Sodium Starch Glycolate, Titanium Dioxide, Triacetin, D&C Yellow NO. 10 Aluminum Lake, D&C Red NO. 28, FD&C Blue NO. 1, FD&C Red NO. 40, FD&C Red NO. 40 Aluminum Lake.

Indications: DIALOSE PLUS is indicated for the treatment of constipation characterized by lack of moisture in the intestinal contents, resulting in hardness of stool and decreased intestinal motility. DIALOSE PLUS combines the advantages of the stool softener, docusate sodium, with the peristaltic activating effect of yellow phenolphthalein.

Directions: *Adults:* One or two tablets daily as needed, at bedtime or on arising
Children 6 to under 12 years: One tablet daily as needed
Children under 6 years: As directed by physician.
It is helpful to increase the daily intake of fluids by taking a glass of water with each dose.

Warnings: Unless directed by a physician: Do not use when abdominal pain, nausea, or vomiting are present. Do not use for a period longer than one week. If skin rash appears do not use this product or any other preparation containing phenolphthalein. Frequent or prolonged use may result in dependence on laxatives. Do not take this product if you are presently taking a prescription drug or mineral oil.
As with any drug, if you are pregnant or nursing a baby, seek the advice of a health professional before using this Keep out of the reach of children.

How Supplied: Bottles of 100 yellow tablets. Also available in 100 tablet unit dose boxes (10 strips of 10 tablets each). NDC 16837-871.

Shown in Product Identification Guide, page 509

INFANTS' MYLICON® Drops
[my 'li-con]
Antiflatulent

Ingredients: Each 0.6 mL of drops contains: Active: simethicone, 40 mg. Inactive: carbomer 934P, citric acid, flavors, hydroxypropyl methylcellulose, purified water, Red 3, saccharin calcium, sodium benzoate, sodium citrate.

Indications: For relief of the symptoms of excess gas in the digestive tract. Such gas is frequently caused by excessive swallowing of air or by eating foods that disagree. The defoaming action of INFANTS' MYLICON® Drops relieves flatulence by dispersing and preventing the formation of mucus-surrounded gas pockets in the gastrointestinal tract. INFANTS' MYLICON® Drops act in the stomach and intestines to change the surface tension of gas bubbles enabling them to coalesce, thereby freeing and eliminating the gas more easily by belching or passing flatus.

Directions: Infants (under 2 years): 0.3 ml four times daily after meals and at bedtime, or as directed by a physician. The dosage can also be mixed with 1 oz of cool water, infant formula or other suitable liquids to ease administration.
Adults and children: 0.6 ml four times daily, after meals and at bedtime, or as directed by a physician.

Warnings: Do not exceed 12 doses per day except under the advice and supervision of a physician. Keep this and all drugs out of the reach of chldren.

How Supplied: INFANTS' MYLICON® Drops are available in bottles of 15 ml (0.5 fl oz) and 30 ml (1.0 fl oz) pink, pleasant tasting liquid. NDC 16837-630.

Shown in Product Identification Guide, page 509

CHILDREN'S MYLANTA UPSET STOMACH RELIEF CALCIUM CARBONATE/ANTACID LIQUID AND TABLETS

Description: Children's Mylanta is a specially formulated antacid to quickly and effectively relieve the upset stomach kids sometime experience.

Active Ingredient: Each tablet or 5 ml teaspoonful contains 400 mg of calcium carbonate.

Inactive Ingredients: Tablets: Citric acid, confectioner's sugar, D&C Red #27 (Bubble Gum and Fruit Punch), D&C Yellow #10 (Fruit Punch), flavors, magnesium stearate, sorbitol, starch.
Liquid: Butylparaben, cellulose, flavor propylparaben, purified water, D&C Red #22, D&C Red #28, simethicone, sodium saccharin, sorbitol, xanthan gum, may contain tartaric acid.

Acid Neutralizing Capacity:

Tablet	Liquid
8 mEq	8 mEq

Indications: For the relief of acid indigestion, sour stomach, or heartburn and upset stomach associated with these conditions, or overindulgence in food and drink.

Directions: Find the right dose on the chart below. If possible use weight as your dosing guide; otherwise use age. Repeat dosing as needed. DO NOT USE MORE THAN THREE TIMES PER DAY.

WEIGHT (LB)	AGE (YR)	TABLET	LIQUID (TSP)
Under 24	Under 2	Consult Physician	
24–47	2–5	1	1
48–95	6–11	2	2

Warnings: Keep this and all drugs out of the reach of children. Do not take more than 3 tablets or 3 teaspoonfuls (2–5 years) or 6 tablets or 6 teaspoonfuls (6–11 years) in a 24-hour period, or use the maximum dosage of this product for more than two weeks, except under the advice and supervision of a physician.

Drug Interaction Precaution: Antacids may interact with certain prescription drugs. If your child is presently taking a prescription drug, do not give this product without checking with your physician or other health professional.

How Supplied: Children's Mylanta Upset Stomach Relief is supplied as a liquid and chewable tablets in bubble gum and fruit punch flavors.

NDC 16837-810 Bubble Gum tablets
NDC 16837-811 Fruit Punch tablets
NDC 16837-820 Bubble Gum liquid
NDC 16837-821 Fruit Punch liquid

Shown in Product Identification Guide, page 509

FAST-ACTING MYLANTA® AND MAXIMUM-STRENGTH FAST-ACTING MYLANTA®

[*my-lan'ta*]

Aluminum, Magnesium and Simethicone Liquid Antacid/Anti-Gas

Description: Fast-acting MYLANTA® and Maximum Strength Fast-Acting MYLANTA® are well-balanced, pleasant-tasting, antacid/anti-gas medications that provide consistent, effective relief of symptoms associated with gastric hyperacidity and excess gas. Non-constipating and very low sodium Fast-Acting MYLANTA® and Maximum Strength Fast-Acting MYLANTA® contain two proven antacids, aluminum hydroxide and magnesium hydroxide, plus simethicone for gas relief.

Active Ingredients: Each 5 mL teaspoon contains:

	MYLANTA®	MYLANTA® Double Strength
Aluminum Hydroxide	200 mg	400 mg
Magnesium Hydroxide	200 mg	400 mg
Simethicone	20 mg	40 mg

Inactive Ingredients: LIQUIDS: Butylparaben, carboxymethylcellulose sodium, flavors, hydroxypropyl methylcellulose, microcrystalline cellulose, propylparaben, purified water, saccharin sodium, and sorbitol.

Sodium Content: Each 5 mL teaspoon contains the following amount of sodium:

	MYLANTA®	MYLANTA® Double Strength
Liquid	0.68 mg (0.03 mEq)	1.14 mg (0.05 mEq)

Acid Neutralizing Capacity
Two teaspoonfuls have the following acid neutralizing capacity:

	Fast Acting MYLANTA®	Maximum Strength Fast Acting MYLANTA®
Liquid	25.4 mEq	50.8 mEq

Indications: Fast-Acting MYLANTA® and Maximum Strength Fast-Acting MYLANTA® are indicated for the relief of acid indigestion, heartburn, sour stomach, and symptoms of gas and upset stomach associated with those conditions. Fast-Acting MYLANTA® and Maximum Strength Fast-Acting MYLANTA® are also indicated as antacids for the symptomatic relief of hyperacidity associated with the diagnosis of peptic ulcer, gastritis, peptic esophagitis, heartburn and hiatal hernia and as antiflatulents to alleviate the symptoms of mucus-entrapped gas, including postoperative gas pain.

Advantages: Fast-Acting MYLANTA and Maximum Strength Fast-Acting MYLANTA are homogenized for a smooth, creamy taste. The choice of three pleasant-tasting liquid flavors and the non-constipating formula encourage patient acceptance, thereby minimizing the skipping of prescribed doses. Fast-Acting MYLANTA and Maximum Strength Fast-Acting MYLANTA are also available in tablets, and both the liquid and tablet forms are very low in sodium. Fast-Acting MYLANTA and Maximum Strength Fast-Acting MYLANTA provide consistent relief in patients suffering from distress associated with hyperacidity, mucus-entrapped gas, or swallowed air.

Directions: **Liquid:** Shake well. 2-4 teaspoonfuls between meals and at bedtime, or as directed by a physician.

Warnings: Keep this and all drugs out of the reach of children. Do not take more than 24 tsps of Fast-Acting MYLANTA® or 12 tsps of Maximum Strength Fast-Acting MYLANTA® in a 24-hour period or use the maximum dose of this product for more than two weeks, except under the advice and supervison of a physician. Do not use this product if you have kidney disease.

Prolonged use of aluminum-containing antacids in patients with renal failure may result in or worsen dialysis osteomalacia. Elevated tissue aluminum levels contribute to the development of the dialysis encephalopathy and osteomalacia syndromes. Small amounts of aluminum are absorbed from the gastrointestinal tract and renal excretion of aluminum is impaired in renal failure. Aluminum is not well removed by dialysis because it is bound to albumin and transferrin, which do not cross dialysis membranes. As a result, aluminum is deposited in bone, and dialysis osteomalacia may develop when large amounts of aluminum are ingested orally by patients with impaired renal function.

Aluminum forms insoluble complexes with phosphate in the gastrointestinal tract, thus decreasing phosphate absorption. Prolonged use of aluminum-containing antacids by normophosphatemic patients may result in hypophosphatemia if phosphate intake is not adequate. In its more severe forms, hypophosphatemia can lead to anorexia, malaise, muscle weakness, and osteomalacia.

Drug Interaction Precaution: Antacids may interact with certain prescription drugs. If you are presently taking a prescription drug, do not take this product without checking with your physician or other health professional.

How Supplied: Fast-Acting MYLANTA® and Maximum Strength Fast-Acting MYLANTA® are available as white liquid suspensions in pleasant-tasting flavors, Original, Cherry Creme and Cool Mint Creme. Liquids are supplied in bottles of 5 oz, 12 oz, and 24 oz. Also available for hospital use in liquid unit dose bottles of 1 oz and bottles of 5 oz.

MYLANTA®
NDC 16837-610 ORIGINAL LIQUID
NDC 16837-629 COOL MINT CREME LIQUID
NDC 16837-621 CHERRY CREME LIQUID

MYLANTA® Double Strength
NDC 16837-652 ORIGINAL LIQUID
NDC 16837-624 COOL MINT CREME LIQUID
NDC 16837-622 CHERRY CREME LIQUID

Professional Labeling

Indications: Stress-induced upper gastrointestinal hemorrhage: Maximum Strength Fast-Acting MYLANTA® is indicated for the prevention of stress-induced upper gastrointestinal hemorrhage. Hyperacidic conditions: As an antacid, for the symptomatic relief of hyperacidity associated with the diagnosis of peptic ulcer and other gastrointestinal conditions where a high degree of acid neutralization is desired.

Directions: Prevention of stress-induced upper gastrointestinal hemorrhage: 1) Aspirate stomach via nasogastric tube* and record pH. 2) Instill 10 mL of Maximum Strength Fast-Acting MYLANTA® followed by 30 mL of water via nasogastric tube. Clamp tube. 3) Wait one hour. Aspirate stomach and record pH. 4a) If pH equals or exceeds 4.0, apply drainage or intermittent suction for one hour, then repeat the cycle. 4b) If pH is less than 4.0, instill double (20 mL) Maximum Strength Fast-Acting MYLANTA® followed by 30 mL of wa-

Continued on next page

J&J • Merck—Cont.

ter. Clamp tube. 5) Wait one hour. If pH equals or exceeds 4.0, see number 7, if pH is still less than 4.0, instill double (40 mL) Maximum Strength Fast-Acting MYLANTA® followed by 30 mL of water. Clamp tube. 6) Wait one hour. If pH equals or exceeds 4.0, see number 7. If pH is still less than 4.0, instill double (80 mL)† Maximum Strength Fast-Acting MYLANTA® followed by 30 mL of water. 7) Drain for one hour and repeat cycle with the effective dosage of Maximum Strength Fast-Acting MYLANTA®.

* If nasogastric tube is not in place, administer 20 mL of Maximum Strength Fast-Acting MYLANTA® orally q2h.

† In a recent clinical study[1] 20 mL of Maximum Strength Fast-Acting MYLANTA®, q2h, was sufficient in more than 85 percent of the patients. No patient studied required more than 80 mL of Maximum Strength Fast-Acting MYLANTA® q2h.

In hyperacid states for symptomatic relief: One or two teaspoonfuls as needed between meals and at bedtime or as directed by a physician. Higher dosage regimens may be employed under the direct supervision of a physician in the treatment of active peptic ulcer disease.

Precautions: Aluminum-magnesium hydroxide containing antacids should be used with caution in patients with renal impairment.

Adverse Effects: Occasional regurgitation and mild diarrhea have been reported with the dosage recommended for the prevention of stress-induced upper gastrointestinal hemorrhage.

References: 1. Zinner MJ, Zuidema GD, Smigh PL, Mignosa M: The prevention of upper gastrointestinal tract bleeding in patients in an intensive care unit. *Surg Gynecol Obster* 153:214–220, 1981. 2. Lucas CE, Sugawa C, Riddle J, et al.: Natural history and surgical dilemma of "stress" gastric bleeding. *Arch Surg* 102:266–273, 1971. 3. Hastings PR, Skillman JJ, Bushnell LS, Silen W: Antacid titration in the prevention of acute gastrointestinal bleeding: a controlled, randomized trial in 100 critically ill patients. *N Engl J Med* 298:1042–1045, 1978. 4. Day SB, MacMillan BG, Altemeier WA: *Curling's Ulcer, An Experience of Nature.* Springfield, IL, Charles C Thomas Co., 1972, p. 205. 5. Skillman JJ, Bushnell LS, Goldman H, Silen W: Respiratory failure, hypotension, sepsis, and jaundice. A clinical syndrome associated with lethal hemorrhage from acute stress ulceration of the stomach. *Am J Surg* 117:523–530, 1969. 6. Priebe HJ, Skillman J, Bushnell LS, et al. Antacid versus cimetidine in preventing acute gastrointestinal bleeding. *N Engl J Med* 302:426–430, 1980. 7. Silen W: The prevention and management of stress ulcers. *Hosp Pract* 15:93–97, 1980. 8. Herrmann V, Kaminski DL: Evaluation of intragastric pH in acutely ill patients. *Arch Surg* 114:511–514, 1979. 9. Martin LF, Staloch DK, Simonowitz DA, et al.: Failure of cimetidine prophylaxis in the critically ill. *Arch Surg* 114:492–496, 1979. 10. Zinner MJ, Turtinen L, Gurll NJ, Reynolds DG: The effect of metiamide on gastric mucosal injury in rat restraint. *Clin Res* 23:484A, 1975. 11. Zinner M, Turtinen BA, Gurll NJ: The role of acid and ischemia in production of stress ulcers during canine hemorrhagic shock. *Surgery* 77:807–816, 1975. 12. Winans CS: Prevention and treatment of stress ulcer bleeding: Antacids or cimetidine? *Drug Ther Bull* (hospital) 12:37–45, 1981.

Shown in Product Identification Guide, page 509

FAST-ACTING MYLANTA AND MAXIMUM STRENGTH FAST ACTING MYLANTA

[mylan 'ta]

Calcium Carbonate and Magnesium Hydroxide Tablets
Antacid

Description: Fast-Acting MYLANTA and Maximum Strength Fast-Acting MYLANTA are well balanced, pleasant tasting antacid medications that provide consistent, effective relief of symptoms associated with gastric hyperacidity. Non-constipating and very low in sodium, Fast-Acting MYLANTA and Maximum Strength Fast-Acting MYLANTA contain two proven antacids, calcium carbonate and magnesium hydroxide.

Active Ingredients
Each tablet contains:

	Fast-Acting MYLANTA	Maximum Strength Fast-Acting MYLANTA
Calcium Carbonate	350mg	700mg
Magnesium Hydroxide	150mg	300mg

Inactive Ingredients
Citric acid, confectioner's sugar, flavors, magnesium stearate, sorbitol, FD&C Blue 1 or D&C Yellow 10 or D&C Red 27

Sodium Content
Each chewable tablet contains the following amount of sodium:

Fast-Acting MYLANTA	Maximum Strength Fast-Acting MYLANTA
0.3mg	0.6mg

Acid Neutralizing Capacity
Two chewable tablets have the following acid neutralizing capacity:

Fast-Acting MYLANTA	Maximum Strength Fast-Acting MYLANTA
24.0mEq	48.0mEq

Indications: Fast-Acting MYLANTA and Maximum Strength Fast-Acting MYLANTA are indicated for the relief of heartburn, acid indigestion, sour stomach and upset stomach associated with these conditions. Fast-Acting MYLANTA and Maximum Strength Fast-Acting MYLANTA are also indicated as antacids for the symptomatic relief of hyperacidity associated with the diagnosis of peptic ulcer, gastritis, peptic esophagitis, heartburn and hiatal hernia.

Directions: Thoroughly chew 2–4 tablets between meals, at bedtime or as directed by a physician.

WARNINGS: Keep this and all drugs out of the reach of children. Do not take more than 20 tablets of Fast-Acting MYLANTA or 10 tablets of MYLANTA Maximum Strength Fast-Acting in a 24-hour period, or use the maximum dosage for more than two weeks. Do not use this product if you have kidney disease, except under the advise and supervision of a physician.

Drug Interaction Precaution: Antacids may interact with certain prescription drugs. If you are presently taking a prescription drug, do not take this product without checking with your physician or other health professional.

How Supplied: Fast-Acting MYLANTA is available as a green Cool Mint Creme chewable tablet. Maximum Strength Fast-Acting MYLANTA is available as a green Cool Mint Creme Chewable tablet and pink Cherry Creme chewable tablet.

Fast-Acting Mylanta
NDC 16837-848 Cool Mint Creme

Maximum Strength Fast-Acting MYLANTA
NDC 16837-869 Cherry Creme
NDC 16837-849 Cool Mint Creme

Shown in Product Identification Guide, page 509

MYLANTA® GAS Relief Tablets
Maximum Strength MYLANTA® GAS Relief Tablets
MYLANTA® Gas Relief Gelcaps

[My-lan '-ta]

Antiflatulent

Active Ingredients: Each chewable tablet contains:

	Simethicone
MYLANTA® GAS Relief	80 mg
Maximum Strength MYLANTA® GAS Relief	125 mg
MYLANTA® GAS Relief Gelcaps	62.5 mg

Inactive Ingredients: TABLETS: Dextrates, flavor, sorbitol, stearic acid, tricalcium phosphate. Cherry: Red 7.
GELCAPS: Benzyl alcohol, butylparaben, castor oil, croscarmellase sodium, D&C Red 28, D&C Yellow 10, dextrose, dibasic calcium phosphate dihydrate, edetate calcium disodium, FD&C Blue 1, FD&C Red 28, gelatin, hydroxypropyl methylcellulose, maltodextrin, methylparaben, microcrystalline cellulose, propylene glycol, propylparaben, silicon dioxide, sodium lauryl sulfate, sodium propionate, sorbitol, stearic acid, titanium dioxide, tribasic calcium phosphate.

Indications: For relief of the symptoms of excess gas in the digestive tract. Such gas is frequently caused by excessive swallowing of air or by eating foods that disagree. MYLANTA® GAS Relief Gelcaps, MYLANTA® GAS Relief, and Maximum Strength MYLANTA® GAS Relief Tablets are high capacity antiflatulents for adjunctive treatment of many conditions in which the retention of gas may be a problem, such as the following: air swallowing, postoperative gaseous distention, peptic ulcer, spastic or irritable colon, diverticulosis. If condition persists, consult your physician.

MYLANTA® GAS Relief Gelcap, MYLANTA® GAS Relief, and Maximum Strength MYLANTA®GAS Relief Tablets have a defoaming action that relieves flatulence by dispersing and preventing the formation of mucus-surrounded gas pockets in the gastrointestinal tract. MYLANTA® GAS Relief Gelcaps, MYLANTA® GAS Relief, and Maximum Strength MYLANTA® GAS Relief Tablets act in the stomach and intestines to change the surface tension of gas bubbles enabling them to coalesce, thereby freeing and eliminating the gas more easily by belching or passing flatus.

Directions:

MYLANTA® GAS Relief Tablets

One tablet four times daily after meals and at bedtime. May also be taken as needed up to six tablets daily or as directed by a physician.

Maximum Strength MYLANTA® GAS Relief Tablets

One tablet four times daily after meals and at bedtime or as directed by a physician.

TABLETS SHOULD BE CHEWED THOROUGHLY

MYLANTA® GAS Relief Gelcaps

Swallow 2-4 gelcaps as needed after meals and at bedtime. Do not exceed 8 gelcaps per day unless directed by a physician.

Warnings: Keep this and all drugs out of the reach of children.

How Supplied: MYLANTA® GAS Relief Tablets are available as white (mint) or pink (cherry) scored, chewable tablets identified "MYL GAS 80." Mint flavor is available in bottles of 60 and 100 tablets and individually wrapped 12 and 30 tablet packages. Cherry flavor is available in packages of 12 individually wrapped tablets. Mint NDC 16837-858. Cherry NDC 16837-859.

Maximum Strength MYLANTA® GAS Relief Tablets are available as white, scored, chewable tablets identified "MYL GAS 125" in individually wrapped 12 and 24 tablet packages and economical 48 tablet bottles. NDC 16837-455.

MYLANTA® Gas Relief Gelcaps are available as blue and yellow gelcaps identified as 'MYLANTA GAS' in individually wrapped 24 tablet packages. NDC 16837–626.

Shown in Product Identification Guide, page 509

MYLANTA® GELCAPS

[*my-lan 'ta*]

Antacid

Description: MYLANTA® GELCAPS are an easy-to-swallow, non-chalky alternative to liquid and tablet antacids. The gelcaps contain two antacid ingredients, calcium carbonate, and magnesium hydroxide, have no chalky taste, are low in sodium and provide fast, effective acid pain relief.

Ingredients: Each gelcap contains: **Active:** Calcium Carbonate 550 mg and Magnesium Hydroxide 125 mg. **Inactive:** Benzyl Alcohol, Butylparaben, Castor Oil, Crospovidone, D&C Red #28, D&C Yellow 10, Disodium Calcium Edetate, FD&C Blue 1, FD&C Red #40, Gelatin, Hydroxypropyl Cellulose, Magnesium Stearate, Methylparaben, Microcrystalline Cellulose, Propylparaben, Sodium Lauryl Sulfate, Sodium Propionate, Starch, Titanium Dioxide. May also contain propylene glycol.

Sodium Content: MYLANTA® GELCAPS contain a very low amount of sodium per daily dose. Typical value is 2.5 mg (.1087 mEq) sodium per gelcap.

Acid Neutralizing Capacity: Two MYLANTA® GELCAPS have an acid neutralizing capacity of 23.0 mEq.

Indications: For the relief of acid indigestion, heartburn, sour stomach and upset stomach associated with these symptoms.

Advantages: MYLANTA® GELCAPS are easy to swallow, provide fast, effective relief, eliminate antacid taste and are low in sodium. Convenience of dosage in the unique gelcap form can promote patient compliance.

Directions: 2–4 gelcaps as needed or as directed by a physician.

Warnings: Keep this and all other drugs out of the reach of children. Do not take more than 24 gelcaps in a 24-hour period or use the maximum dosage for more than two weeks or use if you have kidney disease, except under the advice and supervision of a physician.

Drug Interaction Precaution: Antacids may interact with certain prescription drugs. If you are presently taking a prescription drug, do not take this product without checking with your physician or other health professional.

How Supplied: MYLANTA® GELCAPS are available as a blue and white gelcap in convenient blister packs in boxes of 24 solid gelcaps or in bottles of 50 and 100 solid gelcaps.

NDC 16837-850 1/93

Shown in Product Identification Guide, page 509

PEPCID AC® ACID CONTROLLER™

Description:

ACTIVE INGREDIENT: Famotidine 10 mg per tablet.

INACTIVE INGREDIENTS: Hydroxypropyl cellulose, hydroxypropyl methylcellulose, red iron oxide, magnesium stearate, microcrystalline cellulose, starch, talc, titanium dioxide.

Product Benefits:

- **1 tablet** relieves heartburn and acid indigestion.
- Pepcid AC Acid Controller prevents heartburn and acid indigestion brought on by consuming food and beverages.

It contains famotidine, a prescription-proven medicine.

The ingredient in PEPCID AC Acid Controller, famotidine, has been prescribed by doctors for years to treat millions of patients safely and effectively. The active ingredient in PEPCID AC Acid Controller has been taken safely with many frequently prescribed medications.

Action: It is normal for the stomach to produce acid, especially after consuming food and beverages. However, acid in the wrong place (the esophagus), or too much acid, can cause burning pain and discomfort that interfere with everyday activities.

- **Heartburn—Caused by acid in the esophagus**

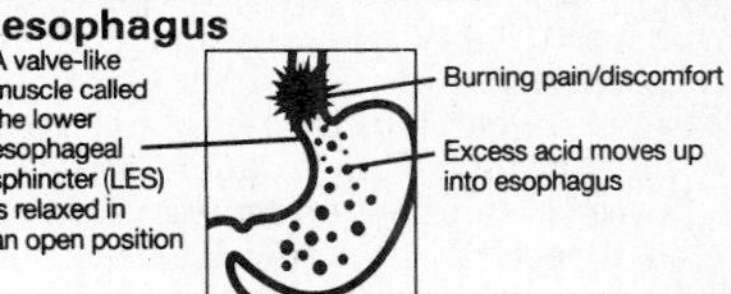

In clinical studies, PEPCID AC Acid Controller was significantly better than placebo pills in relieving and preventing heartburn.

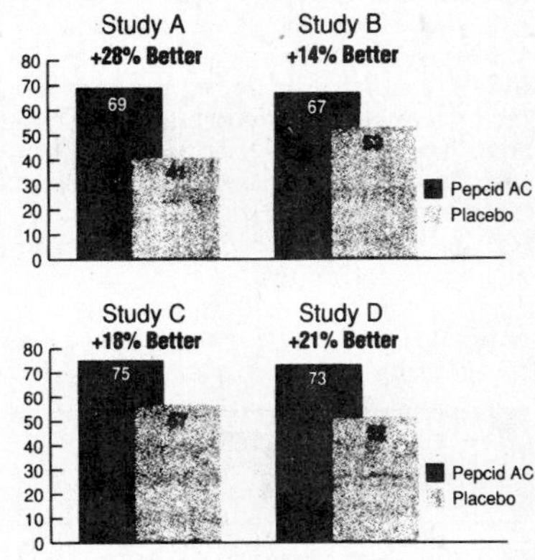

Uses:

- **<u>For Relief</u>** of heartburn, acid indigestion, and sour stomach;
- **<u>For Prevention</u>** of these symptoms brought on by consuming food and beverages.

How to help avoid symptoms

- Do not lie down soon after eating.
- If your are overweight, lose weight.
- If you smoke, stop or cut down.
- Avoid or limit foods such as caffeine, chocolate, fatty foods and alcohol.
- Do not eat just before bedtime.

Continued on next page

J&J • Merck—Cont.

Warnings:

- Do not take the maximum daily dosage (2 tablets) for more than 2 weeks continuously except under the advice and supervision of a doctor.
- As with any drug, if you are pregnant or nursing a baby, seek the advice of a health professional before using this product.
- If you have trouble swallowing, or persistent abdominal pain, see your doctor promptly. You may have a serious condition that may need different treatment.
- Keep this and all drugs out of the reach of children.
- In case of accidental overdose, seek professional assistance or contact a poison control center immediately.

Caution:

Heartburn and acid indigestion are common, but you should see your doctor promptly if:

- You have trouble swallowing or persistent abdominal pain. You may have a serious condition that may need different treatment.
- You have used the maximum dosage every day for two weeks continously.

Important: As with any drug, if you are pregnant or nursing a baby, seek the advice of a health professional before using this product. This product should not be given to children under 12 years old, unless directed by a doctor. Keep this and all drugs out of the reach of children. In case of accidental overdose, seek professional assistance or contact a poison control center immediately.

Directions:

- For **Relief** of symptoms **swallow 1 tablet with water.**
- For **Prevention** of symptoms brought on by consuming food and beverages **swallow 1 tablet with water 1 hour before eating a meal you expect to cause symptoms.**
- Can be used up to twice daily (up to 2 tablets in 24 hours).
- This product should not be given to children under 12 years old unless directed by a doctor.

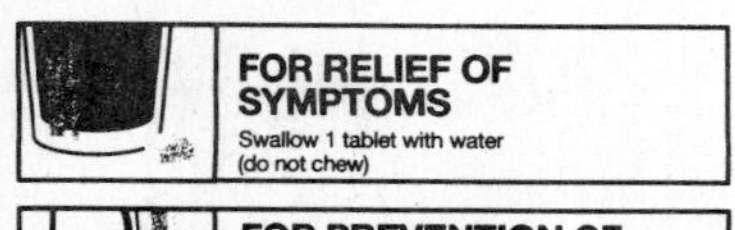

How Supplied:

Pepcid AC Acid Controller is available as a rose-colored tablet identified as 'PEPCID AC'.

Pepcid AC is available in blister packs in boxes of 6, 12, 18, 30, 50, and 80 tablets. NDC 16837-872

- Read the directions and warnings before use.
- Keep the carton. It contains important information.

Store at temperatures up to 30°C (86°F). Protect from moisture.

DO NOT USE IF THE INDIVIDUAL BLISTER UNIT IS OPEN OR BROKEN.

Shown in Product Identification Guide, page 509

Konsyl Pharmaceuticals, Inc.

4200 S. HULEN
FORT WORTH, TX 76109

Direct Inquiries to:
Bill Steiber
(817) 763-8011, Ext. 23
FAX: (817) 731-9389

KONSYL® Fiber Tablets (Calcium Polycarbophil 625mg)

Description: KONSYL Fiber Tablets is a bulk forming fiber laxative for restoring and maintaining regularity. Promotes normal function of the bowel by increasing bulk volume and water content of stool. KONSYL Fiber Tablets contain 625 mg calcium polycarbophil equivalent to 500 mg polycarbophil.

Inactive Ingredients: Caramel, Crospovidone, Ethycellulose, Hydroxypropyl Methylcellulose, Magnesium Stearate, Microcrystalline Cellulose, Polyethylene Glycol, Povidone, Silicon Dioxide.

Actions: KONSYL Fiber Tablets provide bulk that promotes normal elimination. KONSYL Fiber Tablets provide convenience of a bulk forming laxative in a tablet form. The product is easy-to-swallow and non-irritative in the gastrointestinal tract.

Indications: KONSYL Fiber Tablets are indicated in the management of chronic constipation, irritable bowel syndrome, as adjunctive therapy in the constipation of diverticular disease, bowel management of patients with hemorrhoids, and for constipation during pregnancy, convalescence, and senility. KONSYL Fiber Tablets are also used for other indications as prescribed by physician.

Contraindications: Intestinal obstruction, fecal impaction.

Warnings: KEEP THIS AND ALL DRUGS OUT OF THE REACH OF CHILDREN. TAKING THIS PRODUCT WITHOUT ADEQUATE FLUID MAY CAUSE IT TO SWELL AND BLOCK YOUR THROAT OR ESOPHAGUS AND MAY CAUSE CHOKING. DO NOT TAKE THIS PRODUCT IF YOU HAVE DIFFICULTY IN SWALLOWING. IF YOU EXPERIENCE CHEST PAIN, VOMITING, OR DIFFICULTY IN SWALLOWING OR BREATHING AFTER TAKING THIS PRODUCT, SEEK IMMEDIATE MEDICAL ATTENTION.

Interaction Precaution: Contains calcium. If you are taking any form of tetracycline antibiotic, this product should be taken at least 1 hour before or 2 hours after you have taken the antibiotic. Store at controlled room temperature 59°–86°F (15°–30°C). Protect from moisture.

Dosage and Administration: TAKE THIS PRODUCT (CHILD OR ADULT DOSE) WITH AT LEAST 8 OUNCES (A FULL GLASS) OF WATER OR OTHER FLUID. TAKING THIS PRODUCT WITHOUT ENOUGH LIQUID MAY CAUSE CHOKING. SEE WARNINGS. **ADULTS:** 2 TABLETS 1 TO 4 TIMES A DAY. **CHILDREN** (6 TO 12 YEARS OLD): 1 TABLET 1 TO 3 TIMES A DAY. CHILDREN UNDER 6 YEARS CONSULT A PHYSICIAN. DOSAGE WILL VARY ACCORDING TO DIET, EXERCISE, PREVIOUS LAXATIVE USE OR SEVERITY OF CONSTIPATION. THE RECOMMENDED ADULT STARTING DOSE IS 2 TO 4 TABLETS DAILY. MAY BE INCREASED UP TO 8 TABLETS DAILY.

KONSYL FIBER TABLETS GENERALLY PRODUCE RESULTS WITHIN 12–72 HOURS.

How Supplied: Tablets, containers of 90 tablets.

Is this product OTC? Yes

KONSYL® POWDER (psyllium hydrophilic mucilloid) Sugar Free, Sugar Substitute Free. 6.0 grams of psyllium per TEASPOON

Description: Konsyl is a bulk-forming natural therapeutic fiber for restoring and maintaining regularity. Konsyl contains 100% psyllium hydrophilic mucilloid, a highly efficient dietary fiber derived from the husk of the psyllium seed. Konsyl contains no chemical stimulants and is non-addictive. Each dose contains 6.0 grams of psyllium compared to 3.4 grams of psyllium in most other products.

Inactive Ingredients: None. Each 6 gram dose provides 3 calories. Konsyl has a very low sodium content. Since Konsyl is sugar free, it is excellent for diabetics who require a bowel normalizer.

Actions: Konsyl provides bulk that promotes normal elimination. The product is uniform, instantly miscible, palatable, and non-irritative in the gastrointestinal tract.

Indications: Konsyl is indicated in the management of chronic constipation, irritable bowel syndrome, as adjunctive therapy in the constipation of diverticular disease, bowel management of patients with hemorrhoids, and for constipation during pregnancy, convalescence, and senility. Konsyl is also indicated for other indications as prescribed by physician.

Contraindications: Intestinal obstruction, fecal impaction.

Warnings: **KEEP THIS AND ALL DRUGS OUT OF THE REACH OF**

CHILDREN. TAKING THIS PRODUCT WITHOUT ADEQUATE FLUID MAY CAUSE IT TO SWELL AND BLOCK YOUR THROAT OR ESOPHAGUS AND MAY CAUSE CHOKING. DO NOT TAKE THIS PRODUCT IF YOU HAVE DIFFICULTY IN SWALLOWING. IF YOU EXPERIENCE CHEST PAIN, VOMITING OR DIFFICULTY IN SWALLOWING OR BREATHING AFTER TAKING THIS PRODUCT, SEEK IMMEDIATE MEDICAL ATTENTION.

Precautions: May cause allergic reaction in people sensitive to inhaled or ingested psyllium powder.

Dosage and Administration:
MIX THIS PRODUCT (CHILD OR ADULT DOSE) WITH AT LEAST 8 OUNCES (A FULL GLASS) OF WATER OR OTHER FLUID. TAKING THIS PRODUCT WITHOUT ENOUGH LIQUID MAY CAUSE CHOKING. SEE WARNINGS.
ADULTS: Place one rounded teaspoon (6.0 grams) into a dry shaker cup or container that can be closed. Add 8 oz. of juice, cold water or your favorite beverage. Shake, don't stir, for 3–5 seconds. Drink promptly. If mixture thickens, add more liquid and shake. Follow with an 8 oz. glass of juice or water to aid product action. Konsyl can be taken one to three times daily, depending on need and response. Konsyl generally produces results within 12–72 hours. Take Konsyl at any convenient time, morning or evening; before or after meals. When taking Konsyl, one should drink several 8 oz. glasses of water a day to aid product action.
CHILDREN: (6–12 years old) Use 1/2 adult dose in 8 oz. of liquid, 1–3 times daily.
Children under six years, consult a physician.

New Users: Easy Does It. Medical research shows that higher fiber intake is important for good digestive health. To help the body adjust and avoid minor gas and bloating sometimes associated with high fiber intake, it may be necessary to take one half dose over several days and then slowly increase the dosage over several days. Always follow with 8 oz. of liquid.

How Supplied: Powder, containers of 10.6 oz. (300 g), 15.9 oz. (450 g) and 30 single dose (6.0 g) packets.

Is this product OTC? Yes.

Kyolic Ltd.

Division of Wakunaga of America Co., Ltd.
23501 MADERO
MISSION VIEJO, CA 92691

Direct Inquiries to:
(800) 421-2998

BE SURE®

Prevents flatulence
Digestive enzymes: 1–2 capsules to be taken with offending foods. Comes in boxes of 30 and bottles of 60 capsules.

GINKGO-GO!™
Dietary Supplement

Active Ingredient: Each caplet—Ginkgo Biloba Extract 50:1 (120 mg).

Suggested Use: As a dietary supplement, take one caplet daily with food for enhancement of memory, alertness and mental acuity.

How Supplied: Boxes of 15 caplets.

KYOLIC®
Odor Modified Garlic Supplement

Active Ingredient: Each caplet contains 600 mg Aged Garlic Extract™.

Suggested Use: As a dietary supplement, take 1 or more caplets daily with food.

How Supplied: Boxes of 30 Caplets.
Shown in Product Identification Guide, page 522

PROBIATA™
Probiotic Dietary Supplement

Active Ingredient: L. acidophilus

Suggested Use: Take one tablet, twice daily with meals. Replenishes healthy intestinal flora to avoid disorders such as diarrhea, constipation and yeast discomfort caused by antibiotic usage.

How Supplied: Bottles of 30 tablets.
Shown in Product Identification Guide, page 522

Lavoptik Company, Inc.

661 WESTERN AVENUE N.
ST. PAUL, MN 55103

Direct Inquiries to:
661 Western Avenue North
St. Paul, MN 55103-1694
(612) 489-1351

For Medical Emergencies Contact:
B. C. Brainard
(612) 489-1351
FAX: (612) 489-0760

LAVOPTIK® Eye Cups

Description: Device—Sterile disposable eye cups.

How Supplied: Individually bagged eye cups are packed 12 per box, NDC 10651-01004.

LAVOPTIK® Eye Wash

Description: Isotonic LAVOPTIK Eye Wash is a buffered solution designed to help physically remove contaminants from the surface of the eye and lids. Formulated to buffer contaminants toward the safe range and help restore normal salts and water ratios in the tears.

Contents: Each 100 ml	
Sodium Chloride	0.49 gram
Sodium Biphosphate	0.40 gram
Sodium Phosphate	0.45 gram
Preservative Agent	
Benzalkonium Chloride	0.005 gram

Precautions: If you experience severe eye pain, headache, rapid change in vision (side or straight ahead); sudden appearance of floating objects, acute redness of the eyes, pain on exposure to light or double vision consult a physician at once. If symptoms persist or worsen after use of this product, consult a physician. If solution changes color or becomes cloudy do not use. Keep this and all medicines out of reach of children. Keep container tightly closed. Do not use if safety seal is broken at time of purchase.

Administration: 6 ounce size with Eye Cup.
Rinse cup with clean water immediately before and after each use, avoid contamination of rim and inside surfaces of cup. Apply cup, half-filled with LAVOPTIK Eye Wash tightly to the eye. Tilt head backward. Open eyelids wide, rotate eyeball and blink several times to insure thorough washing. Discard washings. Repeat other eye. Tightly cap bottle.
32 ounce size.
Break seal as you remove cap and pour directly on contaminated area.

How Supplied: 6 ounce bottle with eyecup, NDC 10651-01040.
32 ounce bottle, NDC 10651-01019.

Lederle Consumer Health
A Division of Whitehall-Robins Healthcare
FIVE GIRALDA FARMS
MADISON, NJ 07940

Direct Inquiries to:
Lederle Consumer Product Information
(800) 282-8805

CALTRATE® 600
[*căl-trāte*]
High Potency Calcium Supplement
Nature's Most Concentrated Form of Calcium®
No Sugar, No Salt, No Lactose, No Preservatives, Tablet Shape Specially Designed for Easier Swallowing

Caltrate 600 is a dietary supplement that meets USP standards for purity, potency and dissolution.

Nutrition Facts
Serving Size 1 Tablet

Each Tablet Contains	% Daily Value
Calcium 600 mg	60%

Recommended Intake: One or two tablets daily or as directed by your physician.

Warning: Keep out of reach of children.

Ingredients: Calcium Carbonate, Maltodextrin, Cellulose, Mineral Oil, Hydroxypropyl Methylcellulose, Titanium Dioxide, Sodium Lauryl Sulfate, Gelatin, Crospovidone, Stearic Acid and Magnesium Stearate.

How Supplied: Bottle of 60
Store at Room Temperature.

CALTRATE® 600 + D
[*căl-trāte*]
High Potency Calcium Supplement With Vitamin D
Nature's Most Concentrated Form of Calcium®
No Sugar, No Salt, No Lactose, No Preservatives, Tablet Shape Specially Designed for Easier Swallowing

CALTRATE® 600 + D is a dietary supplement that meets USP standards for purity, potency and dissolution.

Nutrition Facts
Serving Size 1 Tablet

Each Tablet Contains	% Daily Value
Vitamin D 200 IU	50%
Calcium 600 mg	60%

Recommended Intake: One or two tablets daily or as directed by your physician.

Warning: Keep out of reach of children.

Ingredients: Calcium Carbonate, Maltodextrin, Cellulose, Mineral Oil, Hydroxypropyl Methylcellulose, Titanium Dioxide, Vitamin D, Sodium Lauryl Sulfate, FD&C Yellow No. 6, Gelatin, Crospovidone, Stearic Acid and Magnesium Stearate.

How Supplied: Bottle of 60
Store at Room Temperature.

CALTRATE® PLUS™
[*căl-trāte*]
High Potency Calcium Supplement With Vitamin D & Minerals
Nature's Most Concentrated Form of Calcium®
No Sugar, No Salt, No Lactose, No Preservatives, Tablet Shape Specially Designed for Easier Swallowing

Caltrate Plus is a dietary supplement that meets USP standards for purity, potency and dissolution.

Nutrition Facts
Serving Size 1 Tablet

Each Tablet Contains	% Daily Value
Vitamin D 200 IU	50%
Calcium 600 mg	60%
Magnesium 40 mg	10%
Zinc 7.5 mg	50%
Copper 1 mg	50%
Manganese 1.8 mg	*
Boron 250 mcg	*

*Daily Value Not Established

Recommended Intake: One or two tablets daily or as directed by your physician.

Warning: Keep out of reach of children.

Ingredients: Calcium Carbonate, Maltodextrin, Magnesium Oxide, Cellulose, Mineral Oil, Hydroxypropyl Methylcellulose, Zinc Oxide, Titanium Dioxide, Manganese Sulfate, Vitamin D, Sodium Lauryl Sulfate, Sodium Borate, Cupric Oxide, FD&C Red No. 40, FD&C Yellow No. 6, FD&C Blue No. 1, Gelatin, Crospovidone, Stearic Acid and Magnesium Stearate.

How Supplied: Bottle of 60
Store at Room Temperature.

CALTRATE® Plus™ Chewables
[*căl-trāte*]
Calcium Carbonate
Nutrient Enriched Calcium Supplement With Vitamin D & Minerals
Contains the most concentrated form of calcium you can buy
No Salt, No Lactose, No Preservatives
EACH TABLET CONTAINS:

		For Adults-Percentage of U.S. Recommended Daily Allowance (U.S. RDA)
Vitamin D	200 IU	50%
Calcium	600 mg	60%
Magnesium	40 mg	10%
Zinc	7.5 mg	50%
Copper	1 mg	50%
Manganese	1.8 mg	*
Boron	250 mcg	*

*U.S. RDA Not Established

Recommended Intake: One or two tablets daily or as directed by your physician.

Warnings: Keep out of the reach of children.

Ingredients:
Assorted Fruit Flavors (• Cherry • Orange • Fruit Punch): Dextrose, Calcium Carbonate, Mineral Oil, Magnesium Stearate, Magnesium Oxide, Maltodextrin, Adipic Acid, Modified Food Starch, Cellulose, Zinc Oxide, Manganese Sulfate, Sodium Borate, Artificial Flavors, Sucrose, FD&C Red #40, Cupric Oxide, FD&C Yellow #6, FD&C Blue #2, Gelatin, Vitamin D, Crospovidone, Stearic Acid
Spearmint Flavor: Dextrose, Calcium Carbonate, Mineral Oil, Magnesium Stearate, Magnesium Oxide, Maltodextrin, Cellulose, Zinc Oxide, Modified Food Starch, Manganese Sulfate, Contains color additives including FD&C Yellow #5 (Tartrazine), Sodium Borate, Sucrose, Cupric Oxide, FD&C Blue #1, Natural Spearmint Flavor, Gelatin, Vitamin D, Crospovidone, Stearic Acid

How Supplied:
Bottles of 60 with Assorted Fruit Flavors
Bottles of 60 with Spearmint Flavor
Store at Room Temperature.
Official Date of New Package Insert:

CENTRUM®
[*sĕn-trŭm*]
High Potency Multivitamin-Multimineral Formula, Advanced Formula
From A to Zinc®

Nutrition Facts
Serving Size 1 Tablet

Each Tablet Contains	%DV
Vitamin A 5000 IU (40% as Beta Carotene)	100%
Vitamin C 60 mg	100%
Vitamin D 400 IU	100%
Vitamin E 30 IU	100%
Thiamin 1.5 mg	100%
Riboflavin 1.7 mg	100%
Niacinamide 20 mg	100%
Vitamin B_6 2 mg	100%
Folic Acid 400 mcg	100%
Vitamin B_{12} 6 mcg	100%
Biotin 30 mcg	10%

Pantothenic Acid 10 mg	100%
Calcium 162 mg	16%
Iron 18 mg	100%
Phosphorus 109 mg	11%
Iodine 150 mcg	100%
Magnesium 100 mg	25%
Zinc 15 mg	100%
Copper 2 mg	100%
Potassium 80 mg	2%
Vitamin K 25 mcg	*
Selenium 20 mcg	*
Manganese 3.5 mg	*
Chromium 65 mcg	*
Molybdenum 160 mcg	*
Chloride 72 mg	*
Nickel 5 mcg	*
Tin 10 mcg	*
Silicon 2 mg	*
Vanadium 10 mcg	*
Boron 150 mcg	*

*Daily Value (%DV) not established.

Recommended Intake: Adults, 1 tablet daily.

Warning: Close tightly and keep out of reach of children. Contains iron, which can be harmful or fatal to children in large doses. In case of accidental overdose, seek professional assistance or contact a Poison Control Center immediately.

Ingredients: Calcium Phosphate, Magnesium Oxide, Calcium Carbonate, Potassium Chloride, Ascorbi Acid (Vit. C), Ferrous Fumarate, Microcrystalline Cellulose, *dl*-alpha Tocopheryl Acetate (Vit. E), Gelatin, Crospovidone, Niacinamide, Zinc Oxide, Hydroxypropyl Methylcellulose, Calcium Pantothenate, Vitamin A Acetate/Vitamin D, Titanium Dioxide, Manganese Sulfate, Magnesium Stearate, Stearic Acid, Silicon Dioxide, Pyridoxine Hydrochloride (Vit. B_6), Cupric Oxide, Riboflavin (Vit. B_2), Triethyl Citrate, Thiamin Mononitrate (Vit. B_1), Polysorbate 80, Beta Carotene, FD&C Yellow #6, Folic Acid, Sodium Selenate, Potassium Iodide, Chromium Chloride, Sodium Metasilicate, Sodium Molybdate, Borates, Phytonadione (Vit. K), Biotin, Sodium Metavanadate, Stannous Chloride, Nickelous Sulfate and Cyanocobalamin (Vit. B_{12}).

How Supplied: Light peach, engraved CENTRUM C1.
Bottle of 60
Combopack†
†Bottles of 100 plus 30
Store at Room Temperature.

CENTRUM, JR.®

[*sĕn-trŭm*]

Shamu and his Crew®
+ EXTRA C
Children's Chewable Vitamin/Mineral Formula

[See table above.]

CENTRUM, JR.® + EXTRA C Nutrition Facts Serving Size:	**Children 2–4 Years Old** 1/2 tablet		**Children Over 4 Years Old** 1 tablet	
	Amount Per Serving	**% Daily Value**	**Amount Per Serving**	**% Daily Value**
Vitamin A (20% as Beta Carotene)	2500 IU	100%	5000 IU	100%
Vitamin C	150 mg	375%	300 mg	500%
Vitamin D	200 IU	50%	400 IU	100%
Vitamin E	15 IU	150%	30 IU	100%
Thiamin	0.75 mg	107%	1.5 mg	100%
Riboflavin	0.85 mg	106%	1.7 mg	100%
Niacinamide	10 mg	111%	20 mg	100%
Vitamin B_6	1 mg	143%	2 mg	100%
Folic Acid	200 mcg	100%	400 mcg	100%
Vitamin B_{12}	3 mcg	100%	6 mcg	100%
Biotin	22.5 mcg	15%	45 mcg	15%
Pantothenic Acid	5 mg	100%	10 mg	100%
Calcium	54 mg	7%	108 mg	11%
Iron	9 mg	90%	18 mg	100%
Phosphorous	25 mg	3%	50 mg	5%
Iodine	75 mcg	107%	150 mcg	100%
Magnesium	20 mg	10%	40 mg	10%
Zinc	7.5 mg	94%	15 mg	100%
Copper	1 mg	100%	2 mg	100%
Vitamin K	5 mcg	*	10 mcg	*
Manganese	0.5 mg	*	1 mg	*
Chromium	10 mcg	*	20 mcg	*
Molybdenum	10 mcg	*	20 mcg	*

*Daily Value not established.

Ingredients: Calcium Phosphate, Sugar, Ascorbic Acid and Sodium Ascorbate (Vit. C), Calcium Carbonate, Sorbitol, Microcrystalline Cellulose, Magnesium Oxide, Citric Acid, (Food) Starch, Mono- and Diglycerides, Gelatin, Modified Food Starch, Stearic Acid, *dl*-alpha Tocopheryl Acetate (Vit. E), Artificial Flavors, Niacinamide, Zinc Oxide, Iron Carbonyl , FD&C Red #40, FD&C Yellow #6, FD&C Blue #2, Calcium Pantothenate Vitamin A Acetate/Vitamin D, Aspartame**, Silicon Dioxide, Magnesium Sterate, Partially Hydrogenated Coconut Oil, Pyridoxine Hydrochloride (Vit. B_6), Cupric Oxide, Riboflavin (Vit. B_2), Thiamin Mononitrate (Vit. B_1), Dextrose, Manganese Sulfate, Beta Carotene, Folic Acid, Lactose, Acacia, Potassium Iodide, Biotin, Sodium Molybdate, Chromium Chloride, Phytonadione (Vit. K) and Cyanocobalamin (Vit. B_{12}).

Contains Asparatame **Phenylketonurics: Contains Phenylalanine.

Warnings: CLOSE TIGHTLY AND KEEP OUT OF REACH OF CHILDREN. CONTAINS IRON, WHICH CAN BE HARMFUL OR FATAL TO CHILDREN IN LARGE DOSES. IN CASE OF ACCIDENTAL OVERDOSE, SEEK PROFESSIONAL ASSISTANCE OR CONTACT A POISON CONTROL CENTER IMMEDIATELY.

Recommended Intake: Children 2 to 4 years of age: Chew approximately one-half tablet daily. Children over 4 years of age: Chew one tablet daily.

How Supplied: Assorted flavors—Uncoated Tablet Bottle of 60

Tamper-evident feature: Bottle sealed with printed foil under cap. If foil is torn, do not accept.
Store at Room Temperature.

 Centrum Jr. is a dietary supplement.

CENTRUM, JR.®

[*sĕn-trŭm*]

Shamu and his Crew®
+EXTRA CALCIUM
Children's Chewable Vitamin/Mineral Formula

[See table at top of next page.]

Ingredients: Calcium Phosphate, Calcium Carbonate, Sugar, Sorbitol, Magnesium Oxide, Ascorbic Acid (Vit. C), (Food) Starch, Microcrystalline Cellulose, Citric Acid, Mono- and Diglycerides, Gelatin, Modified Food Starch, *dl*-alpha Tocopheryl Acetate (Vit. E), Stearic Acid, Artificial flavors, Niacinamide, Zinc Oxide, Iron Carbonyl, FD&C Red #40, FD&C Yellow #6, FD&C Blue #2, Calcium Pantothenate, Vitamin A Acetate/Vitamin D, Silicon Dioxide, Aspartame**, Magnesium Sterate, Partially Hydrogenated Coconut Oil, Pyridoxine Hydrochloride (Vit. B_6), Cupric Oxide, Riboflavin (Vit. B_2), Thiamin Mononitrate (Vit. B_1), Dextrose, Manganese Sulfate, Beta Carotene, Folic Acid, Lactose, Acacia, Potassium Iodide, Biotin, Sodium Molybdate, Chromium Chloride, Phytonadione (Vit. K) and Cyanocobalamin (Vit. B_{12}).

Contains Asparatame ****Phenylketonurics: Contains Phenylalanine.**

Warnings: CLOSE TIGHTLY AND KEEP OUT OF THE REACH OF

Continued on next page

Lederle Consumer Health—Cont.

CHILDREN. CONTAINS IRON, WHICH CAN BE HARMFUL OR FATAL TO CHILDREN IN LARGE DOSES. IN CASE OF ACCIDENTAL OVERDOSE, SEEK PROFESSIONAL ASSISTANCE OR CONTACT A POISON CONTROL CENTER IMMEDIATELY.

Recommended Intake: Children 2 to 4 years of age: chew approximately one-half tablet daily. Children over 4 years of age: chew one tablet daily.

How Supplied : Assorted Flavors—Uncoated Tablet—Bottle of 60

Tamper-evident feature: Bottle sealed with printed foil under cap. If foil is torn, do not accept.

Store at Room Temperature.

 Centrum, Jr. is a dietary supplement.

CENTRUM, JR.®
[sĕn-trŭm]
Shamu and his Crew®
+ IRON
Children's Chewable Vitamin/Mineral Formula

[See table at right.]

Ingredients: Sugar, Calcium Phosphate, Sorbitol, Calcium Carbonate, Citric Acid, Magnesium Oxide, Ascorbic Acid (Vit. C), (Food) Starch, Microcrystalline, Cellulose, Mono- and Diglycerides, Gelatin, *dl*-alpha Tocopheryl Acetate (Vit. E), Stearic Acid, Artificial Flavors, Modified Food Starch, Niacinamide, Zinc Oxide, Iron Carbonyl, FD&C Red #40, FD&C Yellow #6, FD&C Blue #2, Calcium Pantothenate, Vitamin A Acetate/Vitamin D, Aspartame**, Silicon Dioxide, Magnesium Sterate, Partially Hydrogenated Coconut Oil, Pyridoxine Hydrochloride (Vit. B_6), Cupric Oxide, Riboflavin (Vit. B_2), Thiamin Mononitrate (Vit. B_1), Dextrose, Manganese Sulfate, Beta Carotene, Folic Acid, Lactose, Acacia, Potassium Iodide, Biotin, Sodium Molybdate, Chromium Chloride, Phytonadione (Vit. K) and Cyanocobalamin (Vit. B_{12}).

Contains Aspartame. **Phenylketonurics: Contains Phenylalanine.

Warnings: CLOSE TIGHTLY AND KEEP OUT OF REACH OF CHILDREN. CONTAINS IRON, WHICH CAN BE HARMFUL OR FATAL TO CHILDREN IN LARGE DOSES. IN CASE OF ACCIDENTAL OVERDOSE, SEEK PROFESSIONAL ASSISTANCE OR CONTACT A POISON CONTROL CENTER IMMEDIATELY.

CENTRUM, JR.® +EXTRA CALCIUM

Nutrition Facts Serving Size:	Children 2–4 Years Old ½ tablet		Children Over 4 Years Old 1 tablet	
	Amount Per Serving	% Daily Value	Amount Per Serving	% Daily Value
Vitamin A (20% as Beta Carotene)	2500 IU	100%	5000 IU	100%
Vitamin C	30 mg	75%	60 mg	100%
Vitamin D	200 IU	50%	400 IU	100%
Vitamin E	15 IU	150%	30 IU	100%
Thiamin	0.75 mg	107%	1.5 mg	100%
Riboflavin	0.85 mg	106%	1.7 mg	100%
Niacinamide	10 mg	111%	20 mg	100%
Vitamin B_6	1 mg	143%	2 mg	100%
Folic Acid	200 mcg	100%	400 mcg	100%
Vitamin B_{12}	3 mcg	100%	6 mcg	100%
Biotin	22.5 mcg	15%	45 mcg	15%
Pantothenic Acid	5 mg	100%	10 mg	100%
Calcium	80 mg	10%	160 mg	16%
Iron	9 mg	90%	18 mg	100%
Phosphorous	25 mg	3%	50 mg	5%
Iodine	75 mcg	107%	150 mcg	100%
Magnesium	20 mg	10%	40 mg	10%
Zinc	7.5 mg	94%	15 mg	100%
Copper	1 mg	100%	2 mg	100%
Vitamin K	5 mcg	*	10 mcg	*
Manganese	0.5 mg	*	1 mg	*
Chromium	10 mcg	*	20 mcg	*
Molybdenum	10 mcg	*	20 mcg	*

*Daily Value not established.

CENTRUM, JR.® + IRON

Nutrition Facts Serving Size:	Children 2–4 Years Old ½ tablet		Children Over 4 Years Old 1 tablet	
	Amount Per Serving	% Daily Value	Amount Per Serving	% Daily Value
Vitamin A (20% as Beta Carotene)	2500 IU	100%	5000 IU	100%
Vitamin C	30 mg	75%	60 mg	100%
Vitamin D	200 IU	50%	400 IU	100%
Vitamin E	15 IU	150%	30 IU	100%
Thiamin	0.75 mg	107%	1.5 mg	100%
Riboflavin	0.85 mg	106%	1.7 mg	100%
Niacinamide	10 mg	111%	20 mg	100%
Vitamin B_6	1 mg	143%	2 mg	100%
Folic Acid	200 mcg	100%	400 mcg	100%
Vitamin B_{12}	3 mcg	100%	6 mcg	100%
Biotin	22.5 mcg	15%	45 mcg	15%
Pantothenic Acid	5 mg	100%	10 mg	100%
Calcium	54 mg	7%	108 mg	11%
Iron	9 mg	90%	18 mg	100%
Phosphorous	25 mg	3%	50 mg	5%
Iodine	75 mcg	107%	150 mcg	100%
Magnesium	20 mg	10%	40 mg	10%
Zinc	7.5 mg	94%	15 mg	100%
Copper	1 mg	100%	2 mg	100%
Vitamin K	5 mcg	*	10 mcg	*
Manganese	0.5 mg	*	1 mg	*
Chromium	10 mcg	*	20 mcg	*
Molybdenum	10 mcg	*	20 mcg	*

*Daily Value not established.

Recommended Intake: Children 2 to 4 years of age: Chew approximately one-half tablet daily. Children over 4 years of age: Chew one tablet daily.

How Supplied: Assorted Flavors—Uncoated Tablet—Bottle of 60

Tamper-evident feature: Bottle sealed with printed foil under cap. If foil is torn, do not accept.

Store at Room Temperature.

 Centrum, Jr. is a dietary supplement

CENTRUM® SILVER®
Multivitamin/Multimineral for Adults 50+
Complete From A to Zinc®

Nutrition Facts
Serving Size 1 Tablet

Each Tablet Contains	%DV
Vitamin A 5000 IU (50% as Beta Carotene)	100%
Vitamin C 60 mg	100%
Vitamin D 400 IU	100%
Vitamin E 45 IU	150%
Thiamin 1.5 mg	100%
Riboflavin 1.7 mg	100%
Niacinamide 20 mg	100%
Vitamin B_6 3 mg	150%
Folic Acid 400 mcg	100%
Vitamin B_{12} 25 mcg	416%
Biotin 30 mcg	10%
Pantothenic Acid 10 mg	100%
Calcium 200 mg	20%
Iron 4 mg	22%
Phosphorus 48 mg	5%
Iodine 150 mcg	100%
Magnesium 100 mg	25%
Zinc 15 mg	100%
Copper 2 mg	100%
Potassium 80 mg	2%
Vitamin K 10 mcg	*
Selenium 20 mcg	*
Manganese 3.5 mg	*
Chromium 130 mcg	*
Molybdenum 160 mcg	*
Chloride 72 mg	*
Nickel 5 mcg	*
Silicon 2 mg	*
Vanadium 10 mcg	*
Boron 150 mcg	*

*Daily Value (% DV) not established.

Recommended Intake:
Adults, 1 tablet daily.

Warning: Close tightly and keep out of reach of children. Contains iron, which can be harmful or fatal to children in large doses. In case of accidental overdose, seek professional assistance or contact a Poison Control Center immediately.

Ingredients: Calcium Carbonate, Calcium Phosphate, Magnesium Oxide, Potassium Chloride, Microcrystalline Cellulose, Ascorbic Acid (Vit. C), Gelatin, *dl*-alpha Tocopheryl Acetate (Vit. E), Modified Food Starch, Maltodextrin, Crospovidone, Ferrous Fumarate, Hydroxypropyl Methylcellulose, Niacinamide, Zinc Oxide, Calcium Pantothenate, Manganese Sulfate, Vitamin D, Titanium Dioxide, Vitamin A, Magnesium Stearate, Stearic Acid, Pyridoxine Hydrochloride (Vit. B_6), Riboflavin (Vit. B_2), Silicon Dioxide, Cupric Oxide, Beta Carotene, Dextrose, Thiamin Mononitrate (Vit. B_1), Triethyl Citrate, Polysorbate 80, Chromium Chloride, FD&C Blue #2, FD&C Yellow #6, Folic Acid, Potassium Iodide, FD&C Red #40, Sodium Metasilicate, Sodium Molybdate, Borates, Sodium Selenate, Biotin, Sodium Metavanadate, Cyanocobalamin (Vit. B_{12}), Nickelous Sulfate and Phytonadione (Vit. K).

How Supplied: Bottle of 60
Bottle of 100
Store at Room Temperature.

FERRO-SEQUELS®
[fer″rō-sē′quls]
High potency, timed-release iron supplement.
Specially formulated for optimal absorption with less gastric upset. Easy to swallow tablets. Low sodium, no sugar.

The Ferro-Sequels timed-release system delivers iron slowly and gently to maximize absorption while reducing gastric upset common with regular iron tablets. Ferro-Sequels is the effective and gentle way to treat simple iron deficiency and iron deficiency anemia.

Nutrition Facts
Serving Size 1 Tablet

Each Tablet Contains	% Daily Value
Iron 50 mg	277%

Recommended Intake: One tablet daily or as directed by a health care professional.

Warning: Keep out of reach of children. Contains iron, which can be harmful or fatal to children in large doses. In case of accidental overdose, seek professional assistance or contact a Poison Control Center immediately. As with any supplement, if you are pregnant or nursing a baby, seek the advice of a health care professional before using this product.

Ingredients: Lactose, Ferrous Fumarate, Microcrystalline Cellulose, Hydroxypropyl Methylcellulose, Docusate Sodium, Magnesium Stearate, Sodium Benzoate, Silicon Dioxide, Mineral Oil, Titanium Dioxide, Yellow #10, Blue #1 and Sodium Lauryl Sulfate.
Store at Room Temperature.

How Supplied: Box of 30 tablets
Bottle of 30 tablets
Bottle of 100 tablets
Blister pack of 30 tablets
Store at Room Temperature
LEDERLE CONSUMER HEALTH DIVISION
MADE IN USA

FIBERCON®
[fī-bĕr-cŏn]
Calcium Polycarbophil
Bulk-Forming Fiber Laxative

Indications: Helps restore and maintain regularity and relieve constipation. The product generally produces bowel movement in 12 to 72 hours.

Directions: FIBERCON® works naturally so continued use for one to three days is normally required to produce full benefit. FIBERCON dosage may vary according to diet, exercise, previous laxative use or severity of constipation. **TAKE THIS PRODUCT ACCORDING TO THE DOSAGE CHART WITH A FULL GLASS (8 OUNCES) OF LIQUID. TAKING THIS PRODUCT WITHOUT ENOUGH LIQUID MAY CAUSE CHOKING. SEE WARNINGS.**
Do not take more than the maximum daily dose.

[See table below.]

Warnings: Do not use laxative products when abdominal pain, nausea or vomiting are present unless directed by a doctor. If you have noticed a sudden change in bowel habits that persists over a period of 2 weeks, consult a doctor before using a laxative. Laxative products should not be used for a period longer than 1 week unless directed by a doctor. Rectal bleeding or failure to have a bowel movement after use of a laxative may indicate a serious condition. Discontinue use and consult your doctor. **TAKING THIS PRODUCT WITHOUT ADEQUATE FLUID MAY CAUSE IT TO SWELL AND BLOCK YOUR THROAT OR ESOPHAGUS AND MAY CAUSE CHOKING. DO NOT TAKE THIS PRODUCT IF YOU HAVE DIFFICULTY IN SWALLOWING. IF YOU EXPERIENCE CHEST PAIN, VOMITING, OR DIFFICULTY IN SWALLOWING OR BREATHING AFTER TAKING THIS PRODUCT, SEEK IMMEDIATE MEDICAL ATTENTION.** Keep this and all medicines out of the reach of children. In case of accidental overdose, seek professional assistance or contact a poison control center immediately.

Interaction Precaution: Contains calcium. If you are taking any form of tetracycline antibiotic, FIBERCON should be taken at least 1 hour before or 2 hours after you have taken the antibiotic.

FIBERCON®

Age	Recommended Dose	Daily Maximum
Adults & Children over 12	2 caplets once a day	Up to 4 times a day*
Children (6 to 12 years)	1 caplet once a day	Up to 4 times a day*
Children under 6 years	Consult a physician	

*Refer to directions

Continued on next page

Lederle Consumer Health—Cont.

Ingredients: Each caplet contains 625 mg calcium polycarbophil equivalent to 500 mg polycarbophil.

Inactive Ingredients: Calcium Carbonate, Caramel, Crospovidone, Hydroxypropyl Methylcellulose, Magnesium Stearate, Microcrystalline Cellulose, Mineral Oil, Povidone, Silica Gel and Sodium Lauryl Sulfate.
Store At Controlled Room Temperature 15–30° C (59–86°F).
Protect Contents From Moisture.
TAMPER RESISTANT FEATURE: Bottle sealed with printed foil under cap or in plastic blister with foil backing. Do not accept if foil barrier or plastic blister is broken.

How Supplied: Film-coated caplets, scored, engraved LL and F66.
Package of 36 caplets.
Bottles of 60 caplets.
Bottle of 90 caplets.
LEDERLE CONSUMER HEALTH DIVISION

PROTEGRA®
[*prō-tĕg-ră*]
Antioxidant Vitamin & Mineral Supplement

Nutrition Facts
Serving Size 1 Softgel

Each Softgel Contains	% Daily Value
Vitamin A 5000 IU (100% as Beta Carotene)	100%
Vitamin C 250 mg	417%
Vitamin E 200 IU	667%
Zinc 7.5 mg	50%
Copper 1 mg	50%
Selenium 15 mcg	*
Manganese 1.5 mg	*

* Daily Value not established

Ingredients: Ascorbic Acid (Vit. C), *dl*-alpha Tocopheryl Acetate (Vit E), Gelatin, Cottonseed Oil, Glycerin, Sorbitol, Calcium Phosphate, Lecithin, Zinc Oxide, Beeswax, Maganese Sulfate, Soybean Oil, Beta Carotene, FD&C Red #40, Cupric Oxide, Titanium Dioxide, Sodium Selenate and FD&C Blue #1.
May contain edible ink.

Recommended Intake: Adults: One or two softgels daily or as directed by your physician. PROTEGRA® can be taken by itself or with a multiple vitamin.

How Supplied: Bottle of 50
Store at Controlled Room Temperature 15°–30°C (59°–86°F)
Protect Contents From Moisture
Natural color variations in the softgels may occur.

Warning: Keep out of the reach of children.

STRESSTABS®
[*strĕss-tăbs*]
High Potency Stress Formula Vitamins

Nutrition Facts
Serving Size 1 Tablet

Each Tablet Contains	% Daily Value
Vitamin C 500 mg	833%
Vitamin E 30 IU	100%
Thiamin 10 mg	667%
Riboflavin 10 mg	588%
Niacinamide 100 mg	500%
Vitamin B_6 5 mg	250%
Folic Acid 400 mcg	100%
Vitamin B_{12} 12 mcg	200%
Biotin 45 mcg	15%
Pantothenic Acid 20 mg	200%

Recommended Intake: Adults, 1 tablet daily or as directed by physician.

Warning: Keep out of reach of children

Ingredients: Ascorbic Acid (Vit. C), Microcrystalline Cellulose, Niacinamide, Calcium Carbonate, *dl*-Tocopheryl Acetate (Vit. E), Modified Food Starch, Calcium Pantothenate, Thiamin Mononitrate (Vit. B_1), Riboflavin (Vit. B_2), Mineral Oil, Pyridoxine Hydrochloride (Vit. B_6), Magnesium Stearate, Silicon Dioxide, FD&C Yellow #6, Stearic Acid, Folic Acid, Biotin, and Cyanocobalamin (Vit. B_{12}).

How Supplied: Capsule-shaped tablet (film coated, orange, scored). Engraved LL and S1.
Bottle of 60
Store at Room Temperature.
LEDERLE CONSUMER HEALTH DIVISION

STRESSTABS® + IRON
[*strĕss-tăbs*]
High Potency Stress Formula Vitamins

Nutrition Facts
Serving Size 1 Tablet

Each Tablet Contains	% Daily Value
Vitamin C 500 mg	833%
Vitamin E 30 IU	100%
Thiamin 10 mg	667%
Riboflavin 10 mg	588%
Niacinamide 100 mg	500%
Vitamin B_6 5 mg	250%
Folic Acid 400 mcg	100%
Vitamin B_{12} 12 mcg	200%
Biotin 45 mcg	15%
Pantothenic Acid 20 mg	200%
Iron 18 mg	100%

Recommended Intake: Adults, 1 tablet daily or as directed by the physician.

Warning: Close tightly, and keep out of reach of children. Contains iron, which can be harmful or fatal to children in large doses. In case of accidental overdose, seek professional assistance or contact a Poison Control Center immediately.

Ingredients: Ascorbic Acid (Vit. C), Niacinamide, Microcrystalline Cellulose, *dl*-Tocopheryl Acetate (Vit. E), Ferrous Fumarate, Calcium Carbonate, Modified Food Starch, Calcium Pantothenate, Thiamin Mononitrate (Vit. B_1), Stearic Acid, Riboflavin (Vit. B_2), Magnesium Stearate, Mineral Oil, Silicon Dioxide, Pyridoxine Hydrochloride (Vit. B_6), FD&C Yellow #6, FD&C Red #40, Folic Acid, Biotin, and Cyanocobalamin (Vit. B_{12}).

How Supplied: Capsule-shaped tablets (film coated, orange red, scored). Engraved LL and S2.
Bottle of 60
Store at Room Temperature.
LEDERLE CONSUMER HEALTH DIVISION

STRESSTABS® + ZINC
[*strĕss-tăbs*]
High Potency Stress Formula Vitamins

Nutrition Facts
Serving Size 1 Tablet

Each Tablet Contains	% Daily Value
Vitamin C 500 mg	833%
Vitamin E 30 IU	100%
Thiamin 10 mg	667%
Riboflavin 10 mg	588%
Niacinamide 100 mg	500%
Vitamin B_6 5 mg	250%
Folic Acid 400 mcg	100%
Vitamin B_{12} 12 mcg	200%
Biotin 45 mcg	15%
Pantothenic Acid 20 mg	200%
Zinc 23.9 mg	159%
Copper 3 mg	150%

Recommended Intake: Adults, 1 tablet daily or as directed by the physician.

Warning: Keep out of reach of children.

Ingredients: Ascorbic Acid (Vit. C), Niacinamide, Microcrystalline Cellulose, *dl*-Tocopheryl Acetate (Vit. E), Calcium Carbonate, Modified Food Starch, Calcium Pantothenate, Zinc Oxide, Thiamin Mononitrate (Vit. B_1), Riboflavin (Vit. B_2), Mineral Oil, Silicon Dioxide, Pyridoxine Hydrochloride (Vit. B_6), Stearic Acid, Cupric Oxide, Magnesium Stearate, FD&C Yellow #6, Folic Acid, Biotin, and Cyanocobalamin (Vit. B_{12}).

How Supplied: Capsule-shaped tablet (film coated, peach color, scored). Engraved LL and S3.
Bottle of 60
Store at Room Temperature.
LEDERLE CONSUMER HEALTH DIVISION

3M

BUILDING 515-3N-02
ST PAUL, MN 55144-1000

Direct Inquiries to:
Customer Service
(800) 537-2191

For Medical Emergencies Contact:
(612) 733-2882 (answered 24 hrs.)

Sales and Ordering or Returns:
(800) 832-2189

3M™ TITRALAC™ ANTACID AND TITRALAC™ EXTRA STRENGTH ANTACID

[*T ī' tră lăc*]

Active Ingredients: Calcium Carbonate: *Regular:* 420mg./tablet (168 mg. elemental calcium). *Extra Strength:* 750mg/tablet (300 mg. elemental calcium).

Inactive Ingredients: Glycine, Magnesium Stearate, Saccharin, Spearmint Oil, Starch.

Indications: A spearmint flavored non-chalky antacid tablet which quickly relieves heartburn, sour stomach, acid indigestion and upset stomach associated with these symptoms.

Dosage and Administration: *Regular:* Two tablets every two or three hours as symptoms occur or as directed by a physician. Tablets can be chewed, swallowed or allowed to melt in the mouth. *Extra Strength:* One or two tablets every two or three hours as symptoms occur or as directed by a physician. Tablets can be chewed or allowed to melt in the mouth.

Warnings: *Regular:* Do not take more than 19 tablets in a 24-hour period or use maximum dosage for more than two weeks, except under the advise and supervision of a physician. *Extra Strength:* Do not take more than ten tablets in a 24-hour period or use maximum dosage for more than two weeks, except under the advice and supervision of a physician. **Keep this and all medication out of the reach of children**

Drug Interaction Precaution: Antacids may interact with certain prescription drugs. If you are presently taking a prescription drug, do not take this product without checking with your physician or other health professional.

Dietary Information: Titralac antacid tablets are sugar and aluminum free and have a very low sodium content (1.1 mg/tablet).

How Supplied: *Regular:* Available in bottles of 40, 100, 1000 tablets. *Extra Strength:* Available in bottles of 100 tablets.

Shown in Product Identification Guide, page 509

3M™ TITRALAC™ PLUS ANTACID TITRALAC™ PLUS ANTACID LIQUID AND TABLETS

[*T ī'tră lăc*]

Active Ingredients: *Tablets:* Calcium Carbonate: 420 mg/tablet (168 mg elemental calcium), Simethicone: 21 mg/tablet. *Liquid:* Calcium Carbonate: 1000 mg/2 teaspoons (10 ml.) (400 mg elemental calcium), Simethicone: 40 mg/2 teaspoons (10 ml.)

Inactive Ingredients: *Tablets:* Glycine, Magnesium Stearate, Saccharin, Spearmint Oil, Starch. May also contain Croscarmellose Sodium. *Liquid:* Benzyl Alcohol, Colloidal Silicon Dioxide, Glyceryl Laurate, Methylparaben, Potassium Benzoate, Propylparaben, Saccharin, Sorbitol, Spearmint Flavor, Water, Xanthan Gum.

Indications: A spearmint flavored non-chalky antacid which quickly relieves heartburn, sour stomach, acid indigestion, and accompanying gas often associated with these symptoms.

Dosage and Administration: *Tablets:* Two tablets every two or three hours as symptoms occur or as directed by a physician. Tablets can be chewed, swallowed or allowed to melt in the mouth. *Liquid:* Two teaspoons, between meals and at bedtime or as directed by a physician. Shake well before using.

Warnings: *Tablets:* Do not take more than 19 tablets in a 24-hour period or use maximum dosage for more than two weeks, except under the advice and supervision of a physician. *Liquid:* do not take more than 16 teaspoons in a 24-hour period, or use maximum dosage for more than two weeks, except under the advice and supervision of a physician. Keep this and all medication out of the reach of children.

Drug Interaction Precaution: Antacids may interact with certain prescription drugs. If you are presently taking a prescription drug, do not take this product without checking with your physician or other health professional.

Dietary Information: Tablets and liquid are sugar and aluminum free. Tablets: very low sodium, 1.1 mg/tablet. Liquid: low sodium, 5 mg/2 teaspoons.

How Supplied: *Tablets:* Available in bottles of 100 tablets. *Liquid:* Available in 12 fl. oz. bottles.

Shown in Product Identification Guide, page 509

Marlyn Nutraceuticals

14851 N. SCOTTSDALE RD
SCOTTSDALE, AZ 85254

Direct Inquiries to:
Joe Lehmann
(602) 991-0200
FAX: (602) 991-0551

MARLYN FORMULA 50®

PRODUCT OVERVIEW

Key Facts: MARLYN FORMULA 50 is a combination of amino acids and B6 in a gelatin capsule which provides protein "building blocks" important to growth and development of all protein containing tissue including nails, hair and skin.

Major Uses: Dermatologists recommend Formula 50 not only for splitting, peeling nails but also prescribe it in conjunction with their favorite topical cream for control of nail fungus. OB-Gyn's recommend it for help in controlling excessive hair fall-out after child birth.
The recommended daily dose is six capsules daily.

Safety Information: There are no known contraindications or adverse reactions.

PRESCRIBING INFORMATION

MARLYN FORMULA 50®

Composition: Each capsule contains:
Amino Acids................................0.3 Gm*
Vitamin B6 (pyridoxine HCl)......1.0 mg.
*Approximate analysis of the amino acids: indispensable amino acids (lysine, tryptophan, phenylalanine, methionine, threonine, leucine, isoleucine, valine), 35.30%; semi-dispensable amino acids (arginine, histidine, tyrosine, cystine, glycine), 19.18%; dispensable amino acids (glutamic acid, alanine, aspartic acid, serine, proline), 45.56%.
Amino acids: Protein "building blocks" important to growth and development of all protein containing tissue including nails, hair, and skin.

Dosage and Administration: The recommended daily dose is 6 capsules daily.

Supply: Bottles of 100, 250.

FACED WITH AN Rx SIDE EFFECT?
Turn to the
Companion Drug Index
(Green Pages)
for products that
provide symptomatic
relief.

Mayor Pharmaceutical Laboratories

KareMor International
2401 S. 24TH ST.
PHOENIX, AZ 85034

Direct Inquiries to:
Medical Director
(602) 244-8899

VITAMIST® Intra-Oral Spray Dietary Supplements

Description: Vitamist sprays are patented Intra-Oral applications of vitamin, mineral and amino acid supplementation. A 50 microliter spray delivers high concentrations of nutrients directly into the mouth's sensitive tissue. The buccal mucosa transfers the nutrients into the bloodstream, bypassing the G.I. tract. (U.S. Patent 4,525,341—Foreign patents pending.)

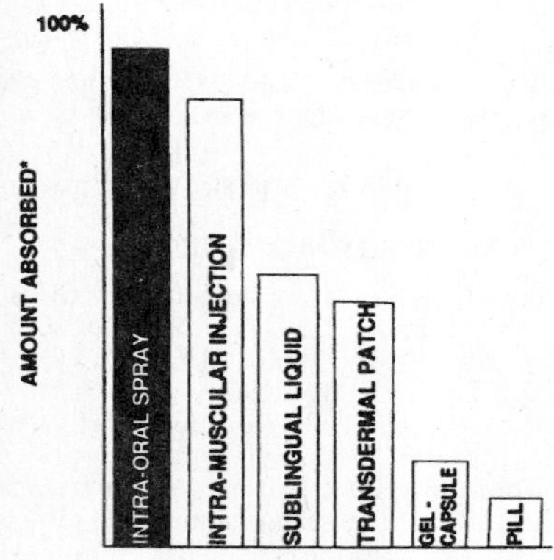

*Representative of the product class.

Product Formulations and Composition:
Anti-Oxidant beta carotene and vitamins A, C and E help irradicate free radicals from system
Multiple essential vitamins and trace minerals in adult/prenatal/children's formulas
Vitamin C + Zinc with lysine and bioflavonoids
Stress double compounded B-complex vitamins in a herbal base
Vitamin B-12 1000% of USRDA per dose
Vitamin E 100% USRDA mixed tocopherols with selenium.
Blue Green Sea Spray Rich in Omega-3 and Omega-6 Fatty acids and GLA
Colloidal Minerals 77 trace and major minerals from natural plant sources
Folacin folic acid prevents neural tube defects.
Herbal Re-leaf minor discomfort, anxiety and distress relief
Melatonin a natural hormone effective in re-establishing waking/sleeping cycles.
Pro-Bio Mist PB/GS pine bark and grape seed source proanthocyanidin.
PMS supplements the nutrient needs during syndrome
Smoke-less® herbal combination with additional nutrients, replace habits
Slendermist® dietary snack replacements with a combination of B vitamins, HCA, L-carnitine and chromium

Dosage and Administration: 8 sprays = 1 dose (except Vit. A formula, 1 spray = 1 dose). Spray directly into mouth 2 sprays 4 times per day.

How Supplied: Vitamist Intra-Oral sprays are supplied in a 13.3 ml vial containing approximately 240 metered sprays from a nonaerosol pump

---

McNeil Consumer Products Company

Division of McNeil-PPC, Inc.
FORT WASHINGTON, PA 19034

Direct Inquiries to:
Consumer Affairs Department
Fort Washington, PA 19034
(215) 233-7000

Children's MOTRIN® Ibuprofen Oral Suspension and Drops

Description: ***Children's MOTRIN® Ibuprofen Oral Suspension*** and ***Children's MOTRIN® Drops*** are alcohol-free, berry-flavored liquid especially developed for children. Each 5 mL (teaspoon) of Children's MOTRIN® Ibuprofen Oral Suspension contains ibuprofen 100 mg. Each 1.25 mL (dropperful) of Children's MOTRIN® Drops contains ibuprofen 50 mg.

Indications: ***Children's MOTRIN® Ibuprofen Oral Suspension*** and ***Children's MOTRIN® Drops*** are indicated for temporary relief of fever, and minor aches and pains due to colds, flu, sore throat, headaches and toothaches. One dose lasts 6–8 hours.

Directions: ***Children's MOTRIN® Ibuprofen Oral Suspension***: Shake well before using. A calibrated dosage cup is provided for accurate dosing of ***Children's MOTRIN® Suspension.*** If possible, use weight to dose; otherwise use age. 2–3 years (24–35 lbs): 1 tsp, 4–5 years (36–47 lbs): 1.5 tsp, 6–8 years (48–59 lbs): 2 tsp, 9–10 years (60–71 lbs): 2.5 tsp, 11 years (72–95 lbs): 3 tsp. ***Children's MOTRIN® Drops*** : Shake well before using. A calibrated dropper is provided for accurate dosing. If possible, use weight to dose; otherwise, use age. 2–3 years (24–35 lbs): 2 dropperfuls (2 × 1.25 mL). Under 2 years consult a physician. Repeat dose every 6–8 hours, if needed. Do not use more than 4 times a day.

Warnings: ASPIRIN SENSITIVE CHILDREN:
- **This product contains no aspirin, but may cause a severe reaction in people allergic to aspirin.**
- **Do not use this product if your child has had an allergic reaction to aspirin such as asthma, swelling, shock or hives.**

CALL YOUR DOCTOR IF:
- Your child is under a doctor's care for any serious condition or is taking any other drug.
- Your child has problems or serious side effects from taking fever reducers or pain relievers.
- Your child does not get any relief within first day (24 hours) of treatment, or pain or fever gets worse.
- Redness or swelling is present in the painful area.
- Sore throat is severe, lasts for more than 2 days or occurs with fever, headache, rash, nausea or vomiting.
- Any new symptoms appear.

DO NOT USE:
- With any other product that contains ibuprofen, or other pain reliever/fever reducers, unless directed by a doctor.
- For more than **3 days** for fever or pain unless directed by a doctor.
- For stomach pain unless directed by a doctor.
- If your child is dehydrated (significant fluid loss) due to continued vomiting, diarrhea or lack of fluid intake.
- If plastic bottle wrap imprinted with "Safety Seal", or foil inner seal on bottle opening imprinted with "Safety Seal" is broken.

IMPORTANT:
- **Keep this and all drugs out of the reach of children. In case of accidental overdose, seek professional assistance or contact a poison control center immediately.**
- If stomach upset occurs while taking this product, give with food or milk. If stomach upset gets worse or lasts, call your doctor.

Inactive Ingredients: ***Children's MOTRIN® Ibuprofen Oral Suspension***: Citric acid, corn starch, artificial flavors, glycerin, polysorbate 80, purified water, sodium benzoate, sucrose, xanthan gum, FD&C Red #40, D&C Yellow #10.
Children's MOTRIN® Drops: Citric acid, cornstarch, artificial flavors, glycerin, polysorbate 80, purified water, sodium benzoate, sorbitol, sucrose, xanthan gum, FD&C Red #40.

How Supplied: ***Children's MOTRIN® Ibuprofen Oral Suspension***: Orange colored liquid in tamper-resistant bottles of 2 and 4 fl. oz.
Children's MOTRIN® Drops: Pink colored liquid in 1/2 fl. oz. bottles.
Store at controlled room temperature 15°–30°C (59°–86°F).

Shown in Product Identification Guide, page 510

CHILDREN'S TYLENOL®
acetaminophen
Chewable Tablets, Elixir, Suspension Liquid and Suspension Drops

Description: ***INFANTS' TYLENOL® Grape Suspension Drops*** are stable, alcohol-free, grape-flavored and purple in color. ***INFANTS' TYLENOL® Cherry Suspension Drops*** are stable, alcohol-free, cherry-flavored and red in color. Each 0.8 ml (one calibrated dropperful) contains 80 mg acetaminophen. ***CHILDREN'S TYLENOL® Elixir*** is stable and alcohol-free, cherry-flavored, and red in color. ***CHILDREN'S TYLENOL® Suspension Liquid*** is stable, alcohol-free, cherry-flavored, and red in color, or bubble gum flavored, and pink in color or grape flavored and purple in color. Each 5 ml (one teaspoonful) contains 160 mg acetaminophen. Each ***CHILDREN'S TYLENOL® Chewable Tablet*** contains 80 mg acetaminophen in a grape, bubble gum, or fruit burst flavor.

Actions: Acetaminophen is a clinically proven analgesic/antipyretic. Acetaminophen produces analgesia by elevation of the pain threshold and antipyresis through action on the hypothalamic heat regulating center. Acetaminophen is equal to aspirin in analgesic and antipyretic effectiveness and it is unlikely to produce many of the side effects associated with aspirin and aspirin containing products.

Indications: ***CHILDREN'S TYLENOL® Chewable Tablets, Elixir, Suspension Liquid*** and ***Suspension Drops*** are designed for treatment of infants and children with conditions requiring temporary relief of fever and discomfort due to colds and "flu," and of simple pain and discomfort due to teething, immunizations and tonsillectomy.

Precautions: If a rare sensitivity reaction occurs, the drug should be stopped.

Usual Dosage: All dosages may be repeated every 4 hours, but not more than 5 times daily. Administer to children under 2 years only on the advice of a physician. ***CHILDREN'S TYLENOL Chewable Tablets:*** 2–3 years: two tablets, 4–5 years: three tablets, 6–8 years: four tablets, 9–10 years: five tablets, 11–12 years: six tablets.
CHILDREN'S TYLENOL® Elixir and ***Suspension Liquid:*** (special cup for measuring dosage is provided) 4–11 months: one-half teaspoon, 12–23 months: three-quarters teaspoon, 2–3 years: one teaspoon, 4–5 years: one and one-half teaspoons, 6–8 years: 2 teaspoons, 9–10 years: two and one-half teaspoons, 11–12 years: three teaspoons.
INFANTS' TYLENOL® Suspension Drops: 0–3 months: 0.4 ml, 4–11 months: 0.8 ml, 12–23 months: 1.2 ml, 2–3 years: 1.6 ml, 4–5 years: 2.4 ml.

Warnings: Do not take for pain more than 5 days or for fever for more than 3 days unless directed by a physician. If pain or fever persists or gets worse, if new symptoms occur, or if redness or swelling is present, consult a physician because these could be signs of a serious condition. Keep this and all drugs out of the reach of children. In case of accidental overdose, contact a physician or poison control center immediately. Prompt medical attention is critical even if you do not notice any signs or symptoms. Do not use with other products containing acetaminophen.
NOTE: In addition to the above:
INFANTS' TYLENOL® Suspension Drops—Do not use if printed carton overwrap or printed plastic bottle wrap is broken or missing or if carton is opened.
CHILDREN'S TYLENOL® Elixir and Suspension Liquid—Do not use if printed carton overwrap is broken or missing or if carton is opened. Do not use if printed plastic bottle wrap or printed foil inner seal is broken. Not a USP elixir.
CHILDREN'S TYLENOL® Chewables—Do not use if carton is opened or if printed foil inner seal is broken. Phenylketonurics: grape contains phenylalanine 3 mg per tablet, bubble gum contains 6 mg per tablet, fruit burst contains 4.5 mg per tablet.

Overdosage Information: Acetaminophen in massive overdosage may cause hepatic toxicity in some patients. In adults and adolescents, hepatic toxicity has rarely been reported following ingestion of acute overdoses of less than 10 grams. Fatalities are infrequent (less than 3–4% of untreated cases) and have rarely been reported with overdoses of less than 15 grams. In children, an acute overdosage of less than 150 mg/kg has not been associated with hepatic toxicity. Early symptoms following a potentially hepatotoxic overdose may include: nausea, vomiting, diaphoresis and general malaise. Clinical and laboratory evidence of hepatic toxicity may not be apparent until 48 to 72 hours postingestion. In adults and adolescents, regardless of the quantity of acetaminophen reported to have been ingested, administer acetylcysteine immediately if 24 hours or less have elapsed from the reported time of ingestion. For full prescribing information, refer to the acetylcysteine package insert. Do not await results of assays for acetaminophen level before initiating treatment with acetylcysteine. The following additional procedures are recommended: The stomach should be emptied promptly by lavage or by induction of emesis with syrup of ipecac. A serum acetaminophen assay should be obtained as early as possible, but no sooner than four hours following ingestion. Liver function studies should be obtained initially and repeated at 24-hour intervals.
Serious toxicity or fatalities are extremely infrequent in children, possibly due to differences in the way they metabolize acetaminophen. In children, the maximum potential amount ingested can be more easily estimated. If more than 150 mg/kg or an unknown amount was ingested, obtain an acetaminophen plasma level. The acetaminophen plasma level should be obtained as soon as possible, but no sooner than 4 hours following the ingestion. Induce emesis using syrup of ipecac. If the plasma level is obtained and falls above the broken line on the acetaminophen overdose nomogram, the acetylcysteine therapy should be initiated and continued for a full course of therapy. If acetaminophen plasma assay capability is not available, and the estimated acetaminophen ingestion exceeds 150 mg/kg, acetylcysteine therapy should be initiated and continued for a full course of therapy.
For additional emergency information, call your regional poison center or call the Rocky Mountain Poison Center toll free, (1-800-525-6115).

Inactive Ingredients: ***CHILDREN'S TYLENOL® Fruit Burst Flavored Chewable Tablets:*** Aspartame, Cellulose (Microcrystalline), Citric Acid, Corn Starch, Flavors, Magnesium Stearate, Mannitol, Red #7. May contain Ethylcellulose or Cellulose Acetate and Povidone.
CHILDREN'S TYLENOL® Grape Flavored Chewable Tablets: Aspartame, Cellulose, Citric Acid, Corn Starch, Flavors, Magnesium Stearate, Mannitol, Blue #1, Red #7, and Red #30. May contain Ethylcellulose or Cellulose Acetate and Povidone.
CHILDREN'S TYLENOL® Bubble Gum Flavored Chewable Tablets: Aspartame, Cellulose, Flavors, Gum Arabic, Magnesium Stearate, Maltodextrin, Mannitol, and Red #7. May contain Ethylcellulose or Cellulose Acetate and Povidone.
CHILDREN'S TYLENOL® Elixir: Benzoic Acid, Citric Acid, Flavors, Glycerin, Polyethylene Glycol, Propylene Glycol, Sodium Benzoate, Sorbitol, Sucrose, Purified Water, Red #33, Red #40.
CHILDREN'S TYLENOL® Suspension Liquid: Butylparaben, Cellulose, Citric Acid, Corn Syrup, Flavors, Glycerin, Propylene Glycol, Purified Water, Sodium Benzoate, Sorbitol, Xanthan Gum. In addition to the above ingredients cherry flavored suspension contains FD&C Red #40, bubble gum flavored suspension contains D&C Red #33, and FD&C Red #40, and grape flavored suspension contains D&C Blue #1 and D&C Red #33.
INFANTS' TYLENOL® Cherry Suspension Drops: Butylparaben, Cellulose, Citric Acid, Corn Syrup, Flavors, Glycerin, Propylene Glycol, Purified Water, Sodium Benzoate, Sorbitol, Xanthan Gum, D&C Red #40.
INFANTS' TYLENOL® Grape Suspension Drops: Butylparaben, Cellulose, Citric Acid, Corn Syrup, Flavors, Glycerin, Propylene Glycol, Purified Water, Sodium Benzoate, Sorbitol, Xanthan Gum, D&C Red #33, and FD&C Blue #1.

Continued on next page

McNeil Consumer—Cont.

How Supplied: Chewable Tablets (pink colored fruit, purple colored grape, pink colored bubble gum, scored, imprinted "TYLENOL")—Bottles of 30 and also blister packaged 60's (fruit burst). **Elixir** (cherry colored red)—bottles of 2 and 4 fl. oz. **Suspension liquid** (cherry colored red)—bottles of 2 and 4 fl. oz. (bubble gum flavored colored pink and grape flavored colored purple)—bottle of 4 fl. oz. **Suspension drops** (grape colored purple)—bottles of 1/2 oz (15 ml) (cherry colored red)—bottles of 1/2 oz and 1 oz, each with calibrated plastic dropper.
All packages listed above have child-resistant safety caps or blisters.

Shown in Product Identification Guide, page 510 and 511

CHILDREN'S TYLENOL® COLD Multi Symptom Chewable Tablets and Liquid

Description: Each ***CHILDREN'S TYLENOL® COLD Multi Symptom Chewable Grape-Flavored Tablet*** contains acetaminophen 80 mg, chlorpheniramine maleate 0.5 mg and pseudoephedrine hydrochloride 7.5 mg. ***CHILDREN'S TYLENOL® COLD Multi Symptom Liquid*** is grape flavored and contains no alcohol. Each teaspoon (5 ml) contains acetaminophen 160 mg, chlorpheniramine maleate 1 mg, and pseudoephedrine hydrochloride 15 mg.

Actions: ***CHILDREN'S TYLENOL® COLD Multi Symptom Chewable Tablets and Liquid*** combine the analgesic-antipyretic acetaminophen with the decongestant pseudoephedrine hydrochloride and the antihistamine chlorpheniramine maleate to help relieve nasal congestion, dry runny noses and prevent sneezing as well as to relieve the fever, aches, pains and general discomfort associated with colds and upper respiratory infections.
Acetaminophen is equal to aspirin in analgesic and antipyretic effectiveness and it is unlikely to produce the side effects often associated with aspirin or aspirin-containing products.

Indications: For temporary relief of nasal congestion, runny nose, sore throat, sneezing, minor aches and pains, headaches and fever due to the common cold, hay fever or other upper respiratory allergies.

Precautions: If a rare sensitivity reaction occurs, the drug should be stopped.

Usual Dosage: All doses may be repeated every 4–6 hours, not to exceed 4 doses in 24 hours.
Administer to children under 6 years only on the advice of a physician. ***CHILDREN'S TYLENOL® COLD Chewable Tablets:*** 2–5 years—2 tablets: 6–11 years—4 tablets.
CHILDREN'S TYLENOL® COLD Liquid Formula: 2–5 years—1 teaspoonful; 6–11 years—2 teaspoonsful. Measuring cup is provided and marked for accurate dosing.

Warning: KEEP THIS AND ALL MEDICATION OUT OF THE REACH OF CHILDREN. IN CASE OF ACCIDENTAL OVERDOSAGE, CONTACT A PHYSICIAN OR POISON CONTROL CENTER IMMEDIATELY. PROMPT MEDICAL ATTENTION IS CRITICAL EVEN IF YOU DO NOT NOTICE ANY SIGNS OR SYMPTOMS. DO NOT USE WITH OTHER PRODUCTS CONTAINING ACETAMINOPHEN. DO NOT EXCEED RECOMMENDED DOSAGE. Do not take for pain for more than 5 days or for fever for more than 3 days unless directed by a doctor. If pain or fever persists or get worse, if new symptoms occur, or if redness or swelling is present, consult a doctor because these could be signs of a serious condition. If sore throat is severe, persists for more than 2 days, is accompanied or followed by fever, headache, rash, nausea, or vomiting, consult a doctor promptly. If nervousness, dizziness, or sleeplessness, occur discontinue use and consult a doctor. May cause excitability especially in children. Do not give this product to children who have a breathing problem such as chronic bronchitis, or who have glaucoma, heart disease, high blood pressure, thyroid disease, or diabetes without first consulting the child's physician. May cause drowsiness. Sedatives and tranquilizers may increase the drowsiness effect. Do not give this product to children who are taking sedatives or tranquilizers, without first consulting the child's doctor.
NOTE: In addition to the above:
CHILDREN'S TYLENOL® COLD CHEWABLES—DO NOT USE IF CARTON IS OPENED, OR IF PRINTED NECK WRAP OR PRINTED FOIL INNER SEAL IS BROKEN. PHENYLKETONURICS: CONTAINS PHENYLALANINE 6 MG PER TABLET.
CHILDREN'S TYLENOL® COLD LIQUID—DO NOT USE IF CARTON IS OPENED, OR IF PRINTED PLASTIC BOTTLE WRAP OR PRINTED FOIL INNER SEAL IS BROKEN.

Drug Interaction Precaution: Do not give this product to a child who is taking a prescription monamine omidase inhibitor (MAOI) (certain drugs for depression, psychiatric or emotional conditions), or for 2 weeks after stopping the MAOI drug. If you are uncertain whether your child's prescription drug contains an MAOI, consult a health professional before giving this product.

Overdosage: Acetaminophen in massive overdosage may cause hepatic toxicity in some patients. In adults and adolescents, hepatic toxicity has rarely been reported following ingestion of acute overdosage of less than 10 grams. Fatalities are infrequent (less than 3–4% of untreated cases) and have rarely been reported with overdoses of less than 15 grams. In children, an acute overdosage of less than 150 mg/kg has not been associated with hepatic toxicity.
Early symptoms following a potentially hepatotoxic overdose may include: nausea, vomiting, diaphoresis and general malaise. Clinical and laboratory evidence of hepatic toxicity may not be apparent until 48 to 72 hours postingestion.
In adults and adolescents, regardless of the quantity of acetaminophen reported to have been ingested, administer acetylcysteine immediately if 24 hours or less have elapsed from the reported time of ingestion. For full prescribing information, refer to the acetylcysteine package insert. Do not await the results of assays for acetaminophen level before initiating treatment with acetylcysteine. The following additional procedures are recommended: The stomach should be emptied promptly by lavage or by induction of emesis with syrup of ipecac. A plasma acetaminophen assay should be obtained as early as possible, but no sooner than four hours following ingestion. Liver function studies should be obtained initially and repeated at 24-hour intervals.
Serious toxicity or fatalities are extremely infrequent in children, possibly due to differences in the way they metabolize acetaminophen. In children, the maximum potential amount ingested can be more easily estimated. If more than 150 mg/kg or an unknown amount was ingested, obtain an plasma acetaminophen level. The acetaminophen plasma level should be obtained as soon as possible, but no sooner than 4 hours following the ingestion. Induce emesis using syrup of ipecac. If the plasma level is obtained and falls above the broken line on the acetaminophen overdose nomogram, the acetylcysteine therapy should be initiated and continued for a full course of therapy. If acetaminophen plasma assay capability is not available, and the estimated acetaminophen ingestion exceeds 150 mg/kg, acetylcysteine therapy should be initiated and continued for a full course of therapy.
For additional emergency information, call your regional poison center or call the Rocky Mountain Poison Center toll-free, (1-800-525-6115).
Chlorpheniramine toxicity should be treated as you would an antihistamine/anticholinergic overdose and is likely to be present within a few hours after acute ingestion.
Symptoms from pseudoephedrine overdose consist most often of mild anxiety, tachycardia and/or mild hypertension. Symptoms usually appear within 4 to 8 hours of ingestion and are transient, usually requiring no treatment.

Inactive Ingredients: Chewable Tablets: Aspartame, Basic Polymethacrylate, cellulose acetate, citric acid, flavors, hydroxypropyl methylcellulose, magnesium stearate, mannitol, microcrystalline cellulose, Blue #1, Red #7. **Liquid:** Benzoic acid, citric acid, flavors, glycerin, malic acid, polyethylene glycol, propylene glycol, sodium benzoate, sorbitol, sucrose, purified water, Blue #1 and Red #40.

How Supplied: **Chewable Tablets** (colored purple, scored, imprinted "Tylenol Cold") on one side and "TC" on opposite side—bottles of 24. **Liquid Formula**—bottles (colored purple) of 4 fl. oz.

Shown in Product Identification Guide, page 511

CHILDREN'S TYLENOL® COLD Multi Symptom PLUS COUGH Chewable Tablets and Liquid

Description: Each ***CHILDREN'S TYLENOL® COLD Multi Symptom Plus Cough Chewable Cherry-Flavored Tablet*** contains:

acetaminophen 80 mg
chlorpheniramine maleate 0.5 mg
dextromethorphan hydrobromide 2.5 mg
pseudoephedrine hydrochloride 7.5 mg

CHILDREN'S TYLENOL® COLD Multi Symptom Plus Cough Liquid is cherry flavored and contains no alcohol. Each teaspoon (5 ml) contains acetaminophen 160 mg, chlorpheniramine maleate 1 mg, dextromethorphan hydrobromide 5 mg and pseudoephedrine hydrochloride 15 mg.

Actions: ***CHILDREN'S TYLENOL® COLD Multi Symptom Plus Cough Chewable Tablets*** and ***Liquid*** combines the analgesic-antipyretic acetaminophen with the decongestant pseudoephedrine hydrochloride, the cough suppressant dextromethorphan hydrobromide, and the antihistamine chlorpheniramine maleate to help relieve coughs, nasal congestion, and sore throat, dry runny noses, and prevent sneezing as well as to relieve the fever, aches, pains and general discomfort associated with colds and upper respiratory infections.

Acetaminophen is equal to aspirin in analgesic and antipyretic effectiveness and it is unlikely to produce the side effects often associated with aspirin or aspirin-containing products.

Indications: For temporary relief of coughs, nasal congestion, runny nose, sore throat, sneezing, minor aches and pains, headaches and fever due to the common cold, hay fever or other upper respiratory allergies.

Precaution: If a rare sensitivity reaction occurs, the drug should be stopped.

Directions: All doses may be repeated every 4–6 hours, not to exceed 4 doses in 24 hours.

Administer to children under 6 years only on the advice of a physician.

CHILDREN'S TYLENOL® COLD Plus Cough Chewable Tablets: 2–5 years—2 tablets, 6–11 years—4 tablets.

CHILDREN'S TYLENOL® COLD Plus Cough Liquid Formula: 2–5 years—1 teaspoonful, 6–11 years—2 teaspoonfuls. Measuring cup is provided and marked for accurate dosing.

Warning: KEEP THIS AND ALL MEDICATION OUT OF THE REACH OF CHILDREN. IN CASE OF ACCIDENTAL OVERDOSE, CONTACT A DOCTOR OR POISON CONTROL CENTER IMMEDIATELY. PROMPT MEDICAL ATTENTION IS CRITICAL EVEN IF YOU DO NOT NOTICE ANY SIGNS OR SYMPTOMS. DO NOT USE WITH OTHER PRODUCTS CONTAINING ACETAMINOPHEN. DO NOT EXCEED RECOMMENDED DOSAGE. Do not take for pain for more than 5 days or for fever for more than 3 days unless directed by a doctor. If pain or fever persists or gets worse, if new symptoms occur, or if redness or swelling is present, consult a doctor because these could be signs of a serious condition. If sore throat is severe, persists for more than 2 days, is accompanied or followed by fever, headache, rash, nausea or vomiting, consult a doctor promptly. If nervousness, dizziness, or sleeplessness occur, discontinue use and consult a doctor. May cause excitability especially in children. Do not give this product to children who have a breathing problem such as chronic bronchitis, or who have glaucoma, heart disease, high blood pressure, thyroid disease, or diabetes, without first consulting the child's doctor. May cause drowsiness. Sedatives and tranquilizers may increase the drowsiness effect. Do not give this product to children who are taking sedatives or tranquilizers, without first consulting the child's doctor. A persistent cough may be a sign of a serious condition. If cough persists for more than 1 week, tends to recur, or is accompanied by fever, rash or persistent headache, consult a doctor. Do not give this product for persistent or chronic cough such as occurs with asthma or if cough is accompanied by excessive phlegm (mucus) unless directed by a doctor.

NOTE: In addition to the above:

Chewable Tablets—DO NOT USE IF CARTON IS OPENED, OR IF PRINTED NECK WRAP OR PRINTED FOIL INNER SEAL IS BROKEN. PHENYLKETONURICS: CONTAINS PHENYLALANINE 4 MG PER TABLET.

Liquid—DO NOT USE IF CARTON IS OPENED, OR IF PRINTED PLASTIC BOTTLE WRAP OR PRINTED FOIL INNER SEAL IS BROKEN.

Drug Interaction Precaution: Do not give this product to a child who is taking a prescription monoamine oxidase inhibitor (MAOI) (certain drugs for depression, psychiatric or emotional conditions), or for 2 weeks after stopping the MAOI drug. If you are uncertain whether your child's prescription drug contains an MAOI, consult a health professional before giving this product.

Overdosage Information: Acetaminophen in massive overdosage may cause hepatic toxicity in some patients. In adults and adolescents, hepatic toxicity has rarely been reported following ingestion of acute overdoses of less than 10 grams. Fatalities are infrequent (less than 3–4% of untreated cases) and have rarely been reported with overdoses of less than 15 grams. In children, an acute overdosage of less than 150 mg/kg has not been associated with hepatic toxicity. Early symptoms following a potentially hepatotoxic overdose may include: nausea, vomiting, diaphoresis and general malaise. Clinical and laboratory evidence of hepatic toxicity may not be apparent until 48 to 72 hours postingestion. In adults and adolescents, regardless of the quantity of acetaminophen reported to have been ingested, administer acetylcysteine immediately if 24 hours or less have elapsed from the reported time of ingestion. For full prescribing information, refer to the acetylcysteine package insert. Do not await the results of assays for plasma acetaminophen level before initiating treatment with acetylcysteine. The following additional procedures are recommended: The stomach should be emptied promptly by lavage or by induction of emesis with syrup of ipecac. A plasma acetaminophen assay should be obtained as early as possible, but no sooner than four hours following ingestion. If plasma level falls above the lower treatment line on the acetaminophen overdose nomogram, acetylcysteine therapy should be continued. Liver function studies should be obtained initially and repeated at 24-hour intervals.

Serious toxicity or fatalities are extremely infrequent in children, possibly due to differences in the way they metabolize acetaminophen. In children, the maximum potential amount ingested can be more easily estimated. If more than 150 mg/kg or an unknown amount was ingested, obtain an plasma acetaminophen level. The plasma acetaminophen level should be obtained as soon as possible, but no sooner than 4 hours following the ingestion. If plasma level falls above the lower treatment line on the acetaminophen overdose nomogram, the acetylcysteine therapy should be initiated and continued for a full course of therapy. If plasma acetaminophen assay capability is not available, and the estimated acetaminophen ingestion exceeds 150 mg/kg, acetylcysteine therapy should be initiated and continued for a full course of therapy.

For additional emergency information, call your regional poison center or call the Rocky Mountain Poison Center toll-free, (1-800-525-6115).

Chlorpheniramine toxicity should be treated as you would an antihistamine/anticholinergic overdose and is likely to be present within a few hours after acute ingestion.

Symptoms from pseudoephedrine overdose consist most often of mild anxiety, tachycardia and/or mild hypertension. Symptoms usually appear within 4 to 8 hours of ingestion and are transient, usually requiring no treatment.

Acute dextromethorphan overdose usually does not result in serious signs and symptoms unless massive amounts have

Continued on next page

McNeil Consumer—Cont.

been ingested. Signs and symptoms of a substantial overdose may include nausea and vomiting, visual disturbances, CNS disturbances, and urinary retention.

Inactive Ingredients: Chewable Tablets: Aspartame, Basic Polymethacrylate, Cellulose Acetate, Colloidal Silicon Dioxide, Flavors, Hydroxypropyl Methylcellulose, Mannitol, Microcrystalline Cellulose, Stearic Acid and Red #7.
Liquid: Citric Acid, Corn Syrup, Flavors, Polyethylene Glycol, Propylene Glycol, Sodium Benzoate, Sodium Carboxymethylcellulose, Sorbitol, Purified Water, Red #33 and Red #40.

How Supplied: Chewable Tablets (colored pink, imprinted "TYLENOL C/C" on one side and "TC/C" on the opposite side)—bottles of 24.
Liquid Formula—(red colored) bottles of 4 fl. oz.

Shown in Product Identification Guide, page 511

Children's TYLENOL® FLU Liquid

Description: ***CHILDREN'S TYLENOL® FLU Liquid*** is bubble-gum flavored and contains no alcohol or aspirin. Each teaspoon (5 mL) contains acetaminophen 160 mg, pseudoephedrine HCl 15 mg, dextromethorphan HBr 7.5 mg, and chlorpheniramine maleate 1 mg.

Actions: ***CHILDREN'S TYLENOL® FLU Liquid*** combines the analgesic-antipyretic acetaminophen with the decongestant pseudoephedrine hydrochloride, the cough suppressant dextromethorphan hydrobromide and the antihistamine chlorpheniramine maleate to help relieve coughs, nasal congestion, and sore throat, dry runny noses, and prevent sneezing as well as to relieve the fever, aches, pains, and general discomfort associated with colds and upper respiratory infections.
Acetaminophen is equal to aspirin in analgesic and antipyretic effectiveness and it is unlikely to produce the side effects often associated with aspirin or aspirin-containing products.

Indications: For the temporary relief of fever, minor aches and pains, headaches, sore throat, nasal congestion, runny nose and coughs due to a cold or "flu".

Dosage Instructions: An Accudose™ measuring cup is provided for accurate dosing of ***CHILDREN'S TYLENOL® FLU Liquid.*** 6–11 years (48–95 lbs): 2 tsp. Administer to children under 6 years only on advice of a physician. All doses may be repeated every 6–8 hours. Not to exceed 4 doses in 24 hours.

Warning: DO NOT USE IF PLASTIC CARTON WRAP, BOTTLE WRAP, OR FOIL INNER SEAL IMPRINTED "SAFETY SEAL"® IS BROKEN OR MISSING. KEEP THIS AND ALL DRUGS OUT OF THE REACH OF CHILDREN. IN CASE OF ACCIDENTAL OVERDOSE, CONTACT DOCTOR OR POISON CONTROL CENTER IMMEDIATELY. PROMPT MEDICAL ATTENTION IS CRITICAL FOR ADULTS AS WELL AS CHILDREN EVEN IF YOU DO NOT NOTICE ANY SIGNS OR SYMPTOMS. DO NOT USE WITH OTHER PRODUCTS CONTAINING ACETAMINOPHEN. DO NOT EXCEED RECOMMENDED DOSAGE. Do not take for pain for more than 5 days or for fever for more than 3 days unless directed by a doctor. If pain of fever persists, or gets worse, if new symptoms occur, or if redness or swelling is present, consult a doctor because these could be signs of a serious condition. If sore throat is severe, persists for more than 2 days, is accompanied or followed by fever, headache, rash, nausea or vomiting, consult a doctor promptly. A persistent cough may be a sign of a serious condition. If cough persists for more than 1 week, tends to recur or is accompanied by fever, rash, or persistent headache, consult a doctor. Do not give this product for persistent or chronic cough such as occurs with asthma, or if cough is accompanied by excessive phlegm (mucus) unless directed by a doctor. If nervousness, dizziness or sleeplessness occur, discontinue use and consult a doctor. May cause excitability especially in children. Do not give this product to children who have a breathing problem such as chronic bronchitis, or who have glaucoma, heart disease, high blood pressure, thyroid disease or diabetes without first consulting the child's doctor. May cause drowsiness; sedatives and tranquilizers may increase the drowsiness effect. Do not give this product to children who are taking sedatives or tranquilizers without first consulting the child's doctor.

Drug Interaction Precaution: Do not give this product to a child who is taking a prescription monoamine oxidase inhibitor (MAOI) (certain drugs for depression, psychiatric or emotional conditions, or Parkinson's disease), or for 2 weeks after stopping the MAOI drug. If you are uncertain whether your child's prescription drug contains an MAOI, consult a health professional before giving this product.

Overdosage Information: Acetaminophen in massive overdosage may cause hepatic toxicity in some patients. In adults and adolescents, hepatic toxicity has rarely been reported following ingestion of acute overdoses of less than 10 grams. Fatalities are infrequent (less than 3–4% of untreated cases) and have rarely been reported with overdoses of less than 15 grams. In children, an acute overdosage of less than 150 mg/kg has not been associated with hepatic toxicity. Early symptoms following a potentially hepatotoxic overdose may include: nausea, vomiting, diaphoresis and general malaise. Clinical and laboratory evidence of hepatic toxicity may not be apparent until 48 to 72 hours postingestion.
In adults and adolescents, regardless of the quantity of acetaminophen reported to have been ingested, administer acetylcysteine immediately if 24 hours or less have elapsed from the reported time of ingestion. For full prescribing information, refer to the acetylcysteine package insert. Do not await the results of assays for plasma acetaminophen level before initiating treatment wit acetylcysteine. The following additional procedures are recommended: the stomach should be emptied promptly by lavage or by induction of emesis with syrup of ipecac. A plasma acetaminophen assay should be obtained as early as possible, but no sooner than four hours following ingestion. If plasma level falls above the lower treatment line on the acetaminophen overdose nomogram, acetylcysteine therapy should be continued. Liver function studies should be obtained initially and repeated at 24–hour intervals.
Serious toxicity or fatalities are extremely infrequent in children, possibly due to differences in the way they metabolize acetaminophen. In children, the maximum potential amount ingested can be more easily estimated. If more than 150 mg/kg or an unknown amount was ingested, obtain an plasma acetaminophen level. The plasma acetaminophen level should be obtained as soon as possible, but no sooner than 4 hours following the ingestion. If plasma level falls above the lower treatment line on the acetaminophen overdose nomogram, the acetylcysteine therapy should be initiated and continued for a full course of therapy. If plasma acetaminophen assay capability is not available, and the estimated acetaminophen ingestion exceeds 150 mg/kg, acetylcysteine therapy should be initiated and continued for a full course of therapy.
For additional emergency information, call your regional poison center or call the Rocky Mountain Poison Center toll-free (1-800-525-6115).
Chlorpheniramine toxicity should be treated as you would an antihistamine anticholinergic overdose and is likely to be present within a few hours after acute ingestion.
Symptoms from pseudoephedrine overdose consist most often of mild anxiety, tachycardia, and/or mild hypertension. Symptoms usually appear within 4 to 8 hours of ingestion and are transient, usually requiring no treatment.
Acute dextromethorphan overdose usually does not result in serious signs and symptoms unless massive amounts have been ingested. Signs and symptoms of a substantial overdose may include nausea and vomiting, visual disturbances, CNS disturbances, and urinary retention.

Inactive Ingredients: Citric Acid, Corn Syrup, Flavors, Polyethylene Glycol, Propylene Glycol, Purified Water, Sodium Benzoate, Sodium Carboxymethylcellulose, Sorbitol, Red #33 and Red #40.

How Supplied: Pink colored liquid in child resistant bottles 4 fl. oz.

Shown in Product Identification Guide, page 511

INFANTS' TYLENOL® COLD
Decongestant & Fever Reducer Drops

Description: ***INFANTS' TYLENOL® COLD Decongestant & Fever Reducer Drops*** are alcohol-free, bubble gum flavored and red in color. Each 0.8 ml (dropperful) contains acetaminophen 80 mg and pseudoephedrine HCl 7.5 mg.

Actions: Acetaminophen is a clinically proven analgesic/antipyretic. Acetaminophen produces analgesia by elevation of the pain threshold and antipyresis through action on the hypothalamic heat regulating center. Acetaminophen is equal to aspirin in analgesic and antipyretic effectiveness and it is unlikely to produce many of the side effects associated with aspirin and aspirin containing products. Pseudoephedrine hydrochloride is a sympathomimetic amine which provides temporary relief of nasal congestion.

Indications: ***INFANTS' TYLENOL® COLD Decongestant & Fever Reducer Drops*** are indicated for the temporary relief of nasal congestion, minor aches and pains, headaches and fever due to the common cold, hay fever or other upper respiratory allergies.

Precautions: If a rare sensitivity reaction occurs, the drug should be stopped.

Usual Dosage: All dosages may be repeated every 4–6 hours, but not more than 4 times daily. Administer to children under 2 years only on the advice of a physician. 0–3 months: 0.4 ml, 4–11 months: 0.8 ml, 12–23 months: 1.2 ml, 2–3 years: 1.6 ml, 4–5 years: 2.4 ml.

Warnings: Do not use if printed carton overwrap or printed plastic bottle wrap is broken or missing or if carton is opened. Keep this and all medication out of the reach of children. In case of accidental overdose, contact a doctor or poison control center immediately. Prompt medical attention is critical even if you do not notice any signs or symptoms. Do not exceed recommended dosage. Do not take for pain for more than 5 days or for fever for more than 3 days unless directed by a doctor. If pain or fever persists or gets worse, if new symptoms occur, or if redness or swelling is present, consult a doctor because these could be signs of a serious condition. If nervousness, dizziness or sleeplessness occur, discontinue use and consult a doctor. Do not give this product to a child who has heart disease, high blood pressure, thyroid disease, or diabetes unless directed by a doctor. Do not use with other products containing acetaminophen.

Drug Interaction Precaution: Do not give this product to a child who is taking a prescription monoamine oxidase inhibitor (MAOI) (certain drugs for depression, psychiatric or emotional conditions), or for 2 weeks after stopping the MAOI drug. If you are uncertain whether your child's prescription drug contains an MAOI, consult a health professional before giving this product.

Overdosage Information: Acetaminophen in massive overdosage may cause hepatic toxicity in some patients. In adults and adolescents, hepatic toxicity has rarely been reported following ingestion of acute overdoses of less than 10 grams. Fatalities are infrequent (less than 3–4% of untreated cases) and have rarely been reported with overdoses of less than 15 grams. In children, an acute overdosage of less than 150 mg/kg has not been associated with hepatic toxicity. Early symptoms following a potentially hepatotoxic overdose may include: nausea, vomiting, diaphoresis and general malaise. Clinical and laboratory evidence of hepatic toxicity may not be apparent until 48 to 72 hours postingestion. In adults and adolescents, regardless of the quantity of acetaminophen reported to have been ingested, administer acetylcysteine immediately if 24 hours or less have elapsed from the reported time of ingestion. For full prescribing information, refer to the acetylcysteine package insert. Do not await results of assays for plasma acetaminophen level before initiating treatment with acetylcysteine. The following additional procedures are recommended. The stomach should be emptied promptly by lavage or by induction of emesis with syrup of ipecac. A plasma acetaminophen assay should be obtained as early as possible, but no sooner than four hours following ingestion. If plasma level falls above the lower treatment line on the acetaminophen overdose nomogram, acetylcysteine therapy should be continued. Liver function studies should be obtained initially and repeated at 24-hour intervals.
Serious toxicity or fatalities are extremely infrequent in children, possibly due to differences in the way they metabolize acetaminophen. In children, the maximum potential amount ingested can be more easily estimated. If more than 150 mg/kg or an unknown amount was ingested, obtain a plasma acetaminophen level. The plasma acetaminophen level should be obtained as soon as possible, but no sooner than 4 hours following the ingestion. If plasma level falls above the lower treatment line on the acetaminophen overdose nomogram, the acetylcysteine therapy should be initiated and continued for a full course of therapy. If plasma acetaminophen assay capability is not available, and the estimated acetaminophen ingestion exceeds 150 mg/kg, acetylcysteine therapy should be initiated and continued for a full course of therapy.
For additional emergency information, call your regional poison center or call the Rocky Mountain Poison Center toll-free, (1-800-525-6115).
Symptoms from pseudoephedrine overdose consist most often of mild anxiety, tachycardia and/or mild hypertension. Symptoms usually appear within 4 to 8 hours of ingestion and are transient, usually requiring no treatment.

Inactive Ingredients: Citric acid, corn syrup, flavors, polyethylene glycol, propylene glycol, purified water, sodium benzoate, saccharin, FD&C red #40.

How Supplied: **Drops** (colored red)—bottles of 1/2 fl. oz.

Shown in Product Identification Guide, page 511

IMODIUM® A–D
(loperamide hydrochloride)

Description: Each 5 ml (teaspoon) of ***IMODIUM® A-D*** liquid contains loperamide hydrochloride 1 mg. ***IMODIUM® A-D*** liquid is stable, cherry-mint flavored, and clear in color.
Each caplet of ***IMODIUM® A-D*** contains 2 mg of loperamide and is scored and colored green.

Actions: ***IMODIUM® A-D*** contains a clinically proven antidiarrheal medication. Loperamide HCl acts by slowing intestinal motility and by affecting water and electrolyte movement through the bowel.

Indication: ***IMODIUM® A-D*** is indicated for the control and symptomatic relief of acute nonspecific diarrhea, including travelers' diarrhea.

Usual Dosage: Adults: Take four teaspoonfuls or two caplets after first loose bowel movement. If needed, take two teaspoonfuls or one caplet after each subsequent loose bowel movement. Do not exceed eight teaspoonfuls or four caplets in any 24 hour period, unless directed by a physician.
9–11 years old (60–95 lbs.): Two teaspoonfuls or one caplet after first loose bowel movement, followed by one teaspoonful or one-half caplet after each subsequent loose bowel movement. Do not exceed six teaspoonfuls or three caplets a day.
6–8 years old (48–59 lbs.): Two teaspoonfuls or one caplet after first loose bowel movement, followed by one teaspoonful or one-half caplet after each subsequent loose bowel movement. Do not exceed four teaspoonfuls or two caplets a day.
Professional Dosage Schedule for children two-five years old (24–47 lbs): One teaspoon after first loose bowel movement, followed by one after each subsequent loose bowel movement. Do not exceed three teaspoonfuls a day.

Warnings: KEEP THIS AND ALL DRUGS OUT OF THE REACH OF CHILDREN. Do not use for more than two days unless directed by a physician. DO NOT USE IF DIARRHEA IS ACCOMPANIED BY HIGH FEVER (GREATER THAN 101°F), OR IF BLOOD OR MUCUS IS PRESENT IN

Continued on next page

McNeil Consumer—Cont.

THE STOOL, OR IF YOU HAVE HAD A RASH OR OTHER ALLERGIC REACTION TO LOPERAMIDE HCl. If you are taking antibiotics or have a history of liver disease, consult a physician before using this product. As with any drug, if you are pregnant or nursing a baby, seek the advice of a health professional before using this product. In case of accidental overdose, seek professional assistance or contact a poison control center immediately.

Overdosage: Overdosage of loperamide HCl in man may result in constipation, CNS depression and nausea. A slurry of activated charcoal administered promptly after ingestion of loperamide hydrochloride can reduce the amount of drug which is absorbed. If vomiting occurs spontaneously upon ingestion, a slurry of 100 grams of activated charcoal should be administered orally as soon as fluids can be retained. If vomiting has not occurred, and CNS depression is evident, gastric lavage should be performed followed by administration of 100 gms of the activated charcoal slurry through the gastric tube. In the event of overdosage, patients should be monitored for signs of CNS depression for at least 24 hours. Children may be more sensitive to central nervous system effects than adults. If CNS depression is observed, naloxone may be administered. If responsive to naloxone, vital signs must be monitored carefully for recurrence of symptoms of drug overdose for at least 24 hours after the last dose of naloxone.

Inactive Ingredients: **Liquid:** Benzoic acid, citric acid, flavors, glycerin, propylene glycol, purified water, sodium benzoate, sorbitol sucrose, contains 0.5% alcohol.
Caplets: Dibasic calcium phosphate, magnesium stearate, microcrystalline cellulose, colloidal silicon dioxide, FD&C Blue #1 and D&C Yellow #10.

How Supplied: Cherry-mint flavored liquid (clear) 2 fl. oz., and 4 fl. oz. tamper resistant bottles with child resistant safety caps and special dosage cups.
Green Scored caplets in 6's and 12's, 18's and 24's blister packaging which is tamper resistant and child resistant.

Shown in Product Identification Guide, page 509

Junior Strength MOTRIN®
Ibuprofen Caplets

Description: ***Junior Strength MOTRIN® Ibuprofen Caplets*** are easy-to-swallow caplets (capsule-shaped tablets). Each caplet contains ibuprofen 100 mg.

Indications: ***Junior Strength MOTRIN® Ibuprofen Caplets*** are indicated for temporary relief of fever, and minor aches and pains due to colds, sore throat, headache and toothaches. One dose lasts 6–8 hours.

Directions: If possible, use weight to dose; otherwise use age. 6–8 years (48–59 lbs): 2 caplets. 9–10 years (60–71 lbs): 2 1/2 caplets. 11 years (72–95 lbs): 3 caplets. Under 6 years of age—consult a physician. Repeat dose every 6–8 hours. Do not use more than 4 times a day.

Warnings: ASPIRIN SENSITIVE CHILDREN:
- This product contains no aspirin, but may cause a severe reaction in people allergic to aspirin.
- Do not use this product if your child has had an allergic reaction to aspirin such as asthma, swelling, shock or hives.

CALL YOUR DOCTOR IF:
- Your child is under a doctor's care for any serious condition or is taking any other drug.
- Your child has problems or serious side effects from taking fever reducers or pain relievers.
- Your child does not get any relief within first day (24 hours) of treatment, or pain or fever gets worse.
- Redness or swelling is present in the painful area.
- Sore throat is severe, lasts for more than 2 days or occurs with fever, headache, rash, nausea or vomiting.
- Any new symptoms appear.

DO NOT USE:
- With any other product that contains ibuprofen, or any other pain reliever/fever reducer, unless directed by a doctor.
- For more than 3 days for fever or pain unless directed by a doctor.
- For stomach pain unless directed by a doctor.
- If your child is dehydrated (significant fluid loss) due to continued vomiting, diarrhea or lack of fluid intake.
- If blister unit is broken or open.

IMPORTANT:
- Keep this and all drugs out of the reach of children. In case of accidental overdose, seek professional assistance or contact a poison control center immediately.
- If stomach upset occurs while taking this product, give with food or milk. If stomach upset gets worse or lasts, call your doctor.

Inactive Ingredients: Carnauba wax, colloidal silicon dioxide, cornstarch, hydroxypropyl methylcellulose, microcrystalline cellulose, polydextrose, polyethylene glycol, propylene glycol, sodium starch glycolate, titanium dioxide, triacetin, D&C Yellow #10, FD&C Yellow #6.

How Supplied: Caplets (white, imprinted "M 100" in orange) in blister packs of 24
Store at controlled room temperature 15°–30°C (59°–86°F).

Shown in Product Identification Guide, page 510

JUNIOR STRENGTH TYLENOL®
acetaminophen
Coated Caplets and Chewable Tablets

Description: Each ***JUNIOR STRENGTH TYLENOL® Coated Caplet or Chewable Tablet*** contains 160 mg acetaminophen in a small, coated, capsule shaped tablet or grape or fruit burst flavored chewable tablet.

Actions: Acetaminophen is a clinically proven analgesic/antipyretic. Acetaminophen produces analgesia by elevation of the pain threshold and antipyresis through action on the hypothalamic heat-regulating center. Acetaminophen is equal to aspirin in analgesic and antipyretic effectiveness and it is unlikely to produce many of the side effects associated with aspirin and aspirin-containing products.

Indications: ***JUNIOR STRENGTH TYLENOL® Caplets*** are designed for easy swallowability in older children and young adults. Both ***JUNIOR STRENGTH TYLENOL® Caplets and JUNIOR STRENGTH TYLENOL® Chewable Tablets*** provide fast, effective temporary relief of fever and discomfort due to colds and "flu," and pain and discomfort due to simple headaches, minor muscle aches, sprains and overexertion.

Precautions: If a rare sensitivity reaction occurs, the drug should be stopped.

Usual Dosage: Caplets should be taken with liquid. Chewable tablets should be well chewed. All dosages may be repeated every 4 hours, but not more than 5 times daily. For ages: 6–8 years: two caplets or tablets, 9–10 years: two and one-half caplets or tablets, 11 years: three caplets or tablets, 12 years: four caplets or tablets.

Warning: Do not use if carton is opened or if a blister unit is broken. Do not take for pain for more than 5 days or for fever for more than 3 days unless directed by a physician. If pain or fever persists or gets worse, if new symptoms occur, or if redness or swelling is present, consult a physician because these could be signs of a serious condition. Keep this and all drugs out of reach of children. In case of accidental overdose, contact a physican or poison control center immediately. Prompt medical attention is critical even if you do not notice any signs or symptoms. Do not use with other products containing acetaminophen. As with any drug, if you are pregnant or nursing a baby, seek the advice of a health professional before using this product. In addition the caplet package states: Not for children who have difficulty swallowing tablets. In addition the Grape Chewable Tablet package states: Phenylketonurics: contains phenylalanine 6 mg per tablet, and the Fruit Burst Chewable Tablet package states: Phenylketonurics: contains phenylalanine 9 mg per tablet.

Overdosage: Acetaminophen in massive overdosage may cause hepatic toxicity in some patients. In adults and adolescents, hepatic toxicity has rarely been reported following ingestion of acute overdosage of less than 10 grams. Fatalities are infrequent (less than 3–4% of untreated cases) and have rarely been reported with overdoses of less than 15 grams. In children, an acute overdosage of less than 150 mg/kg has not been associated with hepatic toxicity.
Early symptoms following a potentially hepatotoxic overdose may include: nausea, vomiting, diaphoresis and general malaise. Clinical and laboratory evidence of hepatic toxicity may not be apparent until 48 to 72 hours postingestion.
In adults and adolescents, regardless of the quantity of acetaminophen reported to have been ingested, administer acetylcysteine immediately if 24 hours or less have elapsed from the reported time of ingestion. For full prescribing information, refer to the acetylcysteine package insert. Do not await the results of assays for acetaminophen level before initiating treatment with acetylcysteine. The following additional procedures are recommended: The stomach should be emptied promptly by lavage or by induction of emesis with syrup of ipecac. A serum acetaminophen assay should be obtained as early as possible, but no sooner than four hours following ingestion. Liver function studies should be obtained initially and repeated at 24-hour intervals.
Serious toxicity or fatalities are extremely infrequent in children, possibly due to differences in the way they metabolize acetaminophen. In children, the maximum potential amount ingested can be more easily estimated. If more than 150 mg/kg or an unknown amount was ingested, obtain an acetaminophen plasma level. The acetaminophen plasma level should be obtained as soon as possible, but no sooner than 4 hours following the ingestion. Induce emesis using syrup of ipecac. If the plasma level is obtained and falls above the broken line on the acetaminophen overdose nomogram, the acetylcysteine therapy should be initiated and continued for a full course of therapy. If acetaminophen plasma assay capability is not available, and the estimated acetaminophen ingestion exceeds 150 mg/kg, acetylcysteine therapy should be initiated and continued for a full course of therapy.
For additional emergency information, call your regional poison center or call the Rocky Mountain Poison Center toll-free, (1-800-525-6115).

Inactive Ingredients: Junior Strength Caplets: Cellulose, Corn Starch, Ethylcellulose, Magnesium Stearate, Sodium Lauryl Sulfate, Sodium Starch Glycolate.
Junior Strength Fruit Burst Chewable Tablets: Aspartame, Cellulose, Citric acid, Corn Starch, Flavors, Magnesium Stearate, Mannitol, Red #7. May contain Ethylcellulose or Cellulose Acetate and Povidone.
Junior Strength Grape Flavored Chewable Tablets: Aspartame, Cellulose, Citric Acid, Corn Starch, Flavors, Magnesium Stearate, Mannitol, Blue #1, Red #7 and Red #30. May contain Ethylcellulose or Cellulose Acetate and Povidone.

How Supplied: Coated Caplets, (colored white, coated, scored, imprinted "TYLENOL 160") Package of 30.
Chewable Tablets (colored purple or pink, imprinted "TYLENOL 160") Package of 24. All packages are safety sealed and use child resistant blister packaging.

Shown in Product Identification Guide, page 511

LACTAID® Original Strength Caplets (lactase enzyme)

LACTAID® Extra Strength Caplets (lactase enzyme)

LACTAID® ULTRA Caplets (lactase enzyme)

PRODUCT OVERVIEW

Key Facts: ***LACTAID®*** is the original lactase dietary supplement that makes milk and dairy foods more digestible. ***LACTAID®*** lactase enzyme hydrolyzes lactose into two digestible simple sugars: glucose and galactose. ***LACTAID® Caplets*** are taken orally for *in vivo* hydrolysis of lactose.

Major Uses: Lactose intolerance, suspected from gastrointestinal discomfort (ie, gas, bloating, cramps, and diarrhea) after drinking milk or ingesting other dairy foods such as cheese and ice cream.

PRESCRIBING INFORMATION

Description: Each ***LACTAID® Original Strength Caplet*** contains 3000 FCC (Food Chemical Codex) units of lactase enzyme (derived from *Aspergillus oryzae*). Each ***LACTAID® Extra Strength Caplet*** contains 4500 FCC units of lactase enzyme (derived from *Aspergillus oryzae*). Each ***LACTAID® ULTRA Caplet*** contains 9000 FCC units of lactase enzyme (derived from Aspergillus oryzae).

Action: ***LACTAID® Caplets*** work to naturally replenish lactase enzyme that aids in dairy food digestion. Lactase enzyme hydrolyzes lactose sugar (a double sugar) into its simple sugar components, glucose and galactose.

Indications: Lactose intolerance, suspected from gastrointestinal discomfort (ie, gas, bloating, flatulence, cramps, and diarrhea) after drinking milk or ingesting other dairy foods such as cheese and ice cream.

Usual Dosage: These convenient, portable caplets are easy to swallow or chew and can be used with milk or any dairy food. Original Strength: Swallow or chew 3 caplets with the first bite of dairy food. Take no more than 6 caplets at a time. Extra Strength: Swallow or chew 2 caplets with first bite of dairy food. Take no more than 4 caplets at a time. Ultra: Swallow or chew 1 caplet with the first bite of dairy food. Take no more than 2 caplets at a time. Don't be discouraged if at first Lactaid does not work to your satisfaction. Because the degree of enzyme deficiency naturally varies from person to person and from food to food, you may have to adjust the number of caplets up or down to find your own level of comfort. Since Lactaid Caplets work only on the food as you eat it, use them every time you enjoy dairy foods.

Warning: If you experience any symptoms which are unusual or seem unrelated to the condition for which you took this product, consult a doctor before taking any more of it. Do not use if carton is opened or if printed plastic neckwrap is broken.

Ingredients: ***LACTAID® Caplets:*** Mannitol, Cellulose, Lactase Enzyme, Dextrose, and Sodium Citrate Magnesium Stearate.
LACTAID® ULTRA Caplets: Lactase enzyme, Cellulose, Dextrose, Sodium Citrate, Magnesium Stearate, Colloidal Silicon Dioxide.

How Supplied: ***LACTAID® Original Strength Caplets*** are available in bottles of 60, and 120 counts. ***LACTAID® Extra Strength Caplets*** are available in bottles of 24, and 50 counts. ***LACTAID® ULTRA Caplets*** are available in single serve packets of 12 and 32 counts. Store at or below room temperature (below 77°F) but do not refrigerate. Keep away from heat.
LACTAID® Caplets are certified kosher from the Orthodox Union.
Also available: 70% lactose reduced Lactaid Milk and 100% lactose-free Lactaid Milk.

Shown in Product Identification Guide, page 510

LACTAID® Drops (lactase enzyme)

PRODUCT OVERVIEW

Key Facts: ***LACTAID®*** is the original dairy digestive supplement that makes milk more digestible. ***LACTAID®*** lactase enzyme hydrolyzes lactose into two digestible simple sugars: glucose and galactose. ***LACTAID® Drops*** are added to milk for *in vitro* hydrolysis of lactose.

Major Uses: Lactose intolerance, suspected from gastrointestinal discomfort (ie, gas, bloating, cramps, and diarrhea) after drinking milk.

PRESCRIBING INFORMATION

Description: ***LACTAID® Drops*** contain sufficient lactase enzyme (derived from *Kluyveromyces lactis*) to hydrolyze lactose in milk.

Action: ***LACTAID® Drops*** are a liquid form of the natural lactase enzyme that makes milk more digestible. The lactase enzyme hydrolyzes the lactose sugar (a

Continued on next page

McNeil Consumer—Cont.

double sugar) into its simple sugar components, glucose and galactose.

Indications: Lactose intolerance, suspected from gastrointestinal discomfort (ie, gas, bloating, cramps, and diarrhea) after drinking milk.

Usual Dosage: ***LACTAID® Drops*** are a liquid form of the natural lactase enzyme that makes milk more digestible. To use, add ***LACTAID® Drops*** to a quart of milk, shake gently and refrigerate for 24 hours. We recommend starting with 5–7 drops per quart of milk but because sensitivity to lactose can vary, you may have to adjust the number of drops you use. If you are still experiencing discomfort after consuming milk with 5–7 ***LACTAID® Drops*** per quart, you may want to add 10 drops per quart or even 15 drops per quart. 15 drops per quart should remove nearly all of the lactose in the milk. Lactaid can be used with any kind of milk: whole, 1%, 2%, non-fat, skim, powdered and chocolate milk.

Warning: If you experience any symptoms which are unusual or seem unrelated to the condition for which you took this product, consult a doctor before taking any more of it. Do not use if carton is opened or if printed plastic bodywrap is broken.

Inactive Ingredients: Glycerin, Water

How Supplied: ***LACTAID® Drops*** are available in .22 fl. oz. (7 mL), (30 quart supply). Store at or below room temperature (below 77°F). Refrigerate after opening.
Lactaid Drops are certified kosher from the Orthodox Union.
Also available: 70% lactose reduced Lactaid Milk and 100% lactose-free Lactaid Milk.

Shown in Product Identification Guide, page 510

NICOTROL®
NICOTINE TRANSDERMAL SYSTEM

Description: ***NICOTROL®*** (nicotine transdermal system) is a multilayered, rectangular, thin film laminated unit containing nicotine as the active ingredient. ***NICOTROL®*** Patch provides systemic delivery of 15 mg of nicotine over 16 hours.

Actions: ***NICOTROL®*** (nicotine trans dermal system) Patch helps smokers quit by reducing nicotine withdrawal symptoms. Many ***NICOTROL®*** Patch users will be able to stop smoking for a few days but often will start smoking again. Most smokers have to try to quit several times before they completely stop.
Your own chances of quitting smoking depend on how much you want to quit, how strongly you are addicted to nicotine and how closely you follow a quitting program like the PATHWAYS TO CHANGE® Program that comes with the ***NICOTROL®*** Patch.
If you find you cannot stop or if you start smoking again after using ***NICOTROL®*** Patch, please talk to a health care professional who can help you find a program that may work better for you. Remember that breaking this addiction doesn't happen overnight.
Because the ***NICOTROL®*** Patch provides some nicotine, the ***NICOTROL®*** Patch will help you stop smoking by reducing nicotine withdrawal symptoms such as nicotine cravings, nervousness and irritability.

Indications: ***NICOTROL®*** Patch is indicated as a stop smoking aid to reduce withdrawal symptoms, including nicotine craving, associated with quitting smoking.

Directions:
- Stop smoking completely when you begin using the ***NICOTROL®*** Patch.
- Refer to enclosed patient information leaflet before using this product.
- Use one ***NICOTROL®*** Patch every day for six weeks. Remove backing from the patch and immediately press onto clean dry hairless skin. Hold for ten seconds. Wash hands.
- The ***NICOTROL®*** Patch should be worn during awake hours and removed prior to sleep.

For Best Results In Quitting Smoking:
1. Firmly commit to quitting smoking.
2. Use enclosed support materials.
3. Use the ***NICOTROL®*** Patches for six weeks.
4. Stop using ***NICOTROL®*** Patches at the end of week six. If you still feel the need for ***NICOTROL®*** Patches talk to your doctor.

Warnings:
- Keep this and all medication out of reach of children and pets. Even used patches have enough nicotine to poison children and pets. Be sure to fold sticky ends together and throw away out of reach of children and pets. In case of accidental overdose, seek professional assistance or contact a poison control center immediately.
- Nicotine can increase your baby's heart rate. First try to stop smoking without the nicotine patch. As with any drug, if you are pregnant or nursing a baby, seek the advice of a health professional before using this product.
- Do not smoke even when you are not wearing the patch. The nicotine in your skin will still be entering your bloodstream for several hours after you take the patch off.
- If you forget to remove the patch at bedtime you may have vivid dreams or other sleep disruptions.

Do Not Use if You:
- Continue to smoke, chew tobacco, use snuff, or use a nicotine gum or other nicotine containing products.

Ask Your Doctor Before Use if You:
- Are under 18 years of age.
- Have heart disease, recent heart attack or irregular heartbeat. Nicotine can increase your heart rate.
- Have high blood pressure not controlled with medication.
  Nicotine can increase blood pressure.
- Take prescription medicine for depression or asthma.
  Your prescription dose may need to be adjusted.
- Are allergic to adhesive tape or have skin problems, because you are more likely to get rashes.

Stop Use and See Your Doctor if You Have:
- Skin redness caused by the patch that does not go away after four days, or if your skin swells or you get a rash.
- Irregular heartbeat or palpitations.
- Symptoms of nicotine overdose such as nausea, vomiting, dizziness, weakness and rapid heartbeat.

Inactive Ingredients: Polyisobutylenes, polybutene non-woven polyester, pigmented aluminized and clear polyesters.

How Supplied: Starter Kit-7 patches, Refill Kit-7 and 14 patches. DO NOT USE IF POUCH IS DAMAGED OR OPEN. Do not Store above 86°F (30°C)
- **Not for sale to those under 18 years of age**
- **Proof of age required.**
- **Not for sale in vending machines or from any source where proof of age cannot be verified.**

Shown in Product Identification Guide, page 510

PEDIACARE® Cough-Cold Liquid and Chewable Tablets
PEDIACARE® NightRest Cough-Cold Liquid
PEDIACARE® Infants' Drops Decongestant
PEDIACARE® Infants' Drops Decongestant Plus Cough

Description: Each 5 ml of ***PEDIACARE® Cough-Cold Liquid*** contains pseudoephedrine hydrochloride 15 mg, chlorpheniramine maleate 1 mg and dextromethorphan hydrobromide 5 mg. Each ***PEDIACARE® Cough-Cold Chewable Tablet*** contains pseudoephedrine hydrochloride 15 mg, chlorpheniramine maleate 1 mg and dextromethorphan hydrobromide 5 mg. Each 0.8 ml oral dropper of ***PEDIACARE® Infants' Drops Decongestant*** contains pseudoephedrine hydrochloride 7.5 mg. Each 0.8 oral dropper of ***PEDIACARE® Infants' Drops Decongestant Plus Cough*** contains pseudoephedrine hydrochloride 7.5 mg and dextromethorphan hydrobromide 2.5 mg. ***PEDIACARE® NightRest Cough-Cold Liquid*** contains pseudoephedrine hydrochloride 15 mg, chlorpheniramine maleate 1 mg and dextromethorphan hydrobromide 7.5 mg per 5 ml. ***PEDIACARE® Cough-Cold Liquid*** and ***NightRest Cough-Cold Liquid*** are stable, cherry flavored and red in color. ***PEDIACARE® Infants' Drops*** are fruit flavored alcohol free and red in

Age Group	0–3 mos	4–11 mos	12–23 mos	2–3 yrs	4–5 yrs	6–8 yrs	9–10 yrs	11 yrs	Dosage
Weight (lbs)	6–11 lb	12–17 lb	18–23 lb	24–35 lb	36–47 lb	48–59 lb	60–71 lb	72–95 lb	
PEDIACARE® Infants' Drops Decongestant*	1/2 dropper (0.4 ml)	1 dropper (0.8 ml)	1 1/2 droppers (1.2 ml)	2 droppers (1.6 ml)					q4–6h
PEDIACARE® Infants' Drops Decongestant Plus Cough*	1/2 dropper (0.4 ml)	1 dropper (0.8 ml)	1 1/2 droppers (1.2 ml)	2 droppers (1.6 ml)					q4–6h
PEDIACARE® Cough-Cold Liquid**				1 tsp	1 1/2 tsp	2 tsp	2 1/2 tsp	3 tsp	q4–6h
and Chewable Tablets**				1 tab	1 1/2 tabs	2 tabs	2 1/2 tabs	3 tabs	q4–6h
PEDIACARE® NightRest Liquid**				1 tsp	1 1/2 tsp	2 tsp	2 1/2 tsp	3 tsp	q6–8h

*Administer to children under 2 years only on the advice of a physician.
**Administer to children under 6 years only on the advice of a physician.

color. ***PEDIACARE® Infants' Drops Decongestant Plus Cough*** are cherry flavored, alcohol free and clear, non-staining in color. ***PEDIACARE® Cough-Cold Chewable Tablets*** are fruit flavored and pink in color.

Actions: ***PEDIACARE*** Products are available in four different formulas, allowing you to select the ideal product to temporarily relieve the patient's symptoms. ***PEDIACARE® Cough-Cold Liquid*** and ***Chewable Tablets*** contain an antihistamine, chlorpheniramine maleate, a nasal decongestant, pseudoephedrine HCl and a cough suppressant, dextromethorphan hydrobromide, to provide temporary relief of nasal congestion, runny nose, sneezing and coughing due to the common cold, hay fever or other upper respiratory allergies. ***PEDIACARE® NightRest Cough-Cold Liquid*** contains a decongestant, pseudoephedrine hydrochloride, an antihistamine, chlorpheniramine maleate, and a cough suppressant, dextromethorphan hydrobromide, to provide temporary relief of coughs, nasal congestion, runny nose and sneezing due to the common cold hayfever or other upper respiratory allergies. ***PEDIACARE® NightRest*** may be used day or night to relieve cough and cold symptoms. ***PEDIACARE® Infants' Drops Decongestant*** contain a decongestant, pseudoephedrine hydrochloride, to provide temporary relief of nasal congestion due to the common cold, hay fever or other upper respiratory allergies. ***PEDIACARE® Infants' Drops Decongestant Plus Cough*** contain a decongestant, pseudoephedrine hydrochloride, and a cough suppressant, dextromethorphan hydrobromide to provide temporary relief of nasal congestion and coughing due to common cold, hay fever or other upper respiratory allergies.

Professional Dosage: A calibrated dosage cup is provided for accurate dosing of the ***PEDIACARE*** Liquid formulas. A calibrated oral dropper is provided for accurate dosing of ***PEDIACARE® Infants' Drops***. All doses of ***PEDIACARE® Cough-Cold Liquid*** and ***Chewable Tablets***, as well as ***PEDIACARE® Infants' Drops*** may be repeated every 4–6 hours, not to exceed 4 doses in 24 hours. ***PEDIACARE® NightRest Liquid*** may be repeated every 6–8 hrs, not to exceed 4 doses in 24 hours.
[See table above.]

Warnings: DO NOT USE IF CARTON IS OPENED, OR IF PRINTED PLASTIC BOTTLE WRAP OR FOIL INNER SEAL IS BROKEN. KEEP THIS AND ALL MEDICATION OUT OF THE REACH OF CHILDREN. IN CASE OF ACCIDENTAL OVERDOSAGE, CONTACT A PHYSICIAN OR POISON CONTROL CENTER IMMEDIATELY.
The following information appears on the appropriate package labels:
PEDIACARE® Cough-Cold Chewable Tablets:
PHENYLKETONURICS: CONTAINS PHENYLALANINE 6MG PER TABLET.
PEDIACARE® Cough-Cold Liquid and Chewable Tablets, Night Rest Cough-Cold Liquid: Do not exceed recommended dosage. If nervousness, dizziness or sleeplessness occur, discontinue use and consult a doctor. If symptoms do not improve within 7 days or are accompanied by fever, consult a doctor. A persistent cough may be a sign of a serious condition. If cough persists for more than one week, tends to recur or is accompanied by fever, rash, or persistent headache, consult a doctor. Do not give this product for persistent or chronic cough such as occurs with asthma or if cough is accompanied by excessive phlegm (mucus) unless directed by a doctor. May cause excitability especially in children. May cause drowsiness. Sedatives and tranquilizers may increase the drowsiness effect. Do not give this product to children who are taking sedatives or tranquilizers without first consulting the child's doctor. Do not give this product to children who have a breathing problem such as chronic bronchitis, or who have glaucoma, heart disease, high blood pressure, thyroid disease or diabetes, without first consulting the child's doctor.
PEDIACARE® Infants' Drops Decongestant: Do not exceed the recommended dosage. If nervousness, dizziness or sleeplessness occur discontinue use and consult a doctor. If symptoms do not improve within 7 days or are accompanied by fever, consult a physician. Do not give this product to a child who has heart disease, high blood pressure, thyroid disease or diabetes unless directed by a doctor. Take by mouth only. Not for nasal use.
PEDIACARE® Infants' Drops Decongestant Plus
Cough: Do not exceed recommended dosage. If nervousness, dizziness, or sleeplessness occur, discontinue use and consult a doctor. If symptoms do not improve within 7 days or are accompanied by fever, consult a doctor. A persistent cough may be a sign of a serious condition. If cough persists for more than one week, tends to recur or is accompanied by fever, rash, or persistent headache, consult a doctor. Do not give this product for persistent or chronic cough such as occurs with asthma or if cough is accompanied by excessive phlegm (mucus) unless directed by a doctor. Do not give this product to a child who has heart disease, high blood pressure, thyroid disease or diabetes unless directed by a doctor. Take by mouth only. Not for nasal use.

Drug Interaction Precaution: Do not give this product to a child who is taking a prescription monoamine oxidase inhibitor (MAOI) (certain drugs for depression, psychiatric or emotional conditions), or for 2 weeks after stopping the MAOI drug. If you are uncertain whether your child's prescription drug contains an MAOI, consult a health professional before giving this product.

Inactive Ingredients: ***PEDIACARE® Cough-Cold Liquid:*** Citric acid, corn syrup, flavors, glycerin, propylene glycol, sodium benzoate, sodium carboxymethylcellulose, sorbitol, purified water and Red #40.
PEDIACARE® NightRest Cough-Cold Liquid: Citric acid, corn syrup, flavors, glycerin, propylene glycol, sodium benzoate, sodium carboxymethylcellulose, sorbitol, purified water and Red #40.
PEDIACARE® Cough-Cold Chewable Tablets: Aspartame, cellulose, citric acid, flavors, magnesium stearate,

Continued on next page

McNeil Consumer—Cont.

magnesium trisilicate, mannitol, corn starch and Red #7.
PEDIACARE® Infants' Drops Decongestant: Benzoic acid, citric acid, flavors, glycerin, polyethylene glycol, propylene glycol, purified water, sodium benzoate, sorbitol, sucrose and Red #40.
PEDIACARE® Infants's Drops Decongestant Plus Cough:Citric acid, flavors, glycerin, purified water, sodium benzoate, and sorbitol.

Overdosage: Acute dextromethorphan overdose usually does not result in serious signs and symptoms unless massive amounts have been ingested. Signs and symptoms of a substantial overdose may include nausea and vomiting, visual disturbances, CNS disturbances, and urinary retention. Symptoms from pseudoephedrine overdose consist most often of mild anxiety, tachycardia and/or mild hypertension. Symptoms usually appear within 4 to 8 hours of ingestion and are transient, usually requiring no treatment. Chlorpheniramine toxicity should be treated as you would an antihistamine/anticholinergic overdose and is likely to be present within a few hours after acute ingestion. Symptoms from pseudoephedrine overdose consist often of mild anxiety, tachycardia and/or mild hypertension. Symptoms usually appear within 4 to 8 hours of ingestion and are transient, usually requiring no treatment.

How Supplied: ***PEDIACARE® Cough-Cold Liquid and NightRest Cough-Cold Liquid*** (colored red)—bottles of 4 fl. oz. (120 ml) with child-resistant safety cap and calibrated dosage cup. ***PEDIACARE Cough-Cold Chewable Tablets*** (pink, scored)—blister packs of 16. ***PEDIACARE® Infants' Drops Decongestant*** (colored red) and ***PEDIACARE® Infants' Drops Decongestant Plus Cough*** (clear)—bottles of 1/2 fl. oz (15 ml) with calibrated dropper.

Shown in Product Identification Guide, page 510

Maximum Strength SINE-AID® Sinus Medication Gelcaps, Caplets and Tablets

Description: Each ***Maximum Strength SINE-AID® Gelcap, Caplet*** or ***Tablet*** contains acetaminophen 500 mg and pseudoephedrine hydrochloride 30 mg.

Actions: ***Maximum Strength SINE-AID® Gelcaps, Caplets*** and ***Tablets*** contain a clinically proven analgesic-antipyretic and a decongestant. Maximum allowable non-prescription levels of acetaminophen and pseudoephedrine provide temporary relief of sinus congestion and pain. Acetaminophen is equal to aspirin in analgesic and antipyretic effectiveness and it is unlikely to produce many of the side effects associated with aspirin and aspirin-containing products. Acetaminophen produces analgesia by elevation of the pain threshold and antipyresis through action on the hypothalamic heat-regulating center. Pseudoephedrine hydrochloride is a sympathomimetic amine that promotes sinus cavity drainage by reducing nasopharyngeal mucosal congestion.

Indications: ***Maximum Strength SINE-AID® Gelcaps, Caplets*** and ***Tablets*** provide effective symptomatic relief from sinus headache pain and congestion. SINE-AID® is particularly well-suited in patients with aspirin allergy, hemostatic disturbances (including anticoagulant therapy), and bleeding diatheses (e.g. hemophilia) and upper gastrointestinal disease (e.g. ulcer, gastritis, hiatus hernia).

Precautions: If a rare sensitivity occurs, the drug should be discontinued. Although pseudoephedrine is virtually without pressor effect in normotensive patients, it should be used with caution in hypertensives.

Directions: Adults & children 12 years of age and older: Two gelcaps, caplets or tablets every four to six hours. Do not exceed eight gelcaps, caplets or tablets in any 24 hour period. Not for use in children under 12 years of age.

Warnings: Do not use if carton is open or if blister unit is broken.
Do not take for pain for more than 7 days or for fever for more than 3 days unless directed by a doctor. If pain or fever persists, or gets worse, if new symptoms occur, or if redness or swelling is present, consult a doctor because these could be signs of a serious condition. **Do not exceed recommended dosage.** If nervousness, dizziness or sleeplessness occur, discontinue use and consult a doctor. Do not take this product if you have heart disease, high blood pressure, thyroid disease, diabetes or difficulty in urination due to enlargement of the prostate gland unless directed by a doctor.
As with any drug, if you are pregnant or nursing a baby, seek the advice of a health professional before using this product. Keep this and all drugs out of the reach of children. In case of accidental overdose, contact a doctor or poison control center immediately. Prompt medical attention is critical for adults as well as for children even if you do not notice any signs or symptoms. Do not use with other products containing acetaminophen.

Alcohol Warning: For this and all other pain relievers, including aspirin, ibuprofen, ketoprofen and naproxen sodium, if you generally consume 3 or more alcohol-containing drinks per day, you should consult your physician for advice on when and how you should take pain relievers.

Drug Interaction Precaution: Do not use this product if you are now taking a prescription monoamine oxidase inhibitor (MAOI) (certain drugs for depression, psychiatric or emotional conditions, or Parkinson's disease), or for 2 weeks after stopping the MAOI drug. If you are uncertain whether your prescription drug contains an MAOI, consult a health professional before taking this product.

Overdosage Information: Acetaminophen in massive overdosage may cause hepatic toxicity in some patients. In adults and adolescents, hepatic toxicity has rarely been reported following ingestion of acute overdoses of less than 10 grams. Fatalities are infrequent (less than 3–4% of untreated cases) and have rarely been reported with overdoses of less than 15 grams. In children, an acute overdosage of less than 150 mg/kg has not been associated with hepatic toxicity. Early symptoms following a potentially hepatotoxic overdose may include: nausea, vomiting, diaphoresis and general malaise. Clinical and laboratory evidence of hepatic toxicity may not be apparent until 48 to 72 hours postingestion. In adults and adolescents, regardless of the quantity of acetaminophen reported to have been ingested, administer acetylcysteine immediately if 24 hours or less have elapsed from the reported time of ingestion. For full prescribing information, refer to the acetylcysteine package insert. Do not await results of assays for plasma acetaminophen level before initiating treatment with acetylcysteine. The following additional procedures are recommended: The stomach should be emptied promptly by lavage or by induction of emesis with syrup of ipecac. A plasma acetaminophen assay should be obtained as early as possible, but no sooner than four hours following ingestion. If plasma level falls above the lower treatment line on the acetaminophen overdose nomogram, acetylcysteine therapy should be continued. Liver function studies should be obtained initially and repeated at 24-hour intervals.
Serious toxicity or fatalities are extremely infrequent in children, possibly due to differences in the way they metabolize acetaminophen. In children, the maximum potential amount ingested can be more easily estimated. If more than 150 mg/kg or an unknown amount was ingested, obtain a plasma acetaminophen level. The plasma acetaminophen level should be obtained as soon as possible, but no sooner than 4 hours following the ingestion. If plasma level falls above the lower treatment line on the acetaminophen overdose nomogram, the acetylcysteine therapy should be initiated and continued for a full course of therapy. If plasma acetaminophen assay capability is not available, and the estimated acetaminophen ingestion exceeds 150 mg/kg, acetylcysteine therapy should be initiated and continued for a full course of therapy.
For additional emergency information, call your regional poison center or call the Rocky Mountain Poison Center toll-free, (1-800-525-6115).
Symptoms from pseudoephedrine overdose consist most often of mild anxiety, tachycardia and/or mild hypertension.

Symptoms usually appear within 4 to 8 hours of ingestion and are transient, usually requiring no treatment.

Alcohol Information: Chronic heavy alcohol abusers may be at increased risk of liver toxicity from excessive acetaminophen use, although reports of this event are rare. Reports almost invariably involve cases of severe chronic alcoholics and the dosages of acetaminophen most often exceed recommended doses and often involve substantial overdose. Professionals should alert their patients who regularly consume large amounts of alcohol not to exceed recommended doses of acetaminophen.

Inactive Ingredients: Gelcaps: Benzyl Alcohol, Butylparaben, Castor Oil, Cellulose, Corn Starch, Edetate Calcium Disodium, Gelatin, Hydroxypropyl Methylcellulose, Iron Oxide Black, Magnesium Stearate, Methylparaben, Propylparaben, Sodium Lauryl Sulfate, Sodium Propionate, Sodium Starch Glycolate, Titanium Dioxide, FD&C Red #40.
Caplets: Cellulose, Corn Starch, Hydroxypropyl Methylcellulose, Magnesium Stearate, Polyethylene Glycol, Sodium Starch Glycolate, Titanium Dioxide, Blue #1 and Red #40.
Tablets: Cellulose, Corn Starch, Magnesium Stearate and Sodium Starch Glycolate.

How Supplied: Gelcaps (colored red and white imprinted "SINE-AID")—blister package of 20 and tamper resistant bottle of 40.
Caplets (colored white imprinted "Maximum SINE-AID")—blister package of 24 and tamper resistant bottle of 50.
Tablets (colored white embossed "SINE-AID")—blister package of 24 and tamper resistant bottle of 50.

Shown in Product Identification Guide, page 510

Extra Strength TYLENOL® acetaminophen Gelcaps, Geltabs, Caplets, Tablets

Extra Strength TYLENOL® acetaminophen Adult Liquid Pain Reliever

Regular Strength TYLENOL® acetaminophen Caplets and Tablets

TYLENOL® Extended Relief acetaminophen extended release Caplets

Product information for all dosage forms of Adult TYLENOL acetaminophen have been combined under this heading.

Description: Each ***Extra Strength TYLENOL® Gelcap, Geltab, Caplet, or Tablet*** contains acetaminophen 500 mg. Each 15 ml (1/2 fl oz or one tablespoonful) of ***Extra Strength TYLENOL® acetaminophen Adult Liquid Pain Reliever*** contains 500 mg acetaminophen (alcohol 7%).
Each ***Regular Strength TYLENOL® Caplet or Tablet*** contains acetaminophen 325 mg.
Each ***TYLENOL® Extended Relief Caplet*** contains acetaminophen 650 mg.

Actions: Acetaminophen is a clinically proven analgesic and antipyretic. Acetaminophen produces analgesia by elevation of the pain threshold and antipyresis through action on the hypothalamic heat-regulating center. Acetaminophen is equal to aspirin in analgesic and antipyretic effectiveness and it is unlikely to produce many of the side effects associated with aspirin and aspirin-containing products.
Tylenol Extended Relief uses a unique, patented bilayer caplet. The first layer dissolves quickly to provide prompt relief while the second layer is time released to provide up to 8 hours of relief.

Indications: For the temporary relief of minor aches and pains associated with the common cold, headache, toothache, muscular aches, back ache, for the minor pain of arthritis, for the pain of menstrual cramps and for the reduction of fever.

Directions: *Extra Strength TYLENOL® Gelcaps, Geltabs, Caplets, or Tablets:* Adults and Children 12 years of Age and Older: Take two gelcaps, geltabs, caplets, or tablets every 4 to 6 hours. Not to exceed 8 gelcaps, geltabs, caplets, or tablets in any 24-hour period. Not for use in children under 12 years of age.
Extra Strength TYLENOL® Adult Liquid Pain Reliever: Adults and Children 12 years of Age and Older: Fill measuring cup once to 2-tablespoon line (1,000 mg) which is equivalent to two 500 mg Extra Strength TYLENOL® Gelcaps, Geltabs, Caplets or Tablets. Take every 4–6 hours. No more than 4 doses in any 24-hour period, or as directed by a doctor. Not for use in children under 12 years of age.
Regular Strength TYLENOL® Caplets or Tablets: Adults and Children 12 years of Age and Older: Take two caplets or tablets every 4 to 6 hours. No more than a total of 12 caplets or tablets in any 24-hour period, or as directed by a doctor. Children (6–11): 1/2 to 1 caplet or tablet every 4 to 6 hours, not to exceed 5 doses in 24 hours. Consult a physician for use by children under 6 years of age.
TYLENOL® Extended Relief Caplets: Adults and Children 12 years of Age and Older: Take two caplets every 8 hours, not to exceed 6 caplets in any 24-hour period. TAKE TWO CAPLETS WITH WATER, SWALLOW EACH CAPLET WHOLE. DO NOT CRUSH, CHEW, OR DISSOLVE THE CAPLET. Not for use in children under 12 years of age.

Precautions: If a rare sensitivity reaction occurs, the drug should be discontinued.

Warnings: Do not use if carton is opened or printed red neck wrap or printed full inner seal is broken. Do not take for pain for more than 10 days or for fever for more than 3 days unless directed by a physician. If pain or fever persists, or gets worse, if new symptoms occur, or if redness or swelling is present, consult a physician because these could be signs of a serious condition. As with any drug, if you are pregnant or nursing a baby, seek the advice of a health professional before using this product. Keep this and all drugs out of the reach of children. In case of accidental overdose, contact a physician or poison control center immediately. Prompt medical attention is critical for adults as well as for children even if you do not notice any signs or symptoms. Do not use with other products containing acetaminophen.

Alcohol Warning: For this and all other pain relievers, including aspirin, ibuprofen, ketoprofen and naproxen sodium, if you generally consume three or more alcohol-containing drinks per day, you should consult your physician for advice on when and how you should take pain relievers.

Overdosage Information: Acetaminophen in massive overdosage may cause hepatic toxicity in some patients. In adults and adolescents, hepatic toxicity has rarely been reported following ingestion of acute overdoses of less than 10 grams. Fatalities are infrequent (less than 3–4% of untreated cases) and have rarely been reported with overdoses of less than 15 grams. In children, an acute overdosage of less than 150 mg/kg has not been associated with hepatic toxicity. Early symptoms following a potentially hepatotoxic overdose may include: nausea, vomiting, diaphoresis and general malaise. Clinical and laboratory evidence of hepatic toxicity may not be apparent until 48 to 72 hours postingestion. In adults and adolescents, regardless of the quantity of acetaminophen reported to have been ingested, administer acetylcysteine immediately if 24 hours or less have elapsed from the reported time of ingestion. For full prescribing information, refer to the acetylcysteine package insert. Do not await results of assays for plasma acetaminophen level before initiating treatment with acetylcysteine. The following additional procedures are recommended: The stomach should be emptied promptly by lavage or by induction of emesis with syrup of ipecac. A plasma acetaminophen assay should be obtained as early as possible, but no sooner than four hours following ingestion. If an acetaminophen extended release product is involved, it may be appropriate to obtain an additional plasma acetaminophen level 4–6 hours following the initial plasma acetaminophen level. If either plasma level falls above the lower treatment line on the acetaminophen overdose nomogram, acetylcysteine therapy should be continued. Liver function studies should be obtained initially and repeated at 24-hour intervals.

Continued on next page

McNeil Consumer—Cont.

Serious toxicity or fatalities are extremely infrequent in children, possibly due to differences in the way they metabolize acetaminophen. In children, the maximum potential amount ingested can be more easily estimated. If more than 150 mg/kg or an unknown amount was ingested, obtain a plasma acetaminophen level. The plasma level should be obtained as soon as possible, but no sooner than 4 hours following the ingestion. If an acetaminophen *extended release* product is involved, it may be appropriate to obtain an additional plasma acetaminophen level 4–6 hours following the initial plasma acetaminophen level. If either plasma level falls above the lower treatment line on the acetaminophen overdose nomogram, the acetylcysteine therapy should be initiated and continued for a full course of therapy. If plasma acetaminophen assay capability is not available, and the estimated acetaminophen ingestion exceeds 150 mg/kg, acetylcysteine therapy should be initiated and continued for a full course of therapy.
For additional emergency information, call your regional poison center or call the Rocky Mountain Poison Center toll-free, (1-800-525-6115).

Alcohol Information: Chronic heavy alcohol abusers may be at increased risk of liver toxicity from excessive acetaminophen use, although reports of this event are rare. Reports almost invariably involve cases of severe chronic alcoholics and the dosages of acetaminophen most often exceed recommended doses and often involve substantial overdose. Professionals should alert their patients who regularly consume large amounts of alcohol not to exceed recommended doses of acetaminophen.

Inactive Ingredients: ***Extra Strength TYLENOL®:*** **Tablets:** Magnesium Stearate, Cellulose, Sodium Starch Glycolate and Starch. **Caplets:** Cellulose, Cornstarch, Hydroxypropyl Methylcellulose, Magnesium Stearate, Polyethylene Glycol, Sodium Starch Glycolate, and Red #40. **Gelcaps:** Benzyl Alcohol, Butylparaben, Castor Oil, Cellulose, Edetate Calcium Disodium, Gelatin, Hydroxypropyl Methylcellulose, Magnesium Stearate, Methylparaben, Propylparaben, Sodium Lauryl Sulfate, Sodium Propionate, Sodium Starch Glycolate, Starch, Titanium Dioxide, Blue #1 and #2, Red #40, and Yellow #10. **Geltabs:** Benzyl Alcohol, Butylparaben, Castor Oil, Cellulose, Corn Starch, Edetate Calcium Disodium, Gelatin, Hydroxypropyl Methylcellulose, Magnesium Stearate, Methylparaben, Propylparaben, Sodium Lauryl Sulfate, Sodium Propionate, Sodium Starch Glycolate, Titanium Dioxide, Blue #1 and #2, Red #40, and Yellow #10.
Extra Strength TYLENOL® Adult Liquid Pain Reliever: Alcohol (7%), Citric Acid, Flavors, Glycerin, Polyethylene Glycol, Purified Water, Sodium Benzoate, Sorbitol, Sucrose, Yellow #6 (Sunset Yellow), Yellow #10 and Blue #1.
Regular Strength TYLENOL®: **Tablets:** Magnesium Stearate, Cellulose, Sodium Starch Glycolate and Starch. **Caplets:** Cellulose, Hydroxypropyl Methylcellulose, Magnesium Stearate, Polyethylene Glycol, Sodium Starch Glycolate, Starch and Red #40.
TYLENOL® Extended Relief Caplets: Corn Starch, Hydroxyethyl Cellulose, Hydroxypropyl Methylcellulose, Magnesium Stearate, Microcrystalline Cellulose, Povidone, Powdered Cellulose, Pregelatinized Starch, Sodium Starch Glycolate, Titanium Dioxide, Triacetin.

How Supplied: ***Extra Strength TYLENOL®:*** **Tablets** (colored white, imprinted "TYLENOL" and "500")—vials of 10, and tamper-resistant bottles of 30, 60, 100, and 200. **Caplets** (colored white, imprinted "TYLENOL 500 mg")—vials of 10, 10 blister packs, and tamper-resistant bottles of 24, 50, 100, 175, and 250 and FastCap package of 72. **Gelcaps** (colored yellow and red, imprinted "Tylenol 500") vials of 10 and tamper-resistant bottles of 24, 50, 100, and 225 and FastCap package of 72. **Geltabs** (colored yellow and red, imprinted "Tylenol 500") tamper-resistant bottles of 24, 50, and 100.
Extra Strength TYLENOL® Adult Liquid Pain Reliever: Mint-flavored liquid (colored green) 8 fl. oz. tamper-resistant bottle with child resistant safety cap and special dosage cup.
Regular Strength TYLENOL®: **Tablets** (colored white, scored, imprinted "TYLENOL" and "325")—tamper-resistant bottles of 24, 50, 100 and 200. **Caplets** (colored white, "TYLENOL 325")—tamper-resistant bottles of 24, 50, 100.
TYLENOL® Extended Relief Caplets: (colored white, engraved "TYLENOL ER") tamper-resistant bottles of 24, 50, and 100's.

Shown in Product Identification Guide, page 512 and 513

TYLENOL® COLD Medication No Drowsiness Formula Caplets and Gelcaps

Multi-Symptom Formula TYLENOL® COLD Medication Tablets and Caplets

TYLENOL® COLD Multi-Symptom Hot Medication Liquid Packets

Product information for all dosage forms of TYLENOL COLD have been combined under this heading.

Description: Each ***TYLENOL® COLD Medication No Drowsiness Formula Caplet and Gelcap*** contains acetaminophen 325 mg, pseudoephedrine hydrochloride 30 mg, and dextromethorphan hydrobromide 15 mg.
Each ***Multi-Symptom Formula TYLENOL® COLD Tablet or Caplet*** contains acetaminophen 325 mg, chlorpheniramine maleate 2 mg, pseudoephedrine hydrochloride 30 mg, and dextromethorphan hydrobromide 15 mg.
Each packet of ***TYLENOL® COLD Multi-Symptom Hot Medication*** contains acetaminophen 650 mg, chlorpheniramine maleate 4 mg, pseudoephedrine hydrochloride 60 mg, and dextromethorphan hydrobromide 30 mg.

Actions: ***TYLENOL® COLD Medication No Drowsiness Formula*** contains a clinically proven analgesic-antipyretic, decongestant and cough suppressant. Acetaminophen produces analgesia by elevation of the pain threshold and antipyresis through action on the hypothalamic heat-regulating center. Acetaminophen is equal to aspirin in analgesic and antipyretic effectiveness and it is unlikely to produce many of the side effects associated with aspirin and aspirin-containing products. Pseudoephedrine is a sympathomimetic amine which provides temporary relief of nasal congestion. Dextromethorphan is a cough suppressant which provides temporary relief of coughs due to minor throat irritations that may occur with the common cold.
Multi-Symptom Formula TYLENOL® COLD Medication and ***TYLENOL® COLD Multi-Symptom Hot Medication*** contain, in addition to the above ingredients, an antihistamine. Chlorpheniramine is an antihistamine which helps provide temporary relief of runny nose, sneezing and watery and itchy eyes.

Indications: ***TYLENOL® COLD Medication No Drowsiness Formula*** provides effective temporary relief of nasal congestion, coughing, and body aches, pains, headache, sore throat and fever due to a cold or "flu."
Multi-Symptom Formula TYLENOL® COLD Medication and ***TYLENOL® COLD Multi-Symptom Hot Medication*** provide effective temporary relief of runny nose, sneezing, watery and itchy eyes, nasal congestion, coughing and body aches, pains, headache, sore throat and fever due to a cold or "flu."

Directions: ***TYLENOL® COLD No Drowsiness Formula and Multi-Symptom Formula TYLENOL® COLD Medication:*** Adults (12 years and older): Two every 6 hours, not to exceed 8 in 24 hours. Children (6–11 years): One every 6 hours, not to exceed 4 in 24 hours. Not for use in children under 6 years of age.
TYLENOL® COLD Multi-Symptom Hot Medication: Adults (12 years and older): dissolve one packet in 6 oz. cup of hot water. Sip while hot. Sweeten to taste, if desired. May repeat every 6 hours, not to exceed 4 doses in 24 hours. Not for use in children under 12 years of age.

Precautions: ***TYLENOL® COLD Medication No Drowsiness Formula, Multi-Symptom Formula TYLENOL® COLD Medication*** and ***TYLENOL® COLD Multi-Symptom Hot Medication:*** If a rare sensitivity reaction occurs, the drug should be stopped. Although pseudoephedrine is virtually without pressor effect in normotensive patients, it should be used with caution in hypertensives.

TYLENOL® COLD Medication No Drowsiness Formula: Do not take this product for more than 7 days or for fever for more than 3 days unless directed by a doctor. If pain or fever persists, or gets worse, if new symptoms occur, or if redness or swelling is present, consult a doctor because these could be signs of a serious condition. If sore throat is severe, persists for more than 2 days, is accompanied or followed by fever, headache, rash, nausea or vomiting, consult a doctor promptly. A persistent cough may be a sign of a serious condition. If cough persists for more than 1 week, tends to recur or is accompanied by fever, rash or persistent headache, consult a doctor. Do not take this product for persistent or chronic cough such as occurs with smoking, asthma, emphysema or if cough is accompanied by excessive phlegm (mucus) unless directed by a doctor. Do not exceed recommended dosage because at higher doses, nervousness, dizziness or sleeplessness may occur. Do not take this product if you have heart disease, high blood pressure, thyroid disease, diabetes or difficulty in urination due to enlargement of the prostate gland unless directed by a doctor. Do not use with other products containing acetaminophen.

DO NOT USE IF CARTON IS OPENED OR IF A BLISTER UNIT IS BROKEN. **KEEP THIS AND ALL MEDICATION OUT OF THE REACH OF CHILDREN. AS WITH ANY DRUG, IF YOU ARE PREGNANT OR NURSING A BABY, SEEK THE ADVICE OF A HEALTH PROFESSIONAL BEFORE USING THIS PRODUCT. IN CASE OF ACCIDENTAL OVERDOSE, CONTACT A DOCTOR OR POISON CONTROL CENTER IMMEDIATELY. PROMPT MEDICAL ATTENTION IS CRITICAL FOR ADULTS AS WELL AS FOR CHILDREN EVEN IF YOU DO NOT NOTICE ANY SIGNS OR SYMPTOMS.**

Multi-Symptom Formula TYLENOL® COLD Medication: Do not take this product for more than 7 days or for fever for more than 3 days unless directed by a doctor. If symptoms do not improve or are accompanied by fever, consult a doctor. If sore throat is severe, persists for more than 2 days, is accompanied or followed by fever, headache, rash, nausea or vomiting, consult a doctor promptly. A persistent cough may be a sign of a serious condition. If cough persists for more than 1 week, tends to recur or is accompanied by fever, rash or persistent headache, consult a doctor. Do not take this product for persistent or chronic cough such as occurs with smoking, asthma, emphysema or if cough is accompanied by excessive phlegm (mucus) unless directed by a doctor. Do not exceed recommended dosage because at higher doses, nervousness, dizziness or sleeplessness may occur. May cause excitability in children. Do not take this product unless directed by a doctor, if you have a breathing problem such as emphysema or chronic bronchitis, or if you have glaucoma or difficulty in urination due to enlargement of the prostate gland. Do not take this product if you have heart disease, high blood pressure, thyroid disease or diabetes unless directed by a doctor. May cause drowsiness; alcohol, sedatives and tranquilizers may increase the drowsiness effect. Avoid alcoholic beverages while taking this product. Do not take this product if you are taking sedatives or tranquilizers without first consulting your doctor. Use caution when driving a motor vehicle or operating machinery. Do not use with other products containing acetaminophen.

DO NOT USE IF CARTON IS OPENED OR IF A BLISTER UNIT IS BROKEN. **KEEP THIS AND ALL MEDICATION OUT OF THE REACH OF CHILDREN. AS WITH ANY DRUG, IF YOU ARE PREGNANT OR NURSING A BABY, SEEK THE ADVICE OF A HEALTH PROFESSIONAL BEFORE USING THIS PRODUCT. IN CASE OF ACCIDENTAL OVERDOSE, CONTACT A DOCTOR OR POISON CONTROL CENTER IMMEDIATELY. PROMPT MEDICAL ATTENTION IS CRITICAL FOR ADULTS AS WELL AS FOR CHILDREN EVEN IF YOU DO NOT NOTICE ANY SIGNS OR SYMPTOMS.**

Warning: ***TYLENOL® COLD Multi-Symptom Hot Medication:*** Do not take this product for more than 7 days or for fever for more than 3 days unless directed by a doctor. If symptoms do not improve or are accompanied by fever, consult a doctor. If sore throat is severe, persists for more than 2 days, is accompanied or followed by fever, headache, rash, nausea or vomiting, consult a doctor promptly. A persistent cough may be a sign of a serious condition. If cough persists for more than 1 week, tends to recur or is accompanied by fever, rash or persistent headache, consult a doctor. Do not take this product for persistent or chronic cough such as occurs with smoking, asthma, emphysema or if cough is accompanied by excessive phlegm (mucus) unless directed by a doctor. Do not exceed recommended dosage because at higher doses, nervousness, dizziness or sleeplessness may occur. May cause excitability especially in children. Do not take this product, unless directed by a doctor, if you have a breathing problem such as emphysema or chronic bronchitis, or if you have glaucoma or difficulty in urination due to enlargement of the prostate gland. Do not take this product if you have heart disease, high blood pressure, thyroid disease or diabetes unless directed by a doctor. May cause drowsiness; alcohol, sedatives and tranquilizers may increase the drowsiness effect. Avoid alcoholic beverages while taking this product. Do not take this product if you are taking sedatives or tranquilizers without first consulting your doctor. Use caution when driving a motor vehicle or operating machinery. Do not use with other products containing acetaminophen.

DO NOT USE IF PRINTED CARTON OVERWRAP IS BROKEN OR MISSING OR IF FOIL PACKET IS TORN OR BROKEN. **KEEP THIS AND ALL MEDICATION OUT OF THE REACH OF CHILDREN. AS WITH ANY DRUG, IF YOU ARE PREGNANT OR NURSING A BABY, SEEK THE ADVICE OF A HEALTH PROFESSIONAL BEFORE USING THIS PRODUCT. IN CASE OF ACCIDENTAL OVERDOSE, CONTACT A DOCTOR OR POISON CONTROL CENTER IMMEDIATELY. PROMPT MEDICAL ATTENTION IS CRITICAL FOR ADULTS AS WELL AS FOR CHILDREN EVEN IF YOU DO NOT NOTICE ANY SIGNS OR SYMPTOMS.**

PHENYLKETONURICS: CONTAINS PHENYLALANINE 11 MG PER PACKET.

Alcohol Warning: For this and all other pain relievers, including aspirin, ibuprofen, ketoprofen and naproxen sodium, if you generally consume 3 or more alcohol-containing drinks per day, you should consult your physician for advice on when and how you should take pain relievers.

Drug Interaction Precaution: ***TYLENOL® COLD Medication No Drowsiness Formula, Multi-Symptom Formula TYLENOL® COLD Medication*** *and* ***TYLENOL® COLD Multi-Symptom Hot Medication:*** Do not take this product if you are presently taking a prescription drug for high blood pressure or you are now taking a prescription monoamine oxidase inhibitor (MAOI) (certain drugs for depression, psychiatric or emotional conditions, or Parkinson's disease), or for 2 weeks after stopping the MAOI drug. If you are uncertain whether your prescription drug contains an MAOI, consult a health professional before taking this product.

Overdosage Information: ***TYLENOL® COLD Medication No Drowsiness Formula, Multi-Symptom Formula TYLENOL® COLD Medication*** *and* ***TYLENOL® COLD Multi-Symptom Hot Medication:*** Acetaminophen in massive overdosage may cause hepatic toxicity in some patients. In adults and adolescents, hepatic toxicity has rarely been reported following ingestion of acute overdoses of less than 10 grams. Fatalities are infrequent (less than 3–4% of untreated cases) and have rarely been reported with overdoses of less than 15 grams. In children, an acute overdosage of less than 150 mg/kg has not been associated with hepatic toxicity.

Early symptoms following a potentially hepatotoxic overdose may include: nausea, vomiting, diaphoresis and general malaise. Clinical and laboratory evidence of hepatic toxicity may not be apparent until 48 to 72 hours postingestion.

Continued on next page

McNeil Consumer—Cont.

In adults and adolescents, regardless of the quantity of acetaminophen reported to have been ingested, administer acetylcysteine immediately if 24 hours or less have elapsed from the reported time of ingestion. For full prescribing information, refer to the acetylcysteine package insert. Do not await results of assays for plasma acetaminophen level before initiating treatment with acetylcysteine. The following additional procedures are recommended. The stomach should be emptied promptly by lavage or by induction of emesis with syrup of ipecac. A plasma acetaminophen assay should be obtained as early as possible, but no sooner than four hours following ingestion. If plasma level falls above the lower treatment line on the acetaminophen overdose nomogram, acetylcysteine therapy should be continued. Liver function studies should be obtained initially and repeated at 24-hour intervals.
Serious toxicity or fatalities are extremely infrequent in children, possibly due to differences in the way they metabolize acetaminophen. In children, the maximum potential amount ingested can be more easily estimated. If more than 150 mg/kg or an unknown amount was ingested, obtain a plasma acetaminophen level. The plasma acetaminophen level should be obtained as soon as possible, but no sooner than 4 hours following the ingestion. If plasma level falls above the lower treatment line on the acetaminophen overdose nomogram, the acetylcysteine therapy should be initiated and continued for a full course of therapy. If plasma acetaminophen assay capability is not available, and the estimated acetaminophen ingestion exceeds 150 mg/kg, acetylcysteine therapy should be initiated and continued for a full course of therapy.
For additional emergency information, call your regional poison center or call the Rocky Mountain Poison Center toll-free, (1-800-525-6115).
Symptoms from pseudoephedrine overdose consist most often of mild anxiety, tachycardia and/or mild hypertension. Symptoms usually appear within 4 to 8 hours of ingestion and are transient, usually requiring no treatment.
Acute dextromethorphan overdose usually does not result in serious signs and symptoms unless massive amounts have been ingested. Signs and symptoms of a substantial overdose may include nausea and vomiting, visual disturbances, CNS disturbances, and urinary retention.
Chlorpheniramine toxicity should be treated as you would an antihistamine/anticholinergic overdose and is likely to be present within a few hours after acute ingestion.

Alcohol Information: ***TYLENOL® COLD Medication No Drowsiness Formula, Multi-symptom Formula TYLENOL® COLD Medication*** and ***TYLENOL® COLD Multi-Symptom Hot Medication:*** Chronic heavy alcohol abusers may be at increased risk of liver toxicity from excessive acetaminophen use, although reports of this event are rare. Reports almost invariably involve cases of severe chronic alcoholics and the dosages of acetaminophen most often exceed recommended doses and often involve substantial overdose. Professionals should alert their patients who regularly consume large amounts of alcohol not to exceed recommended doses of acetaminophen.

Inactive Ingredients: ***TYLENOL® COLD No Drowsiness Formula: Caplets:*** cellulose, corn starch, glyceryl triacetate, hydroxypropyl methylcellulose, iron oxide black, magnesium stearate, sodium starch glycolate, titanium dioxide, Blue #1 and Yellow #10. Gelcap: benzyl alcohol, butylparaben, castor oil, cellulose, corn starch, edetate calcium disodium, gelatin, hydroxypropyl methylcellulose, magnesium stearate, methylparaben, propylparaben, sodium propionate, sodium lauryl sulfate, sodium starch glycolate, titanium dioxide, Red #40 and Yellow #10.
Multi-Symptom Formula TYLENOL® COLD Medication: Tablets: cellulose, cornstarch, magnesium stearate, Sodium Starch Glycolate Yellow #6 and Yellow #10. **Caplets:** cellulose, cornstarch, glyceryl triacetate, hydroxypropyl methylcellulose, iron oxide black, magnesium stearate, sodium starch glycolate, titanium dioxide, Blue #1 and Yellow #6 and #10.
TYLENOL® COLD Multi-Symptom Hot Medication: Aspartame, citric acid, corn starch, sodium citrate, sucrose, Red #40 and Yellow #10.

How Supplied: ***TYLENOL® COLD No Drowsiness Formula: Caplets*** (colored white, imprinted "TYLENOL COLD") blister packs of 24. Gelcaps (colored red and tan, imprinted "TYLENOL COLD") blister packs of 24.
Multi-Symptom Formula TYLENOL® COLD Medication: Tablets (colored yellow, imprinted "TYLENOL Cold") blister packs of 24. **Caplets** (light yellow, imprinted "TYLENOL Cold") blister packs of 24.
TYLENOL® COLD Multi-Symptom Hot Medication: Packets of powder (yellow colored) in cartons of 6 tamper-resistant foil packets.

Shown in Product Identification Guide, page 512

MULTI-SYMPTOM TYLENOL® COLD SEVERE CONGESTION

Description: EACH CAPLET contains acetaminophen 325 mg, pseudoephedrine HCl 30 mg, guaifenesin 200 mg and dextromethorphan HBr 15 mg.

Actions: Multi-Symptom ***TYLENOL® COLD SEVERE CONGESTION Caplets*** contains a clinically proven analgesic-antipyretic, decongestant, expectorant and cough suppressant. Acetaminophen produces analgesia by elevation of the pain threshold and antipyresis through action on the hypothalamic heat-regulating center. Acetaminophen is equal to aspirin in analgesic and antipyretic effectiveness and is unlikely to produce many of the side effects associated with aspirin and aspirin-containing products. Pseudoephedrine is a sympathomimetic amine which provides temporary relief of nasal congestion. Guaifenesin is an expectorant which helps loosen phlegm (mucus) and thin bronchial secretions to make coughs more productive. Dextromethorphan is a cough suppressant which provides temporary relief of coughs due to minor throat irritations that may occur with the common cold.

Indications: Multi-Symptom ***TYLENOL® COLD SEVERE CONGESTION Caplets*** provide temporary relief without drowsiness of nasal congestion, chest congestion, coughing, sore throat, headaches, body aches and fever.

Dosage: Adults and Children 12 years of Age and older: Take two caplets every 6–8 hours, not to exceed 8 caplets in any 24 hour period.
Children 6 to 11 years of age: One caplet every 6–8 hours not to exceed 4 caplets in any 24 hour period. Not for use in children under 6 years of age.

Precautions: If a rare sensitivity reaction occurs, the drug should be discontinued. Although pseudoephedrine is virtually without pressor effect in normotensive patients, it should be used with caution in hypertensives.

Warnings: DO NOT USE IF CARTON IS OPENED OR IF A BLISTER UNIT IS BROKEN. Do not take for pain for more than 7 days or for fever for more than 3 days unless directed by a doctor. If pain or fever persists, or gets worse, if new symptoms occur, or if redness or swelling is present, consult a doctor because these could be signs of a serious condition. If sore throat is severe, persists for more than 2 days, is accompanied or followed by fever, headache, rash, nausea or vomiting, consult a doctor promptly. A persistent cough may be a sign of a serious condition. If cough persists for more than 1 week, tends to recur or is accompanied by fever, rash or persistent headache, consult a doctor. Do not take this product for persistent or chronic cough such as occurs with smoking, asthma, emphysema or if cough is accompanied by excessive phlegm (mucus) unless directed by a doctor. **Do not exceed recommended dosage.** If nervousness, dizziness, or sleeplessness occur, discontinue use and consult a doctor. Do not take this product if you have heart disease, high blood pressure, thyroid disease, diabetes or difficulty in urination due to enlargement of the prostate gland unless directed by a doctor. As with any drug, if you are pregnant or nursing a baby, seek the advice of a health professional before using this product. Keep this and all drugs out of the reach of children., In case of accidental overdose, contact a doctor or poison control center immediately. Prompt medical attention is critical for adults as well as for children even if you do not notice any signs of symptoms. Do not use with other products containing acetaminophen.

Alcohol Warning: For this and all other pain relievers, including aspirin, ibuprofen, ketoprofen and naproxen sodium, if you generally consume 3 or more alcohol-containing drinks per day you should consult your physician for advice on when and how you should take pain relievers.

Overdosage Information: Acetaminophen in massive overdosage may cause hepatic toxicity in some patients. In adults and adolescents, hepatic toxicity has rarely been reported following ingestion of acute overdoses of less than 10 grams. Fatalities are infrequent (less than 3–4% of untreated cases) and have rarely been reported with overdoses of less than 15 grams. In children, an acute overdosage of less than 150 mg/kg has not been associated with hepatic toxicity. Early symptoms following a potentially hepatotoxic overdose may include: nausea, vomiting, diaphoresis and general malaise. Clinical and laboratory evidence of hepatic toxicity may not be apparent until 48 to 72 hours postingestion. In adults and adolescents, regardless of the quantity of acetaminophen reported to have been ingested, administer acetylcysteine immediately if 24 hours or less have elapsed from the reported time of ingestion. For full prescribing information, refer to the acetylcysteine package insert. Do not await results of assays for plasma acetaminophen level before initiating treatment with acetylcysteine. The following additional procedures are recommended. The stomach should be emptied promptly by lavage or by inducing of emesis with syrup of ipecac. A plasma acetaminophen assay should be obtained as early as possible, but no sooner than four hours following ingestion. If plasma level falls above the lower treatment line on the acetaminophen overdose nomogram, acetylcysteine therapy should be continued. Liver function studies should be obtained initially and repeated at 24-hour intervals.
Serious toxicity or fatalities are extremely infrequent in children, possibly due to differences in the way they metabolize acetaminophen. In children, the maximum potential amount ingested can be more easily estimated. If more than 150 mg/kg or an unknown amount was ingested, obtain a plasma acetaminophen level. The plasma acetaminophen level should be obtained as soon as possible, but no sooner than 4 hours following the ingestion. If plasma level falls above the lower treatment line on the acetaminophen overdose nomogram, the acetylcysteine therapy should be initiated and continued for a full course of therapy. If plasma acetaminophen assay capability is not available, and the estimated acetaminophen ingestion exceeds 150 mg/kg, acetlcysteine therapy should be initiated and continued for a full course of therapy.
For additional emergency information, call your regional poison center or call the Rocky Mountain Poison Center toll-free, (1-800-525-6115).
Symptoms from pseudoephedrine overdose consist most often of mild anxiety, tachycardia and/or mild hypertension. Symptoms usually appear within 4 to 8 hours of ingestion and are transient, usually requiring no treatment.
Acute dextromethorphan overdose usually does not result in serious signs and symptoms unless massive amounts have been ingested. Signs and symptoms of a substantial overdose may include nausea and vomiting, visual disturbance, CNS disturbances, and urinary retention.
Chlorpheniramine toxicity should be treated as you would an antihistamine/anticholinergic overdose and is likely to be present within a few hours after acute ingestion. Guaifenesin should be treated as a non-toxic ingestion.

Alcohol Information: Chronic heavy alcohol abusers may be at increased risk of liver toxicity from excessive acetaminophen use, although reports of this event are rare. Reports almost invariably involve cases of severe chronic alcoholics and the dosages of acetaminophen most often exceed recommended doses and often involve substantial overdose. Professionals should alert their patients who regularly consume large amounts of alcohol not to exceed recommended doses of acetaminophen.

Drug Interaction Precaution: Do not use this product if you are now taking a prescription monoamine oxidase inhibitor (MAOI) (certain drugs for depression, psychiatric or emotional conditions, or Parkinson's disease), or for 2 weeks after stopping the MAOI drug. If you are uncertain whether your prescription drug contains an MAOI, consult a health professional before taking this product.

Inactive Ingredients: Carnauba Wax, Cellulose, Colloidal Silicon Dioxide, Corn Starch, Hydroxypropyl Methylcellulose, Iron Oxide, Povidone, Pregelatinized Starch, Propylene Glycol, Sodium Starch Glycolate, Stearic Acid, Titanium Dioxide, Triacetin, Blue #1, Yellow #6 and Yellow #10.

How Supplied: Caplets (colored buttery-tan, with green imprinted "TYLENOL COLD SC") in blister packs of 12 and 24.

Shown in Product Identification Guide, page 512

Multi-Symptom TYLENOL® COUGH Medication

Multi-Symptom TYLENOL® COUGH Medication with Decongestant

Product information for all dosage forms of TYLENOL COUGH have been combined under this heading.

Description: Each 15 ml (3 tsp.) adult dose of ***Multi-Symptom TYLENOL® COUGH Medication*** contains dextromethorphan HBr 30 mg, and acetaminophen 650 mg.
Each 15 ml (3 tsp.) adult dose of ***Multi-Symptom TYLENOL® COUGH Medication with Decongestant*** contains dextromethorphan HBr 30 mg, acetaminophen 650 mg, and pseudoephedrine HCl 60 mg.

Actions: ***Multi-Symptom TYLENOL® COUGH Medication*** contains a clinically proven cough suppressant, and an analgesic-antipyretic. Acetaminophen produces analgesia by elevation of the pain threshold and antipyresis through action on the hypothalamic heat-regulating center. Dextromethorphan is a cough suppressant which provides temporary relief of coughs due to minor throat irritations that may occur with the common cold.
Multi-Symptom TYLENOL® COUGH Medication with Decongestant contains, in addition to the above ingredients, a sympathomimetic amine, pseudoephedrine HCl, which provides temporary relief of nasal congestion.

Indications: ***Multi-Symptom TYLENOL® COUGH Medication*** provides effective, temporary relief of coughing, and the aches, pains and sore throat that may accompany a cough due to a cold.
Multi-Symptom TYLENOL® COUGH Medication with Decongestant provides effective, temporary relief of coughing, nasal congestion and the aches, pains and sore throat that may accompany a cough due to a cold.

Directions: ***Multi-Symptom TYLENOL® COUGH Medication and Multi-Symptom TYLENOL® COUGH Medication with Decongestant:*** Adults (12 years and older): 1 tablespoon or 3 teaspoons every 6–8 hours, not to exceed 4 doses in 24 hours. Children: (ages 6–11) $1^1/_2$ teaspoons every 6–8 hours, not to exceed 4 doses in 24 hours. Not for use in children under 6 years of age.

Precautions: ***Multi-Symptom TYLENOL® COUGH Medication:*** If a rare sensitivity reaction occurs, the drug should be discontinued.
Multi-Symptom TYLENOL® COUGH Medication with Decongestant: If a rare sensitivity reaction occurs, the drug should be discontinued. Although pseudoephedrine is virtually without pressor effect in normotensive patients, it should be used with caution in hypertensives.

Continued on next page

McNeil Consumer—Cont.

Warning: ***Multi-Symptom TYLENOL® COUGH Medication:*** Do not take this product for more than 10 days or for fever for more than 3 days unless directed by a physician. Severe or recurrent pain or high or continued fever may be indicative of serious illness. Under these conditions, consult a doctor. A persistent cough may be a sign of a serious condition. If cough persists for more than 1 week, tends to recur or is accompanied by fever, rash or persistent headache, consult a doctor. Do not take this product for persistent or chronic cough such as occurs with smoking, asthma, emphysema, or if cough is accompanied by excessive phlegm (mucus) unless directed by a doctor. If sore throat is severe, persists for more than 2 days, is accompanied or followed by fever, headache, rash, nausea or vomiting, consult a doctor promptly. Do not use with other products containing acetaminophen.
DO NOT USE IF PRINTED PLASTIC BOTTLE WRAP OR PRINTED FOIL INNER SEAL IS BROKEN. **As with any drug, if you are pregnant or nursing a baby, seek the advice of a health professional before using this product. Keep this and all medication out of the reach of children. In case of accidental overdosage, contact a doctor or poison control center immediately. Prompt medical attention is critical for adults as well as children even if you do not notice any signs or symptoms.**
Multi-Symptom TYLENOL® COUGH Medication with Decongestant: Do not take this product for more than 7 days or for fever for more than 3 days unless directed by a doctor. If symptoms do not improve or are accompanied by fever, consult a doctor. A persistent cough may be a sign of a serious condition. If cough persists for more than 1 week, tends to recur or is accompanied by fever, rash or persistent headache, consult a doctor. Do not take this product for persistent or chronic cough such as occurs with smoking, asthma, emphysema, or if cough is accompanied by excessive phlegm (mucus) unless directed by a doctor. Do not exceed the recommended dosage because at higher doses nervousness, dizziness or sleeplessness may occur. Do not take this product if you have heart disease, high blood pressure, thyroid disease, diabetes or difficulty in urination due to enlargement of the prostate gland unless directed by a doctor. If sore throat is severe, persists for more than 2 days, is accompanied or followed by fever, headache, rash, nausea or vomiting, consult a doctor promptly. Do not use with other products containing acetaminophen.
DO NOT USE IF PRINTED PLASTIC BOTTLE WRAP OR PRINTED FOIL INNER SEAL IS BROKEN. **As with any drug, if you are pregnant or nursing a baby, seek the advice of a health professional before using this product. Keep this and all medication out of the reach of children. In case of accidental overdosage, contact a doctor or poison control center immediately. Prompt medical attention is critical for adults as well as children even if you do not notice any signs or symptoms.**

Alcohol Warning: ***Multi-Symptom TYLENOL® COUGH Medication and Multi-Symptom TYLENOL® COUGH Medication with Decongestant:*** For this and all other pain relievers, including aspirin, ibuprofen, ketoprofen and naproxen sodium; if you generally consume 3 or more alcohol-containing drinks per day, you should consult your physician for advice on when and how you should take pain relievers.

Drug Interaction Precaution: ***Multi-Symptom TYLENOL® COUGH Medication:*** Do not use this product if you are presently taking a prescription monoamine oxidase inhibitor (MAOI) (certain drugs for depression, psychiatric or emotional conditions, or Parkinson's Disease), or for 2 weeks after stopping the MAOI drug. If you are uncertain whether your prescription drug contains an MAOI, consult a health professional before taking this product.
Multi-Symptom TYLENOL® COUGH Medication with Decongestant: Do not use this product if you are presently taking a prescription drug for high blood pressure or you are now taking a prescription monoamine oxidase inhibitor (MAOI) (certain drugs for depression or psychiatric or emotional conditions, or Parkinson's Disease), or for 2 weeks after stopping the MAOI drug. If you are uncertain whether your prescription drug contains an MAOI, consult a health professional before taking this product.

Overdosage Information: ***Multi-Symptom TYLENOL® COUGH Medication and Multi-Symptom TYLENOL® COUGH Medication with Decongestant:*** Acetaminophen in massive overdosage may cause hepatic toxicity in some patients. In adults and adolescents, hepatic toxicity has rarely been reported following ingestion of acute overdoses of less than 10 grams. Fatalities are infrequent (less than 3–4% of untreated cases) and have rarely been reported with overdoses of less than 15 grams. In children, an acute overdosage of less than 150 mg/kg has not been associated with hepatic toxicity.
Early symptoms following a potentially hepatotoxic overdose may include: nausea, vomiting, diaphoresis and general malaise. Clinical and laboratory evidence of hepatic toxicity may not be apparent until 48 to 72 hours postingestion.
In adults and adolescents, regardless of the quantity of acetaminophen reported to have been ingested, administer acetylcysteine immediately if 24 hours or less have elapsed from the reported time of ingestion. For full prescribing information, refer to the acetylcysteine package insert. Do not await results of assays for plasma acetaminophen level before initiating treatment with acetylcysteine. The following additional procedures are recommended. The stomach should be emptied promptly by lavage or by induction of emesis with syrup of ipecac. A plasma acetaminophen assay should be obtained as early as possible, but no sooner than four hours following ingestion. If plasma level falls above the lower treatment line on the acetaminophen overdose nomogram, acetylcysteine therapy should be continued. Liver function studies should be obtained initially and repeated at 24-hour intervals.
Serious toxicity or fatalities are extremely infrequent in children, possibly due to differences in the way they metabolize acetaminophen. In children, the maximum potential amount ingested can be more easily estimated. If more than 150 mg/kg or an unknown amount was ingested, obtain a plasma acetaminophen level. The plasma acetaminophen level should be obtained as soon as possible, but no sooner than 4 hours following the ingestion. If the plasma level falls above the lower treatment line on the acetaminophen overdose nomogram, the acetylcysteine therapy should be initiated and continued for a full course of therapy. If plasma acetaminophen assay capability is not available, and the estimated acetaminophen ingestion exceeds 150 mg/kg, acetycysteine therapy should be initiated and continued for a full course of therapy.
For additional emergency information, call your regional poison center or call the Rocky Mountain Poison Center toll-free (1-800-525-6115).
Acute dextromethorphan overdose usually does not result in serious signs and symptoms unless massive amounts have been ingested. Signs and symptoms of a substantial overdose may include nausea and vomiting, visual disturbances, CNS disturbances, and urinary retention.
Symptoms from pseudoephedrine overdose consist most often of mild anxiety, tachycardia and/or mild hypertension. Symptoms usually appear within 4 to 8 hours of ingestion and are transient, usually requiring no treatment.

Alcohol Information: ***Multi-Symptom TYLENOL® COUGH Medication and Multi-Symptom TYLENOL® COUGH Medication with Decongestant:*** Chronic heavy alcohol abusers may be at increased risk of liver toxicity from excessive acetaminophen use, although reports of this event are rare. Reports almost invariably involve cases of severe chronic alcoholics and the dosages of acetaminophen most often exceed recommended doses and often involve substantial overdose. Professionals should alert their patients who regularly consume large amounts of alcohol not to exceed recommended doses of acetaminophen.

Inactive Ingredients: ***Multi-Symptom TYLENOL® COUGH Medication:*** Alcohol (5%), citric acid, flavors, high fructose corn syrup, polyethylene glycol, propylene glycol, purified water, sodium benzoate, sodium carboxymethylcelluose, sodium saccharin, sorbitol, Red #40.

Multi-Symptom TYLENOL® COUGH Medication with Decongestant: Alcohol (5%), citric acid, flavors, high fructose corn syrup. polyethylene glycol, propylene glycol, purified water, sodium benzoate, sodium carboxymethylcellulose, sodium saccharin, sorbitol, Blue #1, and Red #40.

How Supplied: ***Multi-Symptom TYLENOL® COUGH Medication*** is available in a 4 oz. bottle with child resistant safety cap and tamper resistant packaging.

Multi-Symptom TYLENOL® COUGH Medication with Decongestant is available in a 4 oz. bottle with child resistant safety cap, and tamper resistant packaging.

Shown in Product Identification Guide, page 512

Maximum Strength TYLENOL® FLU Medication No Drowsiness Formula Gelcaps

Maximum Strength TYLENOL® FLU NightTime Medication Gelcaps

Maximum Strength TYLENOL® FLU NightTime Hot Medication Packets

Product information for all dosage forms of TYLENOL FLU have been combined under this heading.

Description: Each ***Maximum Strength TYLENOL® FLU Medication No Drowsiness Formula Gelcap*** contains acetaminophen 500 mg, pseudoephedrine hydrochloride 30 mg, and dextromethorphan hydrobromide 15 mg.

Each ***Maximum Strength TYLENOL® FLU NightTime Medication Gelcap*** contains acetaminophen 500 mg, pseudoephedrine hydrochloride 30 mg, and diphenhydramine hydrochloride 25 mg.

Each packet of ***Maximum Strength TYLENOL FLU NightTime Hot Medication*** contains acetaminophen 1000 mg, pseudoephedrine hydrochloride 60 mg and diphenhydramine hydrochloride 50 mg.

Actions: ***Maximum Strength TYLENOL® FLU Medication No Drowsiness Formula*** contains a clinically proven analgesic-antipyretic, decongestant and cough suppressant. Acetaminophen produces analgesia by elevation of the pain threshold and antipyresis through action on the hypothalamic heat-regulating center. Acetaminophen is equal to aspirin in analgesic and antipyretic effectiveness and it is unlikely to produce many of the side effects associated with aspirin and aspirin-containing products. Pseudoephedrine hydrochloride is a sympathomimetic amine which provides temporary relief of nasal congestion. Dextromethorphan is a cough suppressant which provides temporary relief of coughs due to minor throat irritations that may occur with the common cold.

Maximum Strength TYLENOL® FLU NightTime Medication and ***Maximum Strength TYLENOL® FLU NightTime Hot Medication*** contains the same clinically proven analgesic-antipyretic and decongestant as Maximum Strength TYLENOL FLU Medication No Drowsiness Formula along with an antihistamine. Diphenhydramine is an antihistamine which helps provide temporary relief of runny nose and sneezing.

Indications: ***Maximum Strength TYLENOL® FLU Medication No Drowsiness Formula*** provides effective temporary relief of body aches, headaches, fever, sore throat, coughing and nasal congestion due to a cold or "flu."

Maximum Strength TYLENOL® FLU NightTime Medication and ***Maximum Strength TYLENOL® FLU NightTime Hot Medication*** provides effective temporary relief of body aches, headaches, fever, sore throat, nasal congestion, and runny nose/sneezing due to a cold or "flu" so you can rest.

Directions: ***Maximum Strength TYLENOL® FLU Medication No Drowsiness Formula:*** Adults (12 years and older): Two gelcaps every 6 hours, not to exceed 8 gelcaps in 24 hours. Not for use in children under 12 years of age.

Maximum Strength TYLENOL® FLU NightTime Medication: Adults (12 years and older): Two gelcaps at bedtime. May repeat every 6 hours, not to exceed 8 gelcaps in 24 hours. Not for use in children under 12 years of age.

Maximum Strength TYLENOL® FLU NightTime Hot Medication: Adults (12 years and older): Dissolve one packet in 6 oz. cup of hot water. Sip while hot. Sweeten to taste, if desired. May repeat every 6 hours, not to exceed 4 doses in 24 hours. Not for use in children under 12 years of age.

Precautions: ***Maximum Strength TYLENOL® FLU Medication No Drowsiness Formula, Maximum Strength TYLENOL® FLU NightTime Medication, and Maximum Strength TYLENOL® FLU NightTime Hot Medication:*** If a rare sensitivity reaction occurs, the drug should be stopped. Although pseudoephedrine is virtually without pressor effect in normotensive patients, it should be used with caution in hypertensives.

Warnings: ***Maximum Strength TYLENOL® FLU Medication No Drowsiness Formula:*** Do not take this product for more than 7 days or for fever for more than 3 days unless directed by a doctor. If symptoms do not improve or are accompanied by fever, consult a doctor. A persistent cough may be a sign of a serious condition. If cough persists for more than 1 week, tends to recur or is accompanied by fever, rash or persistent headache, consult a doctor. Do not take this product for persistent or chronic cough such as occurs with smoking, asthma, emphysema or if cough is accompanied by excessive phlegm (mucus) unless directed by a doctor. If sore throat is severe, persists for more than 2 days, is accompanied or followed by fever, headache, rash, nausea or vomiting, consult a doctor promptly. Do not exceed recommended dosage because at higher doses, nervousness, dizziness or sleeplessness may occur. Do not take this product if you have heart disease, high blood pressure, thyroid disease, diabetes, or difficulty in urination due to enlargement of the prostate gland unless directed by a doctor. Do not use with other products containing acetaminophen.

DO NOT USE IF CARTON IS OPENED OR IF A BLISTER UNIT IS BROKEN. KEEP THIS AND ALL MEDICATION OUT OF THE REACH OF CHILDREN. AS WITH ANY DRUG, IF YOU ARE PREGNANT OR NURSING A BABY, SEEK THE ADVICE OF A HEALTH PROFESSIONAL BEFORE USING THIS PRODUCT. IN CASE OF ACCIDENTAL OVERDOSE, CONTACT A DOCTOR OR POISON CONTROL CENTER IMMEDIATELY. PROMPT MEDICAL ATTENTION IS CRITICAL FOR ADULTS AS WELL AS CHILDREN EVEN IF YOU DO NOT NOTICE ANY SIGNS OR SYMPTOMS.

Maximum StrengthTYLENOL® FLU NightTime Medication Gelcaps: Do not exceed the recommended dosage, because at higher doses, nervousness, dizziness or sleeplessness may occur. Do not take this product for more than 7 days or for fever for more than 3 days unless directed by a doctor. If symptoms do not improve or are accompanied by fever, consult a doctor. If sore throat is severe, persists for more than 2 days, is accompanied by fever, headache, rash nausea or vomiting, consult a doctor promptly. May cause excitability, especially in children. Do not take this product, unless directed by a doctor, if you have a breathing problem such as emphysema or chronic bronchitis, or if you have glaucoma or difficulty in urination due to enlargement of the prostate gland. Do not take this product if you have heart disease, high blood pressure, thyroid disease, or diabetes unless directed by a doctor. May cause marked drowsiness: alcohol, sedatives and tranquilizers may increase the drowsiness effect. Avoid alcoholic beverages while taking this product. Do not take this product if you are taking sedatives or tranquilizers without first consulting your doctor. Use caution when driving a motor vehicle or operating machinery. Do not use with other products containing acetaminophen.

DO NOT USE IF CARTON IS OPENED OR IF A BLISTER UNIT IS BROKEN. KEEP THIS AND ALL MEDICATION OUT OF THE REACH OF CHILDREN. AS WITH ANY DRUG, IF YOU ARE PREGNANT OR NURSING A BABY, SEEK THE ADVICE OF A HEALTH PROFESSIONAL BEFORE USING THIS PRODUCT. IN CASE OF ACCIDENTAL OVERDOSE, CONTACT A

Continued on next page

McNeil Consumer—Cont.

DOCTOR OR POISON CONTROL CENTER IMMEDIATELY. PROMPT MEDICAL ATTENTION IS CRITICAL FOR ADULTS AS WELL AS CHILDREN EVEN IF YOU DO NOT NOTICE ANY SIGNS OR SYMPTOMS.

Maximum Strength TYLENOL® FLU NightTime Hot Medication: Do not exceed the recommended dosage, because at higher doses, nervousness, dizziness or sleeplessness may occur. Do not take this product for more than 7 days or for fever for more than 3 days unless directed by a doctor. If symptoms do not improve or are accompanied by fever, consult a doctor. If sore throat is severe, persists for more than 2 days, is accompanied or followed by fever, headache, rash, nausea or vomiting, consult a doctor promptly. May cause excitability especially in children. Do not take this product, unless directed by a doctor, if you have a breathing problem such as emphysema or chronic bronchitis, or if you have glaucoma or difficulty in urination due to enlargement of the prostate gland. Do not take this product if you have heart disease, high blood pressure, thyroid disease or diabetes unless directed by a doctor. May cause marked drowsiness: alcohol, sedatives and tranquilizers may increase the drowsiness effect. Avoid alcoholic beverages while taking this product. Do not take this product if you are taking sedatives or tranquilizers without first consulting your doctor. Use caution when driving a motor vehicle or operating machinery. Do not use with other products containing acetaminophen.

DO NOT USE IF PRINTED CARTON OVERWRAP IS BROKEN OR MISSING OR IF CARTON IS OPENED OR FOIL PACKET IS TORN OR BROKEN. KEEP THIS AND ALL MEDICATION OUT OF THE REACH OF CHILDREN. AS WITH ANY DRUG, IF YOU ARE PREGNANT OR NURSING A BABY, SEEK THE ADVICE OF A HEALTH PROFESSIONAL BEFORE USING THIS PRODUCT. IN CASE OF ACCIDENTAL OVERDOSE, CONTACT A DOCTOR OR POISON CONTROL CENTER IMMEDIATELY. PROMPT MEDICAL ATTENTION IS CRITICAL FOR ADULTS AS WELL AS CHILDREN EVEN IF YOU DO NOT NOTICE ANY SIGNS OR SYMPTOMS.

PHENYLKETONURICS: CONTAINS PHENYLALANINE 67 MG PER PACKET.

Alcohol Warning: ***Maximum Strength TYLENOL® FLU Medication No Drowsiness Formula, Maximum Strength TYLENOL® FLU NightTime Medication, and Maximum Strength TYLENOL® FLU NightTime Hot Medication:*** For this and all other pain relievers, including aspirin, ibuprofen, ketoprofen and naproxen sodium, if you generally consume 3 or more alcohol-containing drinks per day, you should consult your physician for advice on when and how you should take pain relievers.

Drug Interaction Precaution: ***Maximum Strength TYLENOL® FLU Medication No Drowsiness Formula, Maximum Strength TYLENOL® FLU NightTime Medication, and Maximum Strength TYLENOL® FLU NightTime Hot Medication:*** Do not take this product if you are presently taking a prescription drug for high blood pressure or you are now taking a prescription monoamine oxidase inhibitor (MAOI) (certain drugs for depression, psychiatric or emotional conditions, or Parkinson's disease), or for 2 weeks after stopping the MAOI drug. If you are uncertain whether your prescription drug contains an MAOI, consult a health professional before taking this product.

Overdosage Information: ***Maximum Strength TYLENOL® FLU Medication No Drowsiness Formula, Maximum Strength TYLENOL® FLU NightTime Medication, and Maximum Strength TYLENOL® FLU NightTime Hot Medication:*** Acetaminophen in massive overdosage may cause hepatic toxicity in some patients. In adults and adolescents, hepatic toxicity has rarely been reported following ingestion of acute overdoses of less than 10 grams. Fatalities are infrequent (less than 3–4% of untreated cases) and have rarely been reported with overdosage of less than 15 grams. In children, an acute overdosage of less than 150 mg/kg has not been associated with hepatic toxicity. Early symptoms following a potentially hepatotoxic overdose may include: nausea, vomiting, diaphoresis and general malaise. Clinical and laboratory evidence of hepatic toxicity may not be apparent until 48 to 72 hours postingestion. In adults and adolescents, regardless of the quantity of acetaminophen reported to have been ingested, administer acetylcysteine immediately if 24 hours or less have elapsed from the reported time of ingestion. For full prescribing information, refer to the acetylcysteine package insert. Do not await results of assays for plasma acetaminophen level before initiating treatment with acetyleysteine. The following additional procedures are recommended: The stomach should be emptied promptly by lavage or by induction of emesis with syrup of ipecac. A plasma acetaminophen assay should be obtained as early as possible, but not sooner than four hours following ingestion. If plasma level falls above the lower treatment line on the acetaminophen overdose nomogram, acetylcysteine therapy should be continued. Liver function studies should be obtained initially and repeated at 24-hour intervals.

Serious toxicity or fatalities are extremely infrequent in children, possibly due to differences in the way they metabolize acetaminophen. In children, the maximum potential amount ingested can be more easily estimated. If more than 150 mg/kg or an unknown amount was ingested, obtain an plasma acetaminophen level. The plasma acetaminophen level should be obtained as soon as possible, but no sooner than 4 hours following the ingestion. If plasma level falls above the lower treatment line on the acetaminophen overdose nomogram, the acetylcysteine therapy should be initiated and continued for a full course of therapy. If plasma acetaminophen assay capability is not available, and the estimated acetaminophen ingestion exceeds 150 mg/kg, acetylcysteine therapy should be initiated and continued for a full course of therapy.

For additional emergency information call your regional poison center or call the Rocky Mountain Poison Center toll free, (1-800-525-6115).

Symptoms from pseudoephedrine overdose consist most often of mild anxiety, tachycardia and/or mild hypertension. Symptoms usually appear within 4 to 8 hours of ingestion and are transient, usually requiring no treatment.

Acute dextromethorphan overdose usually does not result in serious signs and symptoms unless massive amounts have been ingested. Signs and symptoms of a substantial overdose may include nausea and vomiting, visual disturbances, CNS disturbances, and urinary retention.

Diphenhydramine toxicity should be treated as you would an antihistamine/anticholinergic overdose and is likely to be present within a few hours after acute ingestion.

Alcohol Information: ***Maximum Strength TYLENOL® FLU Medication No Drowsiness Formula, Maximum Strength TYLENOL® FLU NightTime Medication, and Maximum Strength TYLENOL® FLU NightTime Hot Medication:*** Chronic heavy alcohol abusers may be at increased risk of liver toxicity from excessive acetaminophen use, although reports of this event are rare. Reports almost invariably involve cases of severe chronic alcoholics and the dosages of acetaminophen most often exceed recommended doses and often involve substantial overdose. Professionals should alert their patients who regularly consume large amounts of alcohol not to exceed recommended doses of acetaminophen.

Inactive Ingredients: ***Maximum Strength TYLENOL® FLU Medication No Drowsiness Formula:*** Benzyl alcohol, butylparaben, castor oil, cellulose, corn starch edetate calcium disodium, gelatin, hydroxypropyl methylcellulose, iron oxide black, magnesium stearate, methylparaben, propylparaben, sodium lauryl sulfate, sodium propionate, sodium starch glycolate, titanium dioxide, Red #40 and Blue #1.

Maximum Strength TYLENOL® FLU NightTime Medication: Benzyl alcohol, butylparaben, castor oil, cellulose, corn starch, edetate calcium disodium, gelatin, hydroxypropyl methylcellulose, iron oxide black, magnesium stearate, methylparaben, propylparaben, sodium citrate, sodium laurel sulfate, sodium pro-

ionate, sodium starch glycolate, titanium dioxide, Red #28 and Blue #1.
Maximum Strength TYLENOL® FLU Hot Medication Packets: Ascorbic acid (vitamin C), aspartame, citric acid, flavors, sodium citrate, sucrose, Yellow #10, Blue #1, Red #40, and Yellow #6. May also contain: silicon dioxide.

How Supplied: ***Maximum Strength TYLENOL® FLU Medication No Drowsiness Formula:*** **Gelcaps** (colored burgundy and white, imprinted "TYLENOL FLU") in blister packs of 10 and 20.
Maximum Strength TYLENOL® FLU NightTime Medication: **Gelcaps** (colored blue and white, imprinted "TYLENOL FLU NT") in blister packs of 10 and 20.
Maximum Strength TYLENOL® FLU Hot Medication Packets: **Packets of powder** (yellow colored) in cartons of 6 tamper-resistant foil packets.

Shown in Product Identification Guide, page 512

Extra Strength TYLENOL® PM Pain Reliever/Sleep Aid Caplets, Geltabs and Gelcaps

Description: Each ***Extra Strength TYLENOL® PM Caplet, Geltab*** or ***Gelcap*** contains acetaminophen 500 mg and diphenhydramine HCl 25 mg.

Actions: ***Extra Strength TYLENOL® PM Caplets, Geltabs*** and ***Gelcaps*** contain a clinically proven analgesic-antipyretic and an antihistamine. Maximum allowable non-prescription levels of acetaminophen and diphenhydramine provide temporary relief of occasional headaches and minor aches and pains accompanying sleeplessness. Acetaminophen is equal to aspirin in analgesic and antipyretic effectiveness and it is unlikely to produce many of the side effects associated with aspirin containing products. Acetaminophen produces analgesia by elevation of the pain threshold. Diphenhydramine HCl is an antihistamine with sedative properties.

Indications: ***Extra Strength TYLENOL® PM Caplets, Geltabs*** and ***Gelcaps*** provide temporary relief of occasional headaches and minor aches and pains with accompanying sleeplessness.

Precautions: If a rare sensitivity reaction occurs, the drug should be discontinued.

Directions: Adults and Children 12 Years of Age and Older: Two caplets, geltabs or gelcaps at bedtime or as directed by physician. Do not exceed recommended dosage. Not for use in children under 12 years of age.

Warnings: Do not use if carton is opened or printed neck wrap or printed foil inner seal is broken. Do not give to children under 12 years of age. If sleeplessness persists continuously for more than 2 weeks, consult your doctor. Insomnia may be a symptom of serious underlying medical illness. Do not take for pain for more than 10 days or for fever for more than 3 days unless directed by a doctor. If pain or fever persists, or gets worse, if new symptoms occur, or if redness or swelling is present, consult a doctor because these could be signs of a serious condition. Do not take this product, unless directed by a doctor, if you have a breathing problem such as emphysema or chronic bronchitis, or if you have glaucoma or difficulty in urination due to enlargement of the prostate gland. Avoid alcoholic beverages while taking this product. Do not take this product if your are taking sedatives or tranquilizers without first consulting your doctor.
As with any drug, if you are pregnant or nursing a baby, seek the advice of a health professional before using this product. Keep this and all drugs out of the reach of children. In case of accidental overdose, contact a doctor or poison control center immediately. Prompt medical attention is critical for adults as well as for children even if you do not notice any signs or symptoms. Do not use with other products containing acetaminophen.

Alcohol Warning: For this and all other pain relievers, including aspirin, ibuprofen, ketoprofen and naproxen sodium, if you generally consume 3 or more alcohol-containing drinks per day, you should consult your physician for advice on when and how you should take pain relievers.

Caution: This product will cause drowsiness. Do not drive a motor vehicle or operate machinery after use.

Overdosage Information: Acetaminophen in massive overdosage may cause hepatic toxicity in some patients. In adults and adolescents, hepatic toxicity has rarely been reported following ingestion of acute overdoses of less than 10 grams. Fatalities are infrequent (less than 3–4% of untreated cases) and have rarely been reported with overdoses of less than 15 grams. In children, an acute overdosage of less than 150 mg/kg has not been associated with hepatic toxicity. Early symptoms following a potentially hepatotoxic overdose may include: nausea, vomiting, diaphoresis and general malaise. Clinical and laboratory evidence of hepatic toxicity may not be apparent until 48 to 72 hours postingestion. In adults and adolescents, regardless of the quantity of acetaminophen reported to have been ingested, administer acetylcysteine immediately if 24 hours or less have elapsed from the reported time of ingestion. For full prescribing information, refer to the acetylcysteine package insert. Do not await results of assays for plasma acetaminophen level before initiating treatment with acetylcysteine. The following additional procedures are recommended. The stomach should be emptied promptly by lavage or by induction of emesis with syrup of ipecac. A plasma acetaminophen assay should be obtained as early as possible, but no sooner than four hours following ingestion. If plasma level falls above the lower treatment line on the acetaminophen overdose nomogram, acetylcysteine therapy should be continued. Liver function studies should be obtained initially and repeated at 24-hour intervals.
Serious toxicity or fatalities are extremely infrequent in children, possibly due to differences in the way they metabolize acetaminophen. In children, the maximum potential amount ingested can be more easily estimated. If more than 150 mg/kg or an unknown amount was ingested, obtain a plasma acetaminophen level. The plasma acetaminophen level should be obtained as soon as possible, but no sooner than 4 hours following the ingestion. If the plasma level falls above the lower treatment line on the acetaminophen overdose nomogram, the acetylcysteine therapy should be initiated and continued for a full course of therapy. If plasma acetaminophen assay capability is not available, and the estimated acetaminophen ingestion exceeds 150 mg/kg, acetylcysteine therapy should be initiated and continued for a full course of therapy.
For additional emergency information, call your regional poison center or call the Rocky Mountain Poison Center toll-free, (1-800-525-6115).
Diphenhydramine toxicity should be treated as you would an antihistamine/anticholinergic overdose and is likely to be present within a few hours after acute ingestion.

Alcohol Information: Chronic heavy alcohol abusers may be at increased risk of liver toxicity from excessive acetaminophen use, although reports of this event are rare. Reports almost invariably involve cases of severe chronic alcoholics and the dosages of acetaminophen most often exceed recommended doses and often involve substantial overdose. Professionals should alert their patients who regularly consume large amounts of alcohol not to exceed recommended doses of acetaminophen.

Inactive Ingredients: **Caplets:** Cellulose, Cornstarch, Hydroxypropyl Methylcellulose, Magnesium Stearate or Stearic Acid and Colloidal Silicon Dioxide, Polyethylene Glycol, Polysorbate 80, Sodium Citrate, Sodium Starch Glycolate, Titanium Dioxide, Blue #1 and Blue #2.
Geltabs/Gelcaps: Benzyl Alcohol, Butylparaben, Castor Oil, Cellulose, Cornstarch, Edetate Calcium Disodium, Gelatin, Hydroxypropyl Methylcellulose, Magnesium Stearate, Propylparaben, Sodium Lauryl Sulfate, Sodium Citrate, Sodium Propionate, Sodium Starch Glycolate, Titanium Dioxide, Blue #1 and Red #28.

How Supplied: **Caplets** (colored light blue imprinted "Tylenol PM") tamper-resistant bottles of 24, 50, 100, and 150.

Continued on next page

McNeil Consumer—Cont.

Gelcaps (colored blue and white imprinted "TYLENOL PM") tamper-resistant bottles of 24 and 50.
Geltabs (colored blue and white imprinted "TYLENOL PM") tamper-resistant bottles of 24, 50, and 100.

Shown in Product Identification Guide, page 512

TYLENOL® SEVERE ALLERGY Medication Caplets

Maximum Strength TYLENOL® ALLERGY SINUS NIGHTTIME Caplets

Maximum Strength TYLENOL® ALLERGY SINUS Caplets, Gelcaps and Geltabs

Product information for all dosage forms of TYLENOL ALLERGY have been combined under this heading.

Description: Each ***TYLENOL® SEVERE ALLERGY Caplet*** contains acetaminophen 500 mg, and diphenhydramine Hydrochloride 12.5 mg.
Each ***Maximum Strength TYLENOL® ALLERGY SINUS NightTime Caplet*** contains acetaminophen 500 mg, pseudoephedrine hydrochloride 30 mg, and diphenhydramine hydrochloride 25 mg.
Each ***Maximum Strength TYLENOL® ALLERGY SINUS Caplets*** *or* ***Gelcap*** contains acetaminophen 500 mg, chlorpheniramine maleate 2 mg, and pseudoephedrine hydrochloride 30 mg.

Actions: ***TYLENOL® SEVERE ALLERGY Caplets*** contain a clinically proven analgesic-antipyretic and antihistamine. Acetaminophen produces analgesia by elevation of the pain threshold and antipyresis through action on the hypothalamic heat-regulating center. Acetaminophen is equal to aspirin in analgesic and antipyretic effectiveness, and it is unlikely to produce many of the side effects associated with aspirin and aspirin-containing products.
Diphenhydramine is an antihistamine which helps provide temporary relief of itchy, watery eyes, runny nose, sneezing, itching of the nose or throat due to hay fever or other respiratory allergies.
Maximum Strength TYLENOL® ALLERGY SINUS NightTime Caplets contain, in addition to the above ingredients, a decongestant, pseudoephedrine. Pseudoephedrine is a sympathomimetic amine which provides temporary relief of nasal and sinus congestion.
Maximum Strength TYLENOL® ALLERGY SINUS Caplets, Gelcaps and Geltabs contain acetaminophen, pseudoephedrine and the antihistamine, chlorpheniramine. Chlorpheniramine is an antihistamine which helps provide temporary relief of runny nose, sneezing and watery and itchy eyes.

Indications: ***TYLENOL® SEVERE ALLERGY*** provides effective temporary relief of itchy, watery eyes, runny nose, sneezing sore or scratchy throat and itching of the nose or throat due to hay fever or other upper respiratory allergies.
TYLENOL® ALLERGY SINUS Night-Time *and* ***TYLENOL® ALLERGY SINUS*** provide effective temporary relief of runny nose, sneezing, itching of the nose or throat, and itchy, watery eyes due to hay fever or other upper respiratory allergies, nasal and sinus congestion, and sinus pain and headaches.

Precautions: ***TYLENOL® SEVERE ALLERGY:*** If a rare sensitivity reaction occurs, the drug should be stopped.
TYLENOL® ALLERGY SINUS Night-Time and ***TYLENOL® ALLERGY SINUS:*** If a rare sensitivity reaction occurs, the drug should be stopped. Although pseudoephedrine is virtually without pressor effect in normotensive patients, it should be used with caution in hypertensives.

Directions: ***TYLENOL® SEVERE ALLERGY:*** Adults and children 12 years of age and older: Two caplets every four to six hours. Do not exceed 8 caplets in any 24 hour period. Not for use in children under 12 years of age.
TYLENOL® ALLERGY SINUS Night-Time: Adults and children 12 years of age and older: Two caplets at bedtime. Not for use in children under 12 years of age.
TYLENOL® ALLERGY SINUS: Adults and children 12 years of age and older. Two caplets, gelcaps or geltabs every six hours. Do not exceed 8 caplets, gelcaps, or geltabs in any 24 hour period. Not for use in children under 12 years of age.

Warnings: ***TYLENOL® SEVERE ALLERGY:*** Do not use if carton is open or if a blister unit is broken. Do not take for pain for more than 10 days or for fever for more than 3 days unless directed by a doctor. If pain or fever persists, or gets worse, if new symptoms occur, or if redness or swelling is present, consult a doctor because these could be signs of a serious condition. If sore throat is severe, persists for more than 2 days, is accompanied or followed by fever, headache, rash, nausea or vomiting, consult a doctor promptly. May cause excitability especially in children. Do not take this product, unless directed by a doctor, if you have a breathing problem such as emphysema or chronic bronchitis, or if you have glaucoma or difficulty in urination due to enlargement of the prostate gland. May cause marked drowsiness: alcohol, sedatives and tranquilizers may increase the drowsiness effect.
Avoid alcoholic beverages while taking this product. Do not take this product if you are taking sedatives or tranquilizers without first consulting your doctor. Use caution while driving a motor vehicle or operating machinery. As with any drug, if you are pregnant or nursing a baby, seek the advice of a health professional before using this product. Keep this and all drugs out of the reach of children. In case of accidental overdose, contact a doctor or poison control center immediately. Prompt medical attention is critical for adults as well as for children even if you do not notice any signs or symptoms. Do not use with other products containing acetaminophen.
TYLENOL® ALLERGY SINUS Night Time and TYLENOL® ALLERGY SINUS: Do not use if carton is open or if a blister unit is broken. Do not take for pain for more than 7 days or for fever for more than 3 days unless directed by a doctor. If pain or fever persists, or gets worse, if new symptoms occur, or if redness or swelling is present, consult a doctor because these could be signs of a serious condition. Do not exceed recommended dosage. If nervousness, dizziness or sleeplessness occur, discontinue use and consult a doctor.
May cause excitability, especially in children. Do not take this product unless directed by a doctor, if you have a breathing problem such as emphysema or chronic bronchitis, or if you have glaucoma or difficulty in urination due to enlargement of the prostate gland. Do not take this product if you have heart disease, high blood pressure, thyroid disease or diabetes unless directed by a doctor. May cause marked drowsiness: alcohol sedatives and tranquilizers may increase the drowsiness effect. Avoid alcoholic beverages while taking this product. Do not take this product if you are taking sedatives or tranquilizers without first consulting your doctor.
Use caution when driving a motor vehicle or operating machinery. As with any drug, if you are pregnant or nursing a baby, seek the advice of a health professional before using this product. Keep this and all drugs out of the reach of children. In case of accidental overdose, contact a doctor or poison control center immediately. Prompt medical attention is critical for adults as well as for children even if you do not notice any signs or symptoms. Do not use with other products containing acetaminophen.

Alcohol Warning: For this and all other pain relievers, including aspirin ibuprofen, ketoprofen and naproxen sodium. if you generally consume 3 or more alcohol-containing drinks per day, you should consult your physician for advice on when and how you should take pain relievers.

Drug Interaction Precaution: ***TYLENOL® ALLERGY SINUS NightTime and TYLENOL® ALLERGY SINUS:*** Do not use this product if you are now taking a prescription monamine oxidase inhibitor (MAOI) (certain drugs for depression psychiatric or emotional condition, or Parkinson's disease), or for 2 weeks after stopping the MAOI drug. If you are uncertain whether your prescription drug contains an MAOI, consult a health care professional before taking this product.

Overdosage Information: Acetaminophen in massive overdosage may cause hepatic toxicity in some patients. In adults and adolescents, hepatic toxicity has rarely been reported following ingestion of acute overdoses of less than 10 grams. Fatalities are infrequent (less than 3–4% of untreated cases) and have rarely been reported with overdoses of less than 15 grams. In children, an acute overdosage of less than 150 mg/kg has not been associated with hepatic toxicity. Early symptoms following a potentially hepatotoxic overdose may include: nausea, vomiting, diaphoresis and general malaise. Clinical and laboratory evidence of hepatic toxicity may not be apparent until 48 to 72 hours postingestion. In adults and adolescents, regardless of the quantity of acetaminophen reported to have been ingested, administer acetylcysteine immediately if 24 hours or less have elapsed from the reported time of ingestion. For full prescribing information, refer to the acetylcysteine package insert. Do not await results of assays for plasma acetaminophen level before initiating treatment with acetylcysteine. The following additional procedures are recommended: The stomach should be emptied promptly by lavage or by induction of emesis with syrup of ipecac. A plasma acetaminophen assay should be obtained as early as possible, but no sooner than four hours following ingestion. If plasma level falls above the lower treatment line on the acetaminophen overdose nomogram, acetylcysteine therapy should be continued. Liver function studies should be obtained initially and repeated at 24-hour intervals.

Serious toxicity or fatalities are extremely infrequent in children, possibly due to differences in the way they metabolize acetaminophen. In children, the maximum potential amount ingested can be more easily estimated. If more than 150 mg/kg or an unknown amount was ingested, obtain a plasma acetaminophen level. The plasma acetaminophen level should be obtained as soon as possible, but no sooner than 4 hours following the ingestion. If plasma level falls above the lower treatment line on the acetaminophen overdose nomogram, the acetylcysteine therapy should be initiated and continued for a full course of therapy. If plasma acetaminiophen assay capability is not available, and the estimated acetaminophen ingestion exceeds 150 mg/kg, acetylcysteine therapy should be initiated and continued for a full course of therapy.

For additional emergency information, call your regional poison center or call the Rocky Mountain Poison Center toll-free (1–800–525–6115).

Symptoms for pseudoephedrine overdose consist most often of mild anxiety, tachycardia and/or hypertension. Symptoms usually appear within 4 to 8 hours of ingestion and are transient, usually requiring no treatment.

Diphenhydramine and chlorpheniramine toxicity should be treated as you would an antihistamine/anticholinergic overdose and is likely to be present within a few hours after acute ingestion.

Alcohol Information: Chronic heavy alcohol abusers may be at increased risk of liver toxicity from excessive acetaminophen use, although reports of this event are rare. Reports almost invariably involve cases of severe chronic alcoholics and the dosages of acetaminophen most often exceed recommended doses and often involve substantial overdose. Professionals should alert their patients who regularly consume large amounts of alcohol not to exceed recommended doses of acetaminophen.

Inactive Ingredients: ***TYLENOL® SEVERE ALLERGY Caplets:*** Cellulose, Corn Starch, Hydroxpropyl, Cellulose, Hydroxypropyl Methylcellulose, Iron Oxide Black, Magnesium Stearate, Polyethylene Glycol, Sodium Citrate, Sodium Starch Glycolate, Titanium Dioxide, Yellow #6 and Yellow #10.

TYLENOL® ALLERGY SINUS NightTime Caplets: Cellulose, Corn Starch, Hydroxypropyl Methylcellulose, Iron Oxide Black, Magnesium Stearate, Polyethylene Glycol, Polysorbate 80, Sodium Citrate, Sodium Starch Glycolate, Titanium Dioxide, Blue #1, and Yellow #10.

TYLENOL® ALLERGY SINUS: **Caplets:** Carnauba Wax, Cellulose, Cornstarch, Hydroxypropyl Cellulose, Hydroxypropyl Methylcellulose, Iron Oxide Black, Magnesium Stearate, Polyethylene Glycol, Sodium Starch Glycolate, Titanium Dioxide, Blue #1, Yellow #6, and Yellow #10. Gelcaps: Benzyl Alcohol, Butylparaben, Castor Oil Cellulose, Cornstarch, Edetate Calcium Disodium, Gelatin, Hydroxypropyl Methylcellulose, Magnesium Stearate, Methylparaben, propylparaben, Sodium Lauryl Sulfate, Sodium Propionate, Sodium Starch Glycolate, Titanium Dioxide, Blue #1 and #2 and Yellow #10.

How Supplied: ***TYLENOL® SEVERE ALLERGY:*** **Caplets** (dark yellow, imprinted "TYLENOL Severe Allergy") blister packs of 12 and 24.

TYLENOL® ALLERGY SINUS NightTime: **Caplets** (light blue, imprinted "TYLENOL A/S NightTime") child-resistant blister packs of 24.

TYLENOL® ALLERGY SINUS: **Caplets:** (dark yellow, imprinted "TYLENOL Allergy Sinus") Blister packs of 24 and 48.

Gelcaps and Geltabs: (dark green and dark yellow, imprinted "TYLENOL A/S") Blister packs of 24 and 48.

Shown in Product Identification Guide, page 511

Maximum Strength TYLENOL® SINUS Geltabs, Gelcaps, Caplets and Tablets

Description: Each ***Maximum Strength TYLENOL® SINUS Geltab, Gelcap, Caplet or Tablet*** contains acetaminophen 500 mg and pseudoephedrine hydrochloride 30 mg.

Actions: ***Maximum Strength TYLENOL® SINUS*** contains a clinically proven analgesic-antipyretic and a decongestant. Maximum allowable nonprescription levels of acetaminophen and pseudoephedrine provide temporary relief of sinus headache and congestion. Acetaminophen is equal to aspirin in analgesic and antipyretic effectiveness and it is unlikely to produce many of the side effects associated with aspirin and aspirin-containing products.

Acetaminophen produces analgesia by elevation of the pain threshold and antipyresis through action on the hypothalamic heat-regulating center. Pseudoephedrine hydrochloride is a sympathomimetic amine which promotes sinus cavity drainage by reducing nasopharyngeal mucosal congestion.

Indications: ***Maximum Strength TYLENOL® SINUS*** provides for the temporary relief of nasal and sinus congestion and sinus pain and headaches. ***Maximum Strength TYLENOL® SINUS*** is particularly well-suited in patients with aspirin allergy, hemostatic disturbances (including anticoagulant therapy), and bleeding diatheses (e.g., hemophilia) and upper gastrointestinal disease (e.g., ulcer, gastritis, hiatus hernia).

Precautions: If a rare sensitivity occurs, the drug should be discontinued. Although pseudoephedrine is virtually without pressor effect in normotensive patients, it should be used with caution in hypertensives.

Directions: Adults and Children 12 years of Age and Older: Two Tablets, Caplets, Gelcaps, or Geltabs every 4–6 hours. Do not exceed eight Tablets, Caplets, Gelcaps, or Geltabs in any 24-hour period. Not for use in children under 12 years of age.

Warnings: Do not use if carton is opened or if blister unit is broken. Do not take for pain for more than 7 days or for fever for more than 3 days unless directed by a doctor. If pain or fever persists. or get worse, if new symptoms occur, or if redness or swelling is present, consult a doctor because these could be signs of a serious condition. **Do not exceed recommended dosage.** If nervousness, dizziness or sleeplessness occur, discontinue use and consult a doctor. Do not take this product if you have heart disease, high blood pressure, thyroid disease, diabetes, or difficulty in urination due to enlargement of the prostate gland unless directed by a doctor.

As with any drug, if you are pregnant or nursing a baby, seek the advice of a health professional before using this product. Keep this and all drugs out of the reach of children. In case of accidental overdose, contact a doctor or poison control center immediately. Prompt medical attention is critical for adults as well as for children even if you do not notice any signs or symptoms. Do not use with other products containing acetaminophen.

Continued on next page

McNeil Consumer—Cont.

Alcohol Warnings: For this and all other pain relievers, including aspirin, ibuprofen, ketoprofen and naproxen sodium, if you generally consume 3 or more alcohol-containing drinks per day, you should consult your physician for advice on when and how you should take pain relievers.

Drug Interactions Precaution: Do not use this product if you are now taking a prescription monoamine oxidase inhibitor (MAOI) (certain drugs for depression, psychiatric or emotional conditions, or Parkinson's disease), or for 2 weeks after stopping the MAOI drug. If you are uncertain whether your prescription drug contains an MAOI, consult a health professional before taking this product.

Overdosage Information: Acetaminophen in massive overdosage may cause hepatic toxicity in some patients. In adults and adolescents, hepatic toxicity has rarely been reported following ingestion of acute overdoses of less than 10 grams. Fatalities are infrequent (less than 3–4% of untreated cases) and have rarely been reported with overdoses of less than 15 grams. In children, an acute overdosage of less than 150 mg/kg has not been associated with hepatic toxicity. Early symptoms following a potentially hepatotoxic overdose may include: nausea, vomiting, diaphoresis and general malaise. Clinical and laboratory evidence of hepatic toxicity may not be apparent until 48 to 72 hours postingestion. In adults and adolescents, regardless of the quantity of acetaminophen reported to have been ingested, administer acetylcysteine immediately if 24 hours or less have elapsed from the reported time of ingestion. For full prescribing information, refer to the acetylcysteine package insert. Do not await results of assays for plasma acetaminophen level before initiating treatment with acetylcysteine. The following additional procedures are recommended. The stomach should be emptied promptly by lavage or by induction of emesis with syrup of ipecac. A plasma acetaminophen assay should be obtained as early as possible, but no sooner than four hours following ingestion. If plasma level falls above the lower treatment line on the acetaminophen overdose nomogram, acetylcysteine therapy should be continued. Liver function studies should be obtained initially and repeated at 24-hour intervals.
Serious toxicity or fatalities are extremely infrequent in children, possibly due to differences in the way they metabolize acetaminophen. In children, the maximum potential amount ingested can be more easily estimated. If more than 150 mg/kg or an unknown amount was ingested, obtain a plasma acetaminophen level. The plasma acetaminophen level should be obtained as soon as possible, but no sooner than 4 hours following the ingestion. If plasma level falls above the lower treatment line on the acetaminophen overdose nomogram, the acetylcysteine therapy should be initiated and continued for a full course of therapy. If plasma acetaminophen assay capability is not available, and the estimated acetaminophen ingestion exceeds 150 mg/kg, acetylcysteine therapy should be initiated and continued for a full course of therapy.
For additional emergency information, call your regional poison center or call the Rocky Mountain Poison Center toll-free (1-800-525-6115).
Symptoms from pseudoephedrine overdose consist most often of mild anxiety, tachycardia and/or mild hypertension. Symptoms usually appear within 4 to 8 hours after ingestion and are transient, usually requiring no treatment.

Alcohol Information: Chronic heavy alcohol abusers may be at increased risk of liver toxicity from excessive acetaminophen use, although reports of this event are rare. Reports almost invariably involve cases of severe chronic alcoholics and the dosages of acetaminophen most often exceed recommended doses and often involve substantial overdose. Professionals should alert their patients who regularly consume large amounts of alcohol not to exceed recommended doses of acetaminophen.

Inactive Ingredients: Caplets: Carnauba Wax, Cellulose, Corn Starch, Hydroxypropyl Methylcellulose, Magnesium Stearate, Polyethylene Glycol, Polysorbate 80, Sodium Starch Glycolate, Titanium Dioxide, Blue #1, Red #40, Yellow #10.
Tablets: Cellulose, Corn Starch, Magnesium Stearate, Sodium Starch Glycolate,. Blue #1, Yellow #6, and Yellow #10.
Gelcaps: Benzyl Alcohol, Butylparaben, Castor Oil, Cellulose, Corn Starch, Edetate Calcium Disodium, Gelatin, Hydroxypropyl Methylcellulose, Iron Oxide Black, Magnesium Stearate, Methylparaben, Propylparaben, Sodium Lauryl Sulfate, Sodium Propionate, Sodium Starch Glycolate, Titanium Dioxide, Blue #1 and Yellow #10.
Geltabs: Benzyl Alcohol, Butylparaben, Castor Oil, Cellulose, Corn Starch, Edetate Calcium Disodium, Gelatin, Hydroxypropyl Methylcellulose, Iron Oxide Black, Magnesium Stearate, Methylparaben, Propylparaben, Sodium Lauryl Sulfate, Sodium Propionate, Sodium Starch Glycolate, Titanium Dioxide, D&C Yellow #10, FD&C Blue #1

How Supplied: Tablets: (colored light green, imprinted "Maximum Strength TYLENOL SINUS")—in blister packs of 24.
Caplets: (light green coating, printed "TYLENOL SINUS" in dark green) in blister packs of 24 and 48.
Gelcaps: (colored green and white), printed "TYLENOL SINUS" in blister packs of 24 and 48.
Geltabs: (colored green and white), printed "TYLENOL SINUS" in blister packs of 24 and 48.

Shown in Product Identification Guide, page 513

Medeva Pharmaceuticals, Inc.

14801 SOVEREIGN ROAD
FORT WORTH, TX 76155–2645

Direct Inquiries to:
Customer Service Department
P.O. Box 1766
Rochester, NY 14603
(716) 274-5300
(888) 9–MEDEVA

DELSYM® Cough Formula

[del'sĭm]
(dextromethorphan polistirex)
Extended-Release Suspension
12-Hour Cough Relief

Active Ingredient: Each teaspoonful (5 mL) contains dextromethorphan polistirex equivalent to 30 mg dextromethorphan hydrobromide.

Inactive Ingredients: Citric acid, ethylcellulose, FD&C Yellow No. 6, flavor, high fructose corn syrup, methylparaben, polyethylene glycol 3350, polysorbate 80, propylene glycol, propylparaben, purified water, sucrose, tragacanth, vegetable oil, xanthan gum.

Indications: Temporarily relieves cough due to minor throat and bronchial irritation as may occur with the common cold or inhaled irritants.

Warnings: Do not take this product for persistent or chronic cough such as occurs with smoking, asthma, or emphysema, or if cough is accompanied by excessive phlegm (mucus) unless directed by a physician. A persistent cough may be a sign of a serious condition. If cough persists for more than 1 week, tends to recur, or is accompanied by fever, rash, or persistent headache, consult a physician. As with any drug, if you are pregnant or nursing a baby, seek the advice of a health professional before using this product. **Keep this and all drugs out of the reach of children.** In case of accidental overdose, seek professional assistance or contact a Poison Control Center immediately.

Drug Interaction Precaution: Do not use this product if you are now taking a prescription monoamine oxidase inhibitor (MAOI) (certain drugs for depression, psychiatric or emotional conditions, or Parkinson's disease), or for 2 weeks after stopping the MAOI drug. If you are uncertain whether your prescription drug contains an MAOI, consult a health professional before taking this product.

Directions: Shake Bottle Well Before Using. Dose as follows or as directed by a physician.
Adults and Children 12 years of age and over: 2 teaspoonfuls every 12 hours, not to exceed 4 teaspoonfuls in 24 hours.-

Children 6 to under 12 years of age: 1 teaspoonful every 12 hours, not to exceed 2 teaspoonfuls in 24 hours.
Children 2 to under 6 years of age: 1/2 teaspoonful every 12 hours, not to exceed 1 teaspoonful in 24 hours.
Children under 2 years of age: Consult a physician.

How Supplied: 89 mL (3 fl oz) bottles NDC 53014-842-61

Store at 15°–30°C (59°–86°F).
***MEDEVA* Pharmaceuticals**
Medeva Pharmaceuticals, Inc.
Fort Worth, TX 76155 U.S.A.

Menley & James Laboratories, Inc.
Commonwealth Corporate Center

100 TOURNAMENT DRIVE
HORSHAM, PA 19044-3697

Direct Inquiries to:
Consumer Affairs Department
(800) 321-1834

- A.R.M. Allergy Relief Medicine Caplets
- Acnomel Acne Medication Cream
- Acryline 2 Temporary Denture Reliner
- Aqua Care Cream and Lotion
- AsthmaHaler Mist Aerosol Bronchodilator
- AsthmaNefrin Solution Bronchodilator
- B.F.I. Antiseptic First-Aid Powder
- Benzedrex Inhaler
- Congestac Caplets
- Derifil Internal Deodorant
- Hold DM Cough Suppressant Lozenges
- Humibid GC Caplets
- Ornex Caplets
- Plate-weld Temporary Denture Repair Kit
- Serutan Toasted Granules
- S.T. 37 Topical Antiseptic Solution
- Thermotabs Buffered Salt Tablets
- Yodora Cream Deodorant

BENZEDREX® INHALER
Nasal Decongestant

Indications: For the temporary relief of nasal congestion due to the common cold, hay fever, or associated with sinusitis.

Directions: This product delivers in each 800 milliliters of air 0.40 to 0.50 milligrams of propylhexedrine. Adults and children (6–12 years) with adult supervision: 2 inhalations in each nostril not more often than every 2 hours. Children under 6: consult a physician. This inhaler is effective for a minimum of 3 months after first use. KEEP INHALER TIGHTLY CLOSED.
Active Ingredient: Propylhexedrine 250 mg. **Inactive Ingredients:** Lavender Oil, Menthol.

Warnings: Do not exceed recommended dosage. This product may cause temporary discomfort such as burning, stinging, sneezing, or an increase in nasal discharge. The use of this container by more than one person may spread infection. Do not use this product for more than three days. Use only as directed. Frequent or prolonged use may cause nasal congestion to recur or worsen. If symptoms persist, consult a physician. **Keep this and all medication out of the reach of children**. Ill effects may result if taken internally. In case of accidental overdose or ingestion of contents, seek professional assistance or contact a Poison Control Center immediately. As with any drug, if you are pregnant or nursing a baby, seek the advice of a health professional before using this product.
Store at controlled room temperature (59°–86°F).
TAMPER-RESISTANT PACKAGE FEATURE FOR YOUR PROTECTION:
- Inhaler sealed with imprinted cellophane. Do not use if missing or broken.

How Supplied: In single plastic tubes. Comments or questions? Call 1-800-321-1834 Toll Free.

DERIFIL®
Internal Deodorant
Film-Coated Tablets
OSTOMY/INCONTINENT ODOR CONTROL
Each tablet contains
100 mg CHLOROPHYLLIN
COPPER COMPLEX

Indications: Oral deodorant for internal use: 1. An aid to reduce fecal odor due to incontinence, 2. An aid to reduce odor from a colostomy or ileostomy.
See package insert for full information.

Directions: Adults and children 12 years of age and over; Oral dosage is one to two tablets daily in divided doses as required. If odor is not controlled, take up to an additional tablet daily in divided doses as required. The smallest effective dose should be used. Do not exceed 3 tablets daily. Children under 12 years of age: consult a doctor. In ostomies, tablets may either taken by mouth or placed in the appliance.

Warning: If cramps or diarrhea occur, reduce the dosage. If symptoms persist, consult your doctor. KEEP THIS AND ALL MEDICATION OUT OF REACH OF CHILDREN.

How Supplied: Dark, green, round, film-coated tablet with "R" on one side and score on other. Each tablet contains 100 mg Chlorophyllin Copper Complex. Bottles of 30, 100, and 1000 tablets. Blister pack of 40 tablets.

DERIFIL® is available at drug stores and ostomy supply dealers. If the pharmacist or dealer does not have **DERIFIL®** in stock, he can obtain it from his drug wholesaler. Comments or questions? Call 1-800-321-1834 Toll Free.

THERMOTABS®
BUFFERED SALT TABLETS
for heat fatigue

THERMOTABS tablets are especially designed to minimize fatigue, to prevent muscle cramps or heat prostration due to excessive perspiration. THERMOTABS can be used by golfers, tennis players and other athletes as well as at the beach or in homes, offices, stores, kitchens or industries where high temperature causes heat fatigue.
Each Tablet Contains:
ACTIVE INGREDIENTS: Sodium Chloride 450 mg, Potassium Chloride 30 mg.
INACTIVE INGREDIENTS: Calcium Carbonate, Dextrose, Microcrystalline Cellulose, Sodium Starch Glycolate, Stearic Acid.
Sodium content 179 mg per tablet.

Dosage: One tablet with a full glass of water, five to ten times daily, depending on temperature, activity and working conditions.

Warning: If you have or are being treated for heart disease or high blood pressure, consult your physician before using this product. **Keep this and all medication out of the reach of children.** As with any drug, if you are pregnant or nursing a baby, seek the advice of a health professional before using this product. Do not use this product if you are on a sodium-restricted diet unless directed by a doctor.

For Your Protection: Bottle is sealed with imprinted neck seal under cap. Identification code MJ-670 appears on each tablet.

How Supplied: 100 Tablets
Comments or questions? Call 1-800-321-1834 Toll Free.

The Mentholatum Company, Inc

1360 NIAGARA STREET
BUFFALO, NY 14213

Direct Inquiries to:
Director of Consumer Affairs
(716) 882-7660
FAX: (716) 882-6563

For Medical Emergency Contact:
Dr. Henry Chan: (716) 882-7660
FAX: (716) 882-6563

FLETCHER'S® CASTORIA®
The Children's Laxative
Original Flavor
Alcohol Free

Natural, good-tasting Fletcher's Castoria provides gentle, effective relief from the discomfort of constipation for children of

Continued on next page

Mentholatum Co.—Cont.

all ages. Trusted by mothers for generations.

Indications: For relief of occasional constipation. This product generally produces bowel movement in 6 to 12 hours.

Directions: **SHAKE WELL BEFORE USING**
Less than 2 years .... Consult a doctor
2 to 5 years .... 1 to 2 teaspoonfuls
6 to 15 years .... 2 to 3 teaspoonfuls
May be taken up to two times daily.

Warnings: Do not use laxative products when abdominal pain, nausea or vomiting are present unless directed by a doctor. If you have noticed a sudden change in bowel habits that persists over a period of two weeks, consult a doctor before using a laxative. Laxative products should not be used for a period longer than 1 week unless directed by a doctor. Rectal bleeding or failure to have a bowel movement after use of a laxative may indicate a serious condition. Discontinue use and consult your doctor. KEEP THIS AND ALL DRUGS OUT OF THE REACH OF CHILDREN. In case of accidental overdose, seek professional assistance or contact a Poison Control Center immediately. As with any drug, if you are pregnant or nursing a baby, seek the advice of a health professional before using this product.

Contains: Senna Concentrate 33.3 mg/mL.

Also contains: Citric Acid, Flavor, Glycerin, Methlyparaben, Propylparaben, Sodium Benzoate, Sucrose, Water.

How Supplied: 2½ fl oz (74 mL) bottle.

FLETCHER'S® CHERRY FLAVOR
THE CHILDREN'S LAXATIVE

Good tasting Fletcher's® Cherry Flavor provides gentle effective relief from the discomforts of constipation. The convenient dosage cup lets you measure the right amount for your child's age.

Indications: For relief of occasional constipation. The product generally produces bowel movement in 6 to 12 hours.

Directions: **SHAKE WELL BEFORE USING**
Maximum Daily Dose

AGE	DOSAGE
6–11 Years	2–4 teaspoons
2–5 Years	1–2 teaspoons
Under 2 Years	Consult A Doctor

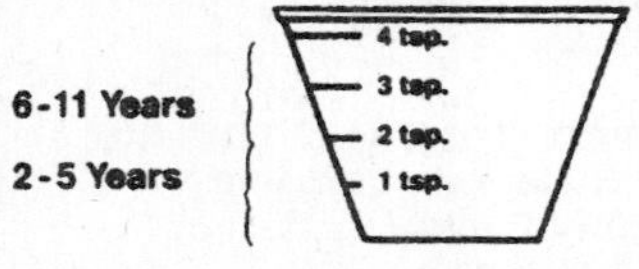

Warnings: Do not use laxative products when abdominal pain, nausea or vomiting are present unless directed by a doctor. If you have noticed a sudden change in bowel habits that persists over a period of two weeks, consult a doctor before using a laxative. Laxative products should not be used for a period longer than 1 week unless directed by a doctor. Rectal bleeding or failure to have a bowel movement after use of a laxative may indicate a serious condition. Discontinue use and consult your doctor. KEEP THIS AND ALL DRUGS OUT OF REACH OF CHILDREN. In case of accidental overdose, seek professional assistance or contact a Poison Control Center immediately. If a skin rash appears, do not use this product or any other preparation containing phenolphthalein. As with any drug if you are pregnant or nursing a baby, seek the advice of a health professional before using this product.

Contains: Yellow Phenolphthalein 0.3%.

Also contains: Citric Acid, FD&C Red No. 40, Flavor, Glycerin, Magnesium Aluminum Silicate, Methylparaben, Sodium Benzoate, Sucrose, Water, Xanthan Gum.

How Supplied: 2½ fl oz (74 mL) bottle.

MENTHACIN®
Arthritis Pain Relieving Cream

Dual Acting Arthritis Therapy
Menthacin® relieves the pain of arthritis in a different way than traditional creams and rubs. Its advanced, dual-acting formula provides:

- **Immediate Pain Relief**
  As soon as you rub it on, Menthacin® provides fast acting, penetrating cooling for immediate relief at the site of the pain.

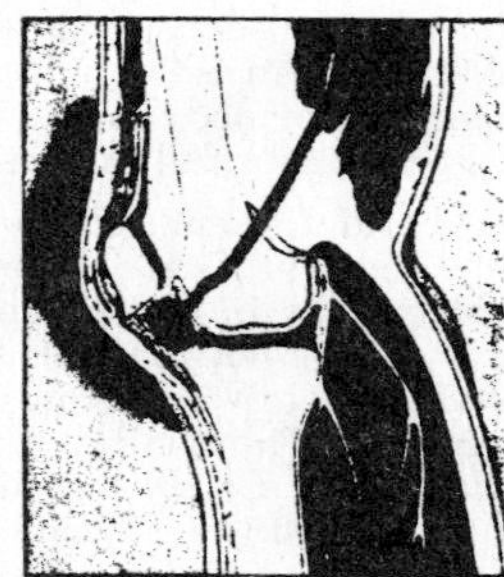

- **Long Lasting Pain Relief**
  Menthacin® contains Capsaicin, which provides long lasting warming pain relief. Over time, with repeated use, Capsaicin works to significantly reduce the sensation of pain within the affected area for long lasting relief.

Indications: For the temporary relief of minor aches and pains of muscles and joints associated with arthritis, simple backache, strains, and sprains.

Directions: Apply to affected area not more than 3 to 4 times daily. Children under 12 years of age, consult a physician. Transient irritation or burning may occur upon application, but generally disappears in several days. Wash hands with soap and water after applying.

Warnings: For external use only. Avoid contact with the eyes or mucous membranes. Do not use with a heating pad. Discontinue use if excessive irritation of the skin develops. If pain persists for 7 days or more, or clears up and occurs again within a few days, discontinue use of this product and consult a physician. Do not apply to wounds or damaged skin. Do not bandage tightly. KEEP THIS AND ALL DRUGS OUT OF THE REACH OF CHILDREN. In case of accidental ingestion, seek professional assistance or contact a Poison Control Center immediately. Store at room temperature.

Contains: Menthol 4%, Capsaicin 0.025%.

Also Contains: Caprylic/Capric Triglyceride, Carbomer 1342, Carbomer 940, Cetyl Alcohol, Diazolidinyl Urea, Glyceryl Stearate (and) Sodium Lauryl Sulfate, Maleated Soybean Oil, Methylparaben, Polysorbate 60, Propylene Glycol, Propylparaben, Sorbitan Stearate, Trolamine, Water.

How Supplied: 1.25 oz (35.4 g) Tube.

MENTHOLATUM®
CHERRY CHEST RUB FOR KIDS®
Nasal Decongestant/Cough Suppressant
Aromatic Colds Care

Mentholatum® Cherry Chest Rub for Kids® is specially made for children 2 years and older. The aromatic medicine penetrates into the nose and throat to break up congestion and ease coughs. It does not contain ingredients known to cause excitability, drowsiness or stomachache. The pleasant cherry aroma tells you it is working.

Indications: For the temporary relief of nasal congestion and coughs associated with a cold.

Directions: Children 2 years of age and older: Rub on the throat and chest as a thick layer. If desired, cover with a warm, dry cloth, but keep clothing loose to let the vapors rise to reach the nose and mouth. Repeat up to three times daily, especially at bedtime, or as directed by a doctor. Children under two years old, consult a doctor.

Warnings: For external use only. Avoid contact with the eyes. Do not take by mouth or place in nostrils. Discontinue use if irritation of the skin occurs. A persistent cough may be a sign of a serious condition. If cough persists for more than a week, tends to recur, or is accompanied by a fever, rash or persistent headache, see your doctor. Do not use this product for persistent or chronic coughs such as occurs with smoking, asthma, emphysema, or if cough is accompanied with excessive phlegm (mucus) unless directed by a doctor. KEEP THIS AND ALL DRUGS OUT OF THE REACH OF CHILDREN. In case of accilental ingestion, seek professional assistance or contact a Poison Control Center immediately.

Contains: Camphor 4.7%, Natural Menthol 2.6%, Eucalyptus Oil 1.2%.
Also Contains: Fragrance, Petrolatum, Steareth-2, Titanium Dioxide.

How Supplied: 1 oz (28 g) jar.

MENTHOLATUM DEEP HEATING®
Extra Strength Formula Provides Warming, Penetrating Pain Relief
- Arthritis
- Sore Muscles
- Back Pain
- Greaseless and Stainless

Directions: Apply to affected area. Repeat 3 to 4 times a day.

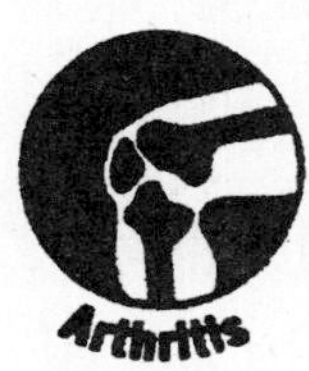

Massage thoroughly into affected joints to relieve arthritis pain and stiffness.

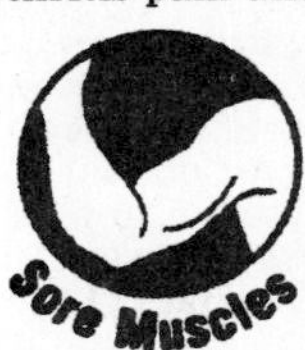

Rub into muscles to relieve the pain of over-exertion or for warming up before you work out.

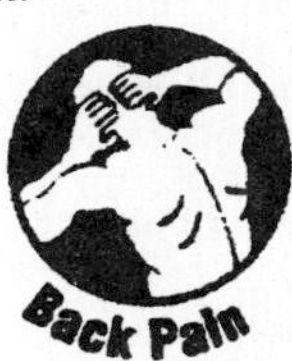

Massage in to relieve the pain of strained back muscles and restore lost mobility.

Indications: For the temporary relief of minor aches and pains of muscles and joints associated with arthritis, simple backache, strains and sprains.

Contains: Methyl Salicylate 30%, Menthol 8%.

Also Contains: Glyceryl Stearate (and) Sodium Lauryl Sulfate, Isoceteth-20, Poloxamer 407, Quaternium-15, Sorbitan Stearate, Water.

Warnings: For external use only. Do not apply to wounds or to damaged or very sensitive skin. Do not wrap, bandage or apply external heat or hot water. If you have impaired circulation or diabetes, use only upon the advice of a physician. KEEP THIS AND ALL DRUGS OUT OF THE REACH OF CHILDREN. In case of accidental ingestion, seek professional assistance or contact a Poison Control Center immediately.

Caution: Use only as directed. If pain persists for more than 10 days, or redness is present, or in conditions affecting children under 12 years of age, consult a physician immediately. Discontinue use if excessive irritation of the skin develops. Avoid getting into the eyes or on mucous membranes.

How Supplied: 1.25 oz (35.4 g) Tube and 3.33 oz (94.4 g) Tube.

MENTHOLATUM® OINTMENT
Decongestant Analgesic
Aromotic Colds Care

Penetrating aromatic vapors act fast to relieve stuffy noses, chest congestion, and the distress of coughs due to colds and sinus congestion.

Indications: Colds Symptoms—Gentle aromatics help relieve stuffy noses, chest congestion, sinus congestion, head colds, chest colds and muscular aches due to coughs and colds.
Chapped Skin—Soothes chapped skin, lips, and other minor skin irritations.

Directions: For adults and children 2 years of age and older. Apply to affected area 3 to 4 times daily.
Stuffy Noses: Apply liberally below each nostril.
Chest Congestion and Muscle Aches: Rub liberally on chest, throat and back and then cover areas with a warm cloth.
Chapped Skin Under Nose, Chapped Lips: Liberally spread a layer over irritated areas.

Warnings: For external use only. Avoid contact with the eyes. Do not place in mouth or nostrils. For conditions that persist or are accompanied by a fever see your doctor. KEEP THIS AND ALL DRUGS OUT OF THE REACH OF CHILDREN. In case of accidental ingestion, seek professional assistance or contact a Poison Control Center immediately.

Contains: Camphor 9%, Natural Menthol 1.3%.

Also Contains: Fragrance, Petrolatum, Titanium Dioxide.

How Supplied: 1 oz (28 g) Jar and 3 oz (85 g) Jar.

RED CROSS® TOOTHACHE FIRST AID MEDICATION

Package includes:
- toothache medication
- cotton pellets
- metal tweezers

Indications: For the temporary relief of throbbing, persistent toothache due to a cavity until a dentist can be seen.

Directions: Rinse the tooth with water to remove any food particles from the cavity. Use tweezers to moisten pellet and place in cavity. Avoid touching tissues other than tooth cavity. Do not apply more than four times daily or as directed by a dentist.

Warnings: Do not swallow. Do not exceed recommended dosage. Not to be used for a period exceeding 7 days. Children under 2 years should not use this product. Children under 12 years should be supervised in the use of this product. If irritation persists, inflammation develops, or if fever or infection develop, discontinue use and see your dentist or physician promptly. Do not use if you are allergic to Eugenol. KEEP THIS AND ALL DRUGS OUT OF THE REACH OF CHILDREN. In case of accidental ingestion, seek professional assistance or contact a Poison Control Center immediately.

Contents: Eugenol 85%. Also contains: Sesame Oil

How Supplied: ⅛ fl oz (3.7 mL) bottle.
The trademarks Red Cross and the Red Cross design are registered trademarks of The Mentholatum Company. Products bearing this trademark have no connection with the American National Red Cross.

Natural M.D.

For product information, please see AML Laboratories.

Niche Pharmaceuticals, Inc.

200 N. OAK STREET
P O BOX 449
ROANOKE, TX 76262

Direct Inquiries to:
Steve F. Brandon
(817) 491-2770
FAX: (817) 491-3533

For Medical Emergencies Contact:
Gerald L. Beckloff, M.D.
(817) 491-2770
FAX: (817) 491-3533

MAGTAB® SR
[*măg-tăb*]
(Magnesium L-lactate dihydrate)
Sustained-release Magnesium Supplement

Description: MagTab® SR is a sustained release oral magnesium supplement. Each pale yellow caplet contains 7mEq (84 Mg) magnesium as magnesium L-lactate dihydrate (835 Mg in a sustained release wax matrix formulation).

Indications/Uses: As a dietary supplement, MagTab® SR is indicated for patients with, or at risk for, magnesium deficiency. Hypomagnesemia and/or

Continued on next page

Niche—Cont.

magnesium deficiency can result from inadequate nutritional intake or absorption, alcoholism, or magnesium depleting drugs such as diuretics.

Warnings/Side Effects: Patients with renal disease should not take magnesium supplements without the advice and direct supervision of a physician. Excessive dosage of magnesium can cause loose stools or diarrhea.

Dosage/How Supplied: As a dietary supplement, take 1 or 2 caplets b.i.d. or as directed by a physician. MagTab® SR is available for oral administration as uncoated yellow caplets, in bottles of 60 and 100.
U.S. Patent Number: 5,002,774

UNIFIBER®
[uni fi' ber]
(Powdered Cellulose)
3 grams Fiber per tablespoon

Description: Unifiber is unique in the fiber field with many patient advantages. It's an all natural bulk fiber supplement that promotes normal bowel function by adding needed bulk to the diet. Unifiber contains powdered cellulose 75%, water 5%, corn syrup 19%, and xanthan gum 1%. Unifiber mixes easily with liquids or soft foods, and is tasteless, non-gelling, and pleasant to take. One tablespoon of Unifiber provides 3 grams of concentrated dietary fiber.

Nutrition Information: Each 4 gram (1T) serving of Unifiber contains 3 grams of fiber, 4 calories, 0% fat, 0% cholesterol, 0% protein, and is free of all electrolytes. Unifiber contains no other inactive ingredient.

Indication/Uses: As a dietary supplement, Unifiber is indicated for patients needing a concentrated source of fiber to help maintain and promote normal bowel function. Published clinical trials report that the daily use of Unifiber by institutionalized elderly patients significantly reduce the need for laxatives, suppositories, enemas, and overall nursing time. Because Unifiber is electrolyte free and contains no excitoxins, it is an ideal fiber supplement for patients on a restricted diet, such as the OB patient, kidney patient on dialysis, or the diabetic patient.

Contradiction: Intestinal obstruction or fecal impaction.

Dosage: Stir one to two tablespoons once or twice daily into a glass of fruit juice, milk, coffee, or water. An advantage of Unifiber is that it can be easily mixed with soft food such as mashed potatoes, applesauce, or pudding. Best results are normally seen in 7–10 days. Liquids should be included in the daily diet.

How Supplied: Unifiber is available over the counter in powder containers of 5 oz (35 servings), 9 oz (63 servings), or 16 oz (113 servings)

Novartis Consumer Health, Inc.
MACK WOODBRIDGE II
581 MAIN STREET
WOODBRIDGE, NJ 07095

Direct Product Inquiries to:
Consumer & Professional Affairs
(800) 452-0051
Fax: (800) 635-2801

Or write to above address.

ACUTRIM® 16 HOUR*
STEADY CONTROL
APPETITE SUPPRESSANT TABLETS
Caffeine Free

ACUTRIM® MAXIMUM STRENGTH
APPETITE SUPPRESSANT TABLETS
Caffeine Free

ACUTRIM LATE DAY® STRENGTH*
APPETITE SUPPRESSANT TABLETS
Caffeine Free

Description: ACUTRIM® tablets are an aid to appetite control in conjunction with a sensible weight loss program.
ACUTRIM® tablets deliver their maximum strength dosage of appetite suppressant at a precisely controlled rate. This timed release is scientifically targeted to effectively distribute the appetite suppressant all day.*
ACUTRIM makes it easier to follow the kind of reduced calorie diet needed for best weight control results.
A diet plan developed by an expert dietician is included in the package for your personal use as a further aid.

Formula: Each ACUTRIM® tablet contains: Active Ingredient—phenylpropanolamine HCl 75 mg (appetite suppressant, time release).
Inactive Ingredients—ACUTRIM® 16 HOUR Steady Control: Cellulose Acetate, Hydroxypropyl Methylcellulose, Stearic Acid—ACUTRIM® MAXIMUM STRENGTH: Cellulose Acetate, D&C Yellow #10, FD&C Blue #1, FD&C Yellow #6, Hydroxypropyl Methylcellulose, Povidone, Propylene Glycol, Stearic Acid, Titanium Dioxide—ACUTRIM LATE DAY® Strength: Cellulose Acetate, FD&C Yellow #6, Hydroxypropyl Methylcellulose, Isopropyl Alcohol, Propylene Glycol, Riboflavin, Stearic Acid, Titanium Dioxide.

Directions: Adult oral dosage is **one tablet** at mid-morning with a full glass of water. SWALLOW EACH TABLET WHOLE; DO NOT DIVIDE, CRUSH, CHEW, OR DISSOLVE THE TABLET. Exceeding the recommended dose has not been shown to result in greater weight loss. This product's effectiveness is directly related to the degree to which you reduce your usual daily food intake. Attempts at weight reduction which involve the use of this product should be limited to periods not exceeding 3 months, because this should be enough time to establish new eating habits. Read and follow important Diet Plan enclosed.

Warnings: FOR ADULT USE ONLY. Do not take more than one tablet per day (24 hours). Exceeding the recommended dose may cause serious health problems. Do not give this product to children under 12 years of age. Persons between 12 and 18 are advised to consult their physician before using this product. If nervousness, dizziness, sleeplessness, palpitations or headache occurs, stop taking this medication and consult your physician. If you are being treated for high blood pressure, depression, or an eating disorder or have heart disease, diabetes, thyroid disease, or an enlarged prostate gland, do not take this product except under the supervision of a physician. As with any drug, if you are pregnant or nursing a baby, seek the advice of a health professional before using this product.

Drug Interaction Precaution: Do not use with (A) a monoamine oxidase inhibitor (MAOI) (certain drugs for depression, psychiatric or emotional conditions, or Parkinson's disease), or for 2 weeks after stopping the MAOI drug. If unsure, ask a health professional. (B) any allergy, asthma, cough-cold, nasal decongestant, or weight control product (containing phenylpropanolamine, phenylephrine, pseudoephedrine, or ephedrine), or any prescription drug, unless directed by a doctor.
Keep this and all medications out of the reach of children. In case of accidental overdose, seek professional assistance or contact a Poison Control Center immediately.

How Supplied: Tamper-evident blister packages of 20 and 40 tablets. Do not use if individual seals are broken.
Do not store above 30°C (86°F).
Protect from moisture.
*Peak strength and extent of duration relate solely to blood levels.

Shown in Product Identification Guide, page 513

ALLEREST®
MAXIMUM STRENGTH AND NO DROWSINESS

Active Ingredients: *Maximum Strength*—Chlorpheniramine maleate 2 mg, pseudoephedrine HCl 30 mg.
No Drowsiness—Acetaminophen 325 mg, pseudoephedrine HCl 30 mg.

Other Ingredients: *Maximum Strength*—Corn starch, FD&C Blue No. 1, hydroxypropyl methylcellulose, lactose, microcrystalline cellulose, polyethylene glycol,

polysorbate 80, stearic acid, titanium dioxide.
No Drowsiness—Corn starch, hydroxypropyl methylcellulose, microcrystalline cellulose, polyethylene glycol, polysorbate 80, stearic acid, titanium dioxide.

Indications: *Maximum Strength*—For the temporary relief of runny nose, sneezing, itching of the nose or throat, and itchy, watery eyes due to hay fever or other upper respiratory allergies. For the temporary relief of nasal and sinus congestion.
No Drowsiness—Temporarily relieves nasal congestion due to hay fever or other upper respiratory allergies, or associated with sinusitis. For temporary relief of minor aches, pains and headache.

Directions: *Maximum Strength*—Dose as follows or as directed by a physician. Adults and children 12 years of age and over: 2 tablets every 4 to 6 hours, not to exceed 8 tablets in 24 hours. Children 6 to under 12 years of age: 1 tablet every 4 to 6 hours, not to exceed 4 tablets in 24 hours. Children under 6 years of age: Consult a physician.
No Drowsiness—Dose as follows while symptoms persist, or as directed by a physician. Adults and children 12 years of age and over: 2 caplets every 4 to 6 hours, not to exceed 8 caplets in 24 hours. Children 6 to under 12 years of age: 1 caplet every 4 to 6 hours, not to exceed 4 caplets in 24 hours. Children under 6 years of age: Consult a physician.

Warnings: *Both Products*—**Do not exceed recommended dosage.** If nervousness, dizziness, or sleeplessness occur, discontinue use and consult a physician. Do not take this product if you have heart disease, high blood pressure, thyroid disease, diabetes, or difficulty in urination due to enlargement of the prostate gland unless directed by a physician. As with any drug, if you are pregnant or nursing a baby, seek the advice of a health professional before using this product. **Keep this and all drugs out of the reach of children.** In case of accidental overdose, seek professional assistance or contact a Poison Control Center immediately.
Maximum Strength—If symptoms do not improve within 7 days or are accompanied by fever, consult a physician. Do not take this product, unless directed by a physician, if you have a breathing problem such as emphysema or chronic bronchitis, or glaucoma. May cause excitability, especially in children. May cause drowsiness; alcohol, sedatives, and tranquilizers may increase the drowsiness effect. Avoid alcoholic beverages while taking this product. Do not take this product if you are taking sedatives or tranquilizers, without first consulting your physician. Use caution when driving a motor vehicle, or operating machinery.
No Drowsiness—Do not take this product for more than 10 days (for adults) or 5 days (for children). If symptoms do not improve or are accompanied by fever that lasts for more than 3 days, or if new symptoms occur, consult a physician. Prompt medical attention is critical for adults as well as for children even if you do not notice any signs or symptoms.

Drug Interaction Precaution: *Both Products*—Do not use this product if you are now taking a prescription monoamine oxidase inhibitor (MAOI) (certain drugs for depression, psychiatric or emotional conditions, or Parkinson's disease), or for 2 weeks after stopping the MAOI drug. If you are uncertain whether your prescription drug contains an MAOI, consult a health professional before taking this product.

How Supplied: *Maximum Strength*—Boxes of 24 tablets.
No Drowsiness—Boxes of 20 caplets.
Store at room temperature 15°–30°C (59°–86°F).
Allerest is a registered trademark of Novartis.

AMERICAINE® HEMORRHOIDAL OINTMENT

[*a-mer ′i-kān*]

Active Ingredient: Benzocaine 20%.

Other Ingredients: Benzethonium chloride, polyethylene glycol 300, polyethylene glycol 3350.

Indications: For the temporary relief of local pain, itching and soreness associated with hemorrhoids and anorectal inflammation.

Directions: *Adults:* When practical, cleanse the affected area with mild soap and warm water and rinse thoroughly. Gently dry by patting or blotting with toilet tissue or a soft cloth before application of this product. Apply externally to the affected area up to 6 times daily. *Children under 12 years of age:* Consult a physician.

Warnings: If condition worsens, or does not improve within 7 days, consult a physician. Do not exceed the recommended daily dosage unless directed by a physician. In case of bleeding, consult a physician promptly. Do not put this product into the rectum by using fingers or any mechanical device or applicator. Certain persons can develop allergic reactions to ingredients in this product. If the symptom being treated does not subside or if redness, irritation, swelling, pain, or other symptoms develop or increase, discontinue use and consult a physician. **Keep this and all drugs out of the reach of children.** In case of accidental ingestion, seek professional assistance or contact a Poison Control Center immediately.

How Supplied: *Hemorrhoidal Ointment* —1 oz. tube.
Store at 15°–30°C (59°–86°F).
AMERICAINE is a registered trademark of Novartis.

Shown in Product Identification Guide, page 513

AMERICAINE® TOPICAL ANESTHETIC SPRAY

[*a-mer ′i-kān*]

Active Ingredient: Benzocaine 20%.

Other Ingredients: Isobutane (propellant), polyethylene glycol 300, propane (propellant).

Indications: For the temporary relief of pain and itching associated with minor cuts, scrapes, burns, sunburn, insect bites, or minor skin irritations.

Directions: Adults and children 2 years of age and older: Apply liberally to affected area not more than 3 to 4 times daily. Children under 2 years of age: Consult a physician.

Warnings: For external use only. Avoid contact with the eyes. If condition worsens, or if symptoms persist for more than 7 days or clear up and occur again within a few days, discontinue use of this product and consult a physician. **Keep this and all drugs out of the reach of children.** In case of accidental ingestion, seek professional assistance or contact a Poison Control Center immediately. Contents under pressure. Do not puncture or incinerate. Flammable mixture; do not use near fire or flame. Do not store at temperature above 49°C. Use only as directed. Intentional misuse by deliberately concentrating and inhaling the contents can be harmful or fatal.

How Supplied: 2 oz. aerosol container. Store at 15°–30°C (59°–86°F).
AMERICAINE is a registered trademark of Novartis.

Shown in Product Identification Guide, page 513

ASCRIPTIN®

[*ă ″skrĭp ′tin*]

Regular Strength
Maximum Strength
Arthritis Pain

Analgesic
Aspirin buffered with Maalox® for stomach comfort

Active Ingredients: Regular Strength and Arthritis Pain Ascriptin®:
Each tablet/caplet contains Aspirin (325 mg), buffered with Maalox® (Alumina-Magnesia) and Calcium Carbonate.
Maximum Strength Ascriptin®:
Each caplet contains Aspirin (500 mg), buffered with Maalox® (Alumina-Magnesia) and Calcium Carbonate.

Continued on next page

Information on Novartis Consumer Health, Inc., products appearing on these pages is effective as of November 1996.

Novartis—Cont.

Inactive Ingredients: Hydroxypropyl Methylcellulose, Magnesium Stearate, Microcrystalline Cellulose, Propylene Glycol, Starch, Talc, Titanium Dioxide, and other ingredients.

Description: Ascriptin is an excellent analgesic, antipyretic agent for general use, and is buffered with Maalox® for stomach comfort. Coated tablets/caplets make swallowing easy.

Indications: Regular Strength/Maximum Strength Ascriptin®: For the temporary relief of minor aches and pains associated with headaches, muscle aches, toothaches, menstrual cramps, and discomfort of the common cold. Also provides relief from the minor aches and pains of arthritis.
Arthritis Pain Ascriptin®: For effective temporary relief of minor aches and pains associated with arthritis. Also provides relief from the minor aches and pains associated with headaches, muscle aches, toothaches, menstrual cramps and discomfort of the common cold.

Directions: Regular Strength and Arthritis Pain Ascriptin®:
Adults: Two tablets/caplets with water every 4 hours while symptoms persist, not to exceed 12 tablets/caplets in 24 hours, or as directed by a doctor. Drink a full glass of water with each dose. **Children under 12 years of age:** Consult a doctor.
Maximum Strength Ascriptin®:
Adults: Two caplets with water every 6 hours while symptoms persist, not to exceed 8 caplets in 24 hours, or as directed by a doctor. Drink a full glass of water with each dose. **Children under 12 years of age:** Consult a doctor.

Warnings: Children and teenagers should not use this medicine for chicken pox or flu symptoms before a doctor is consulted about Reye Syndrome, a rare but serious illness reported to be associated with aspirin. Keep this and all drugs out of the reach of children. Do not take this product for pain for more than 10 days or for fever for more than 3 days unless directed by a doctor. If pain or fever persists or gets worse, if new symptoms occur, or if redness or swelling is present, consult a doctor because these could be signs of a serious condition. Do not take this product if you are allergic to aspirin or if you have asthma unless directed by a doctor. Do not take this product if you have stomach problems (such as heartburn, upset stomach, or stomach pain) that persist or recur, or if you have ulcers or bleeding problems, unless directed by a doctor. As with any drug, if you are pregnant or nursing a baby, seek the advice of a health professional before using this product. **IT IS ESPECIALLY IMPORTANT NOT TO USE ASPIRIN DURING THE LAST 3 MONTHS OF PREGNANCY UNLESS SPECIFICALLY DIRECTED TO DO SO BY A DOCTOR BECAUSE IT MAY CAUSE PROBLEMS IN THE UNBORN CHILD OR COMPLICATIONS DURING DELIVERY.** If ringing in the ears or loss of hearing occurs, consult a doctor before taking any more of this product. **In case of accidental overdose, seek professional assistance or contact a Poison Control Center immediately.**

Drug Interaction Precaution: Do not use if taking a prescription drug for anticoagulation (blood thinning), diabetes, gout or arthritis unless directed by a doctor. Antacids may interact with certain prescription drugs. If you are presently taking a prescription drug, do not take this product without checking with your doctor or other health professional.

Alcohol Warning: If you generally consume 3 or more alcohol-containing drinks per day, you should consult your physician for advice on when and how you should take Ascriptin® and other pain relievers.

Professional Labeling
For professional uses of this product, see Professional Labeling at the end of the product information for Ascriptin® enteric.

How Supplied: Regular Strength: Bottles of 100 tablets, 160 tablets, 225 tablets, and 250 foil packet samples–2 tablets each. Bottles of 500 tablets without child-resistant closures.
Maximum Strength: Bottles of 50 caplets and 85 caplets.
Arthritis Pain: Bottles of 60 caplets, 100 caplets, and 225 caplets. Bottles of 500 caplets without child-resistant closures.

Shown in Product Identification Guide, page 513

ASCRIPTIN® enteric
Pain Reliever
For Aspirin Therapy Users

Ascriptin® enteric is enteric safety coated to help prevent the stomach upset caused by aspirin.

Active Ingredient: Regular Strength Ascriptin® enteric: Aspirin 325 mg. **Adult Low Strength Ascriptin® enteric:** Aspirin 81 mg.

Inactive Ingredients: Hydroxypropyl Methylcellulose, Methacrylic Acid Copolymer, Microcrystalline Cellulose, Polyethylene Glycol, Polysorbate 80, Pregelatinized Starch, Sodium Lauryl Sulfate, Talc, Titanium Dioxide, Triacetin. May also contain Carnauba Wax.

Indications: For the temporary relief of minor aches and pains associated with headaches, muscle aches, toothaches, and menstrual cramps. Ascriptin® enteric also provides relief from the minor aches and pains of arthritis.

Regular Strength Ascriptin® enteric

Directions: Adults: Two tablets every four hours while symptoms persist, not to exceed 12 tablets in 24 hours, or as directed by a doctor. **Children under 12 years of age:** Consult a doctor. Drink a full glass of water with each dose.

Adult Low Strength Ascriptin® enteric

Directions: Adults: 4–8 tablets every four hours while symptoms persist, not to exceed 48 tablets in 24 hours, or as directed by a doctor. **Children under 12 years of age:** Consult a doctor. Drink a full glass of water with each dose.

Warnings: Children and teenagers should not use this medicine for chicken pox or flu symptoms before a doctor is consulted about Reye Syndrome, a rare but serious illness reported to be associated with aspirin. Keep this and all drugs out of the reach of children. Do not take this product for pain for more than 10 days or for fever for more than 3 days unless directed by a doctor. If pain or fever persists or gets worse, if new symptoms occur, or if redness or swelling is present, consult a doctor because these could be signs of a serious condition. Do not take this product if you are allergic to aspirin or if you have asthma unless directed by a doctor. Do not take this product if you have stomach problems (such as heartburn, upset stomach, or stomach pain) that persist or recur, or if you have ulcers or bleeding problems, unless directed by a doctor. As with any drug, if you are pregnant or nursing a baby, seek the advice of a health professional before using this product. **IT IS ESPECIALLY IMPORTANT NOT TO USE ASPIRIN DURING THE LAST 3 MONTHS OF PREGNANCY UNLESS SPECIFICALLY DIRECTED TO DO SO BY A DOCTOR BECAUSE IT MAY CAUSE PROBLEMS IN THE UNBORN CHILD OR COMPLICATIONS DURING DELIVERY.** If ringing in the ears or loss of hearing occurs, consult a doctor before taking any more of this product. **In case of accidental overdose, seek professional assistance or contact a Poison Control Center immediately.**

Drug Interaction Precaution: Do not use if taking a prescription drug for anticoagulation (blood thinning), diabetes, gout, or arthritis unless directed by a doctor.

Alcohol Warning: If you generally consume 3 or more alcohol-containing drinks per day, you should consult your physician for advice on when and how you should take Ascriptin and other pain relievers.

IMPORTANT: See your doctor before taking this product for your heart or for other new uses of aspirin, because serious side effects could occur with self treatment.

Professional Labeling
ASCRIPTIN FOR RECURRENT TIA'S IN MEN

Indications: For reducing the risk of recurrent transient ischemic attacks (TIA's) or stroke in men who have had transient ischemia of the brain due to fibrin platelet emboli. There is inadequate evidence that aspirin or buffered aspirin is effective in reducing TIA's in women at the recommended dosage. There is no evidence that aspirin or buffered aspirin is of benefit in the treatment of completed strokes in men or women.

Clinical Trials: The indication is supported by the results of a Canadian study **(1)** in which 585 patients with threatened stroke were followed in a randomized clinical trial for an average of 26 months to determine whether aspirin or sulfinpyrazone, singly or in combination, was superior to placebo in preventing transient ischemic attacks, stroke, or death. The study showed that, although sulfinpyrazone had no statistically significant effect, aspirin reduced the risk of continuing transient ischemic attacks, stroke, or death by 19 percent and reduced the risk of stroke or death by 31 percent. Another aspirin study carried out in the United States with 178 patients showed a statistically significant number of "favorable outcomes" including reduced transient ischemic attacks, stroke, and death **(2)**.

Precautions: (1) Patients presenting with signs and symptoms of TIA's should have a complete medical and neurologic evaluation. Consideration should be given to other disorders which resemble TIA's. **(2)** Attention should be given to risk factors; it is important to evaluate and treat, if appropriate, other diseases associated with TIA's and stroke such as hypertension and diabetes. **(3)** Concurrent administration of absorbable antacids at therapeutic doses may increase the clearance of salicylates in some individuals. The concurrent administration of nonabsorbable antacids may alter the rate of absorption of aspirin, thereby resulting in a decreased acetylsalicylic acid/salicylate ratio in plasma. The clinical significance on TIA's of these decreases in available aspirin is unknown. Aspirin at dosages of 1,000 milligrams per day has been associated with small increases in blood pressure, blood urea nitrogen, and serum uric acid levels. It is recommended that patients placed on long-term aspirin treatment be seen at regular intervals to assess changes in these measurements.

Adverse Reactions: At dosages of 1,000 milligrams or higher of aspirin per day, gastrointestinal side effects include stomach pain, heartburn, nausea and/or vomiting, as well as increased rates of gross gastrointestinal bleeding.

Dosage and Administration: Adult dosage for men is 1300 mg a day, in divided doses of 650 mg twice a day or 325 mg four times a day.

References:

(1) The Canadian Cooperative Study Group, "A Randomized Trial of Aspirin and Sulfinpyrazone in Threatened Stroke," *New England Journal of Medicine,* 299:53–59, 1978.

(2) Fields, W.S., et al., "Controlled Trial of Aspirin in Cerebral Ischemia," *Stroke,* 8:301–316, 1977.

ASCRIPTIN FOR MYOCARDIAL INFARCTION

Indications:

Recurrent Myocardial Infarction (MI) (Reinfarction) or Unstable Angina Pectoris

Aspirin is indicated to reduce the risk of death and/or nonfatal MI in patients with a previous MI or unstable angina pectoris.

Suspected Acute MI

Aspirin is indicated to reduce the risk of vascular mortality in patients with a suspected acute MI.

Clinical Trials:

Recurrent MI (Reinfarction) and Unstable Angina Pectoris

The indication is supported by the results of six large, randomized multicenter, placebo-controlled studies involving 10,816, predominantly male, post-MI subjects and one randomized placebo-controlled study of 1,266 men with unstable angina (1–7).

Therapy with aspirin was begun at intervals after the onset of acute MI varying from less than 3 days to more than 5 years and continued for periods of from less than 1 year to 4 years. In the unstable angina study, treatment was started within 1 month after the onset of unstable angina and continued for 12 weeks, and patients with complicating conditions such as congestive heart failure were not included in the study.

Aspirin therapy in MI subjects was associated with about a 20-percent reduction in the risk of subsequent death and/or nonfatal reinfarction, a median absolute decrease of 3 percent from the 12- to 22-percent event rates in the placebo groups. In aspirin-treated unstable angina patients the reduction in risk was about 50 percent, a reduction in the event rate of 5-percent from the 10-percent rate in the placebo group over the 12-weeks of the study.

Daily dosage of aspirin in the post-MI studies was 300 milligrams in one study and 900 to 1,500 milligrams in five studies. A dose of 325 milligrams was used in the study of unstable angina.

Suspected Acute MI

The use of aspirin in patients with a suspected acute MI is supported by the results of a large, multicenter 2 × 2 factorial study of 17,187 subjects with suspected acute MI (8). Subjects were randomized within 24 hours of the onset of symptoms so that 8,587 subjects received oral aspirin (162.5 milligrams, enteric-coated) daily for 1 month (the first dose crushed, sucked, or chewed) and 8,600 received oral placebo. Of the subjects, 8,592 were also randomized to receive a single dose of streptokinase (1.5 million units) infused intravenously for about 1 hour, and 8,595 received a placebo infusion. Thus, 4,295 subjects received aspirin plus placebo, 4,300 received streptokinase plus placebo, 4,292 received aspirin plus streptokinase, and 4,300 received double placebo.

Vascular mortality (attributed to cardiac, cerebral, hemorrhagic, other vascular, or unknown causes) occurred in 9.4 percent of the subjects in the aspirin group and in 11.8 percent of the subjects in the oral placebo group in the 35-day followup. This represents an absolute reduction of 2.4 percent in the mean 35-day vascular mortality attributable to aspirin and a 23-percent reduction in the odds of vascular death ($2p < 0.00001$).

Significant absolute reductions in mortality and corresponding reductions in specific clinical events favoring aspirin were found for reinfarction (1.5 percent absolute reduction, 45 percent odds reduction, $2p < 0.00001$), cardiac arrest (1.2 percent absolute reduction, 14.2 percent odds reduction, $2p < 0.01$), and total stroke (0.4 percent absolute reduction, 41.5 percent odds reduction, $2p < 0.01$).

The effect of aspirin over and above its effect on mortality was evidenced by small, but significant, reductions in vascular morbidity in those subjects who were discharged.

The beneficial effects of aspirin on mortality were present with or without streptokinase infusion. Aspirin reduced vascular mortality from 10.4 to 8.0 percent for days 0 to 35 in subjects given streptokinase and reduced vascular mortality from 13.2 to 10.7 percent in subjects given no streptokinase.

The effects of aspirin and thrombolytic therapy with streptokinase in this study were approximately additive. Subjects who received the combination of streptokinase infusion and daily aspirin had significantly lower vascular mortality at 35 days than those who received either active treatment alone (combination 8.0 percent, aspirin 10.7 percent, streptokinase 10.4 percent, and no treatment 13.2 percent). While this study demonstrated that aspirin has an additive benefit in patients given streptokinase, there is no reason to restrict its use to that specific thrombolytic.

Adverse Reactions:

Gastrointestinal Reactions

Doses of 1,000 milligrams per day of aspirin caused gastrointestinal symptoms and bleeding that in some cases were clinically significant. In the Aspirin Myocardial Infarction Study (AMIS) (4) with 4,500 post-infarction subjects, the percentage incidences of gastrointestinal symptoms for the aspirin (1,000 milligrams of a standard, solid-tablet formulation) and placebo-treated subjects, respectively, were: Stomach pain (14.5 percent, 4.4 percent); heartburn (11.9 percent, 4.8 percent); nausea and/or vomit-

Continued on next page

Information on Novartis Consumer Health, Inc., products appearing on these pages is effective as of November 1996.

Novartis—Cont.

ing (7.6 percent, 2.1 percent); hospitalization for gastrointestinal disorder (4.8 percent, 3.5 percent). Symptoms and signs of gastrointestinal irritation were not significantly increased in subjects treated for unstable angina with 325 milligrams buffered aspirin in solution.

Bleeding

In the AMIS and other trials, aspirin-treated subjects had increased rates of gross gastrointestinal bleeding. In the ISIS-2 study (8), there was no significant difference in the incidence of major bleeding (bleeds requiring transfusion) between 8,587 subjects taking 162.5 milligrams aspirin daily and 8,600 subjects taking placebo (31 versus 33 subjects). There were five confirmed cerebral hemorrhages in the aspirin group compared with two in the placebo group, but the incidence of stroke of all causes was significantly reduced from 81 to 47 for the placebo versus aspirin group (0.4 percent absolute change). There was a small and statistically significant excess (0.6 percent) of minor bleeding in people taking aspirin (2.5 percent for aspirin, 1.9 percent for placebo). No other significant adverse effects were reported.

Cardiovascular and Biochemical

In the AMIS trial (4), the dosage of 1,000 milligrams per day of aspirin was associated with small increases in systolic blood pressure (BP) (average 1.5 to 2.1 millimeters Hg) and diastolic BP (0.5 to 0.6 millimeters Hg), depending upon whether maximal or last available readings were used. Blood urea nitrogen and uric acid levels were also increased, but by less than 1.0 milligram percent.

Subjects with marked hypertension or renal insufficiency had been excluded from the trial so that the clinical importance of these observations for such subjects or for any subjects treated over more prolonged periods is not known. It is recommended that patients placed on long-term aspirin treatment, even at doses of 160 milligrams per day, be seen at regular intervals to assess changes in these measurements.

Dosage and Administration:

Recurrent MI (Reinfarction) and Unstable Angina Pectoris

Although most of the studies used dosages exceeding 300 milligrams, two trials used only 300 milligrams, and pharmacologic data indicate that this dose inhibits platelet function fully. Therefore, 300 milligrams or a conventional 325 milligram aspirin dose is a reasonable, routine dose that would minimize gastrointestinal adverse reactions. This use of aspirin applies to both solid, oral dosage forms (buffered and plain aspirin) and buffered aspirin in solution.

Suspected Acute MI

The recommended dose of aspirin to treat suspected acute MI is 160 to 162.5 milligrams taken as soon as the infarct is suspected and then daily for at least 30 days. (One-half of a conventional 325-milligram aspirin tablet or two 80- or 81-milligram aspirin tablets may be taken.) This use of aspirin applies to both solid, oral dosage forms (buffered, plain, and enteric-coated aspirin) and buffered aspirin in solution. If using a solid dosage form, the first dose should be crushed, sucked or chewed. After the 30-day treatment, physicians should consider further therapy based on the labeling for dosage and administration of aspirin for prevention of recurrent MI (reinfarction).

References:

(1) Elwood, P. C. et al., "A Randomized Controlled Trial of Acetylsalicylic Acid in the Secondary Prevention of Mortality from Myocardial Infarction," *British Medical Journal,* 1:436-440, 1974.

(2) The Coronary Drug Project Research Group, "Aspirin in Coronary Heart Disease," *Journal of Chronic Diseases,* 29:625-642, 1976.

(3) Breddin, K. et al., "Secondary Prevention of Myocardial Infarction: A Comparison of Acetylsalicylic Acid, Phenprocoumon or Placebo," *Homeostasis,* 470:263-268, 1979.

(4) Aspirin Myocardial Infarction Study Research Group, "A Randomized, Controlled Trial of Aspirin in Persons Recovered from Myocardial Infarction." *Journal of the American Medical Association,* 243:661-669, 1980.

(5) Elwood, P. C., and P. M. Sweetnam, "Aspirin and Secondary Mortality After Myocardial Infarction," *Lancet,* II:1313-1315, December 22-29, 1979.

(6) The Persantine-Aspirin Reinfarction Study Research Group, "Persantine and Aspirin in Coronary Heart Disease," *Circulation,* 62:449-461, 1980.

(7) Lewis, H. D. et al., "Protective Effects of Aspirin Against Acute Myocardial Infarction and Death in Men with Unstable Angina, Results of a Veterans Administration Cooperative Study," *New England Journal of Medicine,* 309:396-403, 1983.

(8) ISIS-2 (Second International Study of Infarct Survival) Collaborative Group, "Randomized Trial of Intravenous Streptokinase, Oral Aspirin, Both, or Neither Among 17,187 Cases of Suspected Acute Myocardial Infarction: ISIS-2," *Lancet,* 2:349-360, August 13, 1988.

(9) "1984 Report of the Joint National Committee on Detection, Evaluation, and Treatment of High Blood Pressure," United States Department of Health and Human Services and United States Public Health Service, National Institutes of Health, Publication No. NIH 84–1088, 1984.

How Supplied: Regular Strength: Bottles of 100 coated aspirin tablets. **Adult Low Strength:** Bottles of 120 coated aspirin tablets.

Keep tightly closed in a dry place. Do not expose to excessive heat.

Do not use if the imprinted foil seal under the cap is broken or missing.

Questions? Call 1-800-548-3708, weekdays 9 am – 5 pm ET.

Shown in Product Identification Guide, page 513

CALDECORT® ANTI-ITCH CREAM

[kal'de-kort]

Active Ingredient: Hydrocortisone acetate (equivalent to hydrocortisone free base 1%)

Other Ingredients: Cetostearyl alcohol, sodium lauryl sulfate, white petrolatum, propylene glycol, purified water.

Indications: For the temporary relief of itching associated with minor skin irritations, inflammation, and rashes due to eczema, insect bites, poison ivy, poison oak, poison sumac, soaps, detergents, cosmetics and jewelry. Other uses of this product should be only under the advice and supervision of a doctor.

Directions: Adults and children 2 years of age and older: Apply to affected area not more than 3 or 4 times daily. Children under 2 years of age: Do not use, consult a doctor.

IMPORTANT: Unscrew the cap. The tube opening is sealed. Do not use if seal is punctured or not visible and return product to place of purchase. To puncture the seal, reverse the cap and place the puncture-top onto the tube. Push down firmly until seal is open. To close, screw the cap back onto the tube.

Warnings: For external use only. Avoid contact with the eyes. If condition worsens, or if symptoms persist for more than 7 days or clear up and occur again within a few days, stop use of this product and do not begin use of any other hydrocortisone product unless you have consulted a doctor. Do not use for the treatment of diaper rash. Consult a doctor. **Keep this and all drugs out of the reach of children.** In case of accidental ingestion, seek professional assistance or contact a Poison Control Center immediately.

How Supplied: $^1/_2$ oz. tube.

CALDECORT is a registered trademark of Novartis.

CALDESENE® MEDICATED POWDER

[kal'de-sēn]

Active Ingredients: Calcium undecylenate 10%.

Other Ingredients: Fragrance, talc.

Indications: Caldesene Powder is medicated with calcium undecylenate to kill harmful bacteria while forming a protective barrier that repels moisture and helps keep sensitive skin dry. Only Caldesene has this special formula with two way action. Used regularly, Caldesene helps prevent skin infections and protects sensitive skin for both adults and children.

Actions: Caldesene Medicated Powder helps relieve, treat and prevent diaper rash, prickly heat, chafing, with two way action:

- kills bacteria
- protects against wetness.

Directions: Use on baby after every bath or diaper change or as directed by a pediatrician.
Apply powder close to the body away from child's face. (Shake bottle—don't squeeze—to apply powder to your hand or directly into the diaper.) For prickly heat, chafing—Smooth on Caldesene 3 or 4 times a day, or as recommended by your physician, to soothe and comfort sensitive skin and relieve minor irritation.

Warnings: For external use only. Avoid contact with eyes. If condition worsens or does not improve within 7 days, consult a physician. **Keep this and all drugs out of the reach of children.** In case of accidental ingestion, seek professional assistance or contact a Poison Control Center immediately.
Keep powder away from child's face to avoid inhalation, which can cause breathing problems. Do not use on broken skin.

How Supplied: *Medicated Powder*—2 oz (57 g) and 4 oz (113 g) shaker containers.
Store at room temperature 59°–86°F (15°–30°C).
CALDESENE is a registered trademark of Novartis.

Shown in Product Identification Guide, page 513

CRUEX® ANTIFUNGALS

[kru 'ex]

Available in original and Prescription Strength varieties (see below)

Active Ingredients: *Prescription Strength Spray Powder*—Miconazole nitrate 2%. *Prescription Strength Cream*—Clotrimazole 1%. *The original Squeeze Powder*—Undecylenate 10%, as calcium undecylenate. *The original Spray Powder*—Total undecylenate 19%, as undecylenic acid and zinc undecylenate.

Other Ingredients: *Prescription Strength Spray Powder*—Aloe vera gel, aluminum starch octenylsuccinate, isopropyl myristate, propylene carbonate, SD alcohol 40-B (10% w/w), sorbitan monooleate, stearalkonium hectorite. Propellant: Isobutane/propane. *Prescription Strength Cream*—Cetostearyl alcohol, cetyl esters wax, 2-octyldodecanol, polysorbate-60, sorbitan monostearate, purified water and, as a preservative, benzyl alcohol (1%). *The original Squeeze Powder*—Colloidal silicon dioxide, fragrance, isopropyl myristate, talc. *The original Spray Powder*—Fragrance, isobutane (propellant), isopropyl myristate, menthol, talc, trolamine.

Indications: Cures jock itch (tinea cruris). Relieves itching and burning. Cruex powders also absorb perspiration.

Warnings: Do not use on children under 2 years of age unless directed by a doctor. For external use only. Avoid contact with the eyes. If irritation occurs, or if there is no improvement within 2 weeks (of jock itch), discontinue use and consult a doctor. **Keep this and all drugs out of the reach of children.** In case of accidental ingestion, seek professional assistance or contact a Poison Control Center immediately. Use only as directed. *For Sprays only*—Avoid inhaling. Avoid contact with the eyes or other mucous membranes. Contents under pressure. Do not puncture or incinerate. Flammable mixture, do not use near fire or flame. Do not expose to heat or temperatures above 49°C (120°F). Use only as directed. Intentional misuse by deliberately concentrating and inhaling the contents can be harmful or fatal.

Directions: Clean the affected area and dry thoroughly. Apply a thin layer of the product over affected area twice daily (morning and night) or as directed by a doctor. (For Sprays: **Shake spray can well,** and hold 4″ to 6″ from skin when applying.) Supervise children in the use of these products. For jock itch, use daily for 2 weeks. If condition persists longer, consult a doctor. This product is not effective on the scalp or nails.
Important *(Prescription Strength Cream)*: UNSCREW THE CAP. THE TUBE OPENING IS SEALED. DO NOT USE IF SEAL IS PUNCTURED OR NOT VISIBLE AND RETURN PRODUCT TO PLACE OF PURCHASE. TO PUNCTURE THE SEAL, REVERSE THE CAP AND PLACE THE PUNCTURE-TOP ONTO THE TUBE. PUSH DOWN FIRMLY UNTIL SEAL IS OPEN. TO CLOSE, SCREW THE CAP BACK ONTO THE TUBE.

How Supplied: *Prescription Strength Spray Powder*—3 oz. aerosol container. *Prescription Strength Cream*—0.5 oz. tube. *The original Squeeze Powder*—1.5 oz. plastic squeeze bottle. *The original Spray Powder*—1.8 oz., 3.5 oz., and 5.5 oz. aerosol containers.
Store **powders/spray powders** at room temperature, 15°–30°C (59°–86°F). See container bottom for lot number and expiration date. Spray powders: Tamper-resistant aerosol can for your protection. If clogging occurs, remove button and clean nozzle with pin.
Store **Prescription Strength Cream** between 2° and 30° (36°–86°F). See box or tube crimp for lot number and expiration date.
CRUEX is a registered trademark of Novartis.

Shown in Product Identification Guide, page 513

DESENEX® ANTIFUNGALS

[dess 'i-nex]

Available in original and Prescription Strength varieties (see below)

Active Ingredients: *Prescription Strength Spray Powder and Spray Liquid*—Miconazole nitrate 2%. *Prescription Strength Cream*—Clotrimazole 1%. *The original Shake Powder, Spray Powder, and Ointment*—Total undecylenate 25%, as undecylenic acid and zinc undecylenate.

Other Ingredients: *Prescription Strength Spray Powder*—Aloe vera gel, aluminum starch octenylsuccinate, isopropyl myristate, propylene carbonate, SD alcohol 40–B (10% w/w), sorbitan monooleate, stearalkonium hectorite. Propellant: Isobutane/propane. *Prescription Strength Spray Liquid*—Polyethylene glycol 300, polysorbate 20, SD-alcohol 40-B (15% w/w). Propellant: Dimethyl ether. *Prescription Strength Cream*—Cetostearyl alcohol, cetyl esters wax, 2-octyldodecanol, polysorbate-60, sorbitan monostearate, purified water and, as a preservative, benzyl alcohol (1%). *The original Shake Powder*—Fragrance, talc. *The original Spray Powder*—Fragrance, isopropyl myristate, menthol, talc, trolamine. Propellant: Isobutane. *The original Ointment*—Fragrance, glycol stearate SE, lanolin, methylparaben, PEG-8 laurate, PEG-6 stearate, propylparaben, purified water, sorbitol solution, stearic acid, trolamine, white petrolatum.

Indications: Cures athlete's foot (tinea pedis) and ringworm (tinea corporis). For effective relief of the itching, cracking, and burning which can accompany these conditions. Desenex powders also help keep feet dry.

Warnings: Do not use on children under 2 years of age unless directed by a doctor. For external use only. Avoid contact with the eyes. If irritation occurs, or if there is no improvement within 4 weeks (of athlete's foot or ringworm), discontinue use and consult a doctor. **Keep this and all drugs out of the reach of children.** In case of accidental ingestion, seek professional assistance or contact a Poison Control Center immediately. Use only as directed. *For Spray Powders and Spray Liquid*—Avoid inhaling. Avoid contact with the eyes or other mucous membranes. Contents under pressure. Do not puncture or incinerate. Flammable mixture, do not use near fire or flame. Do not expose to heat or temperatures above 49°C (120°F). Use only as directed. Intentional misuse by deliberately concentrating and inhaling the contents can be harmful or fatal.

Directions: Clean the affected area and dry thoroughly. Apply a thin layer of the product over affected area twice daily (morning and night) or as directed by a doctor. (For Sprays: **Shake Spray can well,** and hold 4″ to 6″ from skin when applying.) Supervise children in the use of this product. For athlete's foot, pay special attention to the spaces between the toes. Wear well-fitting, ventilated shoes and change shoes and socks at least

Continued on next page

Information on Novartis Consumer Health, Inc., products appearing on these pages is effective as of November 1996.

Novartis—Cont.

once daily. For athlete's foot or ringworm, use daily for 4 weeks. If condition persists longer, consult a doctor. This product is not effective on the scalp or nails.

Important ***(Prescription Strength Cream):*** UNSCREW THE CAP. THE TUBE OPENING IS SEALED. DO NOT USE IF SEAL IS PUNCTURED OR NOT VISIBLE AND RETURN PRODUCT TO PLACE OF PURCHASE. TO PUNCTURE THE SEAL, REVERSE THE CAP AND PLACE THE PUNCTURE-TOP ONTO THE TUBE. PUSH DOWN FIRMLY UNTIL SEAL IS OPEN. TO CLOSE, SCREW THE CAP BACK ONTO THE TUBE.

How Supplied: *Prescription Strength Spray Powder*—3 oz. aerosol container. *Prescription Strength Liquid Spray*—3.5 oz. aerosol container. *Prescription Strength Cream*—0.5 oz. tube. *The original Shake Powder*—1.5 oz. and 3 oz. plastic bottles. *The original Spray Powder*—2.7 oz. aerosol container. *The original Ointment*—0.5 oz. and 1 oz. tubes. Store **powders/spray powders** and **ointment** at room temperature, 15°–30°C (59°–86°F). For powders, see container bottom for lot number and expiration date. For the original Ointment, see box or tube crimp for lot number and expiration date. Spray powders: Tamper-resistant aerosol can for your protection. If clogging occurs, remove button and clean nozzle with pin.
Store **Prescription Strength Cream** between 2° and 30° (36°–86°F). See box or tube crimp for lot number and expiration date.
DESENEX is a registered trademark of Novartis.

Shown in Product Identification Guide, page 513

REGULAR STRENGTH DOAN'S® Analgesic Caplets
EXTRA STRENGTH DOAN'S® Analgesic Caplets

Active Ingredient: Regular Strength Doan's: Each caplet contains Magnesium Salicylate Tetrahydrate 377 mg. (equivalent to 303.7 mg. of anhydrous Magnesium Salicylate). **Extra Strength Doan's:** Each caplet contains Magnesium Salicylate Tetrahydrate 580 mg. (equivalent to 467.2 mg. of anhydrous Magnesium Salicylate).

Also contains: Regular Strength Doan's: FD&C Blue #1 Aluminum Lake, FD&C Yellow #6 Aluminum Lake, FD&C Yellow #10 Aluminum Lake, Hydroxypropyl Methylcellulose, Magnesium Stearate, Microcrystalline Cellulose, Polyethylene Glycol, Polysorbate 80, Stearic Acid, Titanium Dioxide. **Extra Strength Doan's:** Hydroxypropyl Methylcellulose, Magnesium Stearate, Microcrystalline Cellulose, Polyethylene Glycol, Polysorbate 80, Stearic Acid, Titanium Dioxide.

Indications: For temporary relief of minor backache pain.

Directions: Regular Strength Doan's: Adults—Two caplets every 4 hours while symptoms persist, not to exceed 12 caplets during a 24-hour period or as directed by a doctor. Drink a full glass of water with each dose. Children under 12: consult a doctor. **Extra Strength Doan's:** Adults—Two caplets every 6 hours while symptoms persist, not to exceed 8 caplets during a 24-hour period or as directed by a doctor. Drink a full glass of water with each dose. Children under 12: consult a doctor.

Warnings: Children and teenagers should not use this medicine for chicken pox or flu symptoms before a doctor is consulted about Reye syndrome, a rare but serious illness. As with any drug, if you are pregnant or nursing a baby, seek the advice of a health professional before using this product. Do not take this product for pain for more than 10 days or for fever for more than 3 days unless directed by a doctor. If pain or fever persists or gets worse, if new symptoms occur, or if redness or swelling is present, consult a doctor because these could be signs of a serious condition. Do not take this product if you are allergic to salicylates (including aspirin), have stomach problems (such as heartburn, upset stomach, or stomach pain) that persist or recur, or if you have ulcers or bleeding problems, unless directed by a doctor. If ringing in the ears or a loss of hearing occurs, consult a doctor before taking any more of this product.
Keep this and all drugs out of the reach of children. In case of accidental overdose, seek professional assistance or contact a Poison Control Center immediately.

Drug Interaction Precaution: Do not take this product if you are taking a prescription drug for anticoagulation (thinning of the blood), diabetes, gout, or arthritis unless directed by a doctor.

Alcohol Warning: If you generally consume 3 or more alcohol-containing drinks per day, you should consult your physician for advice on when and how you should take Doan's or other pain relievers.

How Supplied: Blister packages of 24 and 48 caplets.
Store at 15°–30°C (59°–86°F). Protect from moisture.

Extra Strength DOAN'S® P.M. Magnesium Salicylate/ Diphenhydramine Analgesic/Nighttime Sleep Aid Caplets

Active Ingredients: Each caplet contains Magnesium Salicylate Tetrahydrate 580mg. (equivalent to 467.2mg. of anhydrous Magnesium Salicylate) and Diphenydramine HCl 25mg.

Also Contains: Carnauba Wax, Colloidal Silicon Dioxide, Croscarmellose Sodium, FD&C Blue #2 Aluminum Lake, Hydroxypropyl Methylcellulose, Magnesium Stearate, Microcrystalline Cellulose, Polyethylene Glycol, Polysorbate 80, Stearic Acid, Talc, Titanium Dioxide.

Indications: For temporary relief of minor back pain accompanied by sleeplessness.

Directions: Adults and children 12 years of age or older: Take 2 caplets at bedtime if needed, or as directed by a doctor. Drink a full glass of water with each dose.

Warnings: Children and teenagers should not use this medicine for chicken pox or flu symptoms before a doctor is consulted about Reye syndrome, a rare but serious illness. **Keep this and all drugs out of the reach of children.** In case of accidental overdose, seek professional assistance or contact a Poison Control Center immediately. Do not give this product to children under 12 years of age. As with any drug, if you are pregnant or nursing a baby, seek the advice of a health professional before using this product. Do not take this product for pain for more than 10 days or for fever for more than 3 days unless directed by a doctor. If pain or fever persists or gets worse, if new symptoms occur, or if redness or swelling is present, consult a doctor because these could be signs of a serious condition. If sleeplessness persists continuously for more than 2 weeks, consult your doctor. Insomnia may be a symptom of serious underlying medical illness. Do not take this product, unless directed by a doctor, if you have a breathing problem such as emphysema or chronic bronchitis, or if you have glaucoma, difficulty in urination due to enlargement of the prostate gland, stomach problems (such as heartburn, upset stomach, or stomach pain) that persist or recur, ulcers or bleeding problems, or if you are allergic to aspirin or salicylates. If ringing in the ears or a loss of hearing occurs, consult a doctor before taking any more of this product. Avoid alcoholic beverages while taking this product. Do not take this product if you are taking sedatives or tranquilizers without first consulting your doctor.

Drug Interaction Precaution: Do not take this product if you are taking a prescription drug for anticoagulation (thinning of the blood), diabetes, gout, or arthritis unless directed by a doctor.

Alcohol Warning: If you generally consume 3 or more alcohol-containing drinks per day, you should consult your physician for advice on when and how you should take Doan's or other pain relievers.

How Supplied: Blister packages of 20 caplets supplied in child-resistant packaging.

Store at 15°–30°C (59°–86°F). Protect from moisture.

DULCOLAX®
[dul 'co-lax]
brand of bisacodyl USP
Tablets of 5 mg
Suppositories of 10 mg
Laxative

Ingredients: Each enteric coated tablet contains: Active: Bisacodyl USP 5 mg. Also contains: Acacia, acetylated monoglyceride, carnauba wax, cellulose acetate phthalate, corn starch, D&C Red No. 30 aluminum lake, D&C Yellow No. 10 aluminum lake, dibutyl phthalate, docusate sodium, gelatin, glycerin, iron oxides, kaolin, lactose, magnesium stearate, methylparaben, pharmaceutical glaze, polyethylene glycol, povidone, propylparaben, sodium benzoate, sorbitan monooleate, sucrose, talc, titanium dioxide, white wax.
Each suppository contains: Active: Bisacodyl USP 10 mg. Also contains: Hydrogenated vegetable oil.
SODIUM CONTENT: Tablets and suppositories contain less than 0.2 mg per dosage unit and are thus dietetically sodium free.

Indications: For the relief of occasional constipation and irregularity. Physicians should refer to the "Professional Labeling" section for additional indications and information.

Directions:
Tablets
Adults and children 12 years of age and over: Take 2 or 3 tablets (usually 2) in a single dose once daily.
Children 6 to under 12 years of age: Take 1 tablet once daily.
Children under 6 years of age: Consult a physician.
Expect results in 8–12 hours if taken at bedtime or within 6 hours if taken before breakfast.
Suppositories
Adults and children 12 years of age and over: 1 suppository once daily. Remove foil wrapper. Lie on your side and, with pointed end first, push suppository high into the rectum so it will not slip out. Retain it for 15 to 20 minutes. If you feel the suppository must come out immediately, it was not inserted high enough and should be pushed higher.
Children 6 to under 12 years of age: 1/2 suppository once daily.
Children under 6 years of age: Consult a physician.
If the suppository seems soft, hold in foil wrapper under cold water for one or two minutes. In the presence of anal fissures or hemorrhoids, suppository may be coated at the tip with petroleum jelly before insertion.

Warnings: Do not use laxative products when abdominal pain, nausea, or vomiting are present unless directed by a physician. Restoration of normal bowel function by using this product may cause abdominal discomfort including cramps. Laxative products should not be used for a period longer than 1 week unless directed by a physician. Rectal bleeding or failure to have a bowel movement after use of a laxative may indicate a serious condition. If this occurs, discontinue use and consult your physician. As with any drug, if you are pregnant or nursing a baby, seek the advice of a health care professional before using this product. **Keep this and all medication out of the reach of children.** In case of accidental overdose or ingestion, seek professional assistance or contact a Poison Control Center immediately.
For tablets: Do not chew or crush. Do not give to children under 6 years of age unless directed by a physician. Do not take this product within 1 hour after taking an antacid or milk.

How Supplied: Dulcolax, brand of bisacodyl: Yellow, enteric-coated tablets of 5 mg in boxes of 10, 25, 50 and 100; suppositories of 10 mg in boxes of 4, 8, 16 and 50.

Store Dulcolax suppositories and tablets at temperatures below 77°F (25°C). Avoid excessive humidity.

Also Available: Dulcolax® Bowel Prep Kit. Each kit contains:
1 Dulcolax suppository of 10 mg bisacodyl;
4 Dulcolax tablets of 5 mg bisacodyl;
Complete patient instructions.

Professional Labeling

Description and Clinical Pharmacology: Dulcolax is a contact stimulant laxative, administered either orally or rectally, which acts directly on the colonic mucosa to produce normal peristalsis throughout the large intestine. The active ingredient in Dulcolax, bisacodyl, is a colorless, tasteless compound that is practically insoluble in water or alkaline solution. Its chemical name is: bis(p-acetoxyphenyl)-2-pyridylmethane. Bisacodyl is very poorly absorbed, if at all, in the small intestine following oral administration, nor in the large intestine following rectal administration. On contact with the mucosa or submucosal plexi of the large intestine, bisacodyl stimulates sensory nerve endings to produce parasympathetic reflexes resulting in increased peristaltic contractions of the colon. It has also been shown to promote fluid and ion accumulation in the colon, which increases the laxative effect. A bowel movement is usually produced approximately 6 hours after oral administration (8–12 hours if taken at bedtime), and approximately 15 minutes to 1 hour after rectal administration, providing satisfactory cleansing of the bowel which may, under certain circumstances, obviate the need for colonic irrigation.

Indications and Usage: For use as part of a bowel cleansing regimen in preparing the patient for surgery or for preparing the colon for x-ray endoscopic examination. Dulcolax will not replace the colonic irrigations usually given patients before intracolonic surgery, but is useful in the preliminary emptying of the colon prior to these procedures.
Also for use as a laxative in postoperative care (i.e., restoration of normal bowel hygiene), antepartum care, postpartum care, and in preparation for delivery.

Contraindications: Stimulant laxatives, such as Dulcolax, are contraindicated for patients with acute surgical abdomen, appendicitis, rectal bleeding, gastroenteritis, or intestinal obstruction.

Precautions: Long-term administration of Dulcolax is not recommended in the treatment of chronic constipation.

Dosage and Administration:
Preparation for x-ray endoscopy: For barium enemas, no food should be given following oral administration to prevent reaccumulation of material in the cecum, and a suppository should be administered one to two hours prior to examination.
Children under 6 years of age: Oral administration is not recommended due to the requirement to swallow tablets whole. For rectal administration, the suppository dosage is 5 mg (1/2 of 10 mg suppository) in a single daily dose.

Shown in Product Identification Guide, page 513

EUCALYPTAMINT®
Arthritis Pain Relief Formula
Maximum Strength

Description: Maximum Strength topical analgesic that provides hours of effective relief from minor arthritis pain.

Active Ingredient: Menthol (16%).

Inactive Ingredients: Lanolin and Eucalyptus Oil.

Indications: For the temporary relief of minor aches and pains of muscles and joints associated with arthritis.

Directions: Adults and children 2 years of age and older: Gently massage a conservative amount into affected area not more than 3 to 4 times daily.
Children under 2 years of age: Consult a physician.

Warning: FOR EXTERNAL USE ONLY. Avoid contact with eyes. Do not apply to wounds or damaged skin. Do not bandage tightly. Do not use with heating pads or heating devices. If condition worsens, or if symptoms persist for more than 7 days, discontinue use of this product and consult a physician. **Keep this and all drugs out of the reach of children.** In case of accidental ingestion, seek professional assistance or contact a Poison Control Center immediately.

Continued on next page

Information on Novartis Consumer Health, Inc., products appearing on these pages is effective as of November 1996.

Novartis—Cont.

How Supplied: Eucalyptamint Ointment is supplied in a 2 oz. easy to squeeze tube.
Store at room temperature 15°–30°C (59°–86°F). Do not freeze. It is normal for the consistency of Eucalyptamint to vary with temperature changes. If thickening does occur, warm the tube in the palms of your hands or run under warm water.
Eucalyptamint is a registered trademark of Novartis.

EUCALYPTAMINT®
Muscle Pain Relief Formula

Description: A uniquely scented gel creme formulation providing hours of effective pain relief for overworked muscles.

Active Ingredient: Menthol 8%.

Other Ingredients: Carbomer 980, Eucalyptus Oil, Fragrance, Propylene Glycol, SD 3A Alcohol, Triethanolamine, TWEEN 80, Water.

Indications: For the temporary relief of minor aches and pains of muscles and joints associated with simple backache, strains, sprains and sports injuries.

Directions: Adults and children 2 years of age and older. Shake tube with cap facing downward. Gently massage a conservative amount into affected area not more than 3 to 4 times daily. Store on cap. Children under 2 years of age: Consult a physician.

Warning: FOR EXTERNAL USE ONLY. Avoid contact with eyes. Do not apply to wounds or damaged skin. Do not bandage tightly. Do not use with heating pads or heating devices. If condition worsens, or if symptoms persist for more than 7 days, discontinue use of this product and consult a physician. **Keep this and all drugs out of the reach of children.** In case of accidental ingestion, seek professional assistance or contact a Poison Control Center immediately.

How Supplied: Eucalyptamint Muscle Pain Relief Formula is supplied in a 2.25 oz. tube in a Powder Fresh Scent. Store at room temperature 15°–30°C (59°–86°F). Do not freeze. Store tube on cap.

Eucalyptamint is a registered trademark of Novartis.

EX–LAX® Chocolated Laxative Tablets

Active Ingredient: Yellow phenolphthalein, 90 mg phenolphthalein per tablet.

Inactive Ingredients: cocoa, confectioner's sugar, hydrogenated palm kernel oil, lecithin, nonfat dry milk, vanillin. Sodium-free.

Indication: For relief of occasional constipation (irregularity).

Caution: Do not take any laxative when abdominal pain, nausea, or vomiting are present. Frequent or prolonged use of this or any other laxative may result in dependence on laxatives. If skin rash appears, do not use this or any other preparation containing phenolphthalein.

Warnings: Keep this and all drugs out of the reach of children. In case of accidental overdose, seek professional assistance or contact a Poison Control Center immediately. As with any drug, if you are pregnant or nursing a baby, seek the advice of a health care professional before using this product.

Dosage and Administration: Adults and children 12 years old and over: Chew 1 or 2 tablets, preferably at bedtime. Children over 6 years: Chew 1/2 tablet.

How Supplied: Available in boxes of 6, 18, 48, and 72 chewable chocolated tablets.

Shown in Product Identification Guide, page 514

EX–LAX® Laxative Pills

Regular Strength Ex-Lax® Laxative Pills
Extra Gentle Ex-Lax® Laxative Pills
Maximum Relief Formula Ex-Lax® Laxative Pills
Ex-Lax® Gentle Nature® Laxative Pills

Active Ingredients: Regular Strength Ex-Lax Laxative Pills—Yellow phenolphthalein USP, 90 mg. phenolphthalein per pill. **Extra Gentle Ex-Lax Laxative Pills**—Docusate sodium USP, 75 mg; yellow phenolphthalein USP, 65 mg phenolphthalein per pill. **Maximum Relief Formula Ex-Lax Laxative Pills**—Yellow phenolphthalein USP, 135 mg. phenolphthalein per pill. **Ex-Lax Gentle Nature Laxative Pills**—Senna glycosides, equivalent to Sennosides USP 12 mg per pill.

Inactive Ingredients: Regular Strength Ex-Lax Laxative Pills—acacia, alginic acid, carnauba wax, colloidal silicon dioxide, dibasic calcium phosphate, iron oxides, magnesium stearate, microcrystalline cellulose, sodium benzoate, sodium lauryl sulfate, starch, stearic acid, sucrose, talc, titanium dioxide. Sodium-free. **Extra Gentle Ex-Lax Laxative Pills**—acacia, colloidal silicon dioxide, croscarmellose sodium, dibasic calcium phosphate, magnesium stearate, methylparaben, microcrystalline cellulose, povidone, propylparaben, red 7, sodium benzoate, stearic acid, sucrose, talc, titanium dioxide. Sodium content: 6 mg per pill. **Maximum Relief Formula Ex-Lax Laxative Pills**—acacia, alginic acid, blue no. 1, carnauba wax, colloidal silicon dioxide, dibasic calcium phosphate, magnesium stearate, microcrystalline cellulose, povidone, sodium benzoate, sodium lauryl sulfate, starch, stearic acid, sucrose, talc, titanium dioxide. Sodium-free. **Ex-Lax Gentle Nature Laxative Pills**—alginic acid, colloidal silicon dioxide, dibasic calcium phosphate, magnesium stearate, microcrystalline cellulose, pregelatinized starch, sodium lauryl sulfate, stearic acid. Sodium-free.

Indication: For relief of occasional constipation (irregularity).

Caution: Do not take any laxative when abdominal pain, nausea, or vomiting are present. Frequent or prolonged use of this or any other laxative may result in dependence on laxatives. If skin rash appears, do not use this or any other preparation containing phenolphthalein.

Warnings: Keep this and all drugs out of the reach of children. In case of accidental overdose, seek professional assistance or contact a Poison Control Center immediately. As with any drug, if you are pregnant or nursing a baby, seek the advice of a health care professional before using this product.

Dosage and Administration: Regular Strength Ex-Lax Laxative Pills, Extra Gentle Ex-Lax Laxative Pills, and Maximum Relief Formula Ex-Lax Laxative Pills—Adults and children 12 years of age and over: Take 1 or 2 pills with a glass of water, preferably at bedtime. Consult a doctor for children under 12 years of age. **Ex-Lax Gentle Nature Laxative Pills**—Adults and children 12 years of age and over: Take 1 or 2 pills with a glass of water, preferably at bedtime.
Children 6 to under 12 years of age: Take 1 pill with a glass of water, preferably at bedtime.
Children under 6 years of age: Consult a doctor.

How Supplied: Regular Strength Ex-Lax Laxative Pills—Available in boxes of 8, 30, and 60 pills. **Extra Gentle Ex-Lax Laxative Pills**—Available in boxes of 24 pills. **Maximum Relief Formula Ex-Lax Laxative Pills**—Available in boxes of 24 and 48 pills. **Ex-Lax Gentle Nature Laxative Pills**—Available in boxes of 16 pills.

Shown in Product Identification Guide, page 513

EX-LAX® STOOL SOFTENER CAPLETS
docusate sodium 100mg
mild, natural-feeling relief
for sensitive systems
stimulant-free

Active Ingredient: Docusate Sodium, 100 mg per caplet.

Inactive Ingredients: alginic acid, Blue 1, colloidal silicon dioxide, croscarmellose sodium, dibasic calcium phosphate, hydroxypropyl methylcellulose, magnesium stearate, methylparaben, microcrystalline cellulose, polydextrose, polyethylene glycol, silicon dioxide, sodium benzoate, stearic acid, talc, titanium dioxide, triacetin, yellow 10. Sodium content: 8 mg per caplet.

Indications: Relief of occasional constipation (irregularity), especially for sensitive systems. This gentle, stimulant-free formula generally works within 12–72 hours after the first dose.

Warnings: Keep this and all drugs out of the reach of children. In case of accidental overdose, seek professional assistance or contact a Poison Control Center immediately. Do not use laxative products when abdominal pain, nausea, or vomiting are present unless directed by a doctor. If you have noticed a sudden change in bowel habits that persists over a period of 2 weeks, consult a doctor before using a laxative. Laxative products should not be used for a period longer than 1 week unless directed by a doctor. Rectal bleeding or failure to have a bowel movement after use of a laxative may indicate a serious condition. Discontinue use and consult your doctor. As with any drug, if you are pregnant or nursing a baby, seek the advice of a health care professional before using this product.

Drug Interaction Precaution: Do not take this product if you are presently taking mineral oil, unless directed by a doctor.

Store in a dry place at controlled room temperature 15°–30°C (59°–86°F).

Directions: Take Ex-Lax stool softener caplets with a glass of water at any time. Adults and children 12 years of age and over: 1 to 3 caplets daily as needed. Children 2 to under 12 years of age: 1 caplet daily. This dose may be taken as a single daily dose or in divided doses. Children under 2 years of age: consult a doctor.

How Supplied: Available in boxes of 40 caplets.

Shown in Product Identification Guide, page 514

GAS–X®
EXTRA STRENGTH GAS-X®
Antiflatulent, Anti-Gas Chewable Tablets
Extra Strength Softgels

Active Ingredients: GAS-X®—Each chewable tablet contains simethicone 80 mg.
EXTRA STRENGTH GAS-X®—Each chewable tablet contains simethicone, 125 mg and each swallowable softgel contains simethicone, USP, 125 mg.

Inactive Ingredients
Extra Strength Peppermint Creme: calcium phosphate tribasic, colloidal silicon dioxide, dextrose, flavors, maltodextrin, Red 30, Yellow 10.
Extra Strength Cherry Creme: calcium phosphate tribasic, colloidal silicon dioxide, dextrose, flavors, maltodextrin, Red 30.
GAS-X Peppermint Creme: calcium carbonate, dextrose, flavors, maltodextrin. Sodium-free.
GAS-X Cherry Creme: calcium carbonate, dextrose, flavors, maltodextrin, Red 30.
Sodium-free.
Softgels: Blue 1, gelatin, glycerin, peppermint oil, Red 40, sorbitol, titanium dioxide water, Yellow 10.
Sodium-free.

Indications: Relieves the bloating, pressure, and fullness known as "gas".

Actions: GAS-X acts on the body to relieve and reduce uncomplicated "gas" symptoms (see Indications). This action relieves what is felt when "gas" is present.

Warning: Keep this and all drugs out of the reach of children.

Drug Interaction Precautions: No known drug interaction.

Dosage and Administration: For Chewable Tablets: Adults: Chew thoroughly and swallow one or two tablets as needed after meals and at bedtime. Do not exceed six GAS-X chewable tablets or four EXTRA STRENGTH GAS-X chewable tablets in 24 hours. Do not increase dosage unless recommended by your physician.
For Extra Strength GAS-X Softgels: swallow whole with water, follow dosing instructions for Extra Strength Gas-X chewable tablets.

Professional Labeling: GAS-X may be used in the alleviation of postoperative bloating/pressure, and for use in endoscopic examination.

How Supplied: GAS-X Chewable tablets are available in peppermint creme and cherry creme flavored, chewable, scored tablets in boxes of 12 tablets and 36 tablets.
EXTRA STRENGTH GAS-X Chewable tablets are available in peppermint creme and cherry creme flavored, chewable, scored tablets in boxes of 18 tablets and 48 tablets.
Extra Strength Gas-X Softgels are available in easy-to-swallow tasteless softgels in boxes of 10 pills and 30 pills.

Shown in Product Identification Guide, page 514

KONDREMUL®

Active Ingredient: Mineral Oil (55%).

Inactive Ingredients: Acacia, benzoic acid, carrageenan (Irish Moss), ethyl vanillin, glycerin, mapleine triple oil, purified water, vanillin.

Indications: For relief of occasional constipation. This product generally produces bowel movement in 6–8 hours.

Actions: Promotes gentle, predictable regularity of normal bowel movement. Pleasant tasting and smooth acting, it passes through stomach and upper intestine without upset or dehydration. Assures soft stool by retaining moisture balance and mixing thoroughly with bowel content. Permits passage of stool without straining. This product generally produces bowel movement in 6–8 hours.

Warning: Do not take with meals. Do not administer to children under 6 years of age, to pregnant women, to bedridden patients or to persons with difficulty swallowing. Do not use this product when abdominal pain, nausea or vomiting are present, unless directed by a physician. Laxative products should not be used for a period longer than 1 week unless directed by a physician. If you have noticed a sudden change in bowel habits that persists over a period of 2 weeks, consult a physician before using a laxative. Rectal bleeding or failure to have a bowel movement after use of a laxative may indicate a serious condition. Discontinue use and consult a physican. As with any drug, if you are pregnant or nursing a baby, seek the advice of a health care professional before using this product. **Keep this and all drugs out of the reach of children.** In case of accidental overdose, seek professional assistance or contact a Poison Control Center immediately.

Drug Interaction Precaution: Do not take this product if you are presently taking a stool softener laxative.

Directions: Shake well before using. Adults and children over 12 years of age: two to five tablespoonsful (30–75ml). Children 6 to under 12 years of age: two to five teaspoonsful (10–25ml). The dose may be taken as a single dose or in divided doses.
Children under 6 years of age: consult a physician.

How Supplied: 16 oz. bottle.
Store at room temperature 15°–30°C (59°–86°F).
Kondremul is a registered trademark of Novartis.

Shown in Product Identification Guide, page 514

EXTRA STRENGTH MAALOX® ANTACID/ANTI-GAS
Alumina, Magnesia and Simethicone Oral Suspensions and Tablets
Antacid/Anti-Gas

Suspensions and Tablets
- ☐ **Refreshing Lemon Smooth Cherry Cooling Mint**
- ☐ **Physician-proven Maalox® formula for antacid effectiveness.**
- ☐ **Simethicone, at a recognized clinical dose, for antiflatulent action.**

Description: Extra Strength Maalox® Antacid/Anti-Gas, a balanced combination of magnesium and aluminum hy-

Continued on next page

Information on Novartis Consumer Health, Inc., products appearing on these pages is effective as of November 1996.

Novartis—Cont.

droxides plus simethicone, is a nonconstipating antacid/anti-gas product to provide symptomatic relief of acid indigestion, heartburn, sour stomach and gas and upset stomach associated with these symptoms. Available in suspensions in Refreshing Lemon, Smooth Cherry, and Cooling Mint flavors and in tablets in Cooling Mint and assorted (Refreshing Lemon/Smooth Cherry/Cooling Mint) flavors.

Composition: To provide symptomatic relief of hyperacidity plus alleviation of gas symptoms, each teaspoonful/tablet contains:

Active Ingredients	Extra Strength Maalox® Antacid/Anti-Gas Per Tsp. (5 mL)	Per Tablet
Magnesium Hydroxide	450 mg	350 mg
Aluminum Hydroxide (equivalent to dried gel, USP)	500 mg	350 mg
Simethicone	40 mg	30 mg

Inactive Ingredients: Suspensions: calcium saccharin, FD&C Red No. 40 (Smooth Cherry only), flavors, methylparaben, propylparaben, purified water, sorbitol & other ingredients.
Tablets: D&C Red No. 30, D&C Yellow No. 10, dextrose, FD&C Blue No. 1, flavors, magnesium stearate, mannitol, saccharin sodium, sorbitol, starch, sugar.

Directions for Use: Suspensions: 2 to 4 teaspoonfuls, 4 times per day, or as directed by a physician. Tablets: chew 1 to 3 tablets, 4 times per day, or as directed by a physician.

Patient Warnings: Do not take more than 12 teaspoonfuls or 12 tablets in a 24-hour period or use the maximum dosage for more than 2 weeks or use if you have kidney disease except under the advice and supervision of a physician. **Keep this and all drugs out of the reach of children.**

Drug Interaction Precaution: Antacids may interact with certain prescription drugs. If you are presently taking a prescription drug, do not take this product without checking with your physician or other health professional.
To aid in establishing proper dosage schedules, the following information is provided:
[See table on top of next column.]

Professional Labeling
Indications: As an antacid for symptomatic relief of hyperacidity associated with the diagnosis of peptic ulcer, gastritis, peptic esophagitis, gastric hyperacidity, heartburn, or hiatal hernia. As an

Extra Strength Maalox® Antacid/Anti-Gas	Per 2 Tsp. (10 mL) (Minimum Recommended Dosage)	Per Tablet
Acid neutralizing capacity	59.6 mEq	22.1 mEq
Sodium content*	<2 mg	<1.7 mg

*Dietetically insignificant.

antiflatulent to alleviate the symptoms of gas, including postoperative gas pain.

Warnings: Prolonged use of aluminum-containing antacids in patients with renal failure may result in or worsen dialysis osteomalacia. Elevated tissue aluminum levels contribute to the development of the dialysis encephalopathy and osteomalacia syndromes. Small amounts of aluminum are absorbed from the gastrointestinal tract and renal excretion of aluminum is impaired in renal failure. Aluminum is not well removed by dialysis because it is bound to albumin and transferrin, which do not cross dialysis membranes. As a result, aluminum is deposited in bone, and dialysis osteomalacia may develop when large amounts of aluminum are ingested orally by patients with impaired renal function.
Aluminum forms insoluble complexes with phosphate in the gastrointestinal tract, thus decreasing phosphate absorption. Prolonged use of aluminum-containing antacids by normophosphatemic patients may result in hypophosphatemia if phosphate intake is not adequate. In its more severe forms, hypophosphatemia can lead to anorexia, malaise, muscle weakness, and osteomalacia.

Advantages: Among antacids, Extra Strength Maalox® Antacid/Anti-Gas Suspension and Extra Strength Maalox® Antacid/Anti-Gas Tablets are uniquely palatable—an important feature which encourages patients to follow your dosage directions. Extra Strength Maalox® Antacid/Anti-Gas Suspension and Extra Strength Maalox® Antacid/Anti-Gas Tablets have the time-proven, nonconstipating, sodium-free* Maalox® formula—useful for those patients suffering from the problems associated with hyperacidity. Additionally, Extra Strength Maalox® Antacid/Anti-Gas Suspension and Extra Strength Maalox® Antacid/Anti-Gas Tablets contain simethicone to alleviate discomfort associated with entrapped gas.
*Dietetically insignificant.

How Supplied:
Extra Strength Maalox® Antacid/Anti-Gas Suspensions
Available in Refreshing Lemon in the following sizes: 5 fl. oz. (148 mL), 12 fl. oz. (355 mL), and 26 fl. oz. (769 mL).
Smooth Cherry is available in plastic bottles of 12 fl. oz. (355 mL) and 26 fl. oz. (769 mL).
Cooling Mint is available in plastic bottles of 12 fl. oz. (355 mL) and 26 fl. oz. (769 mL).
Extra Strength Maalox® Antacid/Anti-Gas Cooling Mint Tablets are available in bottles of 38 tablets and 75 tablets.
Extra Strength Maalox® Antacid/Anti-Gas assorted flavors tablets are available in bottles of 38 tablets and 75 tablets.

Shown in Product Identification Guide, page 514

MAALOX® ANTI-GAS
(Simethicone)
Tablets (Regular Strength)
Peppermint and Sweet Lemon Flavors

Description: Maalox Anti-Gas relieves the painful symptoms of bloating, pressure, and fullness, commonly referred to as gas. It is formulated with the active ingredient that diffuses the excess gas in the stomach and digestive tract.

Active Ingredient: Simethicone (80 mg per tablet).

Inactive Ingredients: Corn starch, flavor, gelatin, mannitol, sucrose, and tribasic calcium phosphate. Peppermint: D&C red no. 27 aluminum lake. Sweet Lemon: D&C red no. 30 aluminum lake D&C yellow no. 10 aluminum lake.

Indications: For relief of symptoms of excess gas in the digestive tract.
Such gas is frequently caused by excessive swallowing of air or by eating foods that disagree.
Maalox® Anti-Gas acts in the stomach and intestines to change the surface tension of gas bubbles, enabling them to coalesce: thus, the gas is freed and is eliminated more easily by belching or passing flatus.

Directions for Use: Chew 1 to 2 tablets thoroughly. Use after meals or at bedtime, or as directed by a physician. May also be taken as needed, up to 6 tablets daily. If symptoms persist, contact your physician. **DO NOT EXCEED 6 TABLETS A DAY UNLESS DIRECTED BY A PHYSICIAN.**

Warnings: Keep this and all drugs out of the reach of children.

How Supplied: Peppermint: Cartons of 12 tablets. Sweet Lemon: Cartons of 12 tablets.

Shown in Product Identification Guide, page 514

EXTRA STRENGTH MAALOX® ANTI-GAS
(Simethicone) Tablets
Peppermint and Sweet Lemon Flavors

Description: Extra Strength Maalox Anti-Gas relieves the painful symptoms of bloating, pressure, and fullness, commonly referred to as gas. It is formulated with an additional amount of the active ingredient that diffuses the excess gas in the stomach and digestive tract.

Active Ingredient: Simethicone (150 mg per tablet).

Inactive Ingredients: Corn starch, flavor, gelatin, mannitol, sucrose, and tribasic calcium phosphate. Peppermint: D&C red no. 27 aluminum lake. Sweet Lemon: D&C red no. 30 aluminum lake, D&C yellow no. 10 aluminum lake.

Indications: For relief of symptoms of excess gas in the digestive tract.
Such gas is frequently caused by excessive swallowing of air or by eating foods that disagree.
Maalox® Anti-Gas acts in the stomach and intestines to change the surface tension of gas bubbles, enabling them to coalesce: thus, the gas is freed and is eliminated more easily by belching or passing flatus.

Directions for Use: Chew 1 to 2 tablets thoroughly. Use after meals or at bedtime, or as directed by a physician. May also be taken as needed, up to 3 tablets daily. If symptoms persist, contact your physician. **DO NOT EXCEED 3 TABLETS A DAY UNLESS DIRECTED BY A PHYSICIAN.**

Warnings: Keep this and all drugs out of the reach of children.

How Supplied: Peppermint: Cartons of 10 tablets. Sweet Lemon: Cartons of 10 tablets.

Shown in Product Identification Guide, page 514

MAALOX® HEARTBURN RELIEF
Suspension (Antacid)

Description: Maalox® Heartburn Relief provides symptomatic relief of heartburn, acid indigestion and/or sour stomach.

Active Ingredients: Each 5 ml (1 teaspoonful) contains aluminum hydroxide-magnesium carbonate codried gel 140 mg and magnesium carbonate USP 175 mg. It is formulated in a pleasant, cool mint flavor to help provide a cooling and soothing sensation as it goes down the esophagus.

Inactive Ingredients: Calcium carbonate, calcium saccharin, FD&C Blue No. 1, FD&C Yellow No. 5 (tartrazine), flavors, magnesium alginate, methyl- and propylparaben, potassium bicarbonate, purified water, sorbitol and other ingredients.

	Maalox Heartburn Relief Suspension Per 2 tsp. (10 mL) (Minimum Recommended Dosage)
Acid neutralizing capacity	18.7 mEq
Sodium content	<5 mg

Directions for Use: Two to four teaspoonfuls 4 times a day or as directed by a physician.

Patient Warnings: Do not take more than 16 teaspoonfuls in a 24-hour period or use the maximum dosage for more than 2 weeks or use if you have kidney disease except under the advice and supervision of a physician. **Keep this and all drugs out of the reach of children.**

Drug Interaction Precaution: Antacids may interact with certain prescription drugs. If you are presently taking a prescription drug, do not take this product without checking with your physician or other health professional.

Professional Labeling

Indications:
As an antacid for symptomatic relief of hyperacidity associated with the diagnosis of peptic ulcer, gastritis, peptic esophagitis, gastric hyperacidity, heartburn, or hiatal hernia.

Warnings:
Prolonged use of aluminum-containing antacids in patients with renal failure may result in or worsen dialysis osteomalacia. Elevated tissue aluminum levels contribute to the development of the dialysis encephalopathy and osteomalacia syndromes. Small amounts of aluminum are absorbed from the gastrointestinal tract and renal excretion of aluminum is impaired in renal failure. Aluminum is not well removed by dialysis because it is bound to albumin and transferrin, which do not cross dialysis membranes. As a result, aluminum is deposited in bone, and dialysis osteomalacia may develop when large amounts of aluminum are ingested orally by patients with impaired renal function.
Aluminum forms insoluble complexes with phosphate in the gastrointestinal tract, thus decreasing phosphate absorption. Prolonged use of antacids containing aluminum by normophosphatemic patients may result in hypophosphatemia if phosphate intake is not adequate. In its more severe forms, hypophosphatemia can lead to anorexia, malaise, muscle weakness, and osteomalacia.

How Supplied: Maalox® Heartburn Relief is available in (mint flavor only) a 10 fl oz plastic bottle.

MAALOX®
Magnesia and Alumina Oral Suspension Antacid

Liquids
Cooling Mint
Smooth Cherry
Refreshing Lemon

Description: Maalox® Antacid, a balanced combination of magnesium and aluminum hydroxides, is a nonconstipating product to provide symptomatic relief of acid indigestion, heartburn, sour stomach and upset stomach associated with these symptoms.

Active Ingredients	Maalox Suspension 5 mL teaspoon
Magnesium Hydroxide	200 mg
Aluminum Hydroxide (equivalent to dried gel, USP)	225 mg

Inactive Ingredients: Calcium saccharin, flavors, methylparaben, propylparaben, purified water, sorbitol, xanthan gum (Smooth Cherry & Refreshing Lemon only), guar gum (Cooling Mint) and other ingredients.

	Maalox Suspension Per 2 Tsp. (10 mL) (Minimum Recommended Dosage)
Acid neutralizing capacity	26.6 mEq
Sodium content	<3 mg

Directions for Use: Two to four teaspoonfuls, four times a day or as directed by a physician.

Patient Warnings: Do not take more than 16 teaspoonfuls in a 24-hour period or use the maximum dosage for more than 2 weeks or use if you have kidney disease except under the advice and supervision of a physician. **Keep this and all drugs out of the reach of children.**

Drug Interaction Precaution: Antacids may interact with certain prescription drugs. If you are presently taking a prescription drug, do not take this product without checking with your physician or other health professional.

Professional Labeling

Indications: As an antacid for symptomatic relief of hyperacidity associated with the diagnosis of peptic ulcer, gastri-

Continued on next page

Information on Novartis Consumer Health, Inc., products appearing on these pages is effective as of November 1996.

Novartis—Cont.

tis, peptic esophagitis, gastric hyperacidity, heartburn, or hiatal hernia.

Warnings: Prolonged use of aluminum-containing antacids in patients with renal failure may result in or worsen dialysis osteomalacia. Elevated tissue aluminum levels contribute to the development of the dialysis encephalopathy and osteomalacia syndromes. Small amounts of aluminum are absorbed from the gastrointestinal tract and renal excretion of aluminum is impaired in renal failure. Aluminum is not well removed by dialysis because it is bound to albumin and transferrin, which do not cross dialysis membranes. As a result, aluminum is deposited in bone, and dialysis osteomalacia may develop when large amounts of aluminum are ingested orally by patients with impaired renal function.
Aluminum forms insoluble complexes with phosphate in the gastrointestinal tract, thus decreasing phosphate absorption. Prolonged use of aluminum-containing antacids by normophosphatemic patients may result in hypophosphatemia if phosphate intake is not adequate. In its more severe forms, hypophosphatemia can lead to anorexia, malaise, muscle weakness, and osteomalacia.

Advantages: Among antacids, Maalox® Suspension is uniquely palatable—an important feature which encourages patients to follow your dosage directions. Maalox® has the time-proven, nonconstipating Maalox® formula—useful for those patients suffering from the problems associated with hyperacidity.

How Supplied:
Maalox® Cooling Mint Suspension is available in plastic bottles of 5 oz., 12 oz. and 26 oz.
Maalox® Smooth Cherry Suspension is available in plastic bottles of 12 oz. and 26 oz.
Maalox® Refreshing Lemon Suspension is available in plastic bottles of 12 oz. and 26 oz.

Shown in Product Identification Guide, page 514

MAALOX® Antacid/Anti-Gas
Alumina, Magnesia and Simethicone Tablets
Antacid/Anti-Gas
Tablets
Refreshing Lemon, Smooth Cherry, and Cooling Mint Flavors

☐ **Physician-proven Maalox® formula for antacid effectiveness.**
☐ **Simethicone, at a recognized clinical dose, for antiflatulent action.**

Description: Maalox® Antacid/Anti-Gas, a balanced combination of magnesium and aluminum hydroxides plus simethicone, is a nonconstipating antacid/anti-gas product which comes in pleasant tasting flavors.

Composition: To provide symptomatic relief of hyperacidity plus alleviation of gas symptoms, each tablet contains:

Active Ingredients	Maalox® Antacid/Anti-Gas Per Tablet
Magnesium Hydroxide	200 mg
Aluminum Hydroxide (equivalent to dried gel, USP)	200 mg
Simethicone	25 mg

Inactive Ingredients: Maalox® Antacid/Anti-Gas Tablets: D&C Red No. 30, D&C Yellow No. 10, FD&C Blue No. 1, dextrose, flavors, glycerin, magnesium stearate, mannitol, saccharin sodium, sorbitol, starch, sugar, talc. May also contain citric acid.
To aid in establishing proper dosage schedules, the following information is provided:

	Maalox® Antacid/Anti-Gas Per Tablet (Minimum Recommended Dosage)
Acid neutralizing capacity	12.6 mEq
Sodium content*	<1 mg

*Dietetically insignificant.

Directions for Use: Chew 1 to 4 tablets 4 times a day or as directed by a physician.

Patient Warnings: Do not take more than 16 tablets in a 24-hour period or use the maximum dosage for more than 2 weeks or use if you have kidney disease except under the advice and supervision of a physician. **Keep this and all drugs out of the reach of children.**

Drug Interaction Precaution: Antacids may interact with certain prescription drugs. If you are presently taking a prescription drug, do not take this product without checking with your physician or other health professional.

Professional Labeling

Indications: As an antacid for symptomatic relief of hyperacidity associated with the diagnosis of peptic ulcer, gastritis, peptic esophagitis, gastric hyperacidity, heartburn, or hiatal hernia. As an antiflatulent to alleviate the symptoms of gas, including postoperative gas pain.

Warnings: Prolonged use of aluminum-containing antacids in patients with renal failure may result in or worsen dialysis osteomalacia. Elevated tissue aluminum levels contribute to the development of the dialysis encephalopathy and osteomalacia syndromes. Small amounts of aluminum are absorbed from the gastrointestinal tract and renal excretion of aluminum is impaired in renal failure. Aluminum is not well removed by dialysis because it is bound to albumin and transferrin, which do not cross dialysis membranes. As a result, aluminum is deposited in bone, and dialysis osteomalacia may develop when large amounts of aluminum are ingested orally by patients with impaired renal function.
Aluminum forms insoluble complexes with phosphate in the gastrointestinal tract, thus decreasing phosphate absorption. Prolonged use of aluminum-containing antacids by normophosphatemic patients may result in hypophosphatemia if phosphate intake is not adequate. In its more severe forms, hypophosphatemia can lead to anorexia, malaise, muscle weakness, and osteomalacia.

Advantages: Maalox® Antacid/Anti-Gas Tablets are uniquely palatable—an important feature which encourages patients to follow your dosage directions. Maalox® Antacid/Anti-Gas Tablets have the time-proven, nonconstipating, sodium-free* Maalox® formula—useful for those patients suffering from the problems associated with hyperacidity. Additionally, Maalox® Antacid/Anti-Gas Tablets contain simethicone to alleviate discomfort associated with entrapped gas.
*Dietetically insignificant

How Supplied: Maalox® Antacid/Anti-Gas Refreshing Lemon Tablets are available in plastic bottles of 50 tablets and 100 tablets, individual rolls of 12 tablets in a tray of 12 rolls, and 3 roll packs of 36 tablets.
Maalox® Antacid/Anti-Gas Smooth Cherry Tablets are available in plastic bottles of 50 tablets and 100 tablets.
Maalox® Antacid/Anti-Gas Tablets are also available in **assorted flavor** bottles of 50 tablets and 100 tablets, individual rolls of 12 tablets in a tray of 12 rolls and 3 roll packs of 36 tablets.

Shown in Product Identification Guide, page 514

MYOFLEX® PAIN RELIEVING CREAM
[*mī'ō-flex*]

Description: Odorless, greaseless and non-burning topical pain reliever.

Active Ingredient: Trolamine salicylate 10%.

Other Ingredients: Cetyl alcohol, disodium EDTA, fragrance, propylene glycol, purified water, sodium lauryl sulfate, stearyl alcohol, white wax.

Indications: For the temporary relief of minor aches and pains of muscles and joints associated with arthritis, strains and sprains, and simple backache.

Warning: FOR EXTERNAL USE ONLY. Do not apply to irritated skin or if excessive irritation develops. Avoid contact with eyes. If condition worsens, or if symptoms persist for more than 7 days or clear up and occur again within a few days, discontinue use of this product and consult a physician. **Keep this and all drugs out of the reach of children.** In case of accidental ingestion, seek professional assistance or contact a Poison Control Center immediately. As with any drug, if you are pregnant or nursing a baby, seek the advice of a health professional before using this product.

Directions: Use only as directed. **Adults and children 2 years of age and older**: Apply to affected area not more than three to four times daily. Affected areas may be wrapped loosely with two- or three-inch elastic bandage. **Children under 2 years of age**: Consult a physician.

How Supplied: Myoflex is supplied in 2 oz. and 4 oz. easy-squeeze tubes, and 8 oz. and 16 oz. jars.
Store at room temperature 15°–30°C (59°–86°F).

MYOFLEX is a registered trademark of Novartis.

Shown in Product Identification Guide, page 514

---

12 Hour NŌSTRILLA®
[*nō-stril 'a*]
Nasal Decongestant
oxymetazoline HCl, USP

Active Ingredient: oxymetazoline hydrochloride 0.05%.

Inactive Ingredients: benzalkonium chloride as a preservative, glycine, sorbitol solution, water.

Indications: For the temporary relief of nasal congestion due to the common cold, hay fever, or other upper respiratory allergies (allergic rhinitis), or associated with sinusitis.

Actions: NŌSTRILLA metered pump spray for nasal decongestion delivers a measured dose of medication every time. Helps clear your stuffy nose fast so you can breathe easier all day or night.

Warnings: Do not exceed recommended dosage. This product may cause temporary discomfort such as burning, stinging, sneezing, or an increase in nasal discharge. The use of this container by more than one person may spread infection. Do not use this product for more than 3 days. Frequent or prolonged use may cause nasal congestion to recur or worsen. Use only as directed. If symptoms persist, consult a doctor. Do not use this product if you have heart disease, high blood pressure, thyroid disease, diabetes or difficulty in urination due to enlargement of the prostate gland unless directed by a doctor. **Keep this and all drugs out of the reach of children.** In case of accidental ingestion, seek professional assistance or contact a Poison Control Center immediately.

Directions: Adults and children 6 to under 12 years of age (with adult supervision): 2 or 3 sprays in each nostril not more often than every 10 to 12 hours. Do not exceed 2 applications in any 24-hour period. Children under 6 years of age: consult a doctor.
To use pump: Remove protective cap and prime pump by depressing it firmly several times. Hold bottle with thumb at base and nozzle between first and second fingers. With head upright, insert nozzle into nostril. Depress pump two or three times, all the way down, and sniff deeply.

How Supplied: Metered nasal pump spray in white plastic bottles of ½ fl. oz. (15 ml) packaged in tamper-resistant outer cartons.

Shown in Product Identification Guide, page 514

NUPERCAINAL®
Dibucaine
Hemorrhoidal and Anesthetic Ointment

Ingredient: 1% dibucaine USP. Also contains: acetone sodium bisulfite, lanolin, light mineral oil, purified water, and white petrolatum.

Indications: For prompt, temporary relief of pain, itching and burning due to hemorrhoids or other anorectal disorders. May also be used topically for temporary relief of pain and itching associated with sunburn, minor burns, cuts, scrapes, insect bites, or minor skin irritation.

Directions: Adults: When practical, cleanse the affected area with mild soap and warm water and rinse thoroughly. Gently dry by patting or blotting with toilet tissue or a soft cloth before application of this product. Puncture tube seal with cap or sharp object. Apply externally to the affected area up to 3 or 4 times daily. Children 2–12: Do not use except under the advice and supervision of a physician. DO NOT USE ON INFANTS UNDER 2 YEARS OF AGE OR LESS THAN 35 LBS. WEIGHT.

Warnings: IF SWALLOWED, CONSULT A PHYSICIAN OR POISON CONTROL CENTER IMMEDIATELY. **Do not use in or near the eyes.** If condition worsens or does not improve within 7 days, consult a physician. Do not put this product into the rectum by using fingers or any mechanical device. Do not exceed recommended daily dosage unless directed by a physician. Certain persons can develop allergic reactions to ingredients in this product. If the symptom being treated does not subside or if redness, irritation, swelling, pain, bleeding or other symptoms develop or increase, discontinue use and consult a physician promptly. As with any drug, if you are pregnant or nursing a baby, seek the advice of a health care professional before using this product. **Keep this and all medication out of reach of children.**

How Supplied: Nupercainal Hemorrhoidal and Anesthetic Ointment is available in tubes of 1 and 2 ounces. See crimp of tube for lot number and expiration date.
Store between 15°–30°C (59°–86°F).
Nupercainal is a registered trademark of Novartis.
Made in Canada

Shown in Product Identification Guide, page 514

NUPERCAINAL®
HYDROCORTISONE 1% CREAM
Anti-Itch Cream

Active Ingredient: Hydrocortisone Acetate USP (equivalent to Hydrocortisone Free Base 1%).

Inactive Ingredients: Cetostearyl Alcohol, Sodium Lauryl Sulfate, White Petrolatum, Propylene Glycol, Purified Water.

Indications: For the temporary relief of external anal itching. May also be used for the temporary relief of itching associated with minor skin irritations and rashes due to eczema, insect bites, poison ivy, poison oak, poison sumac, soaps, detergents, cosmetics, jewelry, seborrheic dermatitis, or psoriasis. Other uses of this product should be only under the advice and supervision of a physician.

Directions: Adults: When practical, cleanse the affected area with mild soap and warm water and rinse thoroughly. Gently dry by patting or blotting with toilet tissue or a soft cloth before application of this product. Apply to affected area not more than 3 to 4 times daily. **Children under 12 years of age:** Consult a physician.

Warnings: For external use only. Avoid contact with the eyes. If condition worsens, or if symptoms persist for more than 7 days or clear up and occur again within a few days, stop use of this product and do not begin use of any other hydrocortisone product unless you have consulted a physician. Do not use for the treatment of diaper rash; consult a physician. Do not exceed the recommended daily dosage unless directed by a physician. In case of bleeding, consult a physician promptly. Do not put this product into the rectum by using fingers or any mechanical device or applicator. **Keep this and all medication out of reach of children.** In case of accidental ingestion, seek professional assistance or contact a Poison Control Center immediately.

How Supplied: Nupercainal Hydrocortisone Cream is available in a 1 ounce

Continued on next page

Information on Novartis Consumer Health, Inc., products appearing on these pages is effective as of November 1996.

Novartis—Cont.

tube. See crimp of tube for lot number and expiration date.
Store at controlled room temperature 15–30°C (59°–86°F).
Nupercainal is a registered trademark of Novartis.
Made in Canada

NUPERCAINAL®
Suppositories

Ingredients: 2.1 grams cocoa butter, NF and .25 gram zinc oxide. Also contains acetone sodium bisulfite and bismuth subgallate.

Indications: For temporary relief of itching, burning, and discomfort associated with hemorrhoids or other anorectal disorders.

Directions: ADULTS—When practical, cleanse the affected area. Tear one suppository at the "V" cut, peel foil downward and remove foil wrapper before inserting into the rectum. Gently insert the suppository rectally, rounded end first. Use one suppository up to 6 times daily or after each bowel movement. CHILDREN UNDER 12 YEARS OF AGE—Consult a physician.

WARNING: IF ACCIDENTALLY SWALLOWED, CONSULT A PHYSICIAN OR POISON CONTROL CENTER IMMEDIATELY.
If condition worsens or does not improve within 7 days, consult a physician. Do not exceed the recommended daily dosage unless directed by a physician. In case of bleeding consult a physician promptly. As with any drug, if you are pregnant or nursing a baby, seek the advice of a health professional before using this product.
Keep this and all medications out of reach of children.

How Supplied: Nupercainal Suppositories are available in tamper-evident packages of 12.
Do not store above 30°C (86°F).
Nupercainal is a registered trademark of Novartis.

OTRIVIN®
Nasal Decongestant

Active Ingredient: xylometazoline hydrochloride USP (Nasal Spray and Nasal Drops 0.1%, Pediatric Nasal Drops 0.05%).

Inactive Ingredients: Otrivin Nasal Spray/Nasal Drops—benzalkonium chloride, dibasic sodium phosphate, disodium edetate, monobasic sodium phosphate, purified water and sodium chloride.
Otrivin Pediatric Nasal Drops—benzalkonium chloride, dibasic sodium phosphate, disodium edetate, monobasic sodium phosphate, purified water and sodium chloride.

Indications: For the temporary relief of nasal congestion due to the common cold, hay fever or other upper respiratory allergies, or associated with sinusitis.
One application provides long-lasting relief.
Otrivin has been recommended by doctors for many years. Here is how you use it:

Directions: Nasal Spray 0.1%—for adults and children 12 years and over: Spray 2 or 3 times into each nostril not more often than every 8 to 10 hours. **Do not give Nasal Spray 0.1% to children under 12 years of age unless directed by a doctor.**
Nasal Drops 0.1%—for adults and children 12 years and over: 2 or 3 drops in each nostril not more often than every 8 to 10 hours. **Do not give Nasal Drops 0.1% to children under 12 years except under the advice and supervision of a physician.**
Pediatric Nasal Drops 0.05%—children 6 to 12 years of age (with adult supervision): 2 or 3 drops in each nostril not more often than every 8 to 10 hours. Children 2 to 6 years of age (with adult supervision): 2 to 3 drops in each nostril not more often than every 8 to 10 hours. Use dropper provided. Use only recommended amount. Do not exceed 3 doses in any 24 hour period. Children under 2 years of age: consult a doctor.

Warning: Do not exceed recommended dosage. This product may cause temporary discomfort such as burning, stinging, sneezing, or an increase in nasal discharge. Do not use this product for more than 3 days. Use only as directed. Frequent or prolonged use may cause nasal congestion to recur or worsen. If symptoms persist, consult a doctor. Do not use this product if you have heart disease, high blood pressure, thyroid disease, diabetes, or difficulty in urination due to enlargement of the prostate gland unless directed by a doctor. The use of this container by more than one person may spread infection.
Keep this and all drugs out of the reach of children. In case of accidental ingestion, seek professional assistance or contact a Poison Control Center immediately.
Overdosage in young children may cause marked sedation.

Caution: Do not use if the clear overwrap with the name Otrivin® or the printed band on the bottle is missing or damaged.

How Supplied: Nasal Spray—unbreakable plastic spray bottle of 0.66 fl. oz. (20 ml).
Nasal Drops—plastic dropper bottle of 0.83 fl. oz. (25 ml).
Pediatric Nasal Drops—Plastic dropper bottle of 0.83 fl. oz. (25 ml).
Store at 15°–30°C (59°–86°F).
Shown in Product Identification Guide, page 514

PERDIEM®
[pĕr″dē′ŭm]
Bulk Fiber Laxative Plus Natural, Vegetable Stimulant

Description: Perdiem®, with its 100% natural, gentle action, provides relief from occasional constipation. Perdiem® is a unique combination of bulk-forming fiber and natural stimulant. Each rounded teaspoonful (6.0 g) contains approximately 3.25 g psyllium. 0.74 g senna, 1.8 mg of sodium, and 35.5 mg of potassium. Perdiem® is dye free and contains no artificial sweeteners.

Indications: For relief of occasional constipation. This product generally produces bowel movement in 12 to 72 hours.

Active Ingredients: Psyllium and Sennosides.

Inactive Ingredients: Acacia, iron oxides, natural flavors, paraffin, sucrose, talc.

Directions for Use: TAKE THIS PRODUCT (CHILD OR ADULT DOSE) WITH AT LEAST 8 OUNCES (A FULL GLASS) OF COOL WATER OR OTHER FLUID. TAKING THIS PRODUCT WITHOUT ENOUGH LIQUID MAY CAUSE CHOKING. SEE WARNINGS.
Adults and Children 12 years and older: In the evening and/or before breakfast, 1 to 2 rounded teaspoonfuls of Perdiem® (in full or partial doses) should be placed in the mouth and swallowed with at least 8 ounces (a full glass) of cool liquid. Perdiem® should not be chewed.**Children 7 to 11 years:** One (1) rounded teaspoon one to two times daily with at least 8 ounces (a full glass) of cool liquid.
For Severe Cases of Constipation: Perdiem® may be taken more frequently, up to 2 rounded teaspoonfuls every 6 hours not to exceed 5 teaspoonfuls in a 24-hour period. Perdiem® generally takes effect within 12 hours; in severe cases, 24 to 72 hours may be required for optimal relief.

Warnings: TAKING THIS PRODUCT WITHOUT ADEQUATE FLUID MAY CAUSE IT TO SWELL AND BLOCK YOUR THROAT OR ESOPHAGUS AND MAY CAUSE CHOKING. DO NOT TAKE THIS PRODUCT IF YOU HAVE DIFFICULTY IN SWALLOWING. IF YOU EXPERIENCE CHEST PAIN, VOMITING OR DIFFICULTY IN SWALLOWING OR BREATHING AFTER TAKING THIS PRODUCT, SEEK IMMEDIATE MEDICAL ATTENTION.
Patients with esophageal narrowing should not use bulk-forming agents.
If you have noticed a sudden change in bowel habits that persists over a period of 2 weeks, consult a doctor before using a laxative. Laxative products should not be used for a period longer than 1 week unless directed by a doctor. Rectal bleeding or failure to have a bowel movement after use of a laxative may indicate a serious condition. Discontinue use and con-

sult your doctor. Do not use if you have a history of psyllium allergy or experience abdominal pain, nausea, or vomiting unless directed by a doctor.
If you are pregnant or nursing a baby, seek the advice of a health professional before using this product. In case of accidental overdose, seek professional assistance or contact a Poison Control Center immediately. **Keep this and all drugs out of the reach of children.**

How Supplied: Granules: 400–gram (14 oz) canisters, 250-gram (8.8 oz) canisters and 6 single serving packets of 6 g.
Store at room temperature 15–30°C (59–86°F). Avoid exposure to moisture.
Questions? Call 1–800–548–3708 weekdays 9 am–5 pm ET.

Shown in Product Identification Guide, page 515

PERDIEM® FIBER
[*pĕr"dē'ŭm*]
Bulk Fiber Laxative

Description: Perdiem® Fiber is a 100% natural, bulk-forming fiber for the relief of occasional constipation (irregularity). Perdiem Fiber's unique form is easy to swallow and requires no mixing but must be followed by at least 8 ounces of cool liquid. Perdiem® Fiber contains no chemical stimulants. Each rounded teaspoonful (6.0 g) contains 4.03 g psyllium, 1.8 mg sodium, and 36.1 mg of potassium. Perdiem® is dye free and contains no artificial sweeteners.

Active Ingredients: Psyllium.

Inactive Ingredients: Acacia, iron oxides, natural flavors, paraffin, sucrose, talc, titanium dioxide.

Indications: For relief of occasional constipation. This product generally produces bowel movement in 12 to 72 hours.

Directions for Use: TAKE THIS PRODUCT (CHILD OR ADULT DOSE) WITH AT LEAST 8 OUNCES (A FULL GLASS) OF COOL WATER OR OTHER FLUID. TAKING THIS PRODUCT WITHOUT ENOUGH LIQUID MAY CAUSE CHOKING. SEE WARNINGS.
Adults and Children 12 years of age and older: In the evening and/or before breakfast, 1 to 2 rounded teaspoonfuls of Perdiem® Fiber (in full or partial doses) should be placed in the mouth and swallowed with at least 8 ounces (a full glass) of cool liquid. Perdiem® Fiber should not be chewed.**Children 7 to under 11 years:** One (1) rounded teaspoonful with at least 8 ounces (a full glass) of cool liquid.
For Severe Cases of Constipation: Perdiem Fiber may be taken more frequently, up to 2 rounded teaspoonfuls every 6 hours not to exceed 5 teaspoonfuls in a 24-hour period. Perdiem Fiber generally takes effect after 12 hours; in severe cases, 48 to 72 hours may be required for optimal relief.

Warnings: TAKING THIS PRODUCT WITHOUT ADEQUATE FLUID MAY CAUSE IT TO SWELL AND BLOCK YOUR THROAT OR ESOPHAGUS AND MAY CAUSE CHOKING. DO NOT TAKE THIS PRODUCT IF YOU HAVE DIFFICULTY IN SWALLOWING. IF YOU EXPERIENCE CHEST PAIN, VOMITING, OR DIFFICULTY IN SWALLOWING OR BREATHING AFTER TAKING THIS PRODUCT, SEEK IMMEDIATE MEDICAL ATTENTION.
Patients with esophageal narrowing should not use bulk-forming agents. If you have noticed a sudden change in bowel habits that persists over a period of 2 weeks, consult a doctor before using a laxative. Laxative products should not be used for a period longer than 1 week unless directed by a doctor. Rectal bleeding or failure to have a bowel movement after use of a laxative may indicate a serious condition. Discontinue use and consult your doctor. Do not use if you have a history of psyllium allergy or experience abdominal pain, nausea, or vomiting unless directed by a doctor.
In case of accidental overdose, seek professional assistance or contact a Poison Control Center immediately. Keep this and all drugs out of the reach of children.

How Supplied: Granules: 250-gram (8.8 oz) plastic container.

Shown in Product Identification Guide, page 515

PRIVINE®
Naphazoline Hydrochloride, USP
0.05% Nasal Drops
0.05% Nasal Spray
Nasal Decongestant

Active Ingredient: 0.05% Naphazoline hydrochloride, USP.

Other Ingredients: Benzalkonium chloride, dibasic sodium phosphate, disodium edetate, monobasic sodium phosphate, purified water, and sodium chloride.

Privine is a nasal decongestant that comes in two forms: Nasal Drops (in a bottle with a dropper) and Nasal Spray (in a plastic squeeze bottle). Both are for prompt and prolonged relief of nasal congestion due to common colds, sinusitis, hay fever, etc.

Indications: For the temporary relief of nasal congestion due to the common cold, hay fever or other respiratory allergies, or associated with sinusitis.

Warnings: Do not exceed recommended dosage. This product may cause temporary discomfort such as burning, stinging, sneezing, or an increase in nasal discharge. Do not use this product for more than 3 days. Use only as directed. Frequent or prolonged use may cause nasal congestion to recur or worsen. If symptoms persist, consult a doctor. Do not use this product if you have heart disease, high blood pressure, thyroid disease, diabetes, or difficulty in urination due to enlargement of the prostate gland unless directed by a doctor. Do not use this product in children under 12 years of age because it may cause sedation if swallowed. The use of this container by more than one person may spread infection. **Keep this and all drugs out of the reach of children.** In case of accidental ingestion, seek professional assistance or contact a Poison Control Center immediately.

Directions: Nasal Drops: Adults and children 12 years of age and over: 1 or 2 drops in each nostril not more often than every 6 hours. Do not give to children under 12 years of age unless directed by a doctor.

Nasal Spray: Adults and children 12 years of age and over: 1 or 2 sprays in each nostril not more often than every 6 hours. Do not give to children under 12 years of age unless directed by a doctor.

How Supplied: Bottles of 0.66 fl. oz. (20 ml).
Store at 15°–30°C (59°–86°F).

SINAREST® TABLETS AND EXTRA STRENGTH CAPLETS

Active Ingredients: *Tablets*—Acetaminophen 325 mg, chlorpheniramine maleate 2 mg, pseudoephedrine HCl 30 mg.
Extra Strength Caplets—Acetaminophen 500 mg, chlorpheniramine maleate 2 mg, pseudoephedrine HCl 30 mg.

Other Ingredients: *Tablets*—Corn starch, D & C Yellow No. 10, FD & C Yellow No. 6, hydroxypropyl methylcellulose, microcrystalline cellulose, polyethylene glycol, polysorbate 80, polyvinylpyrrolidone, stearic acid, titanium dioxide.
Extra Strength Caplets—Corn starch, hydroxypropyl methylcellulose, microcrystalline cellulose, polyethylene glycol, polysorbate 80, polyvinylpyrrolidone, stearic acid, titanium dioxide.

Indications: *Tablets and Extra Strength Caplets*—Temporarily relieves nasal congestion, runny nose, sneezing, itching of the nose or throat, and itchy, watery eyes due to hay fever or other upper respiratory allergies, or associated with sinusitis. For temporary relief of minor aches, pains, and headache.

Warnings: *Both Products*—**Do not exceed recommended dosage.** If nervousness, dizziness, or sleeplessness occur, discontinue use and consult a physician. Do not take this product for more than 10 days (for adults) or 5 days (for children). If symptoms do not improve or are ac-

Continued on next page

Information on Novartis Consumer Health, Inc., products appearing on these pages is effective as of November 1996.

Novartis—Cont.

companied by fever that lasts for more than 3 days, or if new symptoms occur, consult a physician. Do not take this product, unless directed by a physician, if you have a breathing problem such as emphysema or chronic bronchitis, or if you have heart disease, high blood pressure, thyroid disease, diabetes, glaucoma, or difficulty in urination due to enlargement of the prostate gland. May cause excitability, especially in children. May cause drowsiness; alcohol, sedatives, and tranquilizers may increase the drowsiness effect. Avoid alcoholic beverages while taking this product. Do not take this product if you are taking sedatives or tranquilizers, without first consulting your physician. Use caution when driving a motor vehicle, or operating machinery. As with any drug, if you are pregnant or nursing a baby, seek the advice of a health professional before using this product. **Keep this and all drugs out of the reach of children.** In case of accidental overdose, seek professional assistance or contact a Poison Control Center immediately. Prompt medical attention is critical for adults as well as for children even if you do not notice any signs or symptoms.

Drug Interaction Precaution: *Both Products*—Do not use this product if you are now taking a prescription monoamine oxidase inhibitor (MAOI) (certain drugs for depression, psychiatric or emotional conditions, or Parkinson's disease), or for 2 weeks after stopping the MAOI drug. If you are uncertain whether your prescription drug contains an MAOI, consult a health professional before taking this product.

Directions: *Tablets*—Dose as follows while symptoms persist, or as directed by a physician. Adults and children 12 years of age and over: 2 tablets every 4 to 6 hours, not to exceed 8 tablets in 24 hours. Children 6 to under 12 years of age: 1 tablet every 4 to 6 hours, not to exceed 4 tablets in 24 hours. Children under 6 years of age: Consult a physician.
Extra Strength Caplets—Dose as follows while symptoms persist, or as directed by a physician. Adults and children 12 years of age and over: 2 caplets every 6 hours, not to exceed 8 caplets in 24 hours. Children under 12 years of age: Consult a physician.

How Supplied:
Tablets—Boxes of 20 tablets.
Extra Strength Caplets—Boxes of 24 caplets.
Store at room temperature 15°–30°C (59°–86°F).
Sinarest is a registered trademark of Novartis.

SLOW FE®
Slow Release Iron Tablets

Description: SLOW FE supplies ferrous sulfate for the treatment of iron deficiency and iron deficiency anemia with a significant reduction in the incidence of the common side effects of oral iron preparations. The wax matrix delivery system of SLOW FE is designed to maximize the release of ferrous sulfate in the duodenum and the jejunum where it is best tolerated and absorbed. SLOW FE has been clinically shown to be associated with a lower incidence of constipation, diarrhea and abdominal discomfort when compared to an immediate release iron tablet[1] and a leading sustained release iron capsule.[2]

Formula: Each tablet contains 160 mg. dried ferrous sulfate USP, equivalent to 50 mg. elemental iron. Also contains cetostearyl alcohol, FD&C Blue No. 2 aluminum lake, hydroxypropyl methylcellulose, lactose, magnesium stearate, polysorbate 80, talc, titanium dioxide, yellow iron oxide.

Dosage: ADULTS—one or two tablets daily or as recommended by a physician. A maximum of four tablets daily may be taken. CHILDREN—one tablet daily. Tablets must be swallowed whole.

Warning: Close bottles tightly and keep out of reach of children. Contains iron, which can be harmful or fatal to children in large doses. In case of accidental overdose, seek professional assistance or contact a Poison Control Center immediately. The treatment of any anemic condition should be under the advice and supervision of a physician. As oral iron products interfere with absorption of oral tetracycline antibiotics, these products should not be taken within two hours of each other. As with any drug, if you are pregnant or nursing a baby, seek the advice of a health professional before using this product.
Tamper-Evident Packaging.

How Supplied: Child-resistant blister packages of 30, 60, and child-resistant bottles of 100.
Do Not Store Above 30°C (86°F). Protect From Moisture.

References

1. Brock C et al. Adverse effects of iron supplementation: A comparative trial of a wax-matrix iron preparation and conventional ferrous sulfate tablets. *Clin Ther.* 1985; 7:568-573.
2. Brock C, Curry H. Comparative incidence of side effects of a wax-matrix and a sustained-release iron preparation. *Clin Ther.* 1985; 7:492-496.

Shown in Product Identification Guide, page 515

SLOW FE® WITH FOLIC ACID
(Slow Release Iron, Folic Acid)

Description: Slow Fe + Folic Acid delivers 50 mg. elemental iron (160 mg. dried ferrous sulfate) plus 400 mcg. folic acid using the unique wax matrix delivery system described above (for SLOW FE® Slow Release Iron Tablets). Provides women of childbearing potential with the daily target level of folic acid to reduce the risk of neural tube birth defects. These birth defects are rare, but serious, and occur within 28 days of conception, often before a woman knows she's pregnant.

Formula: Each tablet contains: Active Ingredients: 160 mg. dried ferrous sulfate, USP (equivalent to 50 mg. elemental iron) and 400 mcg. folic acid. Inactive Ingredients: cetostearyl alcohol, hydroxypropyl methylcellulose, lactose, magnesium stearate, polysorbate 80, talc, titanium dioxide, yellow iron oxide.

Dosage: ADULTS—One or two tablets once a day or as recommended by a physician. A maximum of two tablets daily may be taken. CHILDREN UNDER 12—Consult a physician. Tablets must be swallowed whole.

Warning: The treatment of any anemic condition should be under the advice and supervision of a physician. As oral iron products interfere with absorption of oral tetracycline antibiotics, these products should not be taken within two hours of each other. Intake of folic acid from all sources should be limited to 1000 mcg. per day to prevent the masking of Vitamin B_{12} deficiencies. Should you become pregnant while using this product, consult a physician as soon as possible about good prenatal care and the continued use of this product. If you are already pregnant or nursing a baby, seek the advice of a health care professional before using this product. **Keep this product and all drugs out of the reach of children:** Contains iron, which can be harmful or fatal to children in large doses. In case of accidental overdose, contact a physician or a poison control center immediately.

How Supplied: Blister packages of 20 supplied in Child-Resistant packaging.
Do not store above 30°C (86°F). Protect from moisture.
Tablets made in Great Britain

Shown in Product Identification Guide, page 515

CHILDREN'S CHEWABLE SUNKIST® VITAMINS + EXTRA C 60 TABLETS

Nutrition Facts
Serving Size 1 Tablet

Amount Per Tablet
Calories 5
Total Carbohydrate 1 g

Amount Per Tablet	% Daily Value for Children 2–4 Years of Age	% Daily Value for Adults and Children 4 or more Years of Age
Vitamin A 2500 I.U.	100%	50%
Vitamin C 250 mg	630%	420%

ʼitamin D 400 I.U.	100%	100%
/itamin E 15 I.U.	150%	50%
ʼitamin K 5 mcg	*	*
ʼhiamin 1.1 mg	160%	70%
ʼiboflavin 1.2 mg	150%	70%
ʼiacin 14 mg	160%	70%
/itamin B_6 1 mg	140%	50%
ʼolate 0.3 mg	150%	80%
/itamin B_{12} 5 mcg	170%	80%

Daily Value not established.

ngredients: Sorbitol, Sodium Ascorʼate, Ascorbic Acid, Natural Flavors, ʼiono & Diglycerides, Starch, Stearic ʼcid, Hydrolyzed Protein, Vitamin E Acʼtate, Niacinamide, Aspartame Hydroʼenated Vegetable Oils, Magnesium ʼtearate, FD&C Yellow #6, Calcium Silʼcate, Silica, FD&C Red #40, Vitamin A ʼalmitate, Cellulose, FD&C Yellow #5, ʼelatin, Riboflavin, Thiamin, Vitamin B_6, Sucrose, Ascorbyl Palmitate, Folic ʼcid, Beta Carotene, Vitamin D, Vitaʼnin K, Vitamin B_{12}.

ʼirections: Adults and children 2 ʼears and older—Chew one tablet daily. ʼHENYLKETONURICS: CONTAINS ʼHENYLALANINE

ʼow Supplied: Bottles of 60 tablets. ʼtore at controlled room temperature, ʼ5°–30°C (59°–86°F). Protect from moisʼure.

ʼianufactured for and distributed by ʼovartis Consumer Health, Inc., Woodʼridge, NJ 07095 under a trademark liʼense from Sunkist Growers, Inc. Sunʼist® is a registered trademark of Sunʼist Growers, Inc., Sherman Oaks, CA ʼ1423

Shown in Product Identification Guide, page 515

ʼUNKIST® CHILDREN'S ʼHEWABLE MULTIVITAMINS—ʼOMPLETE ʼWITH CALCIUM, IRON & ʼIINERALS

ʼutrition Facts
ʼerving Size 1/2 Tablet or 1 Tablet, ʼepending on age (see Directions)
ʼervings Per Container 120 1/2-tablet ʼervings or 60 single-tablets servings
Amount Per Tablet
ʼodium 8 mg
ʼotal Carbohydrate less than 1g
ʼSee table above.]

SUNKIST® CHILDREN'S CHEWABLE MULTIVITAMINS-COMPLETE Amount Per Tablet	% Daily Value for Children 2–4 Years of Age	% Daily Value for Adults and Children 4 or More Years of Age
Vitamin A 5000 I.U.	100%	100%
Vitamin C 60 mg	80%	100%
Vitamin D 400 I.U.	50%	100%
Vitamin E 30 I.U.	150%	100%
Vitamin K 10 mcg	*	*
Thiamin 1.5 mg	110%	100%
Riboflavin 1.7 mg	110%	100%
Niacin 20 mg	110%	100%
Vitamin B_6 2 mg	140%	100%
Folate 0.4 mg	100%	100%
Vitamin B_{12} 6 mcg	100%	100%
Biotin 40 mcg	15%	15%
Pantothenic Acid 10 mg	100%	100%
Calcium 100 mg	6%	10%
Iron 18 mg	90%	100%
Phosphorus 78 mg	4%	8%
Iodine 150 mcg	110%	100%
Magnesium 20 mg	5%	6%
Zinc 10 mg	60%	60%
Copper 2.0 mg	100%	100%
Manganese 1 mg	*	*

*Daily Value not established.

ʼngredients: Sorbitol, Dicalcium ʼhosphate, Mono & Diglycerides, Ferʼous Fumarate, Natural Flavors, Stearic ʼcid, Carrageenan, Starch, Sodium ʼscorbate, Vitamin E, Magnesium Oxʼde, Hydrolyzed Protein, Ascorbic Acid, ʼiacinamide, Citric Acid, FD&C Yellow ʼ#6, Zinc Oxide, Gelatin, Magnesium ʼtearate, FD&C Red #40, Calcium Panʼothenate, FD&C Yellow #5, Asparʼame, Silica, Calcium Silicate, Vitamin A ʼalmitate, Cellulose, Manganese Sulʼate, Vitamin B_6, Cupric Oxide, Riboflaʼin, Hydrogenated Vegetable Oils, Thiamin, Sucrose, Ascorbyl Palmitate, Folic Acid, Beta Carotene, Potassium Iodide, Biotin, Calcium Stearate, Vitamin K, Vitamin D, Vitamin B_{12}.
PHENYLKETONURICS: CONTAINS PHENYLALANINE

Directions: Ages 2 to 4 years—Chew one-half tablet daily. Ages 4 years and older—Chew one tablet daily.

Warning: Close tightly and keep out of reach of children. Contains iron, which can be harmful or fatal to children in large doses. In case of accidental overdose, seek professional assistance or contact a Poison Control Center immediately.

How Supplied: Bottles of 60 tablets. Store at controlled room temperature, 15°–30°C (59°–86°F). Protect from moisture.

Mfd. for and dist. by Novartis Consumer Health, Inc., Woodbridge, NJ 07095 under a trademark license from Sunkist Growers, Inc. Sunkist® is a registered trademark of Sunkist Growers, Inc. Sherman Oaks, CA 91423.©

Shown in Product Identification Guide, page 515

SUNKIST® VITAMIN C
Citrus Complex
Chewable Tablets

Description: All Sunkist Vitamin C chewable tablets have a delicious orange flavor unlike any other Vitamin C tablet. Each 60 mg chewable tablet contains 100% of the U.S. RDA* of Vitamin C. Each 250 mg chewable tablet contains 417% of the U.S. RDA* of Vitamin C. Each 500 mg chewable tablet contains 833% of the U.S. RDA* of Vitamin C. Sunkist Vitamin C chewable tablets do not contain artificial flavors or colors.

*U.S. Recommended Daily Allowance for adults and children over 4 years of age.

Indication: Dietary supplementation.

How Supplied: 60 mg Chewable Tablets—Rolls of 11.
250 mg and 500 mg Chewable Tablets—Bottles of 60.
Store at controlled room temperature 15°–30°C (59°–86°F).
Sunkist® is a registered trademark of Sunkist Growers, Inc., Sherman Oaks, CA 91423.©

Shown in Product Identification Guide, page 515

TAVIST-1® TABLETS

Description: Active Ingredients: clemastine fumarate, USP 1.34 mg (equivalent to 1 mg clemastine). **Inactive Ingredients:** lactose, povidone, starch, stearic acid, and talc.

Indications: Temporarily reduces runny nose and relieves sneezing, itching of the nose or throat, and itchy, watery eyes due to hay fever or other upper respiratory allergies.

Warnings: May cause drowsiness; alcohol, sedatives, and tranquilizers may increase the drowsiness effect. Avoid alcoholic beverages while taking this product. Do not take this product if you are taking sedatives or tranquilizers without

Continued on next page

Information on Novartis Consumer Health, Inc., products appearing on these pages is effective as of November 1996.

first consulting your doctor. Use caution when driving a motor vehicle or operating machinery. May cause excitability especially in children. Do not take this product if you have glaucoma, a breathing problem such as emphysema or chronic bronchitis, or difficulty in urination due to enlargement of the prostate gland unless directed by a doctor. As with any drug, if you are pregnant or nursing a baby, seek the advice of a health professional before using this product. **Keep this and all drugs out of reach of children.** In case of accidental overdose, seek professional assistance or contact a Poison Control Center immediately.

Directions: Adults and children 12 years of age and over: Take one tablet every 12 hours, not to exceed 2 tablets in 24 hours, or as directed by a doctor. Children under 12 years of age: Consult a doctor.

How Supplied: Tavist-1 tablets (white) imprinted "Tavist-1" on both sides in blister packs of 8, 16, and 32.

Shown in Product Identification Guide, page 515

TAVIST-D® TABLETS

Description: Active Ingredients: clemastine fumarate, USP, 1.34 mg (equivalent to 1 mg clemastine) immediate release and 75 mg phenylpropanolamine hydrochloride, USP, extended release. **Inactive Ingredients:** Colloidal silicon dioxide, dibasic calcium phosphate, lactose, magnesium stearate, methylcellulose, polyethylene glycol, povidone, starch, synthetic polymers, titanium dioxide and Yellow 10.

Indications: For the temporary relief of nasal congestion associated with upper respiratory allergies or sinusitis when accompanied by other symptoms of hay fever or allergies, including runny nose, sneezing, itchy nose or throat or itchy, watery eyes.

Warnings: May cause drowsiness; alcohol, sedatives, and tranquilizers may increase the drowsiness effect. Avoid alcoholic beverages while taking this product. Do not take this product if you are taking sedatives or tranquilizers without first consulting your doctor. Use caution when driving a motor vehicle or operating machinery. May cause excitability especially in children. **Do not exceed recommended dosage because at higher doses nervousness, dizziness, or sleeplessness may occur.** Do not take this product for more than 7 days. If symptoms do not improve or are accompanied by fever, consult a doctor. Do not take this product if you have heart disease, high blood pressure, thyroid disease, diabetes, glaucoma, a breathing problem such as emphysema or chronic bronchitis, or difficulty in urination due to enlargement of the prostate gland unless directed by a doctor. As with any drug, if you are pregnant or nursing a baby, seek the advice of a health professional before using this product. **Keep this and all drugs out of reach of children.** In case of accidental overdose, seek professional assistance or contact a Poison Control Center immediately.

Drug Interaction Precaution: Do not take this product if you are presently taking a decongestant or prescription drug for high blood pressure or depression, without first consulting your doctor.

Directions: Adults and children 12 years of age and over: Take one tablet swallowed whole every 12 hours, not to exceed 2 tablets in 24 hours, or as directed by a doctor. Children under 12 years of age: Consult a doctor.

How Supplied: Tavist-D tablets (white) imprinted "Tavist-D" on both sides, in blister packs of 8, 16, and 32; and Bottles of 50.

Shown in Product Identification Guide, page 515

THERAFLU®
Flu and Cold Medicine
Flu, Cold & Cough Medicine

Description: Each packet of TheraFlu Flu and Cold Medicine contains: acetaminophen 650 mg, pseudoephedrine hydrochloride 60 mg, and chlorpheniramine maleate 4 mg. Each packet of TheraFlu Flu, Cold & Cough Medicine also contains dextromethorphan hydrobromide 20 mg. Other ingredients: ascorbic acid (vitamin C), citric acid, natural lemon flavors, pregelatinized starch, silicon dioxide, sodium citrate, sucrose, titanium dioxide, tribasic calcium phosphate, and Yellow 10.
Sodium content: 25 mg per packet.

Indications: Provides temporary relief of the symptoms associated with flu, common cold and other upper respiratory infections including: headache, body aches, fever, minor sore throat pain, nasal and sinus congestion, runny nose and sneezing. TheraFlu Flu, Cold & Cough Medicine also suppresses coughs due to minor throat and bronchial irritation.

Warnings: Keep this and all drugs out of the reach of children. In case of accidental overdose, seek professional assistance or contact a poison control center immediately. Prompt medical attention is critical for adults as well as children even if you do not notice any signs or symptoms.
Do not exceed recommended dosage. If nervousness, dizziness, or sleeplessness occur, discontinue use and consult a doctor. If symptoms do not improve within 7 days or are accompanied by fever, consult a doctor. May cause excitability especially in children. Do not take this product if you have heart disease, high blood pressure, thyroid disease, diabetes, glaucoma, a breathing problem such as emphysema or chronic bronchitis, or difficulty in urination due to enlargement of the prostate gland, unless directed by a doctor.
Do not take this product for pain for more than 10 days or for fever for more than 3 days unless directed by a doctor. If pain or fever persists or gets worse, if new symptoms occur, or if redness or swelling is present, consult a doctor because these could be signs of a serious condition. If sore throat is severe, persists for more than 2 days, is accompanied or followed by fever, headache, rash, nausea, or vomiting, consult a doctor promptly.
May cause marked drowsiness; alcohol, sedatives, and tranquilizers may increase the drowsiness effect. Avoid alcoholic beverages while taking this product. Do not take this product if you are taking sedatives or tranquilizers, without first consulting your doctor. Use caution when driving a motor vehicle or operating machinery.
A persistent cough may be a sign of a serious condition. If cough persists for more than 1 week, tends to recur, or is accompanied by a fever, rash, or persistent headache, consult a doctor. Do not take the Flu, Cold & Cough formula for persistent or chronic cough such as occurs with smoking, asthma, or emphysema, or if cough is accompanied by excessive phlegm (mucus) unless directed by a doctor.
As with any drug, if you are pregnant or nursing a baby, seek the advice of a health professional before using this product.

Drug Interaction Precaution: Do not take this product if you are now taking a prescription monoamine oxidase inhibitor [MAOI] (certain drugs for depression, psychiatric or emotional conditions, or Parkinson's disease), or for 2 weeks after stopping the MAOI drug. If you are uncertain whether your prescription drug contains an MAOI, consult a health professional before taking this product.

Directions: Adults and children 12 years of age and over—dissolve one packet in 6 oz. hot water; sip while hot. One packet of Flu and Cold formula every 4 to 6 hours; one packet of Flu, Cold and Cough formula every six hours. Not to exceed 4 packets in 24 hours, or as directed by a doctor. Children under 12 years of age: consult a doctor. **Microwave heating instructions:** Add contents of packet and 6 oz. of cool water to a microwave-safe cup and stir briskly. Microwave on high $1^1/_2$ minutes or until hot. Do not boil water or overheat, and remember to stir liquid between reheatings. Sweeten to taste if desired.

How Supplied: TheraFlu Flu and Cold Medicine powder in foil packets, 6 or 12 packets per carton. TheraFlu Flu, Cold & Cough Medicine powder in foil packets, 6 or 12 packets per carton.

Shown in Product Identification Guide, page 515

THERAFLU® MAXIMUM STRENGTH
Flu and Cold Medicine For Sore Throat

Each packet of Theraflu Maximum Strength Sore Throat formula contains: acetaminophen 1000 mg, pseudoephedrine HCl 60 mg, chlorpheniramine maleate 4 mg. **Other Ingredients:** Acesulfame K, natural apple and cinnamon flavors, ascorbic acid, aspartame, Blue 1, citric acid, maltodextrin, Red 40, silicon dioxide, sodium citrate, sucrose, tribasic calcium phosphate, and Yellow 10.
Sodium content: 30 mg per packet.

Indications: Provides temporary relief of minor sore throat pain, body aches, pains, and headaches and reduces fever. Temporarily relieves runny nose, sneezing and nasal congestion due to flu, the common cold, hay fever or other upper respiratory allergies.

Warnings: Keep this and all drugs out of the reach of children. In case of accidental overdose seek professional assistance or contact a doctor or a poison control center immediately. Prompt medical attention is critical for adults as well as children even if you do not notice any signs or symptoms.
Do not exceed recommended dosage. If nervousness, dizziness, or sleeplessness occur, discontinue use and consult a doctor. If symptoms do not improve within 7 days or are accompanied by fever, consult a doctor. May cause excitability, especially in children. Do not take this product if you have heart disease, high blood pressure, thyroid disease, diabetes, glaucoma, a breathing problem such as emphysema or chronic bronchitis, or difficulty in urination due to enlargement of the prostate gland, unless directed by a doctor.
Do not take this product for pain for more than 10 days or for fever for more than 3 days unless directed by a doctor. If pain or fever persists or gets worse, if new symptoms occur, or if redness or swelling is present, consult a doctor because these could be signs of a serious condition. If sore throat is severe, persists for more than 2 days, is accompanied or followed by fever, headache, rash, nausea, or vomiting, consult a doctor promptly.
May cause drowsiness; alcohol, sedatives and tranquilizers may increase the drowsiness effect. Avoid alcoholic beverages while taking this product. Do not take this product if you are taking sedatives or tranquilizers without first consulting your doctor. Use caution when driving a motor vehicle or operating machinery.
As with any drug, if you are pregnant or nursing a baby, seek the advice of a health professional before using this product.

Drug Interaction Precaution: Do not use this product if you are now taking a prescription monoamine oxidase inhibitor [MAOI] (certain drugs for depression, psychiatric or emotional conditions, or Parkinson's Disease), or for 2 weeks after stopping the MAOI drug. If you are uncertain whether your prescription drug contains an MAOI, consult a health professional before taking this product.
Phenylketonurics: Contains Phenylalanine 25 mg per adult dose.

Directions: Adults and children 12 years of age and over: dissolve one packet in 6 oz. of hot water; sip while hot. One packet every 6 hours, not to exceed 4 packets in 24 hours, or as directed by a doctor. Children under 12 years of age: consult a doctor. **Microwave Heating Instructions:** Add contents of packet and 6 oz. of cool water to a microwave-safe cup and stir briskly. Microwave on high 1 $^1/_2$ minutes or until hot. Do not boil water or overheat, and remember to stir liquid between reheatings.
Sweeten to taste if desired. May repeat every 6 hours, but not to exceed 4 doses in 24 hours.

How Supplied: Theraflu Maximum Strength flu and Cold Medicine for Sore Throat powder in foil packets, 6 packets per carton.

Shown in Product Identification Guide, page 515

THERAFLU® MAXIMUM STRENGTH NIGHTTIME
Hot Liquid and Caplet Flu, Cold & Cough Medicine

Description: Each packet of TheraFlu Maximum Strength NightTime Flu, Cold & Cough Hot Liquid Medicine contains: acetaminophen 1000 mg, dextromethorphan HBr 30 mg, pseudoephedrine HCl 60 mg, and chlorpheniramine maleate 4 mg. Other ingredients: ascorbic acid (Vitamin C), citric acid, natural lemon flavors, maltol, pregelatinized starch, silicon dioxide, sodium citrate, sucrose, titanium dioxide, tribasic calcium phosphate, and Yellow 10.
Sodium content: 25 mg per packet.
TheraFlu NIGHTTIME Caplets: each caplet contains acetaminophen 500 mg. pseudo-ephedrine HCl 30 mg. dextromethorphan HBr 15 mg. and chlorpheniramine maleate 2 mg. **Inactive Ingredients:** Blue 1, colloidal silicon dioxide, croscarmellose sodium gelatin, hydroxypropyl cellulose, hydroxypropyl methylcellulose, lactose, magnesium stearate, methylparaben, polydextrose, polyethylene glycol, pregelatinized starch, titanium dioxide, triacetin, Yellow 6, and Yellow 10.
Sodium content: 3 mg per caplet.
TheraFlu Hot Liquid and caplets provide temporary relief of the symptoms associated with flu, common cold and other upper respiratory infections including: headache, body aches, fever, minor sore throat pain, nasal and sinus congestion, runny nose and sneezing. TheraFlu Maximum Strength Flu, Cold, & Cough Medicine also suppresses coughs due to minor throat and bronchial irritation.

Warnings: Keep this and all drugs out of the reach of children. In case of accidental overdose, seek professional assistance or contact a poison control center immediately. Prompt medical attention is critical for adults as well as children even if you do not notice any signs or symptoms.
Do not exceed recommended dosage. If nervousness, dizziness, or sleeplessness occur, discontinue use and consult a doctor. If symptoms do not improve within 7 days or are accompanied by fever, consult a doctor. May cause excitability, especially in children. Do not take this product if you have heart disease, high blood pressure, thyroid disease, diabetes, glaucoma, a breathing problem such as emphysema or chronic bronchitis, or difficulty in urination due to enlargement of the prostate gland, unless directed by a doctor. A persistent cough may be a sign of a serious condition. If cough persists for more than 1 week, tends to recur, or is accompanied by a fever, rash, or persistent headache, consult a doctor. Do not take this product for persistent or chronic cough such as occurs with smoking, asthma, or emphysema, or if cough is accompanied by excessive phlegm (mucus) unless directed by a doctor.
Do not take this product for pain for more than 10 days or for fever for more than 3 days unless directed by a doctor. If pain or fever persists or gets worse, if new symptoms occur, or if redness or swelling is present, consult a doctor because these could be signs of a serious condition. If sore throat is severe, persists for more than 2 days, is accompanied or followed by fever, headache, rash, nausea, or vomiting, consult a doctor promptly.
May cause marked drowsiness; alcohol, sedatives, and tranquilizers may increase the drowsiness effect. Avoid alcoholic beverages while taking this product. Do not take this product if you are taking sedatives or tranquilizers, without first consulting your doctor. Use caution when driving a motor vehicle or operating machinery.
As with any drug, if you are pregnant or nursing a baby, seek the advice of a health professional before using this product.

Drug Interaction Precaution: Do not use this product if you are now taking a prescription monoamine oxidase inhibitor [MAOI] (certain drugs for depression, psychiatric or emotional conditions, or Parkinson's disease), or for 2 weeks after stopping the MAOI drug. If you are uncertain whether your prescription drug contains an MAOI, consult a health professional before taking this product.

Directions: Adults and children 12 years of age and over: dissolve contents of one packet in 6 oz. cup of hot water; sip

Continued on next page

Information on Novartis Consumer Health, Inc., products appearing on these pages is effective as of November 1996.

Novartis—Cont.

while hot. One packet every 6 hours, not to exceed 4 packets in 24 hours, or as directed by a doctor. Children under 12 years of age: consult a doctor. Microwave heating instructions: Add contents of packet and 6 oz. of cool water to a microwave-safe cup and stir briskly. Microwave on high $1^1/_2$ minutes or until water is hot. Do not boil water or overheat, and remember to stir liquid between reheatings. Sweeten to taste if desired. TheraFlu NIGHTTIME Caplets: Adults and children 12 years of age and over: two caplets every 6 hours, not to exceed 8 caplets in 24 hours or as directed by a doctor. Children under 12 years of age: consult a doctor.

How Supplied: TheraFlu Maximum Strength NightTime Flu, Cold, & Cough Medicine powder in foil packets, 6, or 12, packets per carton. TheraFlu maximum strength NIGHTTIME Formula Caplets in blister packs of 12's.

Shown in Product Identification Guide, page 515

THERAFLU® MAXIMUM STRENGTH NO-DROWSINESS FORMULA THERAFLU® MAXIMUM STRENGTH NON-DROWSY FORMULA CAPLETS

Flu, Cold & Cough Medicine

Description: Each packet of TheraFlu Maximum Strength Non-Drowsy Hot Liquid Formula contains: acetaminophen 1000 mg, pseudoephedrine HCl 60 mg, dextromethorphan 30 mg. Other Ingredients: Ascorbic acid (Vitamin C), citric acid, natural lemon flavors, maltol, pregelatinized starch, silicon dioxide, sodium citrate, sucrose, titanium dioxide, tribasic calcium phosphate, and Yellow 10.

Sodium content: 25 mg per packet.

Each TheraFlu Maximum Strength Non-Drowsy caplet contains: Dextromethorphan HBr, 15 mg, pseudoephedrine HCl 30 mg, and acetaminophen 500 mg. Other ingredients: colloidal silicon dioxide, croscarmellose sodium, gelatin, hydroxypropyl cellulose, hydroxypropyl methylcellulose, lactose, magnesium stearate, methylparaben, polydextrose, polyethylene glycol, pregelatinized starch, Red 40, titanium dioxide, triacetin, Yellow 6, Yellow 10.

Sodium content: 3 mg per caplet.

Indications: Provides temporary relief of the symptoms associated with flu, common cold, and other upper respiratory infections including: headache, body aches, fever, minor sore throat pain, nasal and sinus congestion. TheraFlu Maximum Strength Non-Drowsy Formula also suppresses coughs due to minor throat and bronchial irritation.

Warnings: Keep this and all drugs out of the reach of children. In case of accidental overdose, seek professional assistance or contact a poison control center immediately. Prompt medical attention is critical for adults as well as children even if you do not notice any signs or symptoms.

Do not exceed recommended dosage. If nervousness, dizziness, or sleeplessness occur, discontinue use and consult a doctor. If symptoms do not improve within 7 days or are accompanied by fever, consult a doctor. Do not take this product if you have heart disease, high blood pressure, thyroid disease, diabetes, or difficulty in urination due to enlargement of the prostate gland unless directed by a physician.

A persistent cough may be a sign of a serious condition. If cough persists for more than 1 week, tends to recur, or is accompanied by a fever, rash, or persistent headache, consult a doctor. Do not take this product for persistent or chronic cough such as occurs with smoking, asthma, or emphysema, or if cough is accompanied by excessive phlegm (mucus) unless directed by a doctor.

Do not take this product for pain for more than 10 days or for fever for more than 3 days unless directed by a doctor. If pain or fever persists or gets worse, if new symptoms occur, or if redness or swelling is present, consult a doctor, because these could be signs of a serious condition. If sore throat is severe, persists for more than 2 days, is accompanied or followed by fever, headache, rash, nausea, or vomiting, consult a doctor promptly.

As with any drug, if you are pregnant or nursing a baby, seek the advice of a health professional before using this product.

Drug Interaction Precaution: Do not take this product if you are now taking a prescription monoamine oxidase inhibitor [MAOI] (certain drugs for depression, psychiatric or emotional conditions, or Parkinson's disease), or for 2 weeks after stopping the MAOI drug. If you are uncertain whether your prescription drug contains an MAOI, consult a health professional before taking this product.

Directions: Adults and children 12 years of age and over: dissolve one packet in 6 oz. cup of hot water; sip while hot. One packet every 6 hours, not to exceed 4 packets in 24 hours, or as directed by a doctor. Children under 12 years of age: consult a doctor. Microwave Heating Instructions: Add contents of packet and 6 oz. of cool water to a microwave-safe cup and stir briskly. Microwave on high 1 1/2 minutes or until hot. Do not boil or overheat, and remember to stir liquid between reheatings. Sweeten to taste if desired. TheraFlu Maximum Strength Non-Drowsy Caplet: Adults and Children 12 years of age and over: two caplets every 6 hours, not to exceed eight caplets in 24 hours or as directed by a doctor. Children under 12 years of age—Consult a doctor.

How Supplied: TheraFlu Maximum Strength No-Drowsiness Flu, Cold, & Cough Medicine powder in foil packets, 6 or 12 packets per carton. TheraFlu Maximum Strength Non-Drowsy Formula gelatin coated caplets (yellow) in blister packs of 12 and 24.

Shown in Product Identification Guide, page 515

THERAFLU® MAXIMUM STRENGTH SINUS NON-DROWSY FORMULA

Description: Each Theraflu Maximum Strength Sinus Non-Drowsy formula caplet contains: 500 mg acetaminophen, 30 mg pseudophedrine HCl. **Other Ingredients:** Colloidal silicon dioxide, croscarmellose sodium, hydroxypropyl cellulose, lactose, magnesium stearate, methylcellulose, methylparaben, polyethylene glycol, povidone, pregelatinized starch, titanium dioxide.

Sodium content: 3 mg per caplet.

Indications: Each dose provides the maximum allowable levels of these active ingredients in easy-to-swallow coated caplets for temporary relief of these symptoms without drowsiness: Sinus Pain & Headache (Analgesic—acetaminophen 500 mg per caplets). Nasal and Sinus Congestion Pressure (Nasal Decongestant—pseudoephedrine HCl, 30 mg per caplet).

Warnings: Keep this and all drugs out of the reach of children. In case of accidental overdose, contact a doctor or poison control center immediately. Prompt medical attention is critical for adults as well as children even if you do not notice any signs or symptoms.

Do not exceed recommended dosage. If nervousness, dizziness or sleeplessness occur, discontinue use and consult a doctor. If symptoms do not improve within 7 days or are accompanied by fever, consult a doctor. Do not take this product if you have heart disease, high blood pressure, thyroid disease, diabetes or difficulty in urination due to enlargement of the prostate gland, unless directed by a doctor. Do not take this product for pain for more than 10 days or for fever for more than 3 days unless directed by a doctor. If pain or fever persists or gets worse, if new symptoms occur, or if redness or swelling is present, consult a doctor because these could be signs of a serious condition. As with any drug, if you are pregnant or nursing a baby, seek the advice of a health professional before using this product.

Drug Interaction Precaution: Do not use this product if you are now taking a prescription monoamine oxidase inhibitor [MAOI] (certain drugs for depression, psychiatric or emotional conditions or Parkinson's Disease), or for 2 weeks after stopping the MAOI drug. If you are uncertain whether your prescription drug contain an MAOI, consult a health professional before taking this product.

Store in a dry place at controlled room temperature 15°–30°C (59°–86°F).

Directions: Adults and children 12 years of age and over: Two caplets every six hours, not to exceed eight caplets in 24 hours or as directed by a doctor. Children under 12 years of age: Consult a doctor.

How Supplied: Theraflu Maximum Strength Sinus gelatin coated caplets (white) in blister packs of 24.

Shown in Product Identification Guide, page 515

TING® ANTIFUNGAL CREAM, SPRAY LIQUID

Active Ingredient: Tolnaftate, 1%.

Other Ingredients: *Cream*—BHT, fragrance, polyethylene glycol 400, polyethylene glycol 3350, titanium dioxide, white petrolatum. *Spray Liquid*—BHT, fragrance, isobutane (propellant), polyethylene glycol 400, SD alcohol 40-B (41% w/w).

Indications: Cures athlete's foot and jock itch with a clinically proven ingredient. Relieves itching and burning. Prevents the recurrence of athlete's foot with daily use.

Warnings: Do not use on children under 2 years of age unless directed by a doctor. For external use only. Avoid contact with the eyes. If irritation occurs or if there is no improvement within 4 weeks for athlete's foot or within 2 weeks for jock itch, discontinue use and consult a doctor. **Keep this and all drugs out of the reach of children.** In case of accidental ingestion, seek professional assistance or contact a Poison Control Center immediately. *For Spray Liquid only*—Avoid inhaling. Avoid contact with the eyes or other mucous membranes. Contents under pressure; do not puncture or incinerate. Flammable mixture, do not use near fire or flame. Do not expose to heat or temperatures above 49°C (120°F). Use only as directed. Intentional misuse by deliberately concentrating and inhaling contents can be harmful or fatal.

Directions: Clean the affected area and dry thoroughly. Apply a thin layer of the product over affected area twice daily (morning and night) or as directed by a doctor. Supervise children in the use of this product. For athlete's foot: pay special attention to the spaces between the toes, wear well-fitting, ventilated shoes, and change shoes and socks at least once daily. For athlete's foot, use daily for 4 weeks; for jock itch, use daily for 2 weeks. If condition persists longer, consult a doctor. This product is not effective on the scalp or nails. To prevent athlete's foot, apply a thin layer of the product to the feet once or twice daily (morning and/or night) following the above directions.

How Supplied: *Cream*—$^1/_2$ oz (14 g) tube, *Spray Liquid*—3 oz (85 g) aerosol container.
Store at room temperature 15°–30°C (59°–86°F).

TING is a registered trademark of Novartis.

TING® ANTIFUNGAL SPRAY POWDER

Active Ingredient: Miconazole Nitrate, 2%.

Other Ingredients: Aloe vera gel, aluminum starch octenylsuccinate, isopropyl myristate, propylene carbonate, SD alcohol 40-B (10% w/w), sorbitan monooleate, stearalkonium hectorite.

Propellant: Isobutane/propane.

Indications: Proven clinically effective in the treatment of athlete's foot and ring worm (tinea corporis). Relieves the itching, scaling, burning, and discomfort that can accompany athlete's foot. Specially formulated to aid the drying of moist areas of the feet.

Warnings: Do not use on children under 2 years of age, unless directed by a doctor. For external use only. Avoid inhaling. Avoid contact with the eyes or other mucous membranes. If irritation occurs or if there is no improvement within 4 weeks, discontinue use and consult a physician. Contents under pressure. Do not puncture or incinerate. Flammable mixture, do not use near fire or flame. Do not expose to heat or temperatures above 49°C (120°F). Use only as directed. Intentional misuse by deliberately concentrating and inhaling contents can be harmful or fatal. **Keep this and all drugs out of the reach of children**. In case of accidental ingestion, seek professional assistance or contact a Poison Control Center immediately.

Directions: Clean the affected area and dry thoroughly. **Shake can well,** hold 4″ to 6″ from skin. Spray a thin layer of the product over affected area twice daily (morning and night) or as directed by a doctor. Supervise children in the use of this product. Pay special attention to the spaces between the toes. Wear well-fitting, ventilated shoes, and change shoes and socks at least once daily. Use daily for 4 weeks. If condition persists longer, consult a doctor. This product is not effective on the scalp or nails.

How Supplied: Spray Powder 3 oz (85g) aerosol container.
Store at room temperature 15°–30°C (59°–86°F).

TRIAMINIC® AM COUGH AND DECONGESTANT FORMULA

Description: Each teaspoonful (5 mL) of TRIAMINIC AM COUGH AND DECONGESTANT FORMULA contains: pseudoephedrine hydrochloride, USP 15 mg and dextromethorphan hydrobromide, USP 7.5 mg in a palatable, orange/stawberry flavored, dye-free, nondrowsy, alcohol-free liquid. **Other Ingredients:** benzoic acid, citric acid, dibasic sodium phosphate, edetate disodium, flavors, propylene glycol, purified water, sorbitol, sucrose.
Sodium content: 7 mg per teaspoon.

Indications: Temporarily quiets coughs due to minor throat and bronchial irritations and relieves stuffy noses.

Warnings: Keep this and all drugs out of the reach of children. In case of accidental overdose, seek professional assistance or contact a Poison Control Center immediately.
Do not exceed recommended dosage. If nervousness, dizziness, or sleeplessness occur, discontinue use and consult a doctor. If symptoms do not improve within 7 days or are accompanied by fever, consult a doctor. Do not take this product if you have heart disease, high blood pressure, thyroid disease, diabetes, or difficulty in urination due to enlargement of the prostate gland, unless directed by a doctor.
A persistent cough may be a sign of a serious condition. If cough persists for more than 1 week, tends to recur, or is accompanied by fever, rash or persistent headache, consult a doctor. Do not take this product for persistent or chronic cough such as occurs with smoking, asthma, or emphysema or if cough is accompanied by excessive phlegm (mucus) unless directed by doctor.
As with any drug, if you are pregnant or nursing a baby, seek the advice of a health professional before using this product.

Drug Interaction Precaution: Do not use this product if you are now taking a prescription monoamine oxidase inhibitor [MAOI] (certain drugs for depression, psychiatric or emotional conditions, or Parkinson's disease), or for 2 weeks after stopping the MAOI drug. If you are uncertain whether your prescription drug contains an MAOI, consult a health professional before taking this product.

Dosage and Administration: Adults and children 12 and over (96+ lbs)—4 teaspoons every 6 hours. Children 6 to under 12 years (48–95 lbs)—2 teaspoons every 6 hours. Children 2 to under 6 years (24–47 lbs)—1 teaspoon every 6 hours. Do not exceed 4 doses in 24 hours, or as directed by a doctor. Dosing to children under 2 years of age is to be under the direction of a physician. For convenience, a True-Dose® dosage cup is provided with each 4 fl. oz. and 8 fl. oz. bottle.
Professional Labeling: The suggested dosage for pediatric patients is:

4–12 months (12–17 lbs)	1.25 ml ($^1/_4$ tsp) every 6 hours
12–24 months (18–23 lbs)	2.5 ml ($^1/_2$ tsp) every 6 hours

Do not exceed 4 doses in 24 hours.

Continued on next page

Information on Novartis Consumer Health, Inc., products appearing on these pages is effective as of November 1996.

Novartis—Cont.

How Supplied: TRIAMINIC AM COUGH AND DECONGESTANT FORMULA (clear liquid) in 4 fl. oz. plastic bottles with tamper-evident band around child-resistant cap. Dosage cup included. Orange/strawberry flavored. Alcohol-free. Dye-free. Non-drowsy.

Shown in Product Identification Guide, page 515

TRIAMINIC® AM DECONGESTANT FORMULA

Description: Each teaspoonful (5 mL) of TRIAMINIC AM DECONGESTANT FORMULA contains: pseudoephedrine hydrochloride, USP 15 mg in a palatable, orange/strawberry flavored, dye-free, non-drowsy, alcohol-free liquid. **Other ingredients**: benzoic acid, edetate disodium, flavors, purified water, sodium hydroxide, sorbitol, sucrose
Sodium content: 1 mg per teaspoon.

Indications: For temporary relief of nasal congestion due to the common cold, hay fever or upper respiratory allergies, or associated with sinusitis. Reduces swelling of nasal passages; shrinks swollen membranes.

Warnings: Keep this and all drugs out of the reach of children. In case of accidental overdose, seek professional assistance or contact a poison control center immediately.
Do not exceed recommended dosage. If nervousness, dizziness, or sleeplessness occur, discontinue use and consult a doctor. If symptoms do not improve within 7 days or are accompanied by fever, consult a doctor. Do not take this product if you have heart disease, high blood pressure, thyroid disease, diabetes, or difficulty in urination due to enlargement of the prostate gland, unless directed by a doctor.
As with any drug, if you are pregnant or nursing a baby, seek the advice of a health professional before using this product.

Drug Interaction Precaution: Do not use this product if you are now taking a prescription monoamine oxidase inhibitor [MAOI] (certain drugs for depression, psychiatric or emotional conditions, or Parkinson's disease) or for 2 weeks after stopping the MAOI drug. If you are uncertain whether your prescription drug contains an MAOI, consult a health professional before taking this product.

Dosage and Administration: Adults and children 12 and over (96+ lbs)—4 teaspoons every 4–6 hours. Children 6 to under 12 years (48–95 lbs)—2 teaspoons every 4–6 hours. Children 2 to under 6 years (24–47 lbs)—1 teaspoon every 4–6 hours. Do not exceed 4 doses in 24 hours, or as directed by a doctor. Dosing to children under 2 years of age is to be under the direction of a physician. For convenience, a True-Dose® dosage cup is provided with each 4 fl. oz. and 8 fl. oz. bottle.
Professional Labeling: The suggested dosage for pediatric patients is:

4–12 months (12–17 lbs)	1.25 ml (1/4 tsp) every 4 to 6 hours
12–24 months (18–23 lbs)	2.5 ml (1/2 tsp) every 4 to 6 hours

Do not exceed 4 doses in 24 hours.

How Supplied: TRIAMINIC AM DECONGESTANT FORMULA (clear liquid) in 4 fl oz plastic bottles with tamper-evident band around child-resistant cap. Dosage cup included. Orange/strawberry flavored. Alcohol-free. Dye-free. Non-drowsy.

Shown in Product Identification Guide, page 515

TRIAMINIC® EXPECTORANT

[*trī″ah-mĭn′ĭc*]

Description: Each teaspoonful (5 mL) of TRIAMINIC Expectorant contains: guaifenesin, USP 50 mg, and phenylpropanolamine hydrochloride, USP 6.25 mg in a palatable, citrus-flavored alcohol-free liquid. **Other ingredients:** benzoic acid, edetate disodium, flavors, glycerin, polyethylene glycol, propylene glycol, purified water, sorbitol, sucrose, Yellow 6, Yellow 10.
Sodium-free.

Indications: Relieves chest congestion by loosening phlegm to help clear bronchial passageways. Temporarily relieves stuffy nose.

Warnings: Keep this and all drugs out of the reach of children. In case of accidental overdose, seek professional assistance or contact a poison control center immediately.
Do not exceed recommended dosage. If nervousness, dizziness, or sleeplessness occur, discontinue use and consult a doctor. If symptoms do not improve within 7 days or are accompanied by fever, consult a doctor. A persistent cough may be a sign of a serious condition. If cough persists for more than 1 week, tends to recur, or is accompanied by fever, rash, or persistent headache, consult a doctor. Do not take this product: 1) if cough is accompanied by excessive phlegm (mucus), 2) for persistent or chronic cough such as occurs with smoking, asthma, chronic bronchitis or emphysema. 3) if you have heart disease, high blood pressure, thyroid disease, diabetes, difficulty in urination due to enlargement of the prostate gland, or 4) if you are presently taking another product containing phenylpropanolamine, unless directed by a doctor.
As with any drug, if you are pregnant or nursing a baby, seek the advice of a health professional before using this product.

Drug Interaction Precaution: Do not use this product if you are now taking a prescription monoamine oxidase inhibitor [MAOI] (certain drugs for depression, psychiatric or emotional conditions, or Parkinson's disease), or for 2 weeks after stopping the MAOI drug. If you are uncertain whether your prescription drug contains an MAOI, consult a health professional before taking this product.

Dosage and Administration: Adults and children 12 and over (96+ lbs)—4 teaspoons every 4 hours. Children 6 to under 12 years (48–95 lbs)—2 teaspoons every 4 hours. Children 2 to under 6 years (24–47 lbs)—1 teaspoon every 4 hours. Do not exceed 6 doses in 24 hours, or as directed by a doctor. Dosing to children under 2 years of age is to be under the direction of a physician. For convenience, a True-Dose® dosage cup is provided with each 4 fl. oz. and 8 fl. oz. bottle.

Professional Labeling: The suggested dosage for pediatric patients is:

4–12 months (12–17 lbs)	1.25 ml (1/4 tsp) every 4 hours
12–24 months (18–23 lbs)	2.5 ml (1/2 tsp) every 4 hours

Do not exceed 6 doses in 24 hours.

How Supplied: TRIAMINIC Expectorant (yellow), in 4 fl oz and 8 fl oz plastic bottles with tamper-evident band around child-resistant cap. Dosage cup included. Citrus flavored, Alcohol free.

Shown in Product Identification Guide, page 516

TRIAMINIC® INFANT
Oral Decongestant Drops

Description: Each dropperful (0.8mL) of Triaminic Infant Oral Decongestant Drops contains: pseudoephedrine hydrochloride, USP 7.5 mg in a palatable, grape-flavored alcohol-free, dye-free liquid. **Other ingredients:** benzoic acid, edetate disodium, flavors, purified water, sodium chloride, sorbitol solution, sucrose.
Sodium-free.

Indications: For temporary relief of nasal congestion due to the common cold, hay fever or other upper respiratory allergies, or nasal congestion associated with sinusitis. The decongestant is provided in an alcohol-free and antihistamine-free formula.

Warnings: Keep this and all drugs out of the reach of children. In case of accidental overdose, seek professional assistance or contact a poison control center immediately.
Do not exceed recommended dosage. If nervousness, dizziness, or sleeplessness occur, discontinue use and consult a doctor. If symptoms do not improve within 7 days or are accompanied by fever, consult a doctor. Do not give this product to a child who has heart disease, high blood pressure, thyroid disease, or diabetes unless directed by a doctor.

Drug Interaction Precaution: Do not give this product to a child who is taking a prescription monoamine oxidase inhibitor [MAOI] (certain drugs for depression, psychiatric or emotional conditions) or for 2 weeks after stopping the MAOI drug. If you are uncertain whether your child's prescription drug contains an MAOI, consult a health professional before giving this product.

Dosage and Administration: Children 2 to 3 years of age (24–35 lbs.): Two dropperfuls (1.6mL) every 4–6 hours (or as directed by a doctor). Children under 2 years of age: consult a doctor. Do not exceed 4 doses in a 24-hour period. **Give by mouth only.** Not for use in the nose. For convenience, a True-Dose® dosing child-resistant dropper is provided.

Professional Labeling: The suggested dosage for pediatric patients is:

Age	Weight	Amount
4–11 months	12–17 lbs.	1 dropperful (0.8mL)
12–23 months	18–23 lbs.	$1^1/_2$ dropperfuls (1.2mL)
2–3 years	24–35 lbs.	2 dropperfuls (1.6mL)

The dose may be repeated every 4 to 6 hours, not to exceed 4 doses in 24 hours or as directed by a doctor.

How Supplied: Triaminic Infant Oral Decongestant Drops (clear), in a $^1/_2$ fl. oz. (15mL) glass bottle with tamper evident band around cap. True-Dose® dosing child-resistant dropper is also provided. Grape flavored, alcohol-free, antihistamine-free, crystal clear, non-staining formula.

TRIAMINIC® Night Time Maximum Strength Nighttime Cough and Cold Medicine

[*tri "ah-min 'ic*]

Description: Each teaspoonful (5 mL) of Triaminic® Night Time contains: pseudoephedrine hydrochloride USP 15 mg, dextromethorphan hydrobromide, USP 7.5 mg, chlorpheniramine maleate, USP 1 mg, in a palatable, grape-flavored, alcohol-free liquid.

Other ingredients: Other ingredients: benzoic acid, Blue 1, citric acid, dibasic sodium phosphate, flavors, propylene glycol, purified water, Red 33, sorbitol, sucrose.

Sodium content: 23 mg per teaspoon.

Indications: Temporarily relieves cold and allergy symptoms, including coughs due to minor throat and bronchial irritation, runny nose; stuffy nose; sneezing; itching of the nose or throat; and itchy, watery eyes.

Warnings: Keep this and all drugs out of the reach of children. In case of accidental overdose, seek professional assistance or contact a poison control center immediately.

Do not exceed recommended dosage. If nervousness, dizziness, or sleeplessness occur, discontinue use and consult a doctor. If symptoms do not improve within 7 days or are accompanied by fever, consult a doctor. A persistent cough may be a sign of a serious condition. If cough persists for more than 1 week, tends to recur, or is accompanied by fever, rash, or persistent headache, consult a doctor. Do not take this product: 1) if cough is accompanied by excessive phlegm (mucus), 2) for persistent or chronic cough such as occurs with smoking, asthma or emphysema, 3) if you have heart disease, high blood pressure, thyroid disease, diabetes, glaucoma, a breathing problem such as emphysema or chronic bronchitis, or difficulty in urination due to enlargement of the prostate gland, or 4) if you are taking sedatives or tranquilizers, unless directed by a doctor. May cause excitability especially in children. May cause drowsiness; alcohol, sedatives or tranquilizers may increase the drowsiness effect. Avoid alcoholic beverages while taking this product. Use caution when driving a motor vehicle or operating machinery. As with any drug, if you are pregnant or nursing a baby, seek the advice of a health professional before using this product.

Drug Interaction Precaution: Do not use this product if you are now taking a prescription monoamine oxidase inhibitor (MAOI) (certain drugs for depression, psychiatric or emotional conditions, or Parkinson's disease) or for 2 weeks after stopping the MAOI drug. If you are uncertain whether your prescription drug contains an MAOI, consult a health professional before taking this product.

Dosage and Administration: Adults and children 12 and over (96+ lbs.)—4 teaspoons every 6 hours. Children 6 to under 12 years (48–95 lbs.)—2 teaspoons every 6 hours. Do not exceed 4 doses in 24 hours, or as directed by a doctor. Dosing to children under 6 years of age is to be under the direction of a physician. For convenience, a True-Dose® dosage cup is provided with each 4 fl. oz. and 8 fl. oz. bottle.

Professional Labeling: The suggested dosage for pediatric patients is:

4 to under 12 months (12–17 lbs.)	$^1/_4$ teaspoon or 1.25 ml every 6 hours
12 months to under 2 years (18–23 lbs.)	$^1/_2$ teaspoon or 2.5 ml every 6 hours
2 to under 6 years	1 teaspoon or 5 ml every 6 hours

Not to exceed 4 doses in 24 hours

How Supplied: Triaminic® Night Time Cough and Cold Medicine for Children (purple), in 4 fl. oz. and 8 fl. oz. plastic bottles packaged in cartons with tamper-evident band around child-resistant cap. Grape flavored. Alcohol free.

Shown in Product Identification Guide, page 516

TRIAMINIC® Sore Throat Formula

[*trī "ah-mĭn 'ĭc*]

Description: Each teaspoonful (5 mL) of Triaminic Sore Throat Formula contains: acetaminophen, USP 160 mg, pseudoephedrine hydrochloride, USP 15 mg and dextromethorphan hydrobromide, USP 7.5 mg, in a palatable, grape-flavored, alcohol-free liquid. **Other ingredients:** benzoic acid, Blue 1, dibasic sodium phosphate, edetate disodium, flavors, glycerin, polyethylene glycol, propylene glycol, purified water, Red 33, Red 40, sucrose, tartaric acid.

Sodium content: 12 mg per teaspoon.

Indications: Temporarily relieves sore throat pain and other minor aches and pains, quiets coughs due to minor throat and bronchial irritations, relieves stuffy nose, and reduces fever.

Warnings: Keep this and all drugs out of the reach of children. In case of accidental overdose, seek professional assistance or contact a poison control center immediately. Prompt medical attention is critical for adults as well as for children even if you do not notice any signs or symptoms.

Do not exceed recommended dosage. If nervousness, dizziness, or sleeplessness occur, discontinue use and consult a doctor. Do not take this product for more than 7 days (for adults) or 5 days (for children. Do not take for sore throat pain for more than 2 days, and for fever for more than 3 days. If pain or fever persists or gets worse, if new symptoms occur, or if redness or swelling is present, consult a doctor because these could be signs of a serious condition. If sore throat is severe, persists for more than 2 days, is accompanied or followed by fever, headache, rash, nausea, or vomiting, consult a doctor promptly. If symptoms do not improve within 7 days or are accompanied by fever, consult a doctor. A persistent cough may be a sign of a serious condition. If cough persists for more than 1 week, tends to recur, or is accompanied by rash, persistent headache, fever that lasts for more than 3 days, or if new symptoms occur, consult a doctor. Do not take this product: 1) if cough is accompanied by excessive phlegm (mucus), 2) for persistent or chronic cough such as occurs with smoking, asthma or emphysema, or 3) if you have heart disease, high blood pressure, thyroid disease, diabetes, difficulty in urination due to enlargement of the prostate gland, unless directed by a doctor. As with any drug, if you are pregnant or nursing a baby, seek advice from a health professional before using this product.

Drug Interaction Precaution: Do not use this product if you are now taking a prescription monoamine oxidase inhibitor [MAOI] (certain drugs for depression, psychiatric or emotional conditions, or Parkinson's disease) or for 2 weeks after stopping the MAOI drug. If you are uncertain whether your prescription drug

Continued on next page

Information on Novartis Consumer Health, Inc., products appearing on these pages is effective as of November 1996.

Novartis—Cont.

contains an MAOI, consult a health professional before taking this product.

Dosage and Administration: Adults and children 12 and over (96+lbs)—4 teaspoons every 6 hours. Children 6 to under 12 years (48–95 lbs)—2 teaspoons every 6 hours. Children 2 to under 6 years (24–47 lbs)—1 teaspoon every 6 hours. Do not exceed 4 doses in 24 hours, or as directed by a doctor. Dosing to children under 2 years of age is to be under the direction of a physician. For convenience, a True-Dose® dosage cup is provided with each 4 fl. oz and 8 fl. oz. bottle.

Professional Labeling: The suggested dosage for pediatric patients is:

4–12 months	1.25 ml (1/4 tsp)
(12–17 lbs)	every 6 hours
12–24 months	2.5 ml (1/2 tsp)
(18–23 lbs)	every 6 hours
2–6 years	5 ml (1 tsp)
(24–47 lbs)	every 6 hours

Do not exceed 4 doses in 24 hours.

How Supplied: Triaminic Sore Throat Formula (purple), in 4 fl. oz. and 8 fl. oz. plastic bottles with tamper-evident band around child resistant cap. Grape flavored, alcohol-free.

Shown in Product Identification Guide, page 516

TRIAMINIC® SYRUP
[trī″ah-mĭn′ĭc]

Description: Each teaspoonful (5 mL) of TRIAMINIC Syrup contains: phenylpropanolamine hydrochloride, USP 6.25 mg and chlorpheniramine maleate USP 1 mg in a palatable, orange-flavored, alcohol-free liquid. **Other ingredients:** benzoic acid, edetate disodium, flavors, purified water, sodium hydroxide, sorbitol, sucrose, and Yellow 6.
Sodium content: 1 mg per teaspoon.

Indications: Temporarily relieves cold and allergy symptoms, including runny nose; stuffy nose; itching of the nose or throat; and itchy, watery eyes.

Warnings: Keep this and all drugs out of the reach of children. In case of accidental overdose, seek professional assistance or contact a poison control center immediately.
Do not exceed recommended dosage. If nervousness, dizziness or sleeplessness occur, discontinue use and consult a doctor. If symptoms do not improve within 7 days or are accompanied by fever, consult a doctor. Do not take this product: 1) if you have heart disease, high blood pressure, thyroid disease, diabetes, glaucoma, a breathing problem such as emphysema or chronic bronchitis, or difficulty in urination due to enlargement of the prostate gland, 2) if you are taking sedatives or tranquilizers, or 3) if you are presently taking another product containing phenylpropanolamine, unless directed by a doctor. May cause excitability, especially in children. May cause drowsiness; alcohol, sedatives or tranquilizers may increase the drowsiness effect. Avoid alcoholic beverages while taking this product. Use caution when driving a motor vehicle or operating machinery.
As with any drug, if you are pregnant or nursing a baby, seek the advice of a health professional before using this product.

Drug Interaction Precaution: Do not use this product if you are now taking a prescription monoamine oxidase inhibitor [MAOI] (certain drugs for depression, psychiatric or emotional conditions, or Parkinson's disease) or for 2 weeks after stopping the MAOI drug. If you are uncertain whether your prescription drug contains an MAOI, consult a health professional before taking this product.

Dosage and Administration: Adults and children 12 and over (96+ lbs)—4 teaspoons every 4 to 6 hours. Children 6 to under 12 years (48–95 lbs)—2 teaspoons every 4 to 6 hours. Do not exceed 6 doses in 24 hours, or as directed by a doctor. Dosing to children under 6 years of age is to be under the direction of a physician. For convenience, a True-Dose® dosage cup is provided with each 4 fl. oz. and 8 fl. oz. bottle.

Professional Labeling: The suggested dosage for pediatric patients is:

4–12 months	1.25 ml (1/4 tsp)
(12–17 lbs)	every 4 to 6 hours
12–24 months	2.5 ml (1/2 tsp)
(18–23 lbs)	every 4 to 6 hours
2–6 years	5 ml (1 tsp)
(24–47 lbs)	every 4 to 6 hours

Do not exceed 6 doses in 24 hours.

How Supplied: TRIAMINIC Syrup (orange), in 4 fl oz and 8 fl oz plastic bottles with tamper-evident band around child-resistant cap. Dosage cup included. Orange flavored. Alcohol-free.

Shown in Product Identification Guide, page 516

TRIAMINIC®
TRIAMINICOL® Cold & Cough
[trī″ah-mĭn′ĭ-call]

Description: Each teaspoonful (5 mL) of TRIAMINICOL Cold & Cough contains: phenylpropanolamine hydrochloride, USP 6.25 mg, dextromethorphan hydrobromide, USP 5 mg, chlorpheniramine maleate, USP 1 mg in a palatable, cherry flavored alcohol-free liquid. Other ingredients: benzoic acid, flavor, propylene glycol, purified water, Red 40, sodium chloride, sorbitol, sucrose.
Sodium content: 5 mg per teaspoon.

Indications: Temporarily relieves cold and allergy symptoms, including coughs due to minor throat and bronchial irritation, runny nose, stuffy nose, sneezing, itching of the nose or throat and itchy, watery eyes.

Warnings: Keep this and all drugs out of the reach of children. In case of accidental overdose, seek professional assistance or contact a poison control center immediately.
Do not exceed recommended dosage. If nervousness, dizziness, or sleeplessness occur, discontinue use and consult a doctor. If symptoms do not improve within 7 days or are accompanied by fever, consult a doctor. A persistent cough may be a sign of a serious condition. If cough persists for more than 1 week, tends to recur, or is accompanied by fever, rash, or persistent headache, consult a doctor. Do not take this product: 1) if cough is accompanied by excessive phlegm (mucus), 2) for persistent or chronic cough such as occurs with smoking, asthma or emphysema, 3) if you have heart disease, high blood pressure, thyroid disease, diabetes, glaucoma, a breathing problem such as emphysema or chronic bronchitis, or difficulty in urination due to enlargement of the prostate gland, 4) if you are presently taking another product containing, phenylpropanolamine, or 5) if you are taking sedatives or tranquilizers, unless directed by a doctor. May cause excitability, especially in children. May cause drowsiness; alcohol, sedatives and tranquilizers may increase the drowsiness effect. Avoid alcoholic beverages while taking this product. Use caution when driving a motor vehicle or operating machinery.
As with any drug, if you are pregnant or nursing a baby, seek the advice of a health professional before using this product.

Drug Interaction Precaution: Do not use this product if you are now taking a prescription monoamine oxidase inhibitor [MAOI] (certain drugs for depression, psychiatric or emotional conditions, or Parkinson's disease) or for 2 weeks after stopping the MAOI drug. If you are uncertain whether your prescription drug contains an MAOI, consult a health professional before taking this product.

Dosage and Administration: Adults and children 12 and over (96+ lbs)—4 teaspoons every 4 to 6 hours. Children 6 to under 12 years (48–95 lbs)—2 teaspoons every 4 to 6 hours. Unless directed by physician, do not exceed 6 doses in 24 hours or give to children under 6 years of age. For convenience, a True Dose® Dosage cup is provided with each 4 fl. oz. and 8 fl. oz. bottle.

Professional Labeling: The suggested dosage for pediatric patients is:

4–12 months	1.25 ml (1/4 tsp)
(12–17 lbs)	every 4 to 6 hours
12–24 months	2.5 ml (1/2 tsp)
(18–23 lbs)	every 4 to 6 hours
2–6 years	5 ml (1 tsp)
(24–47 lbs)	every 4 to 6 hours

Do not exceed 4 doses in 24 hours

How Supplied: TRIAMINICOL (red), in 4 fl oz and 8 fl oz plastic bottles with tamper-evident band around child-resistant cap. Dosage cup included. Cherry flavored. Alcohol-free.

Shown in Product Identification Guide, page 516

TRIAMINIC® DM SYRUP
[*trī"ah-mĭn 'ĭc*]

Description: Each teaspoonful (5 mL) of TRIAMINIC DM Syrup contains: phenylpropanolamine hydrochloride, USP 6.25 mg and dextromethorphan hydrobromide, USP 5 mg in a palatable, berry-flavored alcohol-free liquid. Other ingredients: benzoic acid, Blue 1, flavors, propylene glycol, purified water, Red 40, sodium chloride, sorbitol, sucrose.
Sodium content: 10 mg per teaspoon.

Indications: Temporarily quiets coughs due to minor throat and bronchial irritation, and relieves stuffy nose.

Warnings: Keep this and all drugs out of the reach of children. In case of accidental overdose, seek professional assistance or contact a poison control center immediately.
Do not exceed recommended dosage.
If nervousness, dizziness, or sleeplessness occur, discontinue use and consult a doctor. If symptoms do not improve within 7 days or are accompanied by fever, consult a doctor. A persistent cough may be a sign of a serious condition. If cough persists for more than 1 week, tends to recur, or is accompanied by fever, rash, or persistent headache, consult a doctor. Do not take this product: 1) if cough is accompanied by excessive phlegm (mucus), 2) for persistent or chronic cough such as occurs with smoking, asthma or emphysema, 3) if you have heart disease, high blood pressure, thyroid disease, diabetes, difficulty in urination due to enlargement of the prostate gland, or 4) if you are presently taking another product containing phenylpropanolamine, unless directed by a doctor.
As with any drug, if you are pregnant or nursing a baby, seek the advice of a health professional before using this product.

Drug Interaction Precaution: Do not use this product if you are now taking a prescription monoamine oxidase inhibitor [MAOI] (certain drugs for depression, psychiatric or emotional conditions, or Parkinson's disease), or for 2 weeks after stopping the MAOI drug. If you are uncertain whether your prescription drug contains an MAOI, consult a health professional before taking this product.

Dosage and Administration: Adults and children 12 and over (96+ lbs)—4 teaspoons every 4 hours. Children 6 to under 12 years (48–95 lbs)—2 teaspoons every 4 hours. Children 2 to under 6 years (24–47 lbs) 1 teaspoon every 4 hours. Do not exceed 6 doses in 24 hours, or as directed by a doctor. Dosing to children under 2 years of age is to be under the direction of a physician. For convenience, a True-Dose® dosage cup is provided with each 4 fl. oz. and 8 fl. oz. bottle.

Professional Labeling: The suggested dosage for pediatric patients is:

4–12 months (12–17 lbs)	1.25 ml (1/4 tsp) every 4 hours
12–24 months (18–23 lbs)	2.5 ml (1/2 tsp) every 4 hours

Do not exceed 6 doses in 24 hours.

How Supplied: TRIAMINIC DM Syrup (dark red), in 4 fl oz and 8 fl oz plastic bottles with tamper-evident band around child-resistant cap. Dosage cup included. Berry flavored. Alcohol-free.

Shown in Product Identification Guide, page 516

TRIAMINICIN® TABLETS
[*trī"ah-mĭn 'ĭ-sĭn*]

Description: Each tablet contains: acetaminophen 650 mg, phenylpropanolamine hydrochloride 25 mg, and chlorpheniramine maleate 4 mg. **Other Ingredients:** colloidal silicon dioxide, croscarmellose sodium, hydroxypropyl cellulose, lactose, magnesium stearate, methylcellulose, methylparaben, polyethylene glycol, povidone, pregelatinized starch, Red 40, titanium dioxide, Yellow 10. Sodium-free.

Indications: Temporarily relieves minor aches, pains, headache, muscular aches, and fever associated with the common cold, nasal congestion associated with sinusitis, or nasal congestion, runny nose, sneezing, itching of the nose or throat and itchy, watery eyes due to hay fever (allergic rhinitis) or other upper respiratory allergies.

Warnings: Keep this and all drugs out of the reach of children. In case of accidental overdose, seek professional assistance or contact a poison control center immediately. Prompt medical attention is critical for adults as well as children even if you do not notice any signs or symptoms.
Do not exceed recommended dosage.
If nervousness, dizziness, or sleeplessness occur, discontinue use and consult a doctor. Do not take this product for pain for more than 10 days or for fever for more than 3 days unless directed by a doctor. If pain or fever persists or gets worse, if new symptoms occur, or if redness or swelling is present, consult a doctor because these could be signs of a serious condition. May cause excitability especially in children. Do not take this product if you have heart disease, high blood pressure, thyroid disease, diabetes, glaucoma, a breathing problem such as emphysema or chronic bronchitis, difficulty in urination due to enlargement of the prostate gland, or you are now taking another product containing phenylpropanolamine, unless directed by a doctor. May cause drowsiness; alcohol, sedatives and tranquilizers may increase the drowsiness effect. Avoid alcoholic beverages while taking this product. Do not take this product if you are taking sedatives or tranquilizers, without first consulting your doctor. Use caution when driving a motor vehicle or operating machinery.
As with any drug, if you are pregnant or nursing a baby, seek the advice of a health professional before using this product.

Drug Interaction Precaution: Do not use this product if you are now taking a prescription monoamine oxidase inhibitor [MAOI] (certain drugs for depression, psychiatric or emotional conditions, or Parkinson's disease), or for 2 weeks after stopping the MAOI drug. If you are uncertain whether your prescription drug contains an MAOI, consult a health professional before taking this product.

Directions: Adults and children 12 years of age and over: 1 tablet every 4 to 6 hours, not to exceed 6 tablets in 24 hours, or as directed by a doctor. Children under 12 years of age: consult a doctor.

How Supplied: TRIAMINICIN Tablets (yellow) imprinted "DORSEY" on one side, "TRIAMINICIN" on the other, in blister packs of 12, 24 and 48, and bottles of 100 tablets.

Shown in Product Identification Guide, page 516

VITRON-C® TABLETS
[*vī'tron c*]

Active Ingredients: Each tablet contains
Ferrous fumarate, USP .... 200 mg equivalent to 66 mg elemental iron (365% U.S. RDA)
Ascorbic acid .... 125 mg (200% U.S. RDA)
Present in part as sodium ascorbate, USP

Other Ingredients: Colloidal silicon dioxide, flavor, glycine, hydroxypropyl methylcellulose, iron oxides, magnesium stearate, microcrystalline cellulose, polyethylene glycol, polysorbate 80, povidone, saccharin sodium, talc, titanium dioxide.

Indications: For iron deficiency anemia.

Directions: Adults—one or two tablets daily or as directed by a physician. Tablet may be swallowed whole, chewed or sucked like a lozenge.

Warning: Close tightly and keep out of reach of children. Contains iron, which can be harmful or fatal to children in large doses. In case of accidental overdose, seek professional assistance or contact a Poison Control Center immediately.
The treatment of any anemic condition should be under the advice and supervision of a physician. As oral iron products interfere with absorption of oral tetracycline antibiotics, these products should not be taken within two hours of each other. As with any drug, if you are pregnant or nursing a baby, seek the advice of

Continued on next page

Information on Novartis Consumer Health, Inc., products appearing on these pages is effective as of November 1996.

Novartis—Cont.

a health professional before using this product.

How Supplied: Bottles of 100 tablets. Store at room temperature 15°–30°C (59°–86°F).

P & S Laboratories

210 WEST 131st STREET
LOS ANGELES, CA 90061

See Standard Homeopathic Company.

The Parthenon Co., Inc.

3311 W. 2400 SOUTH
SALT LAKE CITY, UTAH 84119

Direct Inquiries to:
(801) 972-5184
FAX: (801) 972-4734

For Medical Emergency Contact:
Nick G. Mihalopoulos
(801) 972-5184

DEVROM® CHEWABLE TABLETS

Description: DEVROM® is a safe and effective internal (oral) deodorant. Each tablet contains 200 mg of Bismuth Subgallate powder.

Indications: DEVROM® is indicated for the control of odors from ileostomies, colostomies and fecal incontinence.

Dosage: Take one or two tablets of DEVROM® three times a day with meals or as directed by physician. Chew or swallow whole if desired.

Note: The beneficial ingredient in DEVROM® may coat the tongue which may also darken in color. This condition is harmless and temporary. Darkening of the stool is also possible and equally harmless.

Warning: This product cannot be expected to be effective in the reduction of odor due to faulty personal hygiene.
KEEP THIS BOTTLE AND ALL MEDICATION OUT OF THE REACH OF CHILDREN.

Inactive Ingredients: Mannitol, U.S.P., Lactose, N.F., Corn Starch, N.F., Confectioner's Sugar, N.F., Acacia Powder, N.F., Purified Water, U.S.P., Magnesium Stearate, N.F.
NO PHYSICIAN'S PRESCRIPTION IS NECESSARY

How Supplied: DEVROM® is supplied in bottles of 100 tablets.

DO NOT USE IF PRINTED OUTER SAFETY SEAL OR PRINTED INNER SAFETY SEAL IS BROKEN.

THE PARTHENON CO., INC./
3311 W. 2400 So./
Salt Lake City, Utah 84119

Pfizer Inc Consumer Health Care Group

235 E. 42nd Street
NY, NY 10017

Address Questions & Comments to:
Consumer Relations
(800) 723-7529

For Medical Emergencies/Information Contact:
(800) 723-7529

BENGAY® External Analgesic Products

Description: BENGAY products contain menthol in an alcohol base gel, combinations of methyl salicylate and menthol in cream and ointment bases, as well as a combination of methyl salicylate, menthol and camphor in a non-greasy cream base; all suitable for topical application.
In addition to the Original Formula Pain Relieving Ointment (methyl salicylate, 18.3%; menthol, 16%), BENGAY is offered as BENGAY Greaseless Pain Relieving Cream (methyl salicylate, 15%; menthol, 10%), an Arthritis Formula NonGreasy Pain Relieving Cream (methyl salicylate, 30%; menthol, 8%), an Ultra Strength NonGreasy Pain Relieving Cream (methyl salicylate 30%; menthol 10%; camphor 4%), and Vanishing Scent NonGreasy Pain Relieving Gel (2.5% menthol).

Action and Uses: Methyl salicylate, menthol and camphor are external analgesics which stimulate sensory receptors of warmth and/or cold. This produces a counter-irritant response which provides temporary relief of minor aches and pains of muscles and joints associated with simple backache, arthritis, strains, bruises and sprains.
Several double-blind clinical studies of BENGAY products containing menthol-methyl salicylate have shown the effectiveness of this combination in counteracting minor pain of skeletal muscle stress and arthritis.
Three studies involving a total of 102 normal subjects in which muscle soreness was experimentally induced showed statistically significant beneficial results from use of the active product vs. placebo for lowered Muscle Action Potential (spasms), greater rise in threshold of muscular pain and greater reduction in perceived muscular pain.
Six clinical studies of a total of 207 subjects suffering from minor pain due to osteoarthritis and rheumatoid arthritis showed the active product to give statistically significant beneficial results vs. placebo for greater relief of perceived pain, increased range of motion of the affected joints and increased digital dexterity. In two studies designed to measure the effect of topically applied BENGAY vs. placebo on muscular endurance, discomfort, onset of exercise pain and fatigue, 30 subjects performed a submaximal three-hour run and another 30 subjects performed a maximal treadmill run. BENGAY was found to significantly decrease the discomfort during the submaximal and maximal runs, and increase the time before onset of fatigue during the maximal run.
Applied before workouts, BENGAY relaxes tight muscles and increases circulation to make exercising more comfortable, longer.
To help reduce muscle ache and soreness after exercise, BENGAY can be applied and allowed to work before taking a shower.

Directions: Apply generously and gently massage into painful area until BENGAY disappears. Repeat 3 to 4 times daily.

Warnings: For external use only. Do not use with a heating pad. Keep away from children to avoid accidental poisoning. Do not bandage tightly. Do not swallow. If swallowed, induce vomiting and call a physician. Keep away from eyes, mucous membranes, broken or irritated skin. If skin redness or irritation develops, pain lasts for more than 10 days, or with arthritis—like conditions in children under 12, do not use and call a physician.

Shown in Product Identification Guide, page 516

BONINE® (Meclizine hydrochloride) Chewable Tablets

Action: BONINE (meclizine) is an H_1 histamine receptor blocker of the piperazine side chain group. It exhibits its action by an effect on the Central Nervous System (CNS), possibly by its ability to block muscarinic receptors in the brain.

Indications: BONINE is effective in the management of nausea, vomiting and dizziness associated with motion sickness.

Contraindications: Do not take this product, unless directed by a doctor, if you have a breathing problem such as emphysema or chronic bronchitis, or if you have glaucoma or difficulty in urination due to enlargement of the prostate gland.

Warnings: May cause drowsiness; alcohol, sedatives and tranquilizers may increase the drowsiness effect. Avoid alcoholic beverages while taking this product. Do not take this product if you are taking sedatives or tranquilizers without first consulting your doctor. Do not drive or operate dangerous machinery while taking this medication.

Usage in Children: Clinical studies establishing safety and effectiveness in children have not been done; therefore usage is not recommended in children under 12 years of age.

Usage in Pregnancy: As with any drug, if you are pregnant or nursing a baby, seek advice of a health care professional before taking this product.

Adverse Reactions: Drowsiness, dry mouth, and on rare occasions, blurred vision have been reported.

Dosage and Administration: For motion sickness, take one or two tablets of Bonine once daily, one hour before travel starts, for up to 24 hours of protection against motion sickness. The tablet can be chewed with or without water or swallowed whole with water. Thereafter, the dose may be repeated every 24 hours for the duration of the travel.

How Supplied: BONINE (meclizine HCl) is available in convenient packets of 8 chewable tablets of 25 mg. meclizine HCl.

Inactive Ingredients: FD&C Red #40, Lactose, Magnesium Stearate, Purified Siliceous Earth, Raspberry Flavor, Saccharin Sodium, Starch, Talc.

CORTIZONE-5®
Creme and Ointment

CORTIZONE FOR KIDS™ Creme
Anti-itch
(0.5% hydrocortisone)

Description: CORTIZONE-5® creme and ointment are topical anti-itch preparations containing aloe.

Active Ingredient: Hydrocortisone 0.5%.

Inactive Ingredients: Creme: Aloe Barbadensis Gel, Aluminum Sulfate, Calcium Acetate, Cetearyl Alcohol, Glycerin, Light Mineral Oil, Maltodextrin, Methylparaben, Potato Dextrin, Propylparaben, Purified Water, Sodium Cetearyl Sulfate, Sodium Lauryl Sulfate, White Petrolatum, White Wax.
Ointment: Aloe Barbadensis Extract, White Petrolatum.

Indications: CORTIZONE-5® is recommended for the temporary relief of itching associated with minor skin irritations, inflammation and rashes due to: eczema, insect bites, poison ivy, oak, sumac, soaps, detergents, cosmetics, jewelry, seborrheic dermatitis, psoriasis, external anal and genital itching. Other uses of this product should be only under the advice and supervision of a physician.

Warnings: For external use only. Avoid contact with the eyes. If condition worsens, or if symptoms persist for more than 7 days or clear up and occur again within a few days, stop use of this product and do not begin use of any other hydrocortisone product unless you have consulted a physician. Do not use in genital area if you have a vaginal discharge, consult a physician. Do not use for the treatment of diaper rash, or for the treatment of chicken pox, consult a physician. **Warnings For External Anal Itching Users:** Do not exceed the recommended daily dosage unless directed by a physician. In case of bleeding, consult a physician promptly. Do not put this product into the rectum by using fingers or any mechanical device or applicator.
Keep this and all drugs out of the reach of children. In case of accidental ingestion, seek professional assistance or contact a poison control center immediately.

Dosage and Administration: Adults and children 2 years of age and older: Apply to affected area not more than 3 to 4 times daily. Children under 2 years of age: Do not use, consult a physician.
Directions For External Anal Itching Users: Adults: When practical, cleanse the affected area with mild soap and warm water and rinse thoroughly. Gently dry by patting or blotting with toilet tissue or a soft cloth before application of this product. Children under 12 years of age: Consult a physician.

How to Store: Store at controlled room temperature 15°–30°C (59°–86°F).

How Supplied: CORTIZONE-5® creme: 1 oz. and 2 oz. tubes. CORTIZONE for KIDS™ creme: 1/2 oz. and 1 oz. tubes. CORTIZONE-5® ointment: 1 oz. tube.

Shown in Product Identification Guide, page 516

CORTIZONE–10®
Creme and Ointment

CORTIZONE-10® EXTERNAL ANAL ITCH RELIEF Creme

CORTIZONE-10® SCALP ITCH FORMULA™ Liquid
Anti-itch
(1% hydrocortisone)

Description: CORTIZONE-10® creme with aloe, ointment and liquid are topical anti-itch preparations. Maximum Strength available without a prescription.

Active Ingredient: Hydrocortisone 1%.

Inactive Ingredients: Creme: Aloe Barbadensis Gel, Aluminum Sulfate, Calcium Acetate, Cetearyl Alcohol, Glycerin, Light Mineral Oil, Maltodextrin, Methylparaben, Potato Dextrin, Propylparaben, Purified Water, Sodium Cetearyl Sulfate, Sodium Lauryl Sulfate, White Petrolatum, White Wax.
Ointment: White Petrolatum.
Liquid: Benzyl Alcohol, Propylene Glycol, Purified Water, SD Alcohol 40-2 (60% v/v)

Indications: Cortizone-10® is recommended for the temporary relief of itching associated with minor skin irritations, inflammation and rashes due to: eczema, insect bites, poison ivy, oak, sumac, soaps, detergents, cosmetics, jewelry, seborrheic dermatitis, psoriasis, external anal and genital itching. Other uses of this product should be only under the advice and supervision of a physician.

Warnings: For external use only. Avoid contact with the eyes. If condition worsens, or if symptoms persist for more than 7 days or clear up and occur again within a few days, stop use of this product and do not begin use of any other hydrocortisone product unless you have consulted a physician. Do not use in genital area if you have a vaginal discharge, consult a physician. Do not use for the treatment of diaper rash, consult a physician. **Warnings For External Anal Itching Users:** Do not exceed the recommended daily dosage unless directed by a physician. In case of bleeding, consult a physician promptly. Do not put this product into the rectum by using fingers or any mechanical device or applicator.
Keep this and all drugs out of the reach of children. In case of accidental ingestion, seek professional assistance or contact a poison control center immediately.

Dosage and Administration: Adults and children 2 years of age and older: Apply to affected area not more than 3 to 4 times daily. Children under 2 years of age: Do not use, consult a physician.

Directions For External Anal Itching Users: Adults: When practical, cleanse the affected area with mild soap and warm water. Rinse thoroughly. Gently dry by patting or blotting with toilet tissue or a soft cloth before application of this product. Children under 12 years of age: Consult a physician.

How to Store: Store at controlled room temperature 15°–30°C (59°–86°F).

How Supplied: CORTIZONE-10® creme: 1 oz. and 2 oz. tubes. CORTIZONE-10® ointment: 1 oz. and 2 oz. tubes. CORTIZONE-10® External Anal Itch Relief creme: 1 oz. tube. CORTIZONE-10® Scalp Itch Formula™ liquid: 1.5 fl. oz.

Shown in Product Identification Guide, page 516

DESITIN® CORNSTARCH BABY POWDER
(with Zinc Oxide)

Description: Desitin Cornstarch Baby Powder combines zinc oxide (10%) with topical starch (cornstarch) for topical application. Also contains: fragrance and tribasic calcium phosphate.

Actions and Uses: Desitin Cornstarch Baby Powder with zinc oxide and topical starch (cornstarch) is designed to protect from wetness, help prevent and treat diaper rash, and other minor skin irritations. It offers all the benefits of a talc-free, absorbent cornstarch powder, but with the addition of zinc oxide, the same protective ingredient found in Desitin Ointment. Cornstarch also prevents friction. Zinc oxide provides an additional physical barrier by forming a protective coating over the skin or mucous membranes which serves to reduce further effects of irritants on affected areas.

Directions: Prevention: Change wet and soiled diapers promptly, cleanse the diaper area, and allow to dry.

Continued on next page

Pfizer Inc.—Cont.

Apply powder close to the body away from child's face. Carefully shake the powder into the diaper or into the hand and apply to diaper area. Apply liberally as often as necessary with each diaper change, especially at bedtime, or anytime when exposure to wet diapers may be prolonged.

Treatment: Use liberally in all body creases, and whenever chafing, prickly heat or other minor skin irritations occur.

Warning: For external use only. Do not use on broken skin. Avoid contact with eyes. Keep powder away from child's face to avoid inhalation. If diaper rash worsens or does not improve within 7 days, consult a doctor.

How Supplied: Desitin Cornstarch Baby Powder with Zinc Oxide is available in 14 ounce (397g) containers with sifter-top caps.

Shown in Product Identification Guide, page 516

DAILY CARE® from DESITIN®
Diaper Rash Prevention Ointment Skin Protectant (10% Zinc Oxide)

Description: Daily Care from DESITIN contains Zinc Oxide (10%) in a white petrolatum base suitable for topical application. Also contains: cyclomethicone, dimethicone, fragrance, methylparaben, mineral oil, mineral wax, propylparaben, sodium borate, sorbitan sesquioleate, white wax and purified water.

Actions and Uses: Daily Care helps treat and prevent diaper rash. It helps seal out irritating wetness that can cause diaper rash by creating a protective wetness barrier at every diaper change. Daily Care has a pleasant formula that's easy to apply, easy to clean up and has a fresh scent.

Directions: Prevention—To help prevent diaper rash, change wet and soiled diaper promptly, cleanse the diaper area and allow to dry. Apply Daily Care ointment liberally as often as necessary with each diaper change—especially at bedtime or anytime when exposure to a wet diaper may be prolonged.
Treatment—At the first sign of redness or minor skin irritation, apply Daily Care liberally over the affected area and repeat as necessary. After the rash has cleared, continue to use Daily Care at every diaper change to help protect skin from future diaper rash.

Warnings: For external use only. Avoid contact with eyes. If condition worsens or does not improve within 7 days, consult your doctor. Keep out of reach of children. In case of accidental ingestion, seek professional assistance or contact a Poison Control Center immediately. Store between 2 and 30°C (36 and 86°F).

How Supplied: Daily Care Ointment is available in 2 oz. (57g) and 4 oz. (113g) tubes.

Shown in Product Identification Guide, page 516

DESITIN® OINTMENT

Description: Desitin Ointment combines Zinc Oxide (40%) with Cod Liver Oil in a petrolatum-lanolin base suitable for topical application. Also contains: BHA, fragrances, methylparaben, talc and water.

Actions and Uses: Desitin Ointment is designed to provide relief of diaper rash, superficial wounds and burns, and other minor skin irritations. It helps prevent incidents of diaper rash, protects against urine and other irritants, and soothes chafed skin.
Relief and protection is afforded by Zinc Oxide and Cod Liver Oil. These ingredients together with the petrolatum-lanolin base provide a physical barrier by forming a protective coating over skin or mucous membranes which serves to reduce further effects of irritants on the affected area and relieves burning, pain or itch produced by them.
Several studies have shown the effectiveness of Desitin Ointment in the relief and prevention of diaper rash.
Two clinical studies involving 90 infants demonstrated the effectiveness of Desitin Ointment in curing diaper rash. The diaper rash area was treated with Desitin Ointment at each diaper change for a period of 24 hours, while the untreated site served as controls. A significant reduction was noted in the severity and area of diaper dermatitis on the treated area.
Ninety-seven (97) babies participated in a 12-week study to show that Desitin Ointment helps prevent diaper rash. Approximately half of the infants (49) were treated with Desitin Ointment on a regular daily basis. The other half (48) received the ointment as necessary to treat any diaper rash which occurred. The incidence as well as the severity of diaper rash was significantly less among the babies using the ointment on a regular daily basis.
In a comparative study of the efficacy of Desitin Ointment vs. a baby powder, forty-five (45) babies were observed for a total of eight (8) weeks. Results support the conclusion that Desitin Ointment is a better prophylactic against diaper rash than the baby powder.
In another study, Desitin was found to be dramatically more effective in reducing the severity of medically diagnosed diaper rash than a commercially available diaper rash product in which only anhydrous lanolin and petrolatum were listed as ingredients. Fifty (50) infants participated in the study, half of whom were treated with Desitin and half with the other product. In the group (25) treated with Desitin, seventeen (17) infants showed significant improvement within 10 hours which increased to twenty-three improved infants within 24 hours. Of the group (25) treated with the other product, only three showed improvement at ten hours with a total of four improved within twenty-four hours. These results are statistically valid to conclude that Desitin Ointment reduces severity of diaper rash within ten hours.
Several other studies show that Desitin Ointment helps relieve other skin disorders, such as contact dermatitis.

Directions: Prevention: To prevent diaper rash, apply Desitin Ointment to the diaper area—especially at bedtime when exposure to wet diapers may be prolonged.
Treatment: If diaper rash is present, or at the first sign of redness, minor skin irritation or chafing, simply apply Desitin Ointment three or four times daily as needed. In superficial noninfected surface wounds and minor burns, apply a thin layer of Desitin Ointment, using a gauze dressing, if necessary. For external use only.

How Supplied: Desitin Ointment is available in 1 ounce (28g), 2 ounce (57g), and 4 ounce (114g) tubes, and 9 ounce (255g) and 1 lb. (454g) jars.

Shown in Product Identification Guide, page 516

HEMORID®
Hemorrhoidal Creme, Ointment, and Suppositories

Description: HEMORID® is available in Creme, Ointment and Suppositories

Ingredients:
Creme: Active Ingredients: White Petrolatum 30%, Mineral Oil 20%, Pramoxine Hydrochloride 1%, Phenylephrine Hydrochloride 0.25%. Inactive Ingredients: Aloe Barbadensis Gel, Cetyl Alcohol, Methylparaben, Polysorbate 80, PPG-15 Stearyl Ether, Propylparaben, Purified Water, Sorbitan Monooleate, Stearyl Alcohol.
Ointment: Active Ingredients: White Petrolatum 82.15%, Light Mineral Oil 12.5%, Pramoxine Hydrochloride 1%, Phenylephrine Hydrochloride 0.25%. Inactive Ingredients: Aloe Barbadensis Extract. White Wax.
Suppositories: Active Ingredients: Zinc Oxide USP 11%, Phenylephrine Hydrochloride USP 0.25%, Hard Fat 88.25%.
Inactive Ingredient: Aloe Barbadensis Extract

Indications:
Creme/Ointment: Temporarily shrinks swollen hemorrhoidal tissue and helps relieve the local pain, burning, itching and discomfort associated with hemorrhoids or anorectal inflammation.
Suppositories: Temporarily shrinks swollen hemorrhoidal tissue and helps relieve the local itching, discomfort, and burning associated with hemorrhoids or anorectal inflammation.

Warnings:

Creme/Ointment: Do not use in the eyes or nose. If condition worsens or does not improve within 7 days, consult a physician. Do not exceed the recommended daily dosage, unless directed by a physician. Do not apply to large areas of the body. In case of bleeding, consult a physician promptly. Do not put this product into the rectum by using fingers or any mechanical device or applicator. Certain persons can develop allergic reactions to ingredients in this product. If the symptom being treated does not subside or if redness, irritation, swelling, pain or other symptoms develop or increase, discontinue use and consult a physician. Do not use this product if you have heart disease, high blood pressure, thyroid disease, diabetes or difficulty in urination due to enlargement of the prostate gland, unless directed by a physician. As with any drug, if you are pregnant or nursing a baby, seek the advice of a health professional before using this product. Drug Interaction Precaution: Do not use this product if you are presently taking a prescription drug for high blood pressure or depression, without first consulting your physician. Keep this and all drugs out of the reach of children. In case of accidental ingestion, seek professional assistance or contact a poison control center immediately.

Suppositories: If condition worsens or does not improve within 7 days, consult a physician. Do not exceed the recommended daily dosage, unless directed by a physician. In case of bleeding, consult a physician promptly. Do not use this product if you have heart disease, high blood pressure, thyroid disease, diabetes or difficulty in urination due to enlargement of the prostate gland, unless directed by a physician. As with any drug, if you are pregnant or nursing a baby, seek the advice of a health professional before using this product. Drug Interaction Precaution: Do not use this product if you are presently taking a prescription drug for high blood pressure or depression, without first consulting your physician. Keep this and all drugs out of the reach of children. In case of accidental ingestion, seek professional assistance or contact a poison control center immediately.

Dosage and Administration:

Creme/Ointment: **Adults:** When practical, cleanse the affected area with mild soap and warm water and rinse thoroughly. Gently dry by patting or blotting with toilet tissue or a soft cloth before application of this product. Apply externally to the affected area up to 4 times daily. **Children under 12 years of age:** Consult a physician.

Suppositories: Adults: When practical, cleanse the affected area with mild soap and warm water and rinse thoroughly. Gently dry by patting or blotting with toilet tissue or a soft cloth before application of this product. Detach one suppository from strip of suppositories. Holding one suppository upright, carefully remove the wrapper by peeling down both sides starting from the pointed end. Insert into the rectum pointed end first. Avoid excessive handling of the suppository. May be used up to 4 times daily. **Children under 12 years of age:** Consult a physician.

How to Store: Store at controlled room temperature 15°-30°C (59°–86°F).

How Supplied: HEMORID® Creme: 1 oz. tube. HEMORID® Ointment: 1 oz. tube. HEMORID® Suppositories: 12's.

Shown in Product Identification Guide, page 516

OCUHIST®
Eye Allergy Relief
Itching & Redness Reliever Eye Drops
ANTIHISTAMINE & DECONGESTANT

OcuHist is an antihistamine/decongestant eye drop, clinically proven to temporarily relieve itching and redness of the eye.

Indications: For the temporary relief of itching and redness of the eye due to pollen, ragweed, grass, animal hair and dander.

Directions: Adults and Children 6 years of age or older: Place 1 or 2 drops in the affected eye(s) up to four times a day. Some users may experience a brief tingling sensation.

Active Ingredients: pheniramine maleate 0.3%, naphazoline hydrochloride 0.025%.

Inactive Ingredients: boric acid and sodium borate buffer system preserved with benzalkonium chloride (0.01%) and edetate disodium (0.1%), sodium hydroxide and/or hydrochloric acid (to adjust pH) and purified water. The solution has a pH of 5.5–6.5 and a tonicity of 245—305 mOsm/Kg.

Warnings: If you experience eye pain, changes in vision, continued redness or irritation of the eye, or if the condition worsens or persists for more than 72 hours, discontinue use and consult a physician.

Do not use this product if you have heart disease, high blood pressure, difficulty in urination due to enlargement of the prostate gland or narrow angle glaucoma unless directed by a physician. Accidental oral ingestion in infants and children may lead to coma and marked reduction in body temperature.

To avoid contamination, do not touch tip of container to any surface. Replace cap after using. Do not use if solution changes color or becomes cloudy.

Remove contact lenses before using.

Overuse of this product may produce increased redness of the eye.

Use before expiration date marked on the carton or bottle.

Keep this and all drugs out of the reach of children.

Store between 2° and 30°C (36° and 86°F).

Parents Note: Before using with children under 6 years of age, consult your physician. Keep this and all drugs out of the reach of children. In case of accidental ingestion, seek professional assistance or contact a Poison Control Center immediately.

Caution: Do not use if Pfizer-imprinted neckband on bottle is broken or missing.

Distributed By:

CONSUMER HEALTH CARE GROUP, PFIZER INC, NEW YORK, NEW YORK 10017

Shown in Product Indentification Guide, page 517

RHEABAN® Maximum Strength FAST ACTING CAPLETS
[rē'ăban]
(attapulgite)

Description: Maximum Strength Rheaban is an anti-diarrheal medication containing activated attapulgite and is offered in caplet form.

Each white Rheaban caplets contains 750 mg. of colloidal activated attapulgite. Rheaban provides the maximum level of medication when taken as directed.

Rheaban contains no narcotics, opiates or other habit-forming drugs.

Actions and Uses: Rheaban is indicated for relief of diarrhea and the cramps and pains associated with it. Attapulgite, which has been activated by thermal treatment, is a highly sorptive substance which absorbs nutrients and digestive enzymes as well as noxious gases, irritants, toxins and some bacteria and viruses that are common causes of diarrhea.

In clinical studies to show the effectiveness in relieving diarrhea and its symptoms, 100 subjects suffering from acute gastroenteritis with diarrhea participated in a double-blind comparison of Rheaban to a placebo. Patients treated with the attapulgite product showed significantly improved relief of diarrhea and its symptoms versus the placebo.

Dosage and Administration:
CAPLETS

Adults—2 caplets after initial bowel movement, 2 caplets after each subsequent bowel movement. For a maximum of 12 caplets in 24 hours.

Children 6 to 12 years—1 caplet after initial bowel movement, 1 caplet after each subsequent bowel movement. For a maximum of 6 caplets in 24 hours, or as directed by a physician.

Warnings: Do not exceed 12 caplets in 24 hours. Swallow caplets with water; do not chew. Do not use for more than two days, or in the presence of high fever. Caplets should not be used for infants or children under 6 years of age unless directed by physician. If diarrhea persists, consult a physician.

How Supplied:
Caplets—Box of 12 caplets.

Inactive Ingredients: Carnauba Wax, Croscarmellose Sodium, D&C Yellow No.

Continued on next page

Pfizer Inc.—Cont.

10 Aluminum Lake, FD&C Blue No. 1 Aluminum Lake, Hydroxypropyl Cellulose, Hydroxypropyl Methylcellulose, Methylparaben, Pectin, Pharmaceutical Glaze, Propylene Glycol, Propylparaben, Sucrose, Talc, Titanium Dioxide, Zinc Stearate.

RID® Spray
Lice Control Spray

PRODUCT OVERVIEW

Key Facts: Rid Lice Control Spray is a pediculicide spray for controlling lice and louse eggs on inanimate objects, to help prevent reinfestation. It contains a highly active synthetic pyrethroid that kills lice and their eggs on inanimate objects.

Major Uses: Rid Lice Control Spray effectively kills lice and louse eggs on garments, bedding, furniture and other inanimate objects that cannot be either laundered or dry cleaned.

Safety Information: Rid Lice Control Spray is intended for use on inanimate objects only; it is not for use on humans or animals. It is harmful if swallowed. It should not be sprayed in the eyes or on the skin and should not be inhaled. The product should be used only in well ventilated areas; room(s) should be vacated after treatment and ventilated before reoccupying.

PRESCRIBING INFORMATION

RID® Spray
Lice Control Spray

THIS PRODUCT IS NOT FOR USE ON HUMANS OR ANIMALS

Active Ingredient:

Permethrin*	0.5%
Inert Ingredients	99.5%
	100.00%

*(3-phenoxyphenol)methyl ± cis/trans 3-(2,2-dichloroethenyl) 2,2-dimethylcyclopropane-carboxylate, cis/trans ratio: Minimum 35% (± cis) and maximum 65% (± trans).

Actions: A highly active synthetic pyrethroid for the control of lice and louse eggs on garments, bedding, furniture and other inanimate objects.

Warnings: Avoid contamination of feed and foodstuffs. Remove pets and birds and cover fish aquaria before space spraying on surface applications. HARMFUL IF SWALLOWED. This product is not for use on humans or animals. If lice infestations should occur on humans, consult either your physician or pharmacist for a product for use on humans.

Physical And Chemical Hazards: Contents under pressure. Do not use or store near heat or open flame. Do not puncture or incinerate container. Exposure to temperatures above 130° F (54° C) may cause bursting. Store in cool, dry area. Do not store below 32° F (0° C).

CAUTION: Avoid spraying in eyes. Avoid breathing spray mist. Use only in well ventilated areas. Avoid contact with skin. In case of contact wash immediately with soap and water. Vacate room after treatment and ventilate before reoccupying.

Statement of Practical Treatment: If inhaled: Remove affected person to fresh air. Apply artifical respiration if indicated. Get immediate medical attention.

If in eyes: Flush with plenty of water. Contact physician if irritation persists.

If on skin: Wash affected areas immediately with soap and water.

Direction For Use: It is a violation of Federal law to use this product in a manner inconsistent with its labeling.

Shake well before using.

To kill lice and louse eggs: Spray in an inconspicuous area to test for possible staining or discoloration. Inspect again after drying, then proceed to spray entire area to be treated. Hold container upright with nozzle away from you. Depress valve and spray from a distance of 8 to 10 inches.

Spray each square foot for 3 seconds. Spray only those garments, parts of bedding, including mattresses and furniture that cannot be either laundered or dry cleaned.

Allow all sprayed articles to dry thoroughly before use.

Buyer assumes all risks of use, storage or handling of this material not in strict accordance with directions given herewith.

Disposal Of Container: Wrap container in several layers of newspaper and dispose of in trash. Do not incinerate or puncture.

How Supplied: 5 ounce aerosol can. Also available in combination with RID® Lice Killing Shampoo as the RID® Lice Elimination Kit.

MAXIMUM STRENGTH RID®
Lice Killing Shampoo

PRODUCT OVERVIEW

Key Facts: Maximum Strength Rid® Lice Killing Shampoo contains a liquid pediculicide effective against head, body, and pubic (crab) lice and their eggs. The active ingredients in Rid® are pyrethrum extract and piperonyl butoxide, technical which attack the louse's nervous system. Piperonyl butoxide is a synergist. The pyrethrum extract in Rid® rinses out completely after treatment, and is poorly absorbed through the skin. Each Maximum Strength Rid® Lice Killing Shampoo package also contains a patented nit (egg) removal comb with an exclusive handle design that provides gentle combing action to remove the nits (eggs).**Major Uses:** Rid® has proved to be clinically effective in treating infestations of head lice and their eggs. It is also effective in the treatment of infestations of body lice, pubic (crab) lice and their eggs.

Safety Information: Rid® should be used with caution by ragweed sensitized persons. It is intended for external use on humans only and is harmful if swallowed. It should not be inhaled or allowed to come in contact with the eyes or mucous membranes. Contamination of feed or foodstuffs should be avoided.

PRESCRIBING INFORMATION

MAXIMUM STRENGTH RID®
Lice Killing Shampoo

Description: Rid® contains a liquid pediculicide whose active ingredients are pyrethrum extract 0.33% and piperonyl butoxide, technical 4.00%, equivalent to min. 3.2% (butylcarbityl) (6-propylpiperonyl) ether and 0.8% related compounds. Inert ingredients (95.67%) are: C13–C14 isoparaffin, fragrance, isopropyl alcohol, PEG-25 hydrogenated castor oil, water, xanthan gum.

Actions: Rid® kills head lice (Pediculus humanus capitis), body lice (Pediculus humanus humanus), and pubic (crab) lice (Phthirus pubis), and their eggs. The pyrethrum extract acts as a contact poison and affects the parasite's nervous system, resulting in paralysis and death. The efficacy of the pyrethrum extract is enhanced by a synergist, piperonyl butoxide. The pyrethrum extract rinses out completely after treatment and is not designed to leave long-acting residues. In addition, pyrethrum extract is poorly absorbed through the skin. Of the relatively minor amounts that are absorbed, they are rapidly metabolized to water-soluble compounds and eliminated from the body without ill effects.

Indications: For the treatment of head, pubic (crab), and body lice.

Warnings: Use with caution on persons allergic to ragweed. For external use only. Do not use near the eyes or permit contact with mucous membranes, such as inside the nose, mouth, or vagina, as irritation may occur. Keep out of eyes when rinsing hair. Adults and children: Close eyes tightly and do not open eyes until product is completely rinsed out. Also, protect children's eyes with washcloth, towel, or other suitable material, or by a similar method. If product gets into the eyes, immediately flush with water. If skin irritation or infection is present or develops, discontinue use and consult a doctor. Consult a doctor if infestation of eyebrows or eyelashes occurs.

Storage and Disposal: Do not store below 32°F (0°C) or above 120°F (49° C). Do not reuse empty container. Wrap in several layers of newspaper and discard in trash.

Dosage And Administration: Apply to affected area until all hair is thoroughly wet with product. Allow product to remain on area for 10 minutes but not longer. Add sufficient warm water to form a lather and shampoo as usual. Rinse thoroughly. A fine tooth comb or special lice/nit removing comb may be used to help remove dead lice or their eggs (nits) from hair. A second treatment must be done in 7 to 10 days to kill any newly hatched lice. Since there is no immunity from lice, personal cleanliness and the avoidance of infested persons and their bedding and clothes will aid in preventing infestation. These additional steps are important in order to minimize the chance of possible reinfestation.

- Inspect all family members daily for at least two weeks, and if they become infested, treat with Rid®.
- Wash all personal clothing, nightwear and bedding of any infested person in hot water, at least 130°F, or by dry cleaning.
- Soak all personal articles such as combs, brushes, etc. in Rid® solution or hot, soapy water (at least 130°F) for ten minutes. Inspect and rinse thoroughly before use.
- Tell children not to use any borrowed combs or brushes, nor to wear anyone else's clothes.

LICE WHICH INFEST HUMANS

Head Lice: Head lice live on the scalp and lay small white eggs (nits) on the hair shaft close to the scalp. The nits are most easily found on the nape of the neck or behind the ears. All personal headgear, scarfs, coats, and bed linen should be disinfected by machine washing in hot water and drying, using the hot cycle of a dryer for at least 20 minutes. Personal articles of clothing or bedding that cannot be washed may be dry-cleaned, sealed in a plastic bag for a period of about 2 weeks, or sprayed with a product specifically designed for this purpose. Personal combs and brushes may be disinfected by soaking in hot water (above 130°F) for 5 to 10 minutes. Thorough vacuuming of rooms inhabited by infected patients is recommended.

Pubic (Crab) Lice: Pubic lice may be transmitted by sexual contact; therefore, sexual partners should be treated simultaneously to avoid reinfestation. The lice are very small and look almost like brown or gray dots on the skin. Pubic lice usually cause intense itching and lay small white eggs (nits) on the hair shaft generally close to the skin surface. In hairy individuals, pubic lice may be present on the short hairs of the thighs and trunk, underarms, and occasionally on the beard and mustache. Underwear should be disinfected by machine washing in hot water, then drying, using the hot cycle for at least 20 minutes.

Body Lice: Body lice and their eggs are generally found in the seams of clothing, particularly in the waistline and armpit area. They move to the skin to feed, then return to the seams of the clothing where they lay their eggs. Clothing worn and not laundered before treatment should be disinfected by the same procedure as described for head lice, except that sealing clothing in a plastic bag is not recommended because the nits (eggs) from these lice can remain dormant for a period of up to 30 days.

How Supplied: In 2, 4 and 8 fl. oz. plastic bottles. Exclusive nit (egg) removal comb that removes all nits (eggs) and patient instruction booklet (English and Spanish) are included in each package of Rid®. Also available in combination with Rid® Lice Control Spray as the Rid® Lice Elimination Kit.

MAXIMUM STRENGTH UNISOM SLEEPGELS
Nighttime Sleep Aid

Description: Maximum Strength Unisom SleepGels are liquid-filled, blue soft gelatin capsules.

Active Ingredient: Diphenhydramine Hydrochloride 50 mg.

Inactive Ingredients: FD&C Blue No. 1, Gelatin, Glycerin, Pharmaceutical Glaze, Polyethylene Glycol, Propylene Glycol, Purified Water, Sorbitol, Titanium Dioxide.

Indications: Helps to reduce difficulty falling asleep.

Action: Diphenhydramine Hydrochloride is an ethanolamine antihistamine with anticholinergic and sedative effects.

Administration and Dosage: Adults and children 12 years of age and over: Oral dosage is one softgel (50 mg.) at bedtime if needed, or as directed by a doctor.

Warnings: Do not take this product if you have asthma, glaucoma, emphysema, chronic pulmonary disease, shortness of breath, difficulty in breathing or difficulty in urination due to enlargement of the prostate gland unless directed by a doctor. Do not take this product if pregnant or nursing a baby.

- Do not give to children under 12 years of age.
- If sleeplessness persists continuously for more than two weeks, consult your doctor. Insomnia may be a symptom of serious underlying medical illness.
- Avoid alcoholic beverages while taking this product. Do not take this product if you are taking sedatives or tranquilizers, without first consulting your doctor.
- Keep this and all drugs out of the reach of children.
- In case of accidental overdose, seek professional assistance or contact a Poison Control Center immediately.

Drug Interaction: Monoamine oxidase (MAO) inhibitors prolong and intensify the anticholinergic effects of antihistamines. The CNS depressant effect is heightened by alcohol and other CNS depressant drugs.

Symptoms of Oral Overdosage: Antihistamine overdosage reactions may vary from central nervous system depression to stimulation. Stimulation is particularly likely in children. Atropine-like signs and symptoms, such as dry mouth, fixed and dilated pupils, flushing, and gastrointestinal symptoms, may also occur.

Attention: Use only if softgel blister seals are unbroken.

How Supplied: Boxes of 16 liquid filled softgels in child resistant blisters and boxes of 8 with non-child resistant packaging. Also in a 32 count easy to open child resistant bottle.
Store between 15° and 30°C (59° and 86°F)

UNISOM®
[yu 'na-som]
Nighttime Sleep Aid
(doxylamine succinate)

PRODUCT OVERVIEW

Key Facts: Unisom is an ethanolamine antihistamine (doxylamine) which characteristically shows a high incidence of sedation. It produces a reduced latency to end of wakefulness and early onset of sleep.

Major Uses: Unisom has been shown to be clinically effective as a sleep aid when 1 tablet is given 30 minutes before retiring.

Safety Information: Unisom is contraindicated in pregnancy and nursing mothers. It is also contraindicated in patients with asthma, glaucoma, and enlargement of the prostate. Caution should be used if taken when alcohol is being consumed. Caution is also indicated when taken concurrently with other medications due to the anticholinergic properties of antihistamines.

PRESCRIBING INFORMATION

UNISOM®
[yu 'na-som]
Nighttime Sleep Aid
(doxylamine succinate)

Description: Pale blue oval scored tablets containing 25 mg. of doxylamine succinate, 2-[α-(2-dimethylaminoethoxy)α-methylbenzyl]pyridine succinate.

Action and Uses: Doxylamine succinate is an antihistamine of the ethanolamine class, which characteristically shows a high incidence of sedation. In a comparative clinical study of over 20 antihistamines on more than 3000 subjects, doxylamine succinate 25 mg. was one of the three most sedating antihistamines, producing a significantly reduced latency to end of wakefulness and comparing favorably with established hypnotic drugs such as secobarbital and pentobarbital in sedation activity. It was chosen as the antihistamine, based on dosage, causing the earliest onset of sleep. In another clinical study, doxylamine succinate 25 mg. scored better than secobarbital 100 mg. as a nighttime hypnotic. Two additional, identical clinical studies, involving a total of 121 subjects demon-

Continued on next page

Pfizer Inc.—Cont.

strated that doxylamine succinate 25 mg. reduced the sleep latency period by a third, compared to placebo. Duration of sleep was 26.6% longer with doxylamine succinate, and the quality of sleep was rated higher with the drug than with placebo. An EEG study on 6 subjects confirmed the results of these studies. In yet another study, no statistically significant difference was found between doxylamine succinate and flurazepam in the average time required for 200 patients with mild to moderate insomnia to fall asleep over 5 nights following a nightly dose of doxylamine succinate 25 mg. or flurazepam 30 mg., nor was any statistically significant difference found in the total time the 200 patients slept. Patients on doxylamine succinate awoke an average of 1.2 times per night while those on flurazepam awoke an average of 0.9 times per night. In either case the patients awoke rested the following morning. On a rating scale of 1 to 5, doxylamine succinate was given a 3.0, flurazepam a 3.4 by patients rating the degree of restfulness provided by their medication (5 represents "very well rested"). Although statistically significant, the difference between doxylamine succinate 25 mg. and flurazepam 30 mg. in the number of awakenings and degree of restfulness is clinically insignificant.

Administration and Dosage: One tablet 30 minutes before retiring. Not for children under 12 years of age.

Side Effects: Occasional anticholinergic effects may be seen.

Precautions: Unisom® should be taken only at bedtime.

Contraindications: Do not take this product, unless directed by a doctor, if you have a breathing problem such as emphysema or chronic bronchitis, or if you have glaucoma or difficulty in urination due to enlargement of the prostate gland. This product should not be taken by pregnant women or those who are nursing a baby.

Warnings: Should be taken with caution if alcohol is being consumed. Product should not be taken if patient is concurrently on any other drug, without prior consultation with physician. Should not be taken for longer than two weeks unless approved by physician.

How Supplied: Boxes of 8, 16, 32 or 48 tablets.

Inactive Ingredients: Dibasic Calcium Phosphate, FD&C Blue #1 Aluminum Lake, Magnesium Stearate, Microcrystalline Cellulose, Sodium Starch Glycolate.

UNISOM® WITH PAIN RELIEF®

[yu 'na-som]

Nighttime Sleep Aid and Pain Reliever

PRODUCT OVERVIEW

Key Facts: Unisom With Pain Relief (diphenhydramine sleep aid/acetaminophen pain relief formula) is a product with a dual antihistamine sleep aid/analgesic action to utilize the sedative effects of an antihistamine and relieve mild to moderate pain that may disturb normal sleep patterns. If patients have difficulty in falling asleep but are not experiencing pain at the same time, regular Unisom Sleep Aid which contains doxylamine succinate or Maximum Strength Unisom SleepGels which contains diphenhydramine is indicated.

Major Uses: One Unisom With Pain Relief is indicated 30 minutes before retiring to help reduce difficulty in falling asleep while relieving accompanying minor aches and pains, such as headache, muscle aches or menstrual discomfort.

Safety Information: Do not take this product, unless directed by a doctor, if you have a breathing problem such as emphysema or chronic bronchitis, or if you have glaucoma or difficulty in urination due to enlargement of the prostate gland. Unisom With Pain Relief is contraindicated in pregnancy or in nursing mothers. Excessive dosing may lead to liver damage. Product is intended for patients 12 years and older. Alcoholic beverages should be avoided while taking this product. This product should not be taken without first consulting a physician if sedatives or tranquilizers are being taken.

PRESCRIBING INFORMATION

UNISOM WITH PAIN RELIEF®

[yu 'na-som]

Nighttime Sleep Aid and Pain Reliever

Description: Unisom With Pain Relief® is a pale blue, capsule-shaped, coated tablet.

Active Ingredients: 650 mg. acetaminophen and 50 mg. diphenhydramine HCl per tablet.

Indications: Unisom With Pain Relief (diphenhydramine sleep aid formula) is indicated to help reduce difficulty in falling asleep while relieving accompanying minor aches and pains such as headache, muscle ache or menstrual discomfort. If there is difficulty in falling asleep, but pain is not being experienced at the same time, regular Unisom sleep aid is indicated which contains doxylamine succinate as its active ingredient.

Administration and Dosage: One tablet at bedtime if needed, or as directed by a physician.

Contraindications: Do not take this product, unless directed by a doctor, if you have a breathing problem such as emphysema or chronic bronchitis, or if you have glaucoma or difficulty in urination due to enlargement of the prostate gland. Do not take this product if pregnant or nursing a baby.

Do not take this product for treatment of arthritis except under the advice and supervision of a physican.

Warnings: Do not exceed recommended dosage because severe liver damage may occur. If symptoms persist continuously for more than ten days, consult your physician. Insomnia may be a symptom of serious underlying medical illness. Avoid alcoholic beverages while taking this product. Do not take this product if you are taking sedatives or tranquilizers, without first consulting your doctor. For adults only. Do not give to children under 12 years of age. Keep this and all medications out of reach of children. IN CASE OF ACCIDENTAL OVERDOSE SEEK PROFESSIONAL ADVICE OR CONTACT A POISON CONTROL CENTER IMMEDIATELY.

Caution: This product contains an antihistamine and will cause drowsiness. It should be used only at bedtime.

Drug Interaction: Monoamine oxidase (MAO) inhibitors prolong and intensify the anticholinergic effects of antihistamines. The CNS depressant effect is heightened by alcohol and other CNS depressant drugs.

Attention: Use only if tablet blister seals are unbroken. Child resistant packaging.

How Supplied: Boxes of 8 and 16 tablets in child resistant blisters.

Inactive Ingredients: Corn starch, FD&C Blue #1 Aluminum Lake, FD&C Blue #2 Aluminum Lake, Hydroxypropyl Methylcellulose, Magnesium Stearate, Polyethylene Glycol, Polysorbate 80, Povidone, Stearic Acid, Titanium Dioxide.

VISINE® L. R.™

Oxymetazoline Hydrochloride/ Redness Reliever Eye Drops

Description: Visine L. R. is a sterile, isotonic, buffered ophthalmic solution containing oxymetazoline hydrochloride 0.025%, boric acid, sodium borate, sodium chloride and purified water. It is preserved with benzalkonium chloride 0.01% and edetate disodium 0.1%.

Visine L. R. is produced by a process that assures sterility.

Indications: Visine L. R. is a decongestant ophthalmic solution designed for the relief of redness of the eye due to minor eye irritations. Visine L. R. is specially formulated to relieve redness of the eye in minutes with effective relief that lasts up to 6 hours.

Directions: Adults and children 6 years of age or older: Place 1 or 2 drops in the affected eye(s). This may be repeated as needed every 6 hours or as directed by a physician.

Warnings: If you experience eye pain, changes in vision, continued redness or irritation of the eye, or if the condition worsens or persists for more than 72 hours, discontinue use and consult a physician. If you have glaucoma, do not use this product except under the advice and supervision of a physician. As with any drug, if you are pregnant or nursing a baby, seek the advice of a health professional before using this product. Overuse of this product may produce increased redness of the eye. If solution changes color or becomes cloudy, do not use. To avoid contamination, do not touch tip of container to any surface. Replace cap after using. Remove contact lenses before using.

Parents: Before using with children under 6 years of age, consult your physician. Keep this and all drugs out of the reach of children. In case of accidental ingestion, seek professional assistance or contact a Poison Control Center immediately.

Caution: Should not be used if Visine-imprinted neckband on bottle is broken or missing.

Storage: Store between 2° and 30°C (36° and 86°F).

How Supplied: In 0.5 fl. oz. and 1 fl. oz. plastic dispenser bottle.

Shown in Product Identification Guide, page 517

VISINE A.C®
Seasonal Relief From Pollen and Dust (Formerly Visine® Allergy Relief) Astringent/Redness Reliever Eye Drops

Description: Visine A.C. is a sterile, isotonic, buffered ophthalmic solution containing tetrahydrozoline hydrochloride 0.05%, zinc sulfate 0.25%, boric acid, sodium chloride, sodium citrate and purified water. It is preserved with benzalkonium chloride 0.01% and edetate disodium 0.1%. Visine A.C. is a fast-acting, dual-action ophthalmic solution combining the effects of the vasoconstrictor, tetrahydrozoline hydrochloride, with the astringent effects of zinc sulfate. The vasoconstrictor provides temporary relief of conjunctival edema, hyperemia and discomfort due to airborne irritants such as pollen, dust and ragweed, while zinc sulfate relieves eye discomfort by removing mucus from the eye.

Tetrahydrozoline hydrochloride is a sympathomimetic agent, which brings about decongestion by vasoconstriction. Reddened eyes are rapidly whitened by this effective vasoconstrictor which limits the local vascular response by constricting the small blood vessels. The onset of vasoconstriction becomes apparent within minutes. Zinc sulfate is an ocular astringent which, by precipitating protein, helps to clear mucus from the outer surface of the eye. The effectiveness of Visine A.C. in temporarily relieving conjunctival hyperemia and eye discomfort due to pollen, dust and ragweed has been clinically demonstrated. In one double-blind study of subjects who experienced acute episodes of minor eye irritation, Visine A.C. produced statistically significant beneficial results versus a placebo of normal saline solution in relieving irritation of bulbar conjunctiva, irritation of palpebral conjunctiva and mucus buildup. Treatment with Visine A.C. also significantly improved eye discomfort.

Indications: For temporary relief of discomfort and redness due to minor eye irritations.

Directions: Instill 1 to 2 drops in the affected eye(s) up to 4 times daily.

Note: As drops go to work, some users may notice a brief tingling sensation which will quickly pass.

Warnings: If you experience eye pain, changes in vision, continued redness or irritation of the eye, or if the condition worsens or persists for more than 72 hours, discontinue use and consult a physician. If you have glaucoma, do not use this product except under the advice and supervision of a physician. As with any drug, if you are pregnant or nursing a baby, seek the advice of a health professional before using this product. Overuse of this product may produce increased redness of the eye. If solution changes color or becomes cloudy, do not use. To avoid contamination, do not touch tip of container to any surface. Replace cap after using. Remove contact lenses before using.

Parents Note: Before using with children under 6 years of age, consult your physician. Keep this and all drugs out of the reach of children. In case of accidental ingestion, seek professional assistance or contact a Poison Control Center immediately.

Caution: Should not be used if Visine-imprinted neckband on bottle is broken or missing.

Storage: Store between 2° and 30°C (36° and 86°F).

How Supplied: In 0.5 fl. oz. and 1.0 fl. oz. plastic dispenser bottle.

Shown in Product Identification Guide, page 517

VISINE® MOISTURIZING
Lubricant/Redness Reliever Eye Drops

Description: Visine Moisturizing is a sterile, isotonic, buffered ophthalmic solution containing tetrahydrozoline hydrochloride 0.05%, polyethylene glycol 400 1.0%, boric acid, sodium borate, sodium chloride and purified water. It is preserved with benzalkonium chloride 0.013% and edetate disodium 0.1%.

Visine Moisturizing is an ophthalmic solution combining the effects of the decongestant, tetrahydrozoline hydrochloride, with the demulcent effects of polyethylene glycol. It provides symptomatic relief of conjunctival edema and hyperemia secondary to minor irritations and so-called nonspecific or catarrhal conjunctivitis. Tetrahydrozoline hydrochloride is a sympathomimetic agent, which brings about decongestion by vasoconstriction. Reddened eyes are rapidly whitened by this effective vasoconstrictor, which limits the local vascular response by constricting the small blood vessels. The onset of vasoconstriction becomes apparent within minutes. Additional effects include amelioration of burning, irritation and excessive lacrimation. Relief is afforded by polyethylene glycol.

Polyethylene glycol is an ophthalmic demulcent which has been shown to be effective for the temporary relief of discomfort of minor irritations of the eye due to exposure to wind or sun. It is effective as a protectant and lubricant against further irritation or to relieve dryness of the eye.

The effectiveness of tetrahydrozoline hydrochloride in relieving conjunctival hyperemia and associated symptoms has been demonstrated by numerous clinicals, including several double-blind studies, involving more than 2000 subjects suffering from acute or chronic hyperemia induced by a variety of conditions.

Visine Moisturizing is a product that combines the redness relieving effects of a vasoconstrictor and the soothing, moisturizing and protective effects of a demulcent.

Indications: Relieves redness of the eye due to minor eye irritations. For use as a protectant against further irritation or to relieve dryness.

Directions: Instill 1 to 2 drops in the affected eye(s) up to 4 times daily.

Warnings: If you experience eye pain, changes in vision, continued redness or irritation of the eye, or if the condition worsens or persists for more than 72 hours, discontinue use and consult a physician. If you have glaucoma, do not use this product except under the advice and supervision of a physician. As with any drug, if you are pregnant or nursing a baby, seek the advice of a health professional before using this product. Overuse of this product may produce increased redness of the eye. If solution changes color or becomes cloudy, do not use. To avoid contamination, do not touch tip of container to any surface. Replace cap after using. Remove contact lenses before using.

Parents Note: Before using with children under 6 years of age, consult your physician. Keep this and all drugs out of the reach of children. In case of accidental ingestion, seek professional assistance or contact a Poison Control Center immediately.

Continued on next page

Pfizer Inc.—Cont.

Caution: Should not be used if Visine-imprinted neckband on bottle is broken or missing.

Storage: Store between 2° and 30°C (36° and 86°F).

How Supplied: In 0.5 fl. oz. and 1.0 fl. oz. plastic dispenser bottle.

Shown in Product Identification Guide, page 517

VISINE® ORIGINAL
Tetrahydrozoline Hydrochloride/ Redness Reliever Eye Drops

Description: Visine is a sterile, isotonic, buffered ophthalmic solution containing tetrahydrozoline hydrochloride 0.05%, boric acid, sodium borate, sodium chloride and purified water. It is preserved with benzalkonium chloride 0.01% and edetate disodium 0.1%. Visine is a decongestant ophthalmic solution designed to provide symptomatic relief of conjunctival edema and hyperemia secondary to minor irritations, due to conditions such as smoke, dust, other airborne pollutants, swimming, and so-called nonspecific or catarrhal conjunctivitis. Relief is afforded by tetrahydrozoline hydrochloride, a sympathomimetic agent, which brings about decongestion by vasoconstriction. Reddened eyes are rapidly whitened by this effective vasoconstrictor, which limits the local vascular response by constricting the small blood vessels. The onset of vasoconstriction becomes apparent within minutes.
The effectiveness of Visine in relieving conjunctival hyperemia has been demonstrated by numerous clinicals, including several double-blind studies, involving more than 2,000 subjects suffering from acute or chronic hyperemia induced by a variety of conditions. Visine was found to be efficacious in providing relief from conjunctival hyperemia.

Indications: Relieves redness of the eye due to minor eye irritations.

Directions: Instill 1 to 2 drops in the affected eye(s) up to four times daily.

Warnings: If you experience eye pain, changes in vision, continued redness or irritation of the eye, or if the condition worsens or persists for more than 72 hours, discontinue use and consult a physician. If you have glaucoma, do not use this product except under the advice and supervision of a physician. As with any drug, if you are pregnant or nursing a baby, seek the advice of a health professional before using this product. Overuse of this product may produce increased redness of the eye. If solution changes color or becomes cloudy, do not use. To avoid contamination, do not touch tip of container to any surface. Replace cap after using. Remove contact lenses before using.

Parents Note: Before using with children under 6 years of age, consult your physician. Keep this and all drugs out of the reach of children. In case of accidental ingestion, seek professional assistance or contact a Poison Control Center immediately.

Caution: Should not be used if Visine-imprinted neckband on bottle is broken or missing.

Storage: Store between 2° and 30°C (36° and 86°F).

How Supplied: In 0.5 fl. oz., 0.75 fl. oz., and 1.0 fl. oz. plastic dispenser bottle and 0.5 fl. oz. plastic bottle with dropper.

Shown in Product Identification Guide, page 517

WART-OFF®
Liquid

Active Ingredient: Salicylic Acid 17% w/w.

Inactive Ingredients: Alcohol, 26.35% w/w, Flexible Collodion, Propylene Glycol Dipelargonate.

Indications: For the removal of common warts and plantar warts on the bottom of the foot. The common wart is easily recognized by the rough "cauliflower-like" appearance of the surface. The plantar wart is recognized by its location only on the bottom of the foot, its tenderness, and the interruption of the footprint pattern.

Warnings: For external use only. Keep this and all medications out of the reach of children to avoid accidental poisoning. In case of accidental ingestion, contact a physician or a Poison Control Center immediately. Do not use this product on irritated skin, on any area that is infected or reddened, if you are a diabetic, or if you have poor blood circulation. Do not use on moles, birthmarks, warts with hair growing from them, genital warts, or warts on the face or mucous membranes. If product gets into the eye, flush with water for 15 minutes. Avoid inhaling vapors. If discomfort persists, see your doctor.
Extremely Flammable—Keep away from fire or flame. Cap bottle tightly and store at room temperature away from heat (59°–86°F) (15°–30°C).

Instructions For Use: Read warnings and enclosed instructional brochure. Wash affected area. Dry area thoroughly. Using the special pinpoint applicator, apply one drop at a time to sufficiently cover each wart. Apply Wart-Off to warts only—not to surrounding skin. Let dry. Repeat this procedure once or twice daily as needed (until wart is removed) for up to 12 weeks. Replace cap tightly to prevent evaporation.

How Supplied: 0.45 fluid ounce (13.3mL) bottle with special pinpoint plastic applicator and instructional brochure.

PharmaBotanixx
15225 ALTON PARKWAY
IRVINE, CA 92618

Direct Inquiries to:
(800) 769-4372
FAX: (714) 753-8321

MANUFACTURER'S DECLARATION

1. Traditional Chinese Medicine addresses the body as a whole, not as isolated parts which are either diseased or healthy. In Traditional Chinese Medicine, herbal formulas are developed to treat the underlying problem as well as the symptoms caused by the problem. All Pharmabotanixx formulas are published Traditional Chinese remedies that have been in use for centuries.
2. Formula Ingredients. The ingredients in each formula is published in the Oriental Material Medica, giving the chemical contents of each ingredient. The list of ingredients is reproduced on the label of each bottle/packaging of each product. The botanical identity of the ingredients is provided in a cross reference guide.
3. Every tablet is 500 mg of standardized (HPLC) 5:1 concentrated extract. The weight of each tablet/capsule is indicated on the label and refers to the weight of herbal material.
4. There are no food colorings, fumigants, preservatives, pesticides or other chemical substances. Only natural materials are used in processing, including a flow agent, vegetable binding and vegetable coating. All herb material is of natural origin, there are no synthetic compounds. The herbs are not processed other than grinding to powder, hot water extraction and compressing into tablets.
5. Microbiological testing is conducted on random samples. According to published reports and work done at Silliker Laboratories of California, Inc. located at 1139 East Dominguez, Suite 1, Carson, California 90746, natural herb materials contain from <10 to 50,000 bacteria per gram, which are harmless organisms found throughout the environment. Our analyses show that the Chinese herb formula we use, tested either before or after being made into tablets generally contain less that 10,000 bacteria per gram, an acceptable level. Only trace amounts of coliform bacteria are found (less than 500 MPN) and no salmonella has ever been detected. No sterilization procedures are used for the plant materials either before or after processing. However, the process causes some heat and drying, which has antibacterial action.
6. Bottles are safely sealed with a shrink-band that can indicate tampering. There is also an inner seal, but this is strictly for maintaining freshness and cannot by itself indicate tampering.

7. Labels are stamped with a lot number which indicates the date of packaging. Each label carries conservative values for suggested use. Up to 120 times the amount indicated on the label can be safely used for a typical duration (consuming total amount in any of the bottles).
8. Vitamins, drugs or other chemical agents are not added. There are no requirements for registration, approval or other ation by the Food and Drug Administration (FDA) in the USA or other regulatory agencies.
The tablets are manufactured at the pharmaceutical-grade-factory in Irvine, California. No medical or nutritional claims are made by the manufacturer or distributor. All ingredients are made by the manufacturer under strict "good manufacturing practices" (GMP) which are regulated by the United States Food and Drug Administration (FDA). Pharmabotanixx formulas are sold worldwide.

ACNIXX®

ACNIXX is a complete herbal skin formula to nourish and cleanse for a clearer complexion. Teenagers and adults may take the tablets in the morning or evenings. Topicals and ointments are no longer needed. ACNIXX is a Traditional Chinese formula containing 14 herbs, in a standardized (HPLC) 5:1 concentrated tablet laboratory tested for purity and potency. There are no synthetic ingredients.

Recommended Use: Take 3 to 4 up to three times daily or 3 to 4 tablets may be taken in the AM or PM. After results tablets may be taken as needed or as few as three in the AM or PM.

Contents • 100% Chinese Herbs: Lonicerae Flos, Scutellariae Radix, Violae cum Radice Herba, Paeoniae Alba Radix, Moutan Radicis Cortex, Gardeniae Fructus, Sophorae Flavescentis Radix, Taraxaci Herba, Forsythiae Fructus, Coicis Semen, Rehmanniae Glutinosae Radix, Angelicae Dahuricae Radix, Platycodi Radix, Glycyrrhizae Uralensis Radix.

How Supplied: 60 TABLETS 500 MG EACH

CHOLNIXX

CHOLNIXX is a formula to assist the liver and stomach in the metabolism of lipids. This herbal formula contains the herb Ho Shou Wu (Polygoni Multiflori Radix), revered in Chinese Medicine for its cholesterol lowering effect. After desired results CHOLNIXX may only be needed once per day. There are no synthetic ingredients or harmful side effects. CHOLNIXX contains 10 herbs in a standardized (HPLC) 5:1 concentrated extract tablet laboratory tested for purity and potency.

Recommended Use: Take 3 to 4 tablets one hour before meals two to three times daily. Once results have been achieved 3 to 6 in the AM or PM may be all that is needed.

Content • 100% Chinese Herbs: Crataegi Fructus, Hordei Germinatus Fructus, Rehmanniae Glutinosae Radix, Polygoni Multiflori Radix, Scutellariae Radix, Trichosanthis Radix, Poria Cocos Sclerotium, Alismatis Rhizoma, Rhei Rhizoma, Prunellae Spica.

How Supplied: 120 TABLETS 500 MG EACH

DIANIXX®

Parties? ... Restaurants? DIANIXX stimulates your body's own natural "full" feeling. When you begin eating, you eat less because you already feel full. DIANIXX balances your appetite and the cravings for the wrong foods—Eat right! This traditional Chinese approach to overeating allows you to enjoy food and not over-do it. Don't deprive yourself. Just eat naturally, sensibly and use Dianixx to be in control. No Mahuang/Ephedra or Caffeine. DIANIXX contains 12 herbs in a standardized (HPLC) 5:1 concentrated extract tablet laboratory tested for purity and potency.

Recommended Use: Take 3 or 4 tablets 3 times daily between meals at least 1 hour before eating.

Contents • 100% Chinese Herbs: Poria Cocos Sclerotium, Plantaginis Herba, Gentianae Scabrae Radix, Rhei Rhizoma, Cassiae Torae Semen, Aurantii Immaturus Fructus, Prunellae Spica, Pteris Herba, Elsholtziae Herba, Schizandrae Fructus, Menthae Herba, Glycyrrhizae Uralensis Radix.

How Supplied: 120 TABLETS 500 MG EACH

AN AFFILIATE OF: SUN TEN LABORATORIES, INC.
9250 JERONIMO ROAD • IRVINE, CA • 92718 • 800-769-4372

Shown in Product Identification Guide, page 517

MENIXX®

MENIXX is the original traditional Chinese formula for symptoms commonly associated with menopause. MENIXX is the strongest natural herbal formula available without synthetic additives or side effects. MENIXX® contains 10 herbs in a standardized (HLPC) 5:1 concentrated extract tablet laboratory tested for purity and potency.

Recommended Use: Take 3 to 4 tablets three times daily or 3 to 6 tablets may be taken as needed in the AM or PM.

Contents • 100% Chinese Herbs: Bupleuri Radix, Moutan Radicis Cortex, Gardeniae Fructus, Angelicae Sinensis Radix, Paeoniae Alba Radix, Atractylodis Macrocephalae Rhizoma, Poria Cocos Sclerotium, Menthae Herba, Zingiberis Officinalis Rhizoma, Glycyrrhizae Uralensis Radix.

How Supplied: 120 TABLETS 500 MG EACH

MIGREXX®

MIGREXX is a maximum strength all herbal Chinese medicinal formula for what is known as "dry headaches" or symptoms commonly associated with migraine headaches. MIGREXX contains 16 herbs in a standardized (HPLC) 5:1 concentrated extract tablet laboratory tested for purity and potency.

Recommended Use: Take 4 to 8 tablets as needed up to three times daily. After initial use normally 4 to 8 tablets at onset is needed. MIGREXX begins to work in one hour.

Contents • 100% Chinese Herbs: Ophiopogonis Tuber, Ligustici Wallichii Rhizoma, Corydalis Rhizoma, Notopterygii Rhizoma, Angelica Dahuricae Radix, Viticis Fructus, Ledebouriellae Radix, Asari cum Radice Herba, Chrysanthemi Morifolii Flos, Angelicae Pubescentis Radix, Scutellariae Radix, Angelicae Sinensis Radix, Atractylodis Macrocephalae Rhizoma, Zingiberis Officinalis Rhizoma, Glycyrrhizae Uralensis Radix.

How Supplied: 60 TABLETS 500 MG EACH

NASIXX®

NASIXX is a formula used for symptoms commonly associated with "wet" headaches, allergies, head colds and sinusitis. NASIXX works in about an hour and can also be used to reduce/eliminate snoring when taken before sleep. NASIXX® works without unwanted side effects like grogginess and DOES NOT contain Mahuang/ephedra or harmful stimulants. NASIXX® contains 11 herbs in a standardized (HPLC) 5:1 concentrated extract tablet laboratory tested for purity and potency.

Recommended Use: Take 4 to 8 tablets as needed up to 3 times daily. After initial use 4–8 tablets are needed once per day.

Contents • 100% Chinese Herbs: Magnoliae Liliflorae Flos, Ligustici Wallichii Rhizoma, Notopterygii Rhizoma, Corydalis Tuber, Angelicae Dahuricae Radix, Cimicifugae Rhizoma, Ledebouriellae Radix, Ligustici Sinesis Rhizoma et Radix, Akebiae Caulis, Asari cum Radice Herba, Glycyrrhizae Uralensis Radix.

How Supplied: 60 TABLETS 500 MG EACH

Shown in Product Identification Guide, page 517

Continued on next page

PharmaBotanixx—Cont.

PREMIXX®

PREMIXX is the original Traditional Chinese medicinal formula for the symptoms of premenstrual syndrome (PMS). PREMIXX includes the female ginseng, Tang-Kuei and Bupleurum for a complete formula. The formula may be taken mid-cycle or five days in advance to prevent unwanted symptoms such as bloating, cramping and mood swings. PREMIXX may simply be taken at the onset of symptoms for quick relief. PREMIXX® contains 9 herbs in a standardized (HPLC) 5:1 concentrated extract tablet laboratory tested for purity and potency.

Recommended Use: Take 3 to 4 tablets 3 times daily for five days or take 4–8 tablets as needed.

Contents • 100% Chinese Herbs: Bupleuri Radix, Angelicae Sinensis Radix, Ligustici Wallichii Rhizoma, Poria Cocos Sclerotium, Alismatis Rhizoma, Atractylodis Macrocephalae Rhizoma, Menthae Herba, Zingiberis Officinalis Rhizoma, Glycyrrhizae Uralensis Radix.

How Supplied: 60 TABLETS 500 MG EACH

RHEUMIXX®

RHEUMIXX is a combination of three Traditional Chinese herbal formulas in one convenient product for pain associated with common joint and muscular aches. RHEUMIXX contains nine concentrated herbs to include Olibanum (frankincense) and Myrrha (myrrh) prized since ancient times for their medicinal qualities. RHEUMIXX is a standardized (HPLC) 5:1 concentrated extract tablet laboratory tested for purity and potency.

Recommended Use: Take 3 to 4 tablets three times daily or 6 to 8 tablets as needed.

Contents • 100% Chinese Herbs: Angelicae Pubescentis Radix, Clematis Radix, Asari cum Radice Herba, Olibanum, Myrrha, Corydalis Rhizoma, Millettia Caulis, Achyranthis Bidentatae Radix, Glycyrrhizae Uralensis Radix.

How Supplied: 60 TABLETS 500 MG EACH

STRENIXX®

STRENIXX is a non-stimulant original male potency and vitality formula used exclusively by men for centuries. STRENIXX is a maximum strength herbal Traditional Chinese medicinal to deliver greater focus, stamina and now includes Epimedium for sexual function. Men of all ages rely on STRENIXX and feel the difference. All 9 herbs in STRENIXX are in a standardized (HPLC) 5:1 concentrated herbal extract tablet laboratory tested for purity and potency. No synthetic or chemical additives.

Recommended Use: Take 3 to 4 tablets three times daily for two days. Thereafter tablets may be taken as needed in the AM or PM.

Contents • 100% Chinese Herbs: Astragali Radix, Rehmanniae Glutinosae Radix, Corni Fructus, Epimedii Herba, Dioscoreae Oppositae Rhizoma, Cinnamomi Cassiae Cortex, Poria Cocos Sclerotium, Alismatis Rhixoma, Moutan Radicis Cortex

How Supplied: 60 TABLETS 500 MG EACH

Shown in Product Identification Guide, page 517

VIATEXX®

VIATEXX works to deliver a sustained and focused energy level without harmful stimulants such as Ma Huang/Ephedra or Guarana. This formula contains the key herbs Ginseng and Astragalus that work with your system to counteract the toxins that can contribute to a mid-day slump. This product does not interfere with your needed rest each night. VIATEXX® contains 9 herbs in a standardized (HPLC) 5:1 concentrated extract tablet laboratory tested for purity and potency.

Recommended Use: Take 3 or 4 tablets 3 times daily before meals, or 6 tablets in the A.M. and additional may be taken in the P.M. if needed.

Content • 100% Chinese Herbs: Ginseng Radix, Astragali Radix, Angelicae Sinensis Radix, Bupleuri Radix, Cimicifugae Rhizoma, Citri Reticulatae Pericarpium, Zizyphi Fructus, Zingiberis Officinalis Rhizoma, Glycyrrhizae Uralensis Radix.

How Supplied: 60 TABLETS 500 MG EACH

VINEXX®

Counter the unpleasant side effects of alcohol and jet lag with VINEXX. When VINEXX is taken **before** consuming alcohol, it alleviates the effects better known as a "Hangover". Recent Harvard Medical School studies show that Puerariae Radix (the key ingredient in VINEXX®) is effective in controlling the effects of alcohol. VINEXX® contains 13 herbs in a standardized (HPLC) 5:1 concentrated extract tablet laboratory tested for purity and potency.

Recommended Use: Take 6 to 8 tablets **before** alcohol consumption or prior to air travel. Repeat dosage every 4 to 5 hours.

Contents • 100% Chinese Herbs: Puerariae Radix, Ginseng Radix, Atractylodis Macrocephalae Rhizoma, Poria Cocos Sclerotium, Polypori Umbellati Sclerotium, Alismatis Rhizoma, Amomi Fructus seu Semen, Amomi Cardamomi Fructus, Massa Medicata Fermentata, Saussureae Radix, Citri Reticulatae Periculatae Pericarpium, Citri Reticulatae Viride Pericarpium, Zingiberis Officinalis Rhizoma.

How Supplied: 40 TABLETS 500 MG EACH

ZYZIXX®

ZYZIXX is the original Traditional Chinese formula to assist in anti-stress and sleeplessness. Take before sleep for the rest you need without the side effects of grogginess in the morning. ZYZIXX works as a calmative rather than a sedative. ZYZIXX contains 16 herbs in a standardized (HPLC) 5:1 concentrated extract tablet laboratory tested for purity and potency.

Recommended Use: Take 6 to 8 tablets one hour before sleep. 3 to 4 tablets may be taken as a calmative.

Contents • 100% Chinese Herbs: Rehmanniae Glutinosae Radix, Scrophulariae Radix, Asparagi Radix, Ophiopogonis Tuber, Angelicae Sinensis Radix, Salviae Miltorrhizae Radix, Ginseng Radix, Poria Cocos Sclerotium, Schizandrae Fructus, Biotae Semen, Zizyphi Spinosa Semen, Polygalae Radix, Cinnabaris, Acori Rhizoma, Coptis Rhizoma, Platycodi Radix.

How Supplied: 60 TABLETS 500 MG EACH

Pharmacia & Upjohn

KALAMAZOO, MI 49001

For Medical and Pharmaceutical Information, Including Emergencies:
(616) 833-8244

CORTAID®
Maximum Strength, Sensitive Skin Formula, Intensive Therapy, and FastStick.
Cream, Ointment, Spray and Roll-on Stick
(hydrocortisone 1% and 1/2%)

Anti-itch products

Indications: Use CORTAID for the temporary relief of itching associated with minor skin irritations, inflammation, and rashes due to eczema, psoriasis, seborrheic dermatitis, poison ivy, poison oak, or poison sumac, insect bites, soaps, detergents, cosmetics, jewelry, and for external feminine and anal itching. Other uses of this product should be only under the advice and supervision of a physician.

Description: CORTAID provides safe, effective relief of many different types of itches and rashes and is the brand recommended most by physicians and pharmacists. Maximum Strength CORTAID is the same strength and form of hydrocortisone relief formerly available only with a prescription. CORTAID Sensitive Skin Formula has been specially formulated with aloe and 1/2% hydrocortisone. CORTAID Intensive Therapy Cream's special formula of 1% hydrocortisone is specific for eczema & psoriasis sufferers. CORTAID FastStick provides the relief of Maximum Strength CORTAID in a convenient roll-on-stick—Great for insect bites. CORTAID is available in 1) a greaseless, odorless vanishing cream that leaves no residue; 2) a soothing, lubricating ointment; 3) a quick-drying non-staining, non-aerosol spray and roll-on stick (Maximum Strength only).

Active Ingredients: CORTAID Cream and CORTAID Ointment: 1% or 1/2% hydrocortisone.
CORTAID Spray and FastStick: hydrocortisone 1%.
CORTAID Intensive Therapy: hydrocortisone 1%,

Other Ingredients:
Maximum Strength Products:
Maximum Strength Cream: Aloe vera gel, ceteareth-20, ceteareth alcohol, cetyl palmitate, glycerin, isopropyl myristate, isostearyl neopentanoate, methylparaben, and purified water.
Maximum Strength Ointment: butylparaben, cholesterol, methylparaben, microcrystalline wax, mineral oil, and white petrolatum.
Maximum Strength Spray and FastStick: alcohol, glycerin, methylparaben, and purified water.
Sensitive Skin Products:
Sensitive Skin Formula Cream: aloe vera, butylparaben, cetyl palmitate, glyceryl stearate, methylparaben, polyethylene glycol, stearamidoethyl diethylamine, and purified water.
Sensitive Skin Formula Ointment: aloe vera, butylparaben, cholesterol, methylparaben, mineral oil, white petrolatum, and microcrystalline wax.
Intensive Therapy Products:
Intensive Therapy Cream: cetyl alcohol, citric acid, glyceryl stearate, isopropyl myristate, methylparaben, polyoxyl 40 stearate, polysorbate 60, propylene glycol, propylparaben, purified water, sodium citrate, sorbic acid, sorbitan monostearate, stearyl alcohol and white wax.

Uses: The vanishing action of CORTAID Cream makes it cosmetically acceptable when the skin itch or rash treated is on exposed parts of the body such as the hands or arms. CORTAID Ointment is best used where protection lubrication and soothing of dry and scaly lesions is required. The ointment is also recommended for treating itchy genital and anal areas. CORTAID Spray is a quick-drying, non-staining formulation suitable for covering large areas of the skin. CORTAID FastStick delivers quick-drying, non-staining medicine via a convenient and highly portable roll-on stick.

Warnings: For external use only. Avoid contact with the eyes. If condition worsens, or if symptoms persist for more than 7 days or clear up and occur again within a few days, stop use of this product and do not begin use of any other hydrocortisone product unless you have consulted a physician. Do not use for the treatment of diaper rash. Consult a physician. For external feminine itching, do not use if you have a vaginal discharge. Consult a physician. For external anal itching, do not exceed the recommended daily dosage unless directed by a physician. In case of bleeding, consult a physician promptly. Do not put this product into the rectum by using fingers or any mechanical device or applicator.
Keep this and all drugs out of the reach of children. In case of accidental ingestion, seek professional assistance or contact a poison control center immediately.

Dosage and Administration: *Adults and children 2 years of age and older:* Apply to affected area not more than 3 to 4 times daily. *Children under 2 years of age:* Do not use, consult a physician. *Adults:* For external anal itching, when practical, cleanse the affected area with mild soap and warm water and rinse thoroughly by patting or blotting with an appropriate cleansing pad. Gently dry by patting or blotting with toilet tissue or a soft cloth before application of this product. *Children under 12 years of age:* For external anal itching, consult a physician.

How Supplied:
Cream: 1/2 oz. and 1 oz. tubes
Ointment: 1/2 oz. and 1 oz. tubes
Intensive Therapy Cream: 2 oz. tube
Non-Aerosol Spray: 1.5 fluid oz.
FastStick: 1/2 oz.

Shown in Product Identification Guide, page 517

DOXIDAN® LIQUI-GELS®
Stimulant/Stool Softener Laxative

Indications: DOXIDAN is a safe reliable laxative for the relief of occasional constipation. The combination of a stimulant/stool softener laxative allows positive laxative action on a softened stool for gentle evacuation without straining. DOXIDAN generally produces a bowel movement in 6 to 12 hours.

Active Ingredients: Each soft gelatin Liqui-gel contains 30 mg casanthranol and 100 mg docusate sodium.

Inactive Ingredients: Also contains FD&C Blue #1 and Red #40, gelatin, glycerin, polyethylene glycol, sorbitol, titanium dioxide.

Dosage and Administration: Adults and children 12 years of age and over: one to three Liqui-Gels by mouth in a single daily dose. Children 2 to under 12 years of age: one Liqui-Gel daily. Children under 2 years of age: consult a doctor.

Warnings: Do not use laxative products when abdominal pain, nausea, or vomiting are present unless directed by a doctor. If you have noticed a sudden change in bowel habits that persists over a period of 2 weeks, consult a doctor before using a laxative. Laxative products should not be used for a period longer than 1 week unless directed by a doctor. Rectal bleeding or failure to have a bowel movement after use of a laxative may indicate a serious condition. Discontinue use and consult your doctor. Keep this and all drugs out of the reach of children. In case of accidental overdose, seek professional assistance or contact a poison control center immediately. As with any drug, if you are pregnant or nursing a baby, seek the advice of a health professional before using this product.

Drug Interaction Precaution: Do not take this product if you are presently taking mineral oil, unless directed by a doctor.

How Supplied: Packages of 10, 30, 100 and 1,000 maroon soft gelatin capsules, and Unit Dose 100s (10 × 10 strips).
LIQUI-GELS® Reg TM R P Scherer Corp

Shown in Product Identification Guide, page 517

DRAMAMINE® Tablets
(dimenhydrinate USP)
DRAMAMINE® Chewable Tablets
(dimenhydrinate USP)
DRAMAMINE® Children's Liquid
(dimenhydrinate syrup USP)

Indications: For the prevention and treatment of the nausea, vomiting, or dizziness associated with motion sickness.

Description: Dimenhydrinate is the chlorotheophylline salt of the antihistaminic agent diphenhydramine. Dimenhydrinate contains not less than 53% and not more than 56% of diphenhydramine, and not less than 44% and not more than 47% of 8-chlorotheophylline, calculated on the dried basis.

Active Ingredients:
DRAMAMINE Tablets and Chewable Tablets: Dimenhydrinate 50 mg.
DRAMAMINE Children's: Dimenhydrinate 12.5 mg. per 5 ml.

Inactive Ingredients:
DRAMAMINE Tablets: Acacia, Carboxymethylcellulose Sodium, Corn Starch, Magnesium Stearate, and Sodium Sulfate.
DRAMAMINE Children's: FD&C Red No. 40, Flavor, Glycerin, Methylparaben, Sucrose, and Water.
DRAMAMINE Chewable Tablets: Aspartame, Citric Acid, FD&C Yellow No. 6, Flavor, Magnesium Stearate, Methacrylic Acid Copolymer, Sorbitol.
Phenylketonurics: Contains Phenylalanine 1.5 mg per tablet.
Contains FD&C Yellow No. 5 (tartrazine) as a color additive.

Actions: While the precise mode of action of dimenhydrinate is not known, it is thought to have a depressant action on hyperstimulated labyrinthine function.

Continued on next page

Pharmacia & Upjohn—Cont.

Directions:

DRAMAMINE Tablets and Chewable Tablets: To prevent motion sickness, the first dose should be taken one half to one hour before starting activity.
ADULTS: 1 to 2 tablets every 4 to 6 hours, not to exceed 8 tablets in 24 hours or as directed by a doctor.
CHILDREN 6 TO UNDER 12: $^1/_2$ to 1 tablet every 6 to 8 hours, not to exceed 3 tablets in 24 hours or as directed by a doctor.
CHILDREN 2 to UNDER 6: $^1/_4$ to $^1/_2$ tablet every 6 to 8 hours not to exceed $1^1/_2$ tablets in 24 hours or as directed by a doctor.
Children may also be given DRAMAMINE Cherry Flavored Liquid in accordance with directions for use.

DRAMAMINE Children's: To prevent motion sickness, the first dose should be taken one half to one hour before starting activity. CHILDREN 2 TO UNDER 6: 1 to 2 teaspoonfuls every 6 to 8 hours not to exceed 6 teaspoonfuls in 24 hours or as directed by a doctor. Use of a measuring device is recommended for all liquid medication. CHILDREN 6 TO UNDER 12: 2 to 4 teaspoonfuls every 6 to 8 hours, not to exceed 12 teaspoonfuls in 24 hours or as directed by a doctor. CHILDREN 12 YEARS OR OLDER: 4 to 8 teaspoons (5 ml per teaspoonful) every 4 to 6 hours, not to exceed 32 teaspoonfuls in 24 hours or as directed by a doctor.

Warnings: Do not take this product, unless directed by a doctor, if you have a breathing problem such as emphysema or chronic bronchitis, or if you have glaucoma or difficulty in urination due to enlargement of the prostate gland. Do not give to children under 2 years of age unless directed by a doctor. May cause marked drowsiness; alcohol, sedatives, and tranquilizers may increase the drowsiness effect. Avoid alcoholic beverages while taking this product. Do not take this product if you are taking sedatives or tranquilizers, without first consulting your doctor. Use caution when driving a motor vehicle or operating machinery. Not for frequent or prolonged use except on advice of a doctor. Do not exceed recommended dosage. Keep this and all drugs out of the reach of children. In case of accidental overdose, seek professional assistance or contact a poison control center immediately. As with any drug, if you are pregnant or nursing a baby, seek the advice of a health professional before using this product.

How Supplied: *Tablets* —scored, white tablets available in packets of 12 and 36 and bottles of 100; *Chewables* —scored, orange tablets available in packets of 8 and 24; *Liquid* —Available in bottles of 4 fl oz).

Shown in Product Identification Guide, page 517

DRAMAMINE II™ Less Drowsy Formula (Meclizine hydrochloride)

Indications: For the prevention and treatment of the nausea, vomiting, or dizziness associated with motion sickness.

Description: Meclizine hydrochloride is an antihistamine of the piperazine class with antiemetic action.

Actions: While the precise mode of action of meclizine hydrochloride is not known, it is thought to have a depressant action on hyperstimulated labyrinthine function.

Active Ingredients: Each tablet contains 25 mg. meclizine hydrochloride.

Inactive Ingredients: Colloidal silicon dioxide, croscarmellose sodium, dibasic calcium phosphate, D&C yellow no. 10 aluminum lake, microcrystalline cellulose, magnesium stearate.

Directions: To prevent motion sickness, the first dose should be taken one hour before starting your activity. **Adults:** Take 1 to 2 tablets daily or as directed by a doctor. Do not exceed 2 tablets in 24 hours.

Warnings: Do not take this product, unless directed by a doctor, if you have a breathing problem such as emphysema or chronic bronchitis, or if you have glaucoma or difficulty in urination due to enlargement of the prostate gland. Do not give to children under 12 years of age unless directed by a doctor. May cause drowsiness; alcohol, sedatives, and tranquilizers may increase the drowsiness effect. Avoid alcoholic beverages while taking this product. Do not take this product if you are taking sedatives or tranquilizers without first consulting your doctor. Use caution when driving a motor vehicle or operating machinery. Not for frequent or prolonged use except on the advice of a doctor. Do not exceed recommended dosage. Keep this and all drugs out of reach of children. In case of accidental overdose, seek professional assistance or contact a poison control center immediately. As with any drug, if you are pregnant or nursing a baby, seek the advice of a health professional before using this product.

How Supplied: Dramamine II Less Drowsy Formula is supplied as a yellow tablet in packages of 8.

Shown in Product Identification Guide, page 517

EMETROL® (Phosphorated Carbohydrate Solution)

For the relief of nausea associated with upset stomach

Description: EMETROL is an oral solution containing balanced amounts of dextrose (glucose) and levulose (fructose) and phosphoric acid with controlled hydrogen ion concentration. Availáble in original lemon-mint or cherry flavor.

Ingredients: Each 5 mL teaspoonful contains dextrose (glucose), 1.87 g; levulose (fructose), 1.87 g; phosphoric acid, 21.5 mg; and the following inactive ingredients: glycerin, methylparaben, purified water; D&C yellow No. 10 and natural lemon-mint flavor in lemon-mint Emetrol; FD&C red No. 40 and artificial cherry flavor in cherry Emetrol.

Action: EMETROL quickly relieves nausea by local action on the wall of the hyperactive G.I. tract. No delay in therapeutic action such as that associated with systemic drugs.

Indications: For the relief of nausea due to upset stomach from intestinal flu and food or drink indiscretions. For other conditions, take only as directed by your physician.

Advantages:
1. **Fast Action**—works quickly through local action on contact with the hyperactive G.I. tract.
2. **Effectiveness**—clinically proven to stop nausea.
3. **Safety**—all natural active ingredients won't mask symptoms of organic pathology. No known drug interactions.
4. **Convenience**—no Rx required.
5. **Patient Acceptance**—pleasant tasting lemon-mint or cherry flavor.

Usual Adult Dose: One or two tablespoonfuls. Repeat every 15 minutes until distress subsides.

Usual Children's Dose: One or two teaspoonfuls. Repeat dose every 15 minutes until distress subsides.

Important: Never dilute EMETROL or drink fluids of any kind immediately before or after taking a dose.

Caution: Not to be taken for more than one hour (5 doses) without consulting a physician. If upset stomach continues or recurs frequently, consult a physician promptly as it may be a sign of a serious condition.

WARNING: KEEP THIS AND ALL MEDICATIONS OUT OF THE REACH OF CHILDREN. As with any drug, if you are pregnant or nursing a baby, seek the advice of a health professional before using this product.
This product contains fructose and should not be taken by persons with hereditary fructose intolerance (HFI).

This product contains sugar and should not be taken by diabetics except under the advice and supervision of a physician.

In case of accidental overdose, contact a poison control center, emergency medical facility, or physician immediately for advice.

How Supplied: Each 5 mL teaspoonful of EMETROL contains dextrose (glucose), 1.87 g; levulose (fructose), 1.87 g;

and phosphoric acid, 21.5 mg in a yellow, lemon-mint or red, cherry-flavored syrup.

Yellow, Lemon-Mint
NDC 0009-7573-01—Bottle of 4 fluid ounces (118 mL)
NDC 0009-7573-02—Bottle of 8 fluid ounces (236 mL)
NDC 0009-7573-03—Bottle of 1 pint (473 mL)

Red, Cherry
NDC 0009-7574-01—Bottle of 4 fluid ounces (118 mL)
NDC 0009-7574-02—Bottle of 8 fluid ounces (236 mL)
NDC 0009-7574-03—Bottle of 1 pint (473 mL)

Store at room temperature

NOTICE: Each bottle is protected by a printed band around the cap. Do not use if band is damaged or missing.

Shown in Product Identification Section, page 517

KAO LECTROLYTE™
Electrolyte Replenisher

Usage: To quickly restore fluid and minerals lost with diarrhea and vomiting; for maintenance of hydration and electrolytes.

Features:

- Great tasting electrolyte replenisher preferred over premixed liquid replenishers to help improve compliance.
- Formulated to AAP guidelines for prevention of dehydration
- Convenient, pre-measured power packets for better value and portability
- Available in Grape, Bubble gum–favorite flavors among toddlers; and unflavored for infants.

Dosage: Kao Lectrolyte should be offered frequently in amounts tolerated. Total daily intake should be adjusted to meet individual needs, based on thirst and response to therapy.

Ingredients: Unflavored: Dextrose, Sodium Citrate, Potassium Chloride, Sodium Chloride and Aspertame

Grape: Dextrose, Sodium Citrate, Potassium Chloride, Sodium Chloride, Aspertame, artificial flavor, FD&C Red #40, FD&C Blue #1

Bubble gum: Dextrose, Sodium Citrate, Potassium Chloride, Sodium Chloride, Aspertame, artificial flavor, FD&C Red #40

Each Packet Provides:
Sodium, 12 mEq
Potassium, 5 mEq
Chloride, 10 mEq
Citrate, 7 mEq
Dextrose, 5 grams
Calories, 22.

Shown in Product Identification Guide, page 517

KAOPECTATE®
Anti-Diarrheal, Regular Flavor, Peppermint Flavor and Children's Cherry Flavored Liquids. Maximum Strength Caplets.

Indications: For the fast relief of diarrhea and cramping.

Active Ingredients: Each tablespoon or caplet contains 750 mg attapulgite.

Inactive Ingredients: Liquids: flavors, gluconodelta-lactone, magnesium, aluminum silicate, methylparaben, sorbic acid, sucrose, titanium dioxide, xanthan gum and purified water; Peppermint flavor and Children's Cherry flavor contain FD&C Red #40. Maximum Strength Caplets: Carnauba Wax, Croscarmellose Sodium, Hydroxypropyl Cellulose, Hydroxypropyl Methylcellulose, Methylparaben, Pectin, Propylene Glycol, Propylparaben, Sucrose, Titanium Dioxide, Zinc Stearate. May also contain Talc.

Dosage and Administration: Liquids: For best results, take full recommended dose at first sign of diarrhea and after each subsequent bowel movement. (Maximum 6 times in 24 hours.) Adults and children 12 years of age and over: 2 tablespoons. Children 6 to under 12 years of age: 1 tablespoon. Children 3 to 6 years of age: $^1/_2$ tablespoon. Maximum Strength Tablets: Swallow whole caplets with water; do not chew. For best results, take full recommended dose. Adults: Take 2 caplets after the initial bowel movement and 2 caplets after each subsequent bowel movement, not to exceed 12 caplets in 24 hours. Children 6 to 12 years of age: Take 1 caplet after the initial bowel movement and 1 caplet after each subsequent movement, not to exceed 6 caplets in 24 hours. Children 3 to under 6 years of age: Use Children's Cherry Flavored Liquid or Advanced Formula KAOPECTATE Liquid.

Warnings: Unless directed by a physician, do not use Kaopectate Liquids in infants and children under 3 years of age or Kaopectate Caplets in infants or children under 6 years of age or for more than two days in the presence of high fever. Keep this and all drugs out of the reach of children. In case of accidental overdose, seek professional assistance or contact a poison control center immediately.

How Supplied: Regular flavor available in 8 oz., 12 oz. and 16 oz. bottles. Peppermint flavor available in 8 oz. and 12 oz. bottles. Children's Cherry flavor available in 6 oz. bottle. Maximum Strength Caplets available in blister packs of 12 and 20 caplets.

Shown in Product Identification Guide, page 517

MOTRIN® IB
Caplets, Tablets and Gelcaps (ibuprofen, USP) Pain Reliever/Fever Reducer

WARNING: ASPIRIN-SENSITIVE PATIENTS. Do not take this product if you have had a severe allergic reaction to aspirin, eg—asthma, swelling, shock or hives because even though this product contains no aspirin or salicylates, cross-reactions may occur in patients allergic to aspirin.

Indications: For the temporary relief of headache, muscular aches, minor pain of arthritis, toothache, backache, minor aches and pains associated with the common cold, pain of menstrual cramps, and for reduction of fever.

Directions: Adults: Take 1 caplet, tablet or gelcap every 4 to 6 hours while symptoms persist. If pain or fever does not respond to 1 caplet, tablet or gelcap, 2 caplets, tablets or gelcaps may be used, but do not exceed 6 caplets, tablets or gelcaps in 24 hours, unless directed by a doctor. The smallest effective dose should be used. Take with food or milk, if stomach or stomach pain occurs with use.
Consult a doctor if these symptoms are more than mild or if they persist. Children: Do not give this product to children under 12 except under the advice and supervision of a doctor.

Warnings: Do not take for pain for more than 10 days or for fever for more than 3 days unless directed by a doctor. If pain or fever persists or gets worse, if new symptoms occur, or if the painful area is red or swollen, consult a doctor. These could be signs of serious illness. If you are under a doctor's care for any serious condition, consult a doctor before taking this product. As with aspirin and acetaminophen, if you have any condition which requires you to take prescription drugs or if you have had any problems or serious side effects from taking any nonprescription pain reliever, do not take MOTRIN® IB without first discussing it with your doctor. If you experience any symptoms which are unusual or seem unrelated to the condition for which you took ibuprofen, consult a doctor before taking any more of it.
Although ibuprofen is indicated for the same conditions as aspirin and acetaminophen, it should not be taken with them except under a doctor's direction. Do not combine this product with any other ibuprofen-containing product.
As with any drug, if you are pregnant or nursing a baby, seek the advice of a health professional before using this product. IT IS ESPECIALLY IMPORTANT NOT TO USE IBUPROFEN DURING THE LAST 3 MONTHS OF PREGNANCY UNLESS SPECIFICALLY DIRECTED TO DO SO BY A DOCTOR BECAUSE IT MAY CAUSE PROBLEMS IN THE UNBORN CHILD OR COMPLICATIONS DURING DELIVERY.

Continued on next page

Pharmacia & Upjohn—Cont.

Keep this and all drugs out of the reach of children. In case of accidental overdose, seek professional assistance or contact a poison control center immediately. **Store at room temperature. Avoid excessive heat 40°C (104°F).**

Active Ingredient: Each caplet, tablet or gelcap contains ibuprofen 200 mg.

Other Ingredients: Carnauba wax, cornstarch, hydroxypropyl methylcellulose, propylene glycol, silicon dioxide, pregelatinized starch, stearic acid, titanium dioxide. Gelcaps also contain benzyl alcohol, butylparaben, butyl alcohol, castor oil, colloidal silicon dioxide, edetate calcium disodium, FDC Yellow No. 6, gelatin, iron oxide black, magnesium stearate, methylparaben, microcrystalline cellulose, povidone, propylparaben, SDA 3A starch, propylparaben, SDA 3A alcohol, sodium lauryl sulfate, sodium propionate, and sodium starch glycolate.

How Supplied: Bottles of 24, 50, 100, 130 and 165 Caplets or Tablets. Bottles of 24 and 50 Gelcaps. Vial of 8 caplets.

Shown in Product Identification Guide, page 517

Maximum Strength MYCITRACIN®
Triple Antibiotic First Aid Ointment
MYCITRACIN® Plus Pain Reliever

Indications: Maximum Strength MYCITRACIN and MYCITRACIN Plus Pain Reliever are first aid ointments to help prevent infection in minor burns, cuts, nicks, scrapes, scratches and abrasions.

Description: MYCITRACIN combines three topical antibiotics in a soothing, non-irritating petrolatum base that does not sting, aids healing, and helps prevent infection. MYCITRACIN Plus Pain Reliever also temporarily relieves pain.

Directions: *For adults and children (all ages):* Clean the affected area. Apply a small amount of MYCITRACIN (an amount equal to the surface area of the tip of a finger) on the affected area 1 to 3 times daily. If desired, cover the affected area with a sterile bandage.

Warnings: For external use only. Do not use in the eyes or apply over large areas of the body. In case of deep or puncture wounds, animal bites, or serious burns, consult a physician. Stop use and consult a physician if the condition persists or gets worse. Do not use longer than 1 week unless directed by a physician. Keep this and all medications out of the reach of children. In case of accidental ingestion, seek professional assistance or contact a poison control center immediately.

Active Ingredients:
Maximum Strength MYCITRACIN: ***Each Gram Contains:*** *Bacitracin Zinc 500 units; Neomycin Sulfate equiv. to 3.5 mg neomycin; Polymyxin B Sulfate, 10,000 units;*
MYCITRACIN Plus Pain Reliever: ***Each Gram Contains:*** *Bacitracin Zinc, 500 units; Neomycin Sulfate equiv. to 3.5 mg neomycin; Polymyxin B Sulfate, 10,000 units; Lidocaine, 40 mg.*

Other Ingredients:
Maximum Strength MYCITRACIN: *Also contains butylparaben, cholesterol, methylparaben, microcrystalline wax, mineral oil, and white petrolatum.*
MYCITRACIN Plus Pain Reliever: *Also contains butylparaben, cholesterol, methylparaben, microcrystalline wax, mineral oil, and white petrolatum.*

How Supplied:
$^1/_2$ oz. tubes, 1 oz. tubes and $^1/_{32}$ oz. foil packets (144 per carton)

Shown in Product Identification Guide, page 517

ROGAINE® for Men
Hair Regrowth Treatment
2% Minoxidil Topical Solution

Description: ROGAINE is a colorless liquid medication for use only on the scalp to help regrow hair.
Active Ingredients: Minoxidil 2% w/v
Inactive Ingredients: Alcohol, 60% v/v, propylene glycol, and purified water.

How Supplied: ROGAINE for Men is available in single, twin or triple packs.

Indication: ROGAINE is medically proven to regrow hair. ROGAINE is the only product ever prescribed by doctors for men and women. And, ROGAINE is now available without a prescription in its original, full prescription strength.

Directions: FOR EXTERNAL USE ONLY. Apply one mL 2 times a day directly onto the scalp in the hair loss area. Each applicator contains one dose of medicine. Using more or more often will not improve results. Each bottle should last about 25–30 days, if used as directed. It is not necessary to use fingertips when applying ROGAINE. However, if you use your hands, wash them afterwards. If you miss one or two daily doses of ROGAINE, continue with your next dose. You should not make up for missed doses. Do not apply to other parts of the body. Do not take ROGAINE by mouth.
Keep this and all drugs out of the reach of children. In case of accidental ingestion, seek professional assistance or contact a Poison Control Center Immediately.
Use a mild shampoo if you wash your scalp before applying ROGAINE. There is no need to change your usual hair care routine when using ROGAINE. However, you should apply ROGAINE first and wait for it to dry before applying your styling aids.
Instructions for use of Applicators:
APPLICATOR OPTIONS
Dropper: The child-resistant dropper can be useful for a broad range of hair styles or hair loss because it allows for easy application through the hair and directly onto the scalp.
Sprayer: This may be more useful for broader areas of hair loss.
Using the Applicators
DROPPER
Squeeze the rubber bulb and insert the dropper into the bottle. Release the bulb, allowing the dropper to fill to the 1 mL line. If the level of the solution is above the 1 mL line, squeeze the extra amount back into the bottle. Next, place the tip near the part of the scalp you want to treat and gently squeeze the bulb to gradually release the solution. To prevent the solution from running off the scalp, apply a small amount at a time.
SPRAYER
The sprayer applicator is NOT child resistant. If you have small children, keep the original child-resistant cap and place it back on the bottle after each use. Insert the spray applicator into the bottle and twist on firmly. Next, holding the bottle upright, pump the spray attachment six (6) times to get one full dose (1 mL). Be careful not to inhale the mist.

Warnings: Do not use if
- you have no family history of hair loss.
- hair loss is sudden and/or patchy.
- scalp is red, inflamed, infected, irritated or painful.
- you do not know the reason for your hair loss.
- you are under 18 years of age. Do not use on babies and children.
- you use other topical prescription products on the scalp.

Stop use of ROGAINE and see your doctor if you get:
- chest pain, rapid heatbeat, faintness, or dizziness,
- sudden unexplained weight gain,
- swollen hands or feet,
- redness or irritation.

Side Effects:
The most common side effects are itching and other skin irritations of the treated area of the scalp. ROGAINE contains alcohol, which would cause burning or irritation of the eyes or sensitive skin areas. If ROGAINE accidentally gets into these areas, rinse with large amounts of cold tap water. Contact your doctor if irritation persists.

Additional Information:
Who may use ROGAINE?
ROGAINE may be appropriate for you if you are an adult who is at least 18 years old and experiencing gradually thinning hair or gradual hair loss on the top of the head. The common hereditary thinning or hair loss process begins slowly and may become noticeable only after years of gradual loss. Many of those experiencing hair loss have other family members with gradual thinning hair or hair loss. **If there is no family history of gradual thinning hair or gradual hair loss, or hair loss is patchy, talk to your doctor.**
Who should NOT use ROGAINE?
ROGAINE will not prevent or improve hair loss which may occur with the use of

some prescription and non-prescription medications, certain severe nutritional problems (very low body iron; excessive vitamin A intake), low thyroid states (hypothyroidism), chemotherapy, or diseases which cause scarring of the scalp. Also, ROGAINE will not improve hair loss due to damage from the use of hair care products which cause scarring or deep burns of the scalp or hair grooming methods such as cornrowing or ponytails which require pulling the hair tightly back from the scalp. **You should ask your doctor if you are unsure of the cause of your hair loss.**

Will ROGAINE work for me?
The amount of hair regrowth is different for each person. Not everyone will respond to ROGAINE. The response to ROGAINE cannot be predicted. No one will be able to grow back all their hair. You may respond better if you have been losing your hair for a short period of time or have little initial hair loss.

Will ROGAINE help prevent hair loss?
Yes. ROGAINE is the only brand clinically shown to help stop hair loss.

How soon can I expect results from using ROGAINE?
Since normal hair usually grows only 1/2 to 1 inch per month, hair regrowth with ROGAINE also takes time. Generally new hair growth is slow for a ROGAINE user. Continued use 2 times a day for at least 4 months is usually needed before you notice hair regrowth. Up to 12 months of use may be needed to see your best results from ROGAINE. However, if you do not see hair regrowth in 12 months, stop using ROGAINE and see your doctor. When you first begin to use ROGAINE, your hair loss may continue for up to 2 weeks. This hair loss is temporary. If you continue to lose hair after two weeks, see your doctor.

If ROGAINE is working, what will the hair look like?
At first, hair growth may be soft, downy, colorless hairs. After further use, the new hair should be the same color and thickness as the other hairs on your scalp.

How long do I need to use ROGAINE?
If you respond to ROGAINE, you will need to use it 2 times a day to keep and continue the hair regrowth. Up to 12 months of use may be needed to see your best results with ROGAINE.

What happens if I completely stop using ROGAINE? Will I keep the new hair?
Continuous use of ROGAINE is needed to maintain hair regrowth. If you stop using ROGAINE, the normal hair loss process will start again. You will probably lose your newly regrown hair in three to four months.

Can I have my hair colored or permed or use hair relaxers while using ROGAINE?
We have no information that these treatments change the effect of ROGAINE. However, to avoid possible scalp irritation, you should make sure all of the ROGAINE has been washed off the hair and scalp before using these chemicals.

Can I apply ROGAINE and wash my hair an hour later?
No. For ROGAINE to work best, you should allow ROGAINE to remain on the scalp for about 4 hours before washing.

Can I go swimming or out in the rain?
Yes, as long as you use good judgment. Avoid washing off the ROGAINE. If possible, apply ROGAINE to a dry scalp after swimming, or wait about 4 hours after application before going swimming. Do not let your scalp get wet from the rain after applying ROGAINE.

Can ROGAINE produce unwanted hair growth?
Unwanted hair growth elsewhere on the body has been reported. This may be due to the frequent applying of ROGAINE on the areas of the skin other than the scalp. To prevent unwanted hair growth, limit the application of ROGAINE only to the scalp.

Shown in Product Identification Guide, page 518

ROGAINE® for Women Hair Regrowth Treatment 2% Minoxidil Topical Solution

Description: ROGAINE is a colorless liquid medication for use only on the scalp to help regrow hair.
Active Ingredients: Minoxidil 2% w/v
Inactive Ingredients: Alcohol, 60% v/v, propylene glycol, and purified water.

How Supplied: ROGAINE for Women is available in single, twin, and triple packs.

Indication: ROGAINE is medically proven to regrow hair. ROGAINE is the only product ever prescribed by doctors for men and women. And, ROGAINE is now available without a prescription in its original, full prescription strength.

Directions: FOR EXTERNAL USE ONLY. Apply one mL 2 times a day directly onto the scalp in the hair loss area. Each applicator contains one dose of medicine. Using more or more often will not improve results. Each bottle should last about 25–30 days, if used as directed. It is not necessary to use fingertips when applying ROGAINE. However, if you use your hands, wash them afterwards. If you miss one or two daily doses of ROGAINE, continue with your next dose. You should not make up for missed doses. Do not apply to other parts of the body. Do not take ROGAINE by mouth.
Keep this and all drugs out of the reach of children. In case of accidental ingestion, seek professional assistance or contact a Poison Control Center Immediately.
Use a mild shampoo if you wash your scalp before applying ROGAINE. There is no need to change your usual hair care routine when using ROGAINE. However, you should apply ROGAINE first and wait for it to dry before applying your styling aids.

Instructions for use of Applicators:
APPLICATOR OPTIONS
Dropper: The child-resistant dropper can be useful for a broad range of hair styles or hair loss because it allows for easy application through the hair and directly onto the scalp.
Extender Sprayer: The extender sprayer is designed to help you spray through the hair directly onto the scalp.

Using the Applicators
DROPPER
Squeeze the rubber bulb and insert the dropper into the bottle. Release the bulb, allowing the dropper to fill to the 1 mL line. If the level of the solution is above the 1 mL line, squeeze the extra amount back into the bottle. Next, place the tip near the part of the scalp you want to treat and gently squeeze the bulb to gradually release the solution. To prevent the solution from running off the scalp, apply a small amount at a time.
EXTENDER SPRAYER
The sprayer applicator is NOT child-resistant. If you have small children, keep the original child-resistant cap and place it back on the bottle after each use. Insert the spray applicator into the bottle and twist on firmly. Pull off the small spray head from the plastic tube. Fit the extender spray onto the plastic tub and push down firmly. Remove the cap from the end of the extended spray. Pump the extender spray six (6) times to get one full dose (1 mL). Be careful not to inhale the mist.

Warnings: Do not use if
- you have no family history of hair loss.
- hair loss is sudden and/or patchy.
- scalp is red, inflamed, infected, irritated or painful.
- you do not know the reason for your hair loss.
- you are under 18 years of age. Do not use on babies and children.
- you use other topical prescription products on the scalp.
- you have ever had an allergic reaction to ROGAINE.
- you have normal hair loss associated with childbirth.

Stop use of ROGAINE and see your doctor if you get:
- chest pain, rapid heartbeat, faintness, or dizziness,
- sudden unexplained weight gain,
- swollen hands or feet,
- redness or irritation.

As with any drug, if you are pregnant or nursing a baby, seek the advice of a health professional before using this product.

Side Effects:
The most common side effects are itching and other skin irritations of the treated area of scalp. ROGAINE contains alcohol, which would cause burning or irritation of the eyes or sensitive skin areas. If ROGAINE accidentally gets into these areas, rinse with large amounts of cold tap water. Contact your doctor if irritation persists.

Continued on next page

Pharmacia & Upjohn—Cont.

Additional Information:

Who may use ROGAINE?

ROGAINE may be appropriate for you if your are an adult who is at least 18 years old and experiencing gradually thinning hair or gradual hair loss on the top of the head. The common hereditary thinning or hair loss process begins slowly and may become noticeable only afer years of gradual loss. Many of those experiencing hair loss have other family members with gradual thinning hair or hair loss. **If there is no family history of gradual thinning hair or gradual hair loss, or hair loss is patchy, talk to your doctor.**

Who should NOT use ROGAINE?

ROGAINE will not prevent or improve hair loss which may occur with the use of some prescription and non-prescription medications, certain severe nutritional problems (very low body iron; excessive vitamin A intake), low thyroid states (hypothyroidism), chemotherapy, or diseases which cause scarring of the scalp. Also, ROGAINE will not improve hair loss due to damage from the use of hair care products which cause scarring or deep burns of the scalp or hair grooming methods such as cornrowing or ponytails which require pulling the hair tightly back from the scalp. **You should ask your doctor if you are unsure of the cause of your hair loss.**

Will ROGAINE work for me?

The amount of hair regrowth is different for each person. Not everyone will respond to ROGAINE. The response to ROGAINE cannot be predicted. No one will be able to grow back all their hair. You may respond better if you have been losing your hair for a short period of time or have little initial hair loss.

Will ROGAINE help prevent hair loss?

Yes. ROGAINE is the only brand clinically shown to help stop hair loss.

How soon can I expect results from using ROGAINE?

Since normal hair usually grows only $^1/_2$ to 1 inch per month, hair regrowth with ROGAINE also takes time. Generally new hair growth is slow for a ROGAINE user. Continued use 2 times a day for at least 4 months is usually needed before you notice hair regrowth. Up to 8 months of use may be needed to see your best results from ROGAINE. However, if your do not see hair regrowth in 8 months, stop using ROGAINE and see your doctor. When you first begin to use ROGAINE, your hair loss may continue for up to 2 weeks. This hair loss is temporary. If you continue to lose hair after two weeks, see your doctor.

If ROGAINE is working, what will the hair look like?

At first, hair growth may be soft, downy, colorless hairs. After further use, the new hair should be the same color and thickness as the other hairs on our scalp.

How long do I need to use ROGAINE?

If you respond to ROGAINE, you will need to use it 2 times a day to keep and continue the hair regrowth. Up to 8 months of use may be needed to see your best results with ROGAINE.

What happens if I completely stop using ROGAINE? Will I keep the new hair?

Continuous use of ROGAINE is needed to maintain hair regrowth. If you stop using ROGAINE, the normal hair loss process will start again. You will probably lose your newly regrown hair in three to four months.

Can I have my hair colored or permed or use hair relaxers whle using ROGAINE?

We have no information that these treatments change the effect of ROGAINE. However, to avoid possible scalp irritation, you should make sure all of the ROGAINE has been washed off the hair and scalp before using these chemicals.

Can I apply ROGAINE and wash my hair an hour later?

No. For ROGAINE to work best, you should allow ROGAINE to remain on the scalp for about 4 hours before washing.

Can I go swimming or out in the rain?

Yes, as long as you use good judgment. Avoid washing off the ROGAINE. If possible, apply ROGAINE to a dry scalp after swimming, or wait about 4 hours after application before going swimming. Do not let your scalp get wet from the rain after applying ROGAINE.

Can ROGAINE produce unwanted hair growth?

Unwanted hair growth elsewhere on the body has been reported. This may be due to the frequent applying of ROGAINE on the areas of the skin other than the scalp. To prevent unwanted hair growth, limit the application of ROGAINE only to the scalp.

Shown in Product Identification Guide, page 518

SURFAK® LIQUI-GELS®
Stool Softener Laxative

Indications: Surfak®, a stool softener, is indicated for the relief of occasional constipation. Unlike some other types of laxatives, Surfak contains no harsh stimulants that can upset your stomach or cause cramps. Instead, Surfak works gently by drawing water into the stool, making it softer and easier to pass. With Surfak you can expect to return to regularity in 12 to 72 hours.

Active Ingredients: Each soft gelatin Liqui-gel contains 240 mg docusate calcium.

Inactive Ingredients: Also contains corn oil, FD&C Blue #1 and Red #40, gelatin, glycerin, parabens, sorbitol, and other ingredients.

Dosage and Administration: Adults and children 12 years of age and over: one capsule by mouth daily for several days or until bowel movements are normal. For use in children under 12, consult a physician.

Warnings: Do not use laxative products when abdominal pain, nausea, or vomiting are present unless directed by a doctor. If you have noticed a sudden change in bowel habits that persists over a period of 2 weeks, consult a doctor before using a laxative. Laxative products should not be used for a period longer than 1 week unless directed by a doctor. Rectal bleeding or failure to have a bowel movement after use of a laxative may indicate a serious condition. Discontinue use and consult your doctor. Keep this and all drugs out of the reach of children. In case of accidental overdose, seek professional assistance or contact a poison control center immediately. As with any drug, if you are pregnant or nursing a baby, seek the advice of a health professional before using this product.

Drug Interaction Precaution: Do not take this product if you are presently taking mineral oil, unless directed by a doctor.

How Supplied: Packages of 10, 30, 100 and 500 red soft gelatin capsules and Unit Dose 100s (10 × 10 strips).

LIQUI-GELS® Reg TM R P Scherer Corp

Shown in Product Identification Guide, page 518

Pharmanex Inc.

625 COCHRAN STREET
SIMI VALLEY, CA 93065

Direct Inquiries to:
Customer Service
(800) 999–6229
FAX: (805) 582–9301

Medical Emergency Contact:
Michael Chang, Ph.D.
(805) 582–9300
FAX: (805) 582–9301

BIOGINKGO 27/7™
Extra Strength and

BIOGINKGO 24/6™
***Ginkgo biloba* leaf Extract**
[*bī'o-gĭng'-kō*]
60 mg tablets
Dietary Supplements

Description: **BioGinkgo** is an all-natural, standardized extract of the leaves of *Ginkgo biloba* trees for use as a dietary supplement to improve blood circulation to the brain and extremities, enhance memory and mental function, and protect the body from oxidative cellular damage caused by free radicals.*

Ginkgo biloba extract (GBE) is one of the most widely used botanicals in the world and the focus of extensive scientific research, including over 300 published studies and reports to its credit. Twenty years of research led to the development of a standardized, concentrated extract from the leaves—with a scientifically-supported composition of 22 to 27% flavonoid glycoside content and 5 to 7% terpene lactone content as specified by the German Commission E—an expert panel of physicians, pharmacists, toxicologists, pharmacognosists, and others familiar with medicinal plant research.

BioGinkgo is available in two scientifically-supported formulations:

(1) **BioGinkgo 27/7 Extra Strength** (27% ginkgo flavone glycosides and 7% terpene lactones); contains significantly greater levels of the identified active constituents than the standard strength formulation listed below.

(2) **BioGinkgo 24/6** (24% ginkgo flavone glycosides and 6% terpene lactones).

The natural ginkgolides concentrated in **BioGinkgo** are unique compounds found only in the *Ginkgo biloba* tree. Ginkgolides are potent Platelet Activating Factor (PAF) antagonists; ginkgolide B is the most potent PAF antagonist. Ginkgolide B has been demonstrated to produce beneficial effects in blood circulation and mental function.

BioGinkgo is specifically enriched to provide at least 80% more ginkgolide B than the leading brand of standardized GBE. In an animal study comparing **BioGinkgo 27/7** to the leading GBE, **BioGinkgo 27/7** reached higher levels of plasma concentration of anti-PAF components, and manifested a faster onset and longer duration of action of anti-PAF activity over a 12-hour period.

Ingredients: **BioGinkgo 24/6** and **27/7** are standardized 50:1 extracts of *Ginkgo biloba* leaf extracts supplied in 60 mg tablets and sold as Dietary Supplements for oral administration. Tablets are coated (gold colored coating for **BioGinkgo 24/6** and green colored coating for **BioGinkgo 27/7**) for ease of swallowing. Other ingredients include: lactose anhydrous, microcrystalline cellulose, corn starch, sodium starch glycolate, Opadry® colors (which contain added colors, including the Lakes of Yellow 5, Yellow 6, and Blue 1), colloidal silicon dioxide, and magnesium stearate.

Benefits of *Ginkgo biloba* extract (GBE): GBE promotes healthy blood flow: GBE helps to maintain normal blood circulation in the body, including the brain and the extremities without a "borrowing" effect on adjacent areas of normal flow.* GBE promotes efficient circulation by helping to maintain the elasticity of arteries and capillaries.* Terpene lactones specific to GBE inhibit PAF, which may contribute to circulation blockage.* Ginkgolide B binds to PAF receptors.*

GBE improves memory and enhances mental function: GBE increases the rate at which information is transmitted between nerve cells by increasing blood flow to the brain and the Central Nervous System (CNS).*

GBE promotes antioxidant activity: GBE has potent dietary antioxidant properties. Antioxidants appear to combat free radicals, which may be produced in the body in response to environmental or dietary toxins. Free radicals are considered to be a key factor in the oxidative damage to cellular constituents—including cell membranes and DNA—which is associated with the aging process.* The brain and the rest of the CNS have a high lipid content in the cells membranes. Free radicals may attack the lipids in cell membranes and form lipid peroxides, which damage membrane integrity and produce a gradual loss of membrane semi-permeability. Antioxidants seem to protect against the formation of lipid peroxides.*

Recommended Use: For use by adults as a dietary supplement, take one 60 mg tablet twice per day, in the morning and evening, with fluid after a meal; swallow tablets without chewing them. For optimal results, take **BioGinkgo 24/6** or **27/7** as a dietary supplement daily. Users should allow up to 12 weeks for optimum benefits to manifest themselves, although some people notice benefits in as little as two to three weeks.

Safety: BioGinkgo has not been evaluated in children and should only be used by adults. Because there are no adequate and well-controlled studies in pregnant or lactating women, this product should not be used during pregnancy or lactation without the advice of a physician. No known drug interactions; contact your doctor if you are taking a prescription medicine. GBE appears to be well tolerated. Adverse reactions that have been reported include mild gastrointestinal discomfort in less than 1% of persons in studies conducted, as well as rare reports of allergic skin reactions. Some people may experience a mild, transient headache for the first two or three days of use. Otherwise, there have not been any reports of significant adverse reactions to GBE at the prescribed dosages or in patients ingesting as much as 600 mg of the extract in one dose.

How Supplied: Tablets of **BioGinkgo 27/7** and **24/6** are 60 mg each supplied in packages of 40 count, and can be purchased at major drug, grocery and discount retail outlets in the dietary supplement category.

Storage: Store in a dry, cool place. Avoid excessive heat. Protect from light.

Shelf Life: Expiration date is imprinted on bottom of box and each blister pack.

***These statements regarding BioGinkgo have not been evaluated by the Food and Drug Administration. This product is not intended to diagnose, treat, cure or prevent any disease.**

Shown in Product Identification Guide, page 518

CHOLESTIN™

[*kō-lĕs'-tĭn*]

600 mg capsules

Dietary Supplement

Description: Dietary supplementation with CHOLESTIN is recommended for healthy adult males and postmenopausal women concerned about maintaining healthy blood cholesterol and triglyceride levels, and who—in consultation with their physicians—has determined that dietary supplementation rather than medical treatment is needed for cholesterol control.* CHOLESTIN is intended for use as part of a cholesterol maintenance program that includes a healthy diet that is restricted in saturated fat and cholesterol, and other appropriate measures including regular exercise. **CHOLESTIN is not recommended for treating a disease, and this product should not be substituted for prescribed medications.**

Over twenty clinical trials in China, involving thousands of people, support the use of the ingredient in CHOLESTIN as a dietary supplement to maintain healthy blood lipid levels. Significant effects of dietary supplementation with CHOLESTIN, which contains HMG-CoA reductase inhibitors and unsaturated fatty acids, include lowering of Low Density Lipoprotein (LDL) cholesterol and triglycerides, and increasing High Density Lipoprotein (HDL) cholesterol.* The triglyceride-lowering effect of CHOLESTIN is likely not attributed solely to the presence of HMG-CoA reductase inhibitors.* It has been hypothesized that relatively high concentrations of unsaturated fatty acids found in CHOLESTIN may work in concert with HMG-CoA reductase inhibitors to provide this additional health benefit.

Most of the body's supply of cholesterol (approximately 80%) is synthesized in the liver. This biosynthetic process is rigorously controlled by natural feedback mechanisms. Because the most important, "rate limiting" step in cholesterol biosynthesis is catalyzed by the enzyme HMG-CoA reductase, inhibiting the activity of this enzyme markedly reduces production of cholesterol. When cholesterol biosynthesis in inhibited, liver cells produce more receptors for LDL ("bad") cholesterol and absorb more LDL-cholesterol from the blood. Inhibition of HMG-CoA reductase, in addition to restricting production of cholesterol, thus leads to noticeable reduction of circulating LDL-cholesterol.

Ingredients: Each capsule of CHOLESTIN contains 600 mg of scientifically-standardized, proprietary *Monascus purpureus* Went yeast fermented on premium rice. This yeast is a traditional Chinese health food specifically selected to produce high levels of key compounds found in this product, as well as the yeast's natural fermentation by-products. Among the key constituents naturally found in CHOLESTIN is a mix-

Continued on next page

Pharmanex—Cont.

ture of metabolites which resemble well-characterized HMG-CoA reductase inhibitors, including lovastatin, as well as significant levels of unsaturated fatty acids. CHOLESTIN is produced using a proprietary modern fermentation process, and guarantees a consistent and efficacious dietary supplement by standardizing via HPLC method for maximal levels of the key metabolites.

Recommended Use: As a dietary supplement, it is recommended that two 600 mg capsules of CHOLESTIN be taken twice per day (two capsules with or shortly after the morning meal and two capsules with or shortly after the evening meal). CHOLESTIN should be taken with a meal to minimize the risk of digestive tract discomfort. **Do not take more than four capsules in any 24-hour period, unless recommended by a physician. Immediately discontinue use of CHOLESTIN if you experience any unexplained muscle pain, tenderness or weakness, especially if accompanied by flu symptoms.**

Warnings: Keep out of reach of children.

- **Do not use CHOLESTIN if you are pregnant, can become pregnant, or are breast feeding.**
- CHOLESTIN is not to be used by anyone under 20 years of age.
- Consult with your physician before using CHOLESTIN if you are taking any medication.
- Ingredients in CHOLESTIN (HMG-CoA reductase inhibitors e.g., lovastatin) have been associated with some rare but serious side effects, including serious diseases of the liver and skeletal muscle.
- Do not take CHOLESTIN if:
- you are at risk for liver disease, have active liver disease or any history of liver disease;
- you consume more than 2 drinks of alcohol per day;
- you have a serious infection;
- you have undergone an organ transplantation;
- you have a serious disease or physical disorder or have recently undergone major surgery.

Adverse Effects: Based on foreign clinical studies involving thousands of subjects, only a small number of individuals reported slight discomfort in the digestive tract; otherwise, no adverse effects were observed during eight week study periods.

How Supplied: Capsules of CHOLESTIN 600 mg each are supplied in packages of 48 or 80 count, and can be purchased at major drug, grocery and discount stores in the dietary supplement category.

Storage: Store in a dry, cool place. Avoid excessive heat. Protect from light.

Shelf Life: Expiration date is imprinted on bottom of box and each blister pack.

*** These statements regarding CHOLESTIN have not been evaluated by the Food and Drug Administration. This product is not intended to diagnose, treat, cure or prevent any disease.**

Shown in Product Identification Guide, page 518

CordyMax Cs-4™

Cordyceps sinensis

[*kord' -ə-măk sē-ĕs-fór, kord' -ə- seps sĭ-nĕn'-sĭs*]

525 mg capsules

Dietary Supplement

Description: CordyMax Cs-4 is a standardized, proprietary fermentation product developed from mycelia isolated from the renown mushroom, *Cordyceps sinensis* (Berk.) Sacc., and used as a dietary supplement to promote vitality and overall well-being.* The mycelia strain used to produce CordyMax Cs-4, *Paecilomyces hepiali* Chen, has been scientifically tested on humans and animals over the past 15 years, and is recognized as having activity most similar to natural *Cordyceps sinensis.* For over two-thousand years, *Cordyceps sinensis* has remained the premier agent in the pharmacopeia of Traditional Chinese Medicine to restore vitality and energy, and to serve as a potent tonic conducive to general health.*

In humans and animals, CordyMax Cs-4 substantially increases the serum levels of the enzyme superoxide dismutase (SOD). This enhancement of the enzyme's proven ability to scavenge the free radicals associated with age-related oxidative cellular damage may explain the traditional use of the mushroom as a food additive to improve vitality, energy, and quality of life.* By increasing the body's resistance to daily environmental and occupational stresses, CordyMax Cs-4 promotes a broad spectrum of health benefits, including the dietary management of healthy lung function and a decrease in sensations of tiredness and fatigue.* CordyMax Cs-4 is not reported to stimulate the Central Nervous System.

Ingredients: Each capsule of CordyMax Cs-4 contains 525 mg of the fermentation product of the mycelia (*Paecilomyces hepiali* Chen) isolated from the mushroom *Cordyceps sinensis* (Berk.) Sacc. CordyMax Cs-4 is scientifically standardized by HPLC method to ensure an efficacious and consistent product containing 0.14% adenosine and 5% mannitol (an indicator of polysaccharide content).

Recommended Use: As a dietary supplement: take two 525 mg capsules, two or three times per day with water and food. The effects of CordyMax Cs-4 are gradual; while mild effects are evident within a week, the most significant benefits take 3 to 6 weeks.

Safety: With the exception of one case of allergic skin reaction reported in 1993, no other adverse reactions have been reported from clinicians and hospital records since the commercial introduction of CordyMax Cs-4 in China in 1989, and its use by millions of subjects. During clinical trials in China, some subjects noted a mild sensation of thirst, described as "dry throat," in the first days of dietary supplementation; this sensation later decreased or disappeared. One subject noted slight nausea. All subjects considered these effects quite tolerable, and none of these subjects discontinued supplementation because of these effects. No cases of CNS effects have been reported. No contraindications were identified based on Chinese human studies.

Warnings: CordyMax Cs-4 has not been evaluated in children and should only be used by adults. Because there are no adequate and well-controlled studies in pregnant or lactating women, this product should not be used during pregnancy or lactation without the advice of a physician.

How Supplied: Capsules of CordyMax Cs-4 525 mg each are supplied in packages of 64 or 112 count and can be purchased at major drug, grocery and discount stores in the dietary supplement category.

Storage: Store in a dry, cool place. Avoid excessive heat. Protect from light.

Shelf Life: Expiration date is imprinted on bottom of box and each foil blister pack.

***These statements regarding CordyMax Cs-4 have not been evaluated by the Food and Drug Administration. This product is not intended to diagnose, treat, cure or prevent any disease.**

TĒGREEN 97™

[*tē-grēn 97*]

250 mg capsules

Dietary Supplement

Description: TĒGREEN 97 is a standardized polyphenol extract of the fresh leaves of the tea plant *Camellia sinensis.* The major components of TĒGREEN 97 are polyphenols, which have proven free radical scavenging and antioxidant properties.* The polyphenols with the most active antioxidant activity are the catechins, specifically epigallocatechin gallate (EGCg) and epigallocatechin (EGC).*

Ingredients: The phytochemical composition of green tea leaves varies with age of the leaf, position of the leaf on the harvested shoot, growing region, season and horticultural practices. Each 250 mg capsule of TĒGREEN 97 is produced from high-quality tea leaf buds and the adjacent young leaves, and processed using proprietary manufacturing methods to consistently provide a standardized concentration of polyphenols (97%). Over two-thirds of the polyphenols in TĒGREEN 97 are the important, free radical quenching catechins* as verified by HPLC:

TĒGREEN 97 Polyphenolic Profile

Total polyphenols	>97%	
Catechins fraction	>65%, in which:	
L-EGCg	>40%	(-)-epigallocatechin gallate
GCG	>10%	Gallocatechin gallate
L-EGC	>10%	(-)-epigallocatechin
L-EC	>5%	(-)-epicatechin

Others: proanthocyanidines, lignans and phenolic acids. Minimal amounts of caffeine, less than 2.5%.

Scientific Support: The ingestion of green tea polyphenols promotes general well-being by affecting a very broad spectrum of functions. In large-scale epidemiological studies in Asia (totaling more than 100,000 people for study periods up to 10 years), daily consumption of four or more cups of a green tea beverage was associated with significant overall health benefits, even after adjustments were made for potential confounding factors including age, tobacco and alcohol use, and body weight.

The catechins and other polyphenols in green tea offer antioxidant benefits by combatting free radicals. Free radicals, which are produced in the body as a result of exposure to environmental, occupational or dietary toxins, have been associated with damage to cellular constituents, including cell membranes and DNA.* Following ingestion, green tea polyphenols can be detected in blood, urine and feces, suggesting that the polyphenol compounds are efficiently absorbed and distributed to tissues and cells, where they may be available to protect cells from oxidative damage.*

The dietary supplement use of green tea polyphenols (especially the catechin EGCg) may help: (1) block the formation of toxic compounds, including nitrosamines* (2) suppress the activation of free radicals* (3) detoxify or trap free radicals* (4) inhibit spontaneous and photo-enhanced lipid peroxidation.*

In addition to providing direct protection from the oxidative effects of toxic free radicals, green tea polyphenols may also enhance the body's natural resistance to environmental toxins and stresses by increasing the activity of certain antioxidant and detoxifying enzymes, including glutathione peroxidase, glutathione reductase, glutathione-S-transferase, catalase, and quinone reductase in some cells and tissues.*

Recommended Use: As a dietary supplement: Take one 250 mg capsule daily, which includes >160 mg of catechins, of which >100 mg is EGCg. TĒGREEN 97 can be taken any time of the day, but should be taken with water and food. Each capsule provides the green tea polyphenols typically found in about four cups of high-quality brewed green tea, but with only minimal amounts of caffeine—about 6 mg, or less than the caffeine in one ounce of 5 minute brew green tea. To achieve the health related benefits of a green tea regimen, one may need to consume an amount of green tea or green tea polyphenols equivalent to the amount consumed in the positive population studies - approximately four cups per day.

Warnings: TĒGREEN 97 has not been evaluated in children and should only be used by adults. Because there are no adequate and well-controlled studies in pregnant or lactating women, this product should not be used during pregnancy or lactation without the advise of a physician. The polyphenol content in green tea is not known to be associated with any significant side effects or toxicity; it is recommended that TĒGREEN 97 be taken with food to minimize any possibility of gastric discomfort. Since TĒGREEN 97 contains only minimal amounts of caffeine (approximately 6 mg), it should not produce the stimulant effect in some people caused by the consumption of caffeine-containing beverages.

How Supplied: TĒGREEN 97 capsules are supplied in packages of 30 count, and can be purchased at major drug, grocery and discount stores in the dietary supplement category.

Storage: Store in a dry, cool place. Avoid excessive heat. Protect from light.

Shelf Life: Expiration date is imprinted on bottom of box and each foil blister pack.

*** These statements regarding TĒGREEN 97 have not been evaluated by the Food and Drug Administration. This product is not intended to diagnose, treat, cure or prevent any disease.**

EDUCATIONAL MATERIALS

For more information about Pharmanex Natural Healthcare Products:

Call customer Service at 800-999-6229 or FAX 805-582-9301, Monday through Friday, 8 am to 5 pm, Pacific Time. For specific questions about the ingredients in Pharmanex products, call the Natural Healthcare Hotline and speak with a natural healthcare specialist directly 800-247-5169, Monday through Friday, 9:00 am to 5:00 pm, Mountain Time. Visit our web site and access information from the Internet www.pharmanex.com

---

Pharmaton Natural Health Products Division of Boehringer Ingelheim Pharmaceuticals, Inc.

900 RIDGEBURY ROAD
RIDGEFIELD, CT 06877

Direct Inquiries to:
Customer Service: (800) 243-0127
FAX: (203) 798-5771

For Medical Emergency Contact:
Marvin Wetter, M.D.: (203) 798-4361

GINKOBA™

Ginkgo Biloba Extract
[*Gĭn-kō-bă*]

GINKOBA—Standardized Ginkgo Biloba Extract (50:1).

Over 30 years of extensive research results have shown that GINKOBA is a safe and natural way to supplement your diet. No other extract of the Ginkgo Biloba tree meets the standards of the one in GINKOBA.

NUTRITION FACTS:
Serving Size: 1 tablet
Each Tablet contains:
Calories: 0 Calories from Fat 0

	% Daily Value*
Total Fat 0g	0%
Cholesterol 0mg	0%
Sodium 0mg	0%
Total Carbohydrate 0g	0%
Protein 0g	0%

*Percent Daily Values are based on a 2,000 calorie diet.

Ingredients: Each GINKOBA tablet contains 40 mg of concentrated (50:1) extract from the leaves of the *Ginkgo Biloba* tree. The extract in GINKOBA is precisely standardized to 24% Ginkgo flavonoid glycosides along with other key constituents (Ginkgolides and Bilobalides) in their proven ratios.

Also Contains: Hydroxypropyl methyl cellulose, lactose, talc, polyethylene glycol, magnesium stearate, titanium dioxide, synthetic iron oxides.

Suggested Use: When taken as directed, GINKOBA is a natural way to enhance your mental focus. GINKOBA will help you maintain an overall feeling of healthy well-being, reducing normal forgetfulness and improving conentration.

Recommended Adult Intake: Adults over 12 years old should take one tablet, swallowed whole, with water three times daily at mealtimes.

Cautions: As with other supplements, please keep this product out of the reach of children. In case of accidental overdose, seek the advice of a professional immediately. If you are taking a prescription medicine, are pregnant or

Continued on next page

Pharmaton—Cont.

lactating, please contact your doctor before taking GINKOBA. No information is available on the use of ginkgo biloba extract in children under the age of 12 years old.

The statements presented on this package have not been evaluated by the Food and Drug Administration. This product is not intended to diagnose, treat, cure or prevent any disease.

Store at room temperature and avoid excessive heat above 40°C (104°F) to maintain optimal freshness.

Shown in Product Identification Guide, page 518

GINSANA®
G115 Ginseng Extract
[*Gin-sa-na*]

GINSANA Capsules — Standardized G115® Ginseng Extract (4%).

GINSANA Chewy Squares—Standardized G115® Ginseng Extract.

No other ginseng extract meets the quality standards of the one in GINSANA. Over 25 years of extensive research has shown that GINSANA is a safe and beneficial way to supplement your diet.

NUTRITION FACTS:
Serving Size: 1 capsule
Each Capsule contains:
Calories: 5 Calories from Fat 0

	% Daily Value*
Total Fat 0g	0%
Cholesterol 0mg	0%
Sodium 0mg	0%
Total Carbohydrate 0g	0%
Protein 0g	0%

*Percent Daily Values are based on a 2,000 calorie diet.

Supplement Facts
Serving Size: 1 Square
Amount Per Square: Standardized G115® Ginseng Extract (Panax Ginseng, C.A. Meyer) (root) 50 mg*
* Daily Value not established

Ingredients: Each GINSANA capsule contains 100 mg of highly standardized, concentrated ginseng extract from the roots of the highest quality Korean Panax Ginseng, C.A. Meyer. This special standardization insures a consistent level of the eight most effective ginsenosides in their proven ratios.

Also contains: Sunflower oil, gelatin, glycerin, lecithin, beeswax, chlorophyll.

Ingredients: Each GINSANA Chewy Square contains 50 mg of highly standardized, concentrated ginseng extract from the roots of the highest quality Korean Panax Ginseng, C.A. Meyer.

Also contains: Sucrose, glucose, palm kernel oil, gelatin, citric acid, ascorbic acid, lecithin, natural flavoring and coloring.

Suggested Use: When taken as directed, GINSANA is a natural way to enhance your physical endurance by improving your body's ability to utilize oxygen more efficiently. GINSANA will help you maintain your natural energy and an overall feeling of healthy well-being.

Recommended Adult Intake/Capsules: Adults over 12 years old should take two soft gelatin capsules, swallowed whole, with water in the morning or one capsule in the morning and one in the afternoon. Research on doses above 200 mg per day does not substantiate any better effectiveness. Optimal effectiveness has been shown with 4 weeks of continuous use.

Recommended Adult Intake/Chewy Squares: Adults over 12 years old should take up to four GINSANA Chewy Squares daily.

Precautions: As with other vitamins and supplements, please keep this product out of the reach of children. No serious or significant adverse reactions or drug interactions have been reported to date. However, as with any supplement, contact your doctor if you are taking a prescription medicine, are pregnant or lactating. There have been rare reports of mild allergic skin reactions with the use of the extract in this product. In case of accidental overdose, seek the advice of a professional immediately.

The statements presented on this package have not been evaluated by the Food and Drug Administration. This product is not intended to diagnose, treat, cure or prevent any disease.

Store at room temperature and avoid excess heat above 40°C (104°F) to maintain optimal freshness.

Shown in Product Identification Guide, page 518

VITASANA™
DAILY DIETARY SUPPLEMENT

VITASANA is the first scientifically formulated and clinically tested ginseng multivitamin combination. VITASANA is a unique formula of essential vitamins and minerals you need for good nutrition, plus GINSANA's exclusive G115 ginseng extract for the vitality that's an integral part of your total health. VITASANA is the first multivitamin/ginseng supplement in an easy to swallow Gelcap dosage form.

Recommended Adult Intake: Adults over 12 years old should take two Gelcaps in the morning or one gelcap in the morning and one in the afternoon. Optimal effectiveness has been clinically seen after 4 weeks of continuous use.

The statements presented on this package have not been evaluated by the Food and Drug Administration.
This product is not intended to diagnose, treat, cure or prevent any disease.

Supplement Facts
Serving Size 2 Gelcaps

Each Serving Contains	% Daily Value
Vitamin A 4000 IU (as beta carotene)	80%
Vitamin C 120 mg (as ascorbic acid)	200%
Vitamin D 400 IU (as cholecalciferol)	100%
Vitamin E 30 IU (as dl-alpha tocopherol)	100%
Vitamin B1 2.4 mg (as thiamine mononitrate)	160%
Vitamin B2 3.4 mg (riboflavin)	200%
Vitamin B3 30 mg (niacinamide)1	50%
Vitamin B6 4 mg (as pyridoxine HCl)	200%
Folic Acid 400 mcg	100%
Vitamin B12 2 mcg (as cobalamin conc.)	33%
Calcium 200 mg (as calcium phosphate)	20%
Iron 18 mg (as ferrous sulfate)	100%
Phosphorus 160 mg (as calcium phosphate)	16%
Magnesium 20 mg (as magnesium oxide)	5%
Zinc 2 mg (as zinc sulfate)	13.3%
Copper 2 mg (as copper sulfate)	100%
Manganese 2 mg (as manganese sulfate)	100%
Potassium 16 mg (as potassium chloride)	0.5%

Standardized G115 Ginseng Extract 80 mg (from Panax Ginseng C.A. Meyer) (root)*

*Daily Value not established

Other Ingredients: Microcrystalline Cellulose, Povidone, Croecarmellose Sodium, Magnesium Stearate, Colloidal Silica, Hydroxypropyl mentyl cellulose, Ethylcellulose, Dibutyl Sebecate, Vanillin powder, Polyethylene Glycol.

Warning: Close tightly and keep out of reach of children. Contains iron, which can be harmful or fatal to children in large doses. In case of accidental overdose, seek professional assistance or contact a Poison Control Center Immediately.

Store at room temperature and avoid excessive heat above 40° C (104° F) to maintain optimal freshness.

Shown in Product Identification Guide, page 518

Pharmavite

15451 SAN FERNANDO
MISSION BLVD.
MISSION HILLS, CA 91345

Direct Inquiries to:
Nature's Resource Brand Group
800-423-2405
(FAX) 818-837-6129

Medical Emergency Contact:
Mr. Paul Bolar
800-423-2405
(FAX) 818-837-6109

STANDARDIZED ECHINACEA HERB

Echinacea purpurea

Active Ingredients: Each capsule contains 380 mg of whole *Echinacea purpurea* herb.

Suggested Use: To stimulate natural resistance by boosting the immune system.

Recommended Intake: Take one to three capsules three times daily with water at mealtimes.

Warnings: Keep out of reach of children. Not recommended for individuals with auto-immune conditions. Do not use this product if you are allergic to flowers or of the daisy family (composite flowers).

How Supplied: Capsule, bottle of 50. Store at room temperature.

GINKGO BILOBA LEAF STANDARDIZED EXTRACT

Active Ingredients: Each capsule contains 40 mg of concentrated (50:1) Ginkgo biloba leaf extract standardized to 24% Ginkgo flavone glycosides along with the important terpene lactones (Ginkgolides and Bilobalide), supplied in a base of Alfalfa leaves.

Suggested Use: Increases peripheral circulation, thereby enhancing blood flow to the arms, legs and brain.

Recommended Intake: Take one capsule three times daily with water at mealtimes.

Warnings: Keep out of reach of children.

How Supplied: Capsules, bottle of 50. Store at room temperature.

SAW PALMETTO STANDARDIZED EXTRACT

Serona repens

Active Ingredients: Each capsule contains 80 mg of a liposterolic extract of Saw Palmetto berries standardized to contain between 85% and 95% fatty acids and sterols.

Suggested Use: Helps maintain proper urinary function in mature men.

Recommended Intake: Take two caplets, two times daily with water at mealtimes.

Warnings: Keep out of reach of children.

How Supplied: Capsule, bottle of 50. Store at room temperature.

STANDARDIZED VALERIAN ROOT

Valerina officinalis

Active Ingredients: Each capsule contains 530 mg of whole Valeriana officinalis root.

Suggested Use: Natural support to enhance night time rest.

Recommended Intake: Take one or two capsules with water one hour prior to bedtime.

Warnings: Keep out of reach of children. Do not drive or operate heavy equipment while taking this product.

How Supplied: Capsule, bottle of 50. Store at room temperature.

Procter & Gamble

P. O. BOX 5516
CINCINNATI, OH 45201

Direct Inquiries to:
Charles Lambert
(800) 358-8707

For Medical Emergencies:
Call Collect: (513) 558-4422

CREST® Sensitivity Protection Toothpaste for sensitive teeth and cavity prevention

Active Ingredients: Potassium Nitrate (5%), Sodium Fluoride (0.15% w/v fluoride ion).

Actions: Builds protection against sensitive tooth pain. Contains **Fluoride** for cavity prevention. Gentle on tooth enamel, leaves teeth feeling clean.

WHAT ARE SENSITIVE TEETH?

If you experience flashes of tooth pain or discomfort from cold or hot foods and drinks, or even when you touch your teeth with your toothbrush, you may suffer from **Dentinal Hypersensitivity** (or "sensitive teeth.") **Hypersensitivity** can occur when dentin, which surrounds the pulp cavity and tooth nerve, is not protected. Dentin can become exposed when gums recede and the protective layer covering the root surface is worn away, leaving dentin exposed. Crest Sensitivity Protection helps relieve the pain of sensitive teeth by soothing the nerves in your teeth when the dentin is exposed.

This product has been given the Seal of Acceptance from the Council on Scientific Affairs–ADA.

Uses: When used regularly, builds increasing protection against painful sensitivity of the teeth to cold, heat, acids, sweets, or contact, and aids in the prevention of cavities.

Directions: Adults and children 12 years of age and older: Apply at least a 1-inch strip of the product onto a soft bristle toothbrush. Brush teeth thoroughly for at least 1 minute twice a day (morning and evening) or as recommended by a dentist or physician. Make sure to brush all sensitive areas of the teeth. Do not swallow. Children under 12 years of age: ask a dentist or physician.

Warnings: Sensitive teeth may indicate a serious problem that may need prompt care by a dentist. See your dentist if the problem persists or worsens. Do not use this product longer than four weeks unless recommended by a dentist or physician. **Keep this and all drugs out of the reach of children.**

Inactive Ingredients: Water, Hydrated Silica, Glycerin, Sorbitol, Trisodium Phosphate, Sodium Lauryl Sulfate, Cellulose Gum, Flavor, Xanthan Gum, Sodium Saccharin, Titanium Dioxide.

How Supplied: 6.2 OZ (175g), 2.5 OZ (70g) and 1.0 OZ (28g) tubes in cartons.

HEAD & SHOULDERS® DANDRUFF SHAMPOO

Head & Shoulders Dandruff Shampoo for Normal hair offers effective control of persistent dandruff, and beautiful hair from a pleasant-to-use formula. Double-blind and expert-graded testing have proven that Head & Shoulders Dandruff Shampoo reduces dandruff. It is also gentle enough to use every day for clean, manageable hair.

Active Ingredient: 1% pyrithione zinc suspended in a mild surfactant base. Shampoo also includes mild conditioning agents.

Indications: For effective control of dandruff of the scalp.

Actions: Head & Shoulders reduces the flaking and itching caused by dandruff. The pyrithione zinc active helps kill the microscopic fungus associated with dandruff.

Warnings: For external use only. Avoid contact with eyes. If contact occurs, rinse eyes thoroughly with water. If condition worsens or does not improve after regular use of this product as directed, consult a doctor. Keep this and all drugs out of the reach of children.

Dosage and Administration: For best results, use Head & Shoulders at least twice a week or as directed by a doctor. It is gentle enough to use for every shampoo.

Ingredients: Pyrithione zinc in a shampoo base of water, ammonium laureth sulfate, ammonium lauryl sulfate, sodium lauroyl sarcosinate, glycol

Continued on next page

Procter & Gamble—Cont.

distearate, sodium sulfate, dimethicone, fragrance, DMDM hydantoin, disodium phosphate, sodium phosphate, lauryl alcohol, PEG-12, sodium chloride, polyquaternium-10 and FD&C Blue No. 1.

How Supplied: Head & Shoulders Dandruff Shampoo is available in 2 FL OZ, 6.8 FL OZ, 15 FL OZ unbreakable plastic bottles.

HEAD & SHOULDERS® INTENSIVE TREATMENT DANDRUFF AND SEBORRHEIC DERMATITIS SHAMPOO

Head & Shoulders Intensive Treatment Dandruff and Seborrheic Dermatitis Shampoo offers effective control of persistent dandruff, and beautiful hair from a pleasant-to-use formula. Double-blind and expert-graded testing have proven that Intensive Treatment Dandruff and Seborrheic Dermatitis Shampoo reduces persistent dandruff. It is also gentle enough to use every day for clean, manageable hair.

Active Ingredient: 1% selenium sulfide suspended in a mild surfactant base. Shampoo also includes mild conditioning agents.

Indications: For effective control of seborrheic dermatitis and dandruff of the scalp.

Actions: Selenium sulfide is substantive to the scalp and remains after rinsing. Its mechanism is believed to be antiproliferative, and to also control the microorganisms associated with persistent dandruff flaking and itching.

Warnings: For external use only. Avoid contact with the eyes. If contact occurs, rinse eyes thoroughly with water. If condition worsens or does not improve after regular use of this product as directed, consult a doctor. Keep this and all drugs out of the reach of children.

Caution: If used on bleached, tinted, grey, or permed hair, rinse for 5 minutes.

Dosage and Administration: For best results, use at least twice a week or as directed by a doctor. It is gentle enough to use for every shampoo.

Ingredients: Selenium sulfide in a shampoo base of water, ammonium laureth sulfate, ammonium lauryl sulfate, cocamide MEA, glycol distearate, ammonium xylenesulfonate, dimethicone, fragrance, tricetylmonium chloride, cetyl alcohol, DMDM hydantoin, sodium chloride, stearyl alcohol, hydroxypropyl methylcellulose, FD&C Red No. 4.

How Supplied: Intensive Treatment Dandruff and Seborrheic Dermatitis Shampoo is available in 15 FL OZ unbreakable plastic bottles.

METAMUCIL®
[met uh-mū sil]
(psyllium husk fiber)

Description: Metamucil contains a bulk forming natural therapeutic fiber for restoring and maintaining regularity as recommended by a physician. It contains psyllium husk, a highly efficient fiber from the plant Plantago ovata. Metamucil contains no chemical stimulants and does not disrupt normal bowel function. Each dose contains approximately 3.4 grams of psyllium. Inactive ingredients, sodium, potassium, and phenylalanine content are shown in Table 1 for all forms and flavors. Phenylketonurics should be aware that phenylalanine is present in Metamucil products that contain aspartame. Metamucil Sugar-Free Regular Flavor contains no sugar and no artificial sweeteners.
Metamucil in powdered forms is gluten-free. Wafers contain gluten: Apple Crisp contains 0.7g/dose, Cinnamon Spice contains 0.5g/dose.

Actions: The active ingredient in Metamucil is psyllium, a natural fiber which promotes elimination due to its bulking effect in the colon. This bulking effect is due to both the water-holding capacity of undigested fiber and the increased bacterial mass following partial fiber digestion. These actions result in enlargement of the lumen of the colon, and softer stool, thereby decreasing intraluminal pressure and straining, and speeding colonic transit in constipated patients.

Indications: Metamucil is indicated in the management of chronic constipation, irritable bowel syndrome, as adjunctive therapy in the constipation of diverticular disease, the bowel management of patients with hemorrhoids, for constipation associated with convalescence and senility and for occasional constipation during pregnancy when under the care of a physician. Pregnancy: Category B.

Contraindications: Intestinal obstruction, fecal impaction. Known allergy to any component.

Warnings: Patients are advised they should not use the product without consulting a doctor when abdominal pain, nausea, or vomiting are present or if they have noticed a sudden change in bowel habits that persists over a period of two weeks, or rectal bleeding. Patients are advised to consult a physician if constipation persists for longer than one week, as this may be a sign of a serious medical condition. **PATIENTS ARE CAUTIONED THAT TAKING THIS PRODUCT WITHOUT ADEQUATE FLUID MAY CAUSE IT TO SWELL AND BLOCK THE THROAT OR ESOPHAGUS AND MAY CAUSE CHOKING. THEY SHOULD NOT TAKE THE PRODUCT IF THEY HAVE DIFFICULTY IN SWALLOWING. IF THEY EXPERIENCE CHEST PAIN, VOMITING, OR DIFFICULTY IN SWALLOWING OR BREATHING AFTER TAKING THIS PRODUCT, THEY ARE ADVISED TO SEEK IMMEDIATE MEDICAL ATTENTION.** Psyllium products may cause allergic reaction in people sensitive to inhaled or ingested psyllium. Keep this and all medications out of the reach of children.

Precaution: Notice to Health Care Professionals: To minimize the potential for allergic reaction, health care professionals who frequently dispense powdered psyllium products should avoid inhaling airborne dust while dispensing these products. Handling and Dispensing: To minimize generating airborne dust, spoon product from the canister into a glass according to label directions.
*Laxatives, including bulk fibers, may affect how well other medicines work. If you are taking a prescription medicine by mouth, take this product at least 2 hours before or 2 hours after the prescribed medicine.

Dosage and Administration: The usual adult dosage is 1 rounded teaspoonful or 1 rounded tablespoonful depending on product form. Generally the sugar free products are dosed by the teaspoonful, sucrose-containing products by the tablespoonful. Some forms are available in packets. The appropriate dose should be mixed with 8 oz. of liquid (e.g., cool water, fruit juice, milk) following the labeled instructions. Metamucil wafers should be consumed with 8 oz. of liquid. **THE PRODUCT (CHILD OR ADULT DOSE) SHOULD BE TAKEN WITH AT LEAST 8 OZ (A FULL GLASS) OF WATER OR OTHER FLUID. TAKING THIS PRODUCT WITHOUT ENOUGH LIQUID MAY CAUSE CHOKING (SEE WARNINGS).** Metamucil can be taken orally one to three times a day, depending on the need and response. It may require continued use for 2 to 3 days to provide optimal benefit. It generally produces an effect in 12–72 hours. For children (6 to 12 years old), use 1/2 the adult dose in/with 8 oz. of liquid, 1 to 3 times daily. For children under 6, consult a doctor.

New Users: (Label statement)
Your doctor can recommend the right dosage of Metamucil to best meet your needs. In general, start by taking one dose each day. Gradually increase to three doses per day, if needed or recommended by your doctor. If minor gas or bloating occurs when you increase number of doses, try slightly reducing the size of each dose.

How Supplied: Powder: canisters (OTC) and cartons of single-dose packets (OTC and Institutional). Wafers: cartons of single-dose packets (OTC). (See Table 1).

[See tables at top of next page.]

Shown in Product Identification Guide, page 518

TABLE 1

Forms/ Flavors	Inactive Ingredients	Sodium mg/ Dose	Potas-sium mg/ Dose	Calo-ries per Dose	Carbo-hy-drate g/ Dose	Fat g/ Dose	Phenyl-alanine mg/Dose	Dosage 1–3 Times Daily. Each Dose Contains 3.4 g Psyllium Husk Fiber	How Supplied
Smooth Texture Orange Flavor **METAMUCIL** Powder	Citric acid, D&C Yellow No. 10, FD&C Yellow No. 6, Flavoring, Sucrose	<5	30	35	12	—	—	1 rounded tablespoonful 12 g	Canisters: 13, 20.3, 30.4 and 48 ozs. (Doses: 48, 72 and 114); Cartons: 30 single-dose packets (OTC) 100 single-dose packets (Institutional)
Smooth Texture Sugar-Free Orange Flavor **METAMUCIL** Powder	Aspartame, Citric acid, D&C Yellow No. 10, FD&C Yellow No. 6, Flavoring, Maltodextrin	<5	30	10	5	—	25	1 rounded teaspoonful 5.8 g	Canisters: 10, 15, 23.3 ozs. and 36.8 ozs. (Doses: 48, 72, 114 and 180); Cartons: 30 single-dose packets (OTC), 100 single-dose packets (Institutional)
METAMUCIL Powder	FD&C Yellow No. 6, Flavoring, Maltodextrin								and 114); Cartons: 30 single-dose packets (OTC)
Smooth Texture Sugar-Free Regular Flavor **METAMUCIL** Powder	Citric Acid (less than 1%), Magnesium sulfate*, Maltodextrin	<5	30	10	5	—	—	1 rounded teaspoonful 5.8 g	Canisters: 10, 15 and 23.3 ozs. (Doses: 48, 72 and 114)
Original Texture Regular Flavor **METAMUCIL** Powder	Dextrose	<5	30	14	6	—	—	1 rounded teaspoonful 7 g	Canisters: 13, 19 and 29 ozs. (Doses: 48, 72 and 114)

TABLE 1 (continued)

Forms/ Flavors	Inactive Ingredients	Sodium mg/ Dose	Potas-sium mg/ Dose	Calo-ries per Dose	Carbo-hy-drate g/ Dose	Fat g/ Dose	Phenyl-alanine mg/Dose	Dosage 1–3 Times Daily. Each Dose Contains 3.4 g Psyllium Hydrophilic Mucilloid	How Supplied
Original Texture Orange Flavor **METAMUCIL** Powder	Citric acid, FD&C Yellow No. 6, Flavoring, Sucrose	<5	35	30	10	—	—	1 rounded tablespoonful 11 g	Canisters: 13, 19, 29 and 44.2 ozs. (Doses: 48, 72 and 114)
Apple Crisp **METAMUCIL** Wafers	Ascorbic acid, Brown sugar, Cinnamon, Corn oil, Flavors, Fructose, Lecithin, Modified food starch, Molasses, Oat hull fiber, Sodium bicarbonate, Sucrose, Water, Wheat flour	20	50	100	19	5	—	2 wafers 25 g	Cartons: 12 doses
Cinnamon Spice **METAMUCIL** Wafers	Ascorbic acid, Cinnamon, Corn oil, Flavors, Fructose, Lecithin, Modified food starch, Molasses, Nutmeg, Oat hull fiber, Oats, Sodium bicarbonate, Sucrose, Water, Wheat flour	15	45	100	18	5	—	2 wafers 25 g	Cartons: 12 doses

* Metamucil Sugar-Free Regular Flavor contains 26 mg of magnesium per dose.

Continued on next page

Procter & Gamble—Cont.

OIL OF OLAY®—Daily UV Protectant SPF 15 Beauty Fluid—Original & Fragrance Free Versions (Olay Co., Inc.)

Oil of Olay Daily UV Protectant Beauty Fluid is a light, greaseless lotion that is specially formulated to provide effective moisturization and SPF 15 protection with minimal migration to reduce the likelihood of eye sting. Oil of Olay Daily UV Protectant is PABA free. It is non-comedogenic and is suitable for daily use under facial make-up.

Active Ingredients: Octyl Methoxycinnamate, Phenylbenzimidazole Sulfonic Acid

Inactive Ingredients: Water, Isohexadecane, Butylene Glycol, Triethanolamine, Glycerin, Stearic Acid, Cetyl Alcohol, Cetyl Palmitate, DEA-Cetyl Phosphate, Aluminum Starch Octenylsuccinate, Titanium Dioxide, Imidazolidinyl Urea, Methylparaben, Propylparaben, Carbomer, Acrylates/C10–30 Alkyl Acrylate Crosspolymer, PEG-10 Soya Sterol, Disodium EDTA, Castor Oil, Fragrance, FD&C Red No. 4, FD&C Yellow No. 5.
Available in both lightly scented original version and a 100% color free and fragrance free version.

Indications: Filters out the sun's harmful rays to help prevent skin damage. Provides SPF 15 protection in a light, greaseless moisturizer. Regular use over the years may reduce the chance of skin damage, some types of skin cancer, and other harmful effects due to the sun.

Directions: Adults and children 6 months of age and over: Apply liberally as often as necessary. Children under 6 months of age: Consult a doctor.

WARNINGS: For external use only, not to be swallowed. Avoid contact with the eyes. If contact occurs, rinse eyes thoroughly with water. Discontinue use if signs of irritation or rash appear. If irritation or rash persists, consult a doctor. **KEEP OUT OF REACH OF CHILDREN.**

How Supplied: Available in 4.0 fl. oz. and 6.0 fl. oz. plastic bottles.

PEPTO-BISMOL® ORIGINAL LIQUID, ORIGINAL AND CHERRY TABLETS AND EASY-TO-SWALLOW CAPLETS
For upset stomach, indigestion, diarrhea, heartburn and nausea.

Multi-symptom Pepto-Bismol contains bismuth subsalicylate and is the only leading OTC stomach remedy clinically proven effective for both upper and lower GI symptoms. Pepto-Bismol is in more households than any other stomach remedy, making it a convenient recommendation with a name your patients will know. It has been clinically proven in double-blind placebo-controlled trials for relief of upset stomach symptoms and diarrhea.

Description: Each tablespoon (15 ml) of Pepto-Bismol Liquid contains 262 mg bismuth subsalicylate. Each tablespoonful of liquid contains a total of 130 mg non-aspirin salicylate. Pepto-Bismol liquid contains no sugar and is very low in sodium (less than 3 mg/tablespoonful). Inactive ingredients: benzoic acid, D&C Red No. 22, D&C Red No. 28, flavor, magnesium aluminum silicate, methylcellulose, saccharin sodium, salicylic acid, sodium salicylate, sorbic acid and water.
Each Pepto-Bismol Tablet contains 262 mg bismuth subsalicylate. Each tablet contains a total of 102 mg non-aspirin salicylate (99 mg non-aspirin salicylate for Cherry). Pepto-Bismol tablets contain no sugar and are very low in sodium (less than 2 mg/tablet). Inactive ingredients include: adipic acid (in Cherry only), calcium carbonate, D&C Red No. 27, FD&C Red No. 40 (in Cherry only), flavors, magnesium stearate, mannitol, povidone, saccharin sodium and talc.
Each Pepto-Bismol Caplet contains 262 mg bismuth subsalicylate. Each caplet contains a total of 99 mg non-aspirin salicylate. Caplets contain no sugar and are low in sodium (less than 2 mg/caplet). Inactive ingredients include: calcium carbonate, D&C Red No. 27, magnesium stearate, mannitol, microcrystalline cellulose, polysorbate 80, povidone, silicon dioxide, and sodium starch glycolate.

Indications: Pepto-Bismol controls diarrhea within 24 hours, relieving associated abdominal cramps; soothes heartburn and indigestion without constipating; and relieves nausea and upset stomach.

Actions: For upset stomach symptoms (i.e., indigestion, heartburn, nausea and fullness caused by over-indulgence), the active ingredient is believed to work via a topical effect on the stomach mucosa. For diarrhea, it is believed to work by several mechanisms in the gastrointestinal tract, including: 1) normalizing fluid movement via an antisecretory mechanism, 2) binding bacterial toxins and 3) antimicrobial activity.

Warnings: Children and teenagers who have or are recovering from chicken pox or flu should not use this medicine to treat nausea or vomiting. If nausea or vomiting is present, patients are advised to consult a doctor because this could be an early sign of Reye syndrome, a rare but serious illness.
This product contains non-aspirin salicylates. If taken with aspirin and ringing in the ears occurs, discontinue use. This product does not contain aspirin, but should not be administered to those patients who have a known allergy to aspirin or non-aspirin salicylates as an adverse reaction may occur. Caution is advised in the administration to patients taking medication for anticoagulation, diabetes and gout.
If diarrhea is accompanied by a high fever or continues more than 2 days, patients are advised to consult a physician.
As with any drug, caution is advised in the administration to pregnant or nursing women.
Keep all medicine out of the reach of children.
Note: This medication may cause a temporary and harmless darkening of the tongue and/or stool. Stool darkening should not be confused with melena.

Overdosage: In case of overdose, patients are advised to contact a physician or Poison Control Center. Emesis induced by ipecac syrup is indicated in large ingestions provided ipecac can be administered within one hour of ingestion. Activated charcoal should be administered after gastric emptying. Patients should be evaluated for signs and symptoms of salicylate toxicity.

Dosage and Administration:

Liquid: Shake well before using.
Adults—2 tablespoonsful
(1 dose cup, 30 ml)
Children (according to age)—
9–12 yrs. 1 tablespoonful
(½ dose cup, 15 ml)
6–9 yrs. 2 teaspoonsful
(⅓ dose cup, 10 ml)
3–6 yrs. 1 teaspoonful
(⅙ dose cup, 5 ml)

Repeat dosage every ½ to 1 hour, if needed, to a maximum of 8 doses in a 24-hour period. Drink plenty of clear fluids to help prevent dehydration which may accompany diarrhea.
For children under 3 years of age, consult a physician.

Tablets:
Adults—Two tablets
Children (according to age)—
9–12 yrs. 1 tablet
6–9 yrs. ⅔ tablet
3–6 yrs. ⅓ tablet

Chew or dissolve in mouth. Repeat every ½ to 1 hour as needed, to a maximum of 8 doses in a 24-hour period. Drink plenty of clear fluids to help prevent dehydration, which may accompany diarrhea. For children under 3 years of age, consult a physician.

Caplets:
Adults—Two caplets
Children (according to age)—
9–12 yrs. 1 caplet
6–9 yrs. ⅔ caplet
3–6 yrs. ⅓ caplet

Swallow caplet(s) with water, do not chew. Repeat every ½ to 1 hour as needed, to a maximum of 8 doses in a 24-hour period. Drink plenty of clear fluids to help prevent dehydration, which may accompany diarrhea. For children under 3 years of age, consult a physician.

How Supplied: Pepto-Bismol Liquid is available in: 4, 8, 12, and 16 FL OZ bottles. Pepto-Bismol Tablets are pink, round, chewable tablets imprinted with a debossed triangle and "Pepto-Bismol" on one side. Tablets are available in: boxes of 30 and 48 (Original only). Caplets are available in bottles of 24 and 40. Caplets are imprinted with "Pepto-Bismol" on one side.

Shown in Product Identification Guide, page 518

PEPTO-BISMOL® MAXIMUM STRENGTH LIQUID

For upset stomach, indigestion, diarrhea, heartburn and nausea.

Multi-symptom Pepto-Bismol contains bismuth subsalicylate and is the only leading OTC stomach remedy clinically proven effective for both upper and lower GI symptoms. Pepto-Bismol is in more households than any other stomach remedy, making it a convenient recommendation with a name your patients will know. It has been clinically-proven in double-blind placebo-controlled trials for relief of upset stomach symptoms and diarrhea.

Description: Each tablespoonful (15 ml) of Maximum Strength Pepto-Bismol Liquid contains 525 mg bismuth subsalicylate (236 mg non-aspirin salicylate). Maximum Strength Pepto-Bismol Liquid contains no sugar and is low in sodium (less than 3 mg/tablespoonful). Inactive ingredients include: benzoic acid, D&C Red No. 22, D&C Red No. 28, flavor, magnesium aluminum silicate, methylcellulose, saccharin sodium, salicylic acid, sodium salicylate, sorbic acid and water.

Indications: Maximum Strength Pepto-Bismol soothes upset stomach and indigestion without constipating; controls diarrhea within 24 hours, relieving associated abdominal cramps; and relieves heartburn and nausea.

Actions: For upset stomach symptoms (i.e. indigestion, heartburn, nausea and fullness caused by over-indulgence), the active ingredient is believed to work via a topical effect on the stomach mucosa. For diarrhea, it is believed to work by several mechanisms in the gastrointestinal tract, including: 1) normalizing fluid movement via an antisecretory mechanism, 2) binding bacterial toxins, and 3) antimicrobial activity.

Warnings: Children and teenagers who have or are recovering from chicken pox or flu should not use this medicine to treat nausea or vomiting. If nausea or vomiting is present, patients are advised to consult a doctor because this could be an early sign of Reye syndrome, a rare but serious illness.
This product contains non-aspirin salicylates. If taken with aspirin and ringing in the ears occurs, discontinue use. This product does not contain aspirin, but should not be administered to those patients who have a known allergy to aspirin or other non-aspirin salicylates as an adverse reaction may occur. Caution is advised in the administration to patients taking medication for anticoagulation, diabetes and gout.
If diarrhea is accompanied by a high fever or continues more than 2 days, patients are advised to consult a physician.
As with any drug, caution is advised in the administration to pregnant or nursing women.
Keep all medicine out of the reach of children.
Note: This medication may cause a temporary and harmless darkening of the tongue and/or stool. Stool darkening should not be confused with melena.

Overdosage: In case of overdose, patients are advised to contact a physician or Poison Control Center. Emesis induced by ipecac syrup is indicated in large ingestions provided ipecac can be administered within one hour of ingestion. Activated charcoal should be administered after gastric emptying. Patients should be evaluated for signs and symptoms of salicylate toxicity.

Dosage and Administration: Shake well before using.

Adults—2 tablespoonsful
(1 dose cup, 30 ml)
Children (according to age)—
9–12 yrs. 1 tablespoonful (½ dose cup, 15 ml)
6–9 yrs. 2 teaspoonsful (⅓ dose cup, 10 ml)
3–6 yrs. 1 teaspoonful (⅙ dose cup, 5 ml)

For children under 3 years of age, consult a physician.

Repeat dosage every hour, if needed, to a maximum of 4 doses in a 24-hour period. Drink plenty of clear fluids to help prevent dehydration, which may accompany diarrhea.

How Supplied: Maximum Strength Pepto-Bismol is available in: 4, 8, and 12 FL OZ bottles.

VICKS® 44 COUGH RELIEF

Dextromethorphan HBr/ Cough Suppressant Alcohol 5%

Active Ingredient
per 3 tsp. (15 ml):
Dextromethorphan Hydrobromide 30 mg

Inactive Ingredients: Alcohol, Carboxymethylcellulose Sodium, Citric Acid, FD&C Blue No. 1, FD&C Red No. 40, Flavor, High Fructose Corn Syrup, Polyethylene Oxide, Polyoxyl 40 Stearate, Propylene Glycol, Purified Water, Saccharin Sodium, Sodium Benzoate, Sodium Citrate.
Sodium Content: 31 mg per 15 mL dose.

Use: Temporary relieves coughs due to minor throat and bronchial irritation associated with a cold.

Directions: Use teaspoon (tsp) or dose cup.

Ask a doctor before using in children under 6 yrs. of age.

6–11 yrs.	(48–95 lbs.)	$1^1/_2$ tsp or $7^1/_2$ ml
12 yrs. & older	(Over 95 lbs.)	3 tsp or 15 ml

Repeat every 6–8 hours, not to exceed 4 doses per day or use as directed by a doctor.

Warnings: A persistent cough may be a sign of a serious condition. If cough persists for more than 1 week, tends to recur, or is accompanied by fever, rash, or persistent headache, ask a doctor. Do not take this product for persistent or chronic cough such as occurs with smoking, asthma, emphysema, or if cough is accompanied by excessive phlegm (mucus) unless directed by a doctor.
Keep this and all drugs out of the reach of children.
In case if accidental overdose, seek professional advice or contact a poison control center immediately. As with any drug, if you are pregnant or nursing a baby, seek the advice of a health professional before using this product.

Drug Interaction Precaution: Do not use this product without first asking a doctor if you take a prescription monoamine oxidase inhibitor (MAOI) (certain drugs for depression, psychiatric or emotional conditions, or Parkinson's disease), or for 2 weeks after stopping the MAOI drug or if you are uncertain whether your prescription drug contains an MAOI.

How Supplied: Available in 4 FL OZ (115 ml) plastic bottle. A calibrated dose cup accompanies each bottle.

Continued on next page

Procter & Gamble—Cont.

VICKS® 44D COUGH & HEAD CONGESTION RELIEF
Cough Suppressant/ Nasal Decongestant Alcohol 5%

Active Ingredients per 3 tsp. (15 ml): Dextromethorphan Hydrobromide 30 mg, Pseudoephedrine Hydrochloride 60 mg.

Inactive Ingredients: Alcohol, Carboxymethylcellulose Sodium, Citric Acid, FD&C Blue No. 1, FD&C Red No.40, Flavor, High Fructose Corn Syrup, Polyethylene Oxide, Polyoxyl 40 Stearate, Propylene Glycol, Purified Water, Saaccharin Sodium, Sodium Benzoate, Sodium Citrate.

Uses: Temporary relieves coughs and nasal congestion due to a common cold.

Directions: Use teaspoon (tsp) or dose cup.

Ask a doctor before using in children under 6 yrs. of age.

6–11 yrs.	(48–95 lbs.)	$1^1/_2$ tsp or $7^1/_2$ ml
12 yrs. & older	(Over 95 lbs.)	3 tsp or 15 ml

Repeat every 6 hours, not to exceed 4 doses per day or use as directed by a doctor.

Warnings: Do not exceed recommended dosage.
If nervousness, dizziness, or sleeplessness occur, discontinue use and ask a doctor.

Do not take unless directed by a doctor if you have:
- heart disease
- asthma
- emphysema
- thyroid disease
- diabetes
- high blood pressure
- excessive phlegm (mucus)
- persistent or chronic cough
- cough associated with smoking
- difficulty in urination due to enlarged prostate gland

Keep this and all drugs out of the reach of children. In the case of accidental overdose, seek professional advice or contact a poison control center immediately. As with any drug, if you are pregnant or nursing a baby, seek the advice of a health professional before using this product.

Drug Interaction Precaution: Do not use this product without first asking a doctor if you take a prescription monoamine oxidase inhibitor (MAOI) (certain drugs for depression, psychiatric or emotional conditions, or Parkinson's disease), or for 2 weeks after stopping the MAOI drug or if you are uncertain whether your prescription drug contains an MAOI.

Dosing Duration and When to Ask a Doctor:
- If symptoms do not improve within 7 days or are accompanied by fever.
- If a cough persists for more than 7 days, recurs, or is accompanied by fever, rash or persistent headache. A persistent cough may be the sign of a serious condition.

How Supplied: Available in 4 FL OZ (115 ml) and 8 FL OZ (235 ml) plastic bottles. A calibrated dose cup accompanies each bottle.

VICKS® 44E Cough & Chest Congestion Relief
Cough Suppressant/Expectorant Alcohol 5%

Active Ingredients: per 3 teaspoons (15 ml): Dextromethorphan Hydrobromide 20 mg, Guaifenesin 200 mg

Inactive Ingredients: Alcohol, Carboxymethylcellulose Sodium, Citric Acid, FD&C Blue No. 1, FD&C Red No. 40, Flavor, High Frutose Corn Syrup, Polyethylene Oxide, Polyoxyl 40 Stearate, Propylene Glycol, Purified Water, Saaccharin Sodium, Sodium Benzoate, Sodium Citrate.

Uses: Temporarily relieves coughs due to a common cold. Helps loosen phlegm to rid the bronchial passageways of bothersome mucus.

Directions: Use teaspoon (tsp) or dose cup.

Ask a doctor before using in children under 6 yrs. of age.

6–11 yrs.	(48–95 lbs.)	$1^1/_2$ tsp or $7^1/_2$ ml
12 yrs. & older	(Over 95 lbs.)	3 tsp or 15 ml

A total of 6 doses may be given per day, each 4 hours apart, or use as directed by a doctor.

Warnings: *Do not take unless directed by a doctor if you have:*
- asthma
- emphysema
- excessive phlegm (mucus)
- persistent or chronic cough
- chronic bronchitis
- cough associated with smoking

Keep this and all drugs out of the reach of children.
In the case of accidental overdose, seek professional advice or contact a poison control center immediately. As with any drug, if you are pregnant or nursing a baby, seek the advice of a health professional before using this product. Do not use this product if you are on a sodium-restricted diet unless directed by a doctor.

Drug Interaction Precaution: Do not use this product without first asking a doctor if you take a prescription monoamine oxidase inhibitor (MAOI) (certain drugs for depression, psychiatric or emotional conditions, or Parkinson's disease), or for 2 weeks after stopping the MAOI drug or if you are uncertain whether your prescription drug contains an MAOI.

Dosing Duration & When to Ask a Doctor:
- If a cough persists for more than 7 days, recurs, or is accompanied by fever, rash or persistent headache. A persistent cough may be the sign of a serious condition.

How Supplied: Available in 4 FL OZ (115 ml) and 8 FL OZ (235 ml) plastic bottles. A calibrated dose cup accompanies each bottle.

VICKS® 44M COUGH, COLD & FLU RELIEF
Cough Suppressant/Nasal Decongestant/Antihistamine/ Pain Reliever–Fever Reducer Alcohol 10%

Active Ingredients: per 4 tsp. (20 ml): Dextromethorphan Hydrobromide 30 mg, Pseudoephedrine Hydrochloride 60 mg, Chlorpheniramine Maleate 4 mg, Acetaminophen 650 mg

Inactive Ingredients: Alcohol, Carboxymethylcellulose Sodium, Citric Acid, FD&C Blue No. 1, FD&C Red No. 40, Flavor, High Fructose Corn Syrup, Polyethylene Glycol, Polyethylene Oxide, Propylene Glycol, Purified Water, Saccharin Sodium, Sodium Citrate.
Sodium Content: 35 mg per 20 mL dose.

Uses: Temporarily relieves cough/cold/flu symptoms:
- cough
- nasal congestion
- runny nose
- sneezing
- headache
- fever
- muscular aches
- sore throat pain

Directions: Use teaspoon (tsp) or dose cup.

Ask a doctor before using in children under 12 yrs. of age.

12 yrs. & older	4 tsp or 20 ml

Repeat every 6 hours, not to exceed 4 doses per day, or use as directed by a doctor.

Warnings: Do not exceed recommended dosage.
If nervousness, dizziness, or sleeplessness occur, discontinue use and ask a doctor. May cause marked drowsiness. May cause excitability especially in children.
Do not take unless directed by a doctor if you have:
- heart disease
- asthma
- emphysema
- thyroid disease
- diabetes
- glaucoma
- high blood pressure
- excessive phlegm (mucus)

- breathing problems
- chronic bronchitis
- difficulty in breathing
- persistent or chronic cough
- cough associated with smoking
- difficulty in urination due to enlarged prostate gland

Keep this and all drugs out of the reach of children. In the case of accidental overdose, seek professional advice or contact a poison control center immediately. Prompt medical attention is critical for adults as well as for children even if you do not notice any signs or symptoms. As with any drug, if you are pregnant or nursing a baby, seek the advice of a health professional before using this product.

Alcohol, sedatives, and tranquilizers may increase the drowsiness effect. Avoid alcoholic beverages while taking this product. Use caution when driving a motor vehicle or operating machinery. Do not use this product if you are on a sodium-restricted diet unless directed by a doctor.

Drug Interaction Precaution: Do not use this product without first asking a doctor if you take:
- sedatives
- tranquilizers
- a prescription monoamine oxidase inhibitor (MAOI) (certain drugs for depression, psychiatric or emotional conditions, or Parkinson's disease), or for 2 weeks after stopping the MAOI drug or if you are uncertain whether your prescription drug contains an MAOI.

Dosing Duration: Do not use over 7 days. *Ask a Doctor:*
- If sore throat is severe, persists for more than 2 days, is accompanied or followed by fever, headache, rash, nausea, or vomiting.
- If symptoms do not improve or are accompanied by a fever that lasts more than 3 days, or if new symptoms occur.
- If a cough presists for more than 7 days, recurs, or is accompanied by a rash or persistent headache. A persistent cough may be the sign of a serious condition.

How Supplied: Available in 4 FL OZ (115 ml) and 8 FL OZ (235 ml) plastic bottles. A calibrated dose cup accompanies each bottle.

CHILDREN'S VICKS® DAYQUIL® ALLERGY RELIEF
Antihistamine/Nasal Decongestant

Children's Vicks DayQuil Allergy Relief was specially formulated with two effective ingredients to relieve allergy symptoms and head colds without coughs.

Active Ingredients per 1 TBSP: Chlorpheniramine Maleate 2 mg, Pseudoephedrine HCl 30 mg.

Inactive Ingredients: Citric Acid, FD&C Blue No. 1, FD&C Red No. 40, Flavor, Methylparaben, Potassium Sorbate, Propylene Glycol, Purified Water, Sodium Citrate, Sorbitol and Sucrose.

Uses: Temporarily relieves:
- nasal and sinus congestion
- runny nose
- sneezing
- itchy, watery eyes due to hay fever or other upper respiratory allergies

Directions: Use Tablespoon (TBSP) or dose cup.

Under 6 yrs.	(Under 48 lbs.)	Ask a doctor.
6–11 yrs.	(48–95 lbs.)	1 TBSP or 15 ml
12 yrs. & older	(Over 95 lbs.)	2 TBSP or 30 ml

***Professional Labeling:** Children under 6 years of age: Use only as directed by a physician. Suggested doses for children under 6 years of age:

Age	Weight	Dose
6–11 mo.	17–21 lbs.	1 teaspoon (tsp.) (5 ml)
12–23 mo.	22–27 lbs.	$1^1/_4$ teaspoon (tsp.) (6.25 ml)
2–5 yrs.	28–47 lbs.	$^1/_2$ TABLESPOON (TBSP.) (7.5 ml)

Repeat every 6 hours, not to exceed 4 doses in 24 hours, or use as directed by doctor.

*Based on extrapolation from studies on the safety and efficacy of active ingredients conducted among older children and adults. Use caution in treating children under 2 years of age who were born prematurely.

Warnings: Do not exceed recommended dosage.
If nervousness, dizziness or sleeplessness occur, discontinue use and ask a doctor. May cause drowsiness. May cause excitability, especially in children.

Do not take unless directed by a doctor if you have:
- heart disease
- emphysema
- glaucoma
- thyroid disease
- diabetes
- high blood pressure
- breathing problems
- chronic bronchitis
- difficulty in urination due to enlarged prostate gland

Keep this and all drugs out of the reach of children. In the case of accidental overdose, seek professional advice or contact a poison control center immediately. As with any drug, if you are pregnant or nursing a baby, seek the advice of a health professional before using this product.

Alcohol, sedatives, and tranquilizers may increase the drowsiness effect. Avoid alcoholic beverages while taking this product. Use caution when driving a motor vehicle or operating machinery.

Drug Interaction Precaution: Do not take this product without first asking a doctor if you take:
- sedatives
- tranquilizers
- a prescription monoamine oxidase inhibitor (MAOI) (certain drugs for depression, psychiatric or emotional conditions, or Parkinson's disease), or for weeks after stopping the MAOI drug or if you are uncertain whether your prescription drug contains an MAOI.

Dosing Duration: Do not use over 7 days.
Ask a Doctor: If symptoms do not improve within 7 days or are accompanied by a fever.

How Supplied: Available in 4 FL OZ (115 ml) plastic bottles with child-resistant, tamper-evident cap and a calibrated medicine cup.

CHILDREN'S VICKS® NYQUIL® COLD/COUGH RELIEF
Antihistamine/Nasal Decongestant/Cough Suppressant

Children's NyQuil was specially formulated with three effective ingredients to relieve nighttime cough, nasal congestion, and runny nose so children can rest. Children's NyQuil® is alcohol free and analgesic free and has a pleasant cherry flavor.

Active Ingredients: Per 1 TBSP.: Chlorpheniramine Maleate 2 mg, Pseudoephedrine HCl 30 mg, Dextromethorphan Hydrobromide 15 mg.

Inactive Ingredients: Citric Acid, FD&C Red No. 40, Flavor, Potassium Sorbate, Propylene Glycol, Purified Water, Sodium Citrate, Sucrose.

Uses: Temporarily relieves cold symptoms:
- nasal congestion
- runny nose
- sneezing
- cough

Directions: Use Tablespoon (TBSP) or dose cup.

Under 6 yrs.	(Under 48 lbs.)	Ask a doctor.
6–11 yrs.	(48–95 lbs.)	1 TBSP or 15 ml
12 yrs. & older	(Over 95 lbs.)	2 TBSP or 30 ml

***Professional Labeling:** Children under 6 years of age: Use only as directed by a physician. Suggested doses for children under 6 years of age:

Continued on next page

Procter & Gamble—Cont.

Age	Weight	Dose
6–11 mo.	17–21 lbs.	1 teaspoon (tsp.) (5 ml)
12–23 mo.	22–27 lbs.	$1^1/_4$ teaspoon (tsp.) (6.25 ml)
2–5 yrs.	28–47 lbs.	$^1/_2$ TABLE-SPOON (TBSP.) (7.5 ml)

Repeat every 6 hours, not to exceed 4 doses in 24 hours, or use as directed by doctor.

* Based on extrapolation from studies on the safety and efficacy of active ingredients conducted among older children and adults. Use caution in treating children under 2 years of age who were born prematurely.

Warnings: Do not exceed recommended dosage.
If nervousness, dizziness, or sleeplessness occur, discontinue use and ask a doctor. May cause marked drowsiness. May cause excitability, especially in children.

Do not take unless directed by a doctor if you have:
- heart disease
- asthma
- emphysema
- thyroid disease
- diabetes
- glaucoma
- high blood pressure
- excessive phelgm (mucus)
- breathing problems
- chronic bronchitis
- difficulty in breathing
- persistent or chronic cough
- cough associated with smoking
- difficulty in urination due to enlarged prostate gland

Keep this and all drugs out of the reach of children. In the case of accidental overdose, seek professional advice or contact a poison control center immediately. As with any drug, if you are pregnant or nursing a baby, seek the advice of a health professional before using this product.
Alcohol, sedatives, and tranquilizers may increase the drowsiness effect. Avoid alcoholic beverages while taking this product. Use caution when driving a motor vehicle or operating machinery.

Drug Interaction Precaution: Do not take this product without first asking a doctor if you take:
- sedatives
- tranquilizers
- a prescription monoamine oxidase inhibitor (MAOI) (certain drugs for depression, psychiatric or emotional conditions, or Parkinson's disease), or for 2 weeks after stopping the MAOI drug or if you are uncertain whether your prescription drug contains an MAOI.

Dosing Duration: Do not use over 7 days.
Ask a Doctor:
- If symptoms do not improve within 7 days or are accompanied by a fever.
- If a cough persists for more than 7 days, recurs, or is accompanied by a fever, rash or persistent headache. A persistent cough may be the sign of a serious condition.

How Supplied: Available in 4 FL OZ (115 ml) plastic bottles with child-resistant, tamper-evident cap and a calibrated medicine cup.

VICKS® CHLORASEPTIC® COUGH & THROAT DROPS
Menthol Cough Suppressant/Oral Anesthetic

Active Ingredients: Menthol Flavor: Menthol 8.4 mg, Cherry and Honey Lemon: Menthol 10 mg.

Inactive Ingredients: Menthol Flavor: Corn Syrup, FD&C Blue No. 1, Flavor, Sucrose. Cherry Flavor: Corn Syrup, FD&C Blue No. 2, FD&C Red No. 40, Flavor, Sucrose. Honey Lemon: Citric Acid, Corn Syrup, D&C Yellow No. 10, FD&C Yellow No. 6, Flavor, Sucrose.

Indications: Temporarily relieves sore throat and coughs due to colds or inhaled irritants.

Directions: Adults and children 5 to 12 years: Allow drop to dissolve slowly in mouth. **Cough:** may be repeated every hour as needed or as directed by a doctor. **Sore Throat:** may be repeated every 2 hours as needed or as directed by a doctor.
Children under 5 years of age: consult a doctor.

WARNINGS: A persistent cough may be a sign of a serious condition. If cough persists for more than 1 week, tends to recur, or is accompanied by fever, rash, or persistent headache, consult a doctor. Do not take this product for persistent or chronic cough such as occurs with smoking, asthma, emphysema, or if cough is accompanied by excessive phlegm (mucus), unless directed by a doctor. If sore throat is severe, or is accompanied by difficulty in breathing, or persists for more than 2 days, do not use, and consult a doctor promptly. If sore throat is accompanied or followed by fever, headache, rash, swelling, nausea, or vomiting, consult a doctor promptly. **Keep this and all drugs out of the reach of children.** As with any drug, if you are pregnant or nursing a baby, seek the advice of a health professional before using this product.

How Supplied: Vicks® Chloraseptic® Cough & Throat Drops are available in single sticks of 9 drops each and bags of 25 drops. Each drop is debossed with "V".

VICKS® CHLORASEPTIC® SORE THROAT LOZENGES
Menthol/Benzocaine
Oral Anesthetic
Menthol and Cherry Flavors

Active Ingredients: Benzocaine 6 mg, Menthol 10 mg (per lozenge).

Inactive Ingredients: Menthol Lozenges: Corn syrup, D&C Yellow No. 10, FD&C Blue No. 1, FD&C Yellow No. 6, flavor and sucrose. Cherry Lozenges: Corn syrup, FD&C Blue No. 1, FD&C Red No. 40, flavor and sucrose.

Uses: Temporary relieves:
- sore mouth
- sore throat
- occasional minor mouth irritation and pain
- pain associated with canker sores

Directions: Adults and Children 5 years & older:
Allow 1 lozenge to dissolve slowly in mouth. May be repeated every 2 hours as needed or as directed by a physician or dentist.
Children under 5 years: ask a physician or dentist.

Warnings: *Do not use this product if you have a history of allergy to local anesthetics like:*
- procaine
- butacaine
- benzocaine
- other 'caine' anesthetics

Keep this and all drugs out of the reach of children.
In case of accidental overdose, seek professional advice or contact a poison control center immediately. As with any drug if you are pregnant or nursing a baby, seek the advice of a health professional before using this product.

Dosing Duration and When to Ask a Doctor:
- If sore throat is severe, persists for more than 2 days, or is accompanied by difficulty in breathing.
- If sore throat is accompanied or followed by fever, headache, rash, swelling, nausea, or vomiting.
- If sore mouth symptoms do not improve in 7 days, or if irritation, pain, or redness persists or worsens.

How Supplied: Available in Menthol and Cherry, lozenges in packages of 18. Each green or red lozenge is debossed with "VC".

VICKS® CHLORASEPTIC® SORE THROAT SPRAY
Phenol/oral anesthetic/antiseptic
Menthol and Cherry Flavors

Active Ingredient: Spray—Phenol 1.4%.

Inactive Ingredients: Menthol Liquid: D&C Green No. 5, D&C Yellow No. 10, FD&C Green No. 3, flavor, glycerin, purified water, saccharin sodium. Cherry Liquid: FD&C Red No. 40, flavor, glycerin, purified water, saccharin sodium.

Uses: Temporarily relieves:
- sore mouth
- sore throat pain
- minor irritation or injury of the mouth and gums
- pain due to minor dental procedures, dentures or orthodontic appliances

• pain associated with canker sores

Directions: Adults and Children 12 years & older:
Spray 5 times directly into throat or affected area.
Children 2–12 years: Spray 3 times and swallow. Children under 12 years should be supervised in product use.- Repeat every 2 hours or as directed by a physician or dentist.
Children under 2 years: ask a physician or dentist.

Warnings: Keep this and all drugs out of the reach of children. In case of accidental overdose, seek professional advice or contact a poison control center immediately. As with any drug, if you are pregnant or nursing a baby, seek the advice of a health professional before using this product.
Dosing Duration and When to Ask a Doctor:
- If sore throat is severe, persists for more than 2 days, or is accompanied by difficulty in breathing.
- If sore throat is accompanied or followed by fever, headache, rash, swelling, nausea, or vomiting.
- If sore mouth symptoms do not improve in 7 days, or if irritation, pain, or redness persists or worsens.

How Supplied: Available in Menthol and Cherry flavors in 6 FL OZ (175 mL) plastic bottles with sprayer.

VICKS® Cough Drops
Menthol Cough Suppressant/ Oral Anesthetic
Menthol and Cherry Flavors

Active Ingredient: Menthol 3.3mg (Menthol), 1.7mg (Cherry)

Inactive Ingredients: [Menthol] Ascorbic Acid, Caramel, Corn Syrup, Eucalyptus Oil, Sucrose. [Cherry] Ascorbic Acid, Citric Acid, Corn Syrup, Ecualyptus Oil, FD&C Blue No. 1, FD&C Red No. 40, Flavor, Sucrose.

Directions: Adults and children 5 to 12 years of age:
Menthol: Allow 2 drops to dissolve slowly in mouth.
Cherry: Allow 3 drops to dissolve slowly in mouth.
COUGH: May be repeated every hour as needed or as directed by a doctor.- **SORE THROAT:** May be repeated every 2 hours as needed or as directed by a doctor.
Children under 5 years of age: Ask a doctor.

Warnings: A persistent cough may be a sign of a serious condition. If cough persists for more than 1 week, tends to recur, or is accompanied by fever, rash, or persistent headache, ask a doctor. Do not take this product for persistent or chronic cough such as occurs with smoking, asthma, emphysema, or if cough is accompanied by excessive phlegm (muscus) unless directed by a doctor. If sore throat is severe, or is accompanied by difficulty in breathing, or persists for more than 2 days, do not use, and ask a doctor promptly. If sore throat is accompanied or followed by fever, headache, rash, swelling, nausea, or vomiting, ask a doctor promptly. **Keep this and all drugs out of the reach of children.** As with any drug, if you are pregnant or nursing a baby, seek the advice of a health professional before using this product.

How Supplied: Vicks® Cough Drops are available in boxes of 20 triangular drops. Each red or green drop is debossed with "V."

VICKS® COUGH DROPS
Menthol Cough Suppressant/ Oral Anesthetic

Active Ingredient: Menthol 6.6 mg (menthol), 3.1 mg (cherry)
Menthol and Cherry Flavors.

Inactive Ingredients: Menthol Flavor: Benzyl Alcohol, Camphor, Caramel, Corn Syrup, Eucalyptus Oil, Flavor, Sucrose, Tolu Balsam, Thymol.
Cherry Flavor: Citric Acid, Corn Syrup, FD&C Blue No. 1, FD&C Red No. 40, Flavor, Sucrose.

Uses: Temporarily relieves sore throat and coughs due to colds or inhaled irritants.

Directions: Adults and children 5 to 12 years: [Menthol] Allow drop to dissolve slowly in mouth. [Cherry] Allow 2 drops to dissolve slowly in mouth.
Cough: may be repeated every hour as needed or as directed by a doctor. **Sore Throat:** may be repeated every 2 hours —as needed or as directed by a doctor.
Children under 5 years of age: ask a doctor.

Warnings: A persistent cough may be a sign of a serious condition. If cough persists for more than 1 week, tends to recur, or is accompanied by fever, rash, or persistent headache, ask a doctor. Do not take this product for persistent or chronic cough such as occurs with smoking, asthma, emphysema, or if cough is accompanied by excessive phlegm (mucus), unless directed by a doctor. If sore throat is severe, or is accompanied by difficulty in breathing, or persists for more than 2 days, do not use, and ask a doctor promptly. If sore throat is accompanied or followed by fever, headache, rash, swelling, nausea, or vomiting, ask a doctor promptly. **Keep this and all drugs out of the reach of children.** As with any drug, if you are pregnant or nursing a baby, seek the advice of a health professional before using this product.

How Supplied: Vicks® Cough Drops are available in bags of 30 oval drops. Each red or green drop is debossed with "V".

VICKS® DAYQUIL® ALLERGY RELIEF 12 HOUR EXTENDED RELEASE TABLETS
Nasal Decongestant/Antihistamine

Active Ingredients: Each Extended Release Tablet Contains:
75 mg Phenylpropanolamine Hydrochloride, 12 mg Brompheniramine Maleate

Inactive Ingredients: Dimethyl Polysiloxane Oil, FD&C Blue No. 1 Aluminum Lake, Hydroxypropyl Methylcellulose, Lactose, Magnesium Stearate, Polyethylene Glycol. Talc, Titanium Dioxide.

Uses: For the temporary relief of nasal congestion due to the common cold, hay fever or other upper respiratory allergies, or associated with sinusitis; temporarily relieves runny nose, sneezing, and itchy and watery eyes as may occur in allergic rhinitis (such as hay fever). Temporarily restores freer breathing through the nose.

Directions: Adults and children 12 years of age and older: One tablet every 12 hours. DO NOT EXCEED 1 TABLET EVERY 12 HOURS, OR 2 TABLETS IN A 24-HOUR PERIOD. Children under 12 years of age: ask a doctor.

Warnings: This product may cause excitability, especially in children. Do not take this product if you have heart disease, high blood pressure, thyroid disease, diabetes, glaucoma, or difficulty in urination due to enlargement of the prostate gland, except under the advice and supervision of a doctor. Do not take this product, unless directed by a doctor, if you have a breathing problem such as emphysema or chronic bronchitis. Do not give this product to children under 12 years, except under the advice and supervision of a doctor. May cause drowsiness. Do not exceed recommended dosage because at higher doses nervousness, dizziness, or sleeplessness may occur. If symptoms do not improve within 7 days or are accompanied by fever, ask a doctor before continuing use. Do not take if hypersensitive to any of the ingredients. As with any drug, if you are pregnant or nursing a baby, seek the advice of a health professional before using this product. **CAUTION:** Avoid driving a motor vehicle or operating machinery and avoid alcoholic beverages while taking this product. **DRUG INTERACTION PRECAUTION:** Do not take this product if you are presently taking a prescription antihypertensive or antidepressant drug containing a monoamine oxidase inhibitor, except under the advice and supervision of a doctor. KEEP THIS AND ALL DRUGS OUT OF THE REACH OF CHILDREN. IN CASE OF ACCIDENTAL OVERDOSE, SEEK PROFESSIONAL ASSISTANCE OR CONTACT A POISON CONTROL CENTER IMMEDIATELY.

How Supplied: Available in 24 count blister packages. Each blue tablet is im-

Continued on next page

Procter & Gamble—Cont.

printed with the letter "A" inside the Vicks shield.

VICKS® DAYQUIL® LIQUID
VICKS® DAYQUIL® LIQUICAPS®
Multi-Symptom Cold/Flu Relief
Nasal Decongestant/
Pain Reliever/Cough
Suppressant/Fever Reducer

Active Ingredients: LIQUID—per 2 TBSP or LIQUICAPS—per two softgels, contains: Pseudoephedrine Hydrochloride 60 mg, Acetaminophen 650 mg (Liquid) or 500 mg (softgels), Dextromethorphan Hydrobromide 20 mg.

Inactive Ingredients: Liquid: Citric Acid, FD&C Yellow No. 6, Flavor, Glycerin, Polyethylene Glycol, Propylene Glycol, Purified Water, Saccharin Sodium, Sodium Citrate, Sucrose. Softgels: FD&C Red No. 40, FD&C Yellow No. 6, Gelatin, Glycerin, Polyethylene Glycol, Povidone, Propylene Glycol, Purified Water and Sorbitol Special.

Uses: Temporarily relieves common cold/flu symptoms:
- minor aches
- pains
- headache
- muscular aches
- sore throat pain
- fever
- nasal congestion
- cough

Liquid

Directions: Use measuring spoon or dose cup.

Under 6 years	Ask a doctor.
6–11 years	1 Tablespoon (TBSP) or 15 ml
12 yrs. and older	2 Tablespoons (TBSP) or 30 ml

A total of 4 doses may be given per day, each 4 hours apart, or use as directed by a doctor.

LiquiCaps

Directions: Under 6 years—Ask a doctor.

6–11 years	Swallow 1 softgel with water.
12 yrs. and older	Swallow 2 softgels with water.

A total of 4 doses may be given per day, each four hours apart, or use as directed by a doctor. If taking both DayQuil and NyQuil, limit total to 4 doses per day.

Warnings: Do not exceed recommended dosage. If nervousness, dizziness, or sleeplessness occur, discontinue use and ask a doctor.

Do not take unless directed by a doctor if you have:
- heart disease
- asthma
- emphysema
- thyroid disease
- diabetes
- high blood pressure
- chronic bronchitis
- persistent or chronic cough
- cough associated with smoking
- excessive phlegm (mucus)
- breathing problems
- difficulty in urination due to enlarged prostate gland

DRUG INTERACTION PRECAUTION: Do not take this product without first asking a doctor if you take:
- a prescription monoamine oxidase inhibitor (MAOI) (certain drugs for depression, psychiatric or emotional conditions, or Parkinson's disease), or for 2 weeks after stopping the MAOI drug or if you are uncertain whether your prescription drug contains an MAOI.

Keep this and all drugs out of the reach of children. In the case of accidental overdose, seek professional advice or contact a poison control center immediately. Prompt medical attention is critical for adults as well as for children even if you do not notice any signs or symptoms. As with any drug, if you are pregnant or nursing a baby, seek the advice of a health professional before using this product.

DOSING DURATION: Do not use over 7 days (for adults) or 5 days (for children).
ASK A DOCTOR:
- If sore throat is severe, persists for more than 2 days, is accompanied or followed by fever, headache, rash, nausea, or vomiting.
- If symptoms do not improve or are accompanied by a fever that lasts more than 3 days, or if new symptoms occur.
- If a cough persists for more than 7 days (adults) or 5 days (children), recurs, or is accompanied by a rash or persistent headache. A persistent cough may be the sign of a serious condition.

How Supplied: Available in: **LIQUID** 6 FL OZ (175 ml) plastic bottles with child-resistant, tamper-evident cap and a calibrated medicine cup.
LIQUICAP: in 12-count child-resistant packages and 20-count nonchild-resistant packages. Each softgel is imprinted: "DayQuil."

VICKS® DAYQUIL® SINUS
Pressure & PAIN Relief
WITH IBUPROFEN
IBUPROFEN/PSEUDOEPHEDRINE HCL
Pain Reliever/Fever Reducer/
Nasal Decongestant

Warning: ASPIRIN SENSITIVE PATIENTS. Do not take this product if you have had a severe reaction to aspirin (e.g., asthma, swelling, shock or hives) because even though this product contains no aspirin or salicylates, cross-reactions may occur in patients allergic to aspirin.

Uses: For temporary relief of symptoms associated with the common cold, sinusitis or flu including nasal congestion, headache, fever, body aches, and pains.

Directions: Adults: Take 1 caplet every 4 to 6 hours while symptoms persist. If symptoms do not respond to 1 caplet, 2 caplets may be used but do not exceed 6 caplets in 24 hours, unless directed by a doctor. The smallest effective dose should be used. Take with food or milk if occasional and mild heartburn, upset stomach, or stomach pain occurs with use. Ask a doctor if these symptoms are more than mild or they persist.
Children: Do not give this product to children under 12 years of age except under the advice and supervision of a doctor.

Warnings: Do not take for colds for more than 7 days or for fever for more than 3 days unless directed by a doctor. If the cold or fever persists or gets worse or if new symptoms occur, ask a doctor. These could be signs of serious illness. As with aspirin and actaminophen, if you have any condition which requires you to take prescription drugs or if you have had problems or serious side effects from taking any non-prescription pain reliever, do not take this product without first discussing it with your doctor. IF YOU EXPERIENCE ANY SYMPTOMS WHICH ARE UNUSUAL OR SEEM UNRELATED TO THE CONDITION FOR WHICH YOU TOOK THIS PRODUCT, CONSULT A DOCTOR BEFORE TAKING ANY MORE OF IT. If you are under a doctor's care for any serious condition, ask a doctor before taking this product. **Do not exceed recommended dosage.** If nervousness, dizziness or sleeplessness occur, discontinue use and ask a doctor. Do not take this product if you have high blood pressure, heart disease, diabetes, thyroid disease or difficulty in urination due to enlargement of the prostate gland, unless directed by of a doctor. Do not combine this product with other non-prescription pain relievers. Do not combine this product with any other ibuprofen-containing product. As with any drug, if you are pregnant or nursing a baby, seek the advice of a health professional before using this product. IT IS ESPECIALLY IMPORTANT NOT TO USE THIS PRODUCT DURING THE LAST 3 MONTHS OF PREGNANCY UNLESS SPECIFICALLY DIRECTED TO DO SO BY A DOCTOR BECAUSE IT MAY CAUSE PROBLEMS IN THE UNBORN CHILD OR COMPLICATIONS DURING DELIVERY. Keep this and all drugs out of reach of children. In case of accidental overdose, seek professional assistance or contact a poison control center immediately. DRUG INTERACTION PRECAUTION: Do not take this product if you are taking a prescription monoamine oxidase inhibitor (MAOI) (certain drugs for depression, psychiatric or emotional conditions, or Parkinson's disease), or for 2 weeks after stopping the MAOI drug. If you are uncertain whether your prescription drug contains an MAOI, ask a health professional before taking this product.

Active Ingredients: each caplet contains Ibuprofen 200 mg, Pseudoephedrine Hydrochloride 30 mg.

Inactive Ingredients: Carnuba or Equivalent Wax, Croscarmellose Sodium, Iron Oxide, Methylparaben, Microcrystalline Cellulose, Propylparaben, Silicon Dioxide, Sodium Benzoate, Sodium Lauryl Sulfate, Starch, Stearic Acid, Sucrose, Titanium Dioxide.

How Supplied: Available in 20 count blister package and 40 count bottle. Each white caplet is imprinted: "DAYQUIL Sinus Pain".

VICKS® NYQUIL® HOT THERAPY® ADULT NIGHTTIME COLD/FLU HOT LIQUID MEDICINE

Honey Lemon Hot Liquid Drink
Antihistamine/Cough Suppressant/ Pain Reliever/Nasal Decongestant/ Fever Reducer

Active Ingredients: (per packet) Doxylamine Succinate 12.5 mg, Dextromethorphan Hydrobromide 30 mg, Acetaminophen 1000 mg, Pseudoephedrine Hydrochloride 60 mg.

Inactive Ingredients: Citric Acid, Flavor, and Sucrose.

Uses: For temporary relief of minor aches, pains, headache, muscular aches, sore throat pain, and fever associated with a cold or flu. Temporarily relieves nasal congestion, cough due to minor throat and bronchial irritations, runny nose and sneezing associated with the common cold.

Directions: Adults and Children 12 years and over: Take one dose at bedtime. DISSOLVE ONE PACKET IN 6 OZ. CUP OF HOT WATER. SIP PROMPTLY WHILE HOT. If your cold or flu symptoms keep you confined to bed or at home, a total of 4 doses may be taken per day, each 6 hours apart, or as directed by a doctor. **MICROWAVE HEATING INSTRUCTIONS:** Add contents of packet and 6 ounces of cool water to a microwave-safe cup and stir briskly. Microwave on high 1½ minutes or until hot. Drink promptly. **DO NOT BOIL.** Sweeten to taste if desired.

Warnings: Do not exceed recommended dosage. If nervousness, dizziness, or sleeplessness occurs, discontinue use and ask a doctor. Do not take this product if you have heart disease, high blood pressure, thyroid disease, diabetes, glaucoma, or difficulty in urination due to enlargement of the prostate gland unless directed by a doctor. *Drug Interaction Precaution:* Do not use this product if you are now taking a prescription monoamine oxidase inhibitor (MAOI) (certain drugs for depression, psychiatric or emotional conditions, or Parkinson's disease), or for two weeks after stopping the MAOI drug. If you are uncertain whether your prescription drug contains an MAOI, ask a health professional before taking this product. Do not take this product for persistent or chronic cough such as occurs with smoking, asthma, emphysema, or if cough is accompanied by excessive phlegm (mucus) unless directed by a doctor. May cause excitability especially in children. Do not take this product, unless directed by a doctor, if you have a breathing problem such as emphysema or chronic bronchitis. May cause marked drowsiness; alcohol, sedatives and tranquilizers may increase the drowsiness effect. Avoid alcoholic beverages while taking this product. Do not take this product if you are taking sedatives or tranquilizers without first asking your doctor. Use caution when driving a motor vehicle or operating machinery. Do not take this product for more than 7 days. A persistent cough may be a sign of a serious condition. If cough persists for more than 7 days, tends to recur, or is accompanied by rash, or persistent headache, ask a doctor. If symptoms do not improve or are accompanied by fever that lasts for more than 3 days, or if new symptoms occur, ask a doctor. If sore throat is severe, persists for more than 2 days, is accompanied or followed by fever, headache, rash, nausea or vomiting, ask a doctor promptly. **Keep this and all drugs out of the reach of children.** In case of accidental overdose, seek professional assistance or contact a poison control center immediately. Prompt medical attention is critical for adults as well as for children even if you do not notice any signs or symptoms. As with any drug, if you are pregnant or nursing a baby, seek the advice of a health professional before using this product.

How Supplied: Available in child-resistant packages of 6 single-dose packets.

VICKS® NYQUIL® LIQUICAPS® VICKS® NYQUIL® LIQUID (Original and Cherry)

Multi-Symptom Cold/Flu Relief
Antihistamine/Cough Suppressant/Pain Reliever/ Nasal Decongestant/ Fever Reducer

Active Ingredients (per softgel): Doxylamine Succinate 6.25 mg, Dextromethorphan HBr 10 mg, Acetaminophen 250 mg, Pseudoephedrine HCl 30 mg. **(per 2 TBSP):** Doxylamine succinate 12.5 mg, Dextromethorphan HBr 30 mg, Acetaminophen 1000 mg, Pseudoephedrine HCl 60 mg.

Inactive Ingredients: (per softgel): D&C Yellow No. 10, FD&C Blue No. 1, Gelatin, Glycerin, Polyethylene Glycol, Povidone, Propylene Glycol and Purified Water. May contain Sorbitol Special. **(Liquid):** Alcohol 10%, Citric Acid, Flavor, High Fructase Corn Syrup, Polyethylene Glycol, Propylene Glycol, Purified Water, Saccharin Sodium, Sodium Citrate.
Original flavor also has D&C Yellow No. 10, FD&C Green No. 3, FD&C Yellow No. 6.
Cherry flavor also has FD&C Blue No. 1, FD&C Red No. 40.

Uses: Temporary relieves common cold/flu symptoms:

- minor aches
- pains
- headache
- muscular aches
- sore throat pain
- fever
- runny nose and sneezing
- nasal congestion
- cough due to minor throat and bronchial irritation

Liquid

Directions: Adults Dose (12 yrs. and older):
Take 2 Tablespoons (TBSP) or 30 ml in dose cup provided. A total of 4 doses may be taken per day, each 6 hours apart, or as directed by a doctor. If taking NyQuil and DayQuil, limit total to 4 doses per day.
Ask a doctor for use in children under 12 yrs. of age.

LiquiCaps

Directions: <u>Adults</u> 12 yrs. and older: Swallow two softgels with water. A total of 4 doses may be taken per day, each 4 hours apart or as directed by a doctor. If taking both NyQuil and DayQuil, limit total to 4 doses per day. **NOT RECOMMENDED FOR CHILDREN.**

Warnings: Do not exceed recommended dosage.
If nervousness, dizziness, or sleeplessness occur, discontinue use and ask a doctor. May caused marked drowsiness. May cause excitability, especially in children. *Do not take unless directed by a doctor if you have:*

- heart disease
- asthma
- emphysema
- thyroid disease
- diabetes
- glaucoma
- high blood pressure
- excessive phlegm (muscus)
- breathing problems
- chronic bronchitis
- difficulty in breathing
- persistent or chronic cough
- cough associated with smoking
- difficulty in urination due to enlarged prostate gland

Keep this and all drugs out of the reach of children. In the case of accidental overdose, seek professional advice or contact a poison control center immediately. Prompt medical attention is critical for adults as well as for children even

Continued on next page

Procter & Gamble—Cont.

if you do not notice any signs or symptoms. As with any drug, if you are pregnant or nursing a baby, seek the advice of a health professional before using this product.

Drug Interaction Precaution: Do not take this product without first asking a doctor if you take:

- sedatives
- tranquilizers
- a prescription monoamine oxidase inhibitor (MAOI) (certain drugs for depression, psychiatric or emotional conditions, or Parkinson's disease), or for 2 weeks after stopping the MAOI drug or if you are uncertain whether your prescription drug contains an MAOI.

DOSING DURATION: Do not use over 7 days. *ASK A DOCTOR:*

- If sore throat is severe, persists for more than 2 days, is accompanied or followed by fever, headache, rash, nausea, or vomiting.
- If symptoms do not improve or are accompanied by a fever that lasts more than 3 days, or if new symptoms occur.
- If a cough persists for more than 7 days, recur, or is accompanied by a rash or persistent headache. A persistent cough may be the sign of a serious condition.

Alcohol, sedatives, and tranquilizers may increase the drowsiness effect. Avoid alcoholic beverages while taking this product. Use caution when driving a motor vehicle or operating machinery.

How Supplied: (LiquiCaps®) Available in 12-count child-resistant blister packages and 20-count non-child resistant blister packages. Each softgel is imprinted: "NyQuil".

(Liquid) Available in 6 and 10 FL OZ (175 and 295 ml, respectively) plastic bottles with child-resistant, tamper-evident cap and calibrated medicine cup.

PEDIATRIC VICKS® 44e
Cough & Chest Congestion Relief

Active Ingredients
per 1 tablespoon (TBSP.) (15 ml):
Dextromethorphan Hydrobromide 10 mg, Guaifenesin 100 mg.

CONTAINS NO ALCOHOL

Inactive Ingredients: Carboxymethylcellulose Sodium, Citric Acid, FD&C Red No. 40, Flavor, High Fructose Corn Syrup, Polyethylene Oxide, Polyoxyl 40 Stearate, Propylene Glycol, Purified Water, Saccharin Sodium, Sodium Benzoate, Sodium Citrate.
Sodium Content: 60 mg per 30 mL dose.

Uses: Temporary relief of coughs due to a common cold. Helps loosen phlegm to rid the bronchial passageways of bothersome mucus.

Directions: Use Tablespoon (TBSP) or dose cup.

Under 2 yrs.	(Under 28 lbs.)	Ask a doctor.
2–5 yrs.	(28–47 lbs.)	1/2 TBSP or 7 1/2 ml
6–11 yrs.	(48–95 lbs.)	1 TBSP or 15 ml
12 yrs. & older	(Over 95 lbs.)	2 TBSP or 30 ml

Repeat every 4 hours. Not to exceed 6 doses per day or use as directed by a doctor.

***Professional Dosage:**

Physicians: Suggested doses for children under 2 years of age.

Age	Weight	Dose
* 6–11 mo.	17–21 lbs.	1 teaspoon (tsp.) (5 ml)
*12–23 mo.	22–27 lbs.	1 1/4 teaspoon (tsp.) (6.25 ml)

Repeat every 4 hours. Not to exceed 6 doses per day or use as directed by doctor.

* Based on extrapolation from studies on the safety and efficacy of active ingredients conducted among older children and adults. Use caution in treating children under 2 years who were born prematurely.

Warnings:

Do not take unless directed by a doctor if you have:

- asthma
- emphysema
- excessive phlegm (mucus)
- persistent or chronic cough
- chronic bronchitis
- cough associated with smoking

Keep this and all drugs out of the reach of children.
In the case of accidental overdose, seek professional advice or contact a poison control center immediately. As with any drug, if you are pregnant or nursing a baby, seek the advice of a health professional before using this product. Do not use this product if you are on a sodium-restricted diet unless directed by a doctor.

Drug Interaction Precaution: Do not use this product without first asking a doctor if you are take a prescription monoamine oxidase inhibitor (MAOI) (certain drugs for depression, psychiatric or emotional conditions, or Parkinson's disease), or for 2 weeks after stopping the MAOI drug or if you are uncertain whether your prescription drug contains an MAOI.

Dosing Duration & When to Ask a Doctor:

- If a cough persists for more than 7 days, recurs, or is accompanied by fever, rash or persistent headache. A persistent cough may be the sign of a serious condition.

How Supplied: 4 FL OZ (115 ml) plastic bottles. A calibrated dose cup accompanies each bottle.

PEDIATRIC VICKS® 44m
Cough & Cold Relief
Cough Suppressant/Nasal Decongestant/Antihistamine

Active Ingredients Per 1 tablespoon (TBSP) (15 ml): Dextromethorphan Hydrobromide 15 mg, Pseudoephedrine Hydrochloride 30 mg, Chlorpheniramine Maleate 2 mg

CONTAINS NO ALCOHOL

Inactive Ingredients: Carboxymethylcellulose Sodium, Citric Acid, FD&C Red No. 40, Flavor, High Fructose Corn Syrup, Polyethylene Oxide, Polyoxyl 40 Stearate, Propylene Glycol, Purified Water, Saccharin Sodium, Sodium Benzoate, Sodium Citrate.
Sodium Content: 60 mg per 30 mL dose.

Uses: Temporary relieves cough/cold symptoms:

- cough
- nasal congestion
- runny nose
- sneezing

Directions: Use Tablespoon (TBSP) or dose cup.

Under 6 yrs.	(Under 48 lbs.)	Ask a doctor.
6–11 yrs.	(48–95 lbs.)	1 TBSP or 15 ml
12 yrs. & older	(Over 95 lbs.)	2 TBSP or 30 ml

Repeat every 6 hours, not to exceed 4 doses per day or use as directed by a doctor.

Professional Dosage:

*Physicians: Suggested doses for children under 6 years of age.

Age	Weight	Dose
* 6–11 mo.	17–21 lbs.	1 teaspoon (tsp.) (5 ml)
*12–23 mo.	22–27 lbs.	1 1/4 teaspoon (tsp.) (6.25 ml)
2–5 yrs.	28–47 lbs.	1/2 TABLESPOON (TBSP.) (7.5 ml)

Repeat every 6 hours, no more than 4 doses in 24 hours, or as directed by doctor.

*Based on extrapolation from studies on the safety and efficacy of active ingredients conducted among older children and adults. Use caution in treating children under 2 years of age who were born prematurely.

Warnings: Do not exceed recommended dosage.
If nervousness, dizziness, or sleeplessness occur, discontinue use and ask a doctor. May cause marked drowsiness. May cause excitability especially in children.
Do not take unless directed by a doctor if you have:

- heart disease
- asthma
- emphysema
- thyroid disease
- diabetes
- glaucoma
- high blood pressure
- excessive phlegm (mucus)
- breathing problems
- chronic bronchitis
- difficulty in breathing
- persistent or chronic cough
- cough associated with smoking
- difficulty in urination due to enlarged prostate gland

Keep this and all drugs out of the reach of children. In case of accidental overdose, seek professional advice or contact a poison control center immediately. As with any drug, if you are pregnant or nursing a baby, seek the advice of a health professional before using this product.
Alcohol, sedatives, and tranquilizers may increase the drowsiness effect. Avoid alcoholic beverages while taking this product. Use caution when driving a motor vehicle or operating machinery. Do not use this product if you are on a sodium-restricted diet unless directed by a doctor.
Drug Interaction Precaution: Do not take this product without first asking a doctor if you take:

- sedatives
- tranquilizers
- a prescription monoamine oxidase inhibitor (MAOI) (certain drugs for depression, psychiatric or emotional conditions, or Parkinson's disease), or for 2 weeks after stopping the MAOI drug or if you are uncertain whether your prescription drug contains an MAOI.

Dosing Duration: Do not use over 7 days. *Ask a Doctor:*

- If symptoms do not improve within 7 days or are accompanied by a fever.
- If a cough persists for more than 7 days, recurs, or is accompanied by fever, rash or persistent headache. A persistent cough may be a sign of a serious condition.

How Supplied: 4 FL OZ (115 ml) plastic bottles. A calibrated dose cup accompanies each bottle.

VICKS® SINEX® [NASAL SPRAY] [Ultra Fine Mist] for Sinus Relief
[sī'nĕx]
Nasal Decongestant

Active Ingredient: Phenylephrine Hydrochloride 0.5%.

Inactive Ingredients: Aromatic Vapors (Camphor, Eucalyptol, Menthol), Citric Acid, Disodium EDTA, Purified Water, Tyloxapol.
Preservatives: Benzalkonium Chloride, Chlorhexidine Gluconate.

Use: For temporary relief of sinus/nasal congestion due to colds, hay fever, upper respiratory allergies or sinusitis.

Dosage: Ultra Fine Mist: Remove protective cap. Before using for the first time, prime the pump by firmly depressing its rim several times. Hold container with thumb at base and nozzle between first and second fingers. Without tilting your head, insert nozzle into nostril. Fully depress rim with a firm even stroke and inhale deeply. Adults and Children—age 12 and over: 2 or 3 sprays in each nostril not more often than every 4 hours. Do not give to children under 12 years of age unless directed by a doctor.
Nasal Spray: Adults and Children—age 12 and over: 2 or 3 sprays in each nostril without tilting your head, not more often than every 4 hours. Do not give to children under 12 years of age unless directed by a doctor.

Warnings: Do not exceed recommended dosage. This product may cause temporary discomfort such as burning, stinging, sneezing, or an increase of nasal discharge. The use of this container by more than one person may spread infection. Do not use this product for more than 3 days. Use only as directed. Frequent or prolonged use may cause nasal congestion to recur or worsen. If symptoms persist, ask a doctor. Do not use this product if you have heart disease, high blood pressure, thyroid disease, diabetes, or difficulty in urination due to enlargement of the prostate gland unless directed by a doctor.
Keep this and all drugs out of the reach of children. In case of accidental ingestion, seek professional assistance or contact a poison control center immediately.

How Supplied: Available in 1/2 FL OZ (15 ml) plastic squeeze bottle and 1/2 FL OZ (15 ml) measured dose Ultra Fine mist pump.

VICKS® SINEX®
[sī'nĕx]
12-HOUR [Nasal Spray] [Ultra Fine Mist] for Sinus Relief

Active Ingredient: Oxymetazoline Hydrochloride 0.05%.

Inactive Ingredients: Aromatic Vapors (Camphor, Eucalyptol, Menthol), Disodium EDTA, Potassium Phosphate, Purified Water, Sodium Chloride, Sodium Phosphate, Tyloxapol. Preservatives: Benzalkonium Chloride, Chlorhexidine Gluconate.

Use: For temporary relief of nasal congestion due to colds, hay fever, upper respiratory allergies or sinusitis.

Dosage and Administration:
Ultra Fine Mist: Remove protective cap. Before using for the first time, prime the pump by firmly depressing its rim several times. Hold container with thumb at base and nozzle between first and second fingers. Without tilting head, insert nozzle into nostril. Fully depress rim with a firm even stroke and inhale deeply. Adults and children 6 years of age and over (with adult supervision): 2 or 3 sprays in each nostril not more often than every 10 to 12 hours. Do not exceed 2 applications in any 24-hour period. Children under 6 years of age: ask a doctor.
Squeeze Bottle: Adults and children 6 years of age and over (with adult supervision): 2 or 3 sprays in each nostril without tilting your head, not more often than every 10 to 12 hours. Do not exceed 2 applications in any 24-hour period. Children under 6 years of age: ask a doctor.

Warnings: Do not exceed recommended dosage. This product may cause temporary discomfort such as burning, stinging, sneezing or an increase of nasal discharge. The use of this container by more than one person may spread infection. Do not use this product for more than 3 days. Use only as directed. Frequent or prolonged use may cause nasal congestion to recur or worsen. If symptoms persist, ask a doctor. Do not use this product if you have heart disease, high blood pressure, thyroid disease, diabetes, or difficulty in urination due to enlargement of the prostate gland unless directed by a doctor.
Keep this and all drugs out of the reach of children. In case of accidental ingestion, seek professional assistance or contact a poison control center immediately.

How Supplied: Available in 1/2 FL OZ (15 ml) plastic squeeze bottle and 1/2 FL OZ (15 ml) measured-dose Ultra Fine mist pump.

VICKS® VAPOR INHALER
l-Desoxyephedrine/Nasal Decongestant

Active Ingredient per inhaler: *l*-Desoxyephedrine 50 mg.

Inactive Ingredients: Special Vicks Vapors (bornyl acetate, camphor, lavender oil, menthol).

Indications: For the temporary relief of nasal congestion due to the common cold, hay fever, upper respiratory allergies or sinusitis.

Directions: Adults: 2 inhalations in each nostril not more often than every 2 hours. **Children 6 to under 12 years of age** (with adult supervision): 1 inhalation in each nostril not more often than every 2 hours. Children under 6 years of age: ask a doctor.

Warnings: Do not exceed recommended dosage. This product may cause temporary discomfort such as burning, stinging, sneezing, or an increase of nasal discharge. The use of this container by more than one person may spread infection. Do not use this product for more than 3 days. Frequent or prolonged use may cause nasal congestion to

Continued on next page

Procter & Gamble—Cont.

recur or worsen. If symptoms persist, ask a doctor. Do not use this product if you have heart disease, high blood pressure, thyroid disease, diabetes or difficulty in urination due to enlargement of the prostate gland unless directed by a doctor. **Keep this and all drugs out of the reach of children.** In case of accidental ingestion, seek professional assistance or contact a poison control center immediately.

VICKS® VAPOR INHALER is effective for a minimum of 3 months after first use. Keep tightly closed.

How Supplied: Available as a cylindrical plastic nasal inhaler.
Net weight: 0.007 OZ (200 mg).

VICKS® VAPORUB®
VICKS® VAPORUB® CREAM
[*vā 'pō-rub*]
Nasal Decongestant/Cough Suppressant/Topical Analgesic

Active Ingredients: Camphor (5.2% cream) 4.8% oint.), Menthol (2.8% cream) 2.6% oint.), Eucalyptus Oil 1.2%.

USE on Chest & Throat: For temporary relief of nasal congestion and coughs associated with a cold.

Active Ingredients: Camphor (5.2% cream) 4.8% oint.), Menthol (2.8% cream) 2.6% oint.).

USE: For temporary relief of minor aches and pains of muscles.

Inactive Ingredients: (ointment) Cedarleaf Oil, Nutmeg Oil, Special Petrolatum, Spirits of Turpentine, Thymol. **(cream)** Carbomer 954, Cedarleaf Oil, Cetyl Alcohol, Cetyl Palmitate, Cyclomethicone and Dimethicone Copolyol, Dimethicone, EDTA, Glycerin, Imidazolidinyl Urea, Isopropyl Palmitate, Methylparaben, Nutmeg Oil, PEG-100, Stearate, Propylparaben, Purified Water, Sodium Hydroxide, Spirits of Turpentine, Stearic Acid, Stearyl Alcohol, Thymol, Titanium Dioxide.

Directions: Adults and children 2 years of age and over:
Chest & Throat: rub on a thick layer. [If desired, cover with a dry, soft cloth, but keep clothing loose to let vapors rise to the nose and mouth. (oint.)]
Rub on sore area.
Repeat up to three times daily or as directed by a doctor.
Children under 2 years of age: ask a doctor.
Do not heat. Never expose VapoRub to flame, microwave, or place in any container in which you are heating water. [Such improper use may cause the mixture to splatter. (oint.)]

Warnings: For external use only. Avoid contact with eyes.
Do not use unless directed by a doctor if you have cough associated with:
- smoking
- excessive phlegm (mucus)
- asthma
- emphysema
- a persistent or chronic cough

Do not:
- take by mouth
- place in nostrils
- bandage tightly
- apply to wounds or damaged skin

Ask a doctor:
- If a cough persists for more than 7 days, recurs or is accompanied by a fever, rash or persistent headache. A persistent cough may be the sign of a serious condition.
- If muscle aches/pains persist for more than 7 days or recur.

Keep this and all drugs out of the reach of children. In case of accidental overdose, seek professional assistance or contact a poison control center immediately.

How Supplied: (ointment) Available in 1.5 OZ (40 g), 3.0 OZ (90 g) and 6.0 OZ (170 g) plastic jars. **(cream)** 2.0 OZ (60 g) tube.

VICKS® VAPOSTEAM®
[*vā 'pō "stēm*]
Liquid Medication for Hot Steam Vaporizers. Nasal Decongestant/Cough Suppressant

Active Ingredients: Camphor 6.2%.

Inactive Ingredients: Alcohol 78%, Cedarleaf Oil, Eucalyptus Oil, Laureth 7, Menthol, Nutmeg Oil, Poloxamer 124, Silicone.

Indications: Temporarily relieves cough occurring with a cold.

Directions:
Adults and children 2 years of age and older: Add one tablespoon of solution for each quart of water, directly to the water in a hot steam vaporizer. Breathe in medicated vapors. May be repeated up to 3 times daily or as directed by a doctor.
Children under 2 years of age: ask a doctor.
In Hot/Warm Steam Vaporizers: VAPOSTEAM is formulated to be added directly to the water in your hot/warm steam vaporizer. Do not direct steam from vaporizer too close to face. For best performance, vaporizer should be thoroughly cleaned after each use according to manufacturer's instructions. To promote steaming, follow directions of vaporizer manufacturer.
Never expose VAPOSTEAM to flame, microwave, or place in any container in which you are heating water except for a hot-warm steam vaporizer. Never use VAPOSTEAM in any bowl or washbasin with hot water. Improper use may cause the mixture to splatter and cause burns.

Warnings: For steam inhalation only. **Not to be taken by mouth.** A persistent cough may be a sign of a serious condition. If cough persists for more than one week, tends to recur or is accompanied by fever, rash, or persistent headache, consult a doctor. Do not use this product for persistent or chronic cough such as occurs with smoking, asthma, emphysema, or if cough is accompanied by excessive phlegm (mucus) unless directed by a doctor. **Keep this and all drugs out of the reach of children.**

Accidental Ingestion: In case of accidental ingestion, seek professional assistance or contact a poison control center immediately.

Eye Exposure: In case of eye contact, flush with water. Seek professional assistance or contact a poison control center immediately.

How Supplied: Available in 4 FL OZ (118 mL) and 8 FL OZ (236 mL) bottles.

EDUCATIONAL MATERIAL

Procter & Gamble offers to health care professionals a variety of journal reprints and patient education materials on:
- fiber therapy and related bowel disorders (Metamucil),
- H. pylori research and healthy traveling advice (Pepto-Bismol),
- caffeine reduction (Folgers), and
- pharmacy practice issues (Pharmacy Digest newsletter).

Additionally, selected professional samples of Procter & Gamble Health Care and Skin Care products are available to targeted health care specialists.
For these materials, please call 1-800/358-8707, or write:
Charles Lambert
Manager, Scientific Communications
The Procter & Gamble Company
Two Procter & Gamble Plaza
Cincinnati, OH 45201

The Purdue Frederick Company
100 CONNECTICUT AVENUE
NORWALK, CT 06850-3590

For Medical Information Contact:
Medical Department
(203) 853-0123

BETADINE®
Brand First Aid Antibiotics + Moisturizer Ointment

Actions: Topical broad-spectrum antibiotics in a cholesterolized ointment (moisturizer) base to fight infection while helping to heal damaged skin; antibiotics per gram: polymyxin B sulfate (10,000 IU), bacitracin zinc (500 IU).

Indications: Minor cuts, scrapes, burns

Administration: Clean affected area. Apply small amount on area 1 to 3 times daily. May be covered with a sterile bandage.

Warnings: For External Use Only. Do not use in the eyes or apply over large areas of the body. In case of deep or puncture wounds, animal bites, or serious burns, consult a physician. Stop use and consult a physician if the condition persists or gets worse. Do not use longer than 1 week unless directed by a physician. Keep this and all medications out of the reach of children. In case of accidental ingestion, seek professional assistance or contact a Poison Control Center immediately.

How Supplied: 1/2 oz & 1 oz plastic tubes.

BETADINE® FIRST AID CREAM
(povidone-iodine, 5%)

BETADINE® OINTMENT
(povidone-iodine, 10%)

BETADINE® SKIN CLEANSER
(povidone-iodine, 7.5%)

BETADINE SOLUTION
(povidone-iodine, 10%)
Topical Antiseptic Bactericide/Virucide

Action: Topical microbicides active against organisms commonly encountered in minor skin wounds and burns.

Indications: Cream: For minor cuts, burns or scrapes, to kill bacteria and other germs and enhance healing.
Ointment: As a therapy, used as an adjunct to systemic treatment for skin infections: prophylactically, to prevent contamination of burns, incisions and other topical lesions.
Skin Cleanser: Degerming of skin and removal of dirt or other foreign material.
Solution: Prepping of sites before surgery and other procedures, topical wound or skin-ulcer antisepsis, postoperative application to incisions, oral moniliasis, bacterial and mycotic skin infection, preoperative mouth/throat swab.

Administration: Cream and Ointment: Apply directly to affected area as needed. May be bandaged.
Skin Cleanser: Wet skin, apply sufficient amount to work up lather. Allow lather to remain about 3 min. Rinse thoroughly with water. Repeat 2–3 times a day or as directed by physician.
Solution: Apply full strength as often as needed as a paint/spray/wet soak. May be bandaged.

Warnings: Cream, Ointment, Skin Cleanser: For External Use Only. In case of deep puncture wounds or serious burns, consult physician, If redness, irritation, swelling, or pain persists or increases, or if infection occurs, discontinue use and consult physician. Keep out of reach of children.
Solution: For External Use Only. In preoperative prepping, avoid "pooling" beneath the patient. Prolonged exposure to wet solution may cause irritation or, rarely, severe skin reactions. In rare instance of local irritation or sensitivity, discontinue use. Do not heat prior to application.

How supplied:
Cream: 1/2 oz. tube w/applicator tip
Ointment: 1/32 and 1/8 oz. packettes: 1 oz. tubes; 16 oz. (1 lb.)
Skin Cleanser: 1 and 4 fl. oz. plastic bottles
Solution: 1/2 oz., 4 oz., 8 oz., 16 oz. (1 pt.), 32 oz. (1 qt.), and 1 gal. plastic bottles; 1 oz. packettes; Swab Aid® Pads; swabsticks, aerosol spray

---

SENOKOT® Tablets/Granules
SenokotXTRA® Tablets
(standardized senna concentrate)

SENOKOT® Syrup
SENOKOT® Children's Syrup
(extract of senna concentrate)

SENOKOT-S® Tablets
(standardized senna concentrate and docusate sodium)

Natural Vegetable Laxative

Actions: Senna provides a virtually colon-specific action which is gentle, effective, and predictable, generally producing bowel movement in 6 to 12 hours. Senokot-S tablets contain a stool softener for smoother, easier evacuation.

Indications: Relief of constipation

Dosage and Administration: Take according to product-package instructions or as directed by a doctor. Take preferably at bedtime. For older, debilitated patients, a doctor may consider prescribing $^1/_2$ the initial dose recommended on the package. Senokot Syrup is not to be used for children under 12 years old; use Senokot Children's Syrup in the under-12 age group. For use of Senokot in children under 2 years of age, consult a doctor.

Warnings: Do not use a laxative product when abdominal pain, nausea or vomiting are present unless directed by a doctor. If you have noticed a sudden change in bowel movements that persists over a period of 2 weeks, consult a doctor before using a laxative. Laxative products should not be used for a period longer than 1 week unless directed by a doctor. Rectal bleeding or failure to have a bowel movement after the use of a laxative may indicate a serious condition. Discontinue use and consult your doctor. As with any drug, if you are pregnant or nursing a baby, seek the advice of a health professional before using this product. In case of accidental overdose, seek professional assistance or contact a Poison Control Center immediately. Keep out of children's reach.

How supplied: Senokot Tablets: Boxes of 10 and 20; bottles of 50, 100, and 1000; Unit Strip Packs in boxes of 100 individually sealed tablets.
SenokotXTRA Tablets: Boxes of 12 and 36
Senokot-S Tablets: Packages of 10; bottles of 30, 60 and 1000; Unit Strip boxes of 100.
Senokot Granules: 2, 6, and 12 oz. plastic containers
Senokot Syrup: 2 and 8 fl. oz. bottles.
Senokot Children's Syrup: Chocolate-flavored, alcohol-free syrup in 2.5 fl. oz. plastic bottle packaged with measuring cup.

Richardson-Vicks Inc.

(See Procter & Gamble.)

Roberts Pharmaceutical Corporation

4 INDUSTRIAL WAY WEST
EATONTOWN, NJ 07724

Direct Inquiries to:
Customer Service Department:
(908) 389-1182
(800) 828-2088
FAX: (908) 389-1014

For Medical Emergencies Contact:
Medical Services Department
(800) 992-9306

CHERACOL® Nasal Spray Pump
Cherry Scented

Description: CHERACOL® NASAL SPRAY PUMP is a cherry scented long acting topical nasal decongestant. One application lasts up to 12 hours.

How Supplied: Available in 1 fluid ounce bottles fitted with a metered pump (NDC 54092-880-30).
Manufactured for
Roberts Laboratories Inc.,
a subsidiary of
ROBERTS PHARMACEUTICAL CORPORATION
Eatontown, NJ 07724 USA

CHERACOL® SINUS
12 Hour Formula

Description: Cheracol® SINUS sustained-action tablets combine a nasal decongestant with an antihistamine in a special continuous-acting timed-release tablet to provide temporary relief of nasal congestion due to the common cold, and associated with sinusitis. Also allevi-

Continued on next page

Roberts—Cont.

ates running nose and sneezing due to hay fever.

How Supplied: 10 sustained-action release tablets. NDC 54092-045-10
Manufactured for
Roberts Laboratories Inc., a subsidiary of
ROBERTS PHARMACEUTICAL CORPORATION
Eatontown, NJ 07724, USA

CHERACOL® Sore Throat Spray Anesthetic/Antiseptic Liquid

Description: A pleasant tasting cherry flavored liquid spray with anesthetic and antiseptic properties.

How Supplied: Available in 6 fluid ounce spray pump bottle (NDC 54092-340-06).
Manufactured for
Roberts Laboratories Inc.,
a subsidiary of
ROBERTS PHARMACEUTICAL CORPORATION
Eatontown, NJ 07724 USA

CHERACOL D® Cough Formula Maximum Strength Cough Relief

Description: CHERACOL D® is a non-narcotic cough formula which combines two important medicines in one safe, fast-acting pleasant tasting liquid:

- The highest level of cough suppressant available without prescription.
- A clinically proven expectorant to help loosen phlegm and drain bronchial tubes.

Indications: CHERACOL D® cough formula helps quiet dry, hacking coughs, and helps loosen phlegm and mucus. Recommended for adults and children 6 years of age and older.

Active Ingredients: Each teaspoonful (5 ml) contains dextromethorphan hydrobromide, 10 mg; guaifenesin, 100 mg; **Inactive Ingredients:** alcohol, 4.75%, benzoic acid, FD&C Red #40, flavors, fragrances, fructose, glycerin, propylene glycol, sodium chloride, sucrose, and purified water.

Dosage—Adults and children 12 years of age and over: Oral dosage is 2 teaspoonfuls every 4 hours, not to exceed 12 teaspoonfuls in 24 hours, or as directed by a doctor. **Children 6 to under 12 years of age:** Oral dosage is 1 teaspoonful every 4 hours, not to exceed 6 teaspoonfuls in 24 hours, or as directed by a doctor. **Children under 6 years of age:** Consult a doctor.

Warnings: Keep this and all medication out of the reach of children. Do not give this product to children under 6 years of age except under the advice and supervision of a physician. Do not use this product for persistent or chronic cough such as occurs with smoking, asthma, or emphysema or where cough is accompanied by excessive secretions except under the advice and supervision of a physician. As with any drug, pregnant or nursing women should seek the advice of a health professional before using this product.

Caution: A persistent cough may be a sign of a serious condition. If cough persists for more than 1 week, tends to recur or is accompanied by high fever, rash or persistent headache, consult a physician.

Overdose: In case of accidental overdose contact a physician or a poison control center immediately.

Drug Interaction Precaution: Do not use this product if you are now taking a prescription monoamine inhibitor (maoi) (certain drugs for depression, psychiatric or emotional conditions, or Parkinson's Disease), or for two weeks after stopping the maoi drug. If you are uncertain whether your prescription drug contains an maoi, consult a health professional before taking this product.

How Supplied: Available 4 oz bottle (NDC 54092-400-04), and 6 oz bottle (NDC 54092-400-06).
Manufactured for
Roberts Laboratories Inc.,
a subsidiary of
ROBERTS PHARMACEUTICAL CORPORATION
Eatontown, NJ 07724 USA

Shown in Product Identification Guide, page 515

CHERACOL PLUS® Cough Syrup Multisymptom cough/cold formula

Description: CHERACOL PLUS® Cough Syrup is a pleasant tasting 3-ingredient non-narcotic liquid formulation.

Indications: Cheracol Plus® syrup is an effective 3-ingredient, maximum strength formula for the temporary relief of head cold symptoms and cough (without narcotic side effects).

Active Ingredients: Each tablespoonful (15ml) contains phenylpropanolamine HCl, 25 mg; dextromethorphan hydrobromide, 20 mg; chlorpheniramine maleate, 4 mg; and alcohol, 8%.

Inactive Ingredients: Flavors, glycerin, methylparaben, propylene glycol, propylparaben, FD&C Red No. 40, sodium chloride, sorbitol solution, and purified water.

Dosage and Administration: Adults and children over 12 years of age: 1 tablespoonful (15ml) every 4 hours or as directed by a physician. Do not take more than 6 tablespoonfuls in a 24 hour period. Do not administer to children under 12 years of age.

Uses: Cheracol Plus® multisymptom head cold/cough formula provides cough suppressant and decongestant activity and controls runny nose associated with the common cold ("flu").

Warnings: Do not take this product for persistent or chronic cough such as occurs with smoking, asthma, or emphysema or where cough is accompanied by excessive secretions or if you have high blood pressure, heart or thyroid disease, diabetes, asthma, glaucoma, or difficulty in urination due to enlargement of the prostate gland except under the advice and supervision of a physician. If symptoms do not improve within 7 days or are accompanied by high fever, consult a physician before continuing use. May cause excitability, especially in children. Do not give this product to children under 12 years except under the advice and supervision of a physician. May cause marked drowsiness. Avoid alcoholic beverages, driving a motor vehicle or operating heavy machinery while taking this product. As with any drug, if you are pregnant or nursing a baby consult a health professional before using this product. Keep this and all medication out of the reach of children.

Drug Interaction Precaution: Do not use this product if you are now taking a prescription monoamine oxidase inhibitor (MAOI) (certain drugs for depression, psychiatric or emotional conditions, or Parkinson's disease), or for 2 weeks after stopping the MAOI drug. If you are uncertain whether your prescription drug contains an MAOI, consult a health professional before taking this product.

Overdose: In case of accidental overdose contact a physician or a poison control center immediately.

How Supplied: Available in 4 oz bottle (NDC 54092-401-04), 6 oz bottle (54092-401-06).
Manufactured for
Roberts Laboratories Inc.,
a subsidiary of
ROBERTS PHARMACEUTICAL CORPORATION
Eatontown, NJ 07724 USA

COLACE®
[*kōlās*]
docusate sodium, capsules • syrup • liquid (drops)

Description: Colace® (docusate sodium) is a stool softener.
Colace® Capsules, 50 mg, contain the following inactive ingredients: citric acid, D&C Red No. 33, FD&C Red No. 40, nonporcine gelatin, edible ink, polyethylene glycol, propylene glycol, and purified water.
Colace® Capsules, 100 mg, contain the following inactive ingredients: citric acid, D&C Red No. 33, FD&C Red No. 40, FD&C Yellow No. 6, nonporcine gelatin, edible ink, polyethylene glycol, propylene glycol, titanium dioxide, and purified water.
Colace® Liquid, 1%, contains the following inactive ingredients: citric acid, D&C Red No. 33, methylparaben, poloxamer, polyethylene glycol, propylene glycol,

propylparaben, sodium citrate, vanillin, and purified water.
Colace® Syrup, 20 mg/5 mL, contains the following inactive ingredients: alcohol (not more than 1%), citric acid, D&C Red No. 33, FD&C Red No. 40, flavor (natural), menthol, methylparaben, peppermint oil, poloxamer, polyethylene glycol, propylparaben, sodium citrate, sucrose, and purified water.

Actions and Uses: Colace®, a surface-active agent, helps to keep stools soft for easy, natural passage and is not a laxative, thus, not habit forming. Useful in constipation due to hard stools, in painful anorectal conditions, in cardiac and other conditions in which maximum ease of passage is desirable to avoid difficult or painful defecation, and when peristaltic stimulants are contraindicated.

Note: When peristaltic stimulation is needed due to inadequate bowel motility, see Peri-Colace® (laxative and stool softener).

Contraindications: There are no known contraindications to Colace®.

Warning: As with any drug, pregnant or nursing women should seek the advice of a health professional before using this product. Keep this and all medication out of the reach of children.

Side Effects: The incidence of side effects—none of a serious nature—is exceedingly small. Bitter taste, throat irritation, and nausea (primarily associated with the use of the syrup and liquid) are the main side effects reported. Rash has occurred.

Administration and Dosage: *Orally*—Suggested daily Dosage: *Adults and older children:* 50 to 200 mg *Children 6 to 12:* 40 to 120 mg *Children 3 to 6:* 20 to 60 mg. *Infants and children under 3:* 10 to 40 mg. The higher doses are recommended for initial therapy. Dosage should be adjusted to individual response. The effect on stools is usually apparent 1 to 3 days after the first dose. Colace® liquid or syrup must be given in a 6 oz. to 8 oz. glass of milk or fruit juice or in infant's formula to prevent throat irritation. In *enemas*—Add 50 to 100 mg Colace® (5 to 10 mL Colace® liquid) to a retention or flushing enema.

How Supplied: Colace® capsules, 50 mg
NDC 54092-052-30 Bottles of 30
NDC 54092-052-60 Bottles of 60
NDC 54092-052-52 Cartons of 100 single unit packs
Colace® capsules, 100 mg
NDC 54092-053-30 Bottles of 30
NDC 54092-053-60 Bottle of 60
NDC 54092-053-02 Bottles of 250
NDC 54092-053-10 Bottles of 1000
NDC 54092-053-52 Cartons of 100 single unit packs

Note: Colace® capsules should be stored at controlled room temperature (59°–86°F or 15°–30°C)
Colace® liquid, 1% solution; 10 mg/mL (with calibrated dropper)
NDC 54092-414-16 Bottles of 16 fl oz
NDC 54092-414-30 Bottles of 30 mL
Colace® syrup, 20 mg/5 mL teaspoon; contains not more than 1% alcohol
NDC 54092-415-08 Bottles of 8 fl oz
NDC 54092-415-16 Bottles of 16 fl oz
Manufactured for
Roberts Laboratories Inc.,
a subsidiary of
ROBERTS PHARMACEUTICAL CORPORATION
Eatontown, NJ 07724 USA

Shown in Product Identification Guide, page 518

PERI-COLACE® capsules • syrup (casanthranol and docusate sodium)

Description: Peri-Colace® is a combination of the mild stimulant laxative casanthranol, and the stool-softener Colace® (docusate sodium). Each capsule contains 30 mg of casanthranol and 100 mg of Colace®; the syrup contains 30 mg of casanthranol and 60 mg of Colace® per 15-mL tablespoon (10 mg of casanthranol and 20 mg of Colace® per 5-mL teaspoon) and 10% alcohol.
Peri-Colace® Capsules contain the following inactive ingredients: D&C Red No. 33, FD&C Red No. 40, non-porcine gelatin, edible ink, polyethylene glycol, propylene glycol, titanium dioxide, and purified water.
Peri-Colace® Syrup contains the following inactive ingredients: alcohol (10% v/v), citric acid, flavors, methyl salicylate, methylparaben, poloxamer, polyethylene glycol, propylparaben, sodium citrate, sorbitol solution, sucrose, and purified water.

Action and Uses: Peri-Colace® provides gentle peristaltic stimulation and helps to keep stools soft for easier passage. Bowel movement is induced gently—usually overnight or in 8 to 12 hours. Nausea, griping, abnormally loose stools, and constipation rebound are minimized. Useful in management of chronic or temporary constipation.

Note: To prevent hard stools when laxative stimulation is not needed or undesirable, see Colace® (stool softener).

Warnings: Do not use when abdominal pain, nausea, or vomiting is present. Frequent or prolonged use of this preparation may result in dependence on laxatives.
As with any drug, pregnant or nursing women should seek the advice of a health professional before using this product. Keep this and all medication out of the reach of children.

Side Effects: The incidence of side effects—none of a serious nature—is exceedingly small. Nausea, abdominal cramping or discomfort, diarrhea, and rash are the main side effects reported.

Administration and Dosage:
Adults—1 or 2 capsules, or 1 or 2 tablespoons syrup at bedtime, or as indicated. In severe cases, dosage may be increased to 2 capsules or 2 tablespoons twice daily, or 3 capsules at bedtime. *Children*—1 to 3 teaspoons of syrup at bedtime, or as indicated. Peri-Colace® syrup must be given in a 6 oz. to 8 oz. glass of milk or fruit juice or in infant's formula to prevent throat irritation.

Overdosage: In addition to symptomatic treatment, gastric lavage, if timely, is recommended in cases of large overdosage.

How Supplied: Peri-Colace® Capsules
NDC 54092-054-30 Bottles of 30
NDC 54092-054-60 Bottles of 60
NDC 54092-054-02 Bottles of 250
NDC 54092-054-10 Bottles of 1000
NDC 54092-054-52 Cartons of 100 single unit packs

Note: Peri-Colace® capsules should be stored at controlled room temperatures (59°–86°F or 15°–30°C).
Peri-Colace® Syrup
NDC 54092-418-08 Bottles of 8 fl oz
NDC 54092-418-16 Bottles of 16 fl oz
Manufactured for
Roberts Laboratories Inc.,
a subsidiary of
ROBERTS PHARMACEUTICAL CORPORATION
Eatontown, NJ 07724 USA

Shown in Product Identification Guide, page 518

A. H. Robins Consumer Products

American Home Products Corporation
FIVE GIRALDA FARMS
MADISON, NJ 07940-0871

For information on A.H. Robins Consumer Products see product listings under Whitehall-Robins Healthcare.

TO FIND A BRAND:
Turn to the
Product Name Index
(Pink Pages)

TO FIND A PRODUCT BY ITS GENERIC INGREDIENTS:
Turn to the
Active Ingredients Index
(Yellow Pages)

TO FIND A PRODUCT BY ITS THERAPEUTIC CATEGORY
Turn to the
Product Category Index
(Blue Pages)

Ross Products Division Abbott Laboratories
COLUMBUS, OHIO 43215-1724

Direct Inquiries to:
1-800-227-5767

PEDIATRIC NUTRITIONAL PRODUCTS

Alimentum® Protein Hydrolysate Formula With Iron

Isomil® Soy Formula With Iron

Isomil® DF Soy Formula For Diarrhea

Isomil® SF Sucrose-Free Soy Formula With Iron

PediaSure® Complete Liquid Nutrition

PediaSure® With Fiber Complete Liquid Nutrition

RCF® Ross Carbohydrate Free Soy Formula Base With Iron

Similac® Low-Iron Infant Formula

Similac NeoCare® Infant Formula With Iron

Similac® PM 60/40 Low-Iron Infant Formula

Similac® Special Care® With Iron 24 Premature Infant Formula

Similac® With Iron Infant Formula

For most current information, refer to product labels.

CLEAR EYES®
[*klēr īz*]
Lubricant Eye Redness Reliever Eye Drops

Description: Clear Eyes is a sterile, isotonic buffered solution containing the active ingredients naphazoline hydrochloride (0.012%) and glycerin (0.2%). It also contains boric acid, purified water and sodium borate. Edetate disodium and benzalkonium chloride are added as preservatives. Clear Eyes is a lubricant, decongestant ophthalmic solution specially designed for temporary relief of redness and drying due to minor eye irritation caused by smoke, smog, sun glare or swimming. Clear Eyes contains laboratory-tested and scientifically blended ingredients, including an effective vasoconstrictor which narrows swollen blood vessels and rapidly whitens reddened eyes in a formulation which also contains a lubricant and produces a refreshing, soothing effect. Clear Eyes is a sterile, isotonic solution compatible with the natural fluids of the eye.

Indications: For the temporary relief of redness due to minor eye irritation AND for protection against further irritation or dryness of the eye.

Warnings: To avoid contamination, do not touch tip of container to any surface. Replace cap after using. If you experience eye pain, changes in vision, continued redness or irritation of the eye, or if the condition worsens or persists for more than 72 hours, discontinue use and consult a doctor. If you have glaucoma, do not use this product except under the advice and supervision of a doctor. Overuse of this product may produce increased redness of the eye. If solution changes color or becomes cloudy, do not use. Keep this and all drugs out of the reach of children. In case of accidental ingestion, seek professional assistance or contact a Poison Control Center immediately.

Directions: Instill 1 or 2 drops in the affected eye(s), up to four times daily.

How Supplied: In 0.5-fl-oz (15 mL) and 1.0-fl-oz (30 mL) plastic dropper bottles. (FAN 3178)

CLEAR EYES® ACR
[*klēr īz*]
Astringent/Lubricant Redness Reliever Eye Drops

Description: Clear Eyes ACR is a sterile, isotonic buffered solution containing the active ingredients naphazoline hydrochloride (0.012%), zinc sulfate (0.25%) and glycerin (0.2%). It also contains boric acid, purified water, sodium chloride and sodium citrate. Edetate disodium and benzalkonium chloride are added as preservatives. Clear Eyes ACR is a triple-action formula that: (1) has an extra ingredient to clear away mucus buildup and relieve itching associated with exposure to airborne allergens, (2) immediately removes redness and (3) moisturizes irritated eyes. Clear Eyes ACR contains laboratory-tested and scientifically blended ingredients, including an effective vasoconstrictor which narrows swollen blood vessels and rapidly whitens reddened eyes in a formulation which also contains a lubricant and produces a soothing effect. Clear Eyes ACR also contains an ocular astringent (zinc sulfate) that precipitates the sticky mucus buildup on the eye often associated with exposure to airborne allergens, and this helps clear the mucus from the outer surface of the eye. Clear Eyes ACR is a sterile, isotonic solution compatible with the natural fluids of the eye.

Indications: For the temporary relief of redness due to minor eye irritation AND for protection against further irritation or dryness of the eye.

Warnings: To avoid contamination, do not touch tip of container to any surface. Replace cap after using. If you experience eye pain, changes in vision, continued redness or irritation of the eye, or if the condition worsens or persists for more than 72 hours, discontinue use and consult a doctor. If you have glaucoma, do not use this product except under the advice and supervision of a doctor. Overuse of this product may produce increased redness of the eye. If solution changes color or becomes cloudy, do not use. Keep this and all drugs out of the reach of children. In case of accidental ingestion, seek professional assistance or contact a Poison Control Center immediately.

Directions: Instill 1 or 2 drops in the affected eye(s), up to four times daily.

How Supplied: In 0.5-fl-oz (15 mL) and 1.0-fl-oz (30 mL) plastic dropper bottles. (FAN 3178)

CLEAR EYES ® CLR
[*klēr- īz*]
SOOTHING DROPS
Contact Lens Relief

Description: CLEAR EYES CLR Soothing Drops is a sterile, isotonic solution with a borate buffer system, sodium chloride, hydroxypropyl methylcellulose and glycerin, with sorbic acid (0.25%) and edetate disodium (0.1%) as the preservatives.

Indications (Uses): CLEAR EYES CLR Soothing Drops may be used with daily and extended wear soft (hydrophilic) contact lenses for the following:

- Moistening of daily wear soft lenses while on the eyes during the day.
- Moistening of extended wear soft lenses upon awakening and as needed during the day.
- Moistening of extended wear soft lenses prior to retiring at night.

Placing 1 or 2 drops of CLEAR EYES CLR Soothing Drops on the eye followed by blinking 2 or 3 times will relieve minor irritation, discomfort and blurring which may occur while wearing lenses.

Contraindications (Reasons Not To Use): Patients allergic to any ingredient in CLEAR EYES CLR Soothing Drops should not use this product.

Warnings:

> • PROBLEMS WITH CONTACT LENSES AND LENS CARE PRODUCTS COULD RESULT IN SERIOUS INJURY TO THE EYE. It is essential that you follow your eye care professional's direction and all labeling instructions for proper use of your lenses and lens care products. EYE PROBLEMS, INCLUDING CORNEAL ULCERS, CAN DEVELOP RAPIDLY AND LEAD TO LOSS OF VISION: THEREFORE, IF YOU EXPERIENCE EYE DISCOMFORT, EXCESSIVE TEARING, VISION CHANGES, REDNESS OF THE EYE, IMMEDIATELY REMOVE YOUR LENSES AND PROMPTLY CONTACT YOUR EYE CARE PROFESSIONAL.

All contact lens wearers must see their eye care professional as directed. If your lenses are for extended wear, your eye care professional may prescribe more frequent visits.

- Never touch the dropper tip of the container to any surface, since this may contaminate the solution. If drops turn yellow, discard and use fresh (colorless) drops.

Replace cap after every use.

Precautions:

- Always wash and rinse your hands before handling your lenses.
- Store at room temperature.
- Keep container tightly closed when not in use.
- Use before the expiration date marked on the containers and cartons.
- Keep this and all medications out of the reach of children.

Adverse Reactions (Problems and What To Do): The following problems may occur while wearing contact lenses:

- Eyes stinging, burning or itching (irritation)
- Excessive watering (tearing) of the eyes
- Unusual eye secretions
- Redness of the eyes
- Reduced sharpness of vision (visual acuity)
- Blurred vision
- Sensitivity to light (photophobia)
- Dry eyes

If you notice any of the above problems, immediately remove and examine your lenses.

If the problem stops and the lenses appear to be undamaged, thoroughly clean, rinse and disinfect the lenses and reinsert them. If the problem continues or a lens appears to be damaged, IMMEDIATELY remove your lenses and IMMEDIATELY consult your eye care professional. **Do not reinsert a damaged lens.** If any of the above symptoms occur, a serious condition such as infection, corneal ulcer, neovascularization or iritis may be present. Seek immediate professional identification of the problem and treatment to avoid serious eye damage.

Directions: CLEAR EYES CLR Soothing Drops may be used as needed throughout the day. If minor irritation, discomfort or blurring occur while wearing lenses, place 1 or 2 drops on the eye and blink 2 or 3 times. If discomfort continues, immediately remove lenses and immediately see your eye care professional.

How Supplied: CLEAR EYES CLR Soothing Drops are supplied in sterile 0.5 fl oz (15 mL) and 1.0 fl oz (30 mL) plastic bottles. The containers and cartons are marked with lot number and expiration date.
(FAN 3179)

EAR DROPS BY MURINE®

[*myūr'ēn*]

See Murine Ear Wax Removal System/Murine Ear Drops.

MURINE® EAR WAX REMOVAL SYSTEM/MURINE® EAR DROPS

[*myūr'ēn*]

Carbamide Peroxide
Ear Wax Removal Aid

Description: MURINE EAR DROPS contains the active ingredient carbamide peroxide, 6.5%. It also contains alcohol (6.3%), anhydrous glycerin, polysorbate 20 and other ingredients in a buffered vehicle. The MURINE EAR WAX REMOVAL SYSTEM includes a 1.0-fl-oz soft bulb ear syringe. This system is a complete, medically approved system to safely remove ear wax. Application of carbamide peroxide drops followed by warm-water irrigation is an effective, medically recommended way to help loosen excessive and/or hardened ear wax.

Actions: The carbamide peroxide formula in MURINE EAR DROPS is an aid in the removal of wax from the ear canal. Anhydrous glycerin penetrates and softens wax while the release of oxygen from carbamide peroxide provides a mechanical action resulting in the loosening of the softened wax accumulation. It is usually necessary to remove the loosened wax by gently flushing the ear with warm water, using the soft bulb ear syringe provided.

Indications: The MURINE EAR WAX REMOVAL SYSTEM is indicated for occasional use as an aid to soften, loosen and remove excessive ear wax.

Warnings: DO NOT USE if you have ear drainage or discharge, ear pain, irritation or rash in the ear or are dizzy: Consult a doctor. DO NOT USE if you have an injury or perforation (hole) of the eardrum or after ear surgery, unless directed by a doctor.
DO NOT USE for more than 4 days; if excessive ear wax remains after use of this product, consult a doctor. Avoid contact with the eyes. If accidental contact with eyes occurs, flush eyes with water and consult a doctor. KEEP THIS AND ALL MEDICINES OUT OF THE REACH OF CHILDREN. In case of accidental ingestion, seek professional assistance or contact a Poison Control Center immediately.

Directions: FOR USE IN THE EAR ONLY. Adults and children over 12 years of age: Tilt head sideways and place 5 to 10 drops in ear. Tip of applicator should not enter ear canal. Keep drops in ear for several minutes by keeping head tilted or placing cotton in the ear. Use twice daily for up to 4 days if needed, or as directed by a doctor. Any wax remaining after the 4-day treatment may be removed by gently flushing the ear with warm (body temperature) water, using a soft bulb ear syringe. Children under 12 years of age: Consult a doctor.

Note: DO NOT INSERT SYRINGE TIP INTO EAR CANAL. When the ear canal is irrigated, the tip of the ear syringe should not obstruct the flow of water leaving the ear canal.

How Supplied: The MURINE EAR WAX REMOVAL SYSTEM contains 0.5-fl-oz (15 mL) drops and a 1.0-fl-oz (30 mL) soft bulb ear syringe.
Also available in 0.5-fl-oz (15 mL) drops only, MURINE EAR DROPS.
(FAN 3328)

MURINE TEARS™

[*myūr'ēn 'ti(ə)rs*]

Lubricant Eye Drops

Description: Murine Tears eye lubricant is a sterile, buffered solution containing the active ingredients 0.5% polyvinyl alcohol and 0.6% povidone. Also contains benzalkonium chloride, dextrose, disodium edetate, potassium chloride, purified water, sodium bicarbonate, sodium chloride, sodium citrate and sodium phosphate (mono- and dibasic). Murine Tears is a sterile, hypotonic solution formulated to more closely match the natural tear fluid of the eye for gentle, soothing relief from minor eye irritation while moisturizing and relieving dryness. Use as desired to temporarily relieve minor eye irritation, dryness and burning.

Indications: For the temporary relief or prevention of further discomfort due to minor eye irritations and symptoms related to dry eyes.

Warnings: To avoid contamination, do not touch tip of container to any surface. Replace cap after using. If you experience eye pain, changes in vision, continued redness or irritation of the eye, or if the condition worsens or persists for more than 72 hours, discontinue use and consult a doctor. If solution changes color or becomes cloudy, do not use. Keep this and all drugs out of the reach of children. In case of accidental ingestion, seek professional assistance or contact a Poison Control Center immediately.

Directions: Instill 1 or 2 drops in the affected eye(s) as needed.

How Supplied: In 0.5-fl-oz (15 mL) and 1.0-fl-oz (30 mL) plastic dropper bottles.
(FAN 3249)

MURINE TEARS™ PLUS

[*myūr'ēn 'ti(ə)rs*]

Lubricant Redness Reliever
Eye Drops

Description: Murine Tears Plus is a sterile, non-staining, buffered solution containing the active ingredients 0.5% polyvinyl alcohol, 0.6% povidone and

Continued on next page

If desired, additional information on any Ross product will be provided upon request to Ross Products Division, Abbott Laboratories, Columbus, Ohio 43215-1724.

Ross—Cont.

0.05% tetrahydrozoline hydrochloride. Also contains benzalkonium chloride, dextrose, disodium edetate, potassium chloride, purified water, sodium bicarbonate, sodium chloride, sodium citrate and sodium phosphate (mono- and dibasic). Murine Tears Plus is a sterile, hypotonic, ophthalmic solution formulated to more closely match the natural fluid of the eye. It contains demulcents for gentle, soothing relief from minor eye irritation as well as the sympathomimetic agent, tetrahydrozoline hydrochloride, which produces local vasoconstriction in the eye. Thus, the drug effectively narrows swollen blood vessels locally and provides symptomatic relief of edema and hyperemia of conjunctival tissues due to eye allergies, minor local irritations and conjunctivitis. Use up to four times daily, to remove redness due to minor eye irritation. The effect of Murine Tears Plus is prompt (apparent within minutes).

Indications: For the temporary relief or prevention of further discomfort due to minor eye irritations and symptoms related to dry eyes PLUS removal of redness.

Warnings: To avoid contamination, do not touch tip of container to any surface. Replace cap after using. If you experience eye pain, changes in vision, continued redness or irritation of the eye, or if the condition worsens or persists for more than 72 hours, discontinue use and consult a doctor. If you have glaucoma, do not use this product except under the advice and supervision of a doctor. Overuse of this product may produce increased redness of the eye. If solution changes color or becomes cloudy, do not use. Keep this and all drugs out of the reach of children. In case of accidental ingestion, seek professional assistance or contact a Poison Control Center immediately.

Directions: Instill 1 or 2 drops in the affected eye(s), **up to four times daily.**

How Supplied: In 0.5-fl-oz (15 mL) and 1.0-fl-oz (30 mL) plastic dropper bottles. (FAN 3249)

PEDIALYTE®

[pē'dē-ah-līt"]

Oral Electrolyte Maintenance Solution

Usage: To quickly restore fluid and minerals lost in diarrhea and vomiting; for maintenance of water and electrolytes following corrective parenteral therapy for severe diarrhea.

Features:

- Ready To Use—no mixing or dilution necessary.
- Balanced electrolytes to replace stool losses and provide maintenance requirements.
- Provides glucose to promote sodium and water absorption.
- Unflavored form available for younger infants; Bubble Gum, Fruit and Grape-flavored forms available to enhance compliance in older infants and children.
- Plastic liter bottles are resealable, easy to pour and easy to measure.
- Freezer Pops (2.1-fl-oz Pedialyte per serving) available in assortment of Cherry, Orange, Grape and Blue Raspberry Flavors to encourage compliance with fluid intake recommendations for children 1 year of age and older.
- Widely available in grocery, drug and convenience stores.

Availability:
1 quart 1.8-fl-oz (1 liter) plastic bottles; 8 per case; Unflavored, No. 00336; Fruit flavor, No. 00365; Bubble Gum Flavor, No. 51752; Grape Flavor, No. 00240.
8-fl-oz (237 mL) bottles; 4 six-packs per case; Unflavored, No. 00160. 2.1-fl-oz sleeve Freezer Pops; 8 sixteen-sleeve

Pedialyte, Rehydralyte Administration Guide*

For Infants and Young Children

Age	2 Weeks	3	6 Months	9	1	1½	2	2½ Years	3	3½	4	5	6
Approximate Weight† (lb)	7	13	17	20	23	25	28	30	32	35	38	41	46
(kg)	3.2	6.0	7.8	9.2	10.2	11.4	12.6	13.6	14.6	16.0	17.0	18.7	20.7
PEDIALYTE fl oz/day for maintenance**	13 to 16	28 to 32	34 to 40	38 to 44	41 to 46	45 to 50	48 to 53	51 to 56	54 to 58	56 to 60	57 to 62	59 to 66	62 to 69
REHYDRALYTE fl oz/day for Replacement for 5% Dehydration (including maintenance)**	18 to 21	38 to 42	47 to 53	53 to 59	58 to 63	64 to 69	69 to 74	74 to 79	78 to 82	83 to 87	85 to 90	90 to 97	96 to 104
REHYDRALYTE fl oz/day for Replacement for 10% Dehydration (including maintenance)**	23 to 26	48 to 52	60 to 66	68 to 74	75 to 80	83 to 88	90 to 95	97 to 102	102 to 106	110 to 114	113 to 118	121 to 128	131 to 138

* Administration Guide does not apply to infants less than 1 week of age.

**Fluid intake in guide is total fluid requirement from oral electrolyte solution, formula or other fluids, but does not take into account ongoing stool losses. Fluid loss in the stool should be replaced by consumption of an extra amount of Pedialyte or Rehydralyte equal to stool losses in addition to fluid maintenance requirement in this Administration Guide. Pedialyte Freezer Pops are to be used as a supplement to Pedialyte Oral Electrolyte Maintenance Solution or other appropriate fluids to help prevent dehydration.

† Weight based on the 50th percentile of weight for age of the National Center for Health Statistics (NCHS) reference growth data. Hamill PVV, Drizd TA, Johnson CL, et al: Physical growth: National Center for Health Statistics percentiles. *Am J Clin Nutr* 1979; 32:607-629.

boxes per case; Grape, Cherry, Orange and Blue Raspberry, No. 00245. For hospital use, Pedialyte is available in the Ross Hospital Formula System.

Dosage: See Administration Guide to restore fluid and minerals lost in diarrhea and vomiting (Pedialyte® Oral Electrolyte Maintenance Solution) and management of mild to moderate dehydration secondary to moderate to severe diarrhea (Rehydralyte® Oral Electrolyte Rehydration Solution).

Pedialyte or Rehydralyte should be offered frequently in amounts tolerated. Total daily intake should be adjusted to meet individual needs, based on thirst and response to therapy. The following suggested intakes for maintenance are based on water requirements for ordinary energy expenditure.[1] For dehydrated children, the suggested intakes are for replacement and for maintenance, based on a fluid deficit of 5% or 10% of body weight (including maintenance requirement). The fluid deficit should be replaced as quickly as possible, usually in the first 4 to 6 hours.

[See table on bottom of preceding page.]

Reference:

1. Extrapolated from Barness L: Nutrition and nutritional disorders, in Behrman RE, Kliegman RM, Nelson WE, Vaughan VC III: *Nelson Textbook of Pediatrics,* ed 14. Philadelphia: WB Saunders Co, 1992, pp 105-107.

Composition: Unflavored Pedialyte (Bubble Gum Flavor, Fruit Flavor, and Grape Flavor Pedialyte have similar nutrient values. Fruit Flavor and Grape Flavor Pedialyte contain fructose. Pedialyte Freezer Pops contain aspartame. For specific information, including artificial colors in flavored products, see product labels.)

Ingredients: (Pareve, Ⓤ) Water, dextrose, potassium citrate, sodium chloride and sodium citrate. (Freezer Pops also contain citric acid, sodium carboxymethylcellulose, aspartame, potassium sorbate, and natural and artificial flavor.)

Provides:	Per 8 Fl Oz	Per Liter	Per 32 Fl Oz
Sodium (mEq)	10.6	45	42.4
Potassium (mEq)	4.7	20	18.8
Chloride (mEq)	8.3	35	33.2
Citrate (mEq)	7.1	30	28.4
Dextrose (g)	5.9	25	23.6
Calories	24	100	96

(FAN 3333–01)

PEDIASURE® And PEDIASURE® WITH FIBER

[*pē'dē-ah-shur"*]

Complete Liquid Nutrition For Children 1 to 10 years old.

Usage: As a liquid food providing complete, balanced nutrition for children 1 to 10 years of age. May be used for total nutritional support or as a nutritional supplement with and between meals.

Features: PediaSure and PediaSure With Fiber

- Doctor recommended and hospital used
- Nutrition to help recover from illness
- For unpredictable/"picky" eaters
- Ideal for busy, active lifestyles
- A dietary source of fiber (PediaSure With Fiber only)
- Milk-based enteral supplement
- Lactose free, * easily digested
- Convenient, ready to drink, great tasting

*Not for patients with galactosemia.

PediaSure and PediaSure With Fiber contain 100% or more of the NAS-NRC Recommended Dietary Allowances (RDA) for protein, vitamins and minerals in 1000 mL (approx. 34 fl oz) for children 1 to 6 years of age and in 1300 mL (approx. 44 fl oz) for children 7 to 10 years of age.

Availability: Ready To Use 8-fl-oz (237 mL) cans in 6-packs; 24 cans per case. PediaSure: Vanilla, No. 00373; Chocolate, No. 51812; Strawberry, No. 51810; Banana Cream, No. 51808. PediaSure With Fiber: Vanilla, No. 50652.

Directions for Use: Shake very well. Delicious chilled. Do not add water. Suggest 1 to 3 cans per day for supplemental use. Once opened, cover, refrigerate and use within 48 hours. Consult your health care professional regarding your child's specific needs. Not intended for infants under 1 year of age unless specified by a physician.

Ingredients[†] PediaSure and PediaSure With Fiber (Vanilla flavor): Ⓤ-D Water, hydrolyzed cornstarch, sugar (sucrose), sodium caseinate, high-oleic safflower oil, soy oil, fractionated coconut oil (medium-chain triglycerides), whey protein concentrate, soy fiber (PediaSure With Fiber only), calcium phosphate tribasic, natural and artificial flavor, potassium citrate, magnesium chloride, potassium phosphate dibasic, potassium chloride, soy lecithin, mono- and diglycerides, choline chloride, carrageenan, ascorbic acid, m-inositol, taurine, ferrous sulfate, zinc sulfate, niacinamide, alpha-tocopheryl acetate, L-carnitine, calcium pantothenate, manganese sulfate, thiamine chloride hydrochloride, pyridoxine hydrochloride, riboflavin, cupric sulfate, vitamin A palmitate, folic acid, biotin, potassium iodide, sodium selenite, sodium molybdate, phylloquinone, vitamin D_3 and cyanocobalamin.

NUTRIENTS PER 8 FL OZ:

PROTEIN	7.1	g
FAT	11.8	g
CARBOHYDRATE	26 (26.9‡)	g
L-CARNITINE	0.004	g
TAURINE	0.017	g
WATER	200	g
CALORIES		
PER mL	1.0	
PER FL OZ	29.6	
VITAMINS/MINERALS:		
VITAMIN A	610	IU
VITAMIN D	120	IU
VITAMIN E	5.4	IU
VITAMIN K_1	9.0	mcg
VITAMIN C	24	mg
FOLIC ACID	88	mcg
THIAMIN (VIT B_1)	0.64	mg
RIBOFLAVIN (VIT B_2)	0.50	mg
VITAMIN B_6	0.62	mg
VITAMIN B_{12}	1.4	mcg
NIACIN	4.0	mg
CHOLINE	71	mg
BIOTIN	76	mcg
PANTOTHENIC ACID	2.4	mg
INOSITOL	19	mg
SODIUM	90	mg
POTASSIUM	310	mg
CHLORIDE	240	mg
CALCIUM	230	mg
PHOSPHORUS	190	mg
MAGNESIUM	47	mg
IODINE	23	mcg
MANGANESE	0.59	mg
COPPER	0.24	mg
ZINC	2.8	mg
IRON	3.3	mg
CHROMIUM	7.1	mcg
MOLYBDENUM	8.5	mcg
SELENIUM	5.4	mcg

† For Vanilla product; minor differences exist in other PediaSure flavors. For specific information, see product labels.

‡ Includes soy fiber (a source of dietary fiber that provides 3.4 Calories and 1.2 g of total dietary fiber).

(FAN 3139-02) (PediaSure)
(FAN 3139-01) (PediaSure With Fiber)

REHYDRALYTE®

[*rē-hī'drə-līt"*]

Oral Electrolyte Rehydration Solution

Usage: To restore fluid and minerals lost during moderate to severe diarrhea.

Features:

- Ready To Use—no mixing or dilution necessary.
- Safe, economical alternative to IV therapy.
- 75 mEq of sodium per liter for effective replacement of fluid deficits.
- 2½% glucose solution to promote sodium and water absorption and provide energy.
- Available in pharmacies.

Availability: 8-fl-oz (237 mL) bottles; 4 six-packs per case; No. 00162.

Dosage: (See Administration Guide under Pedialyte®.)

Continued on next page

If desired, additional information on any Ross product will be provided upon request to Ross Products Division, Abbott Laboratories, Columbus, Ohio 43215-1724.

Ross—Cont.

Ingredients: (Pareve, ⓤ) Water, dextrose, potassium citrate, sodium chloride and sodium citrate.

Provides:	Per 8 Fl Oz	Per Liter
Sodium (mEq)	17.7	75
Potassium (mEq)	4.7	20
Chloride (mEq)	15.4	65
Citrate (mEq)	7.1	30
Dextrose (g)	5.9	25
Calories	24	100

(FAN 3333-01)

SELSUN BLUE®

[sel'sun blü]

Dandruff Shampoo (selenium sulfide lotion, 1%)

Description: Selsun Blue is a non-prescription anti-dandruff shampoo containing the active ingredient selenium sulfide, 1%, in a freshly scented, pH-balanced formula to leave hair clean and manageable. Available in Balanced Treatment, Moisturizing Treatment, Medicated Treatment and 2-in-1 Treatment formulas.

Inactive Ingredients:

Balanced Treatment formula—Ammonium laureth sulfate, ammonium lauryl sulfate, citric acid, cocamide DEA, cocamidopropyl betaine, DMDM hydantoin, FD&C blue No. 1, fragrance, hydroxypropyl methylcellulose, magnesium aluminum silicate, purified water, sodium chloride and titanium dioxide.

Moisturizing Treatment formula—Aloe, ammonium laureth sulfate, ammonium lauryl sulfate, citric acid, cocamide DEA, di (hydrogenated) tallow phthalic acid amide, dimethicone, DMDM hydantoin, FD&C blue No. 1, fragrance, hydroxypropyl methylcellulose, purified water, sodium citrate, sodium isostearoyl lactylate and titanium dioxide.

Medicated Treatment formula— Ammonium laureth sulfate, ammonium lauryl sulfate, citric acid, cocamide DEA, cocamidopropyl betaine, DMDM hydantoin, D&C red No. 33, FD&C blue No. 1, fragrance, hydroxypropyl methylcellulose, magnesium aluminum silicate, menthol, purified water, sodium chloride and TEA-lauryl sulfate.

2-in-1 Treatment formula—Ammonium lauryl sulfate, ammonium laureth sulfate, citric acid, cocamide DEA, di (hydrogenated) tallow phthalic acid amide, dimethicone, DMDM hydantoin, hydroxypropyl methycellulose, purified water, sodium citrate and fragrance.

Clinical testing has shown Selsun Blue to be as safe and effective as other leading shampoos in helping control dandruff symptoms with regular use. May be used on color-treated or permed hair, if used as directed.

Directions: Shake well. Shampoo and rinse thoroughly. For best results, use regularly, at least twice a week or as directed by a doctor.

Warnings: For external use only. Avoid contact with the eyes. If contact occurs, rinse eyes thoroughly with water. If condition worsens or does not improve after regular use of this product as directed, consult a doctor. Keep this and all drugs out of the reach of children. In case of accidental ingestion, seek professional assistance or contact a Poison Control Center immediately.

How Supplied: 4 (118 mL), 7 (207 mL) and 11 (325 mL) fl oz plastic bottles.

(FAN 3225)

TRONOLANE®

[tron'ə-lān]

Anesthetic Cream for Hemorrhoids

Description: The active ingredient in Tronolane cream is the topical anesthetic agent, pramoxine hydrochloride, 1% (chemically unrelated to the benzoate esters of the "caine" type), which is chemically designated as a 4-n-butoxyphenyl gammamor-pholinopropyl-ether hydrochloride. Also contains the following inactive ingredients: A nongreasy cream base containing beeswax, cetyl alcohol, cetyl esters wax, glycerin, methylparaben, propylparaben, sodium lauryl sulfate and zinc oxide.

Tronolane cream contains a rapidly acting topical anesthetic producing analgesia that lasts up to 5 hours. Because the drug is chemically unrelated to other anesthetics, cross-sensitization is unlikely. Patients who are already sensitized to the "caine" anesthetics can generally use Tronolane cream.

The emollient/emulsion base of Tronolane cream provides soothing lubrication. Tronolane cream is in a nondrying base that is nongreasy and nonstaining to undergarments.

Indications: Tronolane cream is indicated for the temporary relief of pain, itching, burning and soreness associated with hemorrhoids.

Warnings: If condition worsens or does not improve within 7 days, consult a doctor. Do not exceed the recommended daily dosage, unless directed by a doctor. In case of bleeding, consult a doctor promptly. Do not put this product into the rectum by using fingers or any mechanical device or applicator. Certain persons can develop allergic reactions to ingredients in this product. If the symptom being treated does not subside, or if redness, irritation, swelling, pain or other symptoms develop or increase, discontinue use and consult a doctor. As with any drug, if you are pregnant or nursing a baby, seek the advice of a health care professional before using this product. Keep this and all drugs out of the reach of children. In case of accidental ingestion, seek professional assistance or contact a Poison Control Center.

Dosage and Administration (Directions): Adults—When practical, cleanse the affected area with mild soap and warm water and rinse thoroughly or cleanse by patting or blotting with an appropriate cleansing pad. Gently dry by patting or blotting with toilet tissue or a soft cloth before application of this product. Apply externally to the affected area up to five times daily. Children under 12 years of age—Consult a doctor.

How Supplied: Tronolane cream is available in 1-oz (28g) and 2-oz (57g) tubes.

(FAN 2393)

TRONOLANE®

[tron'ə-lān]

Hemorrhoidal Suppositories

Description: The active ingredients in Tronolane suppositories are zinc oxide, 5%, and hard fat, 95%. Zinc oxide (an astringent) and hard fat (a skin protectant) afford temporary relief of hemorrhoidal itching and burning and protect irritated hemorrhoidal areas.

Indications: Tronolane suppositories are indicated for the temporary relief of the itching, burning and irritation associated with hemorrhoids.

Warnings: If condition worsens or does not improve within 7 days, consult a doctor. Do not exceed the recommended daily dosage, unless directed by a doctor. In case of bleeding, consult a doctor promptly. As with any drug, if you are pregnant or nursing a baby, seek the advice of a health care professional before using this product. **Do not store above 86°F.** Keep this and all drugs out of the reach of children. In case of accidental ingestion, seek professional assistance or contact a Poison Control Center immediately.

Dosage and Administration (Directions): Adults—When practical, cleanse the affected area with mild soap and warm water and rinse thoroughly or cleanse by patting or blotting with an appropriate cleansing pad. Gently dry by patting or blotting with toilet tissue or a soft cloth before application of this product. Remove foil wrapper before inserting into the rectum. Use up to six times daily or after each bowel movement. Children under 12 years of age—Consult a doctor.

How Supplied: Tronolane suppositories are available in 10- and 20-count boxes.

(FAN 2393)

Sandoz Pharmaceuticals Corporation/ Consumer Division

For product information, please see Novartis Consumer Health, Inc.

Scandinavian Natural Health & Beauty Products, Inc. Scandinavian Pharmaceuticals, Inc.

13 NORTH SEVENTH STREET
PERKASIE, PA 18944

Direct Inquiries to:
Catherine Peklak
(215) 453-2505

SALIX SST Lozenges
Saliva Stimulant

Active Ingredients: Sorbitol, malic acid, sodium citrate, dicalcium phosphate, citric acid.

Indications and Usage: SALIX is an aid for mild oral dryness or severe xerostomia conditions such as in autoimmune conditions/Sjogren's, post-irradiation or side effect from dozens of medications. Also helpful in oral candidiasis. Helps defend against dental and denture wear, caries, gum disease, halitosis, swallowing difficulties, reduced oral defense.... SALIX helps provide a regulated stimulation to salivary glands with buffering action to protect the teeth and balance the oral ph.

Note: Primary or secondary saliva cells must be functioning to some degree. The acidic content, although quickly buffered, may irritate conditions of active localized oral tissue inflammation.

Dosage: As needed or up to 1 per hour in severe xerostomia conditions.

Schering-Plough HealthCare Products

LIBERTY CORNER, NJ 07938

Direct Product Requests to:
(908) 604-1983 Telephone Number
(908) 604-1776 Fax Number

For Medical Emergencies Contact:
Clinical Department
(901) 320-2998

A + D® Ointment with Zinc Oxide

Active Ingredients: Dimethicone 1%, Zinc Oxide 10%.

Inactive Ingredients: Aloe Extract, Benzyl Alcohol, Cod Liver Oil (contains Vitamin A and Vitamin D), Fragrance, Glyceryl Oleate, Light Mineral Oil, Ozokerite, Paraffin, Propylene Glycol, Sorbitol, Synthetic Beeswax, Water.

Indications: Helps treat and prevent diaper rash. Protects chafed skin or minor skin irritation associated with diaper rash and helps seal out wetness.

Directions: Change wet and soiled diapers promptly, cleanse the diaper area and allow to dry. Apply ointment liberally as often as necessary, with each diaper change, especially at bedtime or anytime when exposure to wet diapers may be prolonged.

Warning: For external use only. Avoid contact with eyes. If condition worsens or does not improve within 7 days, consult a doctor. Not to be applied over deep or puncture wounds, infections, or lacerations. Consult a doctor. Keep this and all drugs out of the reach of children. In case of accidental ingestion, seek professional assistance or contact a Poison Control Center immediately.

How Supplied: A and D® Ointment with Zinc Oxide is available in 1 ½-ounce (42.5g) and 4-ounce (113g) tubes. Store between 15° and 30°C (59° and 86°F).

Shown in Product Identification Guide, page 518

A + D ® Original Ointment

Active Ingredients: Petrolatum 80.5%, Lanolin 15.5%.

Inactive Ingredients: Cod Liver Oil (Contains Vitamin A and Vitamin D), Fragrance, Light Mineral Oil, Paraffin.

A+D Original Ointment for Diaper Rash:

Indications: Helps treat and prevent diaper rash. Protects chafed skin or minor skin irritation associated with diaper rash and helps seal out wetness.

Directions: Change wet and soiled diapers promptly, cleanse the diaper area, and allow to dry. Apply **A+D Original Ointment** liberally as often as necessary with each diaper change especially at bedtime or anytime when exposure to wet diapers may be prolonged.

A+D Original Ointment for Skin Irritations:

Indications: Helps prevent and temporarily protects chafed, chapped, cracked or windburn skin and lips. Provides temporary protection of minor cuts, scrapes, burns and sunburn.

Directions: Apply **A+D Original Ointment** liberally as often as necessary.

Warnings: For external use only. Avoid contact with eyes. If condition worsens or does not improve within 7 days, consult a doctor. Not to be applied over deep or puncture wounds, infections or lacerations. Consult a doctor. Keep this and all drugs out of the reach of children. In case of acidental ingestion, seek professional assistance or contact a Poinson Control Center immediately.

How Supplied: A and D Ointment is available in 1½-ounce (42.5g) and 4-ounce (113g) tubes and 1-pound (454g) jars.

Store between 15° and 30°C (59° and 86°F)

Shown in Product Identification Guide, page 518

AFRIN® 4 Hour Extra Moisturizing Nasal Spray

Each ml of **AFRIN 4 Hour Extra Moisturizing Nasal Spray** contains Phenylephrine Hydrochloride 0.5%. **Also contains:** Benzalkonium Chloride, Edetate Disodium, Glycerin, Polyethylene Glycol 1450, Povidone, Propylene Glycol, Sodium Phosphate Dibasic, Sodium Phosphate Monobasic, Water.

Indications: For the temporary relief of nasal congestion due to a cold, due to hay fever or other upper respiratory allergies or associated with sinusitis. Reduces swelling of the nasal passages, shrinks swollen membranes. Temporarily restores freer breathing through the nose.

Warning: Do not exceed recommended dosage. This product may cause temporary discomfort such as burning, stinging, sneezing, or an increase in nasal discharge. Do not use this product for more than 3 days. Use only as directed. Frequent or prolonged use may cause nasal congestion to recur or worsen. If symptoms persist, consult a doctor. The use of this container by more than one person may spread infection. Do not use this product if you have heart disease, high blood pressure, thyroid disease, diabetes, or difficulty in urination due to enlargement of the prostate gland

Continued on next page

Information on Schering-Plough HealthCare Products appearing on these pages is effective as of November 1996.

Schering-Plough—Cont.

unless directed by a doctor. As with any drug, if you are pregnant or nursing a baby, seek the advice of a health professional before using this product. Keep this and all medicines out of the reach of children. In case of accidental ingestion seek professional assistance or contact a Poison Control Center immediately.

Directions: Adults and children 12 years of age and over: 2 or 3 sprays in each nostril not more often than every 4 hours. Do not give to children under 12 years of age unless directed by a doctor. To spray, squeeze bottle quickly and firmly. Do not tilt head backward while spraying. Wipe nozzle clean after use.

How Supplied: 15 mL plastic squeeze bottles.
Store between 2° and 30°C (36° and 86°F).

Shown in Product Identification Guide, page 519

AFRIN® 12 Hour
[a'frin]
Nasal Spray 0.05%
Nasal Spray Pump 0.05%
Sinus Nasal Spray 0.05%
Cherry Scented Nasal Spray 0.05%
Menthol Nasal Spray 0.05%
Extra Moisturizing Nasal Spray 0.05%
Nose Drops 0.05%

Description: AFRIN 12 Hour products contain oxymetazoline hydrochloride, the longest acting topical nasal decongestant available.
Each mL of **AFRIN Nasal Spray, Nasal Spray Pump, and Nose Drops** contains Oxymetazoline Hydrochloride, 0.05%. **Also contains:** Benzalkonium Chloride, Edetate Disodium, Polyethlene Glycol 1450, Povidone, Propylene Glycol, Sodium Phosphate Dibasic, Sodium Phosphate Monobasic, Water.
Each mL of **AFRIN Sinus** contains Oxymetazoline Hydrochloride 0.05%. **Also contains:** Benzalkonium Chloride, Benzyl Alcohol, Edetate Disodium, Mentanase-12™ (Camphor, Eucalyptol, Menthol), Polysorbate 80, Propylene Glycol, Sodium Phosphate Dibasic, Sodium Phosphate Monobasic, Water.
AFRIN Extra Moisturizing Nasal Spray is specially formulated to sooth dry, irritated nasal passages.
AFRIN Menthol Nasal Spray contains cooling aromatic vapors of menthol, eucalyptol, camphor and polysorbate in addition to the ingredients of AFRIN Nasal Spray.
AFRIN Cherry Scented Nasal Spray contains artificial cherry flavor in addition to the ingredients in regular AFRIN.

Indications: For the temporary relief of nasal congestion due to a cold, hay fever or other upper respiratory allergies, or associated with sinusitis. Reduces swelling of nasal passages; shrinks swollen membranes. Temporarily restores freer breathing through the nose.

Actions: The sympathomimetic action of AFRIN products constricts the smaller arterioles of the nasal passages, producing a prolonged, gentle and predictable decongesting effect. In just a few minutes a single dose, as directed, provides prompt, temporary relief of nasal congestion that lasts up to 12 hours. AFRIN products last up to 3 or 4 times longer than most ordinary nasal sprays.

Warnings: Do not exceed recommended dosage. This product may cause temporary discomfort such as burning, stinging, sneezing, or an increase in nasal discharge. Do not use this product for more than 3 days. Use only as directed. Frequent or prolonged use may cause nasal congestion to recur or worsen. If symptoms persist, consult a doctor. The use of this container by more than one person may spread infection. Do not use this product if you have heart disease, high blood pressure, thyroid disease, diabetes, or difficulty in urination due to enlargement of the prostate gland unless directed by a doctor. As with any drug, if you are pregnant or nursing a baby, seek the advice of a health professional before using this product. Keep this and all medicines out of the reach of children. In case of accidental ingestion, seek professional assistance or contact a Poison Control Center immediately.

Directions: Adults and children 6 to under 12 years of age (with adult supervision): 2 or 3 sprays in each nostril not more often than every 10 to 12 hours. Do not exceed 2 doses in any 24-hour period. **Children under 6 years of age:** consult a doctor. To spray, squeeze bottle quickly and firmly. Do not tilt head backward while spraying. Wipe nozzle clean after use.

How Supplied: AFRIN Nasal Spray 0.05%, 15 ml and 30 ml plastic squeeze bottles.
AFRIN Nasal Spray Pump 0.05% (1:2000), 15 ml spray pump bottles.
AFRIN Sinus Nasal Spray 0.05%, 15 ml plastic squeeze bottles.
AFRIN Extra Moisturizing Nasal Spray 0.05%, 15 ml and 30 ml plastic squeeze bottles.
AFRIN Cherry Scented Nasal Spray 0.05% (1:2000), 15 ml plastic squeeze bottle.
AFRIN Menthol Nasal Spray 0.05% (1:2000), 15 ml plastic squeeze bottle.
AFRIN Nose Drops 0.05% (1:2000), 20 ml dropper bottle.
Store all nasal sprays and nose drops between 2° and 30°C (36° and 86°F)

Shown in Product Identification Guide, page 519

AFRIN®
Menthol Saline Mist

Ingredients: Water, PEG-32, Propylene Glycol, Sodium Chloride, PVP, Disodium Phsophate, Sodium Phosphate, Benzyl Alcohol, Polysorbate 80, Benzalkonium Chloride, Mentanase™ (Menthol, Camphor, Eucalyptol), Disodium EDTA.

Indications: Provides gentle soothing moisture to relieve dry nasal passages. AFRIN Menthol Saline Mist contains Mentanase™ vapor blend, a unique blend of aromatic ingredients which works instantly to soothe your nasal passages. Use as often as needed to relieve nasal discomfort and irritation caused by colds, allergies, air pollution, smoke dry air (low humidity) and air travel. AFRIN Menthol Saline Mist loosens and thins mucous secretions to clear stuffy, blocked nasal passages. And since it is non-medicated, AFRIN Menthol Saline Mist is safe to use with cold, allergy and sinus medications, it is also safe enough for infants.

Directions: For infants, children and adults: 2 to 6 sprays/drops in each nostril as often as needed or as directed by a doctor. For a fine mist, keep bottle upright; for nose drops, keep bottle upside down; for a stream, keep bottle horizontal. Wipe nozzle clean after use.
Keep out of the reach of children. The use of this dispenser by more than one person may spread infection.

Shown in Product Identification Guide, page 519

AFRIN®
[a'frin]
Saline Mist

Ingredients: Water, PEG-32, Sodium Chloride, PVP, Disodium Phosphate, Sodium Phosphate, Benzalkonium Chloride, Disodium EDTA.

Indications: Provides soothing moisture to dry, inflamed nasal membranes due to colds, allergies, low humidity, and other minor nasal irritations. Afrin Saline Mist loosens and thins mucus secretions to aid removal of mucus from nose and sinuses. Afrin Saline Mist can be used as often as needed, and is safe to use with cold, allergy, and sinus medications. It is also safe for infants.

Directions: For infants, children, and adults, 2 to 6 sprays/drops in each nostril as often as needed or as directed by a physician. For a fine mist, keep bottle upright; for nose drops, keep bottle upside down; for a stream, keep bottle horizontal. Wipe nozzle clean after use.

Keep out of the reach of children.
The use of this dispenser by more than one person may spread infection.

CONTAINS NO ALCOHOL

CHLOR-TRIMETON®
[klor-tri'mĕ-ton]
4 Hour Allergy Tablets
8 Hour Allergy Tablets
12 Hour Allergy Tablets

Active Ingredients: Each 4 Hour Allergy Tablet contains: 4 mg chlorpheniramine maleate, also contains: Corn

Starch, D&C Yellow No. 10 Aluminum Lake, Lactose, Magnesium Stearate.
Each 8 Hour Allergy Tablet contains: 8 mg chlorpheniramine maleate; also contains: Acacia, Butylparaben, Calcium Phosphate, Calcium Sulfate, Carnauba Wax, Corn Starch, D&C Yellow No. 10 Aluminum Lake, FD&C Yellow No. 6 Aluminum Lake, FD&C Yellow No. 6, Lactose, Magnesium Stearate, Neutral Soap, Oleic Acid, Potato Starch, Rosin, Sugar, Talc, White Wax, Zein.
Each 12 Hour Allergy Tablet contains: 12 mg chlorpheniramine maleate; also contains: Acacia, Butylparaben, Calcium Phosphate, Calcium Sulfate, Carnauba Wax, Corn Starch, D&C Yellow No. 10 Aluminum Lake, FD&C Blue No. 2 Aluminum Lake, FD&C Yellow No. 6, FD&C Yellow No. 6 Aluminum Lake, Lactose, Magnesium Stearate, Neutral Soap, Oleic Acid, Potato Starch, Rosin, Sugar, Talc, White Wax, Zein.

Indications: For effective relief of sneezing, itchy, watery eyes, itchy throat, and runny nose due to hay fever and other upper respiratory allergies.

Warnings: May cause excitability especially in children. Do not give the 8 Hour or 12 Hour Allergy Tablets to children under 12 years, or 4 Hour Allergy Tablets to children under 6 years except under the advice and supervision of a doctor. Do not take this product, unless directed by a doctor, if you have a breathing problem such as emphysema or chronic bronchitis, or if you have glaucoma, difficulty in urination due to enlargement of the prostate gland. May cause drowsiness; alcohol may increase the drowsiness effect. Avoid alcoholic beverages while taking this product. Do not take this product if you are taking sedatives or tranquilizers, without first consulting your doctor. Use caution when driving a motor vehicle or operating machinery. As with any drug, if you are pregnant or nursing a baby, seek the advice of a health professional before using this product. Keep this and all drugs out of the reach of children. In case of accidental overdose, seek professional assistance or contact a Poison Control Center immediately.

Dosage and Administration: 4 Hour Allergy Tablets—Adults and Children 12 years of age and over: Oral dosage is one tablet (4 mg) every 4 to 6 hours, not to exceed 6 tablets in 24 hours. Children 6 to under 12 years of age: Oral dosage is one half the adult dose (2 mg) (break tablet in half) every 4 to 6 hours, not to exceed 3 whole tablets (12 mg) in 24 hours, or as directed by a doctor. Children under 6 years of age: consult a doctor.
8 Hour Allergy Tablets—Adults and Children 12 years and over—One tablet every 8 to 12 hours. Do not take more than one tablet every 8 hours or 3 tablets in 24 hours.
12 Hour Allergy Tablets—Adults and children 12 years and over—One tablet every 12 hours. Do not exceed 2 tablets in 24 hours.

How Supplied: CHLOR-TRIMETON 4 Hour Allergy Tablets, box of 24, bottles of 100.
CHLOR-TRIMETON 8 Hour Allergy Tablets, boxes of 15, bottles of 100.
CHLOR-TRIMETON 12 Hour Allergy Tablets, boxes of 10 and 24, bottles of 100.
Store between 2° and 30°C (36° and 86°F). Protect from excessive moisture.

Shown in Product Identification Guide, page 519

CHLOR-TRIMETON®
[*klortri 'mĕ-ton*]
4 Hour Allergy/Decongestant Tablets
12 Hour Allergy/Decongestant Tablets

Active Ingredients: Each 4 Hour Allergy/Decongestant Tablet contains: 4 mg chlorpheniramine maleate, and 60 mg pseudoephedrine sulfate; also contains: Corn Starch, FD&C Blue No. 1, Lactose, Magnesium Stearate, Povidone.
Each 12 Hour Allergy/Decongestant Tablet contains: 8 mg chlorpheniramine maleate and 120 mg pseudoephedrine sulfate; also contains: Acacia, Butylparaben, Calcium Sulfate, Carnauba Wax, Corn Starch, D&C Yellow No. 10 Aluminum Lake, FD&C Blue No. 1 Aluminum Lake, FD&C Yellow No. 6 Aluminum Lake, Gelatin, Lactose, Magnesium Stearate, Neutral Soap, Oleic Acid, Povidone, Rosin, Sugar, Talc, White Wax, Zein.

Indications: For effective temporary relief of sneezing, itchy, watery eyes, itchy throat, and runny nose due to hay fever and other upper respiratory allergies. Helps decongest sinus openings and sinus passages; relieves sinus pressure. Temporarily restores freer breathing through the nose.

Warnings: CHLOR-TRIMETON 4 HOUR ALLERGY/DECONGESTANT: Do not exceed recommended dosage. If nervousness, dizziness, or sleeplessness occur, discontinue use and consult a doctor. If symptoms do not improve within 7 days or are accompanied by fever, consult a doctor. Do not take this product if you have a breathing problem such as emphysema, chronic bronchitis, or if you have glaucoma, heart disease, high blood pressure, thyroid disease, diabetes, or difficulty in urination due to enlargement of the prostate gland unless directed by a doctor. May cause excitability, especially in children. May cause drowsiness; alcohol, sedatives, and tranquilizers may increase the drowsiness effect. Avoid alcoholic beverages while taking this product. Do not take this product if you are taking sedatives or tranquilizers, without first consulting your doctor. Use caution when driving a motor vehicle or operating machinery. As with any drug, if you are pregnant or nursing a baby, seek the advice of a health professional before using this product. Keep this and all drugs out of the reach of children. In case of accidental overdose, seek professional assistance or contact a Poison Control Center immediately.

Drug Interaction Precaution: Do not use this product if you are taking a prescription monoamine oxidase inhibitor (MAOI) (certain drugs for depression, psychiatric or emotional conditions, or Parkinson's disease), or for 2 weeks after stopping the MAOI drug. If you are uncertain whether your prescription drug contains an MAOI, consult a health professional before taking this product.
CHLOR-TRIMETON 12 HOUR ALLERGY/DECONGESTANT: Do not exceed recommended dosage. If nervousness, dizziness, or sleeplessness occur, discontinue use and consult a doctor. If symptoms do not improve within 7 days or are accompanied by fever, consult a doctor. Do not take this product if you have a breathing problem such as emphysema, chronic bronchitis, or if you have glaucoma, heart disease, high blood pressure, thyroid disease, diabetes, or difficulty in urination due to enlargement of the prostate gland, or give this product children under 12 years of age, unless directed by a doctor. May cause excitability especially in children. May cause drowsiness; alcohol, sedatives, and tranquilizers may increase the drowsiness effect. Avoid alcoholic beverages while taking this product. Do not take this product if you are taking sedatives or tranquilizers without first consulting a doctor. Use caution when driving a motor vehicle or operating machinery. As with any drug, if you are pregnant or nursing a baby, seek the advice of a health professional before using this product. Keep this and all drugs out of the reach of children. In case of accidental overdose, seek professional assistance or contact a Poison Control Center immediately.
Drug Interaction Precaution: Do not use this product if you are taking a prescription monoamine oxidase inhibitor (MAOI) (certain drugs for depression, psychiatric or emotional conditions, or Parkinson's disease), or for 2 weeks after stopping the MAOI drug. If you are uncertain whether your prescription drug contains an MAOI, consult a health professional before taking this product.

Dosage and Administration: 4 Hour Allergy/Decongestant Tablets — ADULTS AND CHILDREN 12 YEARS OF AGE AND OVER: Oral dosage is one tablet every 4 to 6 hours, not to exceed 4 tablets in 24 hours, or as directed by a doctor. CHILDREN 6 TO UNDER 12 YEARS OF AGE: Oral dosage is one half the adult dose (break tablet in half) every 4 to 6 hours, not to exceed 2 whole tablets in 24 hours, or as directed by a doctor.

Continued on next page

Information on Schering-Plough HealthCare Products appearing on these pages is effective as of November 1996.

Schering-Plough—Cont.

CHILDREN UNDER 6 YEARS OF AGE: Consult a doctor. **12 Hour Allergy/Decongestant Tablets**—ADULTS AND CHILDREN 12 YEARS AND OVER: one tablet every 12 hours. Do not exceed 2 tablets in 24 hours.

How Supplied: CHLOR-TRIMETON 4 Hour Allergy/Decongestant Tablets—boxes of 24. CHLOR-TRIMETON 12 Hour Allergy/Decongestant Tablets boxes of 10.

Store these CHLOR-TRIMETON Products between 2° and 30°C (36°and 86°F); and protect from excessive moisture.

Shown in Product Identification Guide, page 519

CORICIDIN® Cold & Flu Tablets
[kor-a-see 'din]

CORICIDIN® Cough & Cold Tablets

CORICIDIN Nighttime Cold & Cough Liquid

CORICIDIN 'D'® Decongestant Tablets

Active Ingredients: CORICIDIN Cold & Flu Tablets—2 mg chlorpheniramine maleate, 325 mg acetaminophen.

CORICIDIN® Cough & Cold Tablets—4 mg chlorpheniramine maleate, 30 mg dextromethorphan hydrobromide.

CORICIDIN Nighttime Cold & Cough Liquid—per tablespoon (½ fl. oz.)—325 mg Acetaminophen, 12.5 mg Diphenhydramine Hydrochloride.

CORICIDIN 'D' Decongestant Tablets—2 mg chlorpheniramine maleate, 12.5 mg phenylpropanolamine hydrochloride, 325 mg acetaminophen.

Inactive Ingredients: CORICIDIN Cold & Flu Tablets—Acacia, Butylparaben, Calcium Sulfate, Carnauba Wax, Cellulose, Corn Starch, FD&C Red No. 40 Aluminum Lake, FD&C Yellow No. 6 Aluminum Lake, Lactose, Magnesium Stearate, Povidone, Sugar, Talc, Titanium Dioxide, White Wax.

CORICIDIN® Cough & Cold Tablets—Acacia, Calcium Sulfate, Carnauba Wax, Croscarmellose Sodium, D&C Red No. 27 Aluminum Lake, FD&C Yellow No. 6 Aluminum Lake, Lactose, Magnesium Stearate, Microcrystalline Cellulose, Povidone, Sodium Benzoate, Sugar, Talc, Titanium Dioxide, White Wax.

CORICIDIN® Nighttime Cold & Cough Liquid—Citric Acid, FD&C Blue No. 1, FD&C Red No. 40, Flavor, Glycerin, Polyethylene Glycol, Propylene Glycol, Sodium Citrate, Sodium Saccharin, Sugar, Water.

CORICIDIN 'D' Decongestant Tablets—Acacia, Butylparaben, Calcium Sulfate, Carnauba Wax, Cellulose, Corn Starch, Magnesium Stearate, Povidone, Sugar, Talc, Titanium Dioxide, White Wax.

Indications: CORICIDIN Cold & Flu Tablets temporarily relieve minor aches, pains and headache, and reduce the fever associated with colds or flu; temporarily relieve sneezing, runny nose and itchy watery eyes due to hay fever, other upper respiratory allergies or the common cold. **Unlike other cold remedies, CORICIDIN Cold & Flu Tablets do not contain a decongestant and therefore are suitable for hypertensive patients.**

CORICIDIN Cough & Cold Tablets temporarily relieve coughs due to minor throat irritations as may occur with a cold; temporarily relieve sneezing, runny nose and itchy, watery eyes due to the common cold, hayfever or other respiratory allergies. **Unlike other cold remedies, CORICIDIN Cough & Cold Tablets do not contain a decongestant and therefore are suitable for hypertensive patients.**

CORICIDIN® Nighttime Cold & Cough Liquid temporarily relieves minor aches, pains, headache, sore throat, and fever associated with a cold or flu. Temporarily relieves runny nose, sneezing, and itchy watery eyes due to hay fever or other upper respiratory allergies; temporarily relieves cough associated with the common cold. **Unlike other cold remedies, CORICIDIN Nighttime Cold & Cough Liquid does not contain a decongestant and therefore is suitable for hypertensive patients.**

CORICIDIN 'D' Tablets temporarily relieve minor aches and pains, and reduces the fever associated with a cold or flu. Provides temporary relief of: sneezing and runny nose; nasal congestion due to the common cold and associated with sinusitis; stuffy nose; sinus congestion and pressure. Helps decongest sinus openings and passages. **CORICIDIN 'D' Tablets do contain a decongestant.**

Warnings: CORICIDIN Cold & Flu Tablets—Do not take this product for pain for more than 10 days (adults) or 5 days (children 6 to under 12 years of age) and do not take for fever for more than 3 days unless directed by a doctor. If pain or fever persists or gets worse, if new symptoms occur, or if redness or swelling is present, consult a doctor because these could be signs of a serious condition. May cause excitability especially in children. Do not take this product, unless directed by a doctor, if you have a breathing problem such as emphysema or chronic bronchitis, or if you have glaucoma or difficulty in urination due to enlargement of the prostate gland. May cause drowsiness; alcohol, sedatives, and tranquilizers may increase the drowsiness effect. Avoid alcoholic beverages while taking this product. Do not take this product if you are taking sedatives or tranquilizers without first consulting your doctor. Use caution when driving a motor vehicle or operating machinery. As with any drug if you are pregnant or nursing a baby, seek the advice of a health professional before using this product. Keep this and all drugs out of the reach of children. In case of accidental overdose, seek professional assistance or contact a Poison Control Center immediately. Prompt medical attention is critical for adults as well as for children even if you do not notice any signs or symptoms.

CORICIDIN Cough & Cold Tablets—A persistent cough may be a sign of a serious condition. If cough persists for more than 1 week, tends to recur, or is accompanied by fever, rash or persistent headache, consult a doctor. Do not take this product for persistent or chronic cough such as occurs with smoking, asthma, emphysema, or if cough is accompanied by excessive phlegm (mucus) unless directed by a doctor. May cause excitability, especially in children. Do not take this product, unless directed by a doctor, if you have a breathing problem such as emphysema or chronic bronchitis, or if you have glaucoma or difficulty in urination due to enlargement of the prostate gland. May cause marked drowsiness; alcohol, sedatives, and tranquilizers may increase the drowsiness effect. Avoid alcoholic beverages while taking this product. Do not take this product if you are taking sedatives or tranquilizers, without first consulting your doctor. Use caution when driving a motor vehicle or operating machinery. As with any drug, if you are pregnant or nursing a baby, seek the advice of a health professional before using this product. Keep this and all drugs out of the reach of children. In case of accidental overdose, seek professional assistance or contact a Poison Control Center immediately.

DRUG INTERACTION PRECAUTION: Do not use this product if you are now taking a prescription monoamine oxidase inhibitor (MAOI) (certain drugs for depression, psychiatric or emotional conditions, or Parkinson's disease), or for 2 weeks after stopping the MAOI drug. If you are uncertain whether your prescription drug contains an MAOI, consult a health professional before taking this product.

CORICIDIN® Nighttime Cold & Cough Liquid—Do not take this product for pain for more than 10 days (adults) or 5 days (children 6 to under 12 years of age) and do not take for fever for more than 3 days unless directed by a doctor. If pain or fever persists or gets worse, if new symptoms occur, or if redness or swelling is present, consult a doctor because these could be signs of a serious condition. If sore throat is severe, persists for more than 2 days, is accompanied or followed by fever, headache, rash, or persistent headache, consult a doctor. Do not take this product for persistent or chronic cough such as occurs with smoking, asthma, or emphysema, or if cough is accompanied by excessive phlegm (mucus) unless directed by a doctor. May cause excitability especially in children. Do not take this product, unless directed by a doctor, if you have a breathing problem, such as emphysema or chronic bronchitis, or if you have glaucoma or difficulty in urination due to enlargement of the prostate gland. May cause marked drowsiness; alcohol, sedatives, and tranquilizers may increase the drowsiness effect. Avoid alcoholic beverages while taking this product. Do not take this product if you are taking sedatives or tranquilizers, without first consulting your doctor. Use caution when driving a motor vehicle or operating machinery. As with any drug, if you are pregnant or nursing a baby, seek the advice of a health professional before using this product. Keep this and all drugs out of the reach of children. In case of accidental overdose, seek the advice assistance or contact a Poison Control Center immediately. Prompt medical attention is critical for adults as well as for children even if you do not notice any signs or symptoms.

CORICIDIN 'D' Decongestant Tablets—Do not exceed recommended dosage. If nervousness, dizziness, or sleeplessness occur, discontinue use and consult a doctor. If congestion does not improve within 7 days, consult a doctor. Do not take this product for pain for more than 10 days (adults) or 5 days (children 6 to under 12 years) or for fever for more than 3 days unless directed by a doctor. If pain or fever persists or gets worse, if new symptoms occur, or if redness or swelling is present, consult a doctor because these could be signs of a serious condition. May cause excitability, especially in children. Do not take this product, unless directed by a doctor if you have a breathing problem such as emphysema or chronic bronchitis, or if you have glaucoma, heart disease, high blood pressure, thyroid disease, diabetes, or difficulty in urination due to enlargement of the prostate gland. May cause drowsiness; alcohol, sedatives, and tranquilizers may increase the drowsiness effect. Avoid alcoholic beverages while taking this product. Do not take this product if you are taking sedatives or tranquilizers without first consulting your doctor. Use caution when driving a motor vehicle or operating machinery. As with any drug, if you are pregnant or nursing a baby, seek the advice of a health professional before using this product. Keep this and all drugs out of the reach of children. In case of accidental overdose, seek professional assistance or contact a Poison Control Center immediately. Prompt medical attention is critical for adults as well as for children even if you do not notice any signs or symptoms.

Drug Interaction Precaution: Do not use this product if you are now taking a prescription monoamine oxidase inhibitor (MAOI) (certain drugs for depression, psychiatric or emotional conditions, or Parkinson's disease), or for 2 weeks after stopping the MAOI drug. If you are uncertain whether your prescription drug contains an MAOI, consult a health professional before taking this product. Do not use this product if you are now taking an appetite-controlling medication containing phenylpropanolamine.

Dosage and Administration: CORICIDIN Cold & Flu Tablets—Adults and children 12 years of age and over: oral dosage is 2 tablets every 4 to 6 hours, not to exceed 12 tablets in 24 hours, or as directed by a doctor. **Children 6 to under 12 years of age:** oral dosage is 1 tablet every 4 to 6 hours, not to exceed 5 tablets in 24 hours, or as directed by a doctor. **Children under 6 years of age:** consult a doctor.

CORICIDIN Cough & Cold Tablets—Adults and Children 12 years of age and over: one tablet every 6 hours, not to exceed 4 tablets in 24 hours. This product is not for children under 12 years of age.

CORICIDIN Nighttime Cold & Cough Liquid—Adults and children 12 years of age and over: Oral dosage is two tablespoons (1 fl oz) every 4 hours, not to exceed 6 doses in 24 hours, or as directed by a doctor. **Children 6 to under 12 years of age:** Oral dosage is one tablespoon (½ fl oz) every 4 hours, not to exceed 5 doses in 24 hours, or as directed by a doctor. **Children under 6 years of age:** Consult a doctor.

CORICIDIN 'D' Decongestant Tablets — Adults and children 12 years of age and over: oral dosage is 2 tablets every 4 hours not to exceed 12 tablets in 24 hours, or as directed by a doctor. **Children 6 to under 12 years of age:** oral dosage is 1 tablet every 4 hours not to exceed 5 tablets in 24 hours, or as directed by a doctor. **Children under 6 years of age:** consult a doctor.

How Supplied: CORICIDIN Cold & Flu Tablets— Bottles of 48, and 100 tablets, blisters of 12 and 24.
CORICIDIN Cough & Cold Tablets— blisters of 16.
CORICIDIN Nighttime Cold & Cough Liquid—6 oz. bottles.
CORICIDIN 'D' Decongestant Tablets— Bottles of 48, and 100 tablets, blisters of 12 and 24.
Store between 2° and 30°C (36° and 86°F).

Shown in Product Identification Guide, page 519

CORRECTOL®
Herbal Tea Laxative
Honey Lemon Flavor
Cinnamon Spice Flavor

Active Ingredient: Senna (30 mg Total Sennosides per tea bag)

Inactive Ingredients: Natural Flavors

Indications: For gentle, overnight relief of occasional constipation. **Correctol Herbal Tea Laxative** generally produces a bowel movement in 6–12 hours.

Warnings: Do not reuse individual tea bags. Do not use concurrently with other laxative products or when abdominal pain, nausea, or vomiting are present unless directed by a doctor. If you have noticed a sudden change in bowel habits that persists over two weeks, consult a doctor before using a laxative. Laxative products should not be used for longer than 1 week unless directed by a doctor. Rectal bleeding or failure to have a bowel movement after use of a laxative may indicate a serious condition. Discontinue use and consult a doctor. As with any drug, if you are pregnant nursing a baby, seek the advice of a health professional before using this product. Keep this and all drugs out of the reach of children. In case of accidental overdose, seek professional assistance or contact a Poison Control Center immediately.

Directions: Adults and children 12 years of age and over: 1 cup of tea once a day (maximum: 3 cups of tea per day). **Children under 12 years of age:** consult your doctor. Place one tea bag into a cup and add 6 oz. of boiling water. Let steep for 5 minutes and remove the bag. For iced tea, use 3 oz. of boiling water and add ice cubes after steeping. Sweeten to taste. Take at bedtime for morning results.

In most cases, one 6 oz. cup should be just right. However, you can easily adjust the laxative effect by varying the amount of tea you drink, as long as you don't exceed 3 cups per day. For example, to lessen the laxative effect, brew as directed above but only drink ⅔ of a full 6 oz. cup (4 oz.). To increase the laxative effect, prepare a second 6 oz. cup and drink as much as you feel necessary.

How Supplied: 15 individual tea bags per box.

Shown in Product Identification Guide, page 519

CORRECTOL®
Laxative Tablets and Caplets

Active Ingredient: Bisacodyl, 5 mg.

Inactive Ingredients: Acetylated monoglycerides, calcium sulfate, carnauba wax, corn starch, D&C Red #7 calcium lake, gelatin, hydroxypropyl methylcellulose phthalate, lactose, magnesium stearate, povidone, sugar, talc, titanium dioxide, white wax.

Indications: For gentle, overnight relief of occasional constipation and irregularity. Correctol Laxative generally produces a bowel movement in 6 to 12 hours.

Warnings: Do not chew tablets or caplets. Do not give to children under 6 years of age, or to persons who cannot swallow without chewing, unless directed by a doctor. Do not take this product within 1 hour after taking an antacid or milk. Do not use laxative products when abdominal pain, nausea, or vomiting are present unless directed by a doctor. If you have noticed a sudden change in bowel habits that persists over a period of 2 weeks, consult a doctor before using a laxative. Laxative products should not be used for

Continued on next page

Information on Schering-Plough HealthCare Products appearing on these pages is effective as of November 1996.

Schering-Plough—Cont.

a period longer than 1 week unless directed by a doctor. Rectal bleeding or failure to have a bowel movement after use of a laxative may indicate a serious condition. Discontinue use and consult a doctor. This product may cause abdominal discomfort, faintness, and cramps. As with any drug, if you are pregnant or nursing a baby, seek the advice of a health professional before using this product. Keep this and all drugs out of the reach of children. In case of accidental overdose, seek professional assistance or contact a Poison Control Center immediately. Store at temperatures not above 86°F (30°C).

Directions: Adults and children 12 years of age and older: Take 1 to 3 tablets or caplets in a single dose once daily. **Children 6 to under 12 years of age:** Take 1 tablet or caplet once daily. **Children under 6 years of age:** consult a doctor. **Do not chew or crush tablets or caplets.**

How Supplied: Tablets: Individual foil-backed safety sealed blister packaging in boxes of 5, 10, 30, 60, & 90 tablets. Caplets: Individual foil-backed safety sealed blister packaging in boxes of 30 caplets.

Shown in Product Identification Guide, page 519

CORRECTOL® STOOL SOFTENER
Laxative

Active Ingredient: Docusate sodium 100 mg. per soft gel.
Also Contains—D&C Red No. 33, FD&C Red No. 40, FD&C Yellow No. 6, gelatin, glycerin, polyethylene glycol 400, propylene glycol, sorbitol.

Indications: For relief of occasional constipation. Correctol Stool Softener generally produces a bowel movement in 12 to 72 hours.

Warning: Do not use laxative products when abdominal pain, nausea, or vomiting are present unless directed by a doctor. If you have noticed a sudden change in bowel habits that persists over two weeks, consult a doctor before using a laxative. Laxative products should not be used for longer than 1 week unless directed by a doctor. Rectal bleeding or failure to have a bowel movement after use of a laxative may indicated a serious condition. Discontinue use and consult your doctor. As with any drug, if you are pregnant or nursing a baby, seek the advice of a health professional before using this product. Keep this and all drugs out of the reach of children. In case of accidental overdose, seek professional assistance or contact a Poison Control Center immediately.

Drug Interaction Precaution: Do not take this product if you are presently taking mineral oil, unless directed by a doctor.

Directions: Adults and Children 12 years of age and older: Take 1 to 3 soft gels daily. **Children under 12 years of age:** Take 1 soft gel daily. **Children under 2 years of age:** Consult a doctor.

How Supplied: Tablets—individual foil-backed safety sealed blister packaging in boxes of 30 tablets.
Store below 86°F. Protect from freezing.

Shown in Product Identification Guide, page 519

DI–GEL®
Antacid · Anti-Gas
Tablets/Liquid

DI-GEL Tablets: Active Ingredients: (Per Tablet)—Simethicone 20 mg., Calcium Carbonate 280 mg., Magnesium Hydroxide 128 mg. **Inactive Ingredients:** D & C yellow No. 10 aluminum lake, dextrin, FD&C yellow No. 6 aluminum lake, flavor, magnesium stearate, mannitol, povidone, stearic acid, sucrose, talc.
Dietetically sodium free, calcium rich.

DI-GEL Liquid: Active Ingredients—per teaspoonful (5 ml): Simethicone 20 mg., aluminum hydroxide (equivalent to aluminum hydroxide dried gel USP 200 mg.), magnesium hydroxide 200 mg. **Also contains:** Flavor, hydroxypropyl methylcellulose, methylcellulose, methylparaben, propylparaben, sodium saccharin, sorbitol, water.
Dietetically sodium free.

Indications: For fast, temporary relief of acid indigestion, heartburn, sour stomach and accompanying symptoms of gas.

Actions: When excess acid and bubbles of gas are trapped in the stomach, they can cause heartburn and acid indigestion.
The white layer of Di-Gel goes to work fast to neutralize excess acid. And unlike plain antacids, the Simethicone in the yellow layer breaks up gas bubbles rapidly.

Warnings: Do not take more than 20 teaspoonfuls or 24 tablets in a 24 hour period, or use the maximum dosage of this product for more than 2 weeks, except under the advice and supervision of a physician. If you have kidney disease do not use this product except under the advice and supervision of a physician. Tablets may cause constipation or have a laxative effect. Keep this and all drugs out of the reach of children.

Drug Interaction: Antacids may interact with certain prescription drugs. If you are presently taking a prescription drug, do not take this product without checking with your doctor or other health professional.

Directions: Liquid: Shake well before using. Take 2 to 4 teaspoonfuls every 2 hours or as directed by a doctor. Dispense by spoon only.
TABLETS: Chew 2 to 4 tablets every 2 hours or as directed by a doctor.

How Supplied:
DI-GEL Liquid in Mint Flavor - 6 and 12 fl. oz. bottles, safety sealed and Lemon/Orange Flavor - 12 fl. oz. bottles, safety sealed.
DI-GEL Tablets in Mint and Lemon/Orange Flavor - In boxes of 30 and 90 in handy portable safety sealed blister packaging. Also available in Mint 60-tablet bottles.

DRIXORAL® COLD & ALLERGY
[*dricks-or 'al*]
Sustained-Action Tablets

Description: EACH DRIXORAL® COLD & ALLERGY SUSTAINED-ACTION TABLET CONTAINS: 120 mg of pseudoephedrine sulfate and 6 mg of dexbrompheniramine maleate. Half of the medication is released after the tablet is swallowed and the remaining amount of medication is released hours later providing continuous long-lasting relief for 12 hours. Inactive Ingredients: Acacia, Butylparaben, Calcium Sulfate, Carnauba Wax, Corn Starch, D&C Yellow No. 10 Aluminum Lake, FD&C Blue No. 1 Aluminum Lake, FD&C Yellow No. 6 Aluminum Lake, Gelatin, Lactose, Magnesium Stearate, Neutral Soap, Oleic Acid, Povidone, Rosin, Sugar, Talc, White Wax, Zein.

Indications: The decongestant (pseudoephedrine sulfate) temporarily relieves nasal congestion due to the common cold, hay fever or other upper respiratory allergies, and associated with sinusitis. Helps decongest sinus openings and sinus passages. Reduces swelling of nasal passages; shrinks swollen membranes; and temporarily restores freer breathing through the nose. The antihistamine (dexbrompheniramine maleate) alleviates runny nose, sneezing, itching of the nose or throat and itchy and watery eyes as may occur in allergic rhinitis (such as hay fever).

Warnings: Do not exceed recommended dosage. If nervousness, dizziness, or sleeplessness occur, discontinue use and consult a doctor. If symptoms do not improve within 7 days, or are accompanied by fever, consult a doctor. May cause excitability especially in children. Do not take this product if you have a breathing problem such as emphysema or chronic bronchitis, or if you have glaucoma, heart disease, high blood pressure, thyroid disease, diabetes, or difficulty in urination due to enlargement of the prostate gland or give this product to children under 12 years of age, unless directed by a doctor. May cause drowsiness; alcohol, sedatives, and tranquilizers may increase the drowsiness effect. Avoid alcoholic beverages while taking this product. Do not take this product if you are taking sedatives or tranquilizers without first consulting your doctor. Use caution when driving a motor vehicle or operating machinery. As with any drug, if you are pregnant or nursing a baby, seek the advice of a health professional before using this product. Keep this and all drugs out of the reach of children. In case of accidental overdose, seek professional assistance or contact a Poison Control Center immediately.

Drug Interaction Precaution: Do not use this product if you are now taking a prescription monoamine oxidase inhibitor (MAOI) (certain drugs for depression, psychiatric or emotional conditions, or Parkinson's disease),or for 2 weeks after stopping the MAOI drug. If you are uncertain whether your prescription drug contains an MAOI, consult a health professional before taking this product.

Dosage and Administration: ADULTS AND CHILDREN 12 YEARS AND OVER—one tablet every 12 hours. Do not exceed two tablets in 24 hours.

How Supplied: DRIXORAL® Cold & Allergy Sustained-Action Tablets, green, sugar-coated tablets branded in black with the product name, boxes of 10, 20, and 40, bottle of 100.

Store between 2° and 25°C (36° and 77°F).

Protect from excessive moisture.

Shown in Product Identification Guide, page 519

DRIXORAL® Nasal Decongestant

[*dricks-or 'al*]

Long-Acting Nasal Decongestant

DRIXORAL® Nasal Decongestant Long-Acting Nasal Decongestant Tablets contain 120 mg pseudoephedrine sulfate, a nasal decongestant, in an extended-release tablet providing up to 12 hours of continuous relief . . . without drowsiness. Inactive Ingredients: Acacia, Butylparaben, Calcium Sulfate, Carnauba Wax, Corn Starch, FD&C Blue No. 1 Aluminum Lake, Gelatin, Lactose, Magnesium Stearate, Neutral Soap, Oleic Acid, Povidone, Rosin, Sugar, Talc, White Wax, Zein.

Indications: For temporary relief of nasal congestion due to the common cold, hay fever or other upper respiratory allergies, and associated with sinusitis. Helps decongest sinus openings and sinus passages.

Directions: Adults and Children 12 Years and Over—One tablet every 12 hours. Do not exceed two tablets in 24 hours. **Children under 12 years of age:** Consult a doctor.

Warnings: Do not exceed recommended dosage. If nervousness, dizziness, or sleeplessness occur, discontinue use and consult a doctor. If symptoms do not improve within 7 days or are accompanied by fever, consult a doctor. Do not take this product if you have heart disease, high blood pressure, thyroid disease, diabetes, or difficulty in urination due to enlargement of the prostate gland, or give this product to children under 12 years of age, unless directed by a doctor. As with any drug, if you are pregnant or nursing a baby, seek the advice of a health professional before using this product. Keep this and all drugs out of the reach of children. In case of accidental overdose, seek professional assistance or contact a Poison Control Center immediately.

Drug Interaction Precaution: Do not use this product if you are now taking a prescription monoamine oxidase inhibitor (MAOI) (certain drugs for depression, psychiatric or emotional conditions, or Parkinson's disease), or for 2 weeks after stopping the MAOI drug. If you are uncertain whether your prescription drug contains an MAOI, consult a health professional before taking this product.

How Supplied: DRIXORAL® Nasal Decongestant Long-Acting Non-Drowsy Tablets are available in boxes of 10's and 20's.

Store between 2° and 25°C (36° and 77°F).

Protect from excessive moisture.

DRIXORAL® COLD & FLU

[*dricks-or 'al*]

Extended-Release Tablets

Active Ingredients: 500 mg Acetaminophen, 3 mg Dexbrompheniramine Maleate, 60 mg Pseudoephedrine Sulfate.

Inactive Ingredients: Calcium Phosphate, Carnauba Wax, D&C Yellow No. 10 Aluminum Lake, FD&C Blue No. 1 Aluminum Lake, FD&C Yellow No. 6 Aluminum Lake, Hydroxypropyl Methylcellulose, Magnesium Stearate, Methylparaben, PEG, Propylparaben, Stearic Acid.

DRIXORAL® COLD & FLU Extended-Release Tablets combine a nasal decongestant and an antihistamine with a non-aspirin analgesic in a special 12-hour continuous-acting timed-release tablet.

Indications: The *decongestant* temporarily relieves nasal congestion due to the common cold, hay fever or other upper respiratory allergies, and associated with sinusitis. Reduces swelling of nasal passages; shrinks swollen membranes; and temporarily restores freer breathing through the nose. Also helps decongest sinus openings, sinus passages. The *non-aspirin analgesic* temporarily relieves minor aches, pains, and headache and reduces fever due to the common cold. The *antihistamine* alleviates running nose, sneezing, itching of the nose or throat, and itchy and watery eyes as may occur in allergic rhinitis (such as hay fever).

Directions: ADULTS AND CHILDREN 12 YEARS AND OVER—two tablets every 12 hours. Do not exceed four tablets in 24 hours. **CHILDREN UNDER 12 YEARS OF AGE:** consult a doctor.

Warnings: Do not exceed recommended dosage. If nervousness, dizziness, or sleeplessness occur, discontinue use and consult a doctor. If symptoms do not improve within 7 days , or are accompanied by fever that lasts for more than 3 days or recurs, consult a doctor before continuing use. If pain or fever persists or gets worse, if new symptoms occur, or if redness or swelling is present, consult a doctor because these could be signs of a serious condition. May cause excitability especially in children. Do not take this product if you have a breathing problem such as emphysema or chronic bronchitis, or if you have glaucoma, heart disease, high blood pressure, thyroid disease, diabetes, or difficulty in urination due to enlargement of the prostate gland, or give this product to children under 12 years of age, unless directed by a doctor. May cause drowsiness; alcohol, sedatives, and tranquilizers may increase the drowsiness effect. Avoid alcoholic beverages while taking this product. Do not take this product if you are taking sedatives or tranquilizers without first consulting your doctor. Use caution when driving a motor vehicle or operating machinery. As with any drug, if you are pregnant or nursing a baby, seek the advice of a health professional before using this product. Keep this and all drugs out of the reach of children. In case of accidental overdose, seek professional assistance or contact a Poison Control Center immediately. Prompt medical attention is critical for adults as well as for children even if you do not notice any signs or symptoms.

Drug Interaction Precaution: Do not use this product if you are now taking a prescription monoamine oxidase inhibitor (MAOI) (certain drugs for depression, psychiatric or emotional conditions, or Parkinson's disease), or for 2 weeks after stopping the MAOI drug. If you are uncertain whether your prescription drug contains an MAOI, consult a health professional before taking this product.

How Supplied: DRIXORAL® COLD & FLU Extended-Release Tablets are available in boxes of 12's and 24's.

Store between 2° and 25°C (36° and 77°F).

Protect from excessive moisture.

DRIXORAL® ALLERGY/SINUS

[*dricks-or 'al*]

Nasal decongestant/Pain reliever/ Antihistamine

DRIXORAL® ALLERGY/SINUS Extended-Release Tablets combine a nasal

Continued on next page

Information on Schering-Plough HealthCare Products appearing on these pages is effective as of November 1996.

Schering-Plough—Cont.

decongestant, a non-aspirin analgesic, and an antihistamine in a 12-hour timed-release tablet.

Indications: The *decongestant* temporarily relieves nasal congestion due to sinusitis, the common cold, and hay fever or other upper respiratory allergies. Helps decongest sinus openings, sinus passages; relieves sinus pressure. Reduces swelling of nasal passages; shrinks swollen membranes; and temporarily restores freer breathing through the nose. The *non-aspirin analgesic* temporarily relieves headaches, and minor aches and pains. The *antihistamine* alleviates runny nose, sneezing, itching of the nose or throat, and itchy and watery eyes as may occur in allergic rhinitis (such as hay fever).

Each DRIXORAL® ALLERGY/SINUS Extended-Release Tablet Contains: 60 mg of pseudoephedrine sulfate, 3 mg of dexbrompheniramine maleate, and 500 mg of acetaminophen. These ingredients are released continuously, providing long-lasting relief for 12 hours. Inactive Ingredients: Calcium Phosphate, Carnauba Wax, D&C Yellow No. 10 Aluminum Lake, FD&C Yellow No. 6 Aluminum Lake, Hydroxypropyl Methylcellulose, Magnesium Stearate, Methylparaben, PEG, Propylparaben, Stearic Acid.

Directions: ADULTS AND CHILDREN 12 YEARS AND OVER—two tablets every 12 hours. Do not exceed four tablets in 24 hours. **CHILDREN UNDER 12 YEARS OF AGE:** consult a physician.
Store between 2° and 25°C (36° and 77°F).

Warnings: Do not exceed recommended dosage. If nervousness, dizziness, or sleeplessness occur, discontinue use and consult a doctor. If symptoms do not improve within 7 days, or are accompanied by fever that lasts for more than 3 days or recurs, consult a doctor before continuing use. If pain or fever persists or gets worse, if new symptoms occur, or if redness or swelling is present, consult a doctor because these could be signs of a serious condition. May cause excitability especially in children. Do not take this product if you have a breathing problem such as emphysema or chronic bronchitis, or if you have glaucoma, heart disease, high blood pressure, thryoid disease, diabetes, or difficulty in urination due to enlargement of the prostate gland, or give this product to children under 12 years of age, unless directed by a doctor. May cause drowsiness; alcohol, sedatives, and tranquilizers may increase the drowsiness effect. Avoid alcoholic beverages while taking this product. Do not take this product if you are taking sedatives or tranquilizers without first consulting your doctor. Use caution when driving a motor vehicle or operating machinery. As with any drug, if you are pregnant or nursing a baby, seek the advice of a health professional before using this product. Keep this and all drugs out of the reach of children. In case of accidental overdose, seek professional assistance or contact a Poison Control Center immediately. Prompt medical attention is critical for adults as well as for children even if you do not notice any signs or symptoms.

Drug Interaction Precaution: Do not use this product if you are now taking a prescription monoamine oxidase inhibitor (MAOI) (certain drugs for depression, psychiatric or emotional conditions, or Parkinson's disease), or for 2 weeks after stopping the MAOI drug. If you are uncertain whether your prescription drug contains an MAOI, consult a health professional before taking this product.

How Supplied: DRIXORAL® ALLERGY/SINUS Extended-Release Tablets are available in boxes of 12's and 24's.

DUOFILM® LIQUID
Wart Remover

Active Ingredient: Salicylic Acid 17% (w/w).

Inactive Ingredients: Alcohol 15.8% w/w, castor oil, ether 42.6% w/w, ethyl lactate, and polybutene in flexible collodion.

Indications: For the removal of common and plantar warts. Common warts can be easily recognized by the rough, cauliflower-like appearance of the surface. Plantar warts are found on the bottom of the foot.

Warnings: For external use only. Do not use this product on irritated skin, on any area that is infected or reddened, if you are a diabetic, or if you have poor blood circulation. If discomfort persists, see your doctor. Do not use on moles, birthmarks, warts with hair growing from them, genital warts, or warts on the face or mucous membranes. Keep this and all drugs out of the reach of children. If product gets in eyes, flush with water for 15 minutes. Avoid inhaling vapors. HIGHLY FLAMMABLE. Keep away from fire or flame. Cap bottle tightly when not in use. Store at room temperature away from heat. In case of accidental ingestion, seek professional assistance or contact a Poison Control Center immediately.

Directions: Wash affected area. May soak wart in warm water for 5 minutes. Dry area thoroughly. Apply one thin layer (with brush applicator) at a time to sufficiently cover each wart. Let dry. Repeat this procedure once or twice daily as needed (until wart is removed) for up to 12 weeks.
Note: Adhesive bandage may be used to cover treated area.

How Supplied: DuoFilm Liquid is available in ½ fluid oz. spill-resistant bottles with brush applicator for pinpoint application.

Shown in Product Identification Guide, page 520

DUOFILM® PATCH FOR KIDS
Wart Remover

Active Ingredient: Salicylic Acid 40% in a rubber-based vehicle.

Indications: For the concealment and removal of common warts. Common warts can be easily recognized by the rough, cauliflower-like appearance of the surface.

Warnings: For external use only. Do not use this product on irritated skin, on any area that is infected or reddened, if you are a diabetic, or if you have poor blood circulation. If discomfort persists, see your doctor. Do not use on moles, birthmarks, warts with hair growing from them, genital warts, or warts on the face or mucous membranes. Keep this and all drugs out of the reach of children. In case of accidental ingestion, seek professional assistance or contact a Poison Control Center immediately.

Directions: Parents should supervise use by children. Wash affected area. May soak wart in warm water for five minutes. Dry area thoroughly. Apply Medicated Patch (packet A). If necessary, cut patch to fit wart. Repeat procedure every 48 hours as needed (until wart is removed) for up to 12 weeks.
Note: Self-adhesive cover-up patches (packet B) may be used to conceal Medicated Patch and wart.

How Supplied: DuoFilm Patch includes 18 Medicated Patches and 20 self-adhesive Cover-Up patches for concealment while treatment is ongoing.

Shown in Product Identification Guide, page 520

DUOPLANT® GEL
Plantar Wart Remover

Active Ingredient: Salicylic Acid 17% (w/w).

Inactive Ingredients: Alcohol 57.6% w/w, ether 16.42% w/w, ethyl lactate, hydroxypropyl cellulose, and polybutene in flexible collodion, USP.

Indications: For the removal of plantar and common warts. Plantar warts are found on the bottom of the foot. Common warts can be easily recognized by the rough, cauliflower-like appearance of the surface.

Warnings: For external use only. Do not use this product on irritated skin, on any area that is infected or reddened, if you are a diabetic, or if you have poor blood circulation. If discomfort persists, see your doctor. Do not use on moles, birthmarks, warts with hair growing from them, genital warts, or warts on the face or mucous membranes. Keep this and all drugs out of the reach of children.

If product gets in eyes, flush with water for 15 minutes. Avoid inhaling vapors. DuoPlant Gel is extremely flammable. Keep away from fire or flame. Cap tube tightly and store at room temperature away from heat. In case of accidental ingestion, seek professional assistance or contact a Poison Control Center immediately.

Directions: Wash affected area. May soak wart in warm water for five minutes. Dry area thoroughly. Apply a thin layer to sufficiently cover each wart. Let dry. Repeat this procedure once or twice daily as needed (until wart is removed) for up to 12 weeks.
Note: Adhesive bandage may be used to cover treated area.

How Supplied: DuoPlant Gel is available in ½ oz. tubes with applicator tip for pinpoint application.

Shown in Product Identification Guide, page 520

DURATION
12 Hour Nasal Spray 0.05%

Description: DURATION Nasal Spray contains oxymetazoline hydrochloride, the longest acting topical nasal decongestant available. Each ml of DURATION Nasal Spray contains Oxymetazoline Hydrochloride, USP 0.5 mg (0.05%). **Also Contains:** Benzalkonium Chloride, Edetate Disodium, Polyethylene Glycol 1450, Povidone, Propylene Glycol, Sodium Phosphate Dibasic, Sodium Phosphate Monobasic, Water.

Indications: For prompt, temporary relief for up to 12 hours of nasal congestion due to colds, hay fever and sinusitis, and other upper respiratory allergies.

Actions: The sympathomimetic action of DURATION products constricts the smaller arterioles of the nasal passages, producing a prolonged, gentle and predictable decongesting effect. In just a few minutes a single dose, as directed, provides prompt, temporary relief of nasal congestion that lasts up to 12 hours.

Warnings: Do not exceed recommended dosage. This product may cause temporary discomfort such as burning, stinging, sneezing, or an increase in nasal discharge. Do not use this product for more than 3 days. Use only as directed. Frequent or prolonged use may cause nasal congestion to recur or worsen. If symptoms persist, consult a doctor. The use of this container by more than one person may spread infection. Do not use this product if you have heart disease, high blood pressure, thyroid disease, diabetes, or difficulty in urination due to enlargement of the prostate gland unless directed by a doctor. As with any drug, if you are pregnant or nursing a baby, seek the advice of a health professional before using this product. Keep this and all medicines out of the reach of children. In case of accidental ingestion, seek professional assistance or contact a Poison Control Center immediately.

Directions: Adults and children 6 to under 12 years of age (with adult supervision): 2 or 3 sprays in each nostril not more often than every 10 to 12 hours. Do not exceed 2 doses in any 24-hour period. **Children under 6 years of age:** consult a doctor. To spray squeeze bottle quickly and firmly. Do not tilt head backward while spraying. Wipe nozzle clean after use.

How Supplied: DURATION 12 Hour Nasal Spray 0.05%—1/2 oz and 1 oz plastic squeeze bottles

---

LOTRIMIN® AF ANTIFUNGAL
[lo-tre-min]
Clotrimazole
Cream 1%
Solution 1%
Lotion 1%
Jock Itch Cream 1%

Description: Lotrimin® AF Cream 1% is a white fully vanishing homogeneous cream containing 1% clotrimazole. The cream contains no sensitizing parabens and is totally grease free and nonstaining.
Lotrimin® AF Solution 1% is a nonaqueous liquid, containing polyethylene glycol.
Lotrimin® AF Lotion 1% is a light penetrating buffered emulsion also containing no common sensitizing agents and is greaseless and nonstaining.

Indications: Lotrimin AF Cream, Solution and Lotion cure athlete's foot (tinea pedis), Jock itch (tinea cruris), and ringworm (tinea corporis), For effective relief of the itching, cracking, burning, and discomfort which can accompany these conditions.

Directions: Cleanse skin with soap and water and dry thoroughly. Apply a thin layer over affected area morning and evening or as directed by a physician. For athlete's foot, pay special attention to the spaces between the toes. It is also helpful to wear well-fitting, ventilated shoes and to change shoes and socks at least once daily. Best results in athlete's foot and ringworm are usually obtained with 4 weeks use of this product, and in jock itch, with 2 weeks use. If satisfactory results have not occurred within these times, consult a physician or pharmacist. Children under 12 years of age should be supervised in the use of this product. This product is not effective on the scalp or nails.

Warnings: For external use only. Do not use on children under 2 years of age except under the advice and supervision of a physician. If irritation occurs or if there is no improvement within 4 weeks (for athlete's foot or ringworm) or within 2 weeks (for jock itch), discontinue use and consult a physician or pharmacist. Keep this and all drugs out of the reach of children. In case of accidental ingestion, seek professional assistance or contact a Poison Control Center immediately.

How Supplied: Lotrimin® AF Antifungal Cream is available in a 0.42 oz. tube (12 grams) and a 0.84 oz. tube (24 grams). Lotrimin® AF Jock Itch Cream is available in a 0.42 oz tube (12 grams). Inactive ingredients include: benzyl alcohol, cetearyl alcohol, cetyl esters wax, octyldodecanol, polysorbate, sorbitan monostearate and water.
Lotrimin® AF Antifungal Solution is available in a 0.33 fl. oz. (10 milliliters) bottle. Inactive ingredients include PEG.
Lotrimin® AF Antifungal Lotion is available in a 0.66 fl. oz. (20 milliliters) bottle. Inactive ingredients include benzyl alcohol, cetearyl alcohol, cetyl esters wax, octyldodecanol, polysorbate, sodium biphosphate, sodium phosphate dibasic, sorbitan monostearate and water.

Storage: Keep Lotrimin® AF products between 2° and 30°C (36° and 86°F).

Shown in Product Identification Guide, page 520

LOTRIMIN® AF ANTIFUNGAL
Miconazole Nitrate 2%
Athlete's Foot Spray Liquid
Athlete's Foot Spray Powder
Athlete's Foot Spray Deodorant Powder
Athlete's Foot Powder
Jock Itch Spray Powder

Active Ingredients:
SPRAY LIQUID contains Miconazole Nitrate 2%. Also contains: Alcohol SD-40 (17% w/w), Cocamide DEA, Isobutane, Propylene Glycol, Tocopherol (vitamin E).
SPRAY POWDER (Athlete's Foot/Jock Itch) contains Miconazole Nitrate 2%. Also contains: Alcohol SD-40 (10% w/w), Isobutane, Stearalkonium Hectorite, Talc.
SPRAY DEODORANT POWDER contains Miconazole Nitrate 2%. Also contains: Isobutane, Alcohol SD-40 (10% w/w), Talc, Stearalkonium Hectorite, Fragrance.
POWDER contains Miconazole Nitrate 2%. Also contains: Talc.

Indications: LOTRIMIN AF Athlete's Foot Spray Liquid, Spray Powder, Spray Deodorant Powder and Powder are proven clinically effective in the treatment of athlete's foot (tinea pedis), jock itch (tinea cruris) and ringworm (tinea corporis). For effective relief of the itching, cracking, burning, scaling and discomfort that can accompany these conditions.

Continued on next page

Information on Schering-Plough HealthCare Products appearing on these pages is effective as of November 1996.

Schering-Plough—Cont.

LOTRIMIN AF Powder also aids in the drying of naturally moist areas.

LOTRIMIN AF Jock Itch Spray Powder cures jock itch (tinea cruris). For effective relief of the itching, burning, scaling and discomfort associated with jock itch.

Warnings: For Athlete's Foot Spray Powder, Spray Liquid, Spray Deodorant Powder and Jock Itch Spray Powder: Do not use on children under 2 years of age unless directed by a doctor. For external use only. If irritation occurs or if there is no improvement within 4 weeks (for athlete's foot and ringworm) or 2 weeks (for jock itch), discontinue use and consult a doctor. Flammable. Do not use while smoking or near heat or flame. Avoid spraying in eyes. Contents under pressure. Do not puncture or incinerate. Do not store at temperature above 120°F. Use only as directed. Intentional misuse by deliberately concentrating and inhaling contents can be harmful or fatal. Keep this and all drugs out of the reach of children. In case of accidental ingestion, seek professional assisatnce or contact a Poison Control Center immediately.

Lotrimin AF Powder: Do not use on children under 2 years of age unless directed by a doctor. For external use only. If irritation occurs, or if there is no improvement within 4 weeks (for athlete's foot or ringworm) or within 2 weeks (for jock itch) discontinue use and consult a doctor. Keep this and all drugs out of the reach of children. In case of accidental ingestion, seek professional assistance or contact a Poison Control Center immediately.

Directions: For Athlete's Foot Spray Liquid, Spray Powder, Spray Deodorant Powder and Jock Itch Spray Powder: Wash affected area and dry thoroughly. Shake can well. Spray a thin layer of product over affected area twice daily (morning and night) or as directed by a doctor. Supervise children in the use of this product. For athlete's foot, pay special attention to the spaces between the toes; wear well-fitting, ventilated shoes and change shoes and socks at least once daily. For athlete's foot and ringworm use daily for 4 weeks; for jock itch use daily for 2 weeks. If condition persists longer, consult a doctor. This product is not effective on the scalp or nails.

Powder: Wash affected area and dry throughly. Sprinkle a thin layer of product over affected area twice daily (morning and night) or as directed by a doctor. Supervise children in the use of this product. For athlete's foot, pay special attention to the spaces between the toes; wear well-fitting, ventilated shoes and change shoes and socks at least once daily. For athlete's foot and ringworm use daily for 4 weeks; for jock itch use daily for 2 weeks. If condition persists longer, consult a doctor. This product is not effective on the scalp or nails.
Store between 2° and 30° C (36° and 86°F).

How Supplied: LOTRIMIN AF Athlete's Foot Spray Powder and Jock Itch Spray Powder—3.5 oz. cans. LOTRIMIN AF Spray Liquid—4 oz. can. LOTRIMIN AF POWDER—3 oz. plastic bottle. LOTRIMIN AF Spray Deodorant Powder—3.5 oz. cans.

Shown in Product Identification Guide, page 520

SHADE® SUNBLOCK GEL SPF 30

Active Ingredients: Ethylhexyl p-methoxycinnamate, homosalate, oxybenzone.

Other Ingredients: SD alcohol 40 (73% V/V), water, PVP/VA copolymer, tetrahydroxypropyl ethylenediamine, acrylates/C10-30 alkyl acrylate crosspolymer, acrylates/octylacrylamide copolymer.

Indications: PABA-FREE Shade SPF 30 Oil-Free Clear Gel is clinically tested to protect your skin from the sun's burning UVA and UVB rays. This clean, clear gel vanishes quickly without any greasy residue. It leaves your skin feeling fresh and clean while providing 30 times your natural protection against sunburn. This unique formula blocks UVB rays that are primarily responsible for sunburn and long-term skin damage caused by overexposure to the sun. It also protects your skin against the deeper penetrating UVA rays that have been associated with skin damage resulting in premature aging and wrinkling. Regular use of Shade 30 Oil-Free Clear Gel may help prevent skin cancer caused by long-term overexposure to the sun.

Non-greasy/Non-oily: Fresh, clear, lightweight greaseless formula that absorbs quickly—feels cool. Specially formulated for people with normal to oily skin.

Waterproof: Maintains its degree of protection (SPF 30) for 80 minutes or more in the water.

Non-acnegenic/Non-comedogenic: Won't clog pores or cause blemishes.

Fragrance-free: Free of fragrances that may irritate those with sensitive skin.

Hypoallergenic: Won't irritate or sting sensitive skin like some protective sunscreens. Gentle enough for children's delicate skin.

Warnings: Flammable, do not use near heat or flame.

Directions for Use: Apply liberally to all exposed areas. For best results, let dry 15 minutes before exposure to sun and reapply after prolonged swimming, excessive perspiration and toweling.

Warnings: Avoid contact with eyes. If skin irritation or rash develops, discontinue use. For children under 6 months consult your doctor. Keep this and all drugs out of the reach of children. In case of accidental ingestion, seek professional assistance or contact a Poison Control Center immediately.

How Supplied: 4 oz. plastic bottles.

Shown in Product Identification Guide, page 520

SHADE® SUNBLOCK LOTION SPF 45

Active Ingredients: Ethylhexyl p-Methoxycinnamate, 2-Ethylhexyl Salicylate, Oxybenzone, Homosalate.

Other Ingredients: Water, Sorbitan Isostearate, Sorbitol, Polyglyceryl-3 Distearate, Octadecene/MA Copolymer, Triethanolamine, Stearic Acid, Barium Sulfate, Benzyl Alcohol, Dimethicone, Aloe Extract, Jojoba Oil, Methylparaben, Tocopherol (Vitamin E), Propylparaben, Carbomer, Disodium EDTA, Imidazolidinyl Urea, Phenethyl Alcohol.

Indications: PABA-FREE Shade SPF 45 is clinically tested to protect your skin from the sun's burning UVA and UVB rays. This ultra moisturizing formula keeps your skin feeling soft yet provides 45 times your natural protection against sunburn. It blocks UVB rays that are primarily responsible for sunburn and long-term skin damage caused by overexposure to the sun. It also protects your skin against the deeper penetrating UVA rays that have been associated with skin damage resulting in premature aging and wrinkling. Regular use of Shade 45 may help prevent skin cancer caused by long-term overexposure to the sun.

Moisturizing: Rich moisturizing formula helps keep your skin feeling smooth, soft and supple.

Waterproof: Maintains its degree of protection (SPF 45) for 80 minutes or more in the water.

Non-comedogenic: Won't clog pores.

Non-Irritating: Won't irritate sensitive skin like some protective sunscreens.

Fragrance Free: Free of fragrances that may irritate those with sensitive skin.

Directions: Apply liberally to all exposed areas. For best results, let dry at least 15 minutes before exposure to the sun and reapply often, especially after toweling.

Warnings: Avoid contact with eyes. If skin irritation or rash develops, discontinue use. For children under 6 months, consult your doctor. In case of accidental ingestion, seek professional assistance or contact a Poison Control Center immediately. Keep this and all drugs out of the reach of children.

How Supplied: 4 oz. plastic bottles

Shown in Product Identification Guide, page 520

SHADE® UVAGUARD®
Sunscreen Lotion SPF 15

Active Ingredients: Octyl methoxycinnamate, 7.5%; avobenzone (Parsol® 1789), 3%; oxybenzone, USP, 3%.

Other Ingredients: Benzyl alcohol, carbomer-941, dimethicone, edetate disodium, glyceryl stearate SE, isopropyl myristate, methylparaben, octadecene/MA copolymer, propylparaben, purified water, sorbitan monooleate, sorbitol, stearic acid and trolamine.

Indications: While all sunscreens protect your skin from the sun's burning rays, Shade UVAGUARD® sunscreen, with the patented ingredient Parsol®1789, offers extra protection from the UVA rays that may contribute to skin damage and premature aging of the skin. Shade UVAGUARD is clinically tested to provide 15 times your natural sunburn protection (UVB). And the moisturizing formula of Shade UVAGUARD keeps your skin feeling soft and is PABA-free. Regular use of Shade UVAGUARD may help reduce the chance of acute and long-term skin damage associated with exposure to UVA and UVB rays. Overexposure to the sun may lead to premature aging of the skin and skin cancer.

Water-resistant: Maintains its degree of protection (SPF 15) for 40 minutes or more in water.

Fragrance-free: Free of fragrance that may irritate those with sensitive skin.

Moisturizing: Moisturizing formula helps keep your skin feeling smooth and soft.

Non-comedogenic: Won't clog pores.

Warnings: Do not use if sensitive to cinnamates, benzophenones or any other ingredient in this product. Avoid contact with the eyes, if contact occurs, rinse eyes thoroughly with water. For external use only, not to be swallowed. Discontinue use if signs of irritation or rash appear. Keep this and all drugs out of the reach of children. In case of accidental ingestion, seek professional assistance or contact a Poison Control Center immediately.

Directions for Use: Shake well before using. Before sun exposure, apply evenly and liberally on all exposed areas and reapply after 40 minutes in the water or after excessive sweating. There is no recommended dosage for children under six (6) months of age except under the advice and supervision of a physician.

How Supplied: 4 oz. plastic bottles.

Shown in Product Identification Guide, page 520

ST. JOSEPH®
ADULT CHEWABLE ASPIRIN
Low Strength Caplet (81 mg. each)

Active Ingredient: Each St. Joseph Adult Chewable Aspirin Caplet contains 81 mg. aspirin in a chewable, fruit flavored form.

Inactive Ingredients: Corn Starch, D&C Yellow No. 10 Aluminum Lake, FD&C Yellow No. 6 Aluminum Lake, Flavor, Hydrogenated Vegetable Oil, Maltodextrin, Mannitol, Saccharin.

Indications: St. Joseph® Adult Chewable Aspirin Caplets provide safe, effective, temporary relief from: headaches, muscular aches and pains; and pain associated with a cold, menstrual cramps, backaches and for reducing fever due to colds.

Warnings: Children and teenagers should not use this medicine for chicken pox or flu symptoms before a doctor is consulted about Reye Syndrome, a rare but serious illness reported to be associated with aspirin. Do not take this product for pain for more than 10 days or for fever for more than 3 days unless directed by a doctor. If pain or fever persists or gets worse, if new symptoms occur, or if redness or swelling is present, consult a doctor because these could be signs of serious conditions. Do not take this product for at least 7 days after tonsillectomy or oral surgery unless directed by a doctor. Do not take this product if you are allergic to aspirin, have asthma, have stomach problems (such as heartburn, upset stomach or stomach pain) that persist or recur, or have ulcers or bleeding problems, unless directed by a doctor. If ringing in the ears or loss of hearing occurs, consult a doctor before taking any more of this product. As with any drug, if you are pregnant or nursing a baby, seek the advice of a health professional before using this product. **IT IS ESPECIALLY IMPORTANT NOT TO USE ASPIRIN DURING THE LAST 3 MONTHS OF PREGNANCY UNLESS SPECIFICALLY DIRECTED TO DO SO BY A DOCTOR BECAUSE IT MAY CAUSE PROBLEMS IN THE UNBORN CHILD OR COMPLICATIONS DURING DELIVERY.** Keep this and all drugs out of the reach of children. In case of accidental overdose, seek professional assistance or contact a Poison Control Center immediately.

Drug Interaction Precaution: Do not take this product if you are taking a prescription drug for anticoagulation (thinning the blood), diabetes, gout, or arthritis unless directed by a doctor.

Directions: Adults chew from 4 to 8 caplets (325 to 650 mg) every 4 hours as needed. Do not exceed 48 caplets in 24 hours or as directed by a doctor. Drink a full glass of water with each dose. Do not give to children under 12 years of age unless directed by a doctor.

Professional Labeling: Aspirin for Myocardial Infarction.

Indication: Aspirin is indicated to reduce the risk of death and/or nonfatal myocardial infarction in patients with a previous infarction or unstable angina pectoris.

Clinical Trials: The indication is supported by the results of six large randomized, multicenter, placebo-controlled studies[1–7] involving 10,816 predominantly male post–myocardial infarction (MI) patients and one randomized placebo-controlled study of 1,266 men with unstable angina. Therapy with aspirin was begun at intervals after the onset of acute MI varying from less than three days to more than five years and continued for periods of from less than one year to four years. In the unstable angina study, treatment was started within one month after the onset of unstable angina and continued for 12 weeks, and complicating conditions, such as congestive heart failure, were not included in the study. Aspirin therapy in MI patients was associated with about a 20% reduction in the risk of subsequent death and/or nonfatal reinfarction, a median absolute decrease of 3% from the 12% to 22% event rates in the placebo groups. In the aspirin-treated unstable angina patients, the reduction in risk was about 50%, a reduction in the event rate of 5% from the 10% rate in the placebo group over the 12 weeks of study.
Daily dosage of aspirin in the post–myocardial infarction studies was 300 mg in one study and 900–1,500 mg in five studies. A dose of 325 mg was used in the study of unstable angina.

Adverse Reactions: Gastrointestinal Reactions: Doses of 1,000 mg per day of aspirin caused gastrointestinal symptoms and bleeding that, in some cases, were clinically significant. In the largest postinfarction study (the Aspirin Myocardial Infarction Study [AMIS] with 4,500 people), the percentage of incidences of gastrointestinal symptoms for the aspirin (1,000 mg of a standard, solid-tablet formulation) and placebo-treated subjects, respectively, were stomach pain (14.5%, 4.4%), heartburn, (11.9%, 4.8%), nausea and/or vomiting (7.6%, 2.1%), hospitalization for GI disorder (4.9%, 3.5%). In the AMIS and other trials, aspirin-treated patients had increased rates of gross gastrointestinal bleeding. Symptoms and signs of gastrointestinal irritation were not significantly increased in subjects treated for unstable angina with buffered aspirin in solution.

Cardiovascular and Biochemical: In the AMIS trial, the dosage of 1,000 mg per day of aspirin was associated with small increases in systolic blood pressure (BP) (average 1.5 to 2.1 mm) and diastolic BP (0.5 to 0.6 mm), depending upon whether maximal or last available readings were used. Blood urea nitrogen and

Continued on next page

Information on Schering-Plough HealthCare Products appearing on these pages is effective as of November 1996.

Schering-Plough—Cont.

uric acid levels were also increased, but by less than 1.0 mg percent. Subjects with marked hypertension or renal insufficiency had been excluded from the trial so that the clinical importance of these observations for such subjects or for any subjects treated over more prolonged periods is not known. It is recommended that patients placed on long-term aspirin treatment, even at doses of 300 mg per day, be seen at regular intervals to assess changes in these measurements.

Dosage and Administration: Although most of the studies used dosage exceeding 300 mg, two trials used only 300 mg daily and pharmacologic data indicate that this dose inhibits platelet function fully. Therefore, 300 mg or 325 mg (4 caplets) aspirin dose daily is a reasonable routine dose that would minimize gastrointestinal adverse reactions.

References:

1. Elwood PC, et al: A randomized controlled trial of acetylsalicylic acid in the secondary prevention of mortality from myocardial infarction, *BR Med J.* 1974;1;436–440.
2. The Coronary Drug Project Research Group: Aspirin in coronary heart disease. *J Chronic Dis.* 1976;29:625–642.
3. Breddin K, et al: Secondary prevention of myocardial infarction: a comparison of acetylsalicylic acid, phenprocoumon or placebo. *Homeostasis.* 1979;470:263–268.
4. Aspirin Myocardial Infarction Study Research Group: A randomized, controlled trial of aspirin in persons recovered from myocardial infarction, *JAMA.* 1980;245:661–669.
5. Elwood PC, and Sweetnam, PM: Aspirin and secondary mortality after myocardial infarction. *Lancet.* December 22–29, 1979, pp 1313–1315.
6. The Persantine-Aspirin Reinfarction Study Research Group: Persantine and aspirin in coronary heart disease. *Circulation.* 1980;62:449–460.
7. Lewis HD. et al: Protective effects of aspirin against acute myocardial infarction and death in men with unstable angina: Results of a Veterans Administration Cooperative Study, *N Engl J Med* 1983;309:396–403.

How Supplied: Chewable, orange flavored caplets in plastic bottles of 36 caplets each.

Scot-Tussin Pharmacal Co., Inc.

P.O. BOX 8217
CRANSTON, RI 02920-0217

Direct inquiries to:
(401) 942-8555
(401) 942-8556
(800) 638-SCOT (7268)
FAX (401) 942-5690

For Medical Emergency Contact:
Dr. S. G. Scotti
(800) 638-SCOT (7268)
FAX (401) 942-5690

The following SCOT-TUSSIN® products may be taken by individuals with diabetes, heart condition and/or high blood pressure:
OTC Products Available
NDC 0372-

0002-**Scot-Tussin Sugar-Free Original** (no alcohol); kosher.

0006-**Scot-Tussin Sugar-Free Expectorant** Guaifenesin (Guaifenesin 100 mg./5mL.)
Sugar-free; Alcohol-free; Sorbitol-free; Sodium-free; Decongestant free; Dye-free; Saccharin free; Corn Syrup-free; kosher.

0021-**Vitalize™ Stress Formula** (no alcohol, sugar or dye); kosher.

0036-**Scot-Tussin Sugar-Free DM** Antitussive-Antihistaminic Dextromethorphan, Chlorpheniramine Maleate (Dextromethorphan HBR. 15 mg./5mL., Chlorpheniramine Maleate 2 mg./5mL.)
Sugar-free; Alcohol-free; Sorbitol-free; Sodium-free; Decongestant-free; Dye-free; Saccharin-free; Corn Syrup-free; kosher.

0038-**Hayfebrol™** allergy relief formula (no sugar or alcohol); kosher.

0043-**Scot-Tussin Diabetes Cough Formula Sugar-Free** (Dextromethorphan HBR. 10 mg./5mL)
Sugar-free; Alcohol-free; Sorbitol-free; Sodium-free; Decongestant-free; Dye-free; Saccharin-free; Corn Syrup-free; kosher.

0044-**Scot-Tussin Sugar-Free Cough Chasers Lozenges** Antitussive Dextromethorphan and Sorbitol (Dextromethorphan 2.5 mg./lozenge.)
Sugar-free; Alcohol-free; Sodium-free; Decongestant-free; Dye-free; Saccharin-free; Corn Syrup-free.

0047-**Scot-Tussin Sugar-Free Allergy Relief Formula** Antihistaminic Diphenhydramine HCl (Diphenhydramine HCl 12.5 mg/5 mL.)
Sugar-free; Alcohol-free; Sorbitol-free; Sodium-free; Decongestant-free; Dye-free; Saccharin-free; Corn Syrup-free; kosher.

0049-**Romilar® DM SF**

0050-**Scot-Tussin Senior SF Maximum Strength** Antitussive/Expectorant (Dextromethorphan HBR. 15 mg./5mL., Guaifenesin 200 mg./5mL.)
Sugar-free; Alcohol-free; Sorbitol-free; Sodium-free; Decongestant-free; Dye-free; Saccharin-free; Corn Syrup-free; kosher.

0052-**Vitalize™ with Ginseng High Energy Drink** Sugar-free; Alcohol-free; kosher.

®Romilar U.S. Patent Office Reg. #176-5204
SCOT-TUSSIN
®US Patent Office Reg. #657-674

Similasan Corporation Homeopathic OTC Medications

1321 S. CENTRAL AVENUE
SUITE D
KENT, WA 98032

Direct Inquiries to:
Brian S. Banks
1-800-426-1644
FAX: 206-859-9102

For Medical Emergency Contact:
Alfred Knaus
(206) 859-9072
FAX: (206) 859-9102

SIMILASAN®
Eye Drops #1

Similasan® natural eye drops #1, provide fast relief for dryness and redness due to smog, overwork, contact lens wear etc. The solution is immediately soothing and does not sting upon application. Packaged in a quality glass bottle with a unique dropper.

Suitable for adults and children.

Indications: According to homeopathic principles the ingredients of this medication give you temporary relief from symptoms of:

- Dry, red, irritated eyes
- Inflammation of eyelids
- Sensation of grittiness, hypersensitivity to light, watery eyes
- Tired, strained eyes

Directions for use:

- One to several times daily, place 1–2 drops in each eye.
- Squeeze plastic outlet of bottle with two fingers and allow preparation to drip into the eye.
- Replace cap immediately after using.
- Use before expiration date.

Contraindications: None

Adverse Reactions: None

Drug Interactions: None

Safety packaging:
Use only if bottle seal is intact.

Warning: To avoid contamination of this product, do not touch tip of container to any surface. Replace cap after using. If solution changes color or becomes cloudy, do not use. If you experience eye pain, changes in vision, continued redness or irritation of the eye, or if the condition worsens or persists, consult a physician. Keep this and all medicines out of the reach of children.

Active Ingredients (in homeopathic microdilutions—call for details): 1-800-426-1644. Belladonna HPUS 6X, Euphrasia HPUS 6X, Mercurius sublimatus HPUS 6X
Inactive ingredients: **SoluSept®** 0.001%, Natrium chloratum 0.9%, Purified water
Similasan® and **SoluSept®** are registered Trademarks of Similasan AG, Switzerland
Manufactured by:
Similasan AG, Switzerland
Imported and Distributed by:
Similasan Corp., Kent, WA 98032
1-800-426-1644
Made in Switzerland
NDC 59262-345-11
10 ml/0.33 fl oz

SIMILASAN®
Eye Drops #2

Similasan® natural allergy eye drops provide fast, soothing relief for itching and burning due to allergic reactions caused by pollen, animal hair, dust etc. The solution is immediately soothing and does not sting upon application. Packaged in a quality glass bottle with a unique dropper.
Suitable for adults and children.

Indications: According to homeopathic principles the ingredients of this medication give you temporary relief from symptoms of:
- Hayfever
- Allergic reactions of the eyes and eyelids, such as:
  - — Redness
  - — Itching and burning sensations
  - — Excessive tearing

Directions for use:
- One to several times daily, place 1–2 drops in each eye.
- Squeeze plastic outlet of bottle with two fingers and allow preparation to drip into the eye.
- Replace cap immediately after using.
- Use before expiration date.

Contraindications: None

Adverse Reactions: None

Drug Interactions: None
Safety packaging:
Use only if bottle seal is intact.

Warning: To avoid contamination of this product, do not touch tip of container to any surface. Replace cap after using. If solution changes color or becomes cloudy, do not use. If you experience eye pain, changes in vision, continued redness or irritation of the eye, or if the condition worsens or persists, consult a physician. Keep this and all medicines out of the reach of children.
Active Ingredients (in homeopathic microdilutions—call for details): 1-800-426-1644. Apis HPUS 6X, Euphrasia HPUS 6X, Sabadilla HPUS 6X
Inactive ingredients: SoluSept® 0.001%, Natrium chloratum 0.9%, Purified water
Similasan® and **SoluSept®** are registered Trademarks of Similasan AG, Switzerland
Manufactured by:
Similasan AG, Switzerland
Imported and Distributed by:
Similasan Corp., Kent, WA 98032
1-800-426-1644
Made in Switzerland
NDC 59262-346-11
10 ml/0.33 fl oz

SmithKline Beecham Consumer Healthcare, L.P.
POST OFFICE BOX 1467
PITTSBURGH, PA 15230

For Medical Information Contact:
(800) 245-1040 (Consumer Inquiries)
(800) 378-4055 (Healthcare Professional Inquiries)

Direct Healthcare Professional Sample Requests to:
(800) BEECHAM

CĒPASTAT®
[sē ′pə-stăt]
Sore Throat Lozenges
Cherry Flavor and Extra Strength

Description: Cherry Flavor lozenge:
Active Ingredient: Each lozenge contains Phenol 14.5mg.
Inactive Ingredients: Antifoam Emulsion, D&C Red #33, FD&C Yellow #6, Flavor, Gum Crystal, Menthol, Saccharin Sodium, and Sorbitol.
Extra Strength lozenge:
Active Ingredient: Each lozenge contains Phenol 29mg.
Inactive Ingredients: Antifoam Emulsion, Caramel, Eucalyptus Oil, Gum Crystal, Menthol, Saccharin Sodium, and Sorbitol.

Actions: Phenol is a recognized topical anesthetic. The sugar-free formula should not promote tooth decay as sugar-based lozenges can.

Indications: For the temporary relief of occasional minor irritation, pain, sore mouth and sore throat.

Warnings: If sore throat is severe, persists for more than 2 days, is accompanied or followed by fever, headache, rash, swelling, nausea, or vomiting, consult a doctor promptly. If sore mouth symptoms do not improve in 7 days or if irritation, pain, or redness persists or worsens, see your dentist or doctor promptly. Do not exceed recommended dosage. KEEP THIS AND ALL MEDICINES OUT OF THE REACH OF CHILDREN. In case of accidental overdose, seek professional assistance or contact a poison control center immediately. As with any drug, if you are pregnant or nursing a baby seek the advice of a health professional before using this product.
Note to Diabetics: Each lozenge contributes approximately 8 calories from 2 grams of sorbitol.

Dosage and Administration:
Lozenges–Cherry Flavor
Adults and children 12 years of age and older: Allow the lozenge to dissolve slowly in the mouth. May be repeated every 2 hours, per day, or as directed by a dentist or physician. **Children 6 to under 12 years of age:** Allow lozenge to dissolve slowly in the mouth. May be repeated every 2 hours, not to exceed 300 mg phenol (20 lozenges) per day, or as directed by a dentist or physician. **Children under 6 years of age:** Consult a dentist or physician.
Lozenges–Extra Strength
Adults and children 12 years of age and older: Allow the lozenge to dissolve slowly in the mouth. May be repeated every 2 hours, or as directed by a dentist or physician. **Children 6 to under 12 years of age:** Allow lozenge to dissolve slowly in the mouth. May be repeated every 2 hours, not to exceed 300 mg phenol (10 lozenges) per day, or as directed by a dentist or physician. **Children under 6 years of age:** Consult a dentist or physician.

How Supplied:
Lozenges–Cherry Flavor
Trade package: Boxes of 18 lozenges as 2 pocket packs of 9 lozenges each.
Lozenges–Extra Strength
Trade package: Boxes of 18 lozenges as 2 pocket packs of 9 lozenges each.
Store at room temperature, below 86°F (30°C). Protect contents from humidity.

Shown in Product Identification Guide, page 520

Orange Flavor
CITRUCEL®
[sĭt ′rə-sĕl]
(Methylcellulose)
Bulk-forming Fiber Laxative

Description: Each 19 g adult dose (approximately one heaping measuring tablespoonful) contains Methylcellulose 2 g. Each 9.5 g child's dose (one-half the adult dose) contains Methylcellulose 1 g. Methylcellulose is a nonallergenic fiber. Also contains: Citric Acid, FD&C Yellow No. 6, Orange Flavors (natural and artificial), Potassium Citrate, Riboflavin, Sucrose, and other ingredients. Each adult dose contains approximately 3 mg of sodium, 105 mg of potassium, and contributes 60 calories from Sucrose.

Actions: Promotes elimination by providing additional fiber (bulk) to the diet. This product generally produces bowel movement in 12 to 72 hours.

Indications: For relief of constipation (irregularity). May also be used for relief of constipation associated with other bowel disorders such as irritable bowel syndrome, diverticular disease, and hemorrhoids as well as for bowel management during postpartum, postsurgical, and convalescent periods when recommended by a physician.

Continued on next page

SmithKline Beecham—Cont.

Contraindications: Intestinal obstruction, fecal impaction, known hypersensitivity to formula ingredients.

Warnings: Patients should be instructed to consult their physician before using any laxative if they have noticed a sudden change in bowel habits which persists for two weeks. Unless directed by a physician, patients should be advised not to use laxative products when abdominal pain, nausea, or vomiting is present. Patients should also be advised to discontinue use and consult a physician if rectal bleeding or failure to have a bowel movement occurs after use of any laxative product. Unless recommended by a physician, patients should not exceed the recommended maximum daily dose. Patients should not use laxative products for a period longer than one week unless directed by a physician. **TAKING THIS PRODUCT WITHOUT ADEQUATE FLUID MAY CAUSE IT TO SWELL AND BLOCK YOUR THROAT OR ESOPHAGUS AND MAY CAUSE CHOKING. DO NOT TAKE THIS PRODUCT IF YOU HAVE DIFFICULTY IN SWALLOWING. IF YOU EXPERIENCE CHEST PAIN, VOMITING, OR DIFFICULTY IN SWALLOWING OR BREATHING AFTER TAKING THIS PRODUCT, SEEK IMMEDIATE MEDICAL ATTENTION. KEEP THIS AND ALL DRUGS OUT OF THE REACH OF CHILDREN.**

Dosage and Administration: Adult Dose: *one rounded tablespoonful* (19 g) stirred briskly into at least 8 ounces of cold water up to three times daily at the first sign of constipation. Children age 6 to 12 years of age: *one-half the adult dose* stirred briskly into at least 8 ounces of cold water, once daily at the first sign of constipation. The mixture should be administered promptly and drinking another glass of water is highly recommended (see warnings). Children under 6 years of age: *Use only as directed by a physician.* Continued use for 12 to 72 hours may be necessary for full benefit.

TAKE THIS PRODUCT (CHILD OR ADULT DOSE) WITH AT LEAST 8 OZ. (A FULL GLASS) OF WATER OR OTHER FLUID. TAKING THIS PRODUCT WITHOUT ENOUGH LIQUID MAY CAUSE CHOKING. SEE WARNINGS.

How Supplied: 16 oz. and 30 oz. containers.
Boxes of 20-single-dose packets.
Store below 86°F (30°C). Protect contents from humidity; keep tightly closed.

Shown in Product Identification Guide, page 520

Sugar Free Orange Flavor
CITRUCEL®
[*sĭt 'rə-sĕl*]
(Methylcellulose)
Bulk-forming Fiber Laxative

Description: Each 10.2 g adult dose (approximately one rounded measuring tablespoonful) contains Methylcellulose 2 g. Each 5.1 g child's dose (one-half the adult dose) contains Methylcellulose 1 g. Methylcellulose is a nonallergenic fiber. Also contains: Aspartame, Dibasic Calcium Phosphate, FD&C Yellow No. 6, Malic Acid, Maltodextrin, Orange Flavors (natural and artificial), Potassium Citrate and Riboflavin. Each 10.2 g dose contributes 24 calories from Maltodextrin.

Actions: Promotes elimination by providing additional fiber (bulk) to the diet. This product generally produces bowel movement in 12 to 72 hours.

Indications: For relief of constipation (irregularity). May also be used for relief of constipation associated with other bowel disorders such as irritable bowel syndrome, diverticular disease, and hemorrhoids as well as for bowel management during postpartum, postsurgical, and convalescent periods when recommended by a physician.

Contraindications and Warnings: See entry for "Orange Flavor Citrucel".

Phenylketonurics: CONTAINS PHENYLALANINE 52 mg per adult dose. Individuals with phenylketonuria and other individuals who must restrict their intake of phenylalanine should be warned that each 10.2 g adult dose contains aspartame which provides 52 mg of phenylalanine.

Dosage and Administration: Adult Dose: *one rounded tablespoonful* (10.2 g) stirred briskly into at least 8 ounces of cold water up to three times daily at the first sign of constipation. Children age 6 to 12 years of age: *one-half the adult dose* stirred briskly into at least 8 ounces of cold water, once daily at the first sign of constipation. The mixture should be administered promptly and drinking another glass of water is highly recommended (see warnings). Children under 6 years of age: *Use only as directed by a physician.* Continued use for 12 to 72 hours may be necessary for full benefit.

TAKE THIS PRODUCT (CHILD OR ADULT DOSE) WITH AT LEAST 8 OZ. (A FULL GLASS) OF WATER OR OTHER FLUID. TAKING THIS PRODUCT WITHOUT ENOUGH LIQUID MAY CAUSE CHOKING. SEE WARNINGS.

How Supplied:
8.6 oz and 16.9 oz containers.
Boxes of 20 single-dose packets.
Store below 86°F (30°C). Protect contents from humidity; keep tightly closed.

Shown in Product Identification Guide, page 520

CONTAC
Day & Night Cold/Flu

Composition:

Product Information: Contac Day & Night Cold/Flu includes 15 day caplets and 5 night caplets in each package to provide:

- 5 days of relief from stuffy nose, coughing and aches and pains without drowsiness
- 5 nights of relief from stuffy runny, nose, sneezing and aches and pains to let you rest.

Day Caplets

Product Benefits: Contac Day Caplets provide an ANALGESIC, a DECONGESTANT, and a COUGH SUPPRESSANT.

Indications: For the temporary relief of headache, minor aches and pains, fever, nasal congestion and coughs due to the common cold or flu.

Directions: Adults (12 years and older): Take one Yellow Day Caplet every 6 hours, or as directed by a doctor. DO NOT EXCEED A TOTAL OF 4 CAPLETS (whether all Day or all Night or combination of each) IN 24 HOURS. ALL CAPLETS SHOULD BE TAKEN AT LEAST 6 HOURS APART. Children under 12 years of age: Consult a doctor.

Night Caplets

Product Benefits: Contac Night Caplets provide an ANALGESIC, an ANTIHISTAMINE, and a DECONGESTANT.

Indications: For the temporary relief of headache minor aches and pains, fever, nasal congestion, runny nose, and sneezing due to the common cold and flu.

Directions: Adults (12 years and older): Take one Blue Night Caplet every 6 hours, or as directed by a doctor. DO NOT EXCEED A TOTAL OF 4 CAPLETS (whether all Day or all Night or combination of each) IN 24 HOURS. ALL CAPLETS SHOULD BE TAKEN AT LEAST 6 HOURS APART. Children under 12 years of age: Consult a doctor.

Warnings for Day and Night Caplets: Do not take this product for more than 10 days. If symptoms do not improve or are accompanied by fever that lasts for more than 3 days, or if new symptoms occur, consult a doctor. Do not take this product, unless directed by a doctor, if you have a breathing problem such as emphysema or chronic bronchitis, or if you have heart disease, high blood pressure, thyroid disease, diabetes, glaucoma or difficulty in urination due to enlargement of the prostate gland. **Do not exceed recommended dosage.** If nervousness, dizziness, or sleeplessness occur, discontinue use and consult a doctor. **KEEP THIS AND ALL DRUGS OUT OF THE REACH OF CHILDREN.** Prompt medical attention is critical for adults as well as for children even if you do not notice any signs or symptoms. In case of accidental overdose, seek professional assistance or contact a Poison Control Center immediately. As with any drug, if you are pregnant or nursing a baby, seek the advice of a health professional before using this product.

Additional Warnings for Day Caplets: A persistent cough may be a sign of a serious condition. If cough persists for more than 7 days, tends to recur, or is accompanied by rash, persistent headache, fever that lasts for more than 3 days, or if new symptoms occur, consult a doctor. Do not take this product for persistent or chronic cough such as occurs with smoking, asthma, emphysema, or if cough is accompanied by excessive phlegm (mucus) unless directed by a doctor.

Additional Warnings for Night Caplets: May cause excitability especially in children. May cause marked drowsiness; alcohol, sedatives, and tranquilizers may increase the drowsiness effect. Avoid alcoholic beverages while taking this product. Do not take this product if you are taking sedatives or tranquilizers, without first consulting your doctor. Use caution when driving a motor vehicle or operating machinery.

Drug Interaction Precaution: Do not use this product if you are now taking a prescription monoamine oxidase inhibitor (MAOI) (certain drugs for depression, psychiatric or emotional conditions, or Parkinson's disease), or for 2 weeks after stopping the MAOI drug. If you are uncertain whether your prescription drug contains an MAOI, consult a health professional before taking this product.

Active Ingredients: EACH DAY CAPLET CONTAINS: Acetaminophen 650 mg, Pseudoephedrine Hydrochloride 60 mg. Dextromethorphan Hydrobromide 30 mg. EACH NIGHT CAPLET CONTAINS: Acetaminophen 650 mg, Pseudoephedrine Hydrochloride 60 mg, Diphenhydramine Hydrochloride 50 mg.

Inactive Ingredients: EACH DAY AND NIGHT CAPLET CONTAINS: Hydroxypropyl Methylcellulose, Magnesium Stearate, Microcrystalline Cellulose, Polyethylene Glycol, Polysorbate 80, Silicon Dioxide, Starch, Stearic Acid, Titanium Dioxide. DAY CAPLETS ALSO CONTAIN: D&C Yellow 10, FD&C Yellow 6. NIGHT CAPLETS ALSO CONTAIN: FD&C Blue 1.

How Supplied: Consumer package of 5 Night Caplets and 15 Day Caplets (see previous Day Caplet listing).

Note: There are other CONTAC products. Make sure this is the one you are interested in.

Shown in Product Identification Guide, page 520

CONTAC®
MAXIMUM STRENGTH
Continuous Action Nasal Decongestant/Antihistamine
12 Hour Caplets

Composition: [See table on page 786.]

Product Information: Each CONTAC Maximum Strength timed release caplet provides up to 12 hours of relief. Part of the caplet goes to work right away for fast relief; the rest is released gradually to provide up to 12 hours of prolonged relief. With just *one* caplet in the morning and *one* at bedtime, you feel better all day, sleep better at night, breathing freely without congestion. CONTAC Maximum Strength provides:

- A NASAL DECONGESTANT which helps clear nasal passages, shrinks swollen membranes and helps decongest sinus openings.
- AN ANTIHISTAMINE at the maximum level to help relieve itchy, watery eyes, sneezing, and runny nose.

Indications: For temporary relief of nasal congestion due to the common cold, hay fever or other upper respiratory allergies, and nasal congestion associated with sinusitis.

Directions: Adults and children 12 years of age and older: One caplet every 12 hours, not to exceed 2 caplets in 24 hours, or as directed by a doctor. Children under 12 years of age: consult a doctor.

NOTE: The nonactive portion of the caplet that supplies the active ingredients may occasionally appear in your stool as a soft mass.

TAMPER-RESISTANT PACKAGING FEATURES FOR YOUR PROTECTION:

Each caplet is encased in a plastic cell with a foil back; do not use if cell or foil is broken. The name CONTAC appears on each caplet; do not use this product if the CONTAC name is missing.

This carton is protected by a clear overwrap printed with "safety-sealed"; do not use if overwrap is missing or broken.

Warnings: Do not exceed recommended dosage. If nervousness, dizziness or sleeplessness occur, discontinue use and consult a doctor. If symptoms do not improve within 7 days or are accompanied by fever, consult a physician before continuing use. Do not take this product unless directed by a doctor, if you have a breathing problem such as emphysema, heart disease, high blood pressure, thyroid disease, diabetes, or chronic bronchitis, or if you have glaucoma or difficulty in urination due to enlargement of the prostate gland. Do not take this product if you are taking another medication containing phenylpropanolamine. May cause drowsiness; alcohol, sedatives and tranquilizers may increase the drowsiness effect. Avoid alcoholic beverages while taking this product. Do not take this product if you are taking sedatives or tranquilizers, without first consulting your doctor. Do not drive or operate heavy machinery. May cause excitability, especially in children. Keep this and all drugs out of reach of children. In case of accidental overdose, seek professional assistance or contact a poison control center immediately. As with any drug, if you are pregnant or nursing a baby, seek the advice of a health professional before using this product. Store at controlled room temperature (59°–86°F).

Drug Interaction Precaution: Do not use this product if you are now taking a prescription monoamine oxidase inhibitor (MAOI) (certain drugs for depression, psychiatric or emotional conditions or Parkinson's disease), or for 2 weeks after stopping the MAOI drug. If you are uncertain whether your prescription drug contains an MAOI, consult a health professional before taking this product.

Formula: Active Ingredients: Each Maximum Strength caplet contains Phenylpropanolamine Hydrochloride 75 mg.; Chlorpheniramine Maleate 12 mg. (which is a higher dose of antihistamine than CONTAC capsules). **Inactive Ingredients (listed for individuals with specific allergies):** Acetylated Monoglycerides, Carnauba Wax, Colloidal Silicon Dioxide, Ethylcellulose, Hydroxypropyl Methylcellulose, Lactose, Stearic Acid, Titanium Dioxide.

How Supplied: Consumer packages of 10, and 20 caplets.

Note: There are other CONTAC products. Make sure this is the one you are interested in.

Shown in Product Identification Guide, page 520

CONTAC®
Continuous Action Nasal Decongestant/Antihistamine
12 Hour Capsules

Composition: [See table on next page.]

Product Information: Each CONTAC timed release capsule contains over 600 "tiny time pills." Some go to work right away. The rest are scientifically timed to dissolve slowly to give up to 12 hours of relief.

Indications: Temporarily relieves nasal congestion due to the common cold, hay fever or other upper respiratory allergies and associated with sinusitis. Temporarily relieves runny nose and reduces sneezing, itching of the nose or throat and itchy, watery eyes due to hay fever or other upper respiratory allergies. Helps clear nasal passages; shrinks swollen membranes. Helps decongest sinus openings and passages; temporarily relieves sinus congestion and pressure.

Directions: Adults and children over 12 years of age: One capsule every 12 hours, not to exceed 2 capsules in 24 hours, or as directed by a doctor. Children under 12 years of age: consult a doctor.

Continued on next page

SmithKline Beecham—Cont.

TAMPER-RESISTANT PACKAGING FEATURES FOR YOUR PROTECTION:
Each capsule is encased in a plastic cell with a foil back; do not use if cell or foil is broken. Each CONTAC capsule is protected by a red Perma-Seal™ band which bonds the two capsule halves together; do not use if capsule or band is broken.
This carton is protected by a clear overwrap printed with "safety-sealed"; do not use if overwrap is missing or broken.

Warnings: Do not exceed the recommended dosage. If nervousness, dizziness, or sleeplessness occur, discontinue use and consult a doctor. If symptoms do not improve within 7 days or are accompanied by high fever, consult a doctor. Do not take this product, unless directed by a doctor, if you have a breathing problem such as emphysema or chronic bronchitis, or if you have heart disease, high blood pressure, thyroid disease, diabetes, glaucoma or difficulty in urination due to enlargement of the prostate gland. Do not take this product if you are taking another medication containing phenylpropanolamine. Use caution when driving a motor vehicle or operating machinery. May cause drowsiness; alcohol, sedatives and tranquilizers may increase the drowsiness effect. Avoid alcoholic beverages while taking this product. Do not take this product if you are taking sedatives or tranquilizers, without first consulting your doctor. May cause excitability especially in children. KEEP THIS AND ALL DRUGS OUT OF REACH OF CHILDREN. IN CASE OF ACCIDENTAL OVERDOSE, SEEK PROFESSIONAL ASSISTANCE OR CONTACT A POISON CONTROL CENTER IMMEDIATELY. As with any drug, if you are pregnant or nursing a baby, seek the advice of a health professional before using this product. Store in a dry place at controlled room temperature 15°–30°C (59°–86°F).

Drug Interaction Precaution: Do not use this product if you are now taking a prescription monoamine oxidase inhibitor (MAOI) (certain drugs for depression, psychiatric or emotional conditions, or Parkinson's disease), or for 2 weeks after stopping the MAOI drug. If you are uncertain whether your prescription drug contains an MAOI, consult a health professional before taking this product.

Each Capsule Contains: Phenylpropanolamine Hydrochloride 75 mg. and Chlorpheniramine Maleate 8 mg. Also Contains: Benzyl Alcohol, Butylparaben, D&C Red No. 33, D&C Yellow No. 10, Edetate Calcium Disodium, FD&C Red No. 3, FD&C Yellow No. 6, Gelatin, Methylparaben, Pharmaceutical Glaze, Propylparaben, Sodium Lauryl Sulfate, Sodium Propionate, Starch, Sucrose and other ingredients, may also contain: Polysorbate 80.

How Supplied: Consumer packages of 10, and 20 capsules.

Note: There are other CONTAC products. Make sure this is the one you are interested in.

Shown in Product Identification Guide, page 520

CONTAC®
Severe Cold and Flu Caplets
Analgesic • Decongestant
Antihistamine • Cough Suppressant

Composition: [See table below.]

Product Information: Two caplets every 6 hours to help relieve the discomforts of severe colds with flu-like symptoms.

Product Benefits: CONTAC Severe Cold and Flu contains a Non-Aspirin Analgesic, a Decongestant, an Antihistamine and a Cough Suppressant.

Indications: Provides temporary relief from nasal and sinus congestion, runny nose, sneezing, coughing, fever, headache and minor aches assoicated with the common cold, sore throat and the flu.

Directions: Adults (12 years and over): Two caplets every 6 hours, not to exceed 8 caplets in any 24-hour period, or as directed by a doctor.

TAMPER-RESISTANT PACKAGING FEATURES FOR YOUR PROTECTION:
Caplets are encased in a plastic cell with a foil back; do not use if cell or foil is broken. The letters SCF appear on each caplet; do not use this product if these letters are missing.
This carton is protected by a clean overwrap printed with "safety-sealed"; do not use if overwrap is missing or broken.

Warnings: Do not take this product for more than 10 days. If symptoms do not improve or are accompanied by fever that lasts for more than 3 days, or if new symptoms occur, consult a doctor. If sore throat is severe, persists for more than 2 days, is accompanied or followed by fever, headache, rash, nausea, or vomiting, consult a doctor promptly. A persistent cough may be a sign of a serious condition. If cough persists for more than 7 days, tends to recur, or is accompanied by rash, persistent headache, fever that lasts for more than 3 days, or if new symptoms occur, consult a doctor. Do not take this product for persistent or chronic cough such as occurs with smoking, asthma, emphysema, or if cough is accompanied by excessive phlegm (mucus) unless directed by a doctor. May cause excitability especially in children. Do not take this product, unless directed by a doctor, if you have a breathing problem such as emphysema or chronic bronchitis, or if you have heart disease, high blood pressure, thyroid disease, diabetes, glaucoma or difficulty in urination due to enlargement of the prostate gland. May cause marked drowsiness: alcohol, sedatives, and tranquilizers may increase the drowsiness effect. Avoid taking alcoholic beverages while taking this product. Do not take this product if you are taking sedatives or tranquilizers, without first consulting your doctor. Use caution when driving a motor vehicle or operating machinery. **Do not exceed recommended dosage.** If nervousness, dizziness, or sleeplessness occur, discon-

PDR For Nonprescription Drugs

	CONTACT 12 Hour Cold Caplets	CONTACT 12 Hour Cold Capsules	CONTAC Severe Cold and Flu Caplets (each 2 caplet dose)	CONTAC Severe Cold and Flu Non-Drowsy Caplet (each 2 caplet dose)	CONTAC Day & Night Cold & Flu Day Caplets	CONTAC Day & Night Cold & Flu Night Caplets
Phenylpropanolamine HCl	75.0 mg	75.0 mg	25.0 mg	—	—	—
Chlorpheniramine Maleate	12.0 mg	8.0 mg	4.0 mg	—	—	—
Pseudoephedrine HCl	—	—	—	60.0 mg	60.0 mg	60.0 mg
Acetaminophen	—	—	1000.0 mg	650.0 mg	650.0 mg	650.0 mg
Dextromethorphan Hydrobromide	—	—	30.0 mg	30.0 mg	30.0 mg	—
Diphenhydramine HCl	—	—	—	—	—	50.0 mg

tinue use and consult a doctor. **KEEP THIS AND ALL DRUGS OUT OF THE REACH OF CHILDREN.** Prompt medical attention is critical for adults as well as for children even if you do not notice any signs or symptoms. In case of accidental overdose, seek professional assistance or contact a Poison Control Center immediately. As with any drug, if you are pregnant or nursing a baby, seek the advice of a health professional before using this product.

Drug Interaction Precaution: Do not use this product if you are now taking a prescription monoamine oxidase inhibitor (MAOI) (certain drugs for depression, psychiatric or emotional conditions, or Parkinson's disease), or for 2 weeks after stopping the MAOI drug. If you are uncertain whether your prescription drug contains an MAOI, consult a health professional before taking this product.

Formula: Active Ingredients: Each caplet contains Acetaminophen, 500 mg., Dextromethorphan Hydrobromide, 15 mg.; Phenylpropanolamine Hydrochloride, 12.5 mg.; Chlorpheniramine Maleate, 2 mg. **Inactive Ingredients (listed for individuals with specific allergies):** Cellulose, FD&C Blue 1, Hydroxypropyl Methylcellulose, Polyethylene Glycol, Polysorbate 80, Povidone, Sodium Starch Glycolate, Starch, Stearic Acid, Titanium Dioxide.
Avoid storing at high temperature (greater than 100°F).

How Supplied: Consumer packages of 16 and 30 caplets.

Note: There are other CONTAC products. Make sure this is the one you are interested in.

Shown in Product Identification Guide, page 520

CONTAC
Severe Cold and Flu
Non-Drowsy
Caplets
Decongestant * Analgesic
Cough Suppressant

Product Information: Two caplets every 6 hours to help relieve, without drowsiness, the discomfort of severe colds with flu-like symptoms.
Product Benefits: Contac Severe Cold and Flu Non-Drowsy contains a NON-ASPIRIN ANALGESIC, a DECONGESTANT, and a COUGH SUPPRESSANT.

Indications: Temporarily relieves nasal congestion and coughing due to the common cold. Provides temporary relief of fever, sore throat, headache and minor aches associated with the common cold or the flu.

Directions: Adults (12 years and older): Two caplets every 6 hours, not to exceed 8 caplets in any 24-hour period, or as directed by a doctor. Children under 12 years of age: consult a doctor.

Warnings: Do not take this product for more than 10 days. If symptoms do not improve or are accompanied by fever that lasts for more than 3 days, or if new symptoms occur, consult a doctor. If sore throat is severe, persists for more than 2 days, is accompanied or followed by fever, headache, rash, nausea, or vomiting, consult a doctor promptly. A persistent cough may be a sign of a serious condition. If cough persists for more than 7 days, tends to recur, or is accompanied by rash, persistent headache, fever that lasts for more than 3 days, or if new symptoms occur, consult a doctor. Do not take this product for persistent or chronic cough such as occurs with smoking, asthma, emphysema, or if cough is accompanied by excessive phlegm (mucus) unless directed by a doctor. Do not take this product if you have heart disease, high blood pressure, thyroid disease, diabetes, or difficulty in urination due to enlargement of the prostate gland unless directed by a doctor. **Do not exceed recommended dosage.** If nervousness, dizziness, or sleeplessness occur, discontinue use and consult a doctor. **KEEP THIS AND ALL DRUGS OUT OF THE REACH OF CHILDREN.** In case of accidental overdose, seek professional assistance or contact a Poison Control Center immediately. Prompt medical attention is critical for adults as well as for children even if you do not notice any signs or symptoms. As with any drug, if you are pregnant or nursing a baby, seek the advice of a health professional before using this product.

Drug Interaction Precaution: Do not use this product if you are now taking a prescription monoamine oxidase inhibitor (MAOI) (certain drugs for depression, psychiatric or emotional conditions, or Parkinson's disease), or for 2 weeks after stopping the MAOI drug. If you are uncertain whether your prescription drug contains an MAOI, consult a health professional before taking this product.

Active Ingredients: Acetaminophen 325 mg, Pseudoephedrine Hydrochloride 30 mg and Dextromethorphan Hydrobromide 15 mg.

Inactive Ingredients: Carnauba Wax, Colloidal Silicon Dioxide, Hydroxypropyl Methylcellulose, Magnesium Stearate, Microcrystalline Cellulose, Polyethylene Glycol, Polysorbate 80, Starch, Stearic Acid and Titanium Dioxide.
Store at controlled room temperature (59° to 86°F).
Retain outer carton for complete directions and warnings.

How Supplied: Consumer package of 16 caplets.
Note: There are other Contact products. Make sure this is the one you are interested in.

Shown in Product Identification Guide, page 520

DEBROX® Drops
Ear Wax Removal Aid

Description: Carbamide peroxide 6.5%. Also contains citric acid, glycerin, propylene glycol, sodium stannate, water, and other ingredients.

Actions: DEBROX®, used as directed, cleanses the ear with sustained microfoam. DEBROX Drops foam on contact with earwax due to the release of oxygen (there may be an associated crackling sound). DEBROX Drops provide a safe, nonirritating method of softening and removing ear wax.

Indications: For occasional use as an aid to soften, loosen, and remove excessive earwax.

Directions: FOR USE IN THE EAR ONLY. Adults and children over 12 years of age: tilt head sideways and place 5 to 10 drops into ear. Tip of applicator should not enter ear canal. Keep drops in ear for several minutes by keeping head tilted or placing cotton in the ear. Use twice daily for up to four days if needed, or as directed by a doctor. Any wax remaining after treatment may be removed by gently flushing the ear with warm water, using a soft rubber bulb ear syringe. Children under 12 years of age: consult a doctor.

Warnings: Do not use if you have ear drainage or discharge, ear pain, irritation or rash in the ear, or are dizzy; consult a doctor. Do not use if you have an injury or perforation (hole) of the eardrum or after ear surgery unless directed by a doctor. Do not use for more than four days. If excessive earwax remains after use of this product, consult a doctor. Avoid contact with the eyes.

Cautions: Avoid exposing bottle to excessive heat and direct sunlight. Keep tip on bottle when not in use. Keep this and all drugs out of the reach of children. In case of accidental ingestion, seek professional assistance or contact a poison control center immediately.

How Supplied: DEBROX Drops are available in ½- or 1-fl-oz (15 or 30 ml) plastic squeeze bottles with applicator spouts.

Shown in Product Identification Guide, page 520

ECOTRIN®
Enteric-Coated Aspirin
Antiarthritic, Antiplatelet

Description: 'Ecotrin' is enteric-coated aspirin (acetylsalicylic acid, ASA) available in tablet form in 81 mg, 325 mg and 500 mg dosage units, and in caplet form in 500 mg dosage units.
The enteric coating covers a core of aspirin and is designed to resist disintegration in the stomach, dissolving in the more neutral-to-alkaline environment of the duodenum. Such action helps to pro-

Continued on next page

SmithKline Beecham—Cont.

tect the stomach from injury that may result from ingestion of plain, buffered or highly buffered aspirin (see SAFETY).

Indications: 'Ecotrin' is indicated for:

- conditions requiring chronic or long-term aspirin therapy for pain and/or inflammation, e.g., rheumatoid arthritis, juvenile rheumatoid arthritis, systemic lupus erythematosus, osteoarthritis (degenerative joint disease), ankylosing spondylitis, psoriatic arthritis, Reiter's syndrome and fibrositis,
- antiplatelet indications of aspirin (see the ANTIPLATELET EFFECT section) and
- situations in which compliance with aspirin therapy may be affected because of the gastrointestinal side effects of plain, i.e., non-enteric-coated, or buffered aspirin.

Dosage: For analgesic or anti-inflammatory indications, the OTC maximum dosage for aspirin is 4000 mg per day in divided doses, i.e., up to 650 mg every 4 hours or 1000 mg every 6 hours.

For antiplatelet effect dosage: see the ANTIPLATELET EFFECT section.

Under a physician's direction, the dosage can be increased or otherwise modified as appropriate to the clinical situation. When 'Ecotrin' is used for anti-inflammatory effect, the physician should be attentive to plasma salicylate levels, and may also caution the patient to be alert to the development of tinnitus as an indicator of elevated salicylate levels. It should be noted that patients with a high frequency hearing loss (such as may occur in older individuals) may have difficulty perceiving the tinnitus. Tinnitus would then not be a reliable indicator in such individuals.

Inactive Ingredients: 81 mg: Carnauba Wax, D&C Yellow 10, FD&C Yellow 6, Hydroxypropyl Methylcellulose, Methacrylic Acid Copolymer, Microcrystalline Cellulose, Polyethylene Glycol, Polysorbate 80, Propylene Glycol, Silicon Dioxide, Starch, Stearic Acid, Talc, Titanium Dioxide, Triethyl Citrate.

325 mg and 500 mg: Carnauba wax, Colloidal Silicon Dioxide, FD&C Yellow #6, Hydroxypropyl Methylcellulose, Maltodextrin, Methacrylic Acid Copolymer, Microcrystalline Cellulose, Pregelatinized Starch, Propylene Glycol, Simethicone, Sodium Hydroxide, Sodium Starch Glycolate, Stearic Acid, Talc, Titanium Dioxide, Triethyl Citrate.

Bioavailability: The bioavailability of aspirin from 'Ecotrin' has been demonstrated in a number of salicylate excretion studies. The studies show levels of salicylate (and metabolites) in urine excreted over 48 hours for 'Ecotrin' do not differ statistically from plain, i.e., non-enteric-coated, aspirin.

Plasma studies, in which 'Ecotrin' has been compared with plain aspirin in steady-state studies over eight days, also demonstrate that 'Ecotrin' provides plasma salicylate levels not statistically different from plain aspirin.

Information regarding salicylate levels over a range of doses was generated in a study in which 24 healthy volunteers (12 male and 12 female) took daily (divided) doses of either 2600 mg, 3900 mg, or 5200 mg of 'Ecotrin'. Plasma salicylate levels generally acknowledged to be anti-inflammatory (15 mg/dL) were attained at daily doses of 5200 mg, on Day 2 by females and Day 3 by males. At 3900 mg, anti-inflammatory levels were attained at Day 3 by females and Day 4 by males.

Dissolution of the enteric coating occurs at a neutral-to-basic pH and is therefore dependent on gastric emptying into the duodenum. With continued dosing, appropriate plasma levels are maintained.

Safety: The safety of 'Ecotrin' has been demonstrated in a number of endoscopic studies comparing 'Ecotrin', plain aspirin, buffered aspirin, and highly buffered aspirin preparations. In these studies, all forms of aspirin were dosed to the OTC maximum (3900–4000 mg per day) for up to 14 days. The normal healthy volunteers participating in these studies were gastroscoped before and after the courses of treatment and 14-day drug-free periods followed active drug. Compared to all the other preparations, there was less gastric damage at a statistically significant level during the 'Ecotrin' courses. There was also statistically less duodenal damage when compared with the plain i.e., non-enteric-coated aspirin.

Details of studies demonstrating the safety and bioavailability of 'Ecotrin' are available to health care professionals. Write: Professional Services Department, SmithKline Beecham Consumer Healthcare, P.O. Box 1467, Pittsburgh, Pa. 15230.

Warnings: Children and teenagers should not use this product for chicken pox or flu symptoms before a doctor is consulted about Reye Syndrome, a rare but serious illness reported to be associated with aspirin. Do not take this product for pain for more than 10 days or for fever for more than 3 days, or in conditions affecting children under 12 years of age, unless directed by a doctor. If pain or fever persists or gets worse, if new symptoms occur, or if redness or swelling is present, consult a doctor because these could be signs of a serious condition. Do not take this product if you are allergic to aspirin, have asthma, have stomach problems that persist or recur, or if you have ulcers or bleeding problems unless directed by a doctor. If ringing in the ears or a loss of hearing occurs, consult a doctor before taking any more of this product. **Keep this and all drugs out of the reach of children.** In case of accidental overdose, seek professional assistance or contact a poison control center immediately. As with any medicine, if you are pregnant or nursing a baby, seek the advice of a health professional before using this product. **IT IS ESPECIALLY IMPORTANT NOT TO USE ASPIRIN DURING THE LAST 3 MONTHS OF PREGNANCY UNLESS SPECIFICALLY DIRECTED TO DO SO BY A DOCTOR BECAUSE IT MAY CAUSE PROBLEMS IN THE UNBORN CHILD OR COMPLICATIONS DURING DELIVERY.**

Drug Interaction Precaution: Do not take this product if you are taking a prescription drug for anticoalgulation (thinning of the blood), diabetes, gout, or arthritis unless directed by a doctor.

Professional Warning: There have been occasional reports in the literature concerning individuals with impaired gastric emptying in whom there may be retention of one or more enteric coated aspirin tablets over time. This unusual phenomenon may occur as a result of outlet obstruction from ulcer disease alone or combined with hypotonic gastric peristalsis. Because of the integrity of the enteric coating in an acidic environment, these tablets may accumulate and form a bezoar in the stomach. Individuals with this condition may present with complaints of early satiety or of vague upper abdominal distress. Diagnosis may be made by endoscopy or by abdominal films which show opacities suggestive of a mass of small tablets *(Ref.: Bogacz, K. and Caldron, P.: Enteric-coated Aspirin Bezoar: Elevation of Serum Salicylate Level by Barium Study. Amer. J. Med. 1987:83, 783-6.)*. Management may vary according to the condition of the patient. Options include: gastrotomy and alternating slightly basic and neutral lavage *(Ref.: Baum, J.: Enteric-Coated Aspirin and the Problem of Gastric Retention. J. Rheum., 1984:11, 250-1.)*. While there have been no clinical reports, it has been suggested that such individuals may also be treated with parenteral cimetidine (to reduce acid secretion) and then given sips of slightly basic liquids to effect gradual dissolution of the enteric coating. Progress may be followed with plasma salicylate levels or via recognition of tinnitus by the patient.

It should be kept in mind that individuals with a history of partial or complete gastrectomy may produce reduced amounts of acid and therefore have less acidic gastric pH. Under these circumstances, the benefits offered by the acid-resistant enteric coating may not exist.

Antiarthritic and Anti-inflammatory Indications: For rheumatoid arthritis, juvenile rheumatoid arthritis, systemic lupus erythematosus, osteoarthritis (degenerative joint disease), ankylosing spondylitis, psoriatic arthritis, Reiter's syndrome, and fibrositis.

Antiplatelet Effect: Aspirin may be recommended to reduce the risk of death and/or nonfatal myocardial infarction (MI) in patients with a previous infarction or unstable angina pectoris and its use in reducing the risk of transient ischemic attacks in men.

Aspirin is also indicated to reduce the risk of vascular mortality in patients with suspected acute MI. Indications for these conditions follow:

Aspirin for Myocardial Infarction

Indications: Recurrent Myocardial Infarction (MI) (Reinfarction) or Unstable Angina Pectoris: Aspirin is indicated to reduce the risk of death and/or nonfatal MI in patients with a previous MI or unstable angina pectoris.

Suspected Acute MI: Aspirin is indicated to reduce the risk of vascular mortality in patients with a suspected acute MI.

Clinical Trials: Recurrent MI (Reinfarction) and Unstable Angina Pectoris: The indication is supported by the results of six large, randomized multicenter, placebo-controlled studies involving 10,816, predominantly male, post-myocardial infarction (MI) patients and one randomized placebo-controlled study of 1,266 men with unstable angina (1–7). Therapy with aspirin was begun at intervals after the onset of acute MI varying from less than 3 days to more than 5 years and continued for periods of from less than 1 year to 4 years. In the unstable angina study, treatment was started within 1 month after the onset of unstable angina and continued for 12 weeks, and congestive heart failure were not included in the study.

Aspirin therapy in MI patients was associated with about a 20-percent reduction in the risk of subsequent death and/or non-fatal reinfarction, a median absolute decrease of 3 percent from the 12- to 22-percent event rates in the placebo groups. In aspirin-treated unstable angina patients the reduction in risk was about 50 percent, a reduction in event rate of 5 percent from the 10-percent rate in the placebo group over the 12-weeks of the study.

Daily dosage of aspirin in the post-myocardial infarction studies was 300 milligrams in one study and 900 to 1,500 milligrams in 5 studies. A dose of 325 milligrams was used in the study of unstable angina.

Suspected Acute MI: The use of aspirin in patients with a suspected acute MI is supported by the results of a large, multicenter 2 × 2 factorial study of 17,187 subjects with suspected acute MI (8). Subjects were randomized within 24 hours of the onset of symptoms so that 8,587 subjects received oral aspirin (162.5 milligrams, enteric-coated) daily for 1 month (the first dose crushed, sucked, or chewed) and 8,600 received oral placebo. Of the subjects, 8,592 were also randomized to receive a single dose of streptokinase (1.5 million units) infused intravenously for about 1 hour, and 8,595 received a placebo infusion. Thus, 4,295 subjects received aspirin plus placebo, 4,300 received streptokinase plus placebo, 4,292 received aspirin plus streptokinase, and 4,300 received double placebo.

Vascular mortality (attributed to cardiac, cerebral, hemorrhagic, other vascular, or unknown causes) occurred in 9.4 percent of the subjects in the aspirin group and in 11.8 percent of the subjects in the oral placebo group in the 35-day followup. This represents an absolute reduction of 2.4 percent in the mean 35-day vascular mortality attributable to aspirin and a 23 percent reduction in the odds of vascular death ($2p < 0.0001$).

Significant absolute reductions in mortality and corresponding reductions in specific clinical events favoring aspirin were found for reinfarction (1.5 percent absolute reduction, 45 percent odds reduction, $2p < 0.0001$), cardiac arrest (1.2 percent absolute reduction, 14.2 percent odds reduction, $2p < 0.01$), and total stroke (0.4 percent absolute reduction, 41.5 percent odds reduction, $2p < 0.01$). The effect of aspirin over and above its effect on mortality was evidenced by small, but significant, reductions in vascular morbidity in those subjects who were discharged.

The beneficial effects of aspirin on mortality were present with or without streptokinase infusion. Aspirin reduced vascular mortality from 10.4 to 8.0 percent for days 0 to 35 in subjects given streptokinase and reduced vascular mortality from 13.2 to 10.7 percent in subjects given no streptokinase.

The effects of aspirin and thrombolytic therapy with streptokinase in this study were approximately additive. subjects who received the combination of streptokinase infusion and daily aspirin had significantly lower vascular mortality at 35 days than those who received either active treatment alone (combination 8.0 percent, aspirin 10.7 percent, streptokinase 10.4 percent, and no treatment 13.2 percent). While this study demonstrated that aspirin has an additive benefit in patients given streptokinase, there is no reason to restrict its use to that specific thrombolytic.

Adverse Reactions: Gastrointestinal Reactions: Doses of 1,000 milligrams per day of aspirin caused gastrointestinal symptoms and bleeding that in some cases were clinically significant. In the largest post-infarction study (the Aspirin Myocardial Infarction Study (AMIS) with 4,500 people), the percentage incidences of gastrointestinal symptoms for the aspirin (1,000 milligrams of a standard, solid-tablet formulation) and placebo-treated subjects, respectively, were: stomach pain (14.5 percent; 4.4 percent); heartburn (11.9 percent; 4.8 percent); nausea and/or vomiting (7.6 percent; 2.1 percent); hospitalization for gastrointestinal disorder (4.8 percent; 3.5 percent). Symptoms and signs of gastrointestinal irritation were not significantly increased in subjects treated for unstable angina with 325 milligrams buffered aspirin in solution.

Bleeding: In the AMIS and other trials, aspirin-treated subjects had increased rates of gross gastrointestinal bleeding. In the ISIS-2 study (8), there was no significant difference in the incidence of major bleeding (bleeds requiring transfusion) between 8,587 subjects taking 162.5 milligrams aspirin daily and 8,600 subjects taking placebo (31 versus 33 subjects). There were five confirmed cerebral hemorrhages in the aspirin group compared with two in the placebo group, but the incidence of stroke of all causes was significantly reduced from 81 to 47 for the placebo versus aspirin group (0.4 percent absolute change). There was a small and statistically significant excess (0.6 percent) of minor bleeding in people taking aspirin (2.5 percent for aspirin, 1.9 percent for placebo). No other significant adverse effects were reported.

Cardiovascular and Biochemical: In the AMIS trial, the dosage of 1,000 milligrams per day of aspirin was associated with small increases in systolic blood pressure (BP) (average 1.5 to 2.1 millimeters), depending upon whether maximal or last available readings were used. Blood urea nitrogen and uric acid levels were also increased, but by less than 1.0 milligram percent.

Subjects with marked hypertension or renal insufficiency had been excluded from the trial so that the clinical importance of these observations for such subjects or for any subjects treated over more prolonged periods is not known. It is recommended that patients placed on long-term aspirin treatment, even at doses of 300 milligrams per day, be seen at regular intervals to assess changes in these measurements.

Sodium in Buffered Aspirin for Solution Formulations: One tablet daily of buffered aspirin in solutions adds 553 milligrams of sodium to that in the diet and may not be tolerated by patients with active sodium-retaining states such as congestive heart or renal failure. This amount of sodium adds about 30 percent to the 70- to 90-millieqivalents intake suggested as appropriate for dietary treatment of essential hypertension in the "1984 Report of the Joint National Committee on Detection, Evaluation, and Treatment of High Blood Pressure" (9).

Dosage and Administration: Recurrent MI (Reinfarction) and Unstable Angina Pectoris: Although most of the studies used dosages exceeding 300 milligrams, 2 trials used only 300 milligrams and pharmacologic data indicate that this dose inhibits platelet function fully. Therefore, 300 milligrams or a conventional 325 milligram aspirin dose is a reasonable, routine dose that would minimize gastrointestinal adverse reactions. This use of aspirin applies to both solid, oral dosage forms (buffered and plain aspirin) and buffered aspirin in solution.

Suspected Acute MI: The recommended dose of aspirin to treat suspected acute MI is 160 to 162.5 milligrams taken as soon as the infarct is suspected and then daily for at least 30 days. (One-half of a conventional 325-milligram aspirin tablet or two 80- or 81-milligram aspirin tablets may be taken.) This use of aspirin applies to both solid, oral dosage forms buffered, plain, and enteric-coated aspirin) and buffered aspirin in solution. If using a solid dosage form, the first dose

Continued on next page

SmithKline Beecham—Cont.

should be crushed, sucked, or chewed. After the 30-day treatment, physicians should consider further therapy based on the labeling for dosage and administration of aspirin for prevention of recurrent MI (reinfarction).

References: (1) Elwood, P.C. et al., "A Randomized Controlled Trial of Acetylsalicylic Acid in the Secondary Prevention of Mortality from Myocardial Infarction," British Medical Journal, 1:436–440, 1974.
(2) The Coronary Drug Project Research Group, "Aspirin in Coronary Heart Disease," Journal of Chronic Diseases, 29:625–642, 1976.
(3) Breddin, K. et al., "Secondary Prevention of Myocardial Infarction: A Comparison of Acetylsalicylic Acid, Phenprocoumon or Placebo," Homeostasis, 470:263–268, 1979.
(4) Aspirin Myocardial Infarction Study Research Group, "A Randomized, Controlled Trial of Aspirin in Persons Recovered from Myocardial Infarction," Journal of the American Medical Aassociation, 243:661–669, 1980.
(5) Elwood, P.C., and P.M. Sweetnam, "Aspirin and Secondary Mortality After Myocardial Infarction," Lancet, II:1313–1315, December 22–29, 1979.
(6) The Persantine-Aspirin Reinfarction Study Research Group, "Persantine and Aspirin in Coronary Heart Disease," Circulation, 62:449–461, 1980.
(7) Lewis, H.D. et al., "Protective Effects of Aspirin Against Acute Myocardial Infarction and Death in Men with Unstable Angina, Results of a Veterans Administration Cooperative Study," New England Journal of Medicine, 309:396–403, 1983.
(8) ISIS-2 (Second International Study of Infarct Survival) Collaborative Group, "Randomized Trial of Intravenous Streptokinase, Oral Aspirin, Both, or Neither Among 17,187 Cases of Suspected Acute Myocardial Infarction: ISIS-2," Lancet, 2:349-360, August 13, 1988.
(8) "1984 Report of the Joint National Committee on Detection, Evaluation, and Treatment of High Blood Pressure," United States Department of Health and Human Services and United States Public Health Service, National Institutes of Health, Publication No. NIH 84-1088, 1984.

"ASPIRIN FOR TRANSIENT ISCHEMIC ATTACKS"

Indication:
For reducing the risk of recurrent Transient Ischemic Attacks (TIA's) or stroke in men who have had transient ischemia of the brain due to fibrin platelet emboli. There is inadequate evidence that aspirin or buffered aspirin is effective in reducing TIA's in women at the recommended dosage. There is no evidence that aspirin or buffered aspirin is of benefit in the treatment of completed strokes in men or women.

Clinical Trials:
The indication is supported by the results of a Canadian study (1) in which 585 patients with threatened stroke were followed in a randomized clinical trial for an average of 26 months to determine whether aspirin or sulfinpyrazone, singly or in combination, was superior to placebo in preventing transient ischemic attacks, stroke or death. The study showed that, although sulfinpyrazone had no statistically significant effect, aspirin reduced the risk of continuing transient ischemic attacks, stroke or death by 19 percent and reduced the risk of stroke or death by 31 percent. Another aspirin study carried out in the United States with 178 patients, showed a statistically significant number of "favorable outcomes," including reduced transient ischemic attacks, stroke and death (2).

Precautions: Patients presenting with signs and/or symptoms of TIA's should have a complete medical and neurologic evaluation. Consideration should be given to other disorders that resemble TIA's. Attention should be given to risk factors: it is important to evaluate and treat, if appropriate, other diseases associated with TIA's and stroke, such as hypertension and diabetes.
Concurrent administration of absorbable antacids at therapeutic doses may increase the clearance of salicylates in some individuals. The concurrent administration of nonabsorbable antacids may alter the rate of absorption of aspirin, thereby resulting in a decreased acetylsalicylic acid/salicylate ratio in plasma. The clinical significance of these decreases in available aspirin is unknown.
Aspirin at dosages of 1,000 milligrams per day has been associated with small increases in blood pressure, blood urea nitrogen, and serum uric acid levels. It is recommended that patients placed on long-term aspirin treatment be seen at regular intervals to assess changes in these measurements.

Adverse Reactions:
At dosages of 1,000 milligrams or higher of aspirin per day, gastrointestinal side effects include stomach pain, heartburn, nausea and/or vomiting, as well as increased rates of gross gastrointestinal bleeding.

Dosage and Administration:
Adult dosage for men is 1,300 mg a day, in divided doses of 650 mg twice a day or 325 mg four times a day.

References:
(1) The Canadian Cooperative Study Group, "Randomized Trial of Aspirin and Sulfinpyrazone in Threatened Stroke," *New England Journal of Medicine,* 299:53–59, 1978.
(2) Fields, W. S., et al., "Controlled Trial of Aspirin in Cerebral Ischemia," *Stroke* 8:301–316, 1977."

How Supplied: 'Ecotrin' Tablets
81 mg in bottle of 36
325 mg in bottles of 100* and 250
500 mg in bottles of 60* and 150
'Ecotrin' Caplets
500 mg in bottles of 60.
*Without child-resistant caps.

TAMPER-RESISTANT PACKAGE FEATURES FOR YOUR PROTECTION:
- Bottle has imprinted seal under cap.
- The words ECOTRIN LOW or ECOTRIN REG or ECOTRIN MAX appear on each tablet or caplet (see product illustration printed on carton).
- **DO NOT USE THIS PRODUCT IF ANY OF THESE TAMPER-RESISTANT FEATURES ARE MISSING OR BROKEN.**

Comments or Questions? Call Toll-Free 800-245-1040 weekdays.

Shown in Product Identification Guide, page 520

FEOSOL® Caplets
Hematinic
Iron Supplement

Description: FEOSOL Caplets contain pure iron micro particles called carbonyl iron. Replacing FEOSOL Capsules, this advanced formula is specially designed to be well absorbed, gentle on the stomach and offers enhanced safety in the event of an accidental overdose. Each FEOSOL carbonyl iron caplet delivers 50 mg of pure elemental iron, the same amount of elemental iron contained in the 250 mg ferrous sulfate capsule. At equivalent doses, carbonyl iron and ferrous sulfate were shown to be equally efficacious in correcting hemoglobin, hematocrit and serum iron levels in iron-deficient patients[1].

Safety: According to the American Association of Poison Control Centers, iron containing supplements are the leading cause of pediatric poisoning deaths for children under six in the United States[2]. Widely used as a food additive, carbonyl iron must be gastrically solubilized before it can be absorbed, giving it lower toxicity and enhancing its safety versus any of the ferrous salts[3]. As a result, carbonyl iron presents less chance of harm from accidental overdose. In addition, at equivalent doses, carbonyl iron side effects are no greater than those experienced with ferrous sulfate[4].

Warnings: Do not exceed recommended dosage. The treatment of any anemic condition should be under the advice and supervision of a physician. Since oral iron products interfere with absorption of oral tetracycline antibiotics, these products should not be taken within two hours of each other. Occasional gastrointestinal discomfort (such as nausea) may be minimized by taking with meals. Iron containing medication may occasionally cause constipation or diarrhea.

Keep out of the reach of children. Contains iron, which can be harmful or fatal to children in large doses. In case of accidental overdose, seek professional assistance or contact a poison control center immediately. If you are pregnant or nursing a baby, seek the

advice of a health professional before using this product.

NUTRITION FACTS

Serving Size: 1 Tablet

Amount per Tablet	% Daily Value
Iron 50 mg	280%

Formula Ingredients: Lactose, Sorbitol, Carbonyl Iron, Hydroxypropyl Methylcellulose, Polydextrose, Crospovidone, Polyethylene Glycol, Magnesium Stearate, Stearic Acid, Triacetin, Titanium Dioxide, Maltodextrin, FD&C Blue #2, FD&C Red #40, FD&C Yellow #6.

Directions: Adults—one caplet daily or as directed by a physician. Children under 12 years: Consult a physician.

Tamper-Evident Feature: Each caplet is encased in a plastic cell with a foil back; do not use if cell or foil is broken.

References:

[1]Devasthali SD, Gordeuk VR, Brittenham GM, et al, "Bioavailability of Carbonyl Iron: A randomized, double-blind study." Eur J Haematology, 1991; 46:272–278.
[2]FDA Consumer; March 1996:7
[3]Heubers, JA, Brittenham GM, Csiba E and Finch CA. "Absorption of carbonyl iron." J Lab Clin Med 1986; 108:473–78.
[4]Devasthali SD, Gordeuk VR, Brittenham GM, et al, "Bioavailability of a Carbonyl Iron: A randomized, double-blind study." Eur J Haematology, 1991; 46:272–278.

Store at room temperature, avoid excessive heat (greater than 100°F) or humidity.

How Supplied: Boxes of 30 and 60 caplets in blisters

Comments or Questions? Call Toll-Free 1-800-245-1040 Weekdays.

SmithKline Beecham Consumer Healthcare, L.P.
Pittsburgh, PA 15230 Made in USA

Shown in Product Identification Guide, page 520

FEOSOL® ELIXIR
Iron Supplement

Description: 'Feosol' Elixir, an unusually palatable iron elixir, provides the body with ferrous sulfate—iron in its most efficient form. The standard elixir for simple iron deficiency and iron-deficiency anemia when the need for such therapy has been determined by a physician.

NUTRITION FACTS

Serving Size: 1 teaspoonful
Servings per Container: 94

Amount per teaspoonful	**% Daily Value**
Iron 44 mg	244%

Formula:
INGREDIENTS
Purified Water, Sucrose, Glucose, Alcohol 5%, Ferrous Sulfate, Citric Acid, Saccharin Sodium, FD&C Yellow #6, Flavors.

Directions: Adults—1 teaspoonful daily or as directed by a doctor. Children under 12 years—Consult a physician. Mix with water or fruit juice to avoid temporary staining of teeth; do not mix with milk or wine-based vehicles.

TAMPER-RESISTANT PACKAGE FEATURE:
IMPRINTED SEAL AROUND BOTTLE CAP: DO NOT USE IF BROKEN.

Warnings: Do not exceed recommended dosage. The treatment of any anemic condition should be under the advice and supervision of a physician. Since oral iron products interfere with absorption of oral tetracycline antibiotics, these products should not be taken within two hours of each other. Occasional gastrointestinal discomfort (such as nausea) may be minimized by taking with meals and by beginning with one teaspoonful the first day, two the second, etc., until the recommended dosage is reached. Iron-containing medication may occasionally cause constipation or diarrhea and liquids may cause temporary staining of the teeth (this is less likely when diluted). **Keep away from children. Close tightly. Contains iron, which can be harmful or fatal to children in large doses. In case of accidental overdose, seek professional assistance or contact a Poison Control Center immediately.** If you are pregnant or nursing a baby, seek the advice of a health professional before using this product.
Store at room temperature (59°–86°F). Protect from freezing.

How Supplied: A clear orange liquid in 16 fl. oz. bottle.

Also available: 'Feosol' Tablets, 'Feosol' Caplets

NOTE: There are other Feosol products. Make sure this is the one you are interested in.

Shown in Product Identification Guide, page 521

FEOSOL® TABLETS
Iron Supplement

Description: 'Feosol' Tablets provide the body with ferrous sulfate, iron in its most efficient form, for iron deficiency and iron-deficiency anemia when the need for such therapy has been determined by a physician. The distinctive triangular-shaped tablet has a coating to prevent oxidation and improve palatability.

NUTRITION FACTS

Serving Size: 1 Tablet

Amount per Tablet	**% Daily Value**
Iron 65 mg	361%

Formula: Each tablet contains 200 mg. of dried ferrous sulfate USP (65 mg. of elemental iron), equivalent to 325 mg. (5 grains) of ferrous sulfate USP: calcium sulfate, starch, glucose, hydroxypropyl methylcellulose, talc, stearic acid, polyethylene glycol, sodium lauryl sulfate, mineral oil, titanium dioxide, D&C Yellow 10, FD&C Blue 2.

Directions: Adults and children 12 years and over—One tablet daily or as directed by a physician. Children under 12 years—Consult a physician.

TAMPER-RESISTANT PACKAGE FEATURES:

- Bottle has imprinted seal under cap. Do not use if missing or broken.
- FEOSOL Tablets are triangular shaped (see product illustration printed on carton).

CAUTION: DO NOT USE THIS PRODUCT IF ANY OF THESE TAMPER-RESISTANT FEATURES ARE MISSING OR BROKEN.
Comments or Questions?
Call toll-free 800-245-1040 weekdays.

Warnings: Do not exceed recommended dosage. The treatment of any anemic condition should be under the advice and supervision of a physician. Since oral iron products interfere with absorption of oral tetracycline antibiotics, these products should not be taken within two hours of each other. Occasional gastrointestinal discomfort (such as nausea) may be minimized by taking with meals and by beginning with one tablet the first day, two the second, etc., until the recommended dosage is reached. Iron-containing medication may occasionally cause constipation or diarrhea. **Keep away from children. Close tightly. Contains iron, which can be harmful or fatal to children in large doses. In case of accidental overdose, seek professional assistance or contact a Poison Control Center immediately.** If you are pregnant or nursing a baby, seek the advice of a health professional before using this product.
Store at room temperature (59°–86°F). Not USP for dissolution.

How Supplied: Bottles of 100 tablets. Also available in Caplets and Elixir.

Shown in Product Identification Guide, page 521

GAVISCON® Antacid Tablets
[*găv 'ĭs-kŏn*]

Composition: Each chewable tablet contains the following active ingredients:
Aluminum hydroxide dried gel... 80 mg
Magnesium trisilicate .... 20 mg
and the following inactive ingredients: alginic acid, calcium stearate, flavor, sodium bicarbonate, starch (may contain cornstarch), and sucrose.

Actions: Unique formulation produces soothing foam which floats on stomach contents. Foam containing antacid precedes stomach contents into the esophagus when reflux occurs to help protect the sensitive mucosa from further irrita-

Continued on next page

SmithKline Beecham—Cont.

tion. GAVISCON® acts locally without neutralizing entire stomach contents to help maintain integrity of the digestive process. Endoscopic studies indicate that GAVISCON Antacid Tablets are equally as effective in the erect or supine patient.

Indications: GAVISCON is specifically formulated for the temporary relief of heartburn (acid indigestion) due to acid reflux. GAVISCON is not indicated for the treatment of peptic ulcers.

Directions: Chew two to four tablets four times a day or as directed by a physician. Tablets should be taken after meals and at bedtime or as needed. For best results follow by a half glass of water or other liquid. DO NOT SWALLOW WHOLE.

Warnings: Do not take more than 16 tablets in a 24-hour period or 16 tablets daily for more than 2 weeks, except under the advice and supervision of a physician. Do not use this product except under the advice and supervision of a physician if you are on a sodium-restricted diet. Each GAVISCON Tablet contains approximately 0.8 mEq sodium.

Drug Interaction Precaution: Antacids may interact with certain prescription drugs. If you are presently taking a prescription drug, do not take this product without checking with your physician or other health professional.
Store at a controlled room temperature in a dry place.
Keep this and all drugs out of the reach of children. In case of accidental overdose, seek professional assistance or contact a poison control center immediately.

How Supplied: Available in bottles of 100 tablets and in foil-wrapped 2s in boxes of 30 tablets.

Issued 2/87

Shown in Product Identification Guide, page 521

GAVISCON® EXTRA STRENGTH Antacid Tablets

[găv 'ĭs-kŏn]

Composition: Each chewable tablet contains the following active ingredients:
Aluminum hydroxide .... 160 mg
Magnesium carbonate .... 105 mg
and the following inactive ingredients: alginic acid, calcium stearate, flavor, sodium bicarbonate, and sucrose. May contain stearic acid. Contains sorbitol or mannitol. May contain starch.

Directions: Chew 2 to 4 tablets four times a day or as directed by a physician. Tablets should be taken after meals and at bedtime or as needed. For best results follow by a half glass of water or other liquid. DO NOT SWALLOW WHOLE.

Indications: For the relief of heartburn, sour stomach, acid indigestion and upset stomach associated with these conditions.

Warnings: Do not take more than 16 tablets in a 24-hour period or 16 tablets daily for more than 2 weeks, except under the advice and supervision of a physician. Do not use this product except under the advice and supervision of a physician if you are on a sodium-restricted diet. Each tablet contains approximately 1.3 mEq sodium.

Drug Interaction Precaution: Antacids may interact with certain prescription drugs. If you are presently taking a prescription drug, do not take this product without checking with you physician or other health professional.
Store at a controlled room temperature in a dry place.
Keep this and all drugs out of the reach of children.
In case of accidental overdose, seek professional assistance or contact a poison control center immediately.

How Supplied: Available in bottles of 100 tablets and in foil-wrapped 2s in boxes of 30.

Shown in Product Identification Guide, page 521

GAVISCON® EXTRA STRENGTH Liquid Antacid

[găv 'ĭs-kŏn]

Composition: Each 2 teaspoonfuls (10 mL) contains the following active ingredients:
Aluminum hydroxide................. 508 mg
Magnesium carbonate................ 475 mg
And the following inactive ingredients: benzyl alcohol, edetate disodium, flavor, glycerin, saccharin sodium, simethicone emulsion, sodium alginate, sorbitol solution, water, and xanthan gum.

Indications: For the relief of heartburn, sour stomach, acid indigestion & upset stomach associated with these conditions.

Directions: **SHAKE WELL BEFORE USING.** Take 2 to 4 teaspoonfuls four times a day or as directed by a physician. GAVISCON Extra Strength Relief Formula Liquid should be taken after meals and at bedtime, followed by half a glass of water. Dispense product only by spoon or other measuring device.

Warnings: Except under the advice and supervision of a physician, do not take more than 16 teaspoonfuls in a 24-hour period or 16 teaspoonfuls daily for more than 2 weeks. May have laxative effect. Do not use this product if you have a kidney disease; do not use this product if you are on a sodium-restricted diet. Each teaspoonful contains approximately 0.9 mEq sodium.

Drug Interaction Precaution: Antacids may interact with certain prescription drugs. If you are presently taking a prescription drug, do not take this product without checking with your physician or other health professional.
Keep tightly closed. Avoid freezing. Store at a controlled room temperature.
Keep this and all drugs out of the reach of children.
In case of accidental overdose, seek professional assistance or contact a poison control center immediately.

How Supplied: Available in 12 fl oz (355 mL) bottles.

Shown in Product Identification Guide, page 521

GAVISCON® Liquid Antacid

[găv 'ĭs-kŏn]

Composition: Each tablespoonful (15 ml) contains the following active ingredients:
Aluminum hydroxide .... 95 mg
Magnesium carbonate .... 358 mg
And the following inactive ingredients: benzyl alcohol, D&C Yellow #10, edetate disodium, FD&C Blue #1, flavor, glycerin, saccharin sodium, sodium alginate, sorbitol solution, water, and xanthan gum.

Indications: For the relief of heartburn, sour stomach, acid indigestion & upset stomach associated with these conditions.

Directions: **SHAKE WELL BEFORE USING.** Take 1 or 2 tablespoonfuls four times a day or as directed by a physician. GAVISCON Liquid should be taken after meals and at bedtime, followed by half a glass of water. Dispense product only by spoon or other measuring device.

Warnings: Except under the advice and supervision of a physician, do not take more than 8 tablespoonfuls in a 24-hour period or 8 tablespoonfuls daily for more than 2 weeks. May have laxative effect. Do not use this product if you have a kidney disease; do not use this product if you are on a sodium-restricted diet. Each tablespoonful of GAVISCON Liquid contains approximately 1.7 mEq sodium.

Drug Interaction Precaution: Antacids may interact with certain prescription drugs. If you are presently taking a prescription drug, do not take this product without checking with your physician or other health professional.
Keep tightly closed. Avoid freezing. Store at a controlled room temperature.
Keep this and all drugs out of the reach of children.
In case of accidental overdose, seek professional assistance or contact a poison control center immediately.

How Supplied: Bottles of 12 fluid ounce (355 ml).

Shown in Product Identification Guide, page 521

GAVISCON®-2 Antacid Tablets

[găv 'ĭs-kŏn]

Composition: Each chewable tablet contains the following active ingredients:

Aluminum hydroxide dried gel...160 mg
Magnesium trisilicate .... 40 mg
and the following inactive ingredients: alginic acid, calcium stearate, flavor, sodium bicarbonate, starch (may contain cornstarch), and sucrose.

Indications: GAVISCON® is specifically formulated for the temporary relief of heartburn (acid indigestion) due to acid reflux. GAVISCON is not indicated for the treatment of peptic ulcers.

Directions: Chew one to two tablets four times a day or as directed by a physician. Tablets should be taken after meals and at bedtime or as needed. For best results follow by a half glass of water or other liquid. DO NOT SWALLOW WHOLE.

Warnings: Do not take more than eight tablets in a 24-hour period or eight tablets daily for more than 2 weeks, except under the advice and supervision of a physician. Do not use this product except under the advice and supervision of a physician if you are on a sodium-restricted diet. Each GAVISCON-2 Tablet contains approximately 1.6 mEq sodium.

Drug Interaction Precaution: Antacids may interact with certain prescription drugs. If you are presently taking a prescription drug, do not take this product without checking with your physician or other health professional.
Store at a controlled room temperature in a dry place.
Keep this and all drugs out of the reach of children. In case of accidental overdose, seek professional assistance or contact a poison control center immediately.

How Supplied: Boxes of 48 foil-wrapped tablets.

Issued 2/87

GLY-OXIDE® Liquid

Description: GLY-OXIDE® Liquid contains carbamide peroxide 10%.

Actions: GLY-OXIDE® Liquid has an oxygen-rich formula that works to relieve the pain of canker sores by cleaning and debriding damaged tissue so natural healing can occur. GLY-OXIDE Liquid's dense oxygenating microfoam helps destroy odor-forming germs and flushes out food particles that ordinary brushing can miss.

Administration: Do not dilute. Apply directly from bottle. Replace tip on bottle when not in use.

Indications and Usage: For local treatment and hygienic prevention of minor oral inflammation such as canker sores, denture irritation, and postdental procedure irritation. Place several drops on affected area four times daily, after meals and at bedtime, or as directed by a dentist or physician; expectorate after two or three minutes. Or place 10 drops onto tongue, mix with saliva, swish for several minutes, and expectorate.
As an adjunct to oral hygiene (orthodontics, dental appliances) after regular brushing, swish 10 or more drops vigorously. Continue for two to three minutes; expectorate.
When normal oral hygiene is inadequate or impossible (total care geriatrics, etc), swish 10 or more drops vigorously after meals and expectorate.

Precautions: Severe or persistent oral inflammation, denture irritation, or gingivitis may be serious. If these conditions or unexpected side effects occur, consult a dentist or physician immediately.
Avoid contact with eyes. Protect from heat and direct light. Keep this and all drugs out of the reach of children. In case of accidental overdose, seek professional assistance or contact a poison control center immediately.

How Supplied: GLY-OXIDE® Liquid is available in ½-fl-oz and 2-fl-oz non-spill, plastic squeeze bottles with applicator spouts.

Shown in Product Identification Guide, page 521

MASSENGILL® Douches, Towelettes and Cleansing Wash
[mas 'sen-gil]

PRODUCT OVERVIEW

Key Facts: Massengill is the brand name for a line of douches which are recommended for routine cleansing and for temporary relief of vaginal itching and irritation. Massengill disposable douches are available in two Vinegar & Water formulas (Extra Mild and Extra Cleansing), a Baking Soda formula, four Cosmetic solutions (Country Flowers, Fresh Baby Powder Scent, Mountain Breeze, and Spring Rain Freshness), and a Medicated formula (with povidone-iodine). Massengill also is available in a Non-Medicated liquid concentrate and powder form. Massengill also has products specially designed to safely and gently cleanse the external vaginal area: Massengill Soft Cloth Towelettes (Unscented and Baby Powder), Massengill Medicated Soft Cloth Towelettes and Massingill Feminine Cleansing Wash.

Major Uses: Massengill's Vinegar & Water, Baking Soda & Water, and Cosmetic douches are recommended for routine douching, or for cleansing following menstruation, prescribed use of vaginal medication or use of contraceptives. Massengill Medicated is recommended in a seven day regimen for the symptomatic relief of minor itching and irritation associated with vaginitis due to Candida albicans, Trichomonas vaginalis, and Gardnerella vaginalis. Massengill Feminine Cleansing Wash is a gentle soapfree way to clean the external vaginal area. Massengill Non-medicated Soft Cloth Towelettes are a convenient and portable way to cleanse the external vaginal area and wash odor away. Massengill Medicated Soft Cloth Towelettes provide temporary relief of minor external itching associated with irritation or skin rashes.

Safety Information: Do not douche during pregnancy unless directed by a physician. Douching does not prevent pregnancy. Do not use this product and consult your physician if you are experiencing any of the following symptoms: unusual vaginal discharge, vaginal bleeding, painful and/or frequent urination, lower abdominal/pelvis pain, or you or your sex partner has genital sores or ulcers.
Massengill Vinegar & Water, Baking Soda & Water, and Cosmetic Douches—If vaginal dryness or irritation occurs, discontinue use.
Massengill Medicated — Women with iodine-sensitivity should not use this product. If symptoms persist after seven days, or if redness, swelling or pain develop, consult a physician. Do not use while nursing unless directed by a physician.

PRODUCT INFORMATION

MASSENGILL®
[mas 'sen-gil]
Disposable Douches

MASSENGILL®
Liquid Concentrate
MASSENGILL® Powder

Ingredients: DISPOSABLES: Extra Mild Vinegar and Water—Purified Water and Vinegar.
Extra Cleansing Vinegar and Water—Purified Water, Vinegar, Puraclean™ (Cetylpyridinium Chloride), Diazolidinyl Urea, Disodium EDTA.
*Puraclean is a trademark for cetylpyridinium chloride, a safe, special cleansing ingredient not found in any other vinegar & water douche.
Baking Soda and Water—Sanitized Water, Sodium Bicarbonate (Baking Soda).
Fresh Baby Powder Scent—Water, SD Alcohol 40, Lactic Acid, Sodium Lactate, Octoxynol-9, Cetylpyridinium Chloride, Propylene Glycol (and) Diazolidinyl Urea (and) Methylparaben (and) Propylparaben, Disodium EDTA, Fragrance, FD&C Blue #1.
Country Flowers—Water, SD Alcohol 40, Lactic Acid, Sodium Lactate, Octoxynol-9, Cetylpyridinium Chloride, Propylene Glycol (and) Diazolidinyl Urea (and), Methylparaben (and) Propylparaben, Disodium EDTA, Fragrance, D&C Red #28, FD&C Blue #1.
Mountain Breeze—Water, SD Alcohol 40, Lactic Acid, Sodium Lactate, Octoxynol-9, Cetylpyridinium Chloride, Propylene Glycol (and) Diazolidinyl Urea (and) Methylparaben (and) Propylparaben, Disodium EDTA, Fragrance, D&C Yellow #10, FD&C Blue #1.
Spring Rain Freshness—Water, SD Alcohol 40, Lactic Acid, Sodium Lactate, Octoxynol-9, Cetylpyridinium Chloride, Propylene Glycol (and) Diazolidinyl Urea (and) Methylparaben (and) Propylparaben, Disodium EDTA, Fragrance.
LIQUID CONCENTRATE: Water, SD Alcohol 40, Lactic Acid, Sodium Bicar-

Continued on next page

SmithKline Beecham—Cont.

bonate, Octoxynol-9, Methyl Salicylate, Eucalyptol, Menthol, Thymol, D&C Yellow #10, FD&C Yellow #6 (Sunset Yellow).
POWDER: Sodium Chloride, Ammonium alum, PEG-8, Phenol, Methyl Salicylate, Eucalyptus Oil, Menthol, Thymol, D&C Yellow #10, FD&C Yellow #6 (Sunset Yellow).

Indications: Recommended for routine cleansing at the end of menstruation, after use of contraceptive creams or jellies (check the contraceptive package instructions first) or to rinse out the residue of prescribed vaginal medication (as directed by physician).

Actions: The buffered acid solutions of Massengill Douches are valuable adjuncts to specific vaginal therapy following the prescribed use of vaginal medication or contraceptives and in feminine hygiene.

Directions: DISPOSABLES: Twist off flat, wing-shaped tab from bottle containing premixed solution, attach nozzle supplied and use. The unit is completely disposable.
LIQUID CONCENTRATE: Fill cap 3/4 full, to measuring line, and pour contents into douche bag containing 1 quart of warm water. Mix thoroughly.
POWDER Packettes: Dissolve the contents of 1 packet in a quart of warm water. Mix thoroughly in a separate container or douche bag.
Container: Dissolve two rounded teaspoonfuls in a douche bag containing 1 quart of warm water. Mix thoroughly.

Warning: Douching does not prevent pregnancy. Do not use during pregnancy except under the advice and supervision of your physician. If vaginal dryness or irritation occurs, discontinue use. Use this product only as directed for routine cleansing. You should douche no more than twice a week except on the advice of your doctor.
An association has been reported between douching and pelvic inflammatory disease (PID), a serious infection of your reproductive system which can lead to sterility and/or ectopic (tubal) pregnancy. PID requires immediate medical attention.
PID's most common symptoms are pain and/or tenderness in the lower part of the abdomen and pelvis. You may also experience a vaginal discharge, vaginal bleeding, nausea or fever. Other sexually transmitted diseases (STDs) have similar symptoms and/or frequent urination, genital sores, or ulcers. Douches should not be used for the self treatment of any STDs or PID. If you suspect you have one of these infections or PID, stop using this product and see your doctor immediately.
See the enclosed insert for important health information concerning sexually transmitted diseases and PID.

How Supplied: Disposable—6 oz. disposable plastic bottle.
Liquid Concentrate—4 oz. plastic bottles.
Powder—4 oz., Packettes—12's.

MASSENGILL Feminine Cleansing Wash
[*mas 'sen-gil*]

Ingredients: Water, sodium laureth sulfate, magnesium laureth sulfate, sodium laureth-8 sulfate, magnesium laureth-8 sulfate, sodium oleth sulfate, magnesium oleth sulfate, lauramidopropyl betaine, myristamine oxide, lactic acid, PEG-120 methyl glucose dioleate, fragrance, sodium methylparaben, sodium ethylparaben, sodium propylparaben, methylchloroisothiazolinone, methylisothiazolinone, D&C Red #33.

Indications: For cleansing and refreshing of external vaginal area.

Actions: Massengill feminine cleansing wash safely and gently cleanses the external vaginal area.

Directions: Pour small amount into palm of hand or wash cloth and lather into wet skin. Rinse clean. Safe to use daily. For external use only.

How Supplied: 8 fl. oz plastic flip-top bottle.

MASSENGILL®
[*mas 'sen-gil*]
Fragrance-Free Soft Cloth Towelette and Baby Powder Scent

Ingredients: Unscented
Water, Octoxynol-9, Lactic Acid, Sodium Lactate, Potassium Sorbate, Disodium EDTA, and Cetylpyridinium Chloride.
Baby Powder Scent
Water, Lactic Acid, Sodium Lactate, Potassium Sorbate, Octoxynol-9, Disodium EDTA, Cetylpyridinium Chloride, and Fragrance.

Indications: For cleansing and refreshing the external vaginal area.

Actions: Massengill Baby Powder Scent and Fragrance-Free Soft Cloth Towelettes safely cleanse the external vaginal area. The towelette delivery system makes the application soft and gentle.

Directions: Remove towelette from foil packet, unfold, and gently wipe. Throw away towelette after it has been used once.

How Supplied: Sixteen individually wrapped, disposable towelettes per carton.

MASSENGILL® Medicated
[*mas 'sen-gil*]
Disposable Douche

Active Ingredient: Cepticin™ (povidone-iodine)

Indications: For symptomatic relief of minor vaginal irritation or itching associated with vaginitis due to Candida albicans, Trichomonas vaginalis, and Gardnerella vaginalis.

Action: Povidone-iodine is widely recognized as an effective broad spectrum microbicide against both gram negative and gram positive bacteria, fungi, yeasts and protozoa. While remaining active in the presence of blood, serum or bodily secretions, it possesses virtually none of the irritating properties of iodine.

Warning: Douching does not prevent pregnancy. Do not use during pregnancy or while nursing except under the advice and supervision of your physician. If vaginal dryness or irritation occurs discontinue use. Use this product only as directed. Do not use this product for routine cleansing.
An association has been reported between douching and pelvic inflammatory disease (PID), a serious infection of your reproductive system, which can lead to sterility and/or ectopic (tubal) pregnancy. PID requires immediate medical attention.
PID's most common symptoms are pain and/or tenderness in the lower part of the abdomen and pelvis. You may also experience a vaginal discharge, vaginal bleeding, nausea or fever. Other sexually transmitted diseases (STDs) have similar symptoms and/or frequent urination, genital sores, or ulcers. Douches should not be used for self-treatment of any STDs or PID. If you suspect you have one of these infections or PID, stop using this product and see your doctor immediately.
See the enclosed insert for important health information concerning sexually transmitted diseases and PID.
Women with iodine sensitivity should not use this product.
Keep out of the reach of children.
Avoid storing at high temperature (greater than 100°F).
Protect from freezing.

Dosage and Administration: Dosage is provided as a single unit concentrate to be added to 6 oz. of sanitized water supplied in a disposable bottle. A specially designed nozzle is provided. After use, the unit is discarded. Use one bottle a day for seven days. Although symptoms may be relieved earlier, for maximum relief, treatment should be continued for the full seven days.

How Supplied: 6 oz. bottle of sanitized water with 0.17 oz. vial of povidone-iodine and nozzle.

Shown in Product Identification Guide, page 521

MASSENGILL® Medicated
[mas 'sen-gil]
Soft Cloth Towelette

Active Ingredient: Hydrocortisone (0.5%).

Inactive Ingredients: Diazolidinyl Urea, DMDM Hydantoin, Isopropyl Myristate, Methylparaben, Polysorbate 60, Propylene Glycol, Propylparaben, Sorbitan Stearate, Steareth-2, Steareth-21, Water.
Also available in non-medicated Baby Powder Scent and Unscented formulas to freshen and cleanse the external vaginal area.

Indications: For soothing relief of minor external feminine itching or other itching associated with minor skin irritations, and rashes. Other uses of this product should be only under the advice and supervision of a physician.

Action: Massengill Medicated Soft Cloth Towelettes contain hydrocortisone, a proven anti-inflammatory, anti-pruritic ingredient. The towelette delivery system makes the application soothing, soft, and gentle.

Warnings: For external use only. Avoid contact with eyes. If condition worsens, symptoms persist for more than seven days, or symptoms recur within a few days, do not use this or any other hydrocortisone product unless you have consulted a physician. If experiencing a vaginal discharge, see a physician. Do not use this product for the treatment of diaper rash.
Keep this and all drugs out of the reach of children. As with any drug, if pregnant or nursing a baby, seek the advice of a health professional before using this product. In case of accidental ingestion, seek professional assistance or contact a Poison Control Center immediately.

Directions: Adults and Children two years of age and older—apply to the affected area not more than three to four times daily. Remove towelette from foil packet, gently wipe, and discard. Throw away towelette after it has been used once. Children under 2 years of age: DO NOT USE.

How Supplied: Ten individually wrapped, disposable towelettes per carton.

EDUCATIONAL MATERIAL

"The facts about Vaginal Infections and STDs"
A guide for women on vaginal infections and sexually transmitted diseases (STDs).
Free to physicians, pharmacists and patients in Limited quantities by writing SmithKline Beecham Consumer Healthcare, L.P. or calling 1-800-233-2426.

"A Personal Guide to Feminine Freshness"
A pamphlet on vaginal infections, feminine hygiene and douching. (BiLingual) free to physicians, pharmacists and patients in limited quantities by writing SmithKline Beecham Consumer Healthcare, L.P. or calling 1-800-233-2426

N'ICE® Medicated Sugarless Sore Throat and Cough Lozenges
[nis]

Active Ingredient: Cherry—Each lozenge contains 5.0 mg. menthol in a sorbitol base. Citrus—Each lozenge contains 5.0 mg. menthol in a sorbitol base. Menthol Eucalyptus—Each lozenge contains 5.0 mg. menthol in a sorbitol base. Cool Peppermint—Each lozenge contains 5.0 mg. menthol in a sorbitol base. N'ICE 'N CLEAR Cherry Eucalyptus—Each lozenge contains 7.0 mg. menthol in a sorbitol base. N'ICE 'N CLEAR. Menthol Eucalyptus—Each lozenge contains 5.0 mg. menthol in a sorbitol base.

Inactive Ingredients: Cherry—Flavors, D&C Red 33, Sorbitol, Tartaric Acid, FD&C Yellow 6. Citrus—Citric Acid, Flavors, Saccharin Sodium, Sodium Citrate, Sorbitol, Yellow 10. Cool Peppermint—Blue #2, Flavor, Maltitol Solution, Sorbitol. N'ICE 'N CLEAR Cherry Eucalyptus—Flavors, D&C Red 33, Sorbitol, Tartaric Acid, FD&C Yellow 6. N'ICE 'N CLEAR Menthol Eucalyptus —Citric Acid, Flavors, Sorbitol.

Indications: Temporarily suppresses cough due to minor throat and bronchial irritation associated with a cold or inhaled irritants. Temporarily relieves minor sore throat pain.

Warnings: Do not exceed recommended dosage. Excess consumption may have a laxative effect. A persistent cough may be a sign of a serious condition. If cough persists for more than 1 week, tends to recur, or is accompanied by fever, rash, or persistent headache, consult a doctor. Do not take this product for persistent or chronic cough such as occurs with smoking, asthma, emphysema, or if cough is accompanied by excessive phlegm (mucus) unless directed by a doctor. If sore throat is severe, persists for more than 2 days, is accompanied or followed by fever, headache, rash, nausea, or vomiting, consult a doctor promptly. If sore mouth symptoms do not improve in 7 days or if irritation, pain, or redness persists or worsens, see your dentist or doctor promptly. Do not exceed recommended dosage. KEEP THIS AND ALL DRUGS OUT OF THE REACH OF CHILDREN.

Drug Interaction: No known drug interaction.

Dosage and Administration: Cherry, Citrus, Menthol Eucalyptus, Cool Peppermint, N'ICE 'N CLEAR Cherry Eucalyptus, N'ICE 'N CLEAR Menthol Eucalyptus—Adults and children six and older: Let lozenge dissolve slowly in the mouth. Repeat every hour as needed, or as directed by a doctor, up to 10 lozenges per day. Children under six years of age: Consult a doctor.

Professional Labeling: For the temporary relief of pain associated with tonsillitis, pharyngitis, throat infections or stomatitis.

How Supplied: Available in packages of 16 lozenges. N'ICE Cherry available in packages of 8 and 16 lozenges.

NICODERM® CQ™
Nicotine Transdermal System/Stop Smoking Aid
Available as:
Step 1 - 21 mg/24 hours
Step 2 - 14 mg/24 hours
Step 3 - 7 mg/24 hours

If you smoke: Over 10 cigarettes a Day:Start with Step 1

10 Cigarettes a Day or Less: Start with Step 2

WHAT IS THE NICODERM CQ PATCH AND HOW IS IT USED?
NicoDerm CQ is a small, nicotine containing patch. When you put on a NicoDerm CQ patch, nicotine passes through the skin and into your body. NicoDerm CQ is very thin and uses special material to control how fast nicotine passes through the skin. Unlike the sudden jolts of nicotine delivered by cigarettes, the amount of nicotine you receive remains relatively smooth throughout the 24 or 16 hours period you wear the NicoDerm CQ patch. This helps to reduce cravings you may have for nicotine.

Active Ingredient: Nicotine

Purpose: Stop Smoking Aid

Use: To reduce withdrawal symptoms, including nicotine craving, associated with quitting smoking.

Directions:
- Stop smoking completely when you begin using NicoDerm CQ.

NicoDerm CQ Program

STEP 1 (21 mg)	STEP 2 (14 mg)	STEP 3 (7 mg)
Initial Treatment Period	Step Down Treatment Period	
Weeks 1–6	Weeks 7–8	Weeks 9–10

- Light Smokers (10 cigarettes a day or less): Do not use STEP 1 (21 mg). Use STEP 2 (14 mg) for six weeks and STEP 3 (7 mg) for two weeks and then stop.
- STEPS 2 and 3 allow you to gradually reduce your levels of nicotine. Completing the full program will increase your chances of quitting successfully.
- A the end of 10 weeks (8 weeks for light smokers), stop using NicoDerm CQ. If

Continued on next page

SmithKline Beecham—Cont.

you still feel the need for NicoDerm CQ, talk with your doctor.

- Each day apply a new patch to a different place on skin that is dry, clean and hairless.
- You may wear the patch for 16 or 24 hours.
- If you crave cigarettes when you wake up, wear the patch for 24 hours.
- If you begin to have vivid dreams or other disruptions of your sleep while wearing the patch for 24 hours, try taking the patch off at bedtime (after about 16 hours) and putting on a new one when you get up the next day.
- Remove the used patch and put on a new patch at the same time every day. Do not leave patch on for more than 24 hours because it may irritate your skin and loses strength after 24 hours.
- Wash your hands after applying or removing NicoDerm QC.

WARNINGS:

- Keep this and all medication away from children and pets. Used patches have enough nicotine to poison children and pets. Fold sticky ends together and insert in the disposal tray in the box. For accidental overdose, seek professional assistance or contact a poison control center immediately.
- NicoDerm CQ can increase your baby's heart rate. First try to stop smoking without the nicotine patch. As with any drug, if you are pregnant or nursing a baby, seek the advice of a health professional before using this product.
- Do not smoke even when not wearing the patch. The nicotine in your skin will still be entering your bloodstream for several hours after you take off the patch.

DO NOT USE IF YOU

- Continue to smoke, chew tobacco, use snuff, or use nicotine or other nicotine containing products.

ASK YOUR DOCTOR BEFORE USE IF YOU

- Are under 18 years of age.
- Have heart disease, recent heart attack, or irregular heartbeat. Nicotine can increase your heart rate.
- Have high blood pressure not controlled with medication. Nicotine can increase blood pressure.
- Take prescription medicine for depression or asthma. Your prescription dose may need to be adjusted.
- Are allergic to adhesive tape or have skin problems, because you are more likely to get rashes.

STOP USE AND SEE YOUR DOCTOR IF YOU HAVE

- Skin redness caused by the patch that does not go away after four days, or if your skin swells or you get a rash.
- Irregular heartbeat or palpitations.
- Symptoms of nicotine overdose such as nausea, vomiting, dizziness, weakness and rapid heartbeat.

READ THE LABEL

Read the carton and the User's Guide before using this product. Keep the carton and User's Guide. They contain important information.

Inactive Ingredients: Ethylene vinyl acetate-copolymer, polyisobutylene and high density polyethylene between pigmented and clear polyester backings.
Do not store above 30°C (86°F).

TO INCREASE YOUR SUCCESS IN QUITTING:

1. You must be motivated to quit.
2. Complete the full treatment program, applying a new patch every day.
3. Use with a support program as described in the Users Guide.

USER'S GUIDE:

HOW TO USE NICODERM CQ TO HELP YOU QUIT SMOKING

KEYS TO SUCCESS

1) You must really want to quit smoking for NicoDerm QC to help you.
2) Apply a new patch every day.
3) NicoDerm CQ works best when used together with a support program.
4) If you have trouble using NicoDerm CQ, ask your doctor or pharmacist or call SmithKline Beecham at 1-800-834-5895 weekdays (10:00am - 4:30 pm EST).

SO YOU DECIDED TO QUIT

Congratulations. Your decision to stop smoking is one of the most important things you can do to improve your health. Quitting smoking is a two-part process that involves:
overcoming your physical need for nicotine, and breaking your smoking habit. Nico-Derm CQ helps smokers quit by reducing nicotine withdrawal symptoms. Many NicoDerm CQ users will be able to stop smoking for a few days but often will start smoking again. Most smokers try to quit several times before they completely stop. Your own chances of quitting smoking depend how strongly you are addicted to nicotine, how much you want to quit, and how closely you follow a quitting plan like the one that comes with NicoDerm CQ.

QUITTING SMOKING IS HARD!

If you find you cannot stop or if you start smoking again after using NicoDerm CQ please talk to a health care professional who can help you find a program that may work better for you. Breaking this addiction doesn't happen overnight. Because NicoDerm CQ provides some nicotine, the NicoDerm CQ patch will help you stop smoking by reducing nicotine withdrawal symptoms such as nicotine craving, nervousness and irritability. This User's Guide will give you support as you become a non-smoker. It will answer common questions about NicoDerm CQ and give tips to help you stop smoking, and should be referred to often.

WHERE TO GET HELP

You are more likely to stop smoking by using NicoDerm CQ with a support program that helps you break your smoking habit. There may be support groups in your area for people trying to quit. Call your local chapter of the American Lung Association (1-800-586-4872), American Cancer Society (1-800-227-2345) or American Heart Association (1-800-242-8721) for further information. If you find you cannot stop smoking or if you start smoking again after using NicoDerm CQ, remember breaking this addiction doesn't happen overnight. You may want to talk to a health care professional who can help you improve your chances of quitting the next time you try NicoDerm CQ or another method.

LET'S GET ORGANIZED

Your reason for quitting may be a combination of concerns about health, the effect of smoking on your appearance, and pressure from your family and friends to stop smoking. Or maybe you're concerned about the dangerous effect of second-hand smoke on the people you care about. All of these are good reasons. You probably have others. Decide your most important reasons, and write them down on the wallet card inside the back cover of the User's Guide. Carry this card with you. In difficult moments, when you want to smoke, the card will remind you why you are quitting.

WHAT YOU'RE UP AGAINST

Smoking is addictive in two ways. Your need for nicotine has become both physical and mental. You must overcome both addictions to stop smoking. So while NicoDerm CQ will lessen your body's physical addiction to nicotine, you've got to want to quit smoking to overcome the mental dependence on cigarettes. Once you've decided that you're going to quit, it's time to get started. But first, there are some important cautions you should consider.

SOME IMPORTANT CAUTIONS

This product is only for those who want to stop smoking. If you smoke, chew tobacco, use snuff or use nicotine gum or other nicotine containing products while using NicoDerm CQ, you may get a nicotine overdose. Ask your doctor before using NicoDerm CQ if you have heart disease, had a recent heart attack, irregular heartbeat. Nicotine can increase your blood pressure. If you take a prescription medication for asthma or depression, be sure your doctor knows you are quitting smoking. Your prescription medication dose may need to be adjusted. You should ask your doctor before using NicoDerm CQ if you are allergic to adhesive tape or have skin problems, because you are more likely to get rashes.
Nicotine can increase your baby's heart rate. First try to stop smoking without the nicotine patch. As with any drug, if you are pregnant or nursing a baby, seek the advice of a health professional before using this product. Ask your doctor be-

fore using NicoDerm CQ if you are under 18 years of age.

You should stop use and see your doctor if you have skin redness caused by the patch that does not go away after four days, or if your skin swells or you get a rash, or if you have irregular heartbeat or palpitations.

Also, stop use if you have symptoms of nicotine overdose. These may include nausea, vomiting, diarrhea, dizziness, weakness and rapid heartbeat. Also, seizures have been seen in children who swallowed cigarettes. They may have a similar reaction to nicotine patches.

Keep this and all drugs out of the reach of children and pets. Even used patches have enough nicotine to poison children and pets. Be sure to fold the sticky ends together and insert in the disposal tray provided in the box. In case of accidental overdose, seek professional assistance or contact a poison control center immediately.

LET'S GET STARTED

Becoming a non-smoker starts today. Your first step is to read through the entire User's Guide carefully.

First, check that you bought the right starting dose. If you smoke more than 10 cigarettes a day, begin with Step 1 (21 mg). As the carton indicates, light smokers should not use Step 1 (21 mg). They should start with Step 2 (14 mg). Light smokers are people who smoke 10 cigarettes or less a day. Throughout this User's Guide we will give specific instructions for light smokers.

Next set your personalized quitting schedule.

Take out a calendar that you can use to track your progress. Pick a quit date, and mark this on your calendar using the stickers in the middle of the User's Guide.

For people who smoke over 10 cigarettes a day:

STEP 1. Initial Treatment Period (weeks 1–6): 21 mg patches. Choose your quit date (it should be soon). This is the day you will quit smoking cigarettes entirely and begin using NicoDerm CQ to reduce your cravings for nicotine. Place the Step 1 sticker on this date. For the first six weeks you'll use the highest-strength (21 mg) NicoDerm CQ patches. Be sure to follow the directions on page 10 of the User's Guide.

Completing the full program will increase your chances of quitting successfully. This is done by changing over to the Step 2 (14 mg) patch for 2 weeks followed by a final 2 weeks with the Step 3 (7mg) patch. The four week step down treatment period allows you to gradually reduce the amount of nicotine you get, rather than stopping suddenly, and will increase your chances of quitting.

STEP 2. First step down treatment period (Weeks 7–8): 14 mg patches. Switching to Step 2 (14 mg) patches after 6 weeks begins to gradually reduce your nicotine usage. Place the Step 2 sticker on this date (the first day of week seven). Use the 14 mg patches for two weeks.

STEP 3. Final step down treatment period (Weeks 9–10): 7 mg patches. After eight weeks, nicotine intake is further reduced by moving down to Step 3 (7 mg) patches. Place the Step 3 sticker on this date (the first day of week nine). Use the 7 mg patches for two weeks.

See the chart in the "DIRECTIONS" section above for the recommended usage schedule for NicoDerm CQ. **Stop using NicoDerm CQ at the end of week 10.** If you still feel the need to use NicoDerm CQ after Week 10, talk with your doctor or health professional.

LIGHT SMOKER DIRECTIONS

Do not use Step 1 (21 mg). You should start with Step 2 (14 mg).

For LIGHT SMOKERS–People who smoke 10 cigarettes or less a day: Begin with STEP 2–Initial Treatment Period (Weeks 1–6): 14 mg patches.

Choose your quit date (it should be soon). This is the day you will quit smoking cigarettes entirely and begin using NicoDerm CQ to reduce your cravings for nicotine. Place the Step 2 sticker on this date. For the first six weeks, you'll use the Step 2 (14 mg) NicoDerm CQ patches. Be sure to follow the directions on page 10.

Continue with STEP 3–Step Down Treatment Period (Weeks 7–8): 7 mg patches.

Completing the full program will increase your chances of quitting successfully. This is done by changing over to the Step 3 (7mg) patches for 2 weeks. The two week step down treatment period allows you to gradually reduce the amount of nicotine you get, rather than stopping suddenly, and will increase your chances of quitting. Place the Step 3 sticker on the first day of week seven. Use the 7 mg patches for two weeks.

Light smokers should not use NicoDerm CQ for longer than 8 weeks. If you still feel the need to use NicoDerm CQ after 8 weeks, talk with your doctor.

PLAN AHEAD

Because smoking is an addiction, it is not easy to stop. After you've given up nicotine, you may still have a strong urge to smoke. Plan ahead NOW for these times, so you're not tempted to start smoking again in a moment of weakness. The following tips may help:

- Keep the phone numbers of supportive friends and family members handy.
- Keep a record of your quitting process. Track when you have a craving for nicotine if it occurs. If you smoke at all, write down what you think caused the slip.
- Put together an Emergency Kit that includes items that will help take your mind off occasional urges to smoke. You might include cinnamon gum or lemon drops to suck on, a relaxing cassette tape and something for your hands to play with, like a smooth rock, rubber band or small metal balls.
- Set aside some small rewards, like a new magazine or a gift certificate from your favorite store, which you'll 'give' yourself after passing difficult hurdles.
- Think now about the times when you most often want a cigarette, and then plan what else you might do instead of smoking. For instance, you might plan to take your coffee break in a new location, or take a walk right after dinner, so you won't be tempted to smoke.

HOW NICODERM CQ WORKS

NicoDerm CQ patches provide nicotine to your system—they work as a temporary aid to help you quit smoking by reducing nicotine withdrawal symptoms, including nicotine craving. NicoDerm CQ provides a lower level of nicotine to your blood than cigarettes, and allows you to gradually do away with your body's need for nicotine. Because NicoDerm CQ does not contain the tar or carbon monoxide of cigarette smoke, it does not have the same health dangers as tobacco. However, it still delivers nicotine, the addictive part of cigarette smoke. Nicotine can cause side effects such as headache, nausea, upset stomach and dizziness.

HOW TO USE NICODERM CQ PATCHES

Read all the following instructions, and the instructions on the outer carton, before using NicoDerm CQ. Refer to them often to make sure your're using NicoDerm CQ correctly. Please refer to the audio tape for additional help.

1. Stop smoking completely before you start using NicoDerm CQ.
2. To reduce craving and other withdrawal symptoms, use NicoDerm CQ according to the dosage schedule in the "directions" section above.

Insert used NicoDerm CQ patches in the child resistant disposal tray provided in the box—safely away from children and pets.

When to apply and remove NicoDerm CQ patches.

Each day apply a new patch to a different place on skin that is dry, clean and hairless. **You can wear a NicoDerm CQ patch for either 16 or 24 hours.** If you crave cigarettes when you wake up, wear the patch for 24 hours. If you begin to have vivid dreams or other disruptions of our sleep while wearing the patch 24 hours, try taking the patch off at bedtime (after about 16 hours) and putting on a new one when you get up the next day.

Do not smoke even when you are not wearing the patch.

Remove the used patch and put on a new patch at the same time every day. Applying the patch at about the same time each day (first thing in the morning, for instance) will help you remember when to put on a new patch. Do not leave the same NicoDerm CQ patch on for more than 24 hours because it may irritate your skin and because it loses strength after 24 hours. Do not use NicoDerm CQ continuously for more than 10 weeks (8 weeks for light smokers).

How to apply a NicoDerm CQ patch.

1. Do not remove the NicoDerm CQ patch from its sealed protective pouch until

Continued on next page

SmithKline Beecham—Cont.

you are ready to use it. NicoDerm CQ patches will lose nicotine to the air if you store them out of the pouch.

2. Choose a non-hairy, clean, dry area of skin. Do not put a NicoDerm CQ patch on skin that is burned, broken out, cut or irritated in any way. Make sure your skin is free of lotion and soap before applying a patch.
3. A clear, protective liner covers the sticky silver side of the NicoDerm CQ patch—the side that will be put on your skin. The liner has a slit down the middle to help you remove it from the patch. With the silver side facing you, put half the liner away from the NicoDerm CQ patch starting at the middle slit, as shown in the illustration above. Hold the NicoDerm CQ patch at one of the outside edges (touch the silver side as little as possible), and pull off the other half of the protective liner. Place this liner in the slot in the disposable tray provided in the NicoDerm CQ package where it will be out of reach of children and pets.
4. Immediately apply the sticky side of the NicoDerm CQ patch to your skin. **Press the patch firmly on your skin with the heel of your hand for at least 10 seconds.** Make sure it sticks well to your skin, especially around the edges.
5. Wash your hands when you have finished applying the NicoDerm CQ patch. Nicotine on your hands could get into your eyes and nose, and cause stinging, redness, or more serious problems.
6. After 24 or 16 hours, remove the patch you have been wearing. Fold the used NicoDerm CQ patch in half with the silver side together. Careful dispose of the used patch in the slot of the disposal tray provided in the NicoDerm CQ package where it will be out of the reach of children and pets. Even used patches have enough nicotine to poison children and pets. Wash your hands.
7. Chose a different place on your skin to apply the next NicoDerm CQ patch and repeat Steps 1 to 6. Do not apply a new patch to a previously used skin site for at least one week.

If your NicoDerm CQ patch gets wet during wearing. Water will not harm the NicoDerm CQ patch you are wearing if applied properly. You can bathe, swim or shower for short periods while you are wearing the NicoDerm CQ patch.

If your NicoDerm CQ patch comes off while wearing. NicoDerm CQ patches generally stick well to most people's skin, However, a patch may occasionally come off. If your NicoDerm CQ patch falls off during the day, put on a new patch, making sure you select a non-hairy, non-irritated area of the skin that is clean and dry. If the soap you use has lanolin or moisturizers, the patch may not stick well. Using a different soap may help. Body creams, lotions and sunscreens can also cause problems with keeping your patch on. Do not apply creams or lotions to the place on your skin where you will put the patch. If you have followed the directions and the patch still does not stick to you, try using medical adhesive tape over the patch.

Disposing of NicoDerm CQ patches. Fold the used patch in half with the silver side together. Carefully dispose of the patch in the disposal slot of the tray provided in the NicoDerm CQ package where it will be out of the reach of children and pets. Small amounts of nicotine, even from a used patch can poison children and pets. **Keep all nicotine patches away from children and pets.** Wash. YOUR HANDS AFTER DISPOSING OF THE PATCH.

If your skin reacts to the NicoDerm CQ patch. When you first put on a NicoDerm CQ patch, mild itching, burning or tingling is normal and should go away within an hour. If you remove a NicoDerm CQ patch, the skin under the patch might be somewhat red. Your skin should not stay red for more than a day after removing the patch. **If you get a skin rash after using a NicoDerm CQ patch, or if the skin under the patch becomes swollen or very red, call your doctor. Do not put on a new patch.**

Storage Instructions

Keep each NicoDerm CQ patch in its protective pouch, unopened, until you are ready to use it, because the patch will lose nicotine to the air if it's outside the pouch. Do not store NicoDerm CQ patches above 86°F (30°C) because they are sensitive to heat. Remember, the inside of your car can reach temperatures much higher than this. A slight yellowing of the silver side of the patch is normal. Do not use NicoDerm CQ patches stored in pouches that are damaged or open.

See the chare in the "**DIRECTIONS**" section above for the recommended usage schedule for NicoDerm CQ.

TIPS TO MAKE QUITTING EASIER

Within the first few weeks of giving up smoking, you may be tempted to smoke for pleasure, particularly after completing a difficult task, or at a party or bar. Here are some tips to help get you through the important first stages of becoming a non-smoker:

On Your Quit Date:

- Ask your family, friends and co-workers to support you in your efforts to stop smoking.
- Throw away all your cigarettes, matches, lighters, ashtrays, etc.
- Keep busy on your quit day. Exercise. Go to a movie. Take a walk. Get together with friends.
- Figure out how much money you'll save by not smoking. Most ex-smokers can save more than $1,000 a year on the price of cigarettes alone.
- Write down what you will do with the money you save.
- Know your high risk situations and plan ahead how you will deal with them.
- Visit your dentist and have your teeth cleaned to get rid of the tobacco stains.
- Use a whitening toothpaste to keep your new smile.

Right after Quitting:

- During the first few days after you've stopped smoking, spend as much time as possible at places where smoking is not allowed.
- Drink large quantities of water and fruit juices.
- Try to avoid alcohol, coffee and other beverages you associate with smoking.
- Remember that temporary urges to smoke will pass, even if you don't smoke a cigarette.
- Keep your hands busy with something like a pencil or a paper clip.
- Find other activities which help you relax without cigarettes. Swim, jog, take a walk, play basketball.
- Don't worry too much about gaining weight. Watch what you eat, take time for daily exercise, and change your eating habits if you need to.
- Laughter helps. Watch or read something funny.

WHAT TO EXPECT

Your body is now coming back into balance. During the first few days after you stop smoking, you might feel edgy and nervous and have trouble concentrating. You might get headaches, feel dizzy and a little out of sorts, feel sweaty or have stomach upsets. You might even have trouble sleeping at first. These are typical withdrawal symptoms that will go away with time. Your smoker's cough will get worse before it gets better. But don't worry, that's a good sign. Coughing helps clear the tar deposits out of your lungs.

After a week or two

By now you should be feeling more confident that you can handle those smoking urges. Many of your nicotine withdrawal symptoms have left by now, and you should be noticing some positive signs: less coughing, better breathing and an improved sense of taste and smell, to name a few.

After a month

You probably have the urge to smoke much less often now. But urges may still occur, and when they do, they are likely to be powerful ones that come out of nowhere. Don't let them catch you off guard. Plan ahead for these difficult times. Concentrate on the ways non-smokers are more attractive than smokers. Their skin is less likely to wrinkle. Their teeth are whiter, cleaner. Their breath is fresher. Their hair and clothes smell better. That cough that seems to make even a laugh sound more like a rattle is a thing of the past. Their children and others around them are healthier, too.

What To Do About Relapse.

What should you do if you slip and start smoking again? The answer is simple.

A lapse of one or two or even a few cigarettes should not spoil your efforts! Throw away your cigarettes forgive yourself and continue with the program. Listen to the Audio Tape again and re-read the User's Guide to ensure that you're using NicoDerm CQ correctly and following the other important tips for dealing with the mental and social dependence on nicotine. Your doctor, pharmacist or other health professional can also provide useful counseling on the importance of stopping smoking. You should consider them partners in your quit attempt.

What To Do About Relapse After a Successful Quit Attempt. If you have taken up regular smoking again, don't be discouraged. Research shows that the best thing you can do is to try again, since several quitting attempts may be needed before your're successful. And your

- Admit that you've slipped, but don't treat yourself as a failure.
- Try to identify the 'trigger' that caused you to slip, and prepare a better plan for dealing with this problem next time.
- Talk positively to yourself—tell yourself that you have learned something from this experience.
- Make sure you used NicoDerm CQ patches correctly.

Remember that it takes practice to do anything and quitting smoking is no exception.

WHEN THE STRUGGLE IS OVER

Once you've stopped smoking, take a second and pat yourself on the back. Now do it again. You deserve it. Remember now why you decided to stop smoking in the first place. Look at your list of reasons. Read them again. And smile. Now think about all the money you are saving and what you'll do with it. All the non-smoking places you can go, and what you might do there. All those years you may have added to your life, and what you'll do with them. Remember that temptation may not be gone forever. However, the hard part is behind you, so look forward with a positive attitude and enjoy your new life as a non-smoker.

QUESTIONS & ANSWERS

1. How will I feel when I stop smoking and start using NicoDerm CQ?
You'll need to prepare yourself for some nicotine withdrawal symptoms. These begin almost immediately after you stop smoking, and are usually at their worst during the first three or four days. Understand that any of the following is possible

- craving for nicotine
- anxiety, irritability, restlessness, mood changes, nervousness
- drowsiness
- trouble concentrating
- increased appetite and weight gain
- headaches, muscular pain, constipation, fatigue.

NicoDerm CQ reduces nicotine withdrawal symptoms such as irritability and nervousness, as well as the craving for nicotine you used to satisfy by having a cigarette.

2. Is NicoDerm CQ just substituting one form of nicotine for another?
NicoDerm CQ does contain nicotine. The purpose of NicoDerm CQ is to provide you with enough nicotine to reduce the physical withdrawal symptoms so you can deal with the mental aspects of quitting.

3. Can I be hurt by using NicoDerm CQ? For most adults, the amount of nicotine in the gum is less than from smoking. If you believe you may be sensitive to even this amount of nicotine, you should not use this product without advice from your doctor (see p. 4 of the User's Guide). There are also some important cautions in the User's Guide (See p. 4).

4. Will I gain weight? Many people do tend to gain a few pounds the first 8–10 weeks after they stop smoking. This is a very small price to pay for the enormous gains that you will make in your overall health and attractiveness. If you continue to gain weight after the first two months, try to analyze what you're doing differently. Reduce your fat intake, choose healthy snacks, and increase your physical activity to burn off the extra calories. Drink lots of water. This is good for your body and skin, and also helps to reduce the amount you eat.

5. Is NicoDerm CQ more expensive than smoking? The total cost of NicoDerm CQ for the twelve week program is similar to what a person who smokes one and a half packs of cigarettes a day would spend on cigarettes for the same period of time. Also use of NicoDerm CQ is only a short-term cost, while the cost of smoking is a long-term cost, because of the health problems smoking causes.

6. What if I slip up? Discard your cigarettes, forgive yourself and then get back on track. Don't consider yourself a failure or punish yourself. In fact, people who have already tried to quit are more likely to be successful the next time. **GOOD LUCK!**

For your family's protection, NicoDerm CQ patches are supplied in child resistant pouches. Do not use if individual pouch is damaged or open.
Manufactured by ALZA Corporation, Palo Alto, CA 94304 for SmithKline Beecham Consumer Healthcare, L.P.
Comments or Questions? Call 1–800–834–5895 Weekdays. (10 a.m.–4:30 p.m. EST).

- **Not for sale to those under 18 years of age.**
- **Proof of age required.**
- **Not for sale in vending machines or from any source where proof of age cannot be verified.**

Available as
NicoDerm CQ Step 1 (21 mg/24 hours)–7 Patches*
NicoDerm CQ Step 1 (21 mg/24 hours)–14 Patches*
NicoDerm CQ Step 2 (14 mg/24 hours)–7 Patches*
NicoDerm CQ Step 3 (7 mg/24 hours)–7 Patches**

* User's Guide, Audio Tape & Child Resistant Disposal Tray
** User's Guide, & Child Resistant Disposal Tray

Shown in Product Identification Guide, page 521

NICORETTE
Nicotine Polacrilex Gum/Stop Smoking Aid
Available in 2mg and 4mg Strength

If you smoke:
UNDER 25 CIGARETTES A DAY: Use 2 mg
OVER 24 CIGARETTES A DAY: Use 4 mg

Action: Stop Smoking Aid

Use:
- To reduce withdrawal symptoms, including nicotine craving, associated with quitting smoking.

Directions:
- Stop smoking completely when you begin using Nicorette.
- Read the enclosed User's Guide before using Nicorette.
- Use properly as directed in the User's Guide.
- Don't eat or drink for 15 minutes before using Nicorette or while chewing a piece.
- Use according to the following 12 week schedule:

Weeks 1 to 6	Weeks 7 to 9	Weeks 10 to 12
1 piece every 1 to 2 hours	1 piece every 2 to 4 hours	1 piece every 4 to 8 hours

- Do not exceed 24 pieces a day.
- Stop using Nicorette at the end of week 12. If you still feel the need for Nicorette, talk with your doctor.

Warnings:
- Keep this and all drugs out of the reach of children and pets. In case of accidental overdose, seek professional assistance or contact a poison control center immediately.
- Nicorette can increase your baby's heart rate; if you are pregnant or nursing a bay, seek the advice of a health professional before using this product.

DO NOT USE IF YOU
- Continue to smoke, chew tobacco, use snuff, or use a nicotine patch or other nicotine containing products.

ASK YOUR DOCTOR BEFORE USE IF YOU
- Are under 18 years of age.
- Have heart disease, recent heart attack, or irregular heartbeat. Nicotine can increase your heart rate.
- Have high blood pressure not controlled with medication. Nicotine can increase blood pressure.
- Have stomach ulcer or take insulin for diabetes.
- Take prescription medicine for depression or asthma. Your prescription dose may need to be adjusted.

STOP USE AND SEE YOUR DOCTOR IF YOU HAVE
- Mouth, teeth or jaw problems.

Continued on next page

SmithKline Beecham—Cont.

- Irregular heartbeat, palpitations.
- Symptoms of nicotine overdose such as nausea, vomiting, dizziness, weakness and rapid heartbeat.

READ THE LABEL

Read the carton and the User's Guide before taking this product. Do not discard carton or User's Guide. They contain important information.

[2 mg] Inactive Ingredients: Flavors, glycerin, gum base, sodium carbonate, sorbitol, sodium bicarbonate.

[4 mg] Inactive Ingredients: Flavors, glycerin, gum base, sodium carbonate, sorbitol, D&C Yellow 10.

Do not store above 86°F (30°C). Protect from light.

TO INCREASE YOUR SUCCESS IN QUITTING:

1. **You must be motivated to quit.**
2. **Use Enough** —Chew **at least 9 pieces** of Nicorette per day during the first six weeks.
3. **Use long enough** —Use Nicorette for the full 12 weeks.
4. **Use with a support program** as described in the enclosed User's Guide.

USER'S GUIDE:

HOW TO USE NICORETTE TO HELP YOU QUIT SMOKING

KEYS TO SUCCESS

1) You must really want to quit smoking for Nicorette to help you.
2) You can greatly increase your chances for success by using at least 9 to 12 pieces every day when you start using Nicorette.
3) You should continue to use Nicorette as explained in the User's Guide for 12 full weeks.
4) Nicorette works best when used together with a support program.
5) If you have trouble using Nicorette, ask your doctor or pharmacist or call SmithKline Beecham at 1-800-419-4766 weekdays (10:00am–4:30pm EST).

SO YOU DECIDED TO QUIT

Congratulations. Your decision to stop smoking is an important one. That's why you've made the right choice in choosing Nicorette gum. Your own chances of quitting smoking depend on how much you want to quit, how strongly you are addicted to tobacco, and how closely you follow a quitting program like the one that comes with Nicorette.

QUITTING SMOKING IS HARD!

If you've tried to quit before and haven't succeeded, don't be discouraged! Quitting isn't easy. It takes time, and most people try a few times before they are successful. The important thing is to try again until you succeed. This User's Guide will give you support as you become a non-smoker. It will answer common questions about Nicorette and give tips to help you stop smoking, and should be referred to often.

WHERE TO GET HELP

You are more likely to stop smoking by using Nicorette with a support program that helps you break your smoking habit. There may be support groups in your area for people trying to quit. Call your local chapter of the American Lung Association (1-800-586-4872), American Cancer Society (1-800-227-2345) or American Heart Association (1-800-242-8721) for further information. If you find you cannot stop smoking or if you start smoking again after using Nicorette, remember breaking this addiction doesn't happen overnight. You may want to talk to a health care professional who can help you improve your chances of quitting the next time you try Nicorette or another method.

LET'S GET ORGANIZED

Your reason for quitting may be a combination of concerns about health, the effect of smoking on your appearance, and pressure from your family and friends to stop smoking. Or maybe you're concerned about the dangerous effect of second-hand smoke on the people you care about. All of these are good reasons. You probably have others. Decide your most important reasons, and write them down on the wallet card inside the back cover of the User's Guide. Carry this card with you. In difficult moments, when you want to smoke, the card will remind you why you are quitting.

WHAT YOU'RE UP AGAINST

Smoking is addictive in two ways. Your need for nicotine has become both physical and mental. You must overcome both addictions to stop smoking. So while Nicorette will lessen your body's physical addition to nicotine, you've got to want to quit smoking to overcome the mental dependence on cigarettes. Once you've decided that you're going to quit, it's time to get started. But first, there are some important cautions you should consider.

SOME IMPORTANT CAUTIONS

This product is only for those who want to stop smoking. Do not smoke, chew tobacco, use snuff or nicotine patches while using Nicorette. If you have heart disease, a recent heart attack, irregular heartbeats, palpitations, high blood pressure not controlled with medication, stomach ulcer, or take insulin for diabetes, ask your doctor whether you should use Nicorette. As with any drug, if you are pregnant or nursing a baby, seek the advice of a health professional before using this product. If you take a prescription medication for asthma or depression, be sure your doctor knows you are quitting smoking. Your prescription medication dose may need to be adjusted. Those under 18 should use this product under a doctor's care. Symptoms of nicotine overdose may include vomiting and diarrhea. Young children are more likely to have additional symptoms, including weakness. Also, seizures have been seen in children who swallowed cigarettes. Keep this and all drugs out of the reach of children. In case of accidental overdose, seek professional assistance or contact a poison control center immediately.

LET'S GET STARTED

Becoming a non-smoker starts today. Your first step is to read through the entire User's Guide carefully. **Next, set your personalized quitting schedule.** Take out a calendar that you can use to track your progress, and identify four dates, using the stickers in the User's Guide.

STEP 1: Your quit date (and the day you'll start using Nicorette gum). Choose your quit date (it should be soon). This is the day you will quit smoking cigarettes entirely and begin using Nicorette to satisfy your craving for nicotine. For the first six weeks, you'll use a piece of Nicorette every hour or two. Be sure to follow the directions on pages 8 and 11 of the User's Guide. Place the Step 1 sticker on this date.

STEP 2: The day you'll start reducing your use of Nicorette. After six weeks, you'll begin gradually reducing your Nicorette usage to one piece every two to four hours. Place the Step 2 sticker on this date (the first day of week seven).

STEP 3: The day you'll further reduce your use of Nicorette. Nine weeks after you begin using Nicorette, you will further reduce your nicotine intake by using one piece every four to eight hours. Place the Step 3 sticker on this date (the first day of week ten). For the next three weeks, you'll use a piece of Nicorette every four to eight hours. **End of treatment: The day you'll complete Nicorette therapy. Nicorette** should not be used for longer than twelve weeks. Identify the date thirteen weeks after the date you chose in Step 1 and place the "EX-Smoker" sticker on your calendar.

PLAN AHEAD

Because smoking is an addiction, it is not easy to stop. After you've given up cigarettes, you will still have a strong urge to smoke. Plan ahead NOW for these times, so you're not defeated in a moment of weakness. The following tips may help:

- Keep the phone numbers of supportive friends and family members handy.
- Keep a record of your quitting process. Track the number of Nicorette pieces you use each day, and whether you feel a craving for cigarettes. If you smoke at all, write down what you think caused the slip.
- Put together an Emergency Kit that includes items that will help take your mind off occasional urges to smoke. Include cinnamon gum or lemon drops to suck on, a relaxing cassette tape and something for your hands to play with, like a smooth rock, rubber band or small metal balls.
- Set aside some small rewards, like a new magazine or a gift certificate from your favorite store, which you'll 'give' yourself after passing difficult hurdles.
- Think now about the times when you most often want a cigarette, and then plan what else you might do instead of smoking. For instance, you might plan to take your coffee break in a new location, or take a walk right after dinner, so you won't be tempted to smoke.

HOW NICORETTE GUM WORKS

Nicorette's sugar-free chewing pieces provide nicotine to your system—they work as a temporary aid to help you quit smoking by reducing nicotine withdrawal symptoms. Nicorette provides a lower level of nicotine to your blood than cigarettes, and allows you to gradually do away with your body's need for nicotine. Because Nicorette does not contain the tar or carbon monoxide of cigarette smoke, it does not have the same health dangers as tobacco. However, it still delivers nicotine, the addictive part of cigarette smoke. Nicotine can cause side effects such as headache, nausea, upset stomach and dizziness.

HOW TO USE NICORETTE GUM

Before you can use Nicorette correctly, you have to practice! That sounds silly, but it isn't.

Nicorette isn't like ordinary chewing gum. It's a medicine, and must be chewed a certain way to work right. Chewed like ordinary gum, Nicorette won't work well and can cause side effects. An overdose can occur if you chew more than one piece of Nicorette at the same time, or if you chew many pieces one after another. Read all the following instructions before using Nicorette. Refer to them often to make sure you're using Nicorette gum correctly. If you chew too fast, or do not chew correctly, you may get hiccups, heartburn, or other stomach problems.

1. Stop smoking completely before you start using Nicorette.
2. To reduce craving and other withdrawal symptoms, use Nicorette according to the dosage schedule on page 11 of the User's Guide.
3. Chew each Nicorette piece very slowly several times.
4. Stop chewing when you notice a peppery taste, or a slight tingling in your mouth. (This usually happens after about 15 chews, but may vary from person to person.)
5. "PARK" the Nicorette piece between your cheek and gum and leave it there.
6. When the peppery taste or tingle is almost gone (in about a minute), start to chew a few times slowly again. When the taste or tingle returns, stop again.
7. Park the Nicorette piece again (in a different place in your mouth).
8. Repeat steps 3 to 7 (chew, chew, park) until most of the nicotine is gone from the Nicorette piece (usually happens in about half an hour; the peppery taste or tingle won't return).

Throw away the used Nicorette piece, safely away from children and pets.

See the chart in the "**DIRECTIONS**" section above for the recommended usage schedule for Nicorette.

To improve your chances of quitting, use at least 9 pieces of Nicorette a day. Heavier smokers may need more pieces to reduce their cravings. Don't eat or drink for 15 minutes before using Nicorette or while chewing a piece. The effectiveness of Nicorette may be reduced by some foods and drinks, such as coffee, juices, wine or soft drinks.

HOW TO REDUCE YOUR NICORETTE USAGE

The goal of using Nicorette is to slowly reduce your dependence on nicotine. The schedule for using Nicorette will help you reduce your nicotine craving gradually. Here are some tips to help you cut back during each step:

- After a while, start chewing each Nicorette piece for only 10 to 15 minutes, instead of half an hour. Then gradually begin to reduce the number of pieces used.
- Or, try chewing each piece for longer than half an hour, but reduce the number of pieces you use each day.
- Substitute ordinary chewing gum for some of the Nicorette pieces you would normally use. Increase the number of pieces of ordinary gum as you cut back on the Nicorette pieces.

STOP USING NICORETTE AT THE END OF WEEK 12. If you still feel the need to use Nicorette after Week 12, talk with your doctor.

TIPS TO MAKE QUITTING EASIER

Within the first few weeks of giving up smoking, you may be tempted to smoke for pleasure, particularly after completing a difficult task, or at a party or bar. Here are some tips to help get you through the important first stages of becoming a non-smoker:

On your Quit Date:

- Ask your family, friends, and co-workers to support you in your efforts to stop smoking.
- Throw away all your cigarettes, matches, lighters, ashtrays, etc.
- Keep busy on your quit day. Exercise. Go to a movie. Take a walk. Get together with friends.
- Figure out how much money you'll save by not smoking. Most ex-smokers can save more than $1,000 a year.
- Write down what you will do with the money you save.
- Know your high risk situations and plan ahead how you will deal with them.
- Keep Nicorette gum near your bed, so you'll be prepared for any nicotine cravings when you wake up in the morning.
- Visit your dentist and have your teeth cleaned to get rid of the tobacco stains.

Right after Quitting:

- During the first few days after you've stopped smoking, spend as much time as possible at places where smoking is not allowed.
- Drink large quantities of water and fruit juices.
- Try to avoid alcohol, coffee and other beverages you associate with smoking.
- Remember that temporary urges to smoke will pass, even if you don't smoke a cigarette.
- Keep your hands busy with something like a pencil or a paper clip.
- Find other activities which help you relax without cigarettes. Swim, jog, take a walk, play basketball.
- Don't worry too much about gaining weight. Watch what you eat, take time for daily exercise, and change your eating habits if you need to.
- Laughter helps. Watch or read something funny.

WHAT TO EXPECT

Your body is now coming back into balance. During the first few days after you stop smoking, you might feel edgy and nervous and have trouble concentrating. You might get headaches, feel dizzy and a little out of sorts, feel sweaty or have stomach upsets. You might even have trouble sleeping at first. These are typical withdrawal symptoms that will go away with time. Your smoker's cough will get worse before it gets better. But don't worry, that's a good sign. Coughing helps clear the tar deposits out of your lungs.

After a Week or Two.

By now you should be feeling more confident that you can handle those smoking urges. Many of your withdrawal symptoms have left by now, and you should be noticing some positive signs: less coughing, better breathing and an improved sense of taste and smell, to name a few.

After a Month.

You probably have the urge to smoke much less often now. But urges may still occur, and when they do, they are likely to be powerful ones that come out of nowhere. Don't let them catch you off guard. Plan ahead for these difficult times. Concentrate on the ways nonsmokers are more attractive than smokers. Their skin is less likely to wrinkle. Their teeth are whiter, cleaner. Their breath is fresher. Their hair and clothes smell better. That cough seems to make even a laugh sound more like a rattle is a thing of the past. Their children and others around them are healthier, too.

What To Do About Relapse.

What should you do if you slip and start smoking again? The answer is simple. A lapse of one or two or even a few cigarettes has not spoiled your efforts! Discard your cigarettes, forgive yourself and try again. If you start smoking again, keep your box of Nicarette for your next quit attempt. If you have taken up regular smoking again, don't be discouraged. Research shows that the best thing you can do is to try again. The important thing is to learn from your last attempt.

- Admit that you've slipped, but don't treat yourself as a failure.
- Try to identify the 'trigger' that caused you to slip, and prepare a better plan for dealing with this problem next time.
- Talk positively to yourself—tell yourself that you have learned something from this experience.
- Make sure you used Nicorette gum correctly over the full 12 weeks to reduce your craving for nicotine.
- Remember that it takes practice to do anything, and quitting smoking is no exception.

Continued on next page

SmithKline Beecham—Cont.

WHEN THE STRUGGLE IS OVER
Once you've stopped smoking, take a second and pat yourself on the back. Now do it again. You deserve it. Remember now why you decided to stop smoking in the first place. Look at your list of reasons. Read them again. And smile. Now think about all the money you are saving and what you'll do with it. All the non-smoking places you can go, and what you might do there. All those years you may have added to your life, and what you'll do with them. Remember that temptation may not be gone forever. However, the hard part is behind you, so look forward with a positive attitude and enjoy your new life as a non-smoker.

QUESTIONS & ANSWERS

1. How will I feel when I stop smoking and start using Nicorette? You'll need to prepare yourself for some nicotine withdrawal symptoms. These begin almost immediately after you stop smoking, and are usually at their worst during the first three to four days. Understand that any of the following is possible

- craving for cigarettes
- anxiety, irritability, restlessness, mood changes, nervousness
- drowsiness
- trouble concentrating
- increased appetite and weight gain
- headaches, muscular pain, constipation, fatigue.

Nicorette can help provide relief from withdrawal symptoms such as irritability and nervousness, as well as the craving for nicotine you used to satisfy by having a cigarette.

2. Is Nicorette just substuting one form of nicotine for another? Nicorette does contain nicotine. The purpose of Nicorette is to provide you with enough nicotine to help control the physical withdrawal symptoms so you can deal with the mental aspects of quitting. During the 12 week program, you will gradually reduce your nicotine intake by switching to fewer pieces each day. Remember, don't use Nicorette together with nicotine patches or other nicotine containing products.

3. Can I be hurt by using Nicorette? For most adults, the amount of nicotine in the gum is less than from smoking. Some people will be sensitive to even this amount of nicotine and should not use this product without advice from their doctor. Because Nicorette is a gum-based product, chewing it can cause dental fillings to loosen and aggravate other mouth, tooth and jaw problems. Nicorette can also cause hiccups, heartburn and other stomach problems especially if chewed too quickly or not chewed correctly.

4. Will I gain weight? Many people do tend to gain a few pounds in the first 8–10 weeks after they stop smoking. This is a very small price to pay for the enormous gains that you will make in your overall health and attractiveness. If you continue to gain weight after the first two months, try to analyze what you're doing differently. Reduce your fat intake, choose healthy snacks, and increase your physical activity to burn off the extra calories.

5. Is Nicorette more expensive than smoking? The total cost of Nicorette for the twelve week program is about equal to what a person who smokes one and a half packs of cigarettes a day would spend one cigarettes for the same period of time. Also use of Nicorette is only a short-term cost, while the cost of smoking is a long-term cost, because of the health problems smoking causes.

6. What if I slip up? Discard your cigarettes, forgive yourself and then get back on track. Don't consider yourself a failure or punish yourself. In fact, people who have already tried to quit are more likely to be successful the next time.-

GOOD LUCK!

[End User's Guide]

To remove the gum, tear off a single unit.
Peel off backing starting at corner with loose edge.
Push gum through foil.
Blister Packaged for your protection. Do not use if individual seals are broken.
Manufactured by Pharmacia & Upjohn AB, Stockholm, Sweden for SmithKline Beecham Consumer Healthcare, LP Pittsburgh, PA 15230
Comments or Questions? Call 1-800-419-4766 weekdays.
(10 a.m.–4:30 p.m. EST).

- **Not for sale to those under 18 years of age.**
- **Proof of age required.**
- **Not for sale in vending machines or from any source where proof of age cannot be verified.**

Available as:
Nicorette 2 mg Gum—108 Pieces*
Nicorette 2 mg Gum—48 pieces (refill)
Nicorette 4 mg Gum—108 Pieces*
Nicorette 4 mg Gum—48 pieces (refill)
***User's Guide and Audio Tape included in Kit**

Shown in Product Identification Guide, page 521

NOVAHISTINE® DMX

[*nō″vă-hĭs′tēn*]

Cough/Cold Formula & Decongestant

Active Ingredients: Each 5 ml teaspoonful contains Dextromethorphan Hydrobromide 10 mg., Guaifenesin 100 mg., Pseudoephedrine Hydrochloride 30 mg.

Inactive Ingredients: Alcohol 10%, FD & C Red No. 40, FD & C Yellow No. 6, Flavors, Glycerin, Hydrochloric Acid, Invert Sugar, Saccharin Sodium, Sodium Chloride, Sorbitol and Water.

Indications: For temporary relief from cough and nasal congestion due to the common cold. Helps loosen phlegm (sputum) and thin bronchial secretions to rid the bronchial passageways of bothersome mucus. Helps decongest sinus openings and passages; temporarily relieves sinus congestion and pressure.

Warnings: If symptoms do not improve within 7 days or are accompanied by fever, consult a doctor. A persistent cough may be a sign of a serious condition. If cough persists for more than 7 days, tends to recur, or is accompanied by fever, rash, or persistent headache, consult a doctor. Do not take this product for persistent or chronic cough such as occurs with smoking, asthma, chronic bronchitis or emphysema, or where cough is accompanied by excessive phlegm (mucus) unless directed by a doctor. Do not take this product if you have heart disease, high blood pressure, thyroid disease, diabetes, or difficulty in urination due to enlargement of the prostate gland, unless directed by a doctor. **Do not exceed recommended dosage.** If nervousness, dizziness, or sleeplessness occur, discontinue use and consult a doctor. **KEEP THIS AND ALL DRUGS OUT OF THE REACH OF CHILDREN.** In case of accidental overdose, seek professional assistance or contact a Poison Control Center immediately. As with any drug, if you are pregnant or nursing a baby, seek the advice of a health professional before using this product.

Drug Interaction Precaution: Do not use this product if you are now taking a prescription monoamine oxidase inhibitor (MAOI) (certain drugs for depression, psychiatric or emotional conditions, or Parkinson's Disease), or for 2 weeks after stopping the MAOI drug. If you are uncertain whether your prescription drug contains an MAOI, consult a health professional before taking this product.

Contraindications: NOVAHISTINE DMX is contraindicated in patients with severe hypertension, severe coronary artery disease, and in patients on MAOI therapy. Patient idiosyncrasy to adrenergic agents may be manifested by insomnia, dizziness, weakness, tremor, or arrhythmias.
Nursing mothers: Pseudoephedrine is contraindicated in nursing mothers because of the higher than usual risk for infants from sympathomimetic amines.
Hypersensitivity: NOVAHISTINE DMX is contraindicated in patients with hypersensitivity or idiosyncrasy to sympathomimetic amines, dextromethorphan, or to other formula ingredients.

Adverse Reactions: Adverse reactions occur infrequently with usual oral doses of NOVAHISTINE DMX. When they occur, adverse reactions may include gastrointestinal upset and nausea. Because of the pseudoephedrine in NOVAHISTINE DMX, hyperreactive individuals may display ephedrine-like reactions such as tachycardia, palpitations, headache, dizziness or nausea. Sympathomimetic drugs have been associated with certain untoward reactions including fear, anxiety, tenseness, restlessness, tremor, weakness, pallor, respiratory difficulty, dysuria, insomnia, hal-

lucinations, convulsions, CNS depression, arrhythmias, and cardiovascular collapse with hypotension.
Note: Guaifenesin interferes with the colorimetric determination of 5-hydroxyindoleacetic acid (5-HIAA) and vanillylmandelic acid (VMA).

Directions For Use: Adults and children 12 years and older: 2 teaspoonfuls every 4 hours, not to exceed 8 teaspoonfuls in 24 hours, or as directed by a doctor. Children 6 to under 12 years: 1 teaspoonful every 4 hours, not to exceed 4 teaspoonfuls in 24 hours, or as directed by a doctor. Consult a doctor for the use in children under 6 years of age.

How Supplied: NOVAHISTINE DMX, in 4 fluid ounce bottles. Keep tightly closed. Protect from excessive heat and light. Avoid freezing.

NOVAHISTINE® Elixir

[*nō"vă-hĭs'tēn*]

Cold & Hay Fever Formula

Active Ingredients: Each 5 ml teaspoonful of NOVAHISTINE Elixir contains: Chlorpheniramine Maleate 2 mg. and Phenylephrine Hydrochloride 5 mg.

Inactive Ingredients: Alcohol 5%, D & C Yellow No. 10, FD & C Blue No. 1, Flavors, Glycerin, Sodium Chloride, Sorbitol and Water. Although considered sugar-free, each 5 ml contributes approximately 7 calories from sorbitol.

Indications: For the temporary relief of nasal congestion, runny nose, sneezing, itching of the nose or throat, and itchy watery eyes due to the common cold, hay fever, or other upper respiratory allergies.

Warnings: If symptoms do not improve within 7 days or are accompanied by a fever, consult a doctor. May cause excitability especially in children. Do not take this product, unless directed by a doctor, if you have a breathing problem such as emphysema or chronic bronchitis, or if you have heart disease, high blood pressure, thyroid disease, diabetes, glaucoma, or difficulty in urination due to enlargement of the prostate gland. May cause drowsiness; alcohol, sedatives, and tranquilizers may increase the drowsiness effect. Avoid alcoholic beverages while taking this product. Do not take this product if you are taking sedatives or tranquilizers, without first consulting your doctor. Use caution when driving a motor vehicle or operating machinery. **Do not exceed recommended dosage.** If nervousness, dizziness, or sleeplessness occur, discontinue use and consult a doctor. **KEEP THIS AND ALL DRUGS OUT OF THE REACH OF CHILDREN.** In case of accidental overdose, seek professional assistance or contact a Poison Control Center immediately. As with any drug, if you are pregnant or nursing a baby, seek the advice of a health professional before using this product.

Drug Interaction Precaution: Do not use this product if you are now taking a prescription monoamine oxidase inhibitor (MAOI) (certain drugs for depression, psychiatric or emotional conditions, or Parkinson's Disease), or for 2 weeks after stopping the MAOI drug. If you are uncertain whether your prescription drug contains an MAOI, consult a health professional before taking this product.

Contraindications: NOVAHISTINE Elixir is contraindicated in patients with severe hypertension, severe coronary artery disease, and in patients on MAOI therapy. Patient idiosyncrasy to adrenergic agents may be manifested by insomnia, dizziness, weakness, tremor, or arrhythmias.
NOVAHISTINE Elixir is also contraindicated in patients with narrow-angle glaucoma, urinary retention, peptic ulcer, asthma, emphysema, chronic pulmonary disease, shortness of breath, or difficulty in breathing.
Nursing Mothers: Phenylephrine is contraindicated in nursing mothers.
Hypersensitivity: NOVAHISTINE Elixir is also contraindicated in patients with hypersensitivity or idiosyncrasy to sympathomimetic amines, antihistamines, or to other formula ingredients.

Adverse Reactions: Drugs containing sympathomimetic amines have been associated with certain untoward reactions, including fear, anxiety, tenseness, restlessness, tremor, weakness, pallor, respiratory difficulty, dysuria, insomnia, hallucinations, convulsions, CNS depression, arrhythmias, and cardiovascular collapse with hypotension. Individuals hyperreactive to phenylephrine may display ephedrine-like reactions such as tachycardia, palpitations, headache, dizziness, or nausea.
Phenylephrine is considered safe and relatively free of unpleasant side effects when taken at recommended dosage. Patients sensitive to antihistamine drugs may experience mild sedation. Other side effects from antihistamines may include dry mouth, dizziness, weakness, anorexia, nausea, vomiting, headache, nervousness, polyuria, heartburn, diplopia, dysuria, and very rarely dermatitis.

Directions For Use: Adults (12 years and older): 2 teaspoonfuls every 4 hours, not to exceed 12 teaspoonfuls in 24 hours, or as directed by a doctor. Children 6 to under 12 years: 1 teaspoonful every 4 hours, not to exceed 6 teaspoonfuls in 24 hours, or as directed by a doctor. Consult a doctor for use in chldren under 6 years of age.

How Supplied: NOVAHISTINE Elixir, in 4 fluid ounce bottles. Keep tightly closed. Protect from excessive heat and light. Avoid freezing.

PANADOL®

Acetaminophen Tablets and Caplets

Description: Each Maximum Strength PANADOL Caplet or Tablet contains acetaminophen 500 mg.

Indications: For the fast, temporary relief of minor aches, and pains associated with headaches, backaches, muscle aches, toothache, menstrual pain and colds and flu. Also to reduce fever and for temporary relief of minor arthritis pain.

Directions: Adults and children 12 years and over: 2 tablets or caplets every 4 hours as needed, not to exceed 8 tablets or caplets in 24 hours or as directed by a doctor.
Children under 12 years: Consult a doctor.

Warnings: Do not take this product for pain for more than 10 days or for fever for more than 3 days unless directed by a doctor. If pain or fever persists or gets worse, if new symptoms occur, or if redness or swelling is present, consult a doctor because these could be signs of a serious condition. Keep this and all drugs out of the reach of children. In case of accidental overdose, seek professional assistance or contact a poison control center immediately. Prompt medical attention is critical for adults as well as for children even if you do not notice any signs or symptoms. As with any drug, if you are pregnant or nursing a baby, seek the advice of a health professional before using this product.

Active Ingredient: Acetaminophen 500 mg per tablet or caplet.

Inactive Ingredients: Hydroxypropyl Methylcellulose, Potassium Sorbate, Povidone, Pregelatinized Starch, Starch, Stearic Acid, Talc, and Triacetin.

How Supplied: Tablets (white with "P" and "500" imprint) in bottles of 30 and 60. Caplets (white with "P" and "500" imprint) in bottle of 24.

Shown in Product Identification Guide, page 521

Children's PANADOL®

Acetaminophen Chewable Tablets, Liquid, Drops

Description: Each Children's PANADOL Chewable Tablet contains 80 mg acetaminophen in a fruit-flavored sugar-free tablet. Children's PANADOL Acetaminophen Liquid is fruit-flavored, red in color, and is alcohol-free, sugar-free and aspirin-free. Each ½ teaspoonful contains 80 mg of acetaminophen. Infant's PANADOL Drops are fruit-flavored, red in color, and are alcohol-free, sugar-free and aspirin-free. Each 0.8 mL (one calibrated dropperful) contains 80 mg acetaminophen.

Indications: Acetaminophen, the active ingredient in Children's PANADOL,

Continued on next page

SmithKline Beecham—Cont.

is the analgesic/antipyretic most widely recommended by pediatricians for fast, effective relief of children's fevers. It also relieves the aches and pains of colds and flu, earaches, headaches, teething, immunizations, tonsillectomy, and childhood illnesses.

Children's PANADOL Tablets, Liquid, and Drops are aspirin-free and contain no alcohol or sugar. The pleasant-tasting formulations are not likely to upset or irritate children's stomachs.

Usual Dosage: Dosing is based on single doses in the range of 10–15 mg/kg body weight. Doses may be repeated every four hours up to 4 or 5 times daily, but not to exceed 5 doses in 24 hours. To be administered to children under 2 years only on advice of a physician.

Children's PANADOL Chewable Tablets: 2–3 yr, 24–35 lb, 2 tablets; 4–5 yr, 36–47 lb, 3 tablets; 6–8 yr, 48–59 lb, 4 tablets; 9–10 yr, 60–71 lb, 5 tablets; 11 yr, 72–95 lb, 6 tablets. May be repeated every 4 hours, up to 5 times in a 24-hour period.

Children's PANADOL Liquid: 4–11 mo, 12–17 lb, ½ teaspoonful; 12–23 mo, 18–23 lb, ¾ teaspoonful; 2–3 yr, 24–35 lb, 1 teaspoonful; 4–5 yr, 36–47 lb, 1½ teaspoonfuls; 6–8 yr, 48–59 lb, 2 teaspoonfuls; 9–10 yr, 60–71 lb, 2½ teaspoonfuls; 11 yr, 72–95 lb, 3 teaspoonfuls. May be repeated every 4 hours up to 5 times in a 24-hour period. May be administered alone or mixed with formula, milk, juice, cereal, etc.

Infant's PANADOL Drops: 0–3 mo, 6–11 lb, ½ dropperful (0.4 mL); 4–11 mo, 12–17 lb, 1 dropperful (0.8 mL); 12–23 mo, 18–23 lb, 1½ dropperfuls (1.2 mL); 2–3 yr, 24–35 lb, 2 dropperfuls (1.6 mL); 4–5 yr, 36–47 lb, 3 dropperfuls (2.4 mL); 6–8 yr, 48–59 lb, 4 dropperfuls (3.2 mL). May be repeated every 4 hours, up to 5 times in a 24-hour period. May be administered alone or mixed with formula, milk, juice, cereal, etc.

Warnings: Do not give this product for pain for more than 5 days or for fever for more than 3 days unless directed by a doctor. If pain or fever persists or gets worse, if new symptoms occur, or if redness or swelling is present, consult a doctor because these could be signs of a serious condition. Keep this and all drugs out of the reach of children. In case of accidental overdose, seek professional assistance or contact a poison control center immediately. Prompt medical attention is critical for adults as well as for children even if you do not notice any signs or symptoms. As with any drug, if you are pregnant or nursing a baby, seek the advice of a health professional before using this product.

Composition:

Chewable Tablets: Active Ingredient: Acetaminophen, 80 mg per tablet. Inactive Ingredients: FD&C Red No. 28, FD&C Red No. 40, flavor, Mannitol, Saccharin Sodium, Starch, Stearic Acid and other ingredients.

Liquid: Active Ingredient: Acetaminophen, 80 mg per ½ teaspoon. Inactive Ingredients: Benzoic acid, FD&C Red No. 40, Flavor, Glycerin, Polyethylene Glycol, Potassium Sorbate, Propylene Glycol, Purified Water, Saccharin Sodium, Sorbitol solution. May also contain Sodium Chloride or Sodium Hydroxide.

Drops: Active Ingredient: Acetaminophen, 80 mg per 0.8mL dropper. Inactive Ingredients: Citric Acid, FD&C Red No. 40, Flavors, Glycerin, Parabens, Polyethylene Glycol, Propylene Glycol, Purified Water, Saccharin Sodium, Sodium Chloride, Sodium Citrate.

How Supplied: Chewable Tablets (colored pink and scored)—bottles of 30. Liquid (colored red)—bottles of 2 fl. oz. and 4 fl. oz. Drops (colored red)—bottles of ½ oz. (15 mL).

All packages listed above have child-resistant safety caps and tamper-resistant features.

Shown in Product Identification Guide, page 521

SINGLET® For Adults
Nasal Decongestant/Antihistamine/ Analgesic (pain reliever)/Antipyretic (fever reducer)

Indications: For temporary relief of nasal congestion and sinus and headache pain associated with sinusitis or due to a cold, hay fever or other upper respiratory allergies. Also temporarily relieves nasal congestion, sinus headache, runny nose, sneezing, itching of the nose or throat, and itchy, watery eyes due to hay fever or other upper respiratory allergies. Also temporarily relieves fever due to the common cold.

Directions: Adults (12 years and older): 1 caplet every 4 to 6 hours, **not to exceed 4 caplets in any 24-hour period,** or as directed by a doctor. Children under 12 years of age: Consult a doctor.

Warnings: Do not take this product for more than 10 days. If symptoms do not improve or are accompanied by fever that lasts for more than 3 days, or if new symptoms occur, consult a doctor. Do not take this product, unless directed by a doctor, if you have a breathing problem such as emphysema or chronic bronchitis, or if you have heart disease, high blood pressure, thyroid disease, diabetes, glaucoma or difficulty in urination due to enlargement of the prostate gland. May cause excitability especially in children. May cause drowsiness; alcohol, sedatives, and tranquilizers may increase the drowsiness effect. Avoid alcoholic beverages while taking this product. Do not take this product if you are taking sedatives or tranquilizers, without first consulting your doctor. Use caution when driving a motor vehicle or operating machinery. **Do not exceed recommended dosage.** If nervousness, dizziness, or sleeplessness occur, discontinue use and consult a doctor. **KEEP THIS AND ALL DRUGS OUT OF THE REACH OF CHILDREN.** Prompt medical attention is critical for adults as well as for children even if you do not notice any signs or symptoms. In case of accidental overdose, seek professional assistance or contact a Poison Control Center immediately. As with any drug, if you are pregnant or nursing a baby, seek the advice of a health professional before using this product.

Drug Interaction Precaution: Do not use this product if you are now taking a prescription monoamine oxidase inhibitor (MAOI) (certain drugs for depression, psychiatric or emotional conditions, or Parkinson's disease), or for 2 weeks after stopping the MAOI drug. If you are uncertain whether your prescription drug contains an MAOI, consult a health professional before taking this product.

Active Ingredients: Each caplet contains: Pseudoephedrine Hydrochloride 60 mg, Chlorpheniramine Maleate 4 mg, Acetaminophen 650 mg.

Inactive Ingredients: D&C Red 27, D&C Yellow 10, FD&C Blue 1, Hydroxypropyl Cellulose, Hydroxypropyl Methylcellulose, Magnesium Stearate, Microcrystalline Cellulose, Polyethylene Glycol, Pregelatinized Corn Starch, Sodium Starch Glycolate, Sucrose and Titanium Dioxide.

Protect from excessive heat and moisture.

Comments or Questions? Call toll-free 1-800-245-1040 weekdays

Distributed by: SmithKline Beecham Consumer Healthcare, L.P.
Pittsburgh, PA 15230. Made in U.S.A.
Lot No. 00/00 Exp. 00/00
New NDC# 0135-0107-26

SUCRETS® Maximum Strength
[*su 'krets*]
Wintergreen
SUCRETS® Wild Cherry Regular Strength
SUCRETS® Children's Cherry Flavored
Sore Throat Lozenges
SUCRETS® Regular Strength Original Mint
SUCRETS® Regular Strength Vapor Lemon
SUCRETS® Maximum Strength Vapor Black Cherry
SUCRETS® Assorted

Active Ingredient: Maximum Strength Wintergreen: Dyclonine Hydrochloride 3.0 mg. per lozenge. Wild Cherry, Regular Strength: Dyclonine Hydrochloride 2.0 mg. per lozenge. Children's Cherry: Dyclonine Hydrochloride 1.2 mg. per lozenge. Regular Strength–Original Mint: Hexylresorcinol 2.4 mg. per lozenge. Regular Strength–Vapor Lemon: Dyclonine Hydrochloride 2.0 mg. per lozenge. Maximum Strength–Vapor Black Cherry: Dyclonine Hydrochloride 3.0 mg. per lozenge.

Inactive Ingredients: Maximum Strength Wintergreen: Citric Acid, Corn

Syrup, Silicon Dioxide, Sucrose, Mineral Oil, Yellow 10. Wild Cherry Regular Strength: Blue 1, Corn Syrup, Flavor, Red 40, Silicon Dioxide, Sucrose, Tartaric Acid. Children's Cherry: Blue 1, Citric Acid, Corn Syrup, Red 40, Mineral Oil, Silicon Dioxide, Sucrose. Regular Strength–Original Mint: Blue 1, Corn Syrup, Flavors, Silicon Dioxide, Sucrose, Mineral Oil, Yellow 10. Regular Strength–Vapor Lemon: Citric Acid, Corn Syrup, Flavors, Silicon Dioxide, Sucrose, Mineral Oil, Yellow 10. Maximum Strength–Vapor Black Cherry: Blue 1, Corn Syrup, Flavor, Menthol, Red 40, Silicon Dioxide, Sucrose, Tartaric Acid.

Indications: For temporary relief of occasional minor sore throat pain and mouth irritations.

Actions: Dyclonine Hydrochloride's soothing anesthetic action relieves minor throat irritations.

Warnings: If sore throat is severe, persists for more than 2 days, is accompanied or followed by fever, headache, rash, swelling, nausea, or vomiting, do not use and consult a doctor promptly. If sore mouth symptoms do not improve in 7 days or if irritation, pain, or redness persists or worsens, see your dentist or doctor promptly. Do not exceed recommended dosage. KEEP THIS AND ALL MEDICINES OUT OF THE REACH OF CHILDREN. In case of accidental overdose, seek professional assistance or contact a poison control center immediately.

Drug Interaction: No known drug interaction.

Symptoms and Treatment of Oral Overdosage: Reactions due to large overdosage are systemic and involve the central nervous system and cardiovascular system. Central nervous system reactions are characterized by excitation and/or depression. Nervousness, dizziness, blurred vision or tremors may occur. Reactions involving the cardiovascular system include depression of the myocardium, hypotension or bradycardia. Should a large overdose be suspected seek professional assistance. Call your physician, local poison control center or the Rocky Mountain Poison Control Center at 303-592-1710 (Collect), 24 hours a day.

Dosage and Administration: Adults and children 2 years of age or older: Allow one lozenge to dissolve slowly in the mouth. May be repeated every two hours as needed. **Children under 2 years of age:** Consult a dentist or doctor.

Professional Labeling: For the temporary relief of pain associated with tonsillitis, pharyngitis, throat infections or stomatitis.

How Supplied: Available in plastic packages of 18 lozenges.

Shown in Product Identification Guide, page 521

SUCRETS® 4 HOUR COUGH SUPPRESSANT

[su 'krets]

dextromethorphan hydrobromide

Active Ingredient:
Each cough lozenge contains Dextromethorphan Hydrobromide 15 mg.

Inactive Ingredients:
Menthol Eucalyptus—Corn Syrup, D&C Yellow #10. FD&C Blue #1 Flavor, Magnesium Trisilicate, Menthol, Mineral Oil, Sucrose.
Wild Cherry—Corn Syrup, FD&C Blue #1, FD&C Red #40, Flavor, Magnesium Trisilicate, Menthol, Mineral Oil, Sucrose.

Indications For Use: For effective temporary relief of coughs due to minor sore throat and bronchial irritation associated with colds or inhaled irritants.

Directions: Adults and children twelve years of age and over: Take one (1) cough lozenge every 4 hours as needed. Do not exceed maximum dosage of 6 lozenges in any 24-hour period unless directed by a physician.
Children over six years of age: Take one (1) cough lozenge every 6 hours as needed. Do not exceed maximum dosage of 4 lozenges in any 24-hour period unless directed by a physician.
This product not intended for children under 6 years of age.
Avoid storing at high temperature (greater than 100°F).

Drug Interaction Precaution: Do not use this product (or give this product to your child) if you (or your child) are now taking a prescription monoamine oxidase inhibitor (MAOI) (certain drugs for depression, psychiatric or emotional conditions, or Parkinson's disease), or for 2 weeks after stopping MAOI drug. If you are uncertain whether you or your child's prescription drug contains a MAOI, consult a health professional before taking this product.

Warnings: A persistent cough may be a sign of a serious condition. If cough persists for more than 1 week, tends to recur, or is accompanied by fever, rash or persistent headache, consult a physician. Do not take this product for persistent or chronic cough such as occurs with smoking, asthma, emphysema, or if cough is accompanied by excessive phlegm (mucus) unless directed by a physician. Do not administer to children under 6 years of age unless directed by a physician.
As with any drug, if you are pregnant or nursing a baby, seek the advice of a health professional before using this product.
In case of accidental overdose, seek professional assistance or contact a poison control center immediately.
Keep this and all medication out of the reach of children.

Shown in Product Identification Guide, page 522

TAGAMET HB® 200
Acid Reducer/Cimetidine Tablets 200 mg

Tagamet HB® 200 relieves and prevents heartburn, acid indigestion and sour stomach when used as directed. It contains the same ingredient found in prescription strength Tagamet. Tagamet HB 200 reduces the production of stomach acid.

ACTIVE INGREDIENT Cimetidine Tablets, 200 mg. Acid Reducer.

INACTIVE INGREDIENTS Cellulose, cornstarch, hydroxypropyl methylcellulose, magnesium stearate, polyethylene glycol, polysorbate 80, povidone, sodium lauryl sulfate, sodium starch glycolate, titanium dioxide.

USES Relieves heartburn acid indigestion, and sour stomach. Prevents heartburn acid indigestion and sour stomach brought on by consuming food and beverages.

Directions: For relief of symptoms, take 1 tablet with water. For prevention of symptoms brought on by consuming food and beverages, take 1 tablet with water 30 minutes before eating a meal you expect to cause symptoms.
Tagamet HB 200 can be used up to twice daily (up to 2 tablets in 24 hours). This product should not be given to children under 12 years old unless directed by a doctor.

Warnings:
- Consult your doctor if you are taking theophylline (oral asthma medicine), warfarin (blood thinning medicine), or phenytoin (seizure medicine) before taking Tagamet HB. If you are not sure whether your medication contains one of these drugs or have any other questions about medicines you are taking, call our consumer affairs specialist at 1-800-482-4394.
- Do not take the maximum daily dosage for more than 2 weeks continuously except under the advice and supervision of a doctor.
- As with any drug, if you are pregnant or nursing a baby, seek the advice of a health professional before using this product.
- If you have trouble swallowing, or persistent abdominal pain, see your doctor promptly. You may have a serious condition that may need a different treatment.
- Keep this and all drugs out of the reach of children.
- In case of accidental overdose, seek professional assistance or contact a poison control center immediately.

READ THE LABEL
Read the directions and warnings before taking this medication.
Store at room temperature (59–86°F).
Comments or questions? Call Toll-Free 1-800-482-4394 Weekdays

PHARMACOKINETIC INTERACTIONS
Cimetidine at prescription doses is known to inhibit various P450 metaboliz-

Continued on next page

SmithKline Beecham—Cont.

ing isoenzymes, which could affect metabolism of other drugs and increase their blood concentration. Investigation of pharmacokinetic interactions at the recommended OTC doses of cimetidine have thus far shown only small effects. A pharmacokinetic study conducted in 26 normal male subjects (mean age, 38 years) at steady state using the maximum recommended OTC dose level (200 mg twice a day), showed that Tagamet HB 200, on average, increased the 24 hour AUC of theophylline by 14% and increased peak theophylline levels by 15%. This interaction should be borne in mind in advising patients on the use of Tagamet HB 200. At the prescription doses of cimetidine, clinically significant pharmacokinetic interactions between cimetidine and warfarin, phenytoin, and theophylline have been reported. At prescription doses, pharmacokinetic interactions have been reported for a number of other drugs as well, such as with dihydropyridine calcium channel blockers or some short acting benzodiazepines. At the maximum recommended OTC dose level (200 mg twice a day), a pharmacokinetic study conducted in 21 normal male subjects (mean age, 38 years) showed that Tagamet HB 200, on average, increased the total AUC of triazolam by 26–28% and increased peak triazolam levels by 11–23%. Tagamet HB 200 did not alter the apparent terminal elimination half-life of triazolam.
This labeling information is current as of Nov. 1, 1996.

How Supplied: Tagamet HB 200 (cimetidine Tablets 200 mg) is available in boxes of blister strips in 6, 12, 18 & 30 tablet sizes.

Shown in Product Identification Guide, page 522

TUMS® and Antacid/Calcium Supplement Tablets
TUMS E-X® and TUMS E-X® Sugar Free Antacid/Calcium Supplement Tablets
TUMS ULTRA® Antacid/Calcium Supplement Tablets

Indications: For fast relief of acid indigestion, heartburn, sour stomach, and upset stomach associated with these symptoms.

Professional Labeling: Indicated for the symptomatic relief of hyperacidity associated with the diagnosis of peptic ulcer, gastritis, peptic esophagitis, gastric hyperacidity, and hiatal hernia.

Active Ingredient:
Tums, Calcium Carbonate 500 mg
Tums E-X, Calcium Carbonate 750 mg
Tums ULTRA, Calcium Carbonate 1000 mg

Actions: Tums provides rapid neutralization of stomach acid. Each Tums tablet has an acid-neutralizing capacity (ANC) of 10 mEq. Each Tums E-X tablet has an ANC of 15 mEq and each Tums ULTRA tablet, an ANC of 20 mEq. This high neutralization capacity makes Tums tablets an ideal antacid for management of conditions associated with hyperacidity. It effectively neutralizes free acid yet does not cause systemic alkalosis in the presence of normal renal function. A double-blind placebo-controlled clinical study demonstrated that calcium carbonate taken at a dosage of 16 Tums tablets daily for a two-week period was non-constipating/non-laxative.

Warnings: Tums: Do not take more than 16 tablets in a 24-hour period or use the maximum dosage of this product for more than 2 weeks, except under the advice and supervision of a physician. If symptoms persist for 2 weeks, stop using this product and see a physician. Keep this and all drugs out of the reach of children.
Tums E-X: Do not take more than 10 tablets in a 24-hour period or use the maximum dosage of this product for more than two weeks, except under the advice and supervision of a physician. If symptoms persist for two weeks, stop using this product and see a physician. Keep this and all drugs out of the reach of children.
Additionally, for Tums Ex Sugar Free: Phenylketonurics: Contains phenylalanine, less than 1 mg per tablet.
Tums ULTRA: Do not take more than 8 tablets in 24-hour period or use the maximum dosage of this product for more than two weeks, except under the advice and supervision of a physician. If symptoms persist for two weeks, stop using and see a physician. Keep this and all drugs out of the reach of children.

Drug Interaction Precaution: Antacids may interact with certain prescription drugs. If you are presently taking a prescription drug, do not take this product without checking with your physician or other health professional.

Dosage and Administration:
Tums: Chew 2-4 tablets as symptoms occur. Repeat hourly if symptoms return, or as directed by physician.
Tums E-X: Chew 2-4 tablets as symptoms occur. Repeat hourly if symptoms return, or as directed by a physician.
Tums ULTRA: Chew 2-3 tablets as symptoms occur. Repeat hourly if symptoms return, or as directed by a physician.

AS A DIETARY SUPPLEMENT:
Calcium Supplement Directions
Tums, Tums E-X, & Tums ULTRA:

USES: As a daily source of extra calcium.
Tums is recommended by the National Osteoporosis Foundation.

IMPORTANT INFORMATION ON OSTEOPOROSIS: Regular exercise and a healthy diet with enough calcium helps teen and young adult white and Asian women maintain good bone health and may reduce their risk of osteoporosis later in life. Adequate calcium intake is important, but daily intakes above 2,000 mg are not likely to provide any additional benefit.

DIRECTIONS: Chew 2 tablets twice daily.
Average daily consumption should not exceed:
12 tablets for Tums;
8 tablets for Tums EX;
6 tablets for Tums ULTRA.
[See table below.]

Ingredients (all variants except sugar free): Sucrose, Starch, Talc, Mineral Oil, Flavors (natural and/or artificial), Sodium Polyphosphate. May also contain 1% or less of Adipic Acid, Blue 1 Lake, Yellow 6 Lake, Yellow 10 Lake, Red 27 Lake, Red 30 Lake.

Ingredients (Sugar Free): Sorbitol, Acacia, Natural and Artificial Flavors, Calcium Stearate, Adipic Acid, Yellow 6 Lake, Aspartame.

How Supplied:
Tums: Peppermint flavor is available in 12-tablet rolls, 3-roll wraps, and bottles of 75 and 150. **Assorted Flavors** (Cherry, Lemon, Orange, and Lime), are available in 12-tablet rolls, 3-roll wraps, and bottles of 75, 150, and 400.
Tums E-X: Wintergreen, Assorted Fruit and **Assorted Tropical Fruit Flavors;** 8-tablet rolls, 3-roll wraps and bottles of 48 and 96 tablets. Tropical fruit is also available in bottles of 250 tablets.
Tums EX Sugar Free: Orange Cream; bottles of 48 and 96 tablets.
Tums ULTRA: Assorted Fruit and **Assorted Mint Flavors;** bottles of 36 and 72 tablets.
This labeling information is current as of November 1, 1996.

Shown in Product Identification Guide, page 522

Nutrition Facts

	Tums	Tums E-X	Tums E-X Sugar Free	Tums Ultra
Serving Size	2 Tablets	2 Tablets	2 Tablets	2 Tablets
Amount Per Serving				
Calories	5	10	5	10
Sorbitol (g)	—	—	1	—
Sugars (g)	1	2	—	3
Calcium (mg)	400	600	600	800
% Daily Value	40	60	60	80
Sodium (mg)	—	5	—	10
% Daily Value	—	<1%	—	<1%

Inactive Ingredients: Lactose USP.

Indications: For the relief of symptoms of nausea and dizziness associated with or aggravated by motion. Useful for car sickness and sea sickness. Safe for adults and children and can be used in conjunction with other medications.

Directions: Adults: Dissolve 2–3 tablets under tongue every 4 hours or as needed. Children 6–12 years old: ½ adult dose. Use no more than 6 times per day.

Warnings: Do not use if imprinted cap band is missing or broken. If symptoms persist for more than seven days or worsen, contact a licensed health care professional. As with any drug, if you are pregnant or nursing a baby, seek the advice of a licensed health care professional before using this product. Keep this and all medications out of the reach of children. In case of accidental overdose, contact a poison control center immediately.

How Supplied: Bottles of 50 three grain sublingual tablets (NDC 54973-9147-01). Store at room temperature.

HYLAND'S TEETHING TABLETS

Active Ingredients: *Calcarea Phosphorica* (Calcium Phosphate) 3X HPUS, *Chamomilla* (Chamomile) 3X HPUS, *Coffea Cruda* (Coffee) 3X HPUS, *Belladonna* 3X HPUS (Alkaloids 0.0003%).

Inactive Ingredients: Lactose USP.

Indications: A homeopathic combination for the temporary relief of symptoms of simple restlessness and wakeful irritability due to cutting of teeth.

Directions: 2 to 3 tablets in a teaspoon of water or on the tongue, 4 times per day. If the child is restless or wakeful, 2 tablets every hour for 6 doses or as directed by a licensed health care practitioner.

Warnings: If symptoms persist for more than seven days or worsen, consult a Health Care Professional. As with any drug, if you are pregnant or nursing a baby, seek the advice of a health professional before using this product. Keep this and all medication out of the reach of children.

How Supplied: Bottles of 125—one grain sublingual tablets (NDC 54973-7504-01). Store at room temperature.

HYLAND'S VAGINITIS

Active Ingredients: Natrum Muriaticum 12X HPUS, Candida Albicans 30X HPUS, Kreosotum 12X HPUS, Carbolicum Acidum 12X HPUS.

Inactive Ingredients: Lactose USP.

Indications: For the relief of symptoms of vaginal itching and burning due to vaginal irritation or discharge after diagnosis by your doctor. Symptoms may be accompanied by clear to white vaginal discharge.

Directions: Adults: Dissolve 2–3 tablets under tongue every 4 hours or as needed.

Warnings: Do not use if imprinted cap band is missing or broken. If symptoms persist for more than seven days or worsen, contact a licensed health care professional. As with any drug, if you are pregnant or nursing a baby, seek the advice of a licensed health care professional before using this product. Keep this and all medications out of the reach of children. In case of accidental overdose, contact a poison control center immediately.

How Supplied: Bottles of 100 three grain sublingual tablets (NDC 54973-2962-02). Bottles of 50 three grain sublingual tablets (NDC 54973-2962-01). Store at room temperature.

EDUCATIONAL MATERIAL

Booklets—Brochures
"Homeopathy—What it is, How it Works," A Consumer's Guide to Homeopathic Medicine, Free
"Homeopathy—A Guide for Pharmacists," An ACPE (0.2 CEU) program on the basic principles of homeopathy.

Stellar Health Products, Inc.

71 COLLEGE DRIVE
ORANGE PARK, FL 32065

Direct Inquiries to:
1-800-635-8372

ARTHUR ITIS®
Twin Action External Analgesic Cream Rub
Penetrating Pain Relief

Contains: ACTIVE INGREDIENTS: Trolamine salicytate 10%, capsaicin 0.025%, INDICATIONS: For the temporary relief of minor aches and pains of muscles and joints associated with simple backache, arthritis, strains, bruises and sprains.

Directions: ADULTS & CHILDREN 10 YEARS OF AGE AND OLDER: Apply to affected area 3 to 4 times daily. CHILDREN UNDER 10 YEARS OF AGE: Do not use, consult a physician. In order to be effective this product must be applied 3 to 4 times daily. Application less frequently may not provide optimum relief. Initial relief is usually noted within one or two weeks. If condition does not improve in 4 weeks discontinue use of this product.

Warnings: FOR EXTERNAL USE ONLY. AVOID CONTACT WITH THE EYES. If prone to allergic reaction from aspirin, salicylates and/or capsaicin consult a doctor before using: If condition worsens, or if symptoms persist for more than 7 days or clear up and occur again within a few days, discontinue use of this product and consult a doctor. If redness is present, discontinue use and consult a doctor. Do not apply to wounds or damaged skin. Do not bandage tightly. Do not use with a heating pad (may blister skin).

Warning: USE ONLY AS DIRECTED. KEEP THIS AND ALL DRUGS OUT OF THE REACH OF CHILDREN. As with any drug, if you are pregnant or nursing a baby, seek the advice of a health professional before using this product. In case of accidental ingestion, seek professional assistance or contact a Poison Control Center immediately. You may experience a tingling or stinging sensation in application site. This is related to the mechanism of action of this product. Generally it disappears after a few days of use. This sensation may vary from person to person. Warm water or profuse sweating may increase this burning sensation. Avoid inhaling dried material from the application site which may cause sneezing, nasal irritation, or tearing. Wash hands carefully after applying this product.

How Supplied: Net Wt. 4 oz (113 g) cream & Net wt. 4 oz (113 g) Liquid with E-Z Applicator.
Store at controlled room temperature 15°–30°C (59°–86°F). Distributed by: Stellar Health Products, Inc., Orange Park. FL 32078

DIARRID™
ANTI-DIARRHEAL CAPLETS

DO NOT USE IF SEAL OVER TOP IS TORN OR MISSING

Indication: DIARRID controls the symptoms of diarrhea.

Directions for Use: Swallow whole caplets with water. Drink plenty of clear fluids to help prevent dehydration, which may accompany diarrhea.

Dosage for Relief of Diarrhea:
ADULTS AND CHILDREN 12 YEARS OF AGE AND OLDER: Take 2 caplets after the first loose bowel movement and 1 caplet after each subsequent loose bowel movement but no more than 4 caplets a day for no more than 2 days.
CHILDREN 9–11 YEARS (60–95 LBS): Take 1 caplet after the first loose bowel movement and 1/2 caplet after each subsequent loose bowel movement but no more than 3 caplets a day for no more than 2 days.
CHILDREN 6–8 YEARS (48–59 LBS): Take 1 caplet after the first loose bowel movement and 1/2 caplet after each subsequent loose bowel movement but no

Continued on next page

Stellar Health—Cont.

more than 2 caplets a day for no more than 2 days.
Children under 6 years old (up to 47 lbs.): Consult a physician. Not intended for use in children under 6 years old.

Warnings: KEEP THIS AND ALL DRUGS OUT OF THE REACH OF CHILDREN. Do not use for more than two days unless directed by a physician. DO NOT USE IF DIARRHEA IS ACCOMPANIED BY HIGH FEVER (GREATER THAN 101F), OR IF BLOOD OR MUCUS IS PRESENT IN STOOL, OR IF YOU HAVE A RASH OR OTHER ALLERGIC REACTION TO LOPERAMIDE HCl. If you are taking antibiotics or have a history of liver disease, consult a physician before using this product. As with any drug, if you are pregnant or nursing a baby, seek the advice of a health professional before using this product. In case of accidental overdose, seek professional assistance or contact a poison control center immediately.

Active Ingredient: Loperamide HCl 2mg per caplet.

Inactive Ingredients: Dibasic calcium phosphate, magnesium sterate, morcocrystalline cellulose, colloidal silicon dioxide, and D&C Yellow #10. Store at 15–30 C (59–86 F).

How Supplied: Diarrid™ comes in a 48 count, 12 count, and a 6 count.
Distributed by
Stellar Health Products, Inc.
Orange Park, Florida 32065

Thompson Medical Company, Inc.

222 LAKEVIEW AVENUE
WEST PALM BEACH
FLORIDA 33401

Direct Inquiries to:
Consumer Services: (407) 820-9900
Fax: (407) 832-2297

ASPERCREME®

[*ăs-per-crēme*]
External Analgesic Rub With Aloe

Description: ASPERCREME® is available as an odor-free creme and lotion for use as a topical massage rub that temporarily relieves minor muscle aches and pains.
Aspercreme does not contain aspirin.

Active Ingredient: Salycin® 10% (Thompson Medical's brand of Trolamine Salicylate).

Other Ingredients: Creme: Aloe Vera Gel, Cetyl Alcohol, Glycerin, Methylparaben, Mineral Oil, Potassium Phosphate, Propylparaben, Stearic Acid, Triethanolamine, Water. Lotion: Aloe Vera Gel, Cetyl Alcohol, Glyceryl Stearate, Isopropyl Palmitate, Lanolin, Methylparaben, Potassium Phosphate, Propylene Glycol, Propylparaben, Sodium Lauryl Sulfate, Stearic Acid, Water.

ASPERGEL™

Description: ASPERGEL™ is a topical massage rub that temporarily relieves minor muscle aches and pains. Aspergel is a clear, cool gel that has no embarrassing odor when rubbed in.
Aspergel does not contain aspirin.

Active Ingredient: Salycin® 10% (Thompson Medical's brand of Trolamine Salicylate).

Other Ingredients: Aloe Vera Gel, Hydroxyethylcellulose, PEG-8, Polyglycerylmethacrylate, Propylene Glycol, Purified Water, SD Alcohol 40 (5% w/w).

Actions: External analgesic rub.

Indications: Analgesic rub for temporary relief of minor aches and pains of muscles associated with simple strains and sprains.

Warnings: Use only as directed. If prone to allergic reaction from aspirin or salicylates, consult a physician before using. If redness is present or condition worsens, or if pain persists for more than 7 days or clears up and occurs again within a few days, discontinue use and consult a physician. For external use only. Avoid contact with eyes. As with any drug, if you are pregnant or nursing a baby, seek the advice of a health professional before using this product. **Do not use:** On children under 10 years of age. If skin is irritated or if irritation develops.
KEEP THIS AND ALL MEDICINES OUT OF THE REACH OF CHILDREN.
In case of accidental ingestion seek professional assistance or contact a poison control center immediately.

Dosage and Administration: Apply generously to affected area. Massage into painful area until thoroughly absorbed into skin. Repeat as necessary, but not more than 4 times daily.

How to Store: Store at controlled room temperature 59°–86°F (15°–30°C).

How Supplied: Creme: 1¼ oz., 3 oz. and 5 oz. tubes. Lotion: 6 oz. bottle. Gel: 3 oz. tube.

Shown in Product Identification Guide, page 522

CAPZASIN-P™

[*Căp-zā-sĭn-P*]

CAPZASIN-HP™

[*Căp-zā-sĭn-HP*]
Topical Analgesic Creme

Description: Capzasin-P™ and Capzasin-HP™ contain purified capsaicin, a natural ingredient that penetrates deep to temporarily relieve minor aches and pains of muscles and joints associated with arthritis, simple backache, strains and sprains. Capsaicin is so effective that doctors recommend it more than all other topical analgesic ingredients combined. Capzasin-P™ is available in Creme and Lotion. Capzasin-HP™ is available in Creme.

Capzasin-P™ Creme:

Active Ingredient: Capsaicin 0.025% w/w.

Other Ingredients: Benzyl Alcohol, Cetyl Alcohol, Glyceryl Monostearate, Isopropyl Myristate, Polyoxyl 40 Stearate, Purified Water, Sorbitol Solution, White Petrolatum.

Capzasin-P™ Lotion:

Active Ingredients: Capsaicin 0.025%.

Other Ingredients: Dimethicone Copolyol, DMDM Hydantoin, Hydroxyethylcellulose, Propylene Glycol, Purified Water, SD Alcohol 40 (5% w/w).

Capzasin-HP™ Creme:

Active Ingredient: Capsaicin 0.075%.

Other Ingredients: Benzyl Alcohol, Cetyl Alcohol, Gylceryl Monostearate, Isopropyl Myristate, PEG-100 Stearate, Purified Water, Sorbitol Solution, White Petrolatum.

Actions: External analgesic.

Indications: For the temporary relief of minor aches and pains of muscles and joints associated with arthritis, simple backache, strains and sprains.

Warnings: For external use only. Transient burning may occur upon application, but generally disappears in several days. Avoid contact with the eyes and mucous membranes. If condition worsens, or if symptoms persist for more than 7 days or clear up and occur again within a few days, discontinue use and consult a physician. Do not apply to wounds, damaged, broken (open) or irritated skin, or if excessive irritation develops. Do not bandage tightly. Do not use with a heating pad. As with any drug, if you are pregnant or nursing a baby, seek the advice of a health professional before using this product. **KEEP THIS AND ALL DRUGS OUT OF THE REACH OF CHILDREN.** In case of accidental ingestion, seek professional assistance or contact a poison control center immediately.

Dosage and Administration: Capzasin-P™ Creme/Capzasin-HP™ Creme:
Adults: Apply to affected area not more than 3 to 4 times daily. **WASH HANDS WITH SOAP AND WATER AFTER APPLYING. Children under 12 years of age:** Consult a physician. **READ PACKAGE INSERT BEFORE USING.**
Capzasin-P™ Lotion: **Adults:** Shake well before using. Apply to affected area not more than 3 to 4 times daily. **IF APPLYING TO HANDS, WASH HANDS WITH SOAP AND WATER AFTER APPLICATION.**
Children under 12 years of age: Consult a physician. **READ PACKAGE INSERT BEFORE USING.**
How to Store: Store at controlled room temperature 15°–30°C (59°–86°F)

How Supplied: Capzasin-P™ Creme: 1.5 oz. tube. Capzasin-P™ Lotion: 2.0 oz bottle. Capzasin-HP™ Creme: 1.5 oz. tube.

Shown in Product Identification Guide, page 522

DEXATRIM® Caplets and Tablets
[*dĕx-a-trĭm*]

DEXATRIM® PLUS VITAMINS
[*Dĕx-ă-trĭm Plus Vitamins*]
Prolonged action anorectic for weight control

DEXATRIM® Maximum Strength Plus Vitamin C/Caffeine Free Caplets

Active Ingredient: Phenylpropanolamine HCl 75 mg. (appetite suppressant time release)

Inactive Ingredients: Vitamin C (Ascorbic Acid) 180 mg., Carnauba Wax, Croscarmellose Sodium, Ethylcellulose, FD & C Red No. 40 Aluminum Lake, FD & C Yellow No. 6 Aluminum Lake, Hydroxypropyl Methylcellulose, Magnesium Stearate, Microcrystalline Cellulose, Polyethylene Glycol, Polysorbate 80, Povidone, Silicon Dioxide, Stearic Acid, Titanium Dioxide.

DEXATRIM® Maximum Strength Caffeine Free Caplets

Active Ingredient: Phenylpropanolamine HCl 75 mg. (appetite suppressant time release)

Inactive Ingredients: Carnauba Wax, D&C Yellow No. 10 Aluminum Lake, FD&C Yellow No. 6 Aluminum Lake, Hydroxypropyl Methylcellulose, Iron Oxide, Magnesium Stearate, Microcrystalline Cellulose, Polyethylene Glycol, Polysorbate 80, Povidone, Silicon Dioxide, Stearic Acid, Titanium Dioxide.

Extended Duration DEXATRIM® Maximum Strength Caffeine Free Tablets

Active Ingredient: Phenylpropanolamine HCl 75 mg. (appetite suppressant time release)

Inactive Ingredients: Calcium Sulfate, Carnauba Wax, D&C Yellow No. 10 Aluminum Lake, Ethylcellulose, FD&C Yellow No. 6 Aluminum Lake, Hydroxypropyl Methylcellulose, Iron Oxide, Magnesium Stearate, Propylene Glycol, Povidone, Stearic Acid, Titanium Dioxide, Triacetin.

DEXATRIM® Plus Vitamins:

Active Ingredient: Each Dexatrim Caplet Contains: Phenylpropanolamine HCl 75 mg. (appetite suppressant time release)

Each Vitamin/Mineral Caplet Contains:		% U.S.RDA[1]
Vitamin A (as Acetate & Beta Carotene)	5,000 IU	100%
Vitamin E (di-Alpha Tocopheryl Acetate)	30 IU	100%
Vitamin C (as Ascorbic Acid)	60 mg.	100%
Folic Acid	0.4 mg.	100%
Vitamin B1 (as Thiamine Mononitrate)	1.5 mg.	100%
Vitamin B2 (as Riboflavin)	1.7 mg.	100%
Niacinamide	20 mg.	100%
Vitamin B6 (as Pyridoxine Hydrochloride)	2 mg.	100%
Vitamin B12 (as Cyanocobalamin)	6 mcg.	100%
Vitamin D	400 IU	100%
Biotin	30 mcg.	10%
Pantothenic Acid (as Calcium Pantothenate)	10 mg.	100%
Calcium (as Dibasic Calcium Phosphate)	162 mg.	16%
Phosphorous (as Dibasic Calcium Phosphate)	125 mg.	13%
Iodine (as Potassium Iodide)	150 mcg.	100%
Iron (as Ferrous Fumarate)	18 mg.	100%
Magnesium (as Magnesium Oxide)	100 mg.	25%
Copper (as Cupric Oxide)	2 mg.	100%
Zinc (as Zinc Oxide)	15 mg.	100%
Manganese (as Manganese Sulfate)	2.5 mg.	*
Potassium (as Potassium Chloride)	40 mg.	*
Chloride (as Potassium Chloride)	36.3 mg.	*
Chromium (as Chromium Chloride)	25 mcg	*
Molybdenum (as Sodium Molydbdate)	25 mcg.	*
Selenium (as Sodium Selenate)	25 mcg.	*
Vitamin K1 (as Phytonadione)	25 mcg.	*
Nickel (as Nickel Sulfate)	5 mcg.	*
Tin (as Stannous Chloride)	10 mcg.	*
Silicon (as Sodium Metasilicate & Oxides)	2 mg.	*
Vanadium (as Sodium Metavanadate)	10 mcg.	*
Boron (as Borates)	150 mcg.	*

[1]U.S. RECOMMENDED DAILY ALLOWANCE (U.S. RDA) FOR ADULTS AND CHILDREN 4 OR MORE YEARS OF AGE.
*NO U.S. RDA HAS BEEN ESTABLISHED.

Inactive Ingredients: Vitamin C (Ascorbic Acid) 180 mg., Carnauba Wax, Cellulose, Croscarmellose Sodium, Ethylcellulose, FD & C Blue No. 1, FD & C Red No. 40 Aluminum Lake, FD & C Yellow No. 6, FD & C Yellow No. 6 Aluminum Lake, Hydroxypropyl Methylcellulose, Magnesium Stearate, Methylcellulose, Microcrystalline Cellulose, Polyethylene Glycol, Polysorbate 80, Povidone, Propylene Glycol, Silica, Silicon Dioxide, Starch, Stearic Acid, Titanium Dioxide.

Indication: DEXATRIM® is an aid for effective appetite control to assist weight reduction in conjunction with a sensible weight loss plan. It is available in a time release dosage form. The multi-vitamin, in caplet form, is for dietary supplementation.

Directions: Adult oral dosage is **one caplet** at mid-morning with a full glass of water. **Exceeding the recommended dose has not been shown to result in greater weight loss.** (This product's effectiveness is directly related to the degree to which you reduce your usual daily food intake.) Do not use for more than 3 months, because this should be enough time to establish new eating habits. Read and follow the important Diet Plan enclosed.

DEXATRIM® PLUS VITAMINS:

Directions: Adult oral dosage is **one red caplet marked "dexatrim"** and **one vitamin/mineral caplet marked "COMPLETE VITAMIN"** at mid-morning with a full glass of water. **Exceeding the recommended dose has not been shown to result in greater weight loss.** (This product's effectiveness is directly related to the degree to which you reduce your usual daily food intake.) Do not use for more than 3 months, because this should be enough time to establish new eating habits. Read and follow important Diet Plan enclosed.

Warnings: DO NOT TAKE MORE THAN 1 DEXATRIM CAPLET PER DAY (24 HOURS). Exceeding the recommended dose may cause serious health problems. FOR ADULT USE ONLY. Do not give this product to children under 12 years of age. Persons between 12 and 18 or over 60 are advised to consult their physician before using this product.
There have been reports that stroke, seizure, heart attack, arrhythmia, psychosis, and death might be associated with the ingestion of phenylpropanolamine.
DO NOT USE IF YOU:

- Are being treated for depression, an eating disorder or have heart disease, diabetes, thyroid or any other disease, except under the supervision of a doctor.
- Have any of the following symptoms: Nervousness, dizziness, sleeplessness, palpitations, or headache. If any of these symptoms occur, stop taking this product and consult your doctor.
- Have high blood pressure. Check your blood pressure regularly. If it is high, consult your doctor.
- Are pregnant or nursing a baby without first seeking the advice of a health professional.
- Are hypersensitive to any of this product's ingredients.

Drug Interaction Precaution: If you are taking a cough/cold or allergy medication containing any form of phenylpropanolamine, or any oral nasal decongestant, do not take this product. Do not use this product if you are taking any prescription drug, except under the advice and supervision of a physician. Do not use this product if you are presently taking a prescription monoamine oxidase inhibitor (MAOI) for depression or for two weeks after stopping use of an MAOI without first consulting a physician.
KEEP THIS AND ALL MEDICATIONS OUT OF THE REACH OF CHILDREN. In case of accidental overdose, seek pro-

Continued on next page

Thompson Medical—Cont.

fessional assistance or contact a poison control center immediately.

Dosage and Administration:

Caplet Dosage Forms: DEXATRIM® Maximum Strength Plus Vitamin C/Caffeine Free, DEXATRIM® Maximum Strength/Caffeine Free.
Tablet Dosage Form: DEXATRIM® Maximum Strength Extended Duration Time Tablets.
Administration: One caplet or tablet at midmorning with a full glass of water.

How Supplied: All Dexatrim products are supplied in tamper-evident blister packages. Do not use if individual seals are broken.
DEXATRIM® Maximum Strength Plus Vitamin C/Caffeine Free Caplets: Packages of 20 and 40 with 1250 calorie DEXATRIM Diet Plan.
DEXATRIM® Maximum Strength Extended Duration Time Tablets: Packages of 20 and 40 with 1250 calorie DEXATRIM Diet Plan.
DEXATRIM® PLUS VITAMINS: Packages containing 14 Dexatrim caplets and 14 multi-vitamin/mineral caplets with 1250 calorie DEXATRIM® Plus Vitamins Diet Plan.

References: Schteingart, DE et al. Int J, Obes. 1992; 16: 487–493.
Atkinson RL, et al. Am J Clin Nutr. 1992; 56(4): 755.
Blackburn GL et al. JAMA 1989; 261: 3267–3272.
Morgan JP et al. J Clin Psychopharm. 1989; 9: 33–38.
All referenced materials available on request.

Shown in Product Identification Guide, page 522

ENCARE®
[en'kar]
Vaginal Contraceptive Suppositories

Description: Encare is a safe and effective contraceptive in a convenient vaginal suppository form available without a prescription. Encare is reliable because it offers two-way protection: (1) Encare kills sperm on contact by releasing a precise dose of nonoxynol 9, the spermicide most recommended by doctors. (2) Encare gently disperses a physical barrier of protection against the cervix to help prevent pregnancy.
Encare is colorless and odorless.
It is an effective contraceptive in vaginal suppository form.

Active Ingredient: Each suppository contains 100 mg Nonoxynol 9.

Other Ingredients: Polyethylene Glycols, Sodium Bicarbonate, Sodium Citrate, Tartaric Acid.

Indications: Encare is effective in the prevention of pregnancy.

Action: Encare is 100% free of hormones and free of the serious side effects associated with oral contraceptives.
Encare is convenient and easy to use. Women like Encare because each insert is individually wrapped and can be easily carried in a pocket or purse. Encare is approximately as effective as vaginal foam contraceptives in actual use, yet there is no applicator, so there is nothing to fill, remove, or clean. For added protection, Encare may be used in conjunction with other contraceptive methods, such as a condom or as a second application with a diaphragm.
Because Encare can be inserted as much as an hour before intercourse, it does not interfere with spontaneity. Encare has been used successfully by millions of women throughout Europe and America.

Special Warning: Spermicidal contraceptives should not be used during pregnancy. Some experts believe that there may be an increased risk of birth defects occurring in children whose mothers used a spermicidal contraceptive at the time of conception or during pregnancy. If you believe you may be pregnant, have a pregnancy test before using a spermicidal contraceptive. If you have used a spermicidal contraceptive after becoming pregnant, or used a spermicidal contraceptive when you became pregnant, discuss this issue with your doctor.

Cautions: If your doctor has told you that you should not become pregnant, consult your doctor as to which method, (including Encare), is best for you.
If you or your partner experience irritation, discontinue use. If irritation persists, consult your doctor. This product has not been shown to protect against HIV (AIDS) and other sexually transmitted diseases.
Do not take orally. **KEEP THIS AND ALL DRUGS OUT OF THE REACH OF CHILDREN.** In case of accidental ingestion, call a poison control center, emergency medical facility or a doctor immediately.
Keep away from excessive heat and moisture. Store at controlled room temperature: 15°C–30°C (59°–86°F).

Dosage and Administration: For best protection against pregnancy, it is essential to follow package instructions. At least 10 minutes before intercourse, place one Encare suppository with your fingertip as far as possible into the vagina, towards the small of your back. Best protection will occur when Encare is placed deep into the vagina. You may feel a sensation of warmth as Encare effervesces and distributes the spermicide, nonoxynol 9, within the vagina. This is a natural attribute of the active ingredient.
IMPORTANT: It is essential to insert Encare at least 10 minutes before intercourse. If one chooses, Encare can be inserted up to one hour before intercourse. If intercourse has not taken place within one hour after insertion, use a new Encare suppository. Use a new Encare suppository each time intercourse is repeated. Encare can be used safely and as frequently as needed.
Douching after use of Encare is not recommended, however, should you desire to do so, wait at least six hours after intercourse.
Instructions enclosed in package are in both English and Spanish.

How Supplied: Boxes of 12 and 18.

References: Barwin B. *Contraceptive Delivery System.* 1983; 4: 331–334. Masters WH, et al. *Fertility and Sterility.* 1979; 32: 161–165.
Dimpfl J, et al. *Sexualmedizin.* 1984; 2: 95–98. Schill WB, Wolff HH. *Adrologia.* 1981; 13: 42–49. Stone SC, Cardinale F. *Am J Obstet Gynecol.* 1979; 133: 635–638.

SLEEPINAL®
Night-time Sleep Aid Capsules and Softgels
(Diphenhydramine HCl)

Description: SLEEPINAL is a night-time sleep aid. When taken prior to bedtime, it aids in falling asleep and helps to relieve occasional sleeplessness.

Active Ingredient: Diphenhydramine HCl 50 mg.

Other Ingredients: Capsules: FD&C Blue No. 1, Gelatin, Lactose, Magnesium Stearate, Povidone, Talc.
Softgels: D&C Yellow No. 10, Gelatin, Glycerin, Polyethylene Glycol 400, Povidone , Propylene Glycol, Purified Water, Sorbitol. May also contain: FD&C Blue No. 1, FD&C Green No. 3.

Indications: For relief of occasional sleeplessness.

Action: SLEEPINAL is an antihistamine with anticholinergic and sedative action.

Warnings: Read before using. Do not exceed recommended dosage. Do not give to children under 12 years of age. If sleeplessness persists continuously for more than 2 weeks, consult your physician. Insomnia may be a symptom of serious underlying medical illness. Do not take this product, unless directed by a physician, if you have a breathing problem such as emphysema or chronic bronchitis, or if you have glaucoma or difficulty in urination due to the enlargement of the prostate gland. Avoid alcoholic beverages while taking this product. Do not take this product if you are taking sedatives or tranquilizers, without first consulting your physician. As with any drug, if you are pregnant or nursing a baby, seek the advice of a health professional before using this product.
KEEP THIS AND ALL DRUGS OUT OF THE REACH OF CHILDREN.
In case of accidental overdose, seek professional assistance or contact a poison control center immediately.

Dosage and Administration: Capsules and Softgels: Adults and children 12 years of age and over: Oral dosage, one at bedtime if needed, or as directed by a physician.

How to Store: Store in a dry place at controlled room temperature 15° C–30° C (59° F–86° F). Protect softgels from light, retain product in box until administered.

How Supplied: Capsules and Softgels: Sleepinal is supplied in tamper-evident blister packages. Do not use if individual seals are broken. Packages of 16 and 32 capsules and 8 and 16 softgels.

Shown in Product Identification Guide, page 522

SPORTSCREME®

[*spŏrts-crēme*]

External Analgesic Rub

Description: SPORTSCREME® is available as a creme and lotion for use as a topical massage rub that temporarily relieves minor muscle aches and pains. Sportscreme has a clean, fresh scent.

Active Ingredient: Salycin® 10% (Thompson Medical's brand of Trolamine Salicylate).

Other Ingredients: Cetyl Alcohol, FD&C Blue No. 1, FD&C Yellow No. 5, Fragrance, Glycerin, Methylparaben, Mineral Oil, Potassium Phosphate Monobasic, Propylparaben, Stearic Acid, Triethanolamine, Water.

Actions: External analgesic rub.

Indications: Analgesic rub for temporary relief of minor aches and pains of muscles associated with simple strains and sprains.

Warnings: Use only as directed. If prone to allergic reaction from aspirin or salicylates, consult a physician before using. If redness is present or if condition worsens, or if pain persists for more than 7 days, discontinue use and consult a physician. Do not use on children under ten years of age. Do not apply if skin is irritated or if irritation develops. As with any drug, if you are pregnant or nursing a baby, seek the advice of a health professional before using this product. For external use only. Avoid contact with eyes. KEEP THIS AND ALL MEDICINES OUT OF THE REACH OF CHILDREN. In case of accidental ingestion, seek professional assistance or contact a poison control center immediately.

Dosage and Administration: Apply generously to affected area. Massage into painful area until thoroughly absorbed into skin. Repeat as needed, especially before retiring and in the morning, but not more than 4 times daily.

How to Store: Store at controlled room temperature 15°–30°C (59°–86°F).

How Supplied: Cream: 1.25 oz. and 3 oz. tubes: Lotion: 6 oz. bottle.

Tishcon Corp.

30 NEW YORK AVENUE
WESTBURY, NY 11590

Direct Inquiries to:
Product Information Department
Phone: 1-800-848-8442
Fax: 1-516-338-0829

Product Listing:

Daily Soy™ Capsules
Daily Soy™ Wafers
Driver's Friend™ Coffee Wafers
Dual Release Melatonin
Lipo-Gel™ (alpha-Lipoic Acid) Softsules®
Lumitene™ (Beta Carotene 30 mg) Capsules
Q-Gel™ (Coenzyme Q10) 15 mg Softsules®
Q-Gel™ Forte (Coenzyme Q-10) 30 mg Softsules®
Q-Tab™ (Coenzyme Q10) Tablets
Stimulert® Wafers
Triple Release Vitamin B12

LUMITENE™ BETA CAROTENE 30 mg beadlets (Pharmaceutical grade Dry Beta Carotene beadlets, 10%)

Description: Lumitene™ (beta-carotene) is available in capsules for oral administration. Each capsule is composed of beadlets containing 30 mg beta-carotene, ascorbyl palmitate, corn starch, dl-alpha-tocopherol, gelatin, peanut oil and sucrose. Gelatin capsule shells may contain parabens (methyl and propyl), potassium sorbate, FD&C Blue No. 1, D&C Yellow No. 10, FD&C Red No. 3, FD&C Green No. 3 and titanium dioxide.
Beta-carotene, precursor of vitamin A, is a carotenoid pigment occurring naturally in green and yellow vegetables. Chemically, beta-carotene has the empirical formula $C_{40}H_{56}$ and a calculated molecular weight of 536.85. Trans-beta-carotene is a red, crystalline compound which is insoluble in water. Its structural formula is as follows:

Contraindications: Lumitene™ is contraindicated in patients with known hypersensitivity to beta-carotene.

Warnings: Lumitene™ has not been shown to be effective as a sunscreen.

Precautions: General: Lumitene™ should be used with caution in patients with impaired renal or hepatic function because safe use in the presence of these conditions has not been established.

Information for Patients: Patients receiving Lumitene™ should be advised against taking supplementary vitamin A since Lumitene™ administration will fulfill normal vitamin A requirements. They should be cautioned to continue sun protection, and forewarned that their skin may appear slightly yellow while receiving Lumitene™. *Carcinogenesis, Mutagenesis, Impairment of Fertility:* Long-term studies in animals to determine carcinogenesis have not been completed. *In vitro* and *in vivo* studies to evaluate mutagenic potential were negative. No effects on fertility in male rats were observed at doses as high as 500 mg/kg/day (100 times the recommended human dose).
Pregnancy: Teratogenic Effects: Pregnancy Category C. Beta-carotene has been shown to be fetotoxic (i.e., cause an increase in resorption rate), but not teratogenic when given to rats at doses 300 to 400 times the maximum recommended human dose. No such fetotoxicity was observed at 75 times the maximum recommended human dose or less. A generation reproduction study in rats receiving beta-carotene at a dietary concentration of 0.1% (1000 ppm) has revealed no evidence of impaired fertility or effect on the fetus. There are no adequate and well-controlled studies in pregnant women. Lumitene™ should be used during pregnancy only if the potential benefit justifies the potential risk to the fetus.
Nursing Mothers: It is not known whether this drug is excreted in human milk. Because many drugs are excreted in human milk, caution should be exercised when Lumitene™ is administered to a nursing mother.

Adverse Reactions: Some patients may have occasional loose stools while taking Lumitene™. This reaction is sporadic and may not require discontinuance of medication. Other reactions which have been reported rarely are ecchymoses and arthralgia.

Overdosage: There are no reported cases of overdosage. The oral LD_{50} of beta-carotene (suspended in 5% gum acacia solution) in mice and rats is greater than 20,000 mg/kg. No lethality was observed in mice following administration of 30-mg beadlet capsules (ground and suspended in 5% gum acacia) at a dose of 1200 mg/kg beta-carotene.

Dosage and Administration: Lumitene™ may be administered either as a single daily dose or in divided doses, preferably with meals.

Usage in Children: The usual dosage for children under 14 is 30 to 150 mg (1 to 5 capsules) per day. Capsules may be opened and the contents mixed in orange or tomato juice to aid administration. *Usage in Adults:* The usual adult dosage is 30 to 300 mg (1 to 10 capsules) per day. Dosage should be adjusted depending on the severity of the symptoms and the response of the patient. Several weeks of therapy are necessary to accumulate enough Lumitene™ in the skin to exert its effect. Patients should be instructed not to increase exposure to sunlight until

Continued on next page

Tishcon Corporation—Cont.

they appear carotenemic (first seen as yellowness of palms and soles). This usually occurs after two to six weeks of therapy. Exposure to the sun may then be increased gradually. The protective effect is not total and each patient should establish his or her own limits of exposure.

How Supplied: Lumitene™ is available in blue and green capsules, each containing 30 mg of beta-carotene—bottles of 100 (NDC 1465-4658-08).

Q-GEL™ SOFTSULES®
(Hydrosoluble Coenzyme Q10)

Nutrition Facts: Serving Size: 1 Softsule® daily with a meal.
Amount per Softsule® % Daily Value
Coenzyme Q10 15 mg *
(Ubidecarenone)

Ingredients: Coenzyme Q10, Span 80, Propylene Glycol, Polysorbate 80 (Tween 80), Povidone, Vitamin E Natural (d-alpha tocopherol), Polyethylene Glycol 400, Silicon Dioxide, Medium Chain Triglyceride, Gelatin, Glycerin, Sorbitol, Annato, Titanium Dioxide, Purified Water, Carmine and Pharmaceutical Glaze
*Daily Value in the diet has not been established.

Warning: Close tightly and keep out of the reach of children.

How Supplied: Bottles of 30, 60, 90, 120, and 180 Softsules®
Storage: Keep in a cool, dry place. Do not expose to direct sunlight.

Q-GEL™ SOFTSULES®
(Double Strength Hydrosoluble Coenzyme Q10)

Nutrition Facts: Serving Size: 1 Softsule® daily with a meal.
Amount per Softsule® % Daily Value
Coenzyme Q10 30 mg *
(Ubidecarenone)

Ingredients: Coenzyme Q10, Span 80, Propylene Glycol, Polysorbate 80 (Tween 80), Povidone, Vitamin E Natural (d-alpha Tocopherol), Polyethylene Glycol 400, Silicon Dioxide, Medium Chain Triglyceride, Gelatin, Glycerin, Sorbitol, Annato, Titanium Dioxide, Purified Water, Carmine and Pharmaceutical Glaze
*Daily Value in the diet has not been established.

Warning: Close tightly and keep out of the reach of children.

How Supplied: Bottles of 30, 60, 90, 120, and 180 Softsules®
Storage: Keep in a cool, dry place, Do not expose to direct sunlight.

Triton Consumer Products, Inc.

561 W. GOLF ROAD
ARLINGTON HEIGHTS, IL 60005

Direct Inquiries to:
Karen Shrader
(800) 942-2009

For Medical Emergencies Contact:
(800) 942-2009

MG 217® PSORIASIS/DANDRUFF MEDICATION
Skin Care: Ointment and Lotion
Scalp: Shampoo

Active Ingredients: Ointment—Coal Tar Solution USP 10%. **Lotion**—Coal Tar Solution USP 5%. **Sal-Acid Ointment**—Salicylic acid 3%. **Tar Shampoo**—Coal Tar Solution USP 15%. **Tar-Free Shampoo**—Sulfur 5% and salicylic acid 3%.

Action/Uses: Relief for itching, scaling and flaking of psoriasis, seborrheic dermatitis and/or dandruff.

Warnings: For external use only. Keep out of the reach of children. Avoid contact with eyes. If undue skin irritation occurs, discontinue use.

Administration: Ointment or Lotion—Apply to affected area one to four times daily. **Shampoo**—Wet hair, then massage shampoo into scalp and leave on for several minutes. Rinse thoroughly. Use at least twice a week or as directed by a physician.

How Supplied: Ointment—3.8 oz. jars. **Lotion**—4 oz. bottles. **Sal-Acid Ointment**—2 oz. jars. **Shampoo**—4 oz. and 8 oz. bottles.

UAS Laboratories

5610 ROWLAND RD #110
MINNETONKA, MN 55343

Direct Inquiries To:
Dr. S.K. Dash: (612) 935-1707
Fax: (612) 935-1650

Medical Emergency Contact:
Dr. S.K. Dash: (612) 935-1707
Fax: (612) 935-1650

DDS®-ACIDOPHILUS
Capsule, Tablet & Powder free of dairy products, corn, soy, and preservatives

Description: DDS®-Acidophilus is the source of a special strain of Lactobacillus acidophilus free of dairy products, corn, soy and preservatives. Each capsule or tablet contains one billion viable DDS-1 L.acidophilus at the time of manufacturing. One gram of powder contains two billion viable DDS®- L.acidophilus.

Indications and Usages: An aid in implanting the gut with beneficial Lactobacillus acidophilus under conditions of digestive disorders, acne, yeast infections, and following antibiotic therapy.

Administration: One to two capsules or tablets twice daily before meals. One-fourth teaspoon powder can be substituted for two capsules or tablets.

How Supplied: Bottles of 100 capsules or tablets. 12 bottles per case. Powder is available in 2 oz. bottle; 12 bottles per case.

Storage: Keep refrigerated under 40°F.

EDUCATIONAL MATERIAL

DDS-Acidophilus
Booklet describing superior-strain Acidophilus without dairy products, corn, soy, or preservatives. Two billion viable DDS-L. acidopohilus per gram.

Unipath Diagnostics Company

Lever House
390 PARK AVENUE
NEW YORK, NY 10022

Direct Inquiries to:
(212) 888-1260

CLEARBLUE EASY®
Pregnancy Test Kit

Clearblue Easy is one of the easiest and fastest pregnancy tests available because all a woman has to do is hold the absorbent tip in her urine stream and in 3 minutes she can read the result. A blue line appears in the small window to show that the test is complete and the large window shows the test result. If there is any line in the middle of the large window, the woman is pregnant. If there is no line, she is not pregnant.

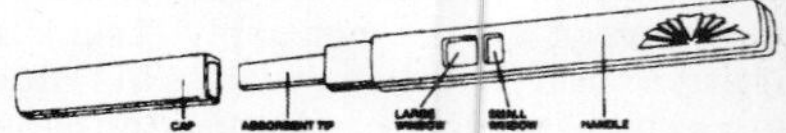

Clearblue Easy is a rapid, one-step pregnancy test for home use, which detects the pregnancy hormone HCG (human chorionic gonadotropin) in the urine. This hormone is produced in increasing amounts during the first part of pregnancy. Clearblue Easy uses sensitive monoclonal antibodies to detect the presence of this hormone from the first day of a missed period.
A negative result means that no pregnancy hormone was detected and the woman is probably not pregnant. If the menstrual period does not start within a week, she may have miscalculated the day her period was due. She should repeat the test using another Clearblue Easy test. If the second test still gives a negative result and she still has not menstruated, she should see her doctor.

Clearblue Easy is specially designed for easy use at home. However, if there are any questions about the test or results, give the Clearblue Easy TalkLine a call at 1-800-883-EASY. A specially trained staff of advisors is available to answer your questions.
Manufactured by Unipath Ltd., Bedford, U.K. Unipath, Clearblue Easy and the fan device are trademarks.
Distributed by
Unipath Diagnostics Company
Lever House
390 Park Avenue
New York, NY 10022

Shown in Product Identification Guide, page 522

CLEARPLAN EASY™
One-Step Ovulation Predictor

CLEARPLAN EASY is one of the easiest home ovulation predictor tests to use because of its unique technological design. It consists of just one piece and involves only one step to get results. To use CLEARPLAN EASY, a woman simply holds the absorbent tip in her urine stream (a woman can test any time of day) for 5 seconds, and after 5 minutes, she can read the results. A blue line will appear in the small window to show her that the test has worked correctly. The large window indicates the presence of luteinizing hormone (LH) in her urine. If there is a line in the large window which is similar to or darker than the line in the small window, she has detected her LH surge.

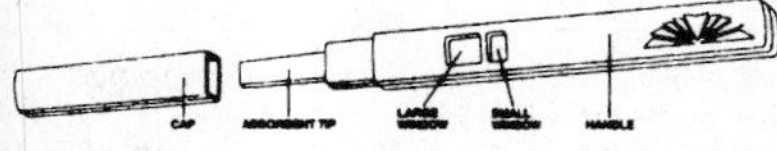

Laboratory tests confirm that CLEARPLAN EASY is over 98% accurate in detecting the LH surge as shown by radioimmunoassay (RIA).
CLEARPLAN EASY employs highly sensitive monoclonal antibody technology to accurately predict the onset of ovulation, and, consequently, the best time each month for a woman to try to become pregnant. The test monitors the amount of LH in a woman's urine. Small amounts of LH are present during most of the menstrual cycle, but the level normally rises sharply about 24 to 36 hours before ovulation (which is when an egg is released from the ovary). CLEARPLAN EASY detects this LH surge preceding ovulation so that a woman knows 24–36 hours beforehand the time she is most able to become pregnant.
A woman will be most fertile during the 1 to 3 days after an LH surge is detected. Sperm can fertilize an egg for many hours after sexual intercourse. So, if sexual intercourse occurs during the 1–3 days after a similar or darker line appears in the large window, the chances of getting pregnant are increased.

CLEARPLAN EASY contains 5 days of tests. If, because a woman's cycles are irregular or if for any other reason a woman does not detect her LH surge after 5 days of testing, she should continue testing with a second CLEARPLAN EASY kit. CLEARPLAN EASY offers users the support of a TalkLine (1-800-883-EASY). This service is operated by trained advisors who are available to answer any questions about using the test or reading the results.

Produced by Unipath Ltd., Bedford, U.K. Unipath, CLEARPLAN EASY and the fan device are trademarks.
Distributed by
Unipath Diagnostics Company
Lever House
390 Park Avenue
New York, NY 10022

Shown in Product Identification Guide, page 522

VÄXA International, Inc.

10307 PACIFIC CENTER COURT
SAN DIEGO, CA 92121-4396

Direct Inquiries to:
(619) 625-8292
FAX: (619) 625-8272
www.vaxa.com/vaxa/vaxa.html

VÄXA'S ARTHRITIN
All Natural Homeopathic Nutraceutical Medicine

Indications: Professionally recommended for relief from Rheumatoid Arthritis and Osteoarthritic pain, inflammation and swelling.

Directions/Dosage: Loading Dosage: (Adults or Children) During Arthritis attacks, take 3–4 capsules every 3 hours, or as directed by a physician.

Maintenance Dosage: (Adults or Children) Take 2–4 capsules every morning and evening.

Each capsule contains:

Active Ingredients: Actea spicata (1c:1.5mg, 3c:1.5mg, 6c:1.5mg, 12c:1.5mg), Apis mellifica (3c:1.5mg, 6c:1.5mg, 12c:1.5mg, 30c:1.5mg), Bryonia alba (1c:1.5mg, 6c:1.5mg, 12c:1.5mg, 30c:1.5mg), Cimicifuga racemosa (1c:1.5mg, 3c:1.5mg, 6c:1.5mg, 12c:1.5mg), Dulcamara (3c:1.5mg, 6c:1.5mg, 12c:1.5mg, 30c:1.5mg), Ledum palustre (6c:1.5mg, 12c:1.5mg, 30c:1.5mg), Rhododendron (6c:1.5mg, 12c:1.5mg, 30c:1.5mg).

Nutraceutical Ingredients: DL-Methionine, Boswellia Serrata, GLA, Perna Canaliculous (with Mucopolysaccharides), 100% Pure Shark Cartilage, DL-Phenylalanine, Chondroitin Sulfate, N-Acetyl Glucosamine (NAG), Glucosamine Sulfate, Harpagophytum Procumbens, Capsaicin, Reishi Mushroom, Cinnamomum Verum, Manganese Ascorbate, Magnesium (from Gluconate/.14% USRDI), Pyridoxine HCL-B6 (500% USRDI), L-Ornithine, Calcium Carbonate (1.2% USRDI), OptiZinc® (6.7% USRDI), Boron, Mixed Glucosaminoglycans, Tanacetum Parthenium, White Willow Bark, Fo-Ti, Yucca.

Warning: As with any medicine, if you are pregnant or nursing, or if conditions persist or worsen, consult a physician. Keep this and all medication out of the reach of children.

How Supplied: Tamper Resistant bottles of 60 capsules. Complements any medical program: Non-Interfering, Natural Homeopathic Nutraceutical.

Guaranteed: Contains no additives, fillers, colors, sugars, flavors or preservatives. 60-day money back guarantee.

VÄXA'S VIREXIN
All Natural Homeopathic Nutraceutical Medicine

Indications: Professionally recommended for relief from Colds, Influenza and Chronic Viral Infections.

Directions/Dosage: Loading Dosage: (Adults or Children) Take 3–4 capsules every 3 hours for two weeks, or as directed by a physician. **Maintenance Dosage:** (Adults or Children) Take 3–4 capsules daily for ongoing prevention and care.

Each capsule contains:

Active Ingredients: Aconitum napellus (3c:2.5mg, 6c:2.5mg, 12c:2.5mg, 30c:2.5mg), Arsenicum album (6c:2.5 mg, 12c:2.5mg, 30c:2.5mg), Asclepias vincetoxinum (3c:2.5mg, 6c:2.5mg, 12c:2.5mg, 30c:2.5mg), Baptisia tinctora (1c:2.5mg, 3c:2.5mg, 6c:2.5mg, 12c:2.5mg), Eupatorium perfoliatum (1c:2.5mg, 3c:2.5mg, 6c:2.5mg, 12c:2.5mg), Gelsemium sempervirens (6c:2.5mg, 12c:2.5mg, 30c:2.5mg), Ranunculus bulbosus (3c:2.5mg, 6c:2.5mg, 12c:2.5mg, 30c:2.5mg).
Nutraceutical Ingredients: Hypericum Perforatum (St. John's Wort: Natural Hypericin), L-Lysine, Radix Sileris, L-Methionine, Caulis Perillae, L-Arginine, L-Cysteine, Cinchona Bark, Myrrh Gum, Glycyrrhiza Glabra, Allium Sativum (allicin), Echinacea, Kombucha Fungus, Dandelion Root, L-Threonine, Inulin, L-Aspartic Acid, Achillea Millefolium, Herba Schizonepetae, Semen Armeniacae, Semen Cuscutae, Pyridoxine HCL-B6 (50% USRDI), L-Glutathione, Golden Seal Root, Calcium Pantothenate-B5 (10% USRDI), Magnesium (from Aspartate/.05% USRDI), OptiZinc®, (1.4% USRDI), Thiotic Acid, Ginkgo Biloba, Niacinamide-B3 (5% USRDI), Biotin (33% USRDI).

Warning: As with any medicine, if you are pregnant or nursing, or if conditions persist or worsen, consult a physician. Keep this and all medication out of the reach of children.

How Supplied: Tamper Resistant bottles of 60 capsules: Non-Interfering, Natural Homeopathic Nutraceutical.

Continued on next page

VAXA International Inc.—Cont.

Guaranteed: Contains no additives, fillers, colors, sugars, flavors or preservatives. 60-day money back guarantee.

Wallace Laboratories

P.O. BOX 1001
HALF ACRE ROAD
CRANBURY, NJ 08512

Direct Inquiries to:
Wallace Laboratories
Div. of Carter-Wallace, Inc.
P.O. Box 1001
Cranbury, NJ 08512
(609) 655-6000

For Medical Emergencies, Contact:
(800) 526-3840

MALTSUPEX®
(malt soup extract)
Powder, Liquid, Tablets

Composition: MALTSUPEX is a nondiastatic extract from barley malt, which is available in powder, liquid, and tablet form. Each MALTSUPEX product has a gentle laxative action and promotes soft, easily passed stools.
Tablet: Each tablet contains 750 mg of Malt Soup Extract. Other ingredients: D&C Yellow No. 10, FD&C Red No. 40, flavor (artificial), hydroxypropyl methylcellulose, methylparaben, polyethylene glycol, propylparaben, povidone, simethicone emulsion, stearic acid, talc, titanium dioxide. Sodium content: Each tablet contains approximately 1 mg of sodium.
Powder: Each level scoop provides approximately 8 g of Malt Soup Extract. Sodium content: Each scoopful contains approximately 5 mg of sodium.
Liquid: Each tablespoonful ($^1/_2$ fl. oz.) contains approximately the equivalent of 16 g Malt Soup Extract Powder. Other ingredients: Sodium propionate and potassium sorbate. Sodium content: Each tablespoon contains approximately 36 mg of sodium.

EFFECTIVE, NON-HABIT-FORMING

Indications: For relief of occasional constipation. This product generally produces a bowel movement in 12 to 72 hours.

Warnings: Do not use laxative products when abdominal pain, nausea or vomiting are present unless directed by a physician. If constipation persists, consult a physician.
If you have noticed a sudden change in bowel habits that persists over a period of 2 weeks, consult a physician before using a laxative.
Keep this and all medications out of the reach of children. In case of accidental overdose, seek professional assistance or contact a poison control center immediately.

AGE	CORRECTIVE*	MAINTENANCE
12 years to ADULTS	Up to 4 scoops twice a day (Take a full glass [8 oz.] of liquid with each dose.)	2 to 4 scoops at bedtime
CHILDREN 6–12 years of age	Up to 2 scoops twice a day (Take a full glass [8 oz.] of liquid with each dose.)	
CHILDREN 2–6 years of age	1 scoop twice a day (Take a full glass [8 oz.] of liquid with each dose.)	
INFANTS	2 scoops twice a day in water, fruit juice, or formula	

* Full corrective dosage should be used for 3 or 4 days or until relief is noted. Then continue on maintenance dosage as needed. Use a clean, dry scoop to remove powder. Replace cover tightly to keep out moisture.

AGE	CORRECTIVE*	MAINTENANCE
12 years to ADULTS	2 tablespoonfuls twice a day (Take a full glass [8 oz.] of liquid with each dose.)	1 to 2 tablespoonfuls at bedtime
CHILDREN 6–12 years of age	1 tablespoonful twice a day (Take a full glass [8 oz.] of liquid with each dose.)	
CHILDREN 2–6 years of age	$^1/_2$ tablespoonful twice a day (Take a full glass [8 oz.] of liquid with each dose.)	
INFANTS	1 tablespoonful twice a day in water, fruit juice, or formula	

* Full corrective dosage should be used for 3 or 4 days or until relief is noted. Then continue on maintenance dosage as needed. Use a clean, dry scoop to remove the liquid. Replace cover tightly after use.

Laxative products should not be used for a period longer than one week unless directed by a physician. Rectal bleeding or failure to have a bowel movement after use of a laxative may indicate a serious condition. Discontinue use and consult a physician.
As with any drug, if you are pregnant or nursing a baby, seek the advice of a health professional before using this product.
MALTSUPEX Liquid only—Do not use this product if you are on a sodium-restricted diet unless directed by a physician. Maltsupex Liquid contains approximately 1.58 mEq (36 mg) of sodium per tablespoon. Maltsupex Tablets contain approximately 0.02 mEq (0.46 mg) of sodium per tablet.
Each scoop of Maltsupex Powder contains approximately 0.22 mEq (5 mg) of sodium per scoop.
Note: Allow for carbohydrate content in diabetic diets and infant formulas.
Liquid: (67%, 14 g/tablespoon, or 56 calories/tablespoon)
Powder: (83%, 6 g or 24 calories per scoop)
Tablets: (Approximately 83%, 0.5 g or 2.5 calories per tablet)

Directions: General—Drink a full glass (8 ounces) of liquid with each dose. The recommended daily dosage of MALTSUPEX may vary. Use the smallest dose that is effective and lower dosage as improvement occurs.

MALTSUPEX **Powder**—Each bottle contains a scoop. Each scoopful (which is the equivalent of a standard measuring tablespoon) should be levelled with a knife.

MALTSUPEX **Tablets:** Adult Dosage: Start with four tablets (3 g) four times daily (with meals and at bedtime) and adjust dosage according to response, not to exceed 48 tablets (36 g) daily. Drink a full glass (8 oz.) of liquid with each dose.

Usual Dosage—Powder:

[See first table above.]

Usual Dosage—Liquid:

[See second table above.]

Preparation Tips: Powder—Add dosage to milk, water, or fruit juice and stir until dissolved. Mixing is easier if added to warm milk or warm water. May be flavored with vanilla or cocoa to make "malteds." Excellent with warm milk at bedtime. Also available in tablet and liquid forms.

Note: Although shade, texture, taste, and height of contents may vary between bottles, action remains the same.

Liquid: Mixing is easier if MALTSUPEX Liquid is added to an ounce or two of warm water and stirred. Then add milk, water, or fruit juice and stir until dissolved. May be flavored with vanilla or cocoa to make "malteds." Excellent with warm milk at bedtime. Also available in tablet and powder forms.

How Supplied: MALTSUPEX is supplied in 8 ounce (NDC 0037-9101-12) and 16 ounce (NDC 0037-9101-08) jars of MALTSUPEX Powder; 8 fluid ounce (NDC 0037-9051-12) and 1 pint (NDC 0037-9051-08) bottles of MALTSUPEX Liquid; and in bottles of 100 MALTSUPEX Tablets (NDC 0037-9201-01).

Storage: Store at controlled room temperature 15°–30°C (59°–86°F). Protect MALTSUPEX powder and tablets from moisture.

MALTSUPEX **Powder** and **Liquid** are Distributed by
WALLACE LABORATORIES
Division of
CARTER-WALLACE, INC.
Cranbury, New Jersey 08512
MALTSUPEX **Tablets** are Manufactured by
WALLACE LABORATORIES
Division of
CARTER-WALLACE, INC.
Cranbury, New Jersey 08512

Rev. 9/96

Shown in Product Identification Guide, page 522 and 523

RYNA®
(Liquid)
RYNA–C® Ⓒ
(Liquid)
RYNA–CX® Ⓒ
(Liquid)

Description:
RYNA® (Liquid)—Each 5 mL (one teaspoonful) contains:
Chlorpheniramine maleate .... 2 mg
Pseudoephedrine hydrochloride....30 mg
Other ingredients: flavor (artificial), glycerin, malic acid, purified water, sodium benzoate, sorbitol in a clear, colorless to slightly yellow-colored, lemon-vanilla flavored demulcent base containing no sugar, dyes, or alcohol.

RYNA-C® (Liquid)—Each 5 mL (one teaspoonful) contains, in addition:
Codeine phosphate ....10 mg
(WARNING: May be habit-forming)
Other ingredients: flavor (artificial), glycerin, malic acid, purified water, saccharin sodium, sodium benzoate, sorbitol in a clear, colorless to slightly yellow, cinnamon flavored demulcent base containing no sugar, dyes, or alcohol.

RYNA-CX® (Liquid)—Each 5 mL (one teaspoonful) contains:
Codeine phosphate ....10 mg
(WARNING: May be habit-forming)
Pseudoephedrine hydrochloride....30 mg
Guaifenesin ....100 mg
Other ingredients: flavors (artificial), glycerin, glycine, malic acid, povidone, propylene glycol, purified water, saccharin sodium, sorbitol in a clear, colorless to slightly yellow or straw-colored, cherry-vanilla-menthol flavored demulcent base containing no sugar, dyes, or alcohol.

Actions:
Chlorpheniramine maleate in RYNA and RYNA-C is an antihistamine that antagonizes the effects of histamine.
Codeine phosphate in RYNA-C and RYNA-CX is a centrally-acting antitussive that relieves cough.
Pseudoephedrine hydrochloride in RYNA, RYNA-C and RYNA-CX is a sympathomimetic nasal decongestant that acts to shrink swollen mucosa of the respiratory tract.
Guaifenesin in RYNA-CX is an expectorant, the action of which promotes or facilitates the removal of secretions from the respiratory tract. By increasing sputum volume and making sputum less viscous, guaifenesin facilitates expectoration of retained secretions.

Indications: RYNA: For the temporary relief of nasal congestion due to the common cold, hay fever, or other upper respiratory allergies. Temporarily relieves runny nose, and alleviates sneezing, itching of the nose or throat, and itchy, watery eyes due to hay fever, or other respiratory allergies such as allergic rhinitis.
RYNA-C: For the temporary relief of nasal congestion due to the common cold, hay fever, or other upper respiratory allergies. Temporarily relieves runny nose and alleviates sneezing, itching of the nose or throat, and itchy, watery eyes due to the common cold, hay fever, or other upper respiratory allergies. Temporarily relieves cough due to minor throat and bronchial irritation as may occur with a cold. Temporarily helps to control the cough reflex that causes coughing. Temporarily reduces the intensity of coughing. Controls the impulse to cough to help you sleep. Calms the cough control center and relieves coughing.
RYNA-CX: Temporarily relieves cough due to minor throat and bronchial irritation as may occur with the common cold. Temporarily helps to control the cough reflex that causes coughing. Temporarily reduces the intensity of coughing. Controls the impulse to cough to help you sleep. Calms the cough control center and relieves coughing. Helps loosen phlegm (mucus) and thin bronchial secretions to rid the bronchial passageways of bothersome mucus, drain bronchial tubes, and make coughs more productive. For the temporary relief of nasal congestion due to the common cold, hay fever, or other upper respiratory allergies.

Warnings:
For RYNA:
Do not give this product to children taking other medication or to children under 6 years except under the advice and supervision of a doctor. **Do not exceed the recommended dosage.** If nervousness, dizziness or sleeplessness occur, discontinue use and call a doctor. If symptoms do not improve within 7 days or are accompanied by fever, consult a doctor. Do not take this product, unless directed by a doctor, if you have a breathing problem such as emphysema or chronic bronchitis, or if you have glaucoma, heart disease, high blood pressure, thyroid disease, diabetes, or difficulty in urination due to enlargement of the prostate gland. May cause excitability, especially in children. May cause drowsiness; alcohol, sedatives, and tranquilizers may increase drowsiness effect. Avoid alcoholic beverages while taking this product. Do not take this product if you are taking sedatives or tranquilizers, without first consulting your doctor. Use caution when driving a motor vehicle or operating machinery. As with any drug, if you are pregnant or nursing a baby, seek the advice of a health care professional before taking this product.

For RYNA-C and RYNA-CX:
Adults and children who have a chronic pulmonary disease or shortness of breath, or children who are taking other drugs, should not take this product unless directed by a doctor. Do not give this product to children under 6 years of age except under the advice and supervision of a doctor. A persistent cough may be a sign of a serious condition. If cough persists for more than one week, tends to recur, or is accompanied by fever, rash or persistent headache, consult a doctor. Do not take this product for persistent or chronic cough such as occurs with smoking, asthma, or emphysema, or if cough is accompanied by excessive phlegm (mucus) unless directed by a doctor. Do not take this product unless directed by a doctor if you have a breathing problem such as emphysema or chronic bronchitis, or if you have glaucoma, heart disease, high blood pressure, thyroid disease, diabetes, or difficulty in urination due to enlargement of the prostate gland. May cause or aggravate constipation. May cause marked drowsiness; alcohol, sedatives, and tranquilizers may increase the drowsiness effect. Avoid alcoholic beverages while taking this product. Do not take this product if you are taking sedatives or tranquilizers, without first consulting your doctor. Use caution when driving a motor vehicle or operating machinery. May cause excitability, especially in children. **Do not exceed recommended dosage.** If nervousness, dizziness or sleepiness occur, discontinue use and consult a doctor. If symptoms do not improve within 7 days or are accompanied by a fever, consult a doctor. As with any drug, if you are pregnant or nursing a baby, seek the advice of a health professional before using this drug.

For RYNA, RYNA-C and RYNA-CX:
Drug Interaction Precaution: Do not use this product if you are now taking a prescription monoamine oxidase inhibitor (MAOI) (certain drugs for depression, psychiatric or emotional conditions, or Parkinson's disease), or for 2 weeks after stopping the MAOI drug. If you are uncertain whether your prescription drug contains an MAOI, consult a health professional before taking this product.

Continued on next page

Wallace—Cont.

Dosage and Administration:
Adults and children 12 years of age and over: 2 teaspoonfuls every 4 to 6 hours, not to exceed 8 teaspoonfuls in 24 hours, or as directed by a doctor.
Children 6 to under 12 years: 1 teaspoonful every 4 to 6 hours, not to exceed 4 teaspoonfuls in 24 hours, or as directed by a doctor.
Children under 6 years of age: Consult a doctor.
RYNA-C and RYNA-CX:
A special measuring device should be used to give an accurate dose of these products to children under 6 years of age. Giving a higher dose than recommended by a doctor could result in serious side effects for the child.

How Supplied:
RYNA: bottles of 4 fl oz (NDC 0037-0638-66).
RYNA-C: bottles of 4 fl oz (NDC 0037-0522-66) and one pint (NDC 0037-0522-68).
RYNA-CX: bottles of 4 fl oz (NDC 0037-0801-66) and one pint (NDC 0037-0801-68).
TAMPER-RESISTANT BAND ON CAP PRINTED "WALLACE LABORATORIES." DO NOT USE IF BAND IS MISSING OR BROKEN.

Storage:
RYNA: Store at controlled room temperature 15°–30°C (59°–86°F).
RYNA-C and RYNA-CX: Store at controlled room temperature 15°–30°C (59°–86°F). Dispense in a tight, light-resistant container.
KEEP THESE AND ALL DRUGS OUT OF THE REACH OF CHILDREN. IN CASE OF ACCIDENTAL OVERDOSE, SEEK PROFESSIONAL ASSISTANCE OR CONTACT A POISON CONTROL CENTER IMMEDIATELY.

WALLACE LABORATORIES
Division of
CARTER-WALLACE, INC.
Cranbury, New Jersey 08512

Rev. 9/94

RYNA-C and RYNA-CX
Shown in Product Identification Guide, page 523

Warner-Lambert Company

Consumer Health Products Group
201 TABOR ROAD
MORRIS PLAINS, NJ 07950

Direct Inquiries to:
1-(800) 223-0182

For Consumer Product Information Call:
1-(800) 524-2854 – Celestial Seasonings Soothers (only)
1-(800) 223-0182

CELESTIAL SEASONINGS® SOOTHERS™ Herbal Throat Drops

Active Ingredients: Menthol and Pectin.

Inactive Ingredients: GOLDEN HERBAL BLEND–Chicory Root Extract; Corn Syrup; Ginseng Root Extract; Horehound Extract; Natural Flavoring; Oils of Angelica Root, Anise Star, Ginger, Lemon Grass, Sage and White Thyme; Peppermint Extract; Sucrose. HONEY-LEMON CHAMOMILE–Chamomile Flower Extract; Citric Acid; Corn Syrup; Honey; Lemon Juice; Natural Flavoring; Oils of Angelica Root, Anise Star, Ginger, Lemon Grass, Sage and White Thyme; Sucrose; Tea Extract. HARVEST CHERRY–Cherry, Elderberry and Pineapple Juices; Citric Acid; Corn Syrup; Natural Flavoring; Oils of Angelica Root, Anise Star, Ginger, Lemon Grass, Sage and White Thyme; Sucrose. HERBAL ORANGE SPICE–Beta Carotene; Citric Acid; Corn Syrup; Natural Flavoring; Oils of Angelica Root, Anise Star, Cassia Bark, Ginger, Lemon Grass, Sage and White Thyme; Orange Juice; Sucrose.

Indications: For temporary relief of occasional minor irritation, pain, sore mouth and sore throat. Provides temporary protection of irritated areas in sore mouth and sore throat.

Warnings: If sore throat is severe, persists for more than 2 days, is accompanied or followed by fever, headache, rash, nausea, or vomiting, consult a doctor promptly. If sore mouth symptoms do not improve in 7 days, see your dentist or doctor promptly. KEEP THIS AND ALL DRUGS OUT OF THE REACH OF CHILDREN.

Dosage and Administration: Adults and children 5 years and over: Dissolve 2 drops (one at a time) slowly in the mouth. May be repeated every 2 hours as needed or as directed by a dentist or doctor. Children under 5 years: Consult a dentist or doctor.

How Supplied: Celestial Seasonings Soothers Throat Drops are available in bags of 24 drops. They are available in three flavors: Golden Herbal Blend, Honey-Lemon Chamomile, Harvest Cherry and Herbal Orange Spice. Boxes of 8 drops are also available in Honey-Lemon Chamomile & Harvest Cherry.

Shown in Product Identification Guide, page 523

HALLS® JUNIORS SUGAR FREE Cough Suppressant Drops

[*Hols*]

Active Ingredient: Menthol 2.5 mg per drop.

Inactive Ingredients: ORANGE: Acesulfame Potassium, Eucalyptus Oil, Isomalt, Natural Flavoring and Yellow 6. GRAPE: Acesulfame Potassium, Blue 1, Eucalyptus Oil, Isomalt, Natural Flavoring and Red 40.

Indications: For temporary relief of minor throat irritation and coughs due to colds or inhaled irritants.

Warnings: A persistent cough may be a sign of a serious condition. If cough persists for more than 1 week, tends to recur, or is accompanied by fever, rash, or persistent headache, consult a doctor. Do not take this product for persistent or chronic cough such as occurs with smoking, asthma, or emphysema, or if cough is accompanied by excessive phlegm (mucus) unless directed by a doctor. If sore throat is severe, persists for more than 2 days, is accompanied or followed by fever, headache, rash, swelling, nausea, or vomiting, consult a doctor promptly. KEEP THIS AND ALL DRUGS OUT OF THE REACH OF CHILDREN.

Dosage and Administration: Adults and children 5 years and over: dissolve 2 drops (one at a time) slowly in mouth. Repeat every hour as needed or as directed by a doctor. Children under 5 years: consult a doctor.

Additional Information:
Exchange Information*:
2 Drops = Free Exchange
22 Drops = 2 Fruits
*The dietary exchanges are based on the *Exchange Lists for Meal Planning,* Copyright © 1989 by the American Diabetes Association, Inc. and the American Dietetic Association.

How Supplied: Halls Juniors Sugar Free Cough Suppressant Drops are available in Grape and Orange flavors in bags of 22 drops each.

Shown in Product Identification Guide, page 523

HALLS® MENTHO-LYPTUS® Cough Suppressant Drops

[*Hols*]

Active Ingredient: MENTHO-LYPTUS: Menthol 7 mg per drop. CHERRY: Menthol 7.6 mg per drop. HONEY LEMON: Menthol 8.6 mg per drop. ICE BLUE PEPPERMINT: Menthol 12 mg per drop. SPEARMINT: 6 mg per drop.

Inactive Ingredients: MENTHO-LYPTUS: Eucalyptus Oil, Flavoring, Glucose Syrup and Sucrose. CHERRY: Blue 2, Eucalyptus Oil, Flavoring, Glucose Syrup, Red 40 and Sucrose. HONEY-LEMON: Beta Carotene, Eucalyptus Oil, Flavoring, Glucose Syrup and Sucrose. ICE BLUE PEPPERMINT: Blue 1, Eucalyptus Oil, Flavoring, Glucose Syrup and Sucrose. SPEARMINT: Beta Carotene, Blue 2, Eucalyptus Oil, Flavoring, Glucose Syrup and Sucrose.

Indications: For temporary relief of minor throat irritation and coughs due to colds or inhaled irritants.

Warnings: A persistent cough may be a sign of a serious condition. If cough persists for more than 1 week, tends to recur, or is accompanied by fever, rash or persistent headache, consult a doctor. Do not take this product for persistent or chronic cough such as occurs with smoking, asthma, or emphysema, or if cough is accompanied by excessive phlegm (mucus) unless directed by a doctor. If sore throat is severe, persists for more than 2 days, is accompanied or followed by fever, headache, rash, swelling, nausea, or vomiting, consult a doctor promptly. KEEP THIS AND ALL DRUGS OUT OF THE REACH OF CHILDREN.

Dosage and Administration: Adults and children 5 years and over: dissolve 1 drop slowly in mouth. Repeat every hour as needed or as directed by a doctor. Children under 5 years: consult a doctor.

How Supplied: Halls Mentho-Lyptus Cough Suppressant Drops are available in single sticks of 9 drops each and in bags of 30 and 60 drops. They are available in five flavors: Regular Mentho-Lyptus, Cherry, Honey-Lemon, Ice Blue Peppermint and Spearmint. Mentho-Lyptus & Cherry flavors are also available in bags of 230 drops.

Shown in Product Identification Guide, page 523

HALLS® SUGAR FREE MENTHO-LYPTUS®
Cough Suppressant Drops
[*Hols*]

Active Ingredient: BLACK CHERRY and CITRUS BLEND: Menthol 5 mg per drop. MOUNTAIN MENTHOL: Menthol 6 mg per drop.

Inactive Ingredients: BLACK CHERRY: Acesulfame Potassium, Blue 1, Citric Acid, Eucalyptus Oil, Flavoring, Isomalt and Red 40. CITRUS BLEND: Acesulfame Potassium, Citric Acid, Eucalyptus Oil, Flavoring, Isomalt and Yellow 5 (Tartrazine). MOUNTAIN MENTHOL: Acesulfame Potassium, Eucalyptus Oil, Flavoring and Isomalt.

Indications: For temporary relief of minor throat irritation and coughs due to colds or inhaled irritants.

Warnings: A persistent cough may be a sign of a serious condition. If cough persists for more than 1 week, tends to recur, or is accompanied by fever, rash, or persistent headache, consult a doctor. Do not take this product for persistent or chronic cough such as occurs with smoking, asthma, or emphysema, or if cough is accompanied by excessive phlegm (mucus) unless directed by a doctor. If sore throat is severe, persists for more than 2 days, is accompanied or followed by fever, headache, rash, swelling, nausea, or vomiting, consult a doctor promptly. KEEP THIS AND ALL DRUGS OUT OF THE REACH OF CHILDREN.

Dosage and Administration: Adults and children 5 years and over: dissolve 1 drop slowly in mouth. Repeat every hour as needed or as directed by a doctor. Children under 5 years: consult a doctor.

Additional Information:

Exchange Information*:
1 Drop = Free Exchange
10 Drops = 1 Fruit

*The dietary exchanges are based on the *Exchange Lists for Meal Planning,* Copyright ©1989 by the American Diabetes Association, Inc. and the American Dietetic Association.

How Supplied: Halls Sugar Free Mentho-Lyptus Cough Suppressant Drops are available in bags of 25 drops. They are available in three flavors: Black Cherry, Citrus Blend and Mountain Menthol.

Shown in Product Identification Guide, page 523

MAXIMUM STRENGTH HALLS® PLUS
Cough Suppressant Drops
[*Hols*]

Active Ingredient: Menthol 10 mg per centerfilled drop.

Inactive Ingredients: MENTHO-LYPTUS: Citric Acid, Eucalyptus Oil, Glucose Syrup, Glycerin, High Fructose Corn Syrup and Sucrose. CHERRY: Blue 2, Eucalyptus Oil, Flavoring, Glucose Syrup, Glycerin, High Fructose Corn Syrup, Red 40 and Sucrose. HONEY-LEMON: Acesulfame Potassium, Eucalyptus Oil, Flavoring, Glucose Syrup, Glycerin, High Fructose Corn Syrup, Honey, Sucrose, Yellow 6 and Yellow 10.

Indications: For temporary relief of minor throat irritation and coughs due to colds or inhaled irritants.

Warnings: A persistent cough may be a sign of a serious condition. If cough persists for more than 1 week, tends to recur, or is accompanied by fever, rash or persistent headache, consult a doctor. Do not take this product for persistent or chronic cough such as occurs with smoking, asthma, or emphysema, or if cough is accompanied by excessive phlegm (mucus) unless directed by a doctor. If sore throat is severe, persists for more than 2 days, is accompanied or followed by fever, headache, rash, swelling, nausea, or vomiting, consult a doctor promptly. KEEP THIS AND ALL DRUGS OUT OF THE REACH OF CHLDREN.

Dosage and Administration: Adults and children 5 years and over: for cough dissolve 1 drop slowly in mouth—repeat every hour as needed or as directed by a doctor; for sore throat dissolve either 1 drop or 2 drops (one at a time) slowly in mouth—repeat every 2 hours as needed or as directed by a doctor. Children under 5 years; consult a doctor.

How Supplied: Maximum Strength Halls Plus Cough Suppressant Drops are available in single sticks of 10 drops each and in bags of 25 drops. They are available in three flavors: Regular Mentho-Lyptus, Cherry and Honey-Lemon.

Shown in Product Identification Guide, page 523

HALLS® Vitamin C Drops
[*Hols*]

Ingredients: ASSORTED CITRUS FLAVORS: Sugar, Glucose Syrup, Citric Acid, Sodium Ascorbate, Natural Flavoring, Ascorbic Acid, Color Added and Red 40.

Description: Halls® Vitamin C Drops are a delicious way to get 100% of the Daily Value of Vitamin C. Each drop provides 60 mg. of Vitamin C (100% of the Daily Value).

Indication: Dietary Supplementation.

How Supplied: Halls® Vitamin C Drops are available in single sticks of 9 drops each and in bags of 30 drops. They are available in an all-natural citrus flavor assortment (lemon, sweet grapefruit and orange).

Shown in Product Identification Guide, page 523

ROLAIDS® Antacid Tablets
Original Peppermint, Spearmint, Cherry and Assorted Fruit flavors

Active Ingredients: Calcium Carbonate 550 mg and Magnesium Hydroxide 110 mg per tablet.

Inactive Ingredients: Peppermint and Spearmint flavors: Flavoring, Light Mineral Oil, Magnesium Stearate, Microcrystalline Cellulose, Polyethylene Glycol, Pregelatinized Starch, Silicon Dioxide and Sucrose.
Cherry flavor: Flavoring, Light Mineral Oil, Magnesium Stearate, Microcrystalline Cellulose, Polyethylene Glycol, Pregelatinized Starch, Red 27 Lake, Silicon Dioxide and Sucrose.
Assorted Fruit flavors: Color (Blue 1 Lake, Red 27 Lake, Yellow 5 Lake [Tartrazine] and Yellow 6 Lake), Flavoring, Light Mineral Oil, Magnesium Stearate, Microcrystalline Cellulose, Polyethylene Glycol, Pregelatinized Starch, Silicon Dioxide and Sucrose.

Indications: For the relief of heartburn, sour stomach or acid indigestion and upset stomach associated with these symptoms.

Actions: Rolaids® provides rapid neutralization of stomach acid. Each tablet

Continued on next page

Warner-Lambert—Cont.

has an acid-neutralizing capacity of 14.7 mEq and the ability to maintain the pH of stomach contents at 3.5 or greater for a significant period of time. Each tablet provides 22% of the adult nutritional Daily Value for calcium and 11% of the adult nutritional Daily Value for magnesium. Each tablet contains less than 1 mg of sodium and is considered to be dietetically sodium free.

Warnings: Do not take more than 12 tablets in a 24 hour period or use the maximum dosage of this product for more than 2 weeks except under the advice and supervision of a physician. KEEP THIS AND ALL DRUGS OUT OF THE REACH OF CHILDREN.

Drug Interaction Precaution: Antacids may interact with certain prescription drugs. If you are presently taking a prescription drug, do not take this product without checking with your physician or other health professional.

Dosage and Administration: Chew 1 to 4 tablets as symptoms occur. Repeat hourly if symptoms return, or as directed by a physician.

How Supplied: Rolaids® is available in 12-tablet rolls, 3-packs containing three 12-tablet rolls and in bottles containing 75 or 150 tablets.

Shown in Product Identification Guide, page 523

Warner-Lambert Consumer HealthCare

Warner-Lambert Company
201 TABOR ROAD
MORRIS PLAINS, NJ 07950

Direct Inquiries to:
1-(800) 223-0182

For Medical Information Contact:
1-(800) 223-0182
1-(800) 378-1783 (e.p.t)
1-(800) 337-7266 (e.p.t–spanish)

ACTIFED® Cold & Allergy Tablets
[*ăk 'tuh-fĕd*]

Active Ingredients: Each tablet contains Pseudoephedrine Hydrochloride 60 mg and Triprolidine Hydrochloride 2.5 mg.

Inactive Ingredients: Corn Starch, Flavor, Hydroxypropyl Methylcellulose, Lactose, Magnesium Stearate, Polyethylene Glycol, Potato Starch, Povidone, Sucrose, and Titanium Dioxide.

Indications: Temporarily relieves nasal congestion due to the common cold. Temporarily dries runny nose and alleviates sneezing, itching of the nose or throat, and itchy, watery eyes due to hay fever or other upper respiratory allergies.

Directions: Adults and children 12 years of age and over: 1 tablet. Children 6 to under 12 years of age: $^1/_2$ tablet. Dosage may be repeated every 4 to 6 hours, not to exceed 4 doses in 24 hours, or as directed by a doctor. Children under 6 years of age: consult a doctor.

Warnings: Do not exceed recommended dosage. If nervousness, dizziness, or sleeplessness occur, discontinue use and consult a doctor. If symptoms do not improve within 7 days or are accompanied by fever, consult a doctor. Do not take this product, unless directed by a doctor, if you have heart disease, high blood pressure, thyroid disease, diabetes, a breathing problem such as emphysema or chronic bronchitis, or if you have glaucoma or difficulty in urination due to enlargement of the prostate gland. May cause excitability especially in children. May cause drowsiness; alcohol, sedatives, and tranquilizers may increase the drowsiness effect. Avoid alcoholic beverages while taking this product. Do not take this product if you are taking sedatives or tranquilizers, without first consulting your doctor. Use caution when driving a motor vehicle or operating machinery. As with any drug, if you are pregnant or nursing a baby, seek the advice of a health professional before using this product. **KEEP THIS AND ALL DRUGS OUT OF THE REACH OF CHILDREN.** In case of accidental overdose, seek professional assistance or contact a Poison Control Center immediately.

Drug Interaction Precaution: Do not use this product if you are now taking a prescription monoamine oxidase inhibitor (MAOI) (certain drugs for depression, psychiatric or emotional conditions, or Parkinson's disease), or for 2 weeks after stopping the MAOI drug. If you are uncertain whether your prescription drug contains an MAOI, consult a health professional before taking this product.

How Supplied: Boxes of 12, 24, 48, and bottles of 100.
Store at 15° to 25°C (59° to 77°F) in a dry place and protect from light.

Shown in Product Identification Guide, page 523

ACTIFED® ALLERGY DAYTIME/NIGHTTIME CAPLETS
[*ăk 'tuh-fĕd*]

This package contains 2 separate products: Actifed® Allergy DAYTIME (white caplets) is an antihistamine-free, non-drowsy product. Actifed® Allergy NIGHTTIME (blue caplets) may cause marked drowsiness. Read directions carefully for both products.

ACTIFED DAYTIME/NIGHTTIME products do not contain triprolidine hydrochloride, the antihistamine found in other ACTIFED products.

ACTIFED® ALLERGY DAYTIME (white caplets) **ANTIHISTAMINE-FREE. NON-DROWSY**

Active Ingredients for Actifed Allergy Daytime Caplet: Each caplet contains Pseudoephedrine Hydrochloride 30 mg.

Inactive Ingredients: Carnauba Wax, Crospovidone, Hydroxypropyl Methylcellulose, Lactose, Magnesium Stearate, Microcrystalline cellulose, Polyethylene Glycol, and Titanium Dioxide.

Indications: The DAYTIME product (white caplets) temporarily relieves nasal congestion due to hay fever or other upper respiratory allergies.

Directions: Adults and children 12 years and over: 2 caplets every 4 to 6 hours during waking hours. **Do not take Actifed Allergy Daytime within 4 hours of Actifed Allergy Nighttime.** Do not exceed a total of 8 caplets (Daytime or Nighttime) in 24 hours. Children under 12 years of age: consult a doctor.

ACTIFED® ALLERGY NIGHTTIME (blue caplets) **MAY CAUSE MARKED DROWSINESS.**

Active Ingredients for Actifed Allergy Nighttime Caplet: Each caplet contains Diphenhydramine Hydrochloride 25 mg and Pseudoephedrine Hydrochloride 30 mg.

Inactive Ingredients: Carnauba Wax, Crospovidone, FD&C Blue No. 1 Aluminum Lake, Hydroxypropyl Methylcellulose, Lactose, Magnesium Stearate, Microcrystalline Cellulose, Polyethylene Glycol, Polysorbate 80, and Titanium Dioxide.

Indications: The NIGHTTIME product (blue caplets) temporarily relieves nasal congestion, dries runny nose and alleviates sneezing, itching of the nose or throat, and itchy, watery eyes due to hay fever or other upper respiratory allergies.

Directions: Adults and children 12 years and over: 2 caplets at bedtime, or as directed by a doctor. Due to potential marked drowsiness, do not take during waking hours unless confined to bed or resting at home; 2 caplets then may be taken every 4 to 6 hours. **Do not take Actifed Allergy Nighttime within 4 hours of Actifed Daytime.** Do not exceed a total of 8 caplets (Daytime and/or Nighttime) in 24 hours. Children under 12 years of age: consult a doctor.

Warnings for both the daytime and nighttime caplets: Do not exceed recommended dosage. If nervousness, dizziness, or sleeplessness occur, discontinue use and consult a doctor. If symptoms do not improve within 7 days or are accompanied by fever, consult a doctor. Do not take this product, if you have heart disease, high blood pressure, thyroid disease, diabetes, difficulty in urination due to enlargement of the prostate gland unless directed by a doctor. As with any drug, if you are pregnant or nursing a baby, seek the advice of a health professional before using this product. **KEEP THIS AND ALL DRUGS OUT OF THE REACH OF CHILDREN.** In case of accidental overdose, seek professional assistance or contact a Poison Control Center immediately.

Additional warnings for the nighttime caplet: May cause excitability especially in children. Do not take this product, unless directed by a doctor, if you have a breathing problem such as emphysema or chronic bronchitis, or if you have glaucoma or difficulty in urination due to enlargement of the prostate gland. May cause marked drowsiness; alcohol, sedatives, and tranquilizers may increase the drowsiness effect. Avoid alcoholic beverages while taking this product. Do not take this product if you are taking sedatives or tranquilizers, without first consulting your doctor. Use caution when driving a motor vehicle or operating machinery.

Drug Interaction Precaution: Do not use this product if you are now taking a prescription monoamine oxidase inhibitor (MAOI) (certain drugs for depression, psychiatric or emotional conditions, or Parkinson's disease), or for 2 weeks after stopping the MAOI drug. If you are uncertain whether your prescription drug contains an MAOI, consult a health professional before taking this product.

How Supplied: Package contains 24 Daytime Caplets and 8 Nighttime Caplets.
Store at 15° to 25°C (59° to 77°F) in a dry place and protect from light.

Shown in Product Identification Guide, page 523

ACTIFED® Cold & Sinus Caplets and Tablets

[*ăk 'tuh-fĕd*]

Active Ingredients: Each tablet/caplet contains Acetaminophen 500 mg, Pseudoephedrine Hydrochloride 30 mg and Triprolidine Hydrochloride 1.25 mg.

Inactive Ingredients: Carnauba Wax, Crospovidone, FD&C Blue No. 1 Aluminum Lake, D&C Yellow No. 10 Aluminum Lake, Hydroxypropyl Methylcellulose, Magnesium Stearate, Microcrystalline Cellulose, Polyethylene Glycol, Polysorbate 80, Povidone, Pregelatinized Starch, Stearic Acid, and Titanium Dioxide.

Indications: Temporarily relieves nasal congestion due to the common cold or associated with sinusitis. Helps decongest sinus openings and passages; temporarily relieves sinus congestion and pressure. For the temporary relief of minor aches, pains, headache, and fever associated with a cold, and runny nose and sneezing, itching of a nose or throat, and itchy, watery eyes due to hay fever.

Directions: Adults and children 12 years of age and over: 2 caplets or tablets. Dosage may be repeated every 6 hours while symptoms persist, not to exceed 8 caplets or tablets in 24 hours, or as directed by a doctor. Children under 12 years of age: consult a doctor.

Warnings: Do not exceed recommended dosage. If nervousness, dizziness, or sleeplessness occur, discontinue use and consult a doctor. Do not take this product for more than 10 days. If symptoms do not improve or are accompanied by fever that lasts for more than 3 days, or if new symptoms occur, consult a doctor. Do not take this product, unless directed by a doctor, if you have heart disease, high blood pressure, thyroid disease, diabetes, a breathing problem such as emphysema or chronic bronchitis, or if you have glaucoma or difficulty in urination due to enlargement of the prostate gland. May cause excitability especially in children. May cause drowsiness; alcohol, sedatives, and tranquilizers may increase the drowsiness effect. Avoid alcoholic beverages while taking this product. Do not take this product if you are taking sedatives or tranquilizers, without first consulting your doctor. Use caution when driving a motor vehicle or operating machinery. As with any drug, if you are pregnant or nursing a baby, seek the advice of a health professional before using this product. **KEEP THIS AND ALL DRUGS OUT OF THE REACH OF CHILDREN.** In case of accidental overdose, seek professional assistance or contact a Poison Control Center immediately. Prompt medical attention is critical for adults as well as for children even if you do not notice any signs or symptoms.

Alcohol Warning: If you generally consume 3 or more alcohol-containing drinks per day, you should consult your physician for advice on when and how you should take Actifed Cold & Sinus and other pain relievers.

Drug Interaction Precaution: Do not use this product if you are now taking a prescription monoamine oxidase inhibitor (MAOI) (certain drugs for depression, psychiatric or emotional conditions, or Parkinson's disease), or for 2 weeks after stopping the MAOI drug. If you are uncertain whether your prescription drug contains an MAOI, consult a health professional before taking this product.

How Supplied: Boxes of 20.
Store at 15° to 25°C (59° to 77°F) in a dry place and protect from light.

Shown in Product Identification Guide, page 523

ACTIFED® SINUS DAYTIME/ NIGHTTIME Tablets and Caplets

[*ak'tuh-fĕd*]

> This package contains 2 separate products: Actifed® Sinus DAYTIME (white tablets or caplets) is an antihistamine-free, non-drowsy product; Actifed® Sinus NIGHTTIME (blue tablets or caplets) may cause marked drowsiness. Read directions carefully for both products.

ACTIFED DAYTIME/NIGHTTIME products do not contain triprolidine hydrochloride, the antihistamine found in other ACTIFED products.

ACTIFED® SINUS DAYTIME (white tablets and caplets)
NON-DROWSY.

Active Ingredients for Actifed Sinus Daytime Tablet or Caplet: Each tablet/caplet contains Acetaminophen 500 mg and Pseudoephedrine Hydrochloride 30 mg.

Inactive Ingredients: Carnauba Wax, Crospovidone, Hydroxypropyl Methylcellulose, Magnesium Stearate, Microcrystalline Cellulose, Polyethylene Glycol, Povidone, Pregelatinized Starch, Stearic Acid, and Titanium Dioxide.

Indications: The DAYTIME product (white caplets) temporarily relieves nasal congestion associated with sinusitis. Helps decongest sinus openings and passages; temporarily relieves sinus congestion and pressure. Temporarily relieves minor aches, pains and headache.

Directions: Adults and children 12 years and over, 2 caplets or tablets every 6 hours during waking hours while symptoms persist, or as directed by a doctor. **Do not take Actifed Sinus Daytime within 6 hours of Actifed Sinus Nighttime.** Do not exceed a total of 8 caplets or tablets (Daytime and/or Nighttime) in 24 hours. Children under 12 years of age: consult a doctor.

ACTIFED® SINUS NIGHTTIME (blue tablets and caplets)
MAY CAUSE MARKED DROWSINESS.

Active Ingredients for Actifed Sinus Nighttime Tablet or Caplet: Each tablet/caplet contains Acetaminophen 500 mg, Diphenhydramine Hydrochloride 25 mg and Pseudoephedrine Hydrochloride 30 mg.

Inactive Ingredients: Carnauba Wax, Crospovidone, FD&C Blue No. 1 Aluminum Lake, Hydroxypropyl Methylcellulose, Magnesium Stearate, Microcrystalline Cellulose, Polyethylene Glycol, Polysorbate 80, Povidone, Pregelatinized Starch, Sodium Starch Glycolate, Stearic Acid, and Titanium Dioxide.

Indications: The NIGHTTIME product (blue caplets) temporarily relieves nasal congestion associated with sinusi-

Continued on next page

This product information was prepared in November 1996. On these and other Warner-Lambert Consumer Healthcare Products, detailed information may be obtained by addressing Warner-Lambert Consumer Healthcare Products, Morris Plains, NJ 07950 USA

Warner-Lambert—Cont.

tis. Helps decongest sinus openings and passages; temporarily relieves sinus congestion and pressure. Temporarily relieves minor aches, pains, and headache associated with a cold, runny nose and sneezing, itching of the nose or throat, and itchy, watery eyes due to hay fever.

Directions: Adults and children 12 years and over: 2 tablets or caplets at bedtime while symptoms persist, or as directed by a doctor. Due to potential marked drowsiness, do not take during waking hours unless confined to bed or resting at home; 2 tablets or caplets then may be taken every 6 hours. **Do not take Actifed Sinus Nighttime within 6 hours of Actifed Sinus Daytime.** Do not exceed a total of 8 tablets or caplets (Daytime and/or Nighttime) in 24 hours. Children under 12 years of age: consult a doctor.

Warnings for both the daytime and nighttime caplets/tablets: Do not exceed recommended dosage. If nervousness, dizziness, or sleeplessness occur, discontinue use and consult a doctor. Do not take this product for more than 10 days. If symptoms do not improve or are accompanied by fever that lasts for more than 3 days, or if new symptoms occur, consult a doctor. Do not take this product if you have heart disease, high blood pressure, thyroid disease, diabetes, or difficulty in urination due to enlargement of the prostate gland. As with any drug, if you are pregnant or nursing a baby, seek the advice of a health professional before using this product. **KEEP THIS AND ALL DRUGS OUT OF THE REACH OF CHILDREN.** In case of accidental overdose, seek professional assistance or contact a Poison Control Center immediately. Prompt medical attention is critical for adults as well as children even if you do not notice any signs or symptoms.

Alcohol Warning: If you generally consume 3 or more alcohol-containing drinks per day, you should consult your physician for advice on when and how you should take Actifed Sinus and other pain relievers.

Additional warnings for the nighttime caplets/tablets: May cause excitability especially in children. Do not take this product, unless directed by a doctor, if you have a breathing problem such as emphysema or chronic bronchitis, or if you have glaucoma or difficulty in urination due to enlargement of the prostate gland. May cause marked drowsiness; alcohol, sedatives, and tranquilizers may increase the drowsiness effect. Avoid alcoholic beverages while taking this product. Do not take this product if you are taking sedatives or tranquilizers, without first consulting your doctor. Use caution when driving a motor vehicle or operating machinery.

Drug Interaction Precaution: Do not use this product if you are now taking a prescription monoamine oxidase inhibitor (MAOI) (certain drugs for depression, psychiatric or emotional conditions, or Parkinson's disease), or for 2 weeks after stopping the MAOI drug. If you are uncertain whether your prescription drug contains an MAOI, consult a health professional before taking this product.

How Supplied: Package contains 18 Daytime Tablets or Caplets and 6 Nighttime Tablets or Caplets.
Store at 15° to 25°C (59° to 77°F) in a dry place and protect from light.

Shown in Product Identification Guide, page 523

ANUSOL®
Hemorrhoidal Suppositories/ Ointment
[*ă'nū-sōl"*]

Description:
Anusol Suppositories: **Active Ingredient:** Topical Starch 51%. Also contains: Benzyl Alcohol, Partially Hydrogenated Soy Bean Oil with Sorbitan Tristearate, Tocopheryl Acetate.
Anusol Ointment: **Active ingredients:** Pramoxine HCl 1%, Mineral Oil and Zinc Oxide 12.5%. Also contains: Benzyl Benzoate, Calcium Phosphate Dibasic, Cocoa Butter, Glyceryl Monooleate, Glyceryl Monostearate, Kaolin, Peruvian Balsam and Polyethylene Wax.

Actions: Anusol Suppositories and Anusol Ointment help to relieve burning, itching and discomfort arising from irritated anorectal tissues. They have a soothing, lubricant action on the intrarectal mucous membrane. Pramoxine Hydrochloride in Anusol Ointment is a rapidly acting local anesthetic for the skin and mucous membranes in the lower portion of the anal canal. Pramoxine HCl is also chemically distinct from procaine, cocaine, and dibucaine and can often be used in the patient previously sensitized to other surface anesthetics. Surface analgesia lasts for several hours.

Indications: Anusol Ointment: Temporarily relieves the pain, soreness, burning and itching associated with hemorrhoids and other anorectal disorders while it forms a temporary protective coating over inflamed tissues to help prevent the drying of tissues. Anusol Ointment is to be applied externally or in the lower portion of the anal canal (The enclosed dispensing cap is designed to control dispersion of the ointment to the affected area in the lower portion of the anal canal only.)
Anusol Suppositories: Gives temporary relief from the itching, burning and discomfort associated with hemorrhoids and other anorectal disorders and provides a coating to protect irritated tissue.

Warnings: Anusol Ointment: If condition worsens or does not improve within 7 days, consult a physician. Certain persons can develop allergic reactions to ingredients in this product. If the symptom being treated does not subside or if redness, irritation, swelling, pain or other symptoms develop or increase, discontinue use and consult a phsyician. In case of bleeding, consult a physician promptly. Do not exceed the recommended daily dosage unless directed by a physician. Do not put this product into the rectum by using fingers or any mechanical device or applicator. KEEP THIS AND ALL DRUGS OUT OF THE REACH OF CHILDREN. In case of accidental ingestion seek professional assistance or contact a Poison Control Center immediately. Anusol Suppositories: Do not exceed recommended daily dosage unless directed by a physician. If condition worsens or does not improve within 7 days, consult a physician. In case of bleeding, consult a physician promptly. KEEP THIS AND ALL DRUGS OUT OF THE REACH OF CHILDREN. In case of accidental ingestion seek professional assistance or contact a Poison Control Center immediately. As with any drug, if you are pregnant or nursing a baby, seek the advice of a health professional before using this product.

Directions: Anusol Suppositories: Adults: When practical, cleanse the affected area with mild soap and warm water and rinse thoroughly. Gently dry by patting or blotting with toilet tissue or soft cloth before application of this product.

1. Detach one suppository from the strip of suppositories.
2. Remove wrapper before inserting into the rectum as follows: Hold suppository upright (with words "pull apart" at top) and carefully separate foil by inserting tip of fingernail at foil split.
3. Peel foil slowly and evenly down both sides, exposing suppository.
4. Avoid excessive handling of suppository which is designed to melt at body temperature. If suppository seems soft, hold in foil wrapper under cold water for 2 or 3 minutes.
5. Insert one (1) suppository rectally up to six (6) times daily or after each bowel movement.

Children under 12 years of age: consult a physician.

Anusol Ointment: Adults: When practical, cleanse the affected area with mild soap and warm water and rinse thoroughly. Gently dry by patting or blotting with toilet tissue or a soft cloth before application of this product. Apply externally to the affected area up to five (5) times daily. To use dispensing cap, attach it to tube, lubricate well, then gently insert part way into the anus. Squeeze tube to deliver medication. Thoroughly cleanse dispensing cap after use. Children under 12 years of age: Consult a physician.

How Supplied: Anusol Suppositories—boxes of 12 or 24 in silver foil strips.
Anusol Ointment—1-oz (28.3g) tubes with plastic applicator.
Ointment: Store between 15° and 30°C (59° and 86°F).

Suppositories: Do not store above 86°F or suppositories may melt.

Shown in Product Identification Guide, page 523

ANUSOL HC-1
Hydrocortisone Anti-Itch Ointment
[*ă'nū-sōl"*]

Active Ingredient: Hydrocortisone Acetate (equivalent to 1% Hydrocortisone).

Inactive Ingredients: Diazolidinyl Urea, Methylparaben, Microcrystalline Wax, Mineral Oil, Propylene Glycol, Propylparaben, Sorbitan Sesquioleate and White Petrolatum.

Indications: For temporary relief of itching associated with minor skin irritations, rashes and for external anal itching. Other uses of this product should be only under the advice and supervision of a physician.

Warnings: For external use only. Avoid contact with the eyes. If condition worsens, or if symptoms persist for more than 7 days or clear up and occur again within a few days, stop use of this product and do not begin use of any other hydrocortisone product unless you have consulted a physician. Do not exceed the recommended daily dosage unless directed by a physician. In case of bleeding, consult a physician promptly. Do not put this product into the rectum by using fingers or any mechanical device or applicator. Do not use for treatment of diaper rash. Consult a physician. KEEP THIS AND ALL DRUGS OUT OF THE REACH OF CHILDREN. In case of accidental ingestion seek professional assistance or contact a Poison Control Center immediately.

Directions: Adults when practical cleanse the affected area with mild soap and warm water and rinse thoroughly. Gently dry by patting or blotting with toilet tissue or soft cloth before application of this product. Apply to affected area not more than 3 to 4 times daily. Children under 12 years of age: consult a physician.

How Supplied: Anusol HC-1 Ointment in 0.7 oz (19.8 g) tube. Store at Room Temperature 59°–86°F.

Shown in Product Identification Guide, page 523

BENADRYL® Allergy Ultratab™ Tablets and Kapseal® Capsules
[*bĕ'nă-drĭl*]

Active Ingredients: Each Tablet/Capsule contains: Diphenhydramine Hydrochloride 25 mg.

Inactive Ingredients: Each Tablet contains: Candelilla Wax, Crospovidone, Dibasic Calcium Phosphate Dihydrate, D&C Red No. 27 Aluminum Lake, Hydroxypropyl Methylcellulose, Magnesium Stearate, Microcrystalline Cellulose, Polyethylene Glycol, Polysorbate 80, Pregelantinized Starch, Stearic Acid, and Titanium Dioxide.
Each Capsule contains: Lactose and Magnesium Stearate. The Kapseals capsule shell contains: D&C Red No. 28, FD&C Red No. 3, Red No. 40, FD&C Blue No. 1, Gelatin, Glyceryl Monooleate, and Titanium Dioxide.

Indications: Temporarily relieves runny nose and sneezing, itching of the nose or throat, and itchy, watery eyes due to hay fever or other upper respiratory allergies, and runny nose and sneezing associated with the common cold.

Warnings: May cause excitability especially in children. Do not take this product, unless directed by a doctor, if you have a breathing problem such as emphysema or chronic bronchitis, or if you have glaucoma or difficulty in urination due to enlargement of the prostate gland. May cause marked drowsiness; alcohol, sedatives, and tranquilizers may increase the drowsiness effect. Avoid alcoholic beverages while taking this product. Do not take this product if you are taking sedatives or tranquilizers, without first consulting your doctor. Use caution when driving a motor vehicle or operating machinery. **Do not use any other products containing diphenhydramine while using this product.** As with any drug, if you are pregnant or nursing a baby, seek the advice of a health professional before using this product. KEEP THIS AND ALL DRUGS OUT OF THE REACH OF CHILDREN. In case of accidental overdose, seek professional assistance or contact a Poison Control Center immediately.

Directions: Adults and children 12 years of age and over: 25 to 50 mg (1 to 2 tablets/capsules) every 4 to 6 hours. Not to exceed 12 tablets/capsules in 24 hours. Children 6 to under 12 years of age: 12.5 mg* to 25 mg (1 tablet/capsule) every 4 to 6 hours, not to exceed 6 tablets/capsules in 24 hours. Children under 6 years of age: consult your doctor.

How Supplied: Benadryl tablets are supplied in boxes of 24 and 48, bottle of 100; capsules are supplied in boxes of 24 and 48.
Store at room temperature 15°–30° C (59°–86° F). Protect from moisture.

* This dosage is not available in this package. Do not attempt to break tablet/capsule. This dosage is available in pleasant tasting Benadryl Allergy Liquid Medication.

Shown in Product Identification Guide, page 524

BENADRYL® ALLERGY/COLD TABLETS
[*bĕ'nă-drĭl*]

Active Ingredients: Each tablet contains: Diphenhydramine Hydrochloride 12.5 mg, Pseudoephedrine Hydrochloride 30 mg and Acetaminophen 500 mg.

Inactive Ingredients: Candelilla Wax, Croscarmellose Sodium, Hydroxypropyl Cellulose, Hydroxypropyl Methylcellulose, Magnesium Stearate, Microcrystalline Cellulose, Polyethylene Glycol, Pregelatinized Starch, Propylene Glycol, Sodium Starch Glycolate, Starch, Stearic Acid, Titanium Dioxide, and Zinc Stearate. Printed with edible blue ink.

Indications: For the temporary relief of minor aches, pains, headache, muscular aches, sore throat, fever, runny nose and sneezing, itching of the nose or throat, and itchy, watery eyes due to hay fever, and nasal congestion due to the common cold.

Warnings: Do not exceed recommended dosage. If nervousness, dizziness, or sleeplessness occur, discontinue use and consult a doctor. Do not take this product for more than 10 days. If symptoms do not improve or are accompanied by fever that lasts for more than 3 days, or if new symptoms occur, consult a doctor. If sore throat is severe, persists for more than 2 days, is accompanied or followed by fever, headache, rash, nausea, or vomiting, consult a doctor promptly. Do not take this product, unless directed by a doctor, if you have a breathing problem such as emphysema or chronic bronchitis, heart disease, high blood pressure, thyroid disease, diabetes, or if you have glaucoma or difficulty in urination due to enlargement of the prostate gland. May cause excitability especially in children. May cause marked drowsiness; alcohol, sedatives, and tranquilizers may increase the drowsiness effect. Avoid alcoholic beverages while taking this product. Do not take this product if you are taking sedatives or tranquilizers, without first consulting your doctor. Use caution when driving a motor vehicle or operating machinery. Do not use any other products containing diphenhydramine while using this product. As with any drug, if you are pregnant or nursing a baby, seek the advice of a health professional before using this product. KEEP THIS AND ALL DRUGS OUT OF THE REACH OF CHILDREN. In case of accidental overdose, seek professional assistance or contact a Poison Control Center immediately. Prompt medical attention is critical for adults as well as for children even if you do not notice any signs or symptoms.

Alcohol Warning: If you generally consume 3 or more alcohol-containing drinks per day, you should consult your physician for advice on when and how

Continued on next page

This product information was prepared in November 1996. On these and other Warner-Lambert Consumer Healthcare Products, detailed information may be obtained by addressing Warner-Lambert Consumer Healthcare Products, Morris Plains, NJ 07950 USA

Warner-Lambert—Cont.

you should take Benadryl Allergy/Cold and other pain relievers.

Drug Interaction Precaution: Do not use this product if you are now taking a prescription monoamine oxidase inhibitor (MAOI) (certain drugs for depression, psychiatric or emotional conditions, or Parkinson's disease), or for 2 weeks after stopping the MAOI drug. If you are uncertain whether your prescription drug contains an MAOI, consult a health professional before taking this product.

Directions: Adults and children 12 years of age and over: two (2) tablets every 6 hours while symptoms persist. Not to exceed 8 tablets in 24 hours. Children under 12 years of age: consult a doctor.

How Supplied: Benadryl® Allergy/Cold tablets are supplied in boxes of 24 tablets. Store at room temperature 59°–86°F. Protect from moisture.

Shown in Product Identification Guide, page 524

BENADRYL® ALLERGY CHEWABLES

[*bĕ 'nă-drĭl*]

Active Ingredients: Each chewable tablet contains: Diphenhydramine Hydrochloride 12.5 mg.

Inactive Ingredients: Aspartame, Dextrates, D&C Red No. 27 Aluminum Lake, FD&C Blue No. 1 Aluminum Lake, Flavors, Magnesium Stearate, Magnesium Trisilicate, and Tartaric Acid.

Indications: Temporarily relieves runny nose and sneezing, itching of the nose or throat, and itchy, water eyes due to hay fever or other upper respiratory allergies, and runny nose and sneezing associated with the common cold.

Warnings: May cause excitability especially in children. Do not take this product, unless directed by a doctor, if you have a breathing problem such as emphysema or chronic bronchitis, or if you have glaucoma or difficulty in urination due to enlargement of the prostate gland. May cause marked drowsiness; alcohol, sedatives, and tranquilizers may increase the drowsiness effect. Avoid alcoholic beverages while taking this product. Do not take this product if you are taking sedatives or tranquilizers, without first consulting your doctor. Use caution when driving a motor vehicle or operating machinery. **Do not use any other products containing diphenhydramine while using this product.** As with any drug, if you are pregnant or nursing a baby, seek the advice of a health professional before using this product. KEEP THIS AND ALL DRUGS OUT OF THE REACH OF CHILDREN. In case of accidental overdose, seek professional assistance or contact a Poison Control Center immediately. **Phenylketonurics: Contains Phenylalanine 4.2 mg. Per Tablet.**

Directions: Chew tablets thoroughly before swallowing. Adults and children 12 years of age and over: 2 to 4 tablets (25 to 50 mg.) every 4 to 6 hours. Not to exceed 24 tablets in 24 hours. Children 6 to under 12 years of age: 1 to 2 tablets (12.5 to 25 mg.) every 4 to 6 hours. Not to exceed 12 tablets in 24 hours. Children under 6 years of age: consult a doctor.

How Supplied: Benadryl® Allergy Chewables are supplied in boxes of 24 tablets. Store at room temperature 59°–77°F. Protect from heat and humidity.

Shown in Product Identification Guide, page 524

BENADRYL®
Allergy Decongestant Tablets

[*bĕ 'nă-drĭl*]

Active Ingredients: Each tablet contains: Diphenhydramine Hydrochloride 25 mg and Pseudoephedrine Hydrochloride 60 mg.

Inactive Ingredients: Each tablet contains: Croscarmellose Sodium, Dibasic Calcium Phosphate Dihydrate, FD&C Blue No. 1 Aluminum Lake, Hydroxypropyl Methylcellulose, Microcrystalline Cellulose, Polyethylene Glycol, Polysorbate 80, Pregelatinized Starch, Stearic Acid, Titanium Dioxide and Zinc Stearate.

Indications: Temporarily relieves nasal congestion; runny nose and sneezing, itching of the nose or throat, and itchy, watery eyes due to hay fever or other upper respiratory allergies, and runny nose, sneezing, and nasal congestion associated with the common cold.

Warning: Do not exceed recommended dosage. If nervousness, dizziness, or sleeplessness occur, discontinue use and consult a doctor. If symptoms do not improve within 7 days or are accompanied by fever, consult a doctor. Do not take this product, unless directed by a doctor, if you have a breathing problem such as emphysema or chronic bronchitis, heart disease, high blood pressure, thyroid disease, diabetes, or if you have glaucoma or difficulty in urination due to enlargement of the prostate gland. May cause excitability especially in children. May cause marked drowsiness; alcohol, sedatives, and tranquilizers may increase the drowsiness effect. Avoid alcoholic beverages while taking this product. Do not take this product if you are taking sedatives or tranquilizers, without first consulting your doctor. Use caution when driving a motor vehicle or operating machinery. Do not use any other products containing diphenhydramine while using this product. As with any drug, if you are pregnant or nursing a baby, seek the advice of a health professional before using this product. KEEP THIS AND ALL DRUGS OUT OF THE REACH OF CHILDREN. In case of accidental overdose, seek professional assistance or contact a Poison Control Center immediately.

Drug Interaction Precaution: Do not use this product if you are now taking a prescription monoamine oxidase inhibitor (MAOI) (certain drugs for depression, psychiatric or emotional conditions, or Parkinson's disease), or for 2 weeks after stopping the MAOI drug. If you are uncertain whether your prescription drug contains an MAOI, consult a health professional before taking this product.

Directions: Adults and children 12 years of age and over: one (1) tablet every 4 to 6 hours, not to exceed 4 tablets in 24 hours. Children under 12 years of age: consult a doctor.

How Supplied: Benadryl Allergy Decongestant Tablets are supplied in boxes of 24.
Store at room temperature 59°–86° F. Protect from moisture.

Shown in Product Identification Guide, page 524

BENADRYL®
Allergy Decongestant Liquid Medication

[*bĕ 'nă-drĭl*]

Active Ingredients: Each teaspoonful (5 mL) contains: Diphenhydramine Hydrochloride) 12.5 mg and Pseudoephedrine Hydrochloride 30 mg.

Inactive Ingredients: Citric Acid, FD&C Blue No. 1, FD&C Red No. 40, Flavors, Glycerin, Poloxamer 407, Polysorbate 20, Purified Water, Saccharin Sodium, Sodium Benzoate, Sodium Chloride, Sodium Citrate and Sorbitol Solution.

Indications: Temporarily relieves nasal congestion, runny nose, and sneezing, itching of the nose or throat, and itchy, watery eyes due to hay fever or other upper respiratory allergies; and runny nose, sneezing, and nasal congestion associated with the common cold.

Directions: Follow dosage recommendations below, or use as directed by your doctor.

Benadryl® Allergy Decongestant Liquid Medication

AGE	DOSAGE
Children under 6 years of age	Consult a doctor.
Children 6 to under 12 years of age	One (1) teaspoonful every 4 to 6 hours. Not to exceed 4 teaspoonfuls in 24 hours.

Adults and children 12 years of age and over	Two (2) teaspoonfuls every 4 to 6 hours. Not to exceed 8 teaspoonfuls in 24 hours.

Warnings: Do not exceed recommended dosage. If nervousness, dizziness, or sleeplessness occur, discontinue use and consult a doctor. If symptoms do not improve within 7 days or are accompanied by fever, consult a doctor. Do not take this product, unless directed by a doctor, if you have a breathing problem such as emphysema or chronic bronchitis, heart disease, high blood pressure, thyroid disease, diabetes, or if you have glaucoma or difficulty in urination due to enlargement of the prostate gland. May cause excitability, especially in children. May cause marked drowsiness; alcohol, sedatives, and tranquilizers may increase the drowsiness effect. Avoid alcoholic beverages while taking this product. Do not take this product if you are taking sedatives or tranquilizers, without first consulting your doctor. Use caution when driving a motor vehicle or operating machinery. **Do not use any other products containing diphenhydramine while using this product.** As with any drug, if you are pregnant or nursing a baby, seek the advice of a health professional before using this product. KEEP THIS AND ALL DRUGS OUT OF THE REACH OF CHILDREN. In case of accidental overdose, seek professional assistance or contact a Poison Control Center immediately.

Drug Interaction Precaution: Do not use this product if you are now taking a prescription monoamine oxidase inhibitor (MAOI) (certain drugs for depression, psychiatric or emotional conditions, or Parkinson's disease), or for 2 weeks after stopping the MAOI drug. If you are uncertain whether your prescription drug contains an MAOI, consult a health professional before taking this product.

How Supplied: Benadryl Allergy Decongestant Liquid Medication is supplied in 4 fl. oz. bottles.
Store at room temperature 59°–86°F.
Protect from freezing.

Shown in Product Identification Guide, page 524

BENADRYL® Allergy Liquid Medication

[*bĕ'nă-drĭl*]

Active Ingredient: Each teaspoonful (5 mL) contains Diphenhydramine Hydrochloride 12.5 mg.

Inactive Ingredients: Each teaspoonful (5 mL) contains: Citric Acid, D&C Red No. 33, FD&C Red No. 40, Flavors, Glycerin, Poloxamer 407, Purified Water, Sodium Benzoate, Sodium Chloride, Sodium Citrate, and Sugar.

Indications: Temporarily relieves runny nose and sneezing, itching of the nose or throat, and itchy, watery eyes due to hay fever or other upper respiratory allergies, and runny nose and sneezing associated with the common cold.

Directions: Follow dosage recommendations below, or use as directed by your doctor.

Benadryl® Allergy Liquid Medication

AGE	DOSAGE
Children under 6 years of age	Consult a doctor.
Children 6 to under 12 years of age	**1 to 2 teaspoonfuls (12.5 to 25 mg.)** every 4 to 6 hours. Not to exceed 12 teaspoonfuls in 24 hours.
Adults and children 12 years of age and over	**2 to 4 teaspoonfuls (25 to 50 mg.)** every 4 to 6 hours. Not to exceed 24 teaspoonfuls in 24 hours.

Warnings: May cause excitability, especially in children. Do not take this product, unless directed by a doctor, if you have a breathing problem such as emphysema, or chronic bronchitis, or if you have glaucoma or difficulty in urination due to enlargment of the prostate gland. May cause marked drowsiness; alcohol, sedatives, and tranquilizers may increase the drowsiness effect. Avoid alcoholic beverages while taking this product. Do not take this product if you are taking sedatives or tranquilizers, without first consulting your doctor. Use caution when driving a motor vehicle or operating machinery. **Do not use any other products containing diphenhydramine while using this product.** As with any drug, if you are pregnant or nursing a baby seek the advice of a health professional before using this product. KEEP THIS AND ALL DRUGS OUT OF THE REACH OF CHILDREN. In case of accidental overdose, seek professional assistance or contact a Poison Control Center immediately.

How Supplied: Benadryl Allergy Liquid Medication is supplied in 4 and 8 fluid ounce bottles.

Store at room temperature 59°–86°F.
Protect from freezing.

Shown in Product Identification Guide, page 524

BENADRYL® Allergy Sinus Headache Caplets

[*bĕ'nă-drĭl*]

Active Ingredients: Each caplet contains Diphenhydramine Hydrochloride 12.5 mg, Pseudoephedrine Hydrochloride 30 mg and Acetaminophen 500 mg.

Inactive Ingredients: Candelilla Wax, Croscarmellose Sodium, D&C Yellow No. 10 Aluminum Lake, FD&C Blue No. 1 Aluminum Lake, FD&C Yellow No. 6 Aluminum Lake, Hydroxypropyl Cellulose, Hydroxypropyl Methylcellulose, Microcrystalline Cellulose, Polyethylene Glycol, Polysorbate 80, Pregelatinized Starch, Sodium Starch Glycolate, Starch, Stearic Acid, Titanium Dioxide, and Zinc Stearate. Printed with edible red ink.

Indications: For the temporary relief of minor aches, pains, and headache, runny nose and sneezing, itching of the nose or throat, and itchy, watery eyes due to hay fever, and nasal congestion due to the common cold, hay fever, or other upper respiratory allergies. Helps decongest sinus openings and passages; temporarily relieves sinus congestion and pressure.

Action: BENADRYL ALLERGY/SINUS/HEADACHE is specially formulated to provide effective relief of your upper respiratory allergy symptoms complicated by sinus and headache problems. It combines the strength of BENADRYL to relieve your runny nose, sneezing, itchy water eyes, itchy nose or throat, with a maximum strength NASAL DECONGESTANT to relieve nasal and sinus congestion, and a maximum strength non-aspirin PAIN RELIEVER to relieve sinus pain and headache.

Warnings: Do not exceed recommended dosage. If nervousness, dizziness, or sleeplessness occur, discontinue use and consult a doctor. Do not take this product for more than 10 days. If symptoms do not improve or are accompanied by fever that lasts for more than 3 days, or if new symptoms occur, consult a doctor. Do not take this product, unless directed by a doctor, if you have a breathing problem such as emphysema or chronic bronchitis, heart disease, high blood pressure, thyroid disease, diabetes, or if you have glaucoma or difficulty in urination due to enlargement of the prostate gland. May cause excitability especially in children. May cause marked drowsiness; alcohol, sedatives, and tranquilizers may increase the drowsiness effect. Avoid alcoholic beverages while taking this product. Do not take this product if you are taking sedatives or tranquilizers, without first consulting your doctor. Use caution when driving a motor vehicle or operating machinery. Do not use any other products containing diphenhydramine while using this prod-

Continued on next page

This product information was prepared in November 1996. On these and other Warner-Lambert Consumer Healthcare Products, detailed information may be obtained by addressing Warner-Lambert Consumer Healthcare Products, Morris Plains, NJ 07950 USA

Warner-Lambert—Cont.

uct. As with any drug, if you are pregnant or nursing a baby, seek the advice of a health professional before using this product. KEEP THIS AND ALL DRUGS OUT OF THE REACH OF CHILDREN. In case of accidental overdose, seek professional assistance or contact a Poison Control Center immediately. Prompt medical attention is critical for adults as well as for children even if you do not notice any signs or symptoms.

Alcohol Warning: If you generally consume 3 or more alcohol-containing drinks per day, you should consult your physician for advice on when and how you should take Benadryl Allergy/Sinus Headache and other pain relievers.

Drug Interaction Precaution: Do not use this product if you are now taking a prescription monoamine oxidase inhibitor (MAOI) (certain drugs for depression, psychiatric or emotional conditions, or Parkinson's disease), or for 2 weeks after stopping the MAOI drug. If you are uncertain whether your prescription drug contains an MAOI, consult a health professional before taking this product.

Directions: Adults and children 12 years of age and over: two (2) caplets every 6 hours while symptoms persist. Not to exceed 8 caplets in 24 hours. Children under 12 years of age: consult a doctor.

How Supplied: Benadryl Allergy Sinus Headache is available in boxes of 24 and 48 caplets. Store at room temperature, (59°–86°F). Protect from moisture.

Shown in Product Identification Guide, page 524

BENADRYL® Dye-Free Allergy Liqui-gels® Softgels

[bĕ'nă-drĭl]

Active Ingredients: Each softgel contains: Diphenhydramine Hydrochloride 25 mg.

Inactive Ingredients: Gelatin, Glycerin, Polyethylene Glycol 400 and Sorbitol.

Indications: Temporarily relieves runny nose and sneezing, itching of the nose or throat, and itchy, watery eyes due to hay fever or other upper respiratory allergies, and runny nose and sneezing associated with the common cold.

Directions: Follow dosage recommendations below, or use as directed by your doctor.

Benadryl® Dye-Free Allergy Liqui-Gels® Softgel

AGE	DOSAGE
Adults and children 12 years of age and over	25 to 50 mg. (1 to 2 softgels) every 4 to 6 hours. Not to exceed 12 softgels in 24 hours.
Children 6 to under 12 years of age **See ** symbol below**	12.5** to 25 mg. (1 softgel) every 4 to 6 hours. Not to exceed 6 softgels in 24 hours.
Children under 6 years of age	Consult a doctor.

**12.5 mg. dosage strength is not available in this package. Do not attempt to break softgels. This dosage is available in bubble gum flavored Benadryl® Dye-Free Allergy Liquid Medication.

Warnings: May cause excitability, especially in children. Do not take this product, unless directed by a doctor, if you have a breathing problem such as emphysema or chronic bronchitis, or if you have glaucoma or difficulty in urination due to enlargement of the prostate gland. May cause marked drowsiness; alcohol, sedatives, and tranquilizers may increase the drowsiness effect. Avoid alcoholic beverages while taking this product. Do not take this product if you are taking sedatives or tranquilizers, without first consulting your doctor. Use caution when driving a motor vehicle or operating machinery. **Do not use any other products containing diphenhydramine while using this product.** As with any drug, if you are pregnant or nursing a baby, seek the advice of a health professional before using this product. KEEP THIS AND ALL DRUGS OUT OF THE REACH OF CHILDREN. In case of accidental overdose, seek professional assistance or contact a Poison Control Center immediately.

How Supplied: Benadryl® Dye-Free Allergy Liqui-Gels® Softgels are supplied in boxes of 24.
Store at 59°–77°F. Protect from heat and humidity.

Liqui-Gels is a registered trademark of R.P. Scherer Corporation.
Protect from heat and humidity.

Shown in Product Identification Guide, page 524

BENADRYL® Dye-Free Allergy Liquid Medication

[bĕ'nă-drĭl]

New Formula
New Dose
Bubble Gum Flavor

Active Ingredients: Each teaspoonful (5 mL.) contains Diphenhydramine HCL 12.5 mg.

Inactive Ingredients: Each teaspoonful (5 mL.) contains: Carboxymethylcellulose Sodium, Citric Acid, Flavor, Glycerin, Saccharin Sodium, Sodium Benzoate, Sodium Citrate, Sorbitol Solution and Purified Water.

Indications: Temporarily relieves runny nose and sneezing, itching of the nose or throat, and itchy, watery eyes due to hay fever or other upper respiratory allergies, and runny nose and sneezing associated with the common cold.

Directions: Follow dosage recommendations below, or use as directed by your doctor.

Benadryl® Dry-Free Allergy Liquid Medication
New Formula
New Dose

AGE	DOSAGE
Children under 6 years of age	Consult a doctor.
Children 6 to under 12 years of age	**1–2 Teaspoonfuls (12.5 to 25 mg)** every 4 to 6 hours. Not to exceed 12 teaspoonfuls in 24 hours.
Adults and children 12 years of age and over	**2–4 teaspoonfuls (25 to 50 mg)** every 4 to 6 hours. Not to exceed 24 teaspoonfuls in 24 hours.

Warnings: May cause excitability especially in children. Do not take this product, unless directed by a doctor, if you have a breathing problem such as emphysema or chronic bronchitis, or if you have glaucoma or difficulty in urination due to enlargement of the prostate gland. May cause marked drowsiness; alcohol, sedatives, and tranquilizers may increase the drowsiness effect. Avoid alcoholic beverages while taking this product. Do not take this product if you are taking sedatives or tranquilizers, without first consulting your doctor. Use caution when driving a motor vehicle or operating machinery. **Do not use any other products containing diphenhydramine while using this product.** As with any drug, if you are pregnant or nursing a baby, seek the advice of a health professional before using this product. KEEP THIS AND ALL DRUGS OUT OF THE REACH OF CHILDREN. In case of accidental overdose, seek professional assistance or contact a Poison Control Center immediately.

How Supplied: Benadryl Dye-Free Allergy Liquid Medication is supplied in 4 fl. oz. bottles.

Store at room temperature 59°–86°F. Protect from freezing.

Shown in Product Identification Guide, page 524

BENADRYL® Itch Relief Stick
Extra Strength
Topical Analgesic/Skin Protectant
[*bĕ'nă-drĭl*]

Active Ingredients: Diphenhydramine Hydrochloride 2%, Zinc Acetate 0.1%.

Inactive Ingredients: Alcohol 73.5% v/v, Glycerin, Povidone, Purified Water, and Tromethamine.

Indications: For the temporary relief of itching and pain associated with insect bites, minor skin irritations, and rashes due to poison oak, poison ivy or poison sumac. Dries the oozing and weeping of poison ivy, poison oak and poison sumac.

Warnings: FOR EXTERNAL USE ONLY. Do not use on chicken pox, measles, blisters, or on extensive areas of skin, except as directed by a physician. Avoid contact with the eyes. If condition worsens or does not improve within 7 days, or if symptoms persist for more than 7 days or clear up and occur again within a few days, discontinue use of this product and consult a physician. Do not use on children under 6 years of age without consulting a physician. **Do not use any other drugs containing diphenhydramine while using this product.** KEEP THIS AND ALL DRUGS OUT OF THE REACH OF CHILDREN. In case of accidental ingestion, seek professional assistance or contact a Poison Control Center immediately. Flammable. Keep away from fire or flame.

Directions: Adults and children 6 years of age and older: Apply to the affected area not more than 3 to 4 times daily. For children under 6 years of age: Consult a physician.
Store at room temperature (59°–86°F).

How Supplied: Benadryl® Itch Relief Stick is available in a .47 fl. oz (14 mL) dauber.

Shown in Product Identification Guide, page 524

BENADRYL® Itch Stopping Cream
Original Strength & Extra Strength
[*bĕ'nă-drĭl*]

Active Ingredients:
Original Strength: Diphenhydramine Hydrochloride 1% and Zinc Acetate 0.1%.
Extra Strength: Diphenhydramine Hydrochloride 2% and Zinc Acetate 0.1%.

Inactive Ingredients: Cetyl Alcohol, Diazolidinyl Urea, Methylparaben, Polyethylene Glycol Monostearate 1000, Propylene Glycol, Propylparaben and Purified Water.

Indications: For the temporary relief of itching and pain associated with insect bites, minor skin irritations and rashes due to poison ivy, poison oak or poison sumac. Dries the oozing and weeping of poison ivy, poison oak and poison sumac.

Actions: Benadryl Itch Stopping Cream:
- Stops your itch at the source by blocking the histamine that causes itch.
- Provides local anesthetic itch and pain relief in a greaseless vanishing cream.

Benadryl gives you the kind of itch and pain relief you can't get from hydrocortisone.

Warnings: FOR EXTERNAL USE ONLY.
Original Strength: Do not use on chicken pox, measles, blisters or on extensive areas of skin, except as directed by a physician. Avoid contact with the eyes. If condition worsens, or does not improve within 7 days or if symptoms persist for more than 7 days, or clear up and occur again within a few days, discontinue use of this product and consult a physician. Do not use on children under 2 years of age without consulting a physician. **Do not use any other drugs containing diphenhydramine while using this product.** KEEP THIS AND ALL DRUGS OUT OF THE REACH OF CHILDREN. In case of accidental ingestion, seek professional assistance or contact a Poison Control Center immediately.
Extra Strength: Do not use on chicken pox, measles, blisters or on extensive areas of skin, except as directed by a physician. Avoid contact with the eyes. If condition worsens, or does not improve within 7 days or if symptoms persist for more than 7 days, or clear up and occur again within a few days, discontinue use of this product and consult a physician. Do not use on children under 12 years of age without consulting a physician. Do not use any other drugs containing diphenhydramine while using this product. KEEP THIS AND ALL DRUGS OUT OF THE REACH OF CHILDREN. In case of accidental ingestion, seek professional assistance or contact a Poison Control Center immediately.

Directions: Original Strength: Adults and children 2 years of age and older: apply to affected area not more than 3 to 4 times daily. Children under 2 years of age: consult a physician. Extra Strength: Adults and children 12 years of age and older: apply to affected area not more than 3 to 4 times daily. Children under 12 years of age: consult a physician.

How Supplied: Benadryl Itch Stopping Cream is available in 1 oz (28.3 g) Original Strength and 1 oz (28.3 g) Extra Strength tubes.
Store at room temperature 59°–86°F.

Shown in Product Identification Guide, page 524

BENADRYL® Itch Stopping Spray
Original Strength & Extra Strength
[*bĕ'nă-drĭl*]

Active Ingredients:
Original Strength: Diphenhydramine Hydrochloride 1% and Zinc Acetate 0.1%.
Extra Strength: Diphenhydramine Hydrochloride 2% and Zinc Acetate 0.1%.

Inactive Ingredients: Alcohol up to 73.6% v/v, Glycerin, Povidone, Purified Water and Tromethamine.

Indications: For the temporary relief of itching and pain associated with insect bites, minor skin irritations and rashes due to poison ivy, poison oak, or poison sumac. Dries the oozing and weeping of poison ivy, poison oak, and poison sumac.

Warnings: FOR EXTERNAL USE ONLY.
Original Strength: Do not use on chicken pox, measles, blisters or on extensive areas of skin, except as directed by a physician. Avoid contact with the eyes. If condition worsens or does not improve within 7 days, or if symptoms persist for more than 7 days or clear up and occur again within a few days, discontinue use of this product and consult a physician. Do not use on children under 2 years of age without consulting a physician. **Do not use any other drugs containing diphenhydramine while using this product.** KEEP THIS AND ALL DRUGS OUT OF THE REACH OF CHILDREN. In case of accidental ingestion, seek professional assistance or contact a Poison Control Center immediately. Flammable. Keep away from fire or flame.
Extra Strength: Do not use on chicken pox, measles, blisters or on extensive areas of skin, except as directed by a physician. Avoid contact with the eyes. If condition worsens or does not improve within 7 days, or if symptoms persist for more than 7 days or clear up and occur again within a few days, discontinue use of this product and consult a physician. Do not use on children under 12 years of age without consulting a physician. Do not use any other drugs containing diphenhydramine while using this product. KEEP THIS AND ALL DRUGS OUT OF THE REACH OF CHILDREN. In case of accidental ingestion, seek professional assistance or contact a Poison Control Center immediately. Flammable. Keep away from fire or flame.

Directions: Original Strength: Adults and children 2 years of age and older: Ap-

Continued on next page

This product information was prepared in November 1996. On these and other Warner-Lambert Consumer Healthcare Products, detailed information may be obtained by addressing Warner-Lambert Consumer Healthcare Products, Morris Plains, NJ 07950 USA

Warner-Lambert—Cont.

ply to affected area not more than 3 to 4 times daily. Children under 2 years of age: Consult a physician. Extra Strength: Adults and children 12 years of age and older: Apply to affected area not more than 3 to 4 times daily. Children under 12 years of age: Consult a physician.

How Supplied: Benadryl Itch Stopping Spray Original and Extra Strength is available in a 2 fl. oz. (59mL) pump spray bottle.
Store at room temperature 59°–86°F.

Shown in Product Identification Guide, page 524

BENADRYL® Itch Stopping Gel Original Strength & Extra Strength
[*bĕ'nă-drĭl*]

Active Ingredients:
Original Strength: Diphenhydramine Hydrochloride 1% and Zinc Acetate 1%.
Extra Strength: Diphenhydramine Hydrochloride 2% and Zinc Acetate 1%.

Inactive Ingredients: SD Alcohol 38B, Camphor, Citric Acid, Diazolidinyl Urea, Glycerin, Hydroxypropyl Methylcellulose, Methylparaben, Propylene Glycol, Propylparaben, Purified Water, Sodium Citrate.

Indications: For the temporary relief of itching and pain associated with insect bites, minor skin irritations and rashes due to poison ivy, poison oak or poison sumac. Dries the oozing and weeping of poison ivy, poison oak and poison sumac.

Actions: Benadryl Itch Stopping Gel stops your itch at the source by blocking the histamine that causes itch. It provides local anesthetic itch and pain relief and it has added drying action for the oozing and weeping associated with some rashes.

Warnings: FOR EXTERNAL USE ONLY.
Original Strength: Do not use on chicken pox, measles, blisters or on extensive areas of skin, except as directed by a physician. Avoid contact with the eyes. If condition worsens or does not improve within 7 days, or if symptoms persist for more than 7 days or clear up and occur again within a few days, discontinue use of this product and consult a physician. Do not use on children under 6 years of age without consulting a physician. **Do not use any other drugs containing diphenhydramine while using this product. KEEP THIS AND ALL DRUGS OUT OF THE REACH OF CHILDREN.** In case of accidental ingestion, seek professional assistance or contact a Poison Control Center immediately.
Extra Strength: Do not use on chicken pox, measles, blisters or on extensive areas of skin, except as directed by a physician. Avoid contact with the eyes. If condition worsens or does not improve within 7 days, or if symptoms persist for more than 7 days or clear up and occur again within a few days, discontinue use of this product and consult a physician. Do not use on children under 12 years of age without consulting a physician. Do not use any other drugs containing diphenhydramine while using this product. **KEEP THIS AND ALL DRUGS OUT OF THE REACH OF CHILDREN.** In case of accidental ingestion, seek professional assistance or contact a Poison Control Center immediately.

Directions: Original Strength: Shake well. Adults and children 6 years of age or older: Apply to affected area not more than 3 to 4 times daily. Children under 6 years of age: Consult a physician.
Extra Strength: Shake well. Adults and children 12 years of age or older: Apply to affected area not more than 3 to 4 times daily. Children under 12 years of age: Consult a physician.

How Supplied: Benadryl Itch Stopping Gel is supplied in 4 fl. oz. (118mL) bottles in both Original and Extra Strength. Store at room temperature 59°–86°F.

Shown in Product Identification Guide, page 524

BENYLIN® Adult Formula Cough Suppressant
[*bĕ'-nă-lĭn*]

Active Ingredient: Each teaspoonful (5 mL) contains: Dextromethorphan Hydrobromide 15 mg.

Inactive Ingredients: Caramel, Citric Acid, D&C Red No. 33, FD&C Red No. 40, Flavors, Glycerin, Poloxamer 407, Polysorbate 20, Purified Water, Saccharin Sodium, Sodium Benzoate, Sodium Carboxymethyl Cellulose, Sodium Citrate, and Sorbitol Solution.

Indication: Temporarily relieves cough due to minor throat and bronchial irritation as may occur with the common cold.

Directions: Follow dosage recommendations below, or as directed by a doctor. Dosage may be repeated every 6 to 8 hours, not to exceed 4 doses in 24 hours.

Benylin® Adult Formula

AGE	DOSAGE
Adults and children 12 years of age and over	2 teaspoonfuls
Children 6 to under 12 years of age	1 teaspoonful
Children 2 to under 6 years of age	1/2 teaspoonful
Children under 2 years of age	Consult a doctor

Warnings: A persistent cough may be a sign of a serious condition. If cough persists for more than one week, tends to recur, or is accompanied by fever, rash or persistent headache, consult a doctor. Do not take this product for persistent or chronic cough such as occurs with smoking, asthma, emphysema, or if cough is accompanied by excessive phlegm (mucus), unless directed by a doctor. As with any drug, if you are pregnant or nursing a baby, seek the advice of a health professional before using this product. KEEP THIS AND ALL DRUGS OUT OF THE REACH OF CHILDREN. In case of accidental overdose, seek professional assistance or contact a Poison Control Center immediately.

Drug Interaction Precaution: Do not use this product if you are now taking a prescription monoamine oxidase inhibitor (MAOI) (certain drugs for depression, psychiatric or emotional conditions, or Parkinson's disease), or for 2 weeks after stopping the MAOI drug. If you are uncertain whether your prescription drug contains an MAOI, consult a health professional before taking this product.

How Supplied: Benylin Adult Formula is supplied in 4 oz. bottles.
Store at room temperature 59–86°F.
See bottom flap for lot number and expiration date.

Shown in Product Identification Guide, page 524

BENYLIN® Cough Suppressant Expectorant
[*bĕ'-nă-lĭn*]

Active Ingredients: Each teaspoonful (5 mL) contains Guaifensin 100 mg and Dextromethorphan Hydrobromide 5 mg.

Inactive Ingredients: Caramel, Citric Acid, D&C Red No. 33, Disodium Edetate, FD&C Red No. 40, Flavors, Poloxamer 407, Polyethylene Glycol, Propyl Gallate, Propylene Glycol, Purified Water, Saccharin Sodium, Sodium Benzoate, Sodium Chloride, Sodium Citrate, and Sorbitol Solution.

Indications: Temporarily relieves cough due to minor throat and bronchial irritation occurring with the common cold. Helps loosen phlegm (mucus) and thin bronchial secretions to drain bronchial tubes and make coughs more productive.

Directions: Follow dosage recommendations below, or as directed by a doctor. Dosage may be repeated every 4 hours, not to exceed 6 doses in 24 hours.

Benylin® Cough Suppressant Expectorant

AGE	DOSAGE
Adults and children 12 years of age and older	Four (4) teaspoonfuls

Children 6 to under 12 years of age	Two (2) teaspoonfuls
Children 2 to under 6 years of age	One (1) teaspoonful
Children under 2 years of age	Consult a doctor

Warning: A persistent cough may be a sign of a serious condition. If cough persists for more than 1 week, tends to recur, or is accompanied by fever, rash, or persistent headache, consult a doctor. Do not take this product for persistent or chronic cough such as occurs with smoking, asthma, chronic bronchitis or emphysema, or where cough is accompanied by excessive phlegm (mucus), unless directed by a doctor. As with any drug, if you are pregnant or nursing a baby, seek the advice of a health professional before using this product. **KEEP THIS AND ALL DRUGS OUT OF THE REACH OF CHILDREN.** In case of accidental overdose, seek professional assistance or contact a Poison Control Center immediately.

Drug Interaction Precaution: Do not use this product if you are now taking a prescription monoamine oxidase inhibitor (MAOI) (certain drugs for depression, psychiatric or emotional conditions, or Parkinson's disease), or for 2 weeks after stopping the MAOI drug. If you are uncertain whether your prescription drug contains an MAOI, consult a health professional before taking this product.

How Supplied: Benylin Expectorant is available in 4 oz. bottles.
Store at room temperature 59°–86°F.

Shown in Product Identification Guide, page 524

BENYLIN® Multisymptom
[*bĕ ′-nă-lĭn*]

Active Ingredients: Each teaspoonful (5 mL) contains Guaifenesin 100 mg, Pseudoephedrine Hydrochloride 15 mg, and Dextromethorphan Hydrobromide 5 mg.

Inactive Ingredients: Caramel, Citric Acid, D&C Red No. 33, Edetate Disodium, FD&C Red No. 40, Flavors, Poloxamer 407, Polyethylene Glycol 1450, Propyl Gallate, Propylene Glycol, Purified Water, Saccharin Sodium, Sodium Benzoate, Sodium Chloride, Sodium Citrate, and Sorbitol Solution.

Indications: For temporary relief of cough due to minor throat and bronchial irritation and nasal congestion occurring with the common cold. Helps loosen phlegm (mucus) and thin bronchial secretions to drain bronchial tubes and make coughs more productive.

Directions: Follow dosage recommendations below or use as directed by a doctor. Dosage may be repeated every 4 hours, not to exceed 4 doses in 24 hours.

Benylin® Multisymptom

AGE	DOSAGE
Adults and children 12 years and over	4 teaspoonfuls
Children 6 to under 12 years of age	2 teaspoonfuls
Children 2 to under 6 years of age	1 teaspoonful
Children under 2 years of age	Consult a doctor

Warnings: Do not exceed recommended dosage. If nervousness, dizziness, or sleeplessness occur, discontinue use and consult a doctor. If symptoms do not improve within 7 days or are accompanied by fever, consult a doctor. Do not take this product if you have heart disease, high blood pressure, thyroid disease, diabetes, or difficulty in urination due to enlargement of the prostate gland unless directed by a doctor. A persistent cough may be a sign of a serious condition. If cough persists for more than 1 week, tends to recur, or is accompanied by a fever, rash or persistent headache, consult a doctor. Do not take this product for persistent or chronic cough such as occurs with smoking, asthma, chronic bronchitis, or emphysema, or where cough is accompanied by excessive phlegm (mucus) unless directed by a doctor. As with any drug, if you are pregnant or nursing a baby, seek the advice of a health professional before using this product. **KEEP THIS AND ALL DRUGS OUT OF THE REACH OF CHILDREN.** In case of accidental overdose, seek professional assistance or contact a Poison Control Center immediately.

Drug Interaction Precaution: Do not use this product if you are now taking a prescription monoamine oxidase inhibitor (MAOI) (certain drugs for depression, psychiatric or emotional conditions, or Parkinson's disease), or for 2 weeks after stopping the MAOI drug. If you are uncertain whether your prescription drug contains an MAOI, consult a health professional before taking this product.

How Supplied: Benylin Multisymptom is available in 4 oz bottles. Store at 59°–86° F.

Shown in Product Identification Guide, page 524

BENYLIN® Pediatric Cough Suppressant
[*bĕ ′-nă-lĭn*]

Active Ingredient: Each teaspoonful (5 mL) contains: Dextromethorphan Hydrobromide 7.5 mg.

Inactive Ingredients: Citric Acid, FD&C Blue No. 1, FD&C Red No. 40, Flavors, Glycerin, Poloxamer 407, Polysorbate 20, Purified Water, Saccharin Sodium, Sodium Benzoate, Sodium Carboxymethyl Cellulose, Sodium Citrate, and Sorbitol Solution.

Indications: Temporarily relieves cough due to minor throat and bronchial irritation occurring with the common cold.

Directions: Follow dosage recommendations below, or as directed by a doctor. Dosage may be repeated every 6 to 8 hours, not to exceed 4 doses in 24 hours.

Benylin® Pediatric

AGE	DOSAGE
Children under 2 years of age	Consult a doctor
Children 2 to under 6 years of age	1 teaspoonful
Children 6 to under 12 years of age	2 teaspoonfuls
Adults and children 12 years of age and over	4 teaspoonfuls

Warnings: A persistent cough may be a sign of a serious condition. If cough persists for more than 1 week, tends to recur, or is accompanied by fever, rash, or persistent headache, consult a doctor. Do not take this product for persistent or chronic cough such as occurs with smoking, asthma, emphysema, or if cough is accompanied by excessive phlegm (mucus), unless directed by a doctor. As with any drug, if you are pregnant or nursing a baby, seek the advice of a health professional before using this product. **KEEP THIS AND ALL DRUGS OUT OF THE REACH OF CHILDREN.** In case of accidental overdose, seek professional assistance or contact a Poison Control Center immediately.

Continued on next page

This product information was prepared in November 1996. On these and other Warner-Lambert Consumer Healthcare Products, detailed information may be obtained by addressing Warner-Lambert Consumer Healthcare Products, Morris Plains, NJ 07950 USA

Warner-Lambert—Cont.

Drug Interaction Precaution: Do not use this product if you are now taking a prescription monoamine oxidase inhibitor (MAOI) (certain drugs for depression, psychiatric or emotional conditions, or Parkinson's disease), or for 2 weeks after stopping the MAOI drug. If you are uncertain whether your prescription drug contains an MAOI, consult a health professional before taking this product.

How Supplied: Benylin Pediatric is supplied in 4 oz bottles.

Shown in Product Identification Guide, page 525

BOROFAX® Skin Protectant
[*bôr 'uh-făks*]

Active Ingredients: Zinc oxide 15% and white petrolatum 68.6%.

Inactive Ingredients: Lanolin, mineral oil, and fragrance.

Indications: Helps treat and prevent diaper rash. Protects chafed skin due to diaper rash and helps seal out wetness.

Directions: Change wet and soiled diapers promptly, cleanse the diaper area, and allow to dry. Apply ointment liberally as often as necessary, with each diaper change, especially at bedtime or anytime when exposure to wet diapers may be prolonged.

Warnings: For external use only. Avoid contact with the eyes. If condition worsens or does not improve within 7 days, consult a doctor. Keep this and all drugs out of the reach of children. In case of accidental ingestion, seek professional assistance or contact a Poison Control Center immediately.

How Supplied: Tube, 1.8 oz (50 g)
Store at 15° to 25°C (59° to 77°F).

Shown in Product Identification Guide, page 525

CALADRYL® Lotion
CALADRYL® Cream For Kids
CALADRYL® Clear Lotion
[*că'lă drĭl"*]

Active Ingredients: Caladryl Lotion and Caladryl Cream For Kids; Calamine 8%, and Pramoxine Hydrochloride 1%. Caladryl Clear Lotion; Pramoxine Hydrochloride 1% and Zinc Acetate 0.1%.

Inactive Ingredients: Caladryl Lotion—SD Alcohol 38B, Camphor, Diazolidinyl Urea, Fragrance, Hydroxypropyl Methylcellulose, Methylparaben, Polysorbate 80, Propylene Glycol, Propylparaben, Water and Xanthan Gum.
Caladryl Cream for Kids—Camphor, Cetyl Alcohol, Cyclomethicone, Diazolidinyl Urea, Fragrance, Methylparaben, Polysorbate 60, Propylene Glycol, Propylparaben, Purified Water, Sorbitan Stearate and Soya Sterol.
Caladryl Clear Lotion—SD Alcohol 38B 2.5% v/v, Camphor, Citric Acid, Diazolidinyl Urea, Fragrance, Glycerin, Hydroxypropyl Methylcellulose, Methylparaben, Polysorbate 40, Propylene Glycol, Propylparaben, Purified Water and Sodium Citrate.

Indications: For the temporary relief of itching and pain associated with rashes due to poison ivy, poison oak or poison sumac, insect bites and minor irritations. Dries the oozing and weeping of poison ivy, poison oak or poison sumac.

Warnings: FOR EXTERNAL USE ONLY. Avoid contact with the eyes. If condition worsens or does not improve within 7 days, or if symptoms persist for more than 7 days or clear up and occur again within a few days, discontinue use of this product and consult a physician. Do not use on children under 2 years of age without consulting a physician. KEEP THIS AND ALL DRUGS OUT OF THE REACH OF CHILDREN. In case of accidental ingestion, seek professional assistance or contact a Poison Control Center immediately.

Directions: Before each application, wash affected area of skin. Adults and children 2 years of age and older: Apply to the affected area not more than 3 to 4 times daily. Children under 2 years of age: Consult a physician.
Additional instructions for only Lotion and Clear Lotion: SHAKE WELL.

How Supplied: Caladryl Cream for Kids—1.5 oz (42.5 g) tubes
Caladryl Clear Lotion—6 fl. oz. (177 mL) bottles
Caladryl Lotion—6 fl. oz. (177 mL) bottles

Shown in Product Identification Guide, page 525

---

e.p.t® PREGNANCY TEST

You can find out whether or not you're pregnant by testing any time of day and as early as the first day of your missed period.
With just one easy step **e.p.t** gives you clear results in just 3 minutes. **e.p.t Pregnancy Test.** The name more women trust™.

Before you begin the test. Please read the instructions carefully. Registered nurses are available to confidentially answer your calls regarding **e.p.t.** If you have any questions about **e.p.t** call toll-free 1-800-378-1783 (8:30 am to 8:00 pm EST) weekdays.

To Use e.p.t
For in-vitro diagnostic use. Only for external use (not for internal use). Remove the test stick from the foil pouch just prior to use and throw away the freshness packet. [See figure below.]

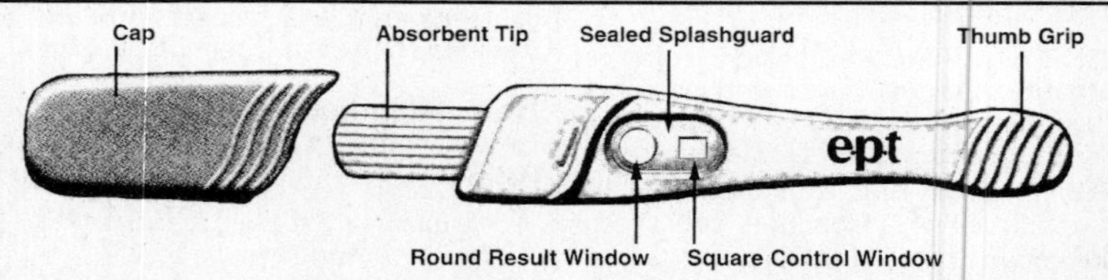

Remove the cap to expose absorbent tip. Hold the test stick by the thumb grip with the exposed **absorbent tip pointing downward. Urinate on the absorbent tip only** until it is thoroughly wet (at least 5 seconds).

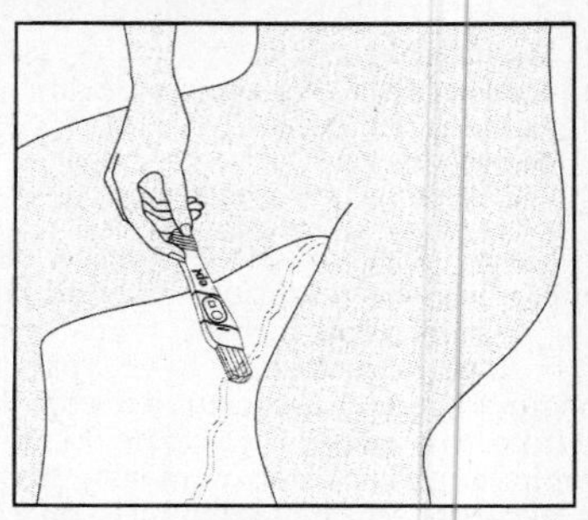

The sealed splashguard will protect the result from excess splashing on the windows. (If you prefer, you can urinate into a clean, dry cup or container.

Dip only the absorbent tip of the stick in the urine for at least 5 seconds.)

Lay the test stick down on a flat surface with the windows on top while you wait for the test result. (If you wish, you can replace the cap to cover the absorbent tip.)
As the test begins to work, you may notice a light pink color moving across the windows.
Important: Lifting the stick before 3 minutes may affect test result.

To Read the Results.
Keep stick on a flat surface while waiting at least 3 minutes to read the result. After 3 minutes, a line will appear in the square Control Window to tell you that the test is finished.
Do not read the result after 20 minutes have passed.

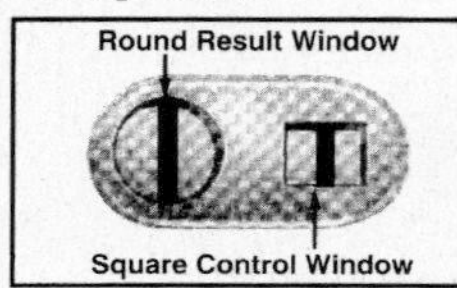

2 Lines—Pregnant If you see one line in each window as illustrated, the test has indicated that you are **pregnant.** (One line can be lighter than the other.
The two lines can be any shade of pink and can be lighter or darker than the color pictured. However, you should see two clear parallel lines as indicated, one in each window.)

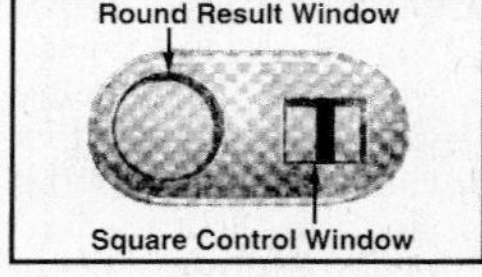

1 Line—Not Pregnant If you see a line in the square Control Window but no line in the

round Result Window, the test has indicated that you are **not pregnant.** Do not read after 20 minutes have passed.
Important: If no line appears in the square Control Window, the test has not functioned properly. Do not read the result. Please call the toll-free number (1-800-378-1783).

Frequently Asked Questions
How does e.p.t work?
e.p.t detects a hormone in your urine known as hCG (human Chorionic Gonadotropin) that your body produces only during pregnancy. e.p.t can detect hCG hormone levels in your urine as early as the first day of your missed period.

When to use e.p.t?
e.p.t can be used as soon as you miss your period as well as any day thereafter. You can use e.p.t any time of day.

What if I don't think the result of the test is correct?
If it is hard to tell whether or not there is a line in the round Result Window, repeat the test after 2–3 days with a new **e.p.t** test stick.
If you follow the instructions carefully, you should not get a false result.

These factors should not affect the test result: Alcohol, analgesics (pain killers), antibiotics, birth control pills or hormone therapies containing clomiphene citrate (such as Clomid or Serophen).

These factors may affect the test result: Certain drugs which contain hCG or that used in combination with hCG (such as Pregnyl, Profasi, Pergonal, APL) and rare medical conditions.
If you repeat the test and continue to get an unexpected result, contact your doctor.
The test may give a false positive result if you have had a miscarriage or have given birth within the past 8 weeks. This is because the test may detect hCG still in your system from a previous pregnancy. You should ask your doctor for help in interpreting the result of your **e.p.t** test if you have recently been pregnant.

What if the line in the Round Result Window is a lighter shade of pink than the line in the square control window?
As long as the 2 lines appear, the result is positive, even if the 2 lines are different shades of pink.

Shown in Product Identification Guide, page 525

LISTERINE® Antiseptic
[*lĭs 'tərēn*]

Active Ingredients: Thymol 0.064%, Eucalyptol 0.092%, Methyl Salicylate 0.060% and Menthol 0.042%.

Inactive Ingredients: Water, Alcohol 26.9%, Benzoic Acid, Poloxamer 407, Sodium Benzoate and Caramel.

Indications: To help prevent and reduce plaque and gingivitis/For bad breath.

Actions: Listerine® Antiseptic has been shown to help prevent and reduce supragingival plaque accumulation and gingivitis when used in a conscientiously applied program of oral hygiene and regular professional care. Its effect on periodontitis has not been determined. Listerine is the only leading nonprescription mouthrinse that has received the American Dental Association's Council on Scientific Affairs Seal of Acceptance for helping to prevent and reduce plaque above the gumline and gingivitis.

Directions: Rinse full strength for 30 seconds with 20 ml (⅔ fl. ounce or 4 teaspoonfuls) morning and night. If bad breath persists, see your dentist.

Warnings: Do not administer to children under twelve years of age. Keep this and all drugs out of the reach of children. Do not swallow. In case of accidental overdose, seek professional assistance or contact a poison control center immediately.

How Supplied: Listerine® antiseptic is supplied in 250 ml, 500 ml, 1.0 liter and 1.5 liter bottles, as well as 3 fl. oz. bottles. It is also available to professionals in 3 fl. oz. bottles and in gallons.

Shown in Product Identification Guide, page 525

COOL MINT LISTERINE®
[*lĭs 'tərēn*]

Active Ingredients: Thymol 0.064%, Eucalyptol 0.092%, Methyl Salicylate 0.060% and Menthol 0.042%.

Inactive Ingredients: Water, Sorbitol Solution, Alcohol 21.6%, Poloxamer 407, Benzoic Acid, Flavoring, Sodium Saccharin, Sodium Citrate, Citric Acid and FD&C Green No. 3.

Indications: To help prevent and reduce plaque and gingivitis/For bad breath.

Actions: Cool Mint Listerine® Antiseptic has been shown to help prevent and reduce supragingival plaque accumulation and gingivitis when used in a conscientiously applied program of oral hygiene and regular professional care. Its effect on periodontitis has not been determined. Listerine is the only leading nonprescription mouthrinse that has received the American Dental Association's Council on Scientific Affairs Seal of Acceptance for helping to prevent and reduce plaque above the gumline and gingivitis.

Directions: Rinse full strength for 30 seconds with 20 ml (⅔ fl. ounce or 4 teaspoonfuls) morning and night. If bad breath persists, see your dentist.

Warnings: Do not administer to children under twelve years of age. Keep this and all drugs out of the reach of children. Do not swallow. In case of accidental overdose, seek professional assistance or contact a poison control center immediately.

How Supplied: Cool Mint Listerine® antiseptic is supplied in 250 ml, 500 ml, 1.0 liter and 1.5 liter bottles, as well as 3 and 58 fl. oz. bottles. It is also available to professionals in gallon bottles.

Shown in Product Identification Guide, page 525

FRESHBURST LISTERINE®
[*lĭs 'tərēn*]

Active Ingredients: Thymol 0.064%, Eucalyptol 0.092%, Methyl Salicylate 0.060% and Menthol 0.042%.

Inactive Ingredients: Water, Sorbitol Solution, Alcohol 21.6%, Poloxamer 407, Benzoic Acid, Flavoring, Sodium Saccharin, Sodium Citrate, Citric Acid, D&C Yellow No. 10 and FD&C Green No. 3.

Indications: To help prevent and reduce plaque and gingivitis/For bad breath.

Actions: FreshBurst Listerine® Antiseptic has been shown to help prevent and reduce supragingival plaque accumulation and gingivitis when used in a conscientiously applied program of oral hygiene and regular professional care. Its effect on periodontitis has not been determined. Listerine is the only leading nonprescription mouthrinse that has received the American Dental Association's Council on Scientific Affairs Seal of Acceptance for helping to prevent and reduce plaque above the gumline and gingivitis.

Directions: Rinse full strength for 30 seconds with 20 ml (⅔ fl. ounce or 4 teaspoonfuls) morning and night. If bad breath persists, see your dentist.

Warnings: Do not administer to children under twelve years of age. Keep this and all drugs out of the reach of children. Do not swallow. In case of accidental overdose, seek professional assistance or contact a poison control center immediately.

How Supplied: FreshBurst Listerine® antiseptic is supplied in 250 ml, 500 ml, 1.0 liter and 1.5 liter bottles, as well as 3 fl. oz. bottles. It is also available to professionals in gallon bottles.

Shown in Product Identification Guide, page 525

Continued on next page

This product information was prepared in November 1996. On these and other Warner-Lambert Consumer Healthcare Products, detailed information may be obtained by addressing Warner-Lambert Consumer Healthcare Products, Morris Plains, NJ 07950 USA

Warner-Lambert—Cont.

LISTERMINT®
Alcohol-Free Mouthrinse
[*lĭs 'tər mĭnt*]

Ingredient: Water, Glycerin, Poloxamer 335, PEG 600, Flavors, Sodium Lauryl Sulfate, Sodium Benzoate, Sodium Saccharin, Benzoic Acid, Zinc Chloride, D&C Yellow No. 10, FD&C Green No. 3.

Indications: Freshens breath; contains no fluoride.

Directions: Rinse with 30 ml (1 fl. oz.) for 30 seconds to freshen breath in the morning and after meals as needed.

Warnings: Do not swallow. Keep out of reach of children.

How Supplied: Listermint® is supplied to consumers in a 32 fl. oz. bottle and is available to professionals in 3 fl. oz. bottles and in gallons.

Shown in Product Identification Guide, page 525

LUBRIDERM®
Dry Skin Care Lotion
[*lū brĭ dĕrm*]

Composition:
Scented—Contains Water, Mineral Oil, Petrolatum, Lanolin, Sorbitol Solution, Stearic Acid, Lanolin Alcohol, Cetyl Alcohol, Glyceryl Stearate/PEG-100 Stearate, Triethanolamine, Dimethicone, Propylene Glycol, Tri(PPG-3 Myristyl Ether) Citrate, Disodium EDTA, Methylparaben, Ethylparaben, Propylparaben, Fragrance, Xanthan Gum, Butylparaben, Methyldibromo Glutaronitrile.
Fragrance Free—Contains Water, Mineral Oil, Petrolatum, Lanolin, Sorbitol Solution, Stearic Acid, Lanolin Alcohol, Cetyl Alcohol, Glyceryl Stearate/PEG-100 Stearate, Triethanolamine, Dimethicone, Propylene Glycol, Tri(PPG-3 Myristyl Ether) Citrate, Disodium EDTA, Methylparaben, Ethylparaben, Propylparaben, Xanthan Gum, Butylparaben, Methyldibromo Glutaronitrile.

Actions and Uses: Lubriderm Lotion is an oil-in-water emulsion indicated for use in softening, soothing and moisturizing dry chapped skin. Lubriderm's water-based formula penetrates dry skin and effectively moisturizes without leaving a greasy feel. Lubriderm helps heal and protect skin from dryness, absorbs rapidly for a clean, natural feel and is non-comedogenic so it won't clog pores.

Administration and Dosage: Apply to hands and body every day. Particularly effective when used after showering or bathing.

Precautions: For external use only.

How Supplied:
Scented: Available in 6, 10 and 16 fl. oz. plastic bottles, and a 2.5 fl. oz. tube.
Fragrance Free: Available in 1, 6, 10 and 16 fl. oz. plastic bottles, and a 2.5 fl. oz. tube.

Shown in Product Identification Guide, page 525

LUBRIDERM® BATH AND SHOWER OIL
[*lū brĭ dĕrm*]

Composition: Contains Mineral Oil, PPG-15 Stearyl Ether, Oleth-2, Nonoxynol-5, Fragrance, D&C Green No. 6.

Actions and Uses: Lubriderm Bath and Shower Oil is a lanolin-free, mineral oil–based, bath oil designed for softening and soothing dry skin during the bath. The formula disperses into countless droplets of oil that coat the skin and help lubricate and soften. It is equally effective in hard or soft water and provides an excellent way to moisturize the skin and help counterbalance the drying effects of harsh soaps and hot water.

Administration and Dosage: Use one or two capfuls in the bath. For shower or sponge bath, apply all over your body by hand or with a sponge and rinse.

Precautions: Avoid getting in eyes; if this occurs, flush with clear water. When using any bath and shower oil, take precautions against slipping. For external use only.

How Supplied: Available in 8 fl. oz. plastic bottles.

Shown in Product Identification Guide, page 525

LUBRIDERM® GelCreme
[*lū brĭ dĕrm*]

Composition: Contains Water, Cetyl Alcohol, Glycerin, Mineral Oil, Cyclomethicone Fluid, Propylene Glycol Dicaprylate/Dicaprate, PEG-40 Stearate, Isopropyl Isostearate, Emulsifying Wax, Lecithin, Carbomer 940, Diazolidinyl Urea, Titanium Dioxide, Sodium Benzoate, BHT, Tri(PPG-3 Myristyl Ether) Citrate, Disodium EDTA, Retinyl Palmitate, Tocopheryl Acetate, Sodium Pyruvate, Iodopropynyl Butylcarbamate, Fragrance, Sodium Hydroxide, Xanthan Gum.

Actions and Uses: Lubriderm Moisture Recovery GelCreme is recommended for patients with extra dry skin. It's patented emollient system contains vitamins, nutrients, and antioxidants to heal and protect dry skin. The unique formulation combines the richness of a creme with the light feel of a gel.

Administration and Dosage: Apply to hands and body every day.

Precautions: For external use only.

How Supplied: Available in .75, 4, and 7.5 fl. oz. plastic bottles.

Shown in Product Identification Guide, page 525

LUBRIDERM® Moisture Recovery Alpha Hydroxy Lotion
[*lū brĭ dĕrm*]

Composition—Contains Water, Isostearic Acid, Stearic Acid, Steareth-21, Sodium Lactate, PPG-12/SMDI Copolymer, Lactic Acid, Steareth-2, Magnesium Aluminum Silicate, Cetyl Alcohol, Imidazolidinyl Urea, Fragrance, Potassium Sorbate, Xanthan Gum.

Actions and Uses: Lubriderm Moisture Recovery Alpha Hydroxy Formula is ideal for patients with extra dry skin. It accelerates the process of exfoliation, allowing newer, healthier looking skin to emerge. The patented alpha hydroxy delivery system provides long lasting, concentrated healing of severely dry skin.

Administration and Dosage: Apply creme to rough, dry skin areas like feet, knees, and elbows. The lotion is ideal for all over body moisturization.

Precautions: For external use only. Avoid contact in and around the eyes.

How Supplied:
Available in .5 and 8 fl. oz. plastic bottles.

Shown in Product Identification Guide, page 525

LUBRIDERM®
Seriously Sensitive® Lotion
[*lū brĭ dĕrm*]

Composition: Contains Water, Butylene Glycol, Mineral Oil, Petrolatum, Glycerin, Cetyl Alcohol, Propylene Glycol Dicaprylate/Dicaprate, PEG-40 Stearate, C11-13 Isoparaffin, Glyceryl Stearate, Tri (PPG-3 Myristyl Ether) Citrate, Emulsifying Wax, Dimethicone, DMDM Hydantoin, Methylparaben, Carbomer 940, Ethylparaben, Propylparaben, Titanium Dioxide, Disodium EDTA, Sodium Hydroxide, Butylparaben, Xanthan Gum.

Action and Uses: Lubriderm Seriously Sensitive Lotion's unique combination of emollients provides sensitive dry skin with the moisture it needs while helping to create a protective layer. It is noncomedogenic, 100% lanolin free, fragrance free, and dye free so its appropriate for skin that is sensitive to these ingredients. It is lightweight, nongreasy, and absorbs quickly.

Administration and Dosage: Apply to hands and body everyday. Particularly effective when used after showering or bathing.

Precautions: For external use only.

How Supplied: Available in 1, 6, 10, and 16 fl. oz. plastic bottles.

Shown in Product Identification Guide, page 525

NEOSPORIN® Ointment
[*nē 'uh-spō 'rŭn*]

Each Gram Contains: Polymyxin B Sulfate 5,000 units, Bacitracin Zinc 400 units and Neomycin 3.5 mg. Also contains a base of Cocoa Butter*, Cottonseen Oil*, Olive Oil*, Sodium Pyruvate*, Tocopheryl Acetate* and White Petrolatum.
*patent pending complex.

Indications: First aid to help prevent infection in minor cuts, scrapes, and burns.

Directions: Clean the affected area. Apply a small amount of this product (an amount equal to the surface area of the tip of a finger) on the area 1 to 3 times daily. May be covered with a sterile bandage.

Warnings: For external use only. Do not use in the eyes or apply over large areas of the body. In case of deep or puncture wounds, animal bites, or serious burns, consult a physician. Stop use and consult a physician if the condition persists or gets worse, or if a rash or other allergic reaction develops. Do not use if you are allergic to any of the ingredients. Do not use longer than 1 week unless directed by a physician. KEEP THIS AND ALL DRUGS OUT OF THE REACH OF CHILDREN. In case of accidental ingestion, seek professional assistance or contact a Poison Control Center immediately.

How Supplied: Tubes, $^1/_2$ oz (14.2 g) (with applicator tip), 1 oz (28.3 g), $^1/_{31}$ oz (0.9 g) foil packets packed 10 per box (Neo To Go™) or 144 per box.
Store at 15° to 25°C (59° to 77°F).

Shown in Product Identification Guide, page 525

NEOSPORIN® PLUS MAXIMUM STRENGTH Cream
[*nē "uh-spō 'rŭn*]

Each Gram Contains: Polymyxin B Sulfate 10,000 units, Neomycin 3.5 mg, and Pramoxine Hydrochloride 10 mg. Also contains: Emulsifying Wax, Methylparaben 0.25% (added as a preservative), Mineral Oil, Poloxamer 188, Propylene Glycol, Purified Water, and White Petrolatum.

Indications: First aid to help prevent infection and provide temporary relief of pain or discomfort in minor cuts, scrapes, and burns.

Directions: Adults and children 2 years of age and older: Clean the affected area. Apply a small amount of this product (an amount equal to the surface area of the tip of a finger) on the area 1 to 3 times daily. May be covered with a sterile bandage. Children under 2 years of age: Consult a physician.

Warnings: For external use only. Do not use in the eyes or apply over large areas of the body. In case of deep or puncture wounds, animal bites, or serious burns, consult a physician. Stop use and consult a physician if the condition persists or gets worse, or if symptoms persist for more than 1 week or clear up and occur again within a few days, or if a rash or other allergic reaction develops. Do not use if you are allergic to any of the ingredients. Do not use longer than 1 week unless directed by a physician. KEEP THIS AND ALL DRUGS OUT OF THE REACH OF CHILDREN. In case of accidental ingestion, seek professional assistance or contact a Poison Control Center immediately.

How Supplied: $^1/_2$ oz (14.2 g) tubes.
Store at 15° to 25°C (59° to 77°F).

Shown in Product Identification Guide, page 525

NEOSPORIN® PLUS MAXIMUM STRENGTH Ointment
[*nē "uh-spō 'rŭn*]

Each Gram Contains: Polymyxin B Sulfate 10,000 units, Bacitracin Zinc 500 units, Neomycin 3.5 mg, and Pramoxine Hydrochloride 10 mg, in a custom blend of White Petrolatum.

Indications: First aid to help prevent infection and provide temporary relief of pain or discomfort in minor cuts, scrapes, and burns.

Directions: Adults and children 2 years of age and older: Clean the affected area. Apply a small amount of this product (an amount equal to the surface area of the tip of a finger) on the area 1 to 3 times daily. May be covered with a sterile bandage. Children under 2 years of age: Consult a physician.

Warnings: For external use only. Do not use in the eyes or apply over large areas of the body. In case of deep or puncture wounds, animal bites, or serious burns, consult a physician. Stop use and consult a physician if the condition persists or gets worse, or if symptoms persist for more than 1 week or clear up and occur again within a few days, or if a rash or other allergic reaction develops. Do not use if you are allergic to any of the ingredients. Do not use longer than 1 week unless directed by a physician. KEEP THIS AND ALL DRUGS OUT OF THE REACH OF CHILDREN. In case of accidental ingestion, seek professional assistance or contact a Poison Control Center immediately.

How Supplied: $^1/_2$ oz (14.2 g) and 1 oz (28.3 g) tubes.
Store at 15° to 25°C (59° to 77°F).

Shown in Product Identification Guide, page 526

NIX® Creme Rinse
Permethrin
Lice Treatment
[*nĭks*]

Each Fluid Ounce Contains: Active Ingredient: Permethrin 280 mg (1%). Also contains: balsam canada, cetyl alcohol, citric acid, FD&C Yellow No. 6, fragrance, hydrolyzed animal protein, hydroxyethylcellulose, polyoxyethylene 10 cetyl ether, propylene glycol, stearalkonium chloride, water, isopropyl alcohol 5.6 g (20%), methylparaben 56 mg (0.2%), and propylparaben 22 mg (0.08%).

Product Benefits: Nix Creme Rinse kills lice and their unhatched eggs with usually only one application. Nix protects against head lice reinfestation for 14 days. The creme rinse formula leaves hair manageable and easy to comb.

Indications: For the treatment of head lice.

Directions for Use: Nix Creme Rinse should be used after hair has been washed with your regular shampoo, rinsed with water and towel dried. A sufficient amount should be applied to saturate hair and scalp (especially behind the ears and on the nape of the neck). Leave on hair for 10 minutes but no longer. Rinse with water. A single application is usually sufficient. If live lice are observed seven days or more after the first application of this product, a second treatment should be given. For proper head lice management, remove nits with the nit comb provided.

Head lice live on the scalp and lay small white eggs (nits) on the hair shaft close to the scalp. The nits are most easily found on the nape of the neck or behind the ears. All personal headgear, scarfs, coats, and bed linen should be disinfected by machine washing in hot water and drying, using the hot cycle of a dryer for at least 20 minutes. Personal articles of clothing or bedding that cannot be washed may be dry-cleaned, sealed in a plastic bag for a period of about 2 weeks, or sprayed with a product specifically designed for this purpose. Personal combs and brushes may be disinfected by soaking in hot water (above 130°F) for 5 to 10 minutes. Thorough vacuuming of rooms inhabited by infected patients is recommended.
Shake well before using.

Warnings: For external use only. Keep out of eyes when rinsing hair. Adults and children: Close eyes and do not open eyes until product is rinsed out. If product gets into the eyes, immediately flush with water. Do not use near the eyes or permit contact with mucous membranes, such as inside the nose, mouth or vagina, as irritation may occur. Children: Also protect children's eyes with a washcloth, towel, or other suitable material or

Continued on next page

This product information was prepared in November 1996. On these and other Warner-Lambert Consumer Healthcare Products, detailed information may be obtained by addressing Warner-Lambert Consumer Healthcare Products, Morris Plains, NJ 07950 USA

Warner-Lambert—Cont.

method. This product should not be used on children less than 2 months of age. Itching, redness, or swelling of the scalp may occur. If skin irritation persists or infection is present or develops, discontinue use and consult a doctor. Consult a doctor if infestation of eyebrows or eyelashes occurs. This product may cause breathing difficulty or an asthmatic episode in susceptible persons. As with any drug, if you are pregnant or nursing a baby, seek the advice of a health professional before using this product. Keep this and all drugs out of the reach of children. In case of accidental ingestion, seek professional assistance or contact a Poison Control Center immediately.

Professional Labeling:
Indications: For the treatment of head lice. For prophylactic use during head lice epidemics.

Warnings: For external use only. Keep out of eyes when rinsing hair. Adults and children: Close eyes and do not open eyes until product is rinsed out. If product gets into the eyes, immediately flush with water. Do not use near the eyes or permit contact with mucous membranes, such as inside the nose, mouth or vagina, as irritation may occur. Children: Also protect children's eyes with a washcloth, towel or other suitable material or method. This product should not be used on pediatric patients less than 2 months of age. Itching, redness, or swelling of the scalp may occur. If skin irritation persists or infection is present or develops, discontinue use and consult a doctor. Consult a doctor if infestation of eyebrows or eyelashes occurs. This product may cause breathing difficulty or an asthmatic episode in susceptible persons. As with any drug, if you are pregnant or nursing a baby, seek the advice of a health professional before using this product. Keep this and all drugs out of the reach of children. In case of accidental ingestion, seek professional assistance or contact a Poison Control Center immediately.

Dosage and Administration

Treatment
Nix Creme Rinse should be used after hair has been washed with patient's regular shampoo, rinsed with water and towel dried. A sufficient amount should be applied to saturate hair and scalp (especially behind the ears and on the nape of the neck). Leave on hair for 10 minutes but not longer. Rinse with water. A single application is usually sufficient. If live lice are observed seven days or more after the first application of this product, a second treatment should be given. For proper head lice management, remove nits with the nit comb provided.

Head lice live on the scalp and lay small white eggs (nits) on the hair shaft close to the scalp. The nits are most easily found on the nape of the neck or behind the ears. All personal headgear, scarfs, coats, and bed linen should be disinfected by machine washing in hot water and drying, using the hot cycle of a dryer for a least 20 minutes. Personal articles of clothing or bedding that cannot be washed my be dry-cleaned, sealed in a plastic bag for a period of about 2 weeks, or sprayed with a product specifically designed for this purpose. Personal combs and brushes may be disinfected by soaking in hot water (above 130°F) for 5 to 10 minutes. Thorough vacuuming of rooms inhabited by infected patients is recommended.

Prophylaxis
Prophylactic use of Nix Creme Rinse is only recommended for individuals exposed to head lice epidemics in which at least 20% of the population at an institution are infested and for immediate household members of infested individuals. Causal use is strongly discouraged. The method of application of Nix Creme Rinse for prophylaxis is identical to that described above for treatment of a lice infestation except nit removal is not required.

Directions for Use
One application of Nix Creme Rinse has been shown to protect greater than 95% of patients against reinfestation for at least two weeks. If epidemic settings, a second prophylactic application is recommended two weeks after the first because the life cycle of a head louse is approximately four weeks.

How Supplied: Bottles of 2 fl. oz. (59 mL) with nit removal comb and Family Pack of 2 bottles, 2 fl. oz. (59 mL) each, with nit removal comb. Store at 15° to 25°C (59° to 77°F).

Shown in Product Identification Guide, page 526

POLYSPORIN® Ointment
[*pŏl 'ē-spō 'rŭn*]

Each Gram Contains: Polymyxin B Sulfate 10,000 units and Bacitracin Zinc 500 units in a special White Petrolatum Base.

Indications: First aid to help prevent infection in minor cuts, scrapes, and burns.

Directions: Clean the affected area. Apply a small amount of this product (an amount equal to the surface area of the tip of a finger) on the area 1 to 3 times daily. May be covered with a sterile bandage.

Warnings: For external use only. Do not use in the eyes or apply over large areas of the body. In case of deep or puncture wounds, animal bites, or serious burns, consult a physician. Stop use and consult a physician if the condition persists or get worse, or if a rash or other allergic reaction develops. Do not use if you are allergic to any of the ingredients. Do not use longer than 1 week unless directed by a physician. KEEP THIS AND ALL DRUGS OUT OF THE REACH OF CHILDREN. In case of accidental ingestion, seek professional assistance or contact a Poison Control Center immediately.

How Supplied: Tubes, $^1/_2$ oz (14.2 g) with applicator tip, 1 oz (28.3 g); $^1/_{32}$ oz (0.9 g) foil packets packed in cartons of 144.
Store at 15° to 25°C (59° to 77°F).

Shown in Product Identification Guide, page 526

POLYSPORIN® Powder
[*pŏl 'ē-spō 'rŭn*]

Each Gram Contains: Polymyxin B Sulfate 10,000 units and Bacitracin Zinc 500 units in a Lactose Base.

Indications: First aid to help prevent infection in minor cuts, scrapes, and burns.

Directions: Clean the affected area. Apply a light dusting of the powder on the area 1 to 3 times daily. May be covered with a sterile bandage.

Warnings: For external use only. Do not use in the eyes or apply over large areas of the body. In case of deep or puncture wounds, animal bites, or serious burns, consult a physician. Stop use and consult a physician if the condition persists or gets worse, or if a rash or other allergic reaction develops. Do not use if you are allergic to any of the ingredients. Do not use longer than 1 week unless directed by a physician. KEEP THIS AND ALL DRUGS OUT OF THE REACH OF CHILDREN. In case of accidental ingestion, seek professional assistance or contact a Poison Control Center immediately.

How Supplied: 0.35 oz (10 g) shaker-vial.

Store at 15° to 25°C (59° to 77°F). Do not store under refrigeration.

Shown in Product Identification Guide, page 526

REPLENS® Vaginal Moisturizer
[*ree 'plenz*]

Ingredients: Purified Water, Glycerin, Mineral Oil, Polycarbophil, Carbomer 934P, Hydrogenated Palm Oil Glyceride, and Sorbic Acid.

Description: Replens relieves the discomfort of vaginal dryness for days with a single application. Replens non-hormonal vaginal moisturizer provides natural feeling moisture to continuously hydrate vaginal tissue. Replens is non-staining, fragrance free, non-greasy, non-irritating and Estrogen-Free.

Actions: When used as directed, Replens provides long-lasting relief from the discomfort of vaginal dryness by providing continuous hydration to the vaginal tissue.

Warnings: Keep out of the reach of children. Replens is not a contraceptive. Does not contain spermicide. If vaginal irritation occurs, discontinue use. If symptoms persist, contact your physician.

Usage: Use as needed. One single application approximately once every 2 to 3 days is recommended.

How Supplied: Replens is available in boxes containing 3 or 8 pre-filled disposable applicators. Each applicator delivers 2.5 grams.
Store at room temperature (59°–86°F). Avoid exposure to extreme heat or cold.

Shown in Product Identification Guide, page 526

SINUTAB® Non-Drying Liquid Caps
[*sĭn 'ū tăb*]

Active Ingredients: Each liquid cap contains: Pseudoephedrine Hydrochloride 30 mg., Guaifenesin 200 mg.

Inactive Ingredients: FD&C Blue No. 1, Gelatin, Glycerin, Polyethylene Glycol 400, Povidone, Propylene Glycol, and Sorbitol. Printed with edible white ink.

Indications: Temporarily relieves nasal congestion associated with sinusitis. Helps loosen phlegm (mucus) and thin bronchial secretions to drain bronchial tubes.

Dosage and Administration: Adults and children 12 years of age and over: swallow 2 liquid caps every 4 hours, not to exceed 8 liquid caps in 24 hours, or as directed by a doctor. Children under 12 years of age: consult a doctor.

Warnings: Do not exceed recommended dosage. If nervousness, dizziness, or sleeplessness occur, discontinue use and consult a doctor. If symptoms do not improve within 7 days or are accompanied by fever, consult a doctor. Do not take this product if you have heart disease, high blood pressure, thyroid disease, diabetes, or difficulty in urination due to enlargement of the prostate gland unless directed by a doctor. A persistent cough may be a sign of a serious condition. If cough persists for more than 1 week, tends to recur, or is accompanied by a fever, rash, or persistent headache, consult a doctor. Do not take this product for persistent or chronic cough such as occurs with smoking, asthma, chronic bronchitis, or emphysema, or where cough is accompanied by excessive phlegm (mucus) unless directed by a doctor. As with any drug, if you are pregnant or nursing a baby, seek the advice of a health professional before using this product.
KEEP THIS AND ALL DRUGS OUT OF THE REACH OF CHILDREN. In case of accidental overdose, seek professional assistance or contact a Poison Control Center immediately.

Drug Interaction Precaution: Do not use this product if you are now taking a prescription monoamine oxidase inhibitor (MAOI) (certain drugs for depression, psychiatric or emotional conditions, or Parkinson's disease), or for 2 weeks after stopping the MAOI drug. If you are uncertain whether your prescription drug contains an MAOI, consult a health professional before taking this product.

How Supplied: Sinutab® Non-Drying supplied in a box of 24 liquid caps.

Shown in Product Identification Guide, page 526

SINUTAB® Sinus Allergy Medication, Maximum Strength Formula, Tablets and Caplets
[*sĭn 'ū tăb*]

Active Ingredients: Each tablet/caplet contains: Acetaminophen 500 mg., Chlorpheniramine Maleate 2 mg., Pseudoephedrine Hydrochloride 30 mg.

Inactive Ingredients:
Tablets contain: Croscarmellose Sodium, Crospovidone, D&C Yellow No. 10 Aluminum Lake, FD&C Yellow No. 6 Aluminum Lake, Microcrystalline Cellulose, Povidone, Pregelatinized Starch, Stearic Acid, and Zinc Stearate.
Caplets contain: Carnauba Wax, Croscarmellose Sodium, Crospovidone, D&C Yellow No. 10 Aluminum Lake, FD&C Yellow No. 6 Aluminum Lake, Hydroxypropyl Cellulose, Hydroxypropyl Methylcellulose, Microcrystalline Cellulose, Polyethylene Glycol, Povidone, Pregelatinized Starch, Stearic Acid, Titanium Dioxide, and Zinc Stearate.

Indications: For the temporary relief of minor aches, pains and headache and nasal congestion associated with sinusitis. Temporarily relieves runny nose, sneezing itching of the nose or throat, and itchy watery eyes due to hay fever or other upper respiratory allergies.

Dosage and Administration: Adults and children 12 years of age and over: 2 tablets or caplets every 6 hours while symptoms persist, not to exceed 8 tablets or caplets in 24 hours, or as directed by a doctor. Children under 12 years of age: consult a doctor.

Warnings: Do not exceed recommended dosage. If nervousness, dizziness, or sleeplessness occur, discontinue use and consult a doctor. Do not take this product for more than 10 days. If symptoms do not improve or are accompanied by fever that lasts for more than 3 days, or if new symptoms occur, consult a doctor. Do not take this product, unless directed by a doctor, if you have heart disease, high blood pressure, thyroid disease, diabetes, a breathing problem such as emphysema or chronic bronchitis, or if you have glaucoma or difficulty in urination due to enlargement of the prostate gland. May cause excitability especially in children. May cause drowsiness; alcohol, sedatives, and tranquilizers may increase the drowsiness effect. Avoid alcoholic beverages while taking this product. Do not take this product if you are taking sedatives or tranquilizers, without first consulting your doctor. Use caution when driving a motor vehicle or operating machinery. As with any drug, if you are pregnant or nursing a baby, seek the advice of a health professional before using this product. **KEEP THIS AND ALL DRUGS OUT OF THE REACH OF CHILDREN.** In case of accidental overdose, seek professional assistance or contact a Poison Control Center immediately. Prompt medical attention is critical for adults as well as for children even if you do not notice any signs or symptoms.

Drug Interaction Precaution: Do not use this product if you are now taking a prescription monoamine oxidase inhibitor (MAOI) (certain drugs for depression, psychiatric or emotional conditions, or Parkinson's disease), or for 2 weeks after stopping the MAOI drug. If you are uncertain whether your prescription drug contains an MAOI, consult a health professional before taking this product.

How Supplied: Sinutab® Sinus Allergy Medication, Maximum Strength Formula, Caplets and Tablets are supplied in child-resistant blister packs in boxes of 24 tablets or caplets.

Store at room temperature (59°–86°F).

Shown in Product Identification Guide, page 526

SINUTAB® Sinus Medication, Maximum Strength Without Drowsiness Formula, Tablets and Caplets
[*sĭn 'ū tăb*]

Active Ingredients: Each tablet/caplet contains: Acetaminophen 500 mg., Pseudoephedrine Hydrochloride 30 mg.

Indications: For the temporary relief of minor aches, pains, and headache and nasal congestion associated with sinusitis.

Dosage and Administration: Adults and children 12 years of age and over: 2 tablets or caplets every 6 hours while symptoms persist, not to exceed 8 tablets or caplets in 24 hours or as directed by a doctor. Children under 12 years of age: consult a doctor.

Warnings: Do not exceed recommended dosage. If nervousness, dizziness, or sleeplessness occur, discontinue use and consult a doctor. Do not take this product for more than 10 days. If symptoms do not improve or are accompanied by fever that lasts for more than 3 days,

Continued on next page

This product information was prepared in November 1996. On these and other Warner-Lambert Consumer Healthcare Products, detailed information may be obtained by addressing Warner-Lambert Consumer Healthcare Products, Morris Plains, NJ 07950 USA

Warner-Lambert—Cont.

or if new symptoms occur, consult a doctor. Do not take this product if you have heart disease, high blood pressure, thyroid disease, diabetes, or difficulty in urination due to enlargement of the prostate gland unless directed by a doctor. As with any drug, if you are pregnant or nursing a baby, seek the advice of a health professional before using this product. **KEEP THIS AND ALL DRUGS OUT OF THE REACH OF CHILDREN.** In case of accidental overdose, seek professional assistance or contact a Poison Control Center immediately. Prompt medical attention is critical for adults as well as for children even if you do not notice any signs or symptoms.

Alcohol Warning: If you generally consume 3 or more alcohol-containing drinks per day, you should consult your physician for advice on when and how you should take Sinutab Sinus and other pain relievers.

Drug Interaction Precaution: Do not use this product if you are now taking a prescription monoamine oxidase inhibitor (MAOI) (certain drugs for depression, psychiatric or emotional conditions, or Parkinson's disease), or for 2 weeks after stopping the MAOI drug. If you are uncertain whether your prescription drug contains an MAOI, consult a health professional before taking this product.

How Supplied: Sinutab® Sinus Medication, Maximum Strength Without Drowsiness Formula, Caplets and Tablets are supplied in child-resistant blister packs in boxes of 24 tablets or caplets and in boxes of 48 caplets.

Shown in Product Identification Guide, page 526

SUDAFED® 12 Hour Caplets

[*sū 'duh-fĕd*]

Description: Sudafed 12 Hour Caplets is a long acting nasal decongestant providing temporary relief of nasal and sinus congestion due to a cold, allergy, or sinusitis for up to 12 hours. Sudafed 12 Hour helps clear nasal congestion and release sinus pressure to restore freer breathing without drowsiness.

Active Ingredient: Each coated extended-release caplet contains Pseudoephedrine Hydrochloride 120 mg in a capsule-shaped tablet.

Inactive Ingredients: Hydroxypropyl Methylcellulose, Magnesium Stearate, Microcrystalline Cellulose, Polyethylene Glycol, Povidone, and Titanium Dioxide. Printed with edible blue ink.

Indications: For temporary relief of nasal congestion due to the common cold, hay fever, or other upper respiratory allergies, and nasal congestion associated with sinusitis; promotes nasal and/or sinus drainage.

Directions: Adults and children 12 years and over—One caplet every 12 hours, not to exceed two caplets in 24 hours. Sudafed 12 Hour is not recommended for children under 12 years of age.

Warnings: Do not exceed recommended dosage because at higher doses, nervousness, dizziness, or sleeplessness may occur. Do not take this product if you have heart disease, high blood pressure, thyroid disease, diabetes, or difficulty in urination due to enlargement of the prostate gland unless directed by a doctor. If symptoms do not improve within 7 days or are accompanied by fever, consult your doctor before continuing use. As with any drug, if you are pregnant or nursing a baby, seek the advice of a health professional before using this product.

Drug Interaction Precaution: Do not take this product if you are presently taking a prescription drug for high blood pressure or depression, without first consulting your doctor.

KEEP THIS AND ALL DRUGS OUT OF THE REACH OF CHILDREN. In case of accidental overdose, seek professional assistance or contact a Poison Control Center immediately.

How Supplied: Boxes of 10 and 20. Store at 15° to 25°C (59° to 77°F) in a dry place and protect from light.

Shown in Product Identification Guide, page 526

SUDAFED® Nasal Decongestant Tablets 30 mg.

[*sū 'duh-fĕd*]

Description: Sudafed Nasal Decongestant tablets provide temporary, maximum strength relief of nasal and sinus congestion due to a cold, allergy, or sinusitis. Sudafed Nasal Decongestant helps clear nasal congestion and relieve sinus pressure to restore freer breathing without drowsy or overdrying side effects.

Active Ingredient: Each tablet contains Pseudoephedrine Hydrochloride 30 mg.

Inactive Ingredients: Acacia, Carnauba Wax, Corn Starch, Dibasic Calcium Phosphate, FD&C Red No. 40 Aluminum Lake, FD&C Yellow No. 6 Aluminum Lake, Magnesium Stearate, Pharmaceutical Glaze, Polysorbate 60, Potato Starch, Povidone, Sodium Benzoate, Stearic Acid, Sucrose, Talc, and Titanium Dioxide. Printed with edible black ink.

Indications: For the temporary relief of nasal congestion due to the common cold, hay fever or other upper respiratory allergies, and nasal congestion associated with sinusitis. Helps decongest sinus openings and passages; temporarily relieves sinus congestion and pressure. Temporarily restores freer breathing through the nose.

Directions: To be given every 4 to 6 hours. Do not exceed 4 doses in 24 hours. Adults and children 12 years of age and over: 2 tablets. Children 6 to under 12 years of age: 1 tablet. Children 2 to under 6 years of age: use Children's Sudafed Liquid. Children under 2 years of age: consult a doctor.

Warnings: Do not exceed recommended dosage. If nervousness, dizziness or sleeplessness occur, discontinue use and consult a doctor. If symptoms do not improve within 7 days, or are accompanied by fever, consult a doctor. Do not take this product if you have heart disease, high blood pressure, thyroid disease, diabetes, or difficulty in urination due to enlargement of the prostate gland unless directed by a doctor. As with any drug, if you are pregnant or nursing a baby, seek the advice of a health professional before using this product. **KEEP THIS AND ALL DRUGS OUT OF THE REACH OF CHILDREN.** In case of accidental overdose, seek professional assistance or contact a Poison Control Center immediately.

Drug Interaction Precaution: Do not use this product if you are now taking a prescription monoamine oxidase inhibitor (MAOI) (certain drugs for depression, psychiatric or emotional conditions, or Parkinson's disease), or for 2 weeks after stopping the MAOI drug. If you are uncertain whether your prescription drug contains an MAOI, consult a health professional before taking this product.

How Supplied: Boxes of 24, 48. Bottles of 100. Institutional Pack. Carton of 500 x 2.
Store at 15° to 25°C (59°–77°F) in a dry place and protect from light.

Shown in Product Identification Guide, page 526

CHILDREN'S SUDAFED® Nasal Decongestant Chewables

[*sū ' duh-fed*]

Description: Children's Sudafed Nasal Decongestant Chewables provides temporary relief for a child's stuffy nose and head due to a cold, allergy, or sinusitis. It also comes in a wonderful orange flavor chewable tablet that makes it easy to give to children. And Children's Sudafed Nasal Decongestant Chewables are part of the only children's line of cold medicines that are all free of drowsy side effects.

Active Ingredient: Each chewable tablet contains Pseudoephedrine Hydrochloride 15 mg.

Inactive Ingredients: Ascorbic Acid, Aspartame, Carnauba Wax, Citric Acid, Crospovidone, FD&C Yellow No. 6, Flavors, Hydroxypropyl Methylcellulose, Magnesium Stearate, Mannitol, Microcrystalline Cellulose, Sodium Chloride, Tartaric Acid.

Indications: For the temporary relief of nasal congestion due to the common cold, hay fever or other upper respiratory allergies, and nasal congestion associated with sinusitis. Promotes nasal and/or sinus drainage; temporarily relieves sinus congestion and pressure.

Directions: Do not exceed 4 doses in a 24-hour period. Children 6 to under 12 years of age: 2 chewable tablets every 4 to 6 hours. Children 2 to under 6 years of age: 1 chewable tablet every 4 to 6 hours. Children under 2 years of age: consult a doctor.

Warnings: Do not exceed recommended dosage. If nervousness, dizziness, or sleeplessness occur, discontinue use and consult a doctor. If symptoms do not improve within 7 days or are accompanied by fever, consult a doctor. Do not give this product to a child who has heart disease, high blood pressure, thyroid disease, or diabetes unless directed by a doctor. **KEEP THIS AND ALL DRUGS OUT OF THE REACH OF CHILDREN.** In case of accidental overdose, seek professional assistance or contact a Poison Control Center immediately. **Phenylketonurics: Contains Phenylalanine 0.78mg Per Tablet.**

Drug Interaction Precaution: Do not give this product to a child who is taking a prescription monoamine oxidase inhibitor (MAOI) (certain drugs for depression, psychiatric or emotional conditions), or for 2 weeks after stopping the MAOI drug. If you are uncertain whether your child's prescription drug contains an MAOI, consult a health professional before giving this product.

How Supplied: Box of 24 chewable tablets. Store at 15° to 25°C (59° to 77°F) in a dry place and protect from light.

Shown in Product Identification Guide, page 526

SUDAFED® CHILDREN'S NASAL DECONGESTANT LIQUID MEDICATION

[*sū ' duh-fĕd*]

Description: Children's Sudafed Nasal Decongestant Liquid provides temporary relief for a child's stuffy nose and head due to a cold or allergy. And Children's Sudafed Nasal Decongestant Liquid is part of the only children's line of cold medicines that are all free of drowsy side effects. It also comes in a wonderful grape flavor that makes it easy to give to children.

Active Ingredient: Each teaspoonful (5 mL) contains Pseudoephedrine Hydrochloride 15 mg.

Inactive Ingredients: Citric Acid, Edetate Disodium, FD&C Red No. 40, FD&C Blue No. 1, Flavors, Glycerin, Poloxamer 407, Polyethylene Glycol 1450, Povidone K-90, Purified Water, Saccharin Sodium, Sodium Benzoate, Sodium Citrate and Sorbitol Solution.

Indications: For the temporary relief of nasal congestion due to the common cold, hay fever or other upper respiratory allergies, and nasal congestion associated with sinusitis. Promotes nasal and/or sinus drainage; temporarily relieves sinus congestion and pressure.

Directions: Follow dosage recommendations below. Dosage may be repeated every 4 to 6 hours, not to exceed 4 doses in 24 hours.

Age	Dosage
Children under 2 years of age	Consult a doctor
Children 2 to under 6 years of age	One (1) teaspoonful
Children 6 to under 12 years of age	Two (2) teaspoonfuls
Adults and children 12 years of age and over	Four (4) teaspoonfuls

Warnings: Do not exceed recommended dosage. If nervousness, dizziness, or sleeplessness occur, discontinue use and consult a doctor. If symptoms do not improve within 7 days or are accompanied by fever, consult a doctor. Do not take this product if you have heart disease, high blood pressure, thyroid disease, diabetes, or difficulty in urination due to enlargement of the prostate gland unless directed by a doctor. As with any drug, if you are pregnant or nursing a baby, seek the advice of a health professional before using this product. **KEEP THIS AND ALL DRUGS OUT OF THE REACH OF CHILDREN.** In case of accidental overdose, seek professional assistance or contact a Poison Control Center immediately.

Drug Interaction Precaution: Do not use this product if you are now taking a prescription monoamine oxidase inhibitor (MAOI) (certain drugs for depression, psychiatric or emotional conditions, or Parkinson's disease), or for 2 weeks after stopping the MAOI drug. If you are uncertain whether your prescription drug contains an MAOI, consult a health professional before taking this product.

How Supplied: Sudafed Children's Nasal Decongestant is supplied in 4 fl. oz. bottles
Store at 15° to 25°C (59° to 77°F) and protect from light.

Shown in Product Identification Guide, page 526

PEDIATRIC SUDAFED® NASAL DECONGESTANT LIQUID ORAL DROPS

[*sū 'duh-fĕd*]

Description: Pediatric Sudafed Nasal Decongestant Drops provides temporary relief for a child's stuffy nose and head due to a cold or allergy. And Sudafed Pediatric Nasal Decongestant Drops is part of the only children's line of cold medicines that are all free of drowsy side effects. It also comes in a wonderful fruit flavor with a calibrated dropper that makes it easy to administer.

Active Ingredient: Each dropperful (0.8 mL) contains Pseudoephedrine Hydrochloride 7.5 mg.

Inactive Ingredients: Carboxymethylcellulose Sodium, Citric Acid, Flavors, Glycerin, Poloxamer 407, Purified Water, Saccharin Sodium, Sodium Benzoate, Sodium Chloride, Sodium Citrate and Sorbitol Solution.

Indications: For the temporary relief of nasal congestion due to the common cold, hay fever or other upper respiratory allergies, and nasal congestion associated with sinusitis. Promotes nasal and/or sinus drainage; temporarily relieves sinus congestion and pressure.

Directions: TAKE BY MOUTH ONLY; NOT FOR NASAL USE. Use enclosed calibrated dropper for accurate dosing. Dosage may be repeated every 4 to 6 hours, not to exceed 4 doses in 24 hours. Follow dosage recommendations below.

Age	Dosage
Children under 2 years of age	Consult a doctor
Children 2 to under 6 years of age	2 Dropperfuls (1.6 mL)

Warnings: Do not exceed recommended dosage. If nervousness, dizziness, or sleeplessness occur, discontinue use and consult a doctor. If symptoms do not improve within 7 days or are accompanied by fever, consult a doctor. Do not give this product to a child who has heart disease, high blood pressure, thyroid disease or diabetes unless directed by a doctor. **KEEP THIS AND ALL DRUGS OUT OF THE REACH OF CHILDREN.** In case of accidental overdose, seek professional assistance or contact a Poison Control Center immediately.

Drug Interaction Precaution: Do not give this product to a child who is taking a prescription monoamine oxidase inhibitor (MAOI) (certain drugs for depression, psychiatric or emotional conditions), or for 2 weeks after stopping the MAOI drug. If you are uncertain whether your child's prescription drug contains an MAOI, consult a health professional before giving this product.

Continued on next page

This product information was prepared in November 1996. On these and other Warner-Lambert Consumer Healthcare Products, detailed information may be obtained by addressing Warner-Lambert Consumer Healthcare Products, Morris Plains, NJ 07950 USA

Warner-Lambert—Cont.

How Supplied: Sudafed Pediatric Nasal Decongestant Oral Drops are supplied in 1/2 fl. oz. bottles.
Store at 15° to 25°C (59° to 77°F).

Shown in Product Identification Guide, page 527

SUDAFED® Cold & Allergy Tablets

[*sū 'duh-fĕd*]

Description: Sudafed Cold & Allergy provides temporary, maximum strength relief of nasal congestion and allergy symptoms. Sudafed Cold & Allergy helps dry a runny nose and relieve sneezing, and itchy, watery eyes due to allergies.

Active Ingredients: Each tablet contains: Chlorpheniramine Maleate 4 mg. and Pseudoephedrine Hydrochloride 60 mg.

Inactive Ingredients: Lactose, Magnesium Stearate, Potato Starch, and Povidone.

Indications: For the temporary relief of runny nose, sneezing and nasal congestion due to the common cold. For the temporary relief of runny nose, sneezing, itching of the nose or throat, itchy, watery eyes, and nasal congestion due to hay fever (allergic rhinitis).

Directions: To be given every 4 to 6 hours. Do not exceed 4 doses in 24 hours, or as directed by a doctor. Adults and children 12 years of age and over: 1 tablet. Children 6 to under 12 years of age: 1/2 tablet. Children under 6 years of age: consult a doctor.

Warnings: Do not exceed recommended dosage. If nervousness, dizziness, or sleeplessness occur, discontinue use and consult a doctor. If symptoms do not improve within 7 days or are accompanied by fever, consult a doctor. Do not take this product, unless directed by a doctor, if you have a breathing problem such as emphysema or chronic bronchitis, heart disease, high blood pressure, thyroid disease, diabetes, or if you have glaucoma or difficulty in urination due to enlargement of the prostate gland. May cause excitability especially in children. May cause drowsiness; alcohol, sedatives, and tranquilizers may increase the drowsiness effect. Avoid alcoholic beverages while taking this product. Do not take this product if you are taking sedatives or tranquilizers, without first consulting your doctor. Use caution when driving a motor vehicle or operating machinery. As with any drug, if you are pregnant or nursing a baby, seek the advice of a health professional before using this product. **KEEP THIS AND ALL DRUGS OUT OF THE REACH OF CHILDREN.** In case of accidental overdose, seek professional assistance or contact a Poison Control Center immediately.

Drug Interaction Precaution: Do not use this product if you are now taking a prescription monoamine oxidase inhibitor (MAOI) (certain drugs for depression, psychiatric or emotional conditions, or Parkinson's disease), or for 2 weeks after stopping the MAOI drug. If you are uncertain whether your prescription drug contains an MAOI, consult a health professional before taking this product.

How Supplied: Boxes of 24 and 48.
Store at 15° to 25° C (59°–77°F) in a dry place and protect from light.

Shown in Product Identification Guide, page 526

SUDAFED® Cold & Cough Liquid Caps

[*sū 'duh-fĕd*]

Description: Sudafed Cold & Cough Liquid Caps provide temporary relief of colds and coughs. Sudafed Cold & Cough helps clear nasal and chest congestion and relieve sinus pressure while relieving headaches, fever, body aches, coughs and sore throats due to colds without drowsy or overdrying side effects.

Active Ingredients: Each liquid cap contains: Acetaminophen 250 mg, Guaifenesin 100 mg, Pseudoephedrine Hydrochloride 30 mg, and Dextromethorphan Hydrobromide 10 mg.

Inactive Ingredients: D&C Yellow No. 10, FD&C Red No. 40, Gelatin, Glycerin, Polyethylene Glycol 400, Povidone, Propylene Glycol, Purified Water, and Sorbitol. Printed with edible white ink.

Indications: For the temporary relief of nasal congestion, minor aches, pains, headache, muscular aches, sore throat, and fever associated with the common cold. Temporarily relieves cough occurring with a cold. Helps loosen phlegm (mucus) and thin bronchial secretions to drain bronchial tubes and make coughs more productive.

Directions: Adults and children 12 years of age and over: 2 liquid caps every 4 hours, while symptoms persist, not to exceed 8 liquid caps in 24 hours, or as directed by a doctor. Children under 12 years of age: consult a doctor.

Warnings: Do not exceed recommended dosage. If nervousness, dizziness, or sleeplessness occur, discontinue use and consult a doctor. Do not take this product for more than 10 days. A persistent cough may be a sign of a serious condition. If symptoms do not improve of if cough persists for more than 7 days, tends to recur, or is accompanied by rash, persistent headache, fever that lasts for more than 3 days, or if new symptoms occur, consult a doctor. Do not take this product for persistent or chronic cough such as occurs with smoking, asthma, chronic bronchitis, or emphysema, or where cough is accompanied by excessive phlegm (mucus) unless directed by a doctor. If sore throat is severe, persists for more than 2 days, is accompanied or followed by fever, headache, rash, nausea, or vomiting, consult a doctor promptly. Do not take this product if you have heart disease, high blood pressure, thyroid disease, diabetes, or difficulty in urination due to enlargement of the prostate gland unless directed by a doctor. As with any drug, if you are pregnant or nursing a baby, seek the advice of a health professional before using this product. **KEEP THIS AND ALL DRUGS OUT OF THE REACH OF CHILDREN.** In case of accidental overdose, seek professional assistance or contact a Poison Control Center immediately. Prompt medical attention is critical for adults as well as for children even if you do not notice any signs or symptoms.

Alcohol Warning: If you generally consume 3 or more alcohol-containing drinks per day, you should consult your physician for advice on when and how you should take Sudafed Cold & Cough and other pain relievers.

Drug Interaction Precaution: Do not use this product if you are now taking a prescription monoamine oxidase inhibitor (MAOI) (certain drugs for depression, psychiatric or emotional conditions, or Parkinson's disease), or for 2 weeks after stopping the MAOI drug. If you are uncertain whether your prescription drug contains an MAOI, consult a health professional before taking this product.

How Supplied: Boxes of 10 and 20.
Store at 15° to 25°C (59°–77°F) in a dry place and protect from light.

Shown in Product Identification Guide, page 526

SUDAFED® COLD & SINUS Liquid Caps

[*sū 'duh-fed*]

Description: Sudafed Cold & Sinus temporarily relieves cold symptoms and sinus pain. Sudafed Cold & Sinus contains Sudafed's maximum strength nasal decongestant to help clear nasal congestion and relieve sinus pressure, plus a pain reliever to alleviate the headache, fever, sore throat, and body aches for relief without drowsy or overdrying side effects.

Active Ingredients: Each liquid cap contains: Acetaminophen 325mg and Pseudoephedrine Hydrochloride 30 mg.

Inactive Ingredients: FD&C Blue No. 1, FD&C Red No. 40, Gelatin, Glycerin, Pharmaceutical Glaze, Polyethylene Glycol, Povidone, Purified Water, Sodium Acetate, Sorbitol Special, and Titanium Dioxide.

Indications: For the temporary relief of nasal congestion, minor aches, pains, headache, muscular aches, sore throat, and fever due to the common cold. Temporarily relieves nasal congestion associated with sinusitis. Reduces swelling of nasal passages; shrinks swollen membranes. Promotes nasal and/or sinus drainage; temporarily relieves sinus congestion and pressure. Temporarily restores freer breathing through the nose.

Directions: Adults and children 12 years of age and over: 2 liquid caps every 4 to 6 hours, while symptoms persist, not to exceed 8 liquid caps in 24 hours, or as directed by a doctor. Children under 12 years of age: consult a doctor.

Warnings: **Do not exceed recommended dosage.** If nervousness, dizziness, or sleeplessness occur, discontinue use and consult a doctor. Do not take this product for more than 10 days. If symptoms do not improve or are accompanied by fever that lasts for more than 3 days, or if new symptoms occur, consult a doctor. If sore throat is severe, persists for more than 2 days, is accompanied or followed by fever, headache, rash, nausea, or vomiting, consult a doctor promptly. Do not take this product if you have heart disease, high blood pressure, thyroid disease, diabetes, or difficulty in urination due to enlargement of the prostate gland unless directed by a doctor. As with any drug, if you are pregnant or nursing a baby, seek the advice of a health professional before using this product. **KEEP THIS AND ALL DRUGS OUT OF THE REACH OF CHILDREN.** In case of accidental overdose, seek professional assistance or contact a Poison Control Center immediately. Prompt medical attention is critical for adults as well as for children even if you do not notice any signs or symptoms.

Alcohol Warning: If you generally consume 3 or more alcohol-containing drinks per day, you should consult your physician for advice on when and how you should take Sudafed Cold & Sinus Liquid Caps and other pain relievers.

Drug Interaction Precaution: Do not use this product if you are now taking a prescription monoamine oxidase inhibitor (MAOI) (certain drugs for depression, psychiatric or emotional conditions, or Parkinson's disease), or for 2 weeks after stopping the MAOI drug. If you are uncertain whether your prescription drug contains an MAOI, consult a health professional before taking this product.

How Supplied: Boxes of 10 and 20 liquid caps. Store at 15° to 25°C (59° to 77°F) in a dry place and protect from light.

Shown in Product Identification Guide, page 526

SUDAFED® NON-DRYING SINUS LIQUID CAPS

[*sū 'duh-fĕd*]

Description: Sudafed Non-Drying Sinus provides temporary, maximum strength relief of nasal congestion and sinus pressure due to sinusitis, colds, or allergies. Sudafed Non-Drying Sinus contains ingredients that help clear nasal congestion, relieve sinus pressure without overdrying sensitive nasal tissue or causing drowsiness and temporarily relieves chest congestion.

Active Ingredients: Each liquid cap contains Guaifenesin 200 mg. and Pseudoephedrine Hydrochloride 30 mg.

Inactive Ingredients: FD&C Blue No. 1, Gelatin, Glycerin, Polyethylene Glycol 400, Povidone, Propylene Glycol and Sorbitol. Printed with edible white ink.

Indications: For the temporary relief of nasal congestion associated with sinusitis. Promotes nasal and/or sinus drainage; temporarily relieves sinus congestion and pressure. Helps loosen phlegm (mucus) and thin bronchial secretions to rid the bronchial passageways of bothersome mucus and make coughs more productive.

Directions: Adults and children 12 years of age and over: swallow 2 liquid caps every 4 hours, not to exceed 8 liquid caps in 24 hours, or as directed by a doctor. Children under 12 years of age: consult a doctor.

Warnings: **Do not exceed recommended dosage.** If nervousness, dizziness, or sleeplessness occur, discontinue use and consult a doctor. If symptoms do not improve within 7 days or are accompanied by fever, consult a doctor. Do not take this product if you have heart disease, high blood pressure, thyroid disease, diabetes, or difficulty in urination due to enlargement of the prostate gland unless directed by a doctor. A persistent cough may be a sign of a serious condition. If cough persists for more than 1 week, tends to recur, or is accompanied by a fever, rash, or persistent headache, consult a doctor. Do not take this product for persistent or chronic cough such as occurs with smoking, asthma, chronic bronchitis, or emphysema, or where cough is accompanied by excessive phlegm (mucus) unless directed by a doctor. As with any drug, if you are pregnant or nursing a baby, seek the advice of a health professional before using this product. **KEEP THIS AND ALL DRUGS OUT OF THE REACH OF CHILDREN.** In case of accidental overdose, seek professional assistance or contact a Poison Control Center immediately.

Drug Interaction Precaution: Do not use this product if you are now taking a prescription monoamine oxidase inhibitor (MAOI) (certain drugs for depression, psychiatric or emotional conditions, or Parkinson's disease), or for 2 weeks after stopping the MAOI drug. If you are uncertain whether your prescription drug contains an MAOI, consult a health professional before taking this product.

How Supplied: Sudafed Non-Drying Sinus is supplied in boxes of 24 liquid caps.
Store at 15° to 25°C (59° to 77°F) in a dry place and protect from light.

Shown in Product Identification Guide, page 527

SUDAFED® Severe Cold Formula Caplets and Tablets

[*sū 'duh-fĕd*]

Description: Sudafed Severe Cold Formula contains maximum strength ingredients to temporarily relieve the worst cold symptoms. Sudafed Severe Cold Formula helps clear nasal congestion and relieve sinus pressure while relieving headaches, fever, body aches, coughs and sore throats due to colds without drowsy or overdrying side effects.

Active Ingredients: Each coated caplet/tablet contains: Acetaminophen 500 mg, Pseudoephedrine Hydrochloride 30 mg, and Dextromethorphan Hydrobromide 15 mg.

Inactive Ingredients: Carnauba Wax, Crospovidone, Hydroxypropyl Methylcellulose, Magnesium Stearate, Microcrystalline Cellulose, Polyethylene Glycol, Povidone, Pregelatinized Starch, Stearic Acid, and Titanium Dioxide.

Indications: For the temporary relief of nasal congestion, minor aches, pains, headache, muscular aches, sore throat, and fever associated with the common cold. Temporarily relieves cough occurring with a cold.

Directions: Adults and children 12 years of age and over: 2 caplets or tablets every 6 hours, while symptoms persist, not to exceed 8 caplets or tablets in 24 hours, or as directed by a doctor. Children under 12 years of age: consult a doctor.

Warnings: **Do not exceed recommended dosage.** If nervousness, dizziness, or sleeplessness occur, discontinue use and consult a doctor. Do not take this product for more than 10 days. A persistent cough may be a sign of a serious condition. If symptoms do not improve or if cough persists for more than 7 days, tends to recur, or is accompanied by rash, persistent headache, fever that lasts for more than 3 days, or if new symptoms occur, consult a doctor. Do not take this product for persistent or chronic cough such as occurs with smoking, asthma or emphysema, or if cough is accompanied by excessive phlegm (mucus) unless directed by a doctor. If sore throat is severe, persists for more than 2 days, is accompanied or followed by fever, headache, rash, nausea, or vomiting, consult a doctor promptly. Do not take this product if you have heart disease, high blood pressure, thyroid disease, diabetes, or

Continued on next page

This product information was prepared in November 1996. On these and other Warner-Lambert Consumer Healthcare Products, detailed information may be obtained by addressing Warner-Lambert Consumer Healthcare Products, Morris Plains, NJ 07950 USA

Warner-Lambert—Cont.

difficulty in urination due to enlargement of the prostate gland unless directed by a doctor. As with any drug, if you are pregnant or nursing a baby, seek the advice of a health professional before using this product. **KEEP THIS AND ALL DRUGS OUT OF THE REACH OF CHILDREN.** In case of accidental overdose, seek professional assistance or contact a Poison Control Center immediately. Prompt medical attention is critical for adults as well as for children even if you do not notice any signs or symptoms.

Alcohol Warning: If you generally consume 3 or more alcohol-containing drinks per day, you should consult your physician for advice on when and how you should take Sudafed Severe Cold Formula and other pain relievers.

Drug Interaction Precaution: Do not use this product if you are now taking a prescription monoamine oxidase inhibitor (MAOI) (certain drugs for depression, psychiatric or emotional conditions, or Parkinson's disease), or for 2 weeks after stopping the MAOI drug. If you are uncertain whether your prescription drug contains an MAOI, consult a health professional before taking this product.

How Supplied: Boxes of 12 and 24.
Store at 15° to 25°C (59°–77°F) in a dry place and protect from light.

Shown in Product Identification Guide, page 526

SUDAFED® Sinus Caplets and Tablets
[*sū 'duh-fĕd*]

Description: Sudafed Sinus contains Sudafed's maximum strength decongestant and a maximum strength pain reliever to temporarily relieve sinus symptoms. Sudafed Sinus helps clear nasal congestion and relieve sinus pressure while relieving sinus headaches due to sinusitis, allergies or colds without drowsy or overdrying side effects.

Active Ingredients: Each coated caplet/tablet contains: Acetaminophen 500 mg and Pseudoephedrine Hydrochloride 30 mg.

Inactive Ingredients: Caplets and Tablets contain Carnauba Wax, Crospovidone, FD&C Yellow No. 6 Aluminum Lake, Hydroxypropyl Methylcellulose, Magnesium Stearate, Microcrystalline Cellulose, Polyethylene Glycol, Polysorbate 80, Povidone, Pregelatinized Starch, Stearic Acid and Titanium Dioxide.

Indications: For the temporary relief of nasal congestion associated with sinusitis. Helps decongest sinus openings and passages; temporarily relieves sinus congestion and pressure. Temporarily relieves headache, minor aches, and pains. Temporarily restores freer breathing through the nose.

Directions: Adults and children 12 years and over: 2 caplets or tablets every 6 hours, while symptoms persist, not to exceed 8 caplets or tablets in 24 hours, or as directed by a doctor. Children under 12 years of age: consult a doctor.

Warnings: Do not exceed recommended dosage. If nervousness, dizziness, or sleeplessness occur, discontinue use and consult a doctor. Do not take this product for more than 10 days. If symptoms do not improve or are accompanied by fever that lasts for more than 3 days, or if new symptoms occur, consult a doctor. Do not take this product if you have heart disease, high blood pressure, thyroid disease, diabetes, or difficulty in urination due to enlargement of the prostate gland unless directed by a doctor. As with any drug, if you are pregnant or nursing a baby, seek the advice of a health professional before using this product. **KEEP THIS AND ALL DRUGS OUT OF THE REACH OF CHILDREN.** In case of accidental overdose, seek professional assistance or contact a Poison Control Center immediately. Prompt medical attention is critical for adults as well as children even if you do not notice any signs or symptoms.

Alcohol Warning: If you generally consume 3 or more alcohol-containing drinks per day, you should consult your physician for advice on when and how you should take Sudafed Sinus and other pain relievers.

Drug Interaction Precaution: Do not use this product if you are now taking a prescription monoamine oxidase inhibitor (MAOI) (certain drugs for depression, psychiatric or emotional conditions, or Parkinson's disease), or for 2 weeks after stopping the MAOI drug. If you are uncertain whether your prescription drug contains an MAOI, consult a health professional before taking this product.

How Supplied: Box of 24.
Store at 15° to 25°C (59° to 77°F) in a dry place and protect from light.

Shown in Product Identification Guide, page 527

TUCKS® Clear Hemorrhoidal Gel
[*tŭks*]

Active Ingredients: Witch Hazel 50% and Glycerin 10.7%.

Inactive Ingredients: Alcohol, Benzyl Alcohol, Carbomer 974 P, Disodium Edetate, Propylene Glycol, Sodium Hydroxide and Water.

Indications: For the temporary relief of external itching, burning and discomfort associated with inflamed hemorrhoidal tissues.

Directions: For External Use Only. Adults: When practical, cleanse the affected area with mild soap and warm water and rinse thoroughly. Gently dry by patting or blotting with toilet tissue or soft cloth before application of this product. Apply externally to the affected area up to 6 times daily or after each bowel movement. Children under 12 years of age: consult a physician.

Warnings: If condition worsens or does not improve within 7 days, consult a physician. Do not exceed recommended daily dosage unless directed by a physician. In case of bleeding, consult a physician promptly. Do not put this product into the rectum by using fingers or any mechanical device or applicator. **Keep this and all drugs out of the reach of children.** In case of accidental ingestion, seek professional assistance or contact a Poison Control Center immediately.

How Supplied: Tucks Clear Gel is supplied in 0.7 oz (19.8g) tubes.
Store at room temperature 15°–30°C (59°–86°F).

Shown in Product Identification Guide, page 527

TUCKS®
Pre-moistened Hemorrhoidal/Vaginal Pads
[*tŭks*]

Active Ingredients: Soft pads are pre-moistened with a solution containing Witch Hazel 50%.

Inactive Ingredients: Water, Glycerin, Alcohol, Propylene Glycol, Sodium Citrate, Diazolidinyl Urea, Citric Acid, Methylparaben, Propylparaben.

Indications: For the temporary relief of external itching, burning and irritation associated with hemorrhoids.

Other Uses:
Hygienic Wipe: Tucks Pads are effective for everyday personal hygienic use on outer rectal and vaginal areas. Used in place of toilet tissue, Tucks Pads gently and thoroughly remove irritation-causing matter. They are especially handy during menstrual periods.
Moist Compress: For additional relief, Tucks Pads can be folded and used as a compress on inflamed tissue. Tucks Pads are particularly helpful in relieving discomfort following childbirth, rectal or vaginal surgery.

Directions: For external use only. *As a hemorrhoidal treatment* —Adults: When practical, cleanse the affected area with mild soap and warm water, and rinse thoroughly. Gently dry by patting or blotting with toilet tissue or soft cloth before each application of this product. Gently apply to affected area by patting and then discard. Can be used up to six times daily or after each bowel movement. Children under 12 years of age: consult a physician.
As a hygienic wipe —Use as a wipe instead of toilet tissue.
As a moist compress —For soothing relief, fold pad and place in contact with irritated tissue. Leave in place for 5 to 15 minutes. Repeat as needed.

Warnings: If condition worsens or does not improve within 7 days, consult a physician. Do not exceed recommended daily dosage unless directed by a physician. In case of bleeding, consult a physician promptly. Do not put this product in the rectum by using fingers or any mechanical device or applicator. **Keep this and all drugs out of the reach of children.** In case of accidental ingestion, seek professional assistance or contact a Poison Control Center immediately.

How Supplied: Jars of 40 and 100 pads. Also available Tucks Take-Alongs®, individual, foil-wrapped, nonwoven (6 Two-Packs) pads.

Shown in Product Identification Guide, page 527

ZANTAC® 75
Acid Reducer/Ranitidine Tablets 75 mg
[*zan' tak*]

Active Ingredient: Each tablet contains: 84 mg ranitidine hydrochloride (equivalent to 75 mg ranitidine).

Inactive Ingredients: Hydroxypropyl methylcellulose, magnesium stearate, microcrystalline cellulose, synthetic red iron oxide, titanium dioxide and triacetin. Zantac 75 is sodium and sugar free.

Uses: For the relief of heartburn, acid indigestion and sour stomach.

Directions:
- Swallow 1 tablet with water. (Do not chew.)
- Can be used up to twice daily (up to 2 tablets in 24 hours).
- This product should not be given to children under 12 years old unless directed by a doctor.

Warnings:
- Do not take the maximum daily dose for more than 14 consecutive days, unless directed by your doctor.
- As with any drug, if you are pregnant or nursing a baby, seek the advice of a health professional before using this product.
- If you have trouble swallowing or persistent abdominal pain, see your doctor promptly. You may have a serious condition that may need different treatment.
- Keep this and all drugs out of the reach of children.
- In case of accidental overdose, seek professional assistance or contact a poison control center immediately.

Read the Label: Read the directions, consumer information leaflet and warnings before use. Keep the carton. It contains important information.

How Supplied: Zantac 75 is available in convenient blister packs in boxes of 4, 10, 20, and 30 tablets. Store between 2°C and 30°C (36°F and 86°F). Avoid excessive heat or humidity.
DO NOT USE IF THE INDIVIDUAL BLISTER UNIT IS OPEN OR BROKEN.

Zantac is a registered trademark of the Glaxo Wellcome group of companies.

Questions or Comments? Call us Toll-Free at 1-800-223-0182 weekdays between 9:00 am and 5:00 pm EST.

Shown in Product Identification Guide, page 527

Wellness International Network, Ltd.

1501 LUNA ROAD, BLDG. 102
CARROLLTON, TX 75006

Direct Inquiries to:
Director, Product Development
(972) 245-1097
FAX: (972) 389-3060

BIO-COMPLEX 5000™
Gentle Foaming Cleanser

Uses: BIO-COMPLEX 5000™ Gentle Foaming Cleanser, with alpha-hydroxy acids, aloe vera, and botanical infusions, is an advanced cleansing gel designed for all skin types. BIO-COMPLEX 5000 Gentle Foaming Cleanser protects the skin and works to restore elasticity while gently removing surface impurities, make-up, and pollution.

Inactive Ingredients: Aloe Vera Gel, Infusion of Sage, Infusion of Chamomile, Ammonium Lauryl Sulfate, Lauramidopropyl Betaine, Glycerin, Lauramide DEA, Cetyl Betaine, Tocopherol, Citric Acid, Lactic Acid, Malic Acid, Ascorbic Acid, Methylchloroisothiazolinone, Methylisothiazolinone, Propylparaben, Methylparaben.

Directions: Splash warm water onto face. Place a small amount of gel on fingertips. Apply evenly to face and neck in circular motions, massaging skin gently but thoroughly. Rinse completely and pat dry with a soft towel.

How Supplied: 8 fluid ounce/236 ml. bottle.

BIO-COMPLEX 5000™
Revitalizing Conditioner

Uses: BIO-COMPLEX 5000™ Revitalizing Conditioner, with vitamins, antioxidants, and sunscreen, helps restore moisture to dried-out, heat-styled hair. This advanced conditioner enhances hair with silkening agents and detangles hair after shampooing. Hair is left clean, soft, manageable, and protected against styling aids and environmental elements. BIO-COMPLEX 5000 Revitalizing Conditioner is excellent for all hair types, especially damaged or over-processed hair.

Inactive Ingredients: Water, Stearyl Alcohol, Propylene Glycol, Stearamidopropyl Dimethalymine, Cyclomethicone, Polyquaternium - 11, Stearalkonium Chloride, Cetearyl Alcohol, PEG - 40 Hydrogenated Castor Oil, Citric Acid, Tocopherol, Ascorbic Acid, Retinyl Palmitate, Octyl Methoxycinnamate, Awapuhi Fragrance, Ceteth - 20, Soluble Animal Keratin, Imidazolidinyl Urea, Propylparaben, Methylparaben.

Directions: After shampooing with BIO-COMPLEX 5000™ Revitalizing Shampoo, apply to wet hair. Massage through hair, paying special attention to the ends. Leave on 2–3 minutes. Rinse thoroughly. Towel dry and style as usual.

How Supplied: 12 fluid ounce bottle.

BIO-COMPLEX 5000™
Revitalizing Shampoo

Uses: BIO-COMPLEX 5000™ Revitalizing Shampoo, with vitamins, anti-oxidants, and sunscreen, cleanses and moisturizes hair for excellent manageability. Specially formulated with the essence of awapuhi, a Hawaiian ginger plant extract known for its healing qualities, this formula contains the mildest blend of surfactants and a wealth of natural conditioning ingredients to provide body, luster, and healthier-looking hair.

Inactive Ingredients: Water, Ammonium Lauryl Sulfate, Tea Lauryl Sulfate, Cetyl Betaine, Lauramide DEA, Cocamidopropyl Betaine, Glycerin, Ascorbic Acid, Tocopherol, Retinyl Palmitate, Citric Acid, Hydrolyzed Wheat Protein, Awapuhi Fragrance, Octyl Methoxycinnamate, PEG - 7 Glyceryl Cocoate, Methylchloroisothiazolinone, Methylisothiazolinone, Caramel.

Directions: Apply a small amount to wet hair and massage gently into scalp, creating a generous lather. Rinse and repeat if necessary. To further intensify this reconstructive process, follow with BIO-COMPLEX 5000™ Revitalizing Conditioner.

How Supplied: 12 fluid ounce bottle.

BIOLEAN®
Herbal & Amino Acid Food Supplement

Uses: BIOLEAN® is a unique combination of Chinese herbal extracts and pharmaceutical grade amino acids specifically designed to help raise overall health, participate in individual life extension programs, and enhance athletic performance. It has been shown to be extremely effective in promoting the healthy loss of excess body fat while helping to maintain lean body mass and potent energy levels. BIOLEAN, when used as a daily nutritional supplement, has also been shown to stimulate immune function in individuals with blunted sympathetic nervous systems, especially overweight and obese persons. It acts as a positive stimulator to immune functions involved in protection from environmental and dietary carcinogens.
Components in BIOLEAN are known to cause fat loss through thermogenic activity and altered fuel metabolism resulting

Continued on next page

Wellness International—Cont.

from sympathomimetic response to stimulation of beta receptors in adipose and muscle cells. The positive immune response, though not completely understood, is at least partially attributable to beta stimulation in adipocytes and the adaptogenic and tonifying activity of certain of the herbal extracts. This has been demonstrated in their long history of use in traditional Chinese herbal medicine as well as current scientific research which points to, among other possibilities, the extremely potent antioxidant properties found in some of the component plants, most notably in the Green Tea and Schizandrae extracts. BIOLEAN may increase athletic performance and endurance through three pathways: 1) increased oxygen uptake in the lungs as a result of expanding bronchial passages; 2) enhanced mental acuity and response resulting from sympathetic nervous system stimulus; and 3) increasing the employment of fatty acids as fuel in muscle mitochondria while simultaneously sparing muscle glycogen and nitrogen.
The herbal extracts in BIOLEAN are produced in a unique and exclusive process which is proprietary to this product. Instead of creating extracts based on a set quantity of one particular active within many which may be present in any particular plant, BIOLEAN components are concentrated to maintain the natural and complete spectrum of biologically active factors, in the same ratio presented by the unprocessed plant.

Directions: Adults take one white capsule and one to three tablets with low-calorie food mid to late morning. If using BIOLEAN for the first time, take one capsule and one tablet on days 1 and 2, one capsule and two tablets on days 3 and 4, and one capsule and three tablets beginning day 5. Needs vary with the individual. Some persons may require less than three tablets daily or wish to spread the taking of the tablets throughout morning and early afternoon to achieve optimum results. Do not exceed recommended daily amounts. It is recommended that you drink at least eight glasses of water daily.

Warnings: Phenylketonurics: Contains Phenylalanine. Not for use by children. Consult your physician before using this product if you are taking asthma medications, appetitie suppressing drugs, antidepressants, or cardiovascular medication. Do not consume if you are pregnant or lactating, or have high blood pressure, cardiovascular disease, diabetes, prostatic hypertrophy, glaucoma, hyperthyroidism, psychosis, or thyroid disease. If symptoms of allergy develop, discontinue use. It is recommended that you minimize your caffeine intake while consuming this product. Do not consume on the same day that you consume BIOLEAN free.

Ingredients: *Capsules:* 400 mg. of the following mix: L-Phenylalanine, L-Tyrosine, L-Carnitine. *Tablets:* 650 mg. of the following herbal mix: Ma Huang, Green Tea, Schizandrae Berry, Rehmannia Root, Hawthorne Berry, Jujube Seed, Alisma Root, Angelicae Dahuricae Root, Epemidium, Poria Cocos, Rhizoma Rhei, Stephania Root, Angelicae Sinensis Root, Codonopsis Root, Eucommium Bark, Notoginseng Root.

How Supplied: One box contains 28 packets, one capsule and three tablets per packet.

BIOLEAN Accelerator™
Herbal & Amino Acid Formulation

Uses: BIOLEAN Accelerator™ is a unique combination of Chinese herbal extracts and pharmaceutical grade amino acids specifically designed to complement both BIOLEAN® and BIOLEAN Free™ by extending and accelerating their actions. BIOLEAN and BIOLEAN Free are, in the traditional view of Chinese herbal medicine, strong Yang blends. This means that they are energy or heat-producing at their core. The addition of the amino acids and certain of the herbal components lends a very definite restorative, or Yin element, as well. BIOLEAN Accelerator is a strong Yin herbal formula, intended to augment the lesser replenishing Yin elements of the other two herbal and amino acid supplements. Though the physiological actions of many herbs are complex and not totally understood, the formula in BIOLEAN Accelerator extends the adaptogenic, thermogenic, restorative, and detoxifying results experienced with BIOLEAN and BIOLEAN Free, with an emphasis on the restorative and adaptogenic effects. The herbal formula is a combination of tonifiers traditionally used in China for the lungs, liver, and kidneys.

Directions: For maximum effectiveness, use in conjunction with original BIOLEAN or BIOLEAN Free. (Do not consume BIOLEAN and BIOLEAN Free on the same day.) Take one tablet in the morning with original BIOLEAN or BIOLEAN Free. BIOLEAN Accelerator™ may also be taken in the afternoon with or without additional BIOLEAN or BIOLEAN Free if desired. Maximum absorption will be attained if taken with low-calorie food.

Warnings: Phenylketonurics: Contains Phenylalanine. Not for use by children. Consult your physician before using this product if you are taking appetite suppressing drugs or antidepressants. If symptoms of allergy develop, discontinue use.

Ingredients: Each tablet contains 250 mg. herbal mix (Black Sesame Seed, Raw Chinese Foxglove Root, Chinese Wolfberry Fruit, Achyranthes Root, Cornelian Cherry Fruit, Chinese Yam, Eclipta Herb, Rose Hips, Privet Fruit, Mulberry Fruit-Spike, Polygonati Rhizome, Cooked Chinese Foxglove Root, Poria Cocos, Cuscuta Seed, Foxnut Seed, Alisma Rhizome, Moutan Bark, Phellodendron Bark, Anemarrhena Rhizome, Schisandra Berry, Royal Jelly), L-Tyrosine, L-Phenylalanine.

How Supplied: One bottle contains 56 tablets.

BIOLEAN Free™
Herbal & Amino Acid Food Supplement

Uses: BIOLEAN Free™ is a strategic blend of herbs, spices, vitamins, minerals, and amino acids specifically formulated to enhance fat utilization and energy production through various metabolic pathways. It has been shown to reduce body fat through its thermogenic effects and to enhance both physical and mental performance.
Thermogenesis refers to the body's ability to convert substrates such as proteins, fats, and carbohydrates into heat energy. This is carried out most efficiently in the Brown Adipose Tissue of our body which uses fatty acids as its preferred fuel. Other fat cells, namely White Adipose Tissue, are concerned primarily with the storage of fat rather than its conversion to energy. The thermogenic pathway is complex and relies upon a series of reactions to occur. BIOLEAN Free utilizes many compounds which act at various locations in this pathway to ensure the maximum efficiency of the thermogenic process. Quebracho is one of these very special compounds. This South American plant contains quebrachine, aspidiospermine, and other alkaloids that possess the ability to block alpha-2 adrenergic receptors in the body. This produces an enhanced sympathetic nervous system effect which, in turn, increases lipolysis (fat breakdown) within fat cells. The fatty acids released by this process can then be transported into the mitochondria to be used as a fuel. Ginger, cinnamon, horseradish, turmeric, cayenne, and mustard are spices that stimulate thermogenesis in different ways. Some stimulate lipid mobilization in adipose tissue; others raise the resting metabolic rate; and some increase cAMP levels by inducing more beta receptors on fat cells and by increasing the concentration of adenylate cyclase. cAMP increases the breakdown of triglycerides to free fatty acids which are later used as fuel by the mitochondria in the cell. Methylxanthines (such as those found in green tea and yerba maté) also increase cAMP levels, but do this by inhibiting the enzyme, phosphodiesterase. These compounds have been noted to increase mental alertness, improve vitality, satisfy the appetite, and increase energy. In addition to its methylxanthine content, green tea has recently been shown to possess strong antioxidant properties. Yerba maté is a plant that has been shown to

produce the positive effects above without causing the insomnia seen with other methylxanthine-containing plants (such as coffee and kola nut). BIOLEAN Free also contains vitamin B-3, vitamin B-6, chromium, and vanadium which aid in the proper metabolism of fats, proteins, and carbohydrates. L-tyrosine also aids in metabolism and promotes satiety through hypothalamic release of CCK. Methionine is a precursor of L-carnitine which aids in the transport of fatty acids into the mitochondria for thermogenesis. Other herbs have been utilized in BIOLEAN Free. Ginseng and ho shou wu possess adaptogenic properties. Adaptogens help the body adapt to physiological and environmental stresses. Ginseng accomplishes this through its stabilizing effect on the hypothalamic-pituitary-adrenal-sympathetic nervous system. It can mediate an increase adrenal response to stress.

Ho shou wu has a stabilizing effect on the endocrine system and has restorative properties. It is also an antioxidant with a high flavonoid content. *Centella asiatica* contains asiaticoside and has been shown to increase activity levels and ease the body's ability to overcome fatigue when taken with ginseng and cayenne. Individually, *centella* has been shown to increase memory and mental acuity in studies abroad. Uva ursi contains the glycoside arbutin and promotes urinary health and body strength through its purifying effects. Ginkgo biloba is a tree whose leaves have been used for centuries as an herbal medicine. It contains flavonoids and is therefore a strong antioxidant. It reduces the tendency of platelets to stick together by inhibiting Platelet Activating Factor. It has been shown to increase blood flow to the heart, brain, and other organs.

Directions: Adults (18 years and older) may take 4 caplets in the mid to late morning with a low-calorie food. Needs may vary with each individual. Some persons may require less than 4 caplets, or may prefer taking 3 caplets mid morning and 1 additional caplet mid afternoon to achieve optimum results. Do not exceed recommended daily amounts. It is recommended that you drink at least eight glasses of water daily.

Warnings: Not for use by children, pregnant women, or lactating women. Consult your physician before using this product if you are taking appetite suppressing drugs or cardiovascular medication. Also consult your physician if you have hypertension, heart disease, arrhythmias, prostatic hypertrophy, glaucoma, liver disease, renal disease, or diabetes. Do not use if you have hyperthyroidism, psychosis, Parkinson's Disease, or are taking Monoamine oxidase inhibitors. BIOLEAN Free should not be taken on the same day as original BIOLEAN®. It is recommended that you minimize your caffeine intake while consuming this product. If allergic symptoms develop, discontinue use. Store in a cool, dry place. Keep out of reach of children.

Ingredients: Each caplet contains the following: Standardized botanical extracts containing 720 mg of the following mixture: Green Tea, Yerba Maté, Korean Ginseng, Uva Ursi, and Quebracho. Non-irradiated pure herbs and spices containing 360 mg of the following mixture: Jamaican Ginger, Ceylon Cinnamon, Chinese Horseradish, Alleppy Turmeric, Nigerian Cayenne, English Mustard, *Centella Asiatica,* Ho Shou Wu, Ginkgo Biloba. Also included are 125 mg of L-Tyrosine, 25 mg of Methionine, 25 mg of Potassium (citrate), 10 mg of Vitamin B-3, 4 mg of Vitamin B-6, 100 mcg of Chromium Chelavite™, 100 mcg of Vanadium.

How Supplied: One box contains 28 packets, four tablets per packet.

BIOLEAN LipoTrim™
All-Natural Dietary Supplement

Uses: LipoTrim™ is a highly active, synergistic combination of garcinia cambogia extract and chromium polynicotinate specifically created for use with the other products in the BIOLEAN® System. The method of action is by inhibition of lipogenesis and regulation of blood glucose levels. Serum glucose derived from dietary carbohydrates and not immediately converted to energy or glycogen tends to be converted into fat stores and cholesterol. In individuals with excess body fat stores or slow basal metabolism, this tendency is thought to be higher. The garcinia cambogia extract present in LipoTrim is verified by HPLC analysis to be no less that 50%(-) hydroxycitrate (HCA). HCA inhibits ATP-citrate lyase which retards Acetyl CoA synthesis, severely restricting conversion of excess glucose into fatty acids and cholesterol. Animal studies have shown post-meal fatty acid synthesis reduction of 40–80% for an 8–12 hour period. When glucose to fat/cholesterol conversion is retarded, glycogen conversion continues, increasing liver stores and causing satiety signals to be sent to the brain resulting in appetite suppression. In situations of intense physical exercise, increased glycogen stores have been shown to result in enhanced endurance and recovery. By restricting the activity of insulin, chromium has been shown to exhibit a regulating effect on blood glucose levels thus extending the benefits of HCA.

Directions: As a dietary supplement, take one capsule three times daily, 30 minutes before each meal. LipoTrim should be used in conjunction with a healthy diet and exercise plan.

Warnings: Do not consume if you are pregnant or lactating. Not for use by young children. Consult your physician before using this product if your diet consists of less than 1,000 calories per day.

Ingredients: CitriMax™* (garcinia cambogia), ChromeMate®* (chromium polynicotinate).

How Supplied: One bottle contains 84 easy-to-swallow capsules.

*CitriMax™ is a trademark of InterHealth.
ChromeMate® is a registered trademark of InterHealth.

BIOLEAN Meal™
Nutritional Meal Replacement Drink

Uses: BIOLEAN Meal™ is formulated specifically for use with the other products in the BIOLEAN® System. It has a natural chocolate flavor which mixes instantly, without need for blending, to form a creamy drink which is equally delicious in water, milk, or milk substitutes, including rice and soy base. BIOLEAN Meal is a low-calorie, nonfat, low-lactose powder designed to provide an optimum, alternative blend of protein, carbohydrates, and dietary fiber to individuals who have unhealthy or insufficient dietary habits, are on a fat-loss program, or desire to enhance their athletic ability.

BIOLEAN Meal has been biologically engineered to contain a 1:1 ratio of casein proteins to whey proteins. This represents a significant improvement in taste, solubility, nutritional content, and BV (biological value) compared to caseinates, soy defatted whole egg, and egg white protein, the latter historically being the standard of comparison for all protein sources. There are several factors contributing to this higher BV. Bovine milk has a ratio of casein to whey of 4:1, whereas human milk is 2:3. The amino acid composition, absorption, and utilization of whey protein is superior to other sources of supplemental dietary protein. This is especially true for individuals with limited or compromised GI function which often accompanies situations involving physical and emotional stress, illness, disease, and trauma. Athletes with increased protein requirements will also benefit from a higher BV protein source. Whey protein has the highest ratio of essential to nonessential amino acids and contains the highest quantity of Branched Chain Amino Acids (BCAA), especially leucine, which is double that of egg protein. Leucine is consumed in large amounts during periods of exercise, trauma, infection, and caloric restriction. Muscle recovery, fuel production, and immune function are dependent upon adequate supply and replacement of leucine. Research has also shown that tissue stores of glutathione are increased by the regular intake of whey protein.

The immune enhancing effects of whey protein, combined with the high nutritive value of milk protein isolate, promotes the loss of body fat and the retention and growth of lean body mass (mus-

Continued on next page

Wellness International—Cont.

cle, bone, and internal organs) as well as supporting all other normal physiological processes such as immune function and cellular replacement, especially during periods of added stress brought on by dieting, illness, and athletic activity.

Directions: Add contents to 8 ounces of water or nonfat milk and stir or shake until completely mixed. For a thicker drink, blend for 10 seconds and drink immediately. For pudding, blend for 30 seconds and refrigerate.

Warnings: Phenylketonurics: Contains Phenylalanine.

Ingredients: Myotein (Proprietary bioengineered protein blend of specially isolated fat and lactose free milk proteins and whey protein concentrate), Fructose, Maltodextrin, Nonfat Milk Solids, Naturally Processed Cocoa, Natural Flavor Complex (Chocolate, Vanilla, and Vanilla Cream), Cellulose Gel, Guar Gum, Corn Starch, Aspartame.

How Supplied: One box contains 14 packets. Serving size equals one packet.

Food For Thought™
Choline-Enriched Nutritional Drink

Uses: A unique and tasty blend of essential vitamins and minerals, Food For Thought™ is specifically designed for anyone desiring to function at peak mental capacity. This nutritious beverage mix is choline-enriched and is ideal for work, school, or any time performance is needed.

Directions: Add 6 ounces of chilled water or fruit juice to one packet of mix. Stir briskly. Consume 1–2 times per day. Keep in a cool, dry place. For maximum results, combine this product with one serving of Winrgy™.

Warnings: Not for use by children, pregnant or lactating women. Persons taking medications should seek medical advice before taking this product. Persons with ulcers or a history of ulcers should consult their physician before using a choline supplement. Do not consume more than four servings per day. Avoid the use of antacids containing aluminum with this product.

Ingredients: Fructose, Choline Bitartrate, Calcium Pantothenate, Natural Flavor, Glycine, Ascorbic Acid, Vitamin E Acetate, Niacinamide, Lysine, Silicon Dioxide, Zinc Gluconate, Chromium Aspartate, Niacin, Magnesium Gluconate, Pyridoxine Hydrochloride, Thiamin Mononitrate, Riboflavin, Copper Gluconate, Vitamin B12.

How Supplied: One box contains 28 packets of drink mix. Serving size equals one packet.

STEPHAN™ BIO-NUTRITIONAL
Daytime Hydrating Creme

Uses: Hypo-allergenic STEPHAN™ BIO-NUTRITIONAL Daytime Hydrating Creme hydrates the skin and preserves the moisture level of the upper layers of the epidermis. It is an excellent day cream for both men and women who wish to combat the visible signs of aging skin, the appearance of wrinkles or lines, and the inelastic look of facial features and contours. These light emulsions are absorbed rapidly, leaving an invisible protective film which hydrates the epidermis, regulates moisture levels, and leaves skin feeling supple and soft.

Inactive Ingredients: Water, Stearic Acid, Isodecyl Neopentanoate, Isostearyl Stearoyl Stearate, DEA Cetyl Phosphate, C12-15 Alkyl Benzoate, Squalane, Dimethicone, Aloe Vera Gel, Tocopherol, Cetyl Esters, Carbomer, Fragrance, Benzophenone-3, Triethanolamine, Imidazolidinyl Urea, Propylparaben, Methylparaben, Annatto.

Directions: Apply evenly on a completely cleansed face and neck. May be used around the eye area, avoiding direct contact with the eyes. Suitable for all skin types. For best results, use in conjunction with the complete STEPHAN BIO-NUTRITIONAL Skin Care line.

Warnings: For external use only. Avoid contact with eyes.

How Supplied: Net Wt. 1.75 oz.

STEPHAN™ BIO-NUTRITIONAL
Eye-Firming Concentrate

Uses: Hypo-allergenic STEPHAN™ BIO-NUTRITIONAL Eye-Firming Concentrate is specially formulated to revitalize the delicate area around the eyes. This non-oily fluid pampers sensitive eyes while reducing the look of puffiness and dark circles, and smoothing and softening the appearance of fine lines in the eye area.

Inactive Ingredients: Infusion of Chamomile, Cornflower Extract, Horsetail Extract, Sugar Cane Extract, Citrus Extract, Apple Extract, Green Tea Extract, Methyl Gluceth-20, Panthenol, Cyanocobalamin, Propylene Glycol, Laureth-4, Hydrolyzed Wheat Protein, Tissue Respiratory Factors, Plant Pseudocollagen, Aloe Vera Gel, Triethanolamine, Dimethicone Copolyol, PEG-30 Glyceryl Laurate, Phenethyl Alcohol, Carbomer, Xanthan Gum, Benzophenone-4, Disodium EDTA, Methylchloroisothiazolinone, Methylisothiazolinone, Methylparaben, Propylparaben.

Directions: Apply in the morning, or any time of the day, in small quantities to the skin around the eyes with light, tapping motions, avoiding direct contact with the eyes. In the evening, apply gently to the entire eye contour area. For best results, use in conjunction with the complete STEPHAN BIO-NUTRITIONAL Skin Care line.

Warnings: For external use only. Avoid direct contact with eyes.

How Supplied: 1 fl. oz.

STEPHAN™ BIO-NUTRITIONAL
Nightime Moisture Creme

Uses: Hypo-allergenic STEPHAN™ BIO-NUTRITIONAL Nightime Moisture Creme is a heavier, richer cream for mature, dry, or sun-damaged skin. This advanced formula is excellent for dehydrated skin, promoting suppleness and moisture, while improving the appearance of fine lines and wrinkles.

Inactive Ingredients: Water, Caprylic/Capric Triglyceride, Propylene Glycol, Stearic Acid, Polysorbate 60, Cetyl Alcohol, Octyl Palmitate, Beeswax, Sorbitan Stearate, Canola Oil, Avocado Oil, Safflower Oil, Squalane, Liposomes, Soluble Collagen, Dimethicone, Bisabolol, Aloe Vera Gel, Fragrance, C12-15 Alkyl Benzoate, Hydroxyethylcellulose, Octyl Methoxycinnamate, Disodium EDTA, Sodium Borate, Benzophenone-3, Allantoin, Phenoxyethanol, Methylparaben, Propylparaben, Butylparaben, Ethylparaben, FD&C Yellow No. 10, Caramel.

Directions: In the evening, apply by lightly massaging onto a thoroughly cleansed face and neck. Avoid direct contact with eyes. For drier skin, it may be used during the day as a moisturizer, under make-up, or after sun bathing. For best results, use in conjunction with the complete STEPHAN BIO-NUTRITIONAL Skin Care line.

Warning: For external use only. Avoid contact with eyes.

How Supplied: Net Wt. 1.75 oz.

STEPHAN™ BIO-NUTRITIONAL
Refreshing Moisture Gel

Uses: Hypo-allergenic STEPHAN™ BIO-NUTRITIONAL Refreshing Moisture Gel is specially formulated to refine pores and promote a clear, clean, and smooth-looking complexion. It is designed to deeply cleanse and super-stimulate the skin. This gel is suitable for all skin types, especially problem areas. A quick "pick-me-up," STEPHAN BIO-NUTRITIONAL Refreshing Moisture Gel immediately restores the radiant, firm, and youthful appearance of the face while acting as a cumulative, revitalizing beauty treatment.

Inactive Ingredients: Water, Propylene Glycol, Glycerin, Hydroxyethylcellulose, Sugar Cane Extract, Citrus Extract, Apple Extract, Green Tea Extract, Hydrolyzed Wheat Protein, Tissue Respiratory Factors, Panthenol, Aloe Vera Gel, Laureth-4, Magnesium Aluminum Silicate, Tetrasodium EDTA, Benzophenone-3, Imidazolidinyl Urea, Methylchloroisothiazolinone, Methylisothiazolinone, Methylparaben, Propylparaben, Phenethyl Alcohol, FD&C Yellow No. 10, FD&C Red No. 40, FD&C Yellow No. 5.

Directions: After thoroughly cleansing in the morning or evening, apply a liberal layer to the face, neck, and eye area, avoiding eye contact. Remove after 20–30 minutes with warm water. Suitable for all skin types. For best results, use in conjunction with the complete STEPHAN BIO-NUTRITIONAL Skin Care line.

Warnings: For external use only. Avoid contact with eyes.

How Supplied: Net Wt. 1.75 oz.

STEPHAN™ BIO-NUTRITIONAL
Ultra Hydrating Fluid

Uses: Hypo-allergenic STEPHAN™ BIO-NUTRITIONAL Ultra Hydrating Fluid is a complete treatment formulated to soften fine lines and preserve youthful-looking, radiant skin. By utilizing ingredients focused on revitalization, STEPHAN BIO-NUTRITIONAL Ultra Hydrating Fluid possesses a progressive firming effect, helping to combat the aged look of skin due to external negative conditions.

Inactive Ingredients: Water, Glycerin, Panthenol, Sodium Hyaluronate, Phenethyl Alcohol, Aloe Vera Gel, Methyl Gluceth-20, PEG-30 Glyceryl Laurate, Methylsilanol Hydroxyproline Aspartate, Xanthan Gum, Methylchloroisothiazolinone, Methylisothiazolinone.

Directions: Gently apply all over the face, neck, and eye contour area, preferably in the morning. Use as a part of a regular daily skin care routine or as an occasional preventive treatment. For best results, use in conjunction with the complete STEPHAN BIO-NUTRITIONAL Skin Care line.

Warnings: For external use only. Avoid direct contact with eyes.

How Supplied: 1 fl. oz.

STEPHAN™ Clarity
Nutritional Supplement

Uses: STEPHAN™ Clarity, designed for use by both men and women, contains selected tissue proteins in the form of nutrients important to memory and concentration.
This is achieved by utilizing such ingredients as lecithin and glutamic acid. Lecithin is a popular supplement widely embraced for the treatment and prevention of memory loss. Known for properties that have been scientifically proven to increase the firing of neurons in the nervous system, glutamic acid is an amino acid which influences the body by serving as brain fuel. It also metabolizes sugars and fats, as well as detoxifies.
Ginkgo biloba, a third primary ingredient in STEPHAN™ Clarity, is a special additive which increases flow of blood to the brain and is noted for improving concentration and learning ability. Together with the support of carefully selected vitamins, minerals, amino acids, and herbs, STEPHAN™ Clarity is a natural and effective way to better one's health.

Directions: Take one to two capsules per day.

Warnings: Phenylketonurics: Contains Phenylalanine.

Ingredients: Lecithin, Bee Pollen, Glutamic Acid, Vitamin C, Ribonucleic Acid, Ginkgo Biloba (as 8:1 extract), Aspartic Acid, Vitamin E, Vitamin B-3, Leucine, Arginine, Lysine, Phenylalanine, Serine, Valine, Proline, Isoleucine, Alanine, Glycine, Threonine, Tyrosine, Vitamin B-5, Vitamin B-1, Histidine, Methionine, Cysteine, Adenosine Triphosphate, Vitamin B-6, Vitamin B-2, Vitamin A, Folic Acid, Biotin, Vitamin D-3, Vitamin B-12.

How Supplied: One bottle contains 60 easy-to-swallow capsules.

DHEA Plus™
Pharmaceutical-Grade Formulation

Uses: By utilizing the latest and most advanced breakthrough applications in age management, DHEA Plus™ uniquely combines dehydroepiandrosterone (DHEA), Bioperine® and ginkgo biloba leaf to safely and effectively aid the body.
These age management factors are mainly attributed to the properties of DHEA, a natural substance obtained from the barbasco root, also known as Mexican Wild Yam, which is synthesized in a pharmaceutical laboratory to be utilized for specific health applications. Once supplemental DHEA is orally consumed, it is quickly absorbed into the bloodstream through the intestines and binds to a sulfate compound which creates DHEA-S. DHEA-S is the ultimate substance for which the body uses to manufacture hormones. Natural DHEA levels, abundant in the bloodstream and present at an even higher level in the tissues of the brain, are known to decline with age in both sexes. Scientific research proves that adequate levels of DHEA in the body can actually slow the aging process. Further studies have shown that it often prevents, improves and, many times, reverses conditions such as cancer, heart disease, memory loss, obesity and osteoporosis.
Bioperine, a pure piperine extract, enhances the body's natural thermogenic activity and is another important ingredient in DHEA Plus. Thermogenesis is the metabolic process that generates energy at the cellular level. While thermogenesis plays an integral role in our body's ability to properly utilize daily foods and nutrients into the body, it also sets in motion the mechanisms that lead to digestion and subsequent gastrointestinal absorption.
Known for possessing antioxidant activity, or flavonoid effects, ginkgo biloba proves to decrease platelet aggregation and increase vasodilation which appears to extend blood flow to the peripheral arteries and the brain. Some improvement in cognitive abilities has been noted as well as inhibition of lipid peroxidation, thereby stabilizing the cell wall against free-radical attack.

Directions: Adults take one capsule daily with food.

Warnings: This product should only be consumed by adults and is not intended for use by children. Do not consume if you are pregnant or lactating. Consult your physician before using this product if you are taking prescription medications. Persons with a history of prostate cancer should seek medical advice before using this product.

Ingredients: Dehydroepiandrosterone (DHEA), Bioperine*, Ginkgo Biloba.

How Supplied: One bottle contains 60 capsules.

*Bioperine is a registered trademark of Sabinsa Corporation.

STEPHAN™ Elasticity
Nutritional Supplement

Uses: A nutritional food supplement for men and women, STEPHAN™ Elasticity contains a scientifically balanced mixture of specific tissue proteins established as important for skin tone and texture.
Utilizing such scientifically respected ingredients as vitamin A and selenium, STEPHAN™ Elasticity is also supported by various other vitamins, minerals, and amino acids dedicated to epidermal appearance.
Due to its antioxidant properties, vitamin A has been dubbed the "skin vitamin." It is commonly used as a means of preventing premature aging of the skin. In addition, synthetic derivatives of vitamin A are often used to treat acne and psoriasis.
Selenium is also considered beneficial to the skin. It was recently reported that low blood selenium in the context of low blood vitamin A increases the risk for certain types of skin cancer.

Directions: Take one capsule per day.

Warning: Phenylketonurics: Contains Phenylalanine.

Ingredients: Equisetum Arvense, Protein Isolates (Alanine, Arginine, Aspartic Acid, Cysteine, Glutamic Acid, Glycine, Histidine, Isoleucine, Leucine, Lysine, Methionine, Phenylalanine, Proline, Serine, Threonine, Tyrosine, Valine), Fucus, Vitamine E (Dl-Alpha), Zinc (Amino Acid Chelate), Vitamin C, Ribonucleic Acid, Calcium (Amino Acid Che-

Continued on next page

Wellness International—Cont.

late), Magnesium (Amino Acid Chelate), Iron (Amino Acid Chelate), Manganese (Amino Acid Chelate), Selenium (Amino Acid Chelate), Chromium (Amino Acid Chelate), Adenosine Triphosphate, Vitamin A (Acetate).

How Supplied: One bottle contains 60 easy-to-swallow capsules.

STEPHAN™ Elixir Nutritional Supplement

Uses: Formulated with an exclusive blend of specific proteins, STEPHAN™ Elixir is ideal for both men and women. These tissue proteins are supported by vitamins, minerals, amino acids, and herbs recognized as important for general health and well-being.

Among the scientifically researched and proven ingredients utilized in STEPHAN™ Elixir are vitamin E and cysteine. Vitamin E protects against the ravages of aging in several ways. It is essential for the normal functioning of the body and is especially important for normal neurological functions in humans. It also serves as a potent antioxidant and has been dubbed the body's "first line of defense" against free-radical attack by helping to guard against free radicals, the type of cellular damage that has been linked to the initiation of cancer and heart disease.

Cysteine has also been found to inactivate free radicals and thus protect and preserve the cells. This sulfur-containing amino acid is a precursor of glutathione, a tripeptide, that is claimed to safeguard the body against various toxins and pollutants, therefore extending the life span.

Directions: Take one capsule per day.

Warnings: Phenylketonurics: Contains Phenylalanine.

Ingredient: Soya Isolate (Alanine, Arginine, Aspartic Acid, Cysteine, Glutamic Acid, Glycine, Histidine, Isoleucine, Leucine, Lysine, Methionine, Phenylalanine, Proline, Serine, Threonine, Tyrosine, Valine), Bee Pollen, Vitamin C, Malic Acid, Ginkgo Biloba (8:1 extract), Citric Acid, Ribonucleic Acid, Vitamin E, Vitamin B-3, Zinc (Amino Acid Chelate), Iron (Amino Acid Chelate), Calcium Pantothenate, Vitamin B-1, Vitamin B-5, Adenosine Triphosphate, Vitamin B-6, Vitamin B-2, Vitamin A, Folic Acid, Selenium (Amino Acid Chelate), Biotin, Vitamin D-3, Vitamin B-12.

How Supplied: One bottle contains 60 easy-to-swallow capsules.

STEPHAN™ Essential Nutritional Supplement

Uses: STEPHAN™ Essential is a nutritional food supplement which contains specific tissue proteins supported by vitamins, minerals, herbs, and amino acids that are proactive to cardiovascular and circulatory management. L-carnitine, vitamin E, and linoleic acid are only some of these very important components.

Scientifically researched and a major contributor to the effects of STEPHAN™ Essential, L-carnitine is necessary for the transport of long-chain fatty acids into the mitochondria, the metabolic furnaces of the cells. These fatty acids prove a major source for the production of energy in the heart and skeletal muscles, structures that are particularly vulnerable to L-carnitine deficiency. Appropriate levels of L-carnitine in the body have been shown to protect against cardiovascular disease, muscle disease, diabetes, and kidney disease.

While vitamin E has proven beneficial in serving to boost the immune system and protect against cardiovascular disease, it has also been established as an important therapy for disorders related to neurologic symptoms. Omega 3–Oil, another important addition to STEPHAN™ Essential, can lower serum cholesterol levels and decrease platelet stickiness, proving beneficial in the prevention of coronary heart disease.

STEPHAN™ Essential may be consumed by both men and women.

Directions: Take one to two capsules per day.

Warnings: Phenylketonurics: Contains Phenylalanine.

Ingredients: Bee Pollen, L-Carnitine, Omega 3 Oil, Glutamic Acid, Ribonucleic Acid, Aspartic Acid, Vitamin E, Leucine, Arginine, Lysine, Magnesium (Amino Acid Chelate), Phenylalanine, Serine, Valine, Proline, Isoleucine, Alanine, Glycine, Threonine, Tyrosine, Histidine, Methionine, Cysteine, Adenosine Triphosphate, Selenium (Amino Acid Chelate).

How Supplied: One bottle contains 60 easy-to-swallow capsules.

STEPHAN™ Feminine Nutritional Supplement

Uses: Specifically designed for women, STEPHAN™ Feminine contains selected tissue proteins supported by vitamins, minerals, and amino acids regarded as important to the ever-changing female body. This is achieved through such scientifically researched ingredients as magnesium and boron.

STEPHAN™ Feminine utilizes magnesium as an important ingredient responsible for regulating the flow of calcium between cells. Studies reveal that women with high-calcium diets report fewer PMS symptoms including less irritability and depression, as well as fewer headaches, backaches, and cramps. Magnesium thus ensures individuals are receiving maximum benefits from calcium intake.

Researchers also report many promising results on the effects of dietary boron. Conclusions show that supplementary boron markedly reduces the excretion of both calcium and magnesium while increasing production of an active form of estrogen and testosterone.

Directions: Take one to two capsules per day.

Warnings: Phenylketonurics: Contains Phenylalanine.

Ingredients: Magnesium Oxide, Glutamic Acid, Ribonucleic Acid, Aspartic Acid, Vitamin E, Leucine, Arginine, Lysine, Phenylalanine, Serine, Valine, Proline, Isoleucine, Alanine, Glycine, Threonine, Tyrosine, Histidine, Methionine, Cysteine, Boron (Amino Acid Chelate), Adenosine Triphosphate, Selenium.

How Supplied: One bottle contains 60 easy-to-swallow capsules.

STEPHAN™ Flexibility Nutritional Supplement

Uses: A nutritional supplement for both men and women, STEPHAN™ Flexibility is rich with exclusive proteins which are supported by vitamins, minerals, and amino acids recognized as beneficial to the health of joint and soft tissues.

Glycine, an amino acid, is one very significant ingredient utilized in STEPHAN™ Flexibility. In a pilot study investigating the possibility of glycine's effect on spastic control, a 25% improvement was noted on subjects with chronic multiple sclerosis. Furthermore, all patients benefited to some degree, and no toxicity or other adverse side effects were noted.

Another important amino acid in STEPHAN Flexibility is L-histidine. Reports suggest that supplementary L-histidine may actually boost the activity of suppressor T cells. Because rheumatoid arthritis is one of the many autoimmune diseases in which T-cell activity is subnormal, these conclusions lend further support that L-histidine may prove beneficial in its treatment.

Vitamin E can also be found in STEPHAN Flexibility because of its ability to relieve muscular cramps. According to one popular study, supplemental vitamin E caused remarkable relief from persistent nocturnal leg and foot cramps in 82% of the 125 patients tested.

Directions: Take one to two capsules per day.

Warnings: Phenylketonurics: Contains Phenylalanine.

Ingredients: Vitamin C, Ribonucleic Acid, Vitamin E, Vitamin B-3, Glutamic Acid, Zinc (Amino Acid Chelate), Calcium (Amino Acid Chelate), Aspartic Acid, Bee Pollen, Leucine, Arginine, Lysine, Vitamin B-5, Vitamin B-1, Phenylalanine, Serine, Valine, Proline, Isoleucine, Alanine, Glycine, Threonine, Tyrosine, Histidine, Cysteine, Adenosine Triphosphate, Vitamin B-6, Boron

(Amino Acid Chelate), Vitamin B-2, Methionine, Vitamin A, Folic Acid, Selenium (Amino Acid Chelate), Biotin, Vitamin D-3, Vitamin B-12.

How Supplied: One bottle contains 60 easy-to-swallow capsules.

STEPHAN™ Lovpil
Nutritional Supplement

Uses: STEPHAN™ Lovpil is a nutritional food supplement for men and women of all ages that is formulated with vitamins, minerals, herbs, amino acids, and selected proteins recognized as important for general health and sexual vitality.
Damiana, typically thought of as an aphrodisiac by those who are familiar with its effects, is an important ingredient utilized in STEPHAN Lovpil. A major herbal remedy in Mexican medical folklore, damiana is often used for the treatment of both impotency and sterility. However, its proven stimulating properties of male virility and libido make it an ideal addition to STEPHAN Lovpil's formulation.
A number of scientific studies have shown a direct relationship between low sperm count and diets deficient in arginine. Well established as being significant to normal sperm production, arginine is, therefore, an important contributor to STEPHAN Lovpil.
A third imperative ingredient is vitamin C. Scientific studies have uncovered that ascorbic acid may actually protect human sperm from oxidative DNA damage, which could in turn help prevent birth defects.

Directions: Take one capsule per day.

Warnings: Phenylketonurics: Contains Phenylalanine.

Ingredients: Calcium Carbonate, Vitamin C, Damiana Powder, Ribonucleic Acid, Soya Isolate (Isoleucine, Phenylalanine, Leucine, Threonine, Lysine, Methionine, Valine, Alanine, Glycine, Histidine, Arginine, Proline, Aspartic Acid, Serine, Cysteine, Tyrosine, Glutamic Acid), Zinc (Amino Acid Chelate), Manganese (Amino Acid Chelate), Adenosine Triphosphate, Vitamin A (Acetate), Folic Acid, Vitamin D (Cholecalciferol), Selenium (Methionine), Vitamin B12.

How Supplied: One bottle contains 60 easy-to-swallow capsules.

STEPHAN™ Masculine
Nutritional Supplement

Uses: A nutritional food supplement formulated for the adult male, STEPHAN™ Masculine contains a special blend of nutrients with vitamins, minerals, herbs, and amino acids.
Scientifically researched ingredients have been carefully selected to help ensure STEPHAN™ Masculine's effectiveness. Zinc is one such ingredient. Proven to be closely interrelated with the male sex hormone, testosterone, zinc deficiency often results in regression of the male sex glands, decreased sexual interest, mental lethargy, emotional problems and even poor appetite. It has been found that in males with only a mild zinc deficiency, zinc supplementation was accompanied by increased sperm count and plasma testosterone.
Selenium proves an important proponent of STEPHAN™ Masculine as well. Men in particular need this special mineral due to the fact that almost half of their body's supply is concentrated in the testicles and portions of the seminal ducts. Selenium is an antioxidant that helps protect cells from the kind of damage that could initiate the growth of cancerous tumors.

Directions: Take one to two capsules per day.

Ingredients: L-Histidine, Calcium (Carbonate), Bee Pollen, Parsley, Ribonucleic Acid, Zinc (Amino Acid Chelate), Magnesium (Amino Acid Chelate), Adenosine Triphosphate.

How Supplied: One bottle contains 60 easy-to-swallow capsules.

PHYTO-VITE™
Advanced Antioxidant, Vitamin, and Chelated Mineral Formulation

Uses: Phyto-Vite™ is a state-of-the-art nutritional supplement providing chelated minerals, vitamins, and a diverse group of antioxidants. It was formulated to meet the nutritional needs of our society where studies estimate only 9% consume foods in the quantities necessary to protect against the oxidative damage caused by free radicals.
The antioxidant coverage provided by Phyto-Vite is both comprehensive and diverse. First, it includes optimal amounts of vitamins A, C, and E as well as the pro-vitamins alpha and beta carotene. Vitamin A, in addition to its antioxidant capabilities, is also felt to improve immune function, protein synthesis, RNA synthesis, and steroid hormone synthesis. In this product, vitamin A is derived from two sources: retinyl palmitate and lemongrass. Additional vitamin A activity is provided by the alpha and beta carotene found in *Dunaliella salina.* These carotenoids are strong antioxidants in their own right; however, they can also be converted to vitamin A. This occurs only when the body is deficient in this vitamin. Consequently, vitamin A toxicity cannot be caused by alpha or beta carotene. Vitamin C has long been associated with wound healing, collagen formation, and maintaining the structural integrity of capillaries, cartilage, dentine, and bone. Its antioxidant effects are felt to play a major role in the prevention of cardiovascular disease and some cancers. Phyto-Vite utilizes esterified vitamin C which has been shown to provide a quicker uptake and a decreased rate of excretion when compared with conventional vitamin C. This allows for higher, more sustained levels of this vitamin in the body. Phyto-Vite also contains 400 I.U. of vitamin E, from natural sources. The antioxidant effects of vitamin E have been shown to stabilize cell membranes, increase HDL cholesterol, and decrease platelet aggregation.
Many flavonoids are incorporated into Phyto-Vite. These substances possess antioxidant activity themselves and also potentiate the effects of vitamins C and E. This later effect is produced by decreasing the degradation of vitamin C and E into inactive metabolites. Ginkgo biloba has flavonoid activity as well as other significant effects. Among these are a decrease in platelet aggregation and an increase in vasodilation which appears to increase blood flow to the peripheral arteries and the brain. Some improvement in cognitive abilities has been noted. It also helps to inhibit lipid peroxidation, thereby stabilizing the cell wall against free radical attack.
A phytonutrient blend has been incorporated into Phyto-Vite to further enhance its antioxidant effects. Phytonutrient is a term given to the thousands of chemical compounds found in fruits and vegetables. Some of these compounds, including sulforaphane in broccoli and isothiocyanate in cabbage, have been shown to inhibit cancer in laboratory animals and human cell cultures. Others have shown great promise in aiding the cardiovascular system. Currently, much research is ongoing to isolate and identify more of these compounds, but it has already been clearly established that phytonutrients work best when the entire plant source is used rather than just the isolated compound. The phytonutrients found in Phyto-Vite are obtained from alfalfa (lutein), broccoli (indoles), cabbage (isothiocyanates), cayenne (capsanthin and capsorubin), green onion (thioallyl compounds), parsley (chlorophyll), spirulina (gamma linolenic acid), tomato (lycopene), soy isoflavones (genistein, lecithin, and daidzein), aged garlic concentrate, and Pure-Gar-A-8000™ (allicin).
The antioxidant minerals copper, zinc, manganese, and selenium have also been incorporated into Phyto-Vite. These minerals have been chelated via a patented process in which the mineral is wrapped within an amino acid. Once inside the body, the minerals can then be utilized in the millions of metabolic reactions that take place in the body. With this process, overall mineral absorption can approach 95% instead of the 5 to 10% absorption seen with other mineral supplements.
Phyto-Vite also provides two antioxidant enzymes (catalase and peroxidase). These help to reduce the body's free radical burden by neutralizing free radicals in the pharynx or stomach.
There are three other features that make Phyto-Vite unique among supplements. First, a small amount of canola oil was included to aid in the proper absorption of fat soluble vitamins, even on an empty

Continued on next page

Wellness International—Cont.

stomach. Canola oil also provides essential fatty acids. Second, the product is formed into prolonged-release tablets which allow flexibility in dosing frequency. It can be taken all at once or staggered throughout the day. Dissolution testing has been performed to insure that the product will dissolve properly. Lastly, Phyto-Vite tablets are covered with a Betacoat™. This is a beta carotene coating that is designed to provide antioxidant coverage to the tablet itself. This helps to protect the integrity and activity of the product.

Directions: As a dietary supplement take six tablets per day with eight ounces of liquid. Tablets may be taken all at once or staggered throughout the day.

Warnings: If pregnant or lactating, consult physician before using.

Ingredients: Vitamin A (5,000 IU), Alpha and Beta Carotene (20,000 IU), Vitamin C (500 mg), Vitamin E (400 IU), Citrus Bioflavonoids with Hesperidin (50 mg), Rutin and Quercetin (50 mg), Bilberry Standardized Extract (10 mg), Grape Seed Proanthocyanidins (5 mg), Red Grape Polyphenols (5 mg), Ginkgo Biloba Standardized Extract (20 mg), Copper (2 mg), Zinc (15 mg), Manganese (5 mg), Selenium (200 mcg), Catalase and Peroxidase Enzymes (3,500 units), Phytonutrient Blend (800 mg), Vitamin B-1 (15 mg), Vitamin B-2 (17 mg), Vitamin B-3 (100 mg), Vitamin B-5 (75 mg), Vitamin B-6 (20 mg), Vitamin B-12 (60 mcg), Biotin (300 mcg), Folic Acid (400 mcg), Choline (50 mg), Inositol (50 mg), PABA (25 mg), Vitamin D-3 (400 IU), Vitamin K (70 mcg), Boron (1 mg), Calcium (500 mg), Magnesium (400 mg), Phosphorus (250 mg), Chromium (200 mcg), Iodine (150 mcg), Iron (4 mg), Potassium (70 mg), Essential Fatty Acids (100 mg).

How Supplied: One bottle contains 180 Betacoat™ tablets.

STEPHAN™ Protector
Nutritional Supplement

Uses: STEPHAN™ Protector is a nutritional food supplement that combines specific proteins, vitamins, minerals, and amino acids recognized as important for the health of areas associated with the human immune system.

Among these specially selected and scientifically researched ingredients are astragalus, kelp and arginine. Known for its strengthening effects of both the immune and digestive systems, astragalus can be combined with other herbs to increase phagocytosis, interferon production and the number of macrophages. It, in combination, enhances T-cell transformation and functions as an adaptogen to relieve stress-induced immune system suppression.

Research clearly indicates that kelp supplies dozens of important nutrients for improved cardiovascular health and is used to balance the thyroid gland. Arginine stimulates the thymus gland and promotes production of lymphocytes, crucial for immunity, in that gland. The arginine lymphocytes are not only produced in better quantity, but they have also proven more active and effective in fighting illness.

STEPHAN Protector may be used by men and women of all ages.

Directions: Take one capsule per day.

Warnings: Phenylketonurics: Contains Phenylalanine.

Ingredients: Bee Pollen, Astragalus, Kelp, Glutamic Acid, Ribonucleic Acid, Aspartic Acid, Leucine, Arginine, Lysine, Phenylalanine, Serine, Proline, Valine, Isoleucine, Alanine, Glycine, Threonine, Tyrosine, Histidine, Methionine, Cysteine, Adenosine Triphosphate.

How Supplied: One bottle contains 60 easy-to-swallow capsules.

STEPHAN™ Relief
Nutritional Supplement

Uses: Designed for both men and women, STEPHAN™ Relief has been formulated with a special combination of nutrients, vitamins, minerals, amino acids, and herbs which are recognized as important to the digestive and excretory systems.

Parsley, one of the ingredients found in STEPHAN™ Relief and a member of the carrot family, can be used as a carminative and an aid to digestion. While the root has a mild diuretic property, parsley has also been reported, in large doses, to lower blood pressure.

A second important ingredient in STEPHAN™ Relief is psyllium. This gel-forming fiber is used in many bulk laxatives to promote bowel regularity. In recent years, because of its ability to lower cholesterol, psyllium has gained widespread popularity and can be found in some ready-to-eat cereals.

Directions: Take one to two capsules per day.

Ingredients: Fucus, Parsley (extract 4:1), Psyllium, Leucine, Isoleucine, Valine, Bee Pollen, Ribonucleic Acid, Calcium Pantothenate, Adenosine Triphosphate.

How Supplied: One bottle contains 60 easy-to-swallow capsules.

Sleep-Tite™
Herbal Sleep Aid

Uses: Sleep-Tite™ is a non-addicting herbal sleep aid formulated to promote a deeper, more restorative sleep without the use of pharmaceutically synthesized hormones. With the body's overall health, and proper functioning, dependent upon efficient sleep patterns in order to achieve cellular, organ, tissue, and emotional repair, this powerful tool's primary function is to rejuvenate and restore by assisting the body in initiating and maintaining sleep.

Sleep-Tite is a blend of 10 highly effective, all-natural herbs. California poppy, passion flower, valerian, kava kava, and skullcap have been used for centuries as a remedy for insomnia because of their calming effects and ability to relieve muscle tension. Hops and celery seed produce a generalized calming effect and are especially helpful for indigestion, gastrointestinal, and smooth muscle relaxation. Chamomile also has a relaxing effect on the body and the gastrointestinal tract, but with the added benefit of producing anti-inflammatory effects on joints. Feverfew has been used as a treatment for fever, migraines, and arthritic complaints dating back to ancient Greece. Recently, a study published in ***Lancet*** demonstrated that feverfew inhibited the body's production of prostaglandin and serotonin. These biochemicals can cause inflammation, fever, and the vasoactive response that triggers migraine headaches.

By utilizing this unique blend of herbs to aid in the effective initiation and maintenance of sleep patterns, Sleep-Tite can be consumed by adults, thereby promoting physical and emotional well-being in a safe, active manner.

Directions: Adults (18 years and older) may take two Sleep-Tite caplets approximately 30 to 60 minutes prior to bedtime. Needs may vary with each individual. Some persons may require less than two caplets to achieve optimum results. Do not exceed recommended nightly amounts.

Warnings: Not for use by children, pregnant women, or lactating women. Consult your physician before using this product if you have any medical condition or are taking antidepressant, sedative, or hypnotic medications. Do not take this product if using Monoamine Oxidase (M.A.O.) Inhibitors. This product may cause drowsiness and should not be taken with alcohol or while operating a vehicle or other machinery. If allergic symptoms develop, discontinue use. Store in a cool, dry place. Keep out of reach of children.

Ingredients: European Valerian Rhizome and Root 4:1 Extract (*Valerian officinalis*), Fijian Kava Kava Root 5:1 Extract (*Piper methysticum*), American Hops Strobiles 4:1 Extract (*Humulus lupulus*), Central American Passion Flower Herb 4:1 Extract (*Passiflora incarnata*), Argentine Chamomile Flower 5:1 Extract (*Matricaria chamomilla*), California Poppy Herb 5:1 Extract (*Eschscholzia californica*), Chinese Fu Ling Sclerotium 5:1 Extract (*Poria cocos*), Israeli Feverfew Herb 5:1 Extract (*Tanacetum parthenium*), Celery Seed 4:1 Extract (*Apium graveolens*), American Skullcap Herb (*Scutellaria lateriflora*).

How Supplied: One box contains 28 packets. Two caplets per packet.

STEPHAN™ Tranquility
Nutritional Supplement

Uses: Designed for both men and women, STEPHAN™ Tranquility is a nutritional food supplement which contains a blend of vitamins, minerals, and amino acids recognized as important to areas involved in stress management.
Myo-Inositol is among these specially researched ingredients. It has long been claimed to lower blood concentrations of triglycerides and cholesterol, as well as to generally protect against cardiovascular disease. In addition, Myo-Inositol intake can influence the phosphatidylinositol levels in the membranes of brain cells. Compounds derived from this process could conceivably have some beneficial effect on insomnia and anxiety proving a safer alternative than most to treat these common problems.
Another key ingredient used in STEPHAN Tranquility is valerian root, a folk remedy used throughout the years for several disorders including insomnia, hysteria, palpitations, nervousness and menstrual problems. Valerian root contains valepotriates which are said to be the source of its sedative effects. Studies reveal that valeranon, an essential oil component of this herb, produces a pronounced smooth-muscle effect on the intestine.

Directions: Take one to two capsules per day.

Warnings: Phenylketonurics: Contains Phenylalanine.

Ingredients: Lecithin, Choline Bitartrate, Myo-Inositol, Vitamin C, Valerian (As 4:1 extract), Ribonucleic Acid, Vitamin E, Vitamin B-3, Glutamic Acid, Aspartic Acid, Calcium (Amino Acid Chelate), Leucine, Arginine, Lysine, Phenylalanine, Serine, Valine, Proline, Isoleucine, Alanine, Glycine, Threonine, Tyrosine, Vitamin B-5, Vitamin B-1, Histidine, Magnesium, Methionine, Cysteine, Adenosine Triphosphate, Vitamin B-6, Vitamin B-2, Vitamin A, Folic Acid, Biotin (Amino Acid Chelate), Vitamin D-3, Vitamin B-12.

How Supplied: One bottle contains 60 easy-to-swallow capsules.

Winrgy™
Nutritional Drink with Vitamin C

Uses: A delicious, vitamin C-enriched beverage, Winrgy™ is formulated with a special blend of nutrients designed to offer a nutritional alternative to coffees and colas.

Directions: Add 6 ounces of chilled water or fruit juice to one packet of mix. Stir briskly. Consume 1–2 times per day. Keep in a cool, dry place. For maximum results, combine this product with one serving size of Food For Thought.™

Warnings: Phenylketonurics: Contains Phenylalanine. Not for use by children, pregnant or lactating women. Persons taking medications should seek medical advice before taking this product. Do not consume more than four servings per day. Avoid the use of antacids containing aluminum with this product.

Ingredients: Fructose, L-Phenylalanine, Natural Flavors, Citric Acid, Taurine, Glycine, Ascorbic Acid, Caffeine, Niacinamide, Vitamin E Acetate, Calcium Pantothenate, Silicon Dioxide, Potassium Aspartate, Manganese Aspartate, Chromium Aspartate, Pyridoxine Hydrochloride, Zinc Gluconate, Riboflavin, Thiamin Mononitrate, Copper Gluconate, Folic Acid, Vitamin B12.

How Supplied: One box contains 28 packets. Serving size equals one packet.

Whitehall-Robins Healthcare
American Home Products Corporation
FIVE GIRALDA FARMS
MADISON, NJ 07940

Direct Inquiries to:
Whitehall Consumer Product Information 800-322-3129
Robins Consumer Product Information 800-762-4672

ADVIL®
[ad 'vĭl]
Ibuprofen Tablets, USP
Ibuprofen Caplets
(Oval-Shaped Tablets)
Ibuprofen Gel Caplets
(Oval-Shaped Gelatin Coated Tablets)

WARNING: ASPIRIN-SENSITIVE PATIENTS. Do not take this product if you have had a severe allergic reaction to aspirin, e.g.—asthma, swelling, shock or hives, because even though this product contains no aspirin or salicylates, cross-reactions may occur in patients allergic to aspirin.

Active Ingredient: Each tablet or caplet contains Ibuprofen 200 mg.

Inactive Ingredients: Tablets and Caplets Acetylated Monoglyceride, Beeswax and/or Carnauba Wax, Croscarmellose Sodium, Iron Oxides, Lecithin, Methylparaben, Microcrystalline Cellulose, Pharmaceutical Glaze, Povidone, Propylparaben, Silicon Dioxide, Simethicone, Sodium Benzoate, Sodium Lauryl Sulfate, Starch, Stearic Acid, Sucrose, Titanium Dioxide. Gel Caplets Croscarmellose Sodium, FD&C Red 40, FD&C Yellow 6, Gelatin, Glycerin, Hydroxypropyl Methylcellulose, Iron Oxides, Lecithin, Pharmaceutical Glaze, Propyl Gallate, Silicon Dioxide, Simethicone, Sodium Lauryl Sulfate, Starch, Stearic Acid, Titanium Dioxide, Triacetin.

Indications: For the temporary relief of minor aches and pains associated with the common cold, headache, toothache, muscular aches, backache, for the minor pain of arthritis, for the pain of menstrual cramps and for reduction of fever.

Dosage and Administration: Adults: Take one tablet or caplet every 4 to 6 hours while symptoms persist. If pain or fever does not respond to one tablet or caplet, two tablets or caplets may be used but do not exceed six tablets or caplets in 24 hours unless directed by a doctor. The smallest effective dose should be used. Take with food or milk if occasional and mild heartburn, upset stomach, or stomach pain occurs with use. Consult a doctor if these symptoms are more than mild or if they persist. Children: Do not give this product to children under 12 years of age except under the advice and supervision of a doctor.

Warnings: Do not take for pain for more than 10 days or for fever for more than 3 days unless directed by a doctor. If pain or fever persists or gets worse, if new symptoms occur, or if the painful area is red or swollen, consult a doctor. These could be signs of serious illness. If you are under a doctor's care for any serious condition, consult a doctor before taking this product. As with aspirin and acetaminophen, if you have any condition which requires you to take prescription drugs or if you have had any problems or serious side effects from taking any nonprescription pain reliever, do not take this product without first discussing it with your doctor. **IF YOU EXPERIENCE ANY SYMPTOMS WHICH ARE UNUSUAL OR SEEM UNRELATED TO THE CONDITION FOR WHICH YOU TOOK IBUPROFEN, CONSULT A DOCTOR BEFORE TAKING ANY MORE OF IT.** Although ibuprofen is indicated for the same conditions as aspirin and acetaminophen, it should not be taken with them except under a doctor's direction. Do not combine this product with any other ibuprofen-containing product. As with any drug, if you are pregnant or nursing a baby, seek the advice of a health professional before using this product. **IT IS ESPECIALLY IMPORTANT NOT TO USE IBUPROFEN DURING THE LAST 3 MONTHS OF PREGNANCY UNLESS SPECIFICALLY DIRECTED TO DO SO BY A DOCTOR BECAUSE IT MAY CAUSE PROBLEMS IN THE UNBORN CHILD OR COMPLICATIONS DURING DELIVERY.** Keep this and all drugs out of the reach of children. In case of accidental overdose, seek professional assistance or contact a poison control center immediately.

How Supplied: Coated tablets in bottles of 4, 8, 24, 50 (non-child resistant size), 72 (E-Z Cap) 100, 165 and 250. Coated caplets in bottles of 24, 50 (non-child resistant size), 72 (E-Z Cap) 100, 165, and 250. Coated tablets in thermoform packaging of 8.
Gel caplets in bottles of 4, 8, 24, 50, 100, 165 and 250.

Continued on next page

Whitehall-Robins—Cont.

Storage: Store at room temperature; avoid excessive heat (40°C, 104°F).

ADVIL® Cold and Sinus
Ibuprofen/Pseudoephedrine HCl
Caplets* and Tablets
Pain Reliever/Fever Reducer/Nasal Decongestant

***Oval-Shaped tablets**

WARNING: **ASPIRIN-SENSITIVE PATIENTS. Do not take this product if you have had a severe allergic reaction to aspirin, eg, asthma, swelling, shock or hives, because even though this product contains no aspirin or salicylates, cross-reactions may occur in patients allergic to aspirin.**

Indications: For temporary relief of symptoms associated with the common cold, sinusitis or flu, including nasal congestion, headache, fever, body aches, and pains.

Directions: *Adults:* Take 1 caplet or tablet every 4 to 6 hours while symptoms persist. If symptoms do not respond to 1 caplet or tablet, 2 caplets or tablets may be used, but do not exceed 6 caplets or tablets in 24 hours unless directed by a doctor. The smallest effective dose should be used. Take with food or milk if occasional and mild heartburn, upset stomach, or stomach pain occurs with use. Consult a doctor if these symptoms are more than mild or if they persist. *Children:* Do not give this product to children under 12 years of age except under the advice and supervision of a doctor.

Warnings: Do not take for colds for more than 7 days or for fever for more than 3 days unless directed by a doctor. If the cold or fever persists or gets worse, or if new symptoms occur, consult a doctor. These could be signs of serious illness. As with aspirin and acetaminophen, if you have any condition which requires you to take prescription drugs or if you have had any problems or serious side effects from taking any nonprescription pain reliever, do not take this product without first discussing it with your doctor. IF YOU EXPERIENCE ANY SYMPTOMS WHICH ARE UNUSUAL OR SEEM UNRELATED TO THE CONDITION FOR WHICH YOU TOOK THIS PRODUCT, CONSULT A DOCTOR BEFORE TAKING ANY MORE OF IT. If you are under a doctor's care for any serious condition, consult a doctor before taking this product.

Do not exceed recommended dosage. If nervousness, dizziness, or sleeplessness occur, discontinue use and consult a doctor. Do not take this product if you have high blood pressure, heart disease, diabetes, thyroid disease or difficulty in urination due to enlargement of the prostate gland, except under the advice and supervision of a doctor.

Drug Interaction Precaution: Do not use if you are now taking a prescription monoamine oxidase inhibitor (MAOI) (certain drugs for depression, psychiatric or emotional conditions, or Parkinson's disease), or for 2 weeks after stopping the MAOI drug. If you are uncertain whether your prescription drug contains an MAOI, consult a health professional before taking this product. Do not combine this product with other non-prescription pain relievers. Do not combine this product with any other ibuprofen-containing product. As with any drug, if you are pregnant or nursing a baby, seek the advice of a health professional before using this product.

IT IS ESPECIALLY IMPORTANT NOT TO USE THIS PRODUCT DURING THE LAST 3 MONTHS OF PREGNANCY UNLESS SPECIFICALLY DIRECTED TO DO SO BY A DOCTOR BECAUSE IT MAY CAUSE PROBLEMS IN THE UNBORN CHILD OR COMPLICATIONS DURING DELIVERY. Keep this and all drugs out of the reach of children. In case of accidental overdose, seek professional assistance or contact a poison control center immediately.

Active Ingredients: Each caplet or tablet contains Ibuprofen 200 mg and Pseudoephedrine HCl 30 mg.

Inactive Ingredients: Carnauba or Equivalent Wax, Croscarmellose Sodium, Iron Oxides, Methylparaben, Microcrystalline Cellulose, Propylparaben, Silicon Dioxide, Sodium Benzoate, Sodium Lauryl Sulfate, Starch, Stearic Acid, Sucrose, Titanium Dioxide.

How Supplied: Advil® Cold and Sinus is an oval-shaped tan-colored caplet or tan-colored tablet supplied in consumer bottles of 40 and blister packs of 20. Medical samples are available in a 2's pouch dispenser.

Storage: Store at room temperature; avoid excessive heat (40°C, 104°F).

CHILDREN'S ADVIL®
[ad' vil]
Ibuprofen

Description: Children's Advil® Ibuprofen Oral Suspension is an alcohol-free, fruit-flavored liquid specially developed for children. Each 5 mL (teaspoon) contains ibuprofen 100 mg.

Inactive Ingredients: Artificial flavors, Carboxymethylcellulose Sodium, Citric Acid, Edetate Disodium, FD&C Red No. 40, Glycerin, Microcrystalline Cellulose, Polysorbate 80, Purified Water, Sodium Benzoate, Sorbitol Solution, Sucrose, Xanthan Gum.

Indications: Children's Advil® Ibuprofen Oral Suspension is indicated for the temporary relief of fever, and minor aches and pains due to colds, flu, sore throat, headaches and toothaches. One dose lasts 6–8 hours.

WARNINGS:
ASPIRIN SENSITIVE CHILDREN
- **This product contains no aspirin, but may cause a severe reaction in people allergic to aspirin**
- **Do not use this product if your child has had an allergic reaction to aspirin such as asthma, swelling, shock or hives.**

CALL YOUR DOCTOR IF:
- Your child is under a doctor's care for any serious condition or is taking any other drug.
- Your child has problems or serious side effects from using fever reducers or pain relievers.
- Your child does not get any relief within one day (24 hours) of treatment or if pain or fever gets worse.
- Redness or swelling is present in the painful area.
- Sore throat is severe, lasts for more than two days or occurs with fever, headache, rash, nausea or vomiting.
- Any new symptoms appear.

DO NOT USE:
- With any other product that contains ibuprofen, or any other pain reliever/fever reducer, unless directed by a doctor.
- For more than 3 days for fever or pain unless directed by a doctor.
- For stomach pain unless directed by a doctor.
- If your child is dehydrated (significant fluid loss) due to continued vomiting, diarrhea or lack of fluid intake.
- If imprinted plastic carton or bottle wrap is broken or missing.

IMPORTANT:
- Keep this and all drugs out of the reach of children. In case of accidental overdose, seek professional assistance or contact a poison control center immediately.
- If stomach upset occurs while taking this product, give with food or milk. If stomach upset gets worse or lasts, call your doctor.

Directions: Shake well before using. Find right dose on chart. If possible, use weight to dose; otherwise, use age. Measure dose with calibrated cup provided. Repeat dose every 6–8 hours, if needed. Do not use more than 4 times a day.

DOSING CHART

WEIGHT (lb.)	AGE (yr.)	DOSE (tsp.)
Under 24	Under 2	Consult a Doctor
24–35	2–3	1 tsp.
36–47	4–5	1½ tsp.
48–59	6–8	2 tsp.
60–71	9–10	2½ tsp.
72–95	11	3 tsp.

Store at controlled room temperature 15°–30°C (59°–86°F).

How Supplied: bottles of 2 fl. oz. and 4 fl. oz.
Revised: 6/25/96

AXID® AR
[ak' sid]
Nizatidine

Active Ingredient: Nizatidine 75 mg per tablet.

Inactive Ingredients: Colloidal Silicon Dioxide, Hydroxypropylmethylcellulose, Synthetic Iron Oxides, Magnesium Stearate, Microcrystalline Cellulose, Polyethylene Glycol, Pregelatinized Starch, Propylene Glycol, Corn Starch, Titanium Dioxide.

Product Benefits: Taken one-half to one hour before eating, one tablet of AXID® AR prevents heartburn, acid indigestion, and sour stomach caused by food and beverages. Unlike antacids which neutralize acid after symptoms have occurred, AXID AR reduces the production of acid in the stomach so you can prevent symptoms.

Action: The stomach normally produces acid following eating and drinking. Sometimes, acid backing up into the esophagus can cause heartburn which can interfere with everyday activities.

In clinical studies AXID AR was significantly better than placebo in preventing heartburn.
[See figure above.]

Use: For prevention of heartburn, acid indigestion and sour stomach brought on by consuming food and beverages.

How to help avoid symptoms:
- Avoid lying down soon after eating.
- Avoid or limit foods such as caffeine, chocolate, fried foods, and alcohol.
- Avoid eating right before bedtime.
- If you are overweight, lose weight.
- If you smoke, stop or cut down.

Warnings: While the symptoms of heartburn are common, you should see your doctor promptly if:
- You have trouble swallowing or persistent abdominal pain. You may have a serious condition that may need different treatment.
- You have taken the maximum dosage (2 tablets per 24 hours) for 2 weeks continuously.

Important:
- As with any drug, if you are pregnant or nursing a baby, seek the advice of a health professional before using this product.
- This product should not be given to children under 12 years old unless directed by a doctor.
- Keep this and all drugs out of the reach of children.
- In case of accidental overdose, seek professional assistance or contact a poison control center immediately.

Directions: To prevent heartburn, swallow one tablet with water one-half to one hour before consuming food and beverages that you expect to cause symptoms. AXID AR can be used up to twice daily (up to 2 tablets in 24 hours); the maximum daily dosage.

Benefit of AXID AR Compared to Placebo

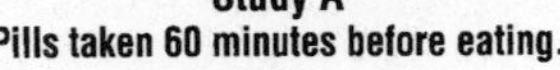

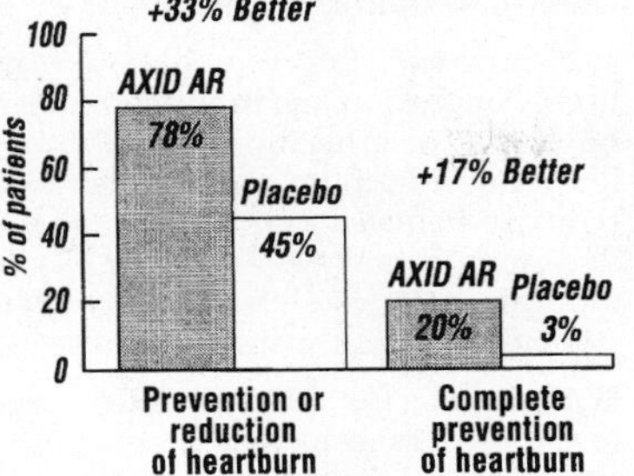

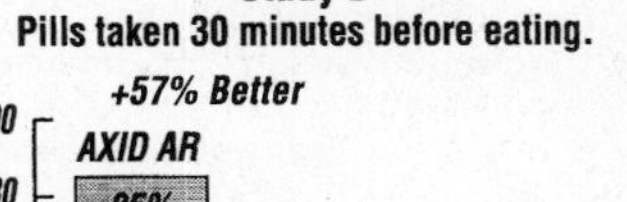

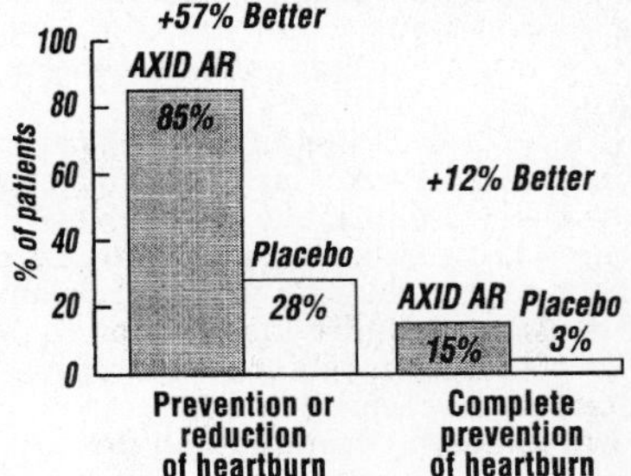

How Supplied: AXID AR Acid Reducer is available in boxes of 6 individual packets and bottles of 12, 18, and 30 tablets.
Store at 20°–25° C (68°–77°F). Protect from light. Replace cap tightly after opening bottle. The bottle is sealed with printed foil under cap. Do not use if foil is torn.

DIMETAPP Allergy Dye-Free Elixir
[dī'mĕ-tap]

Description: (Brompheniramine Maleate) Antihistamine Dye-Free Elixir

Active Ingredients: Each 5 mL (1 teaspoonful) contains: Brompheniramine Maleate, USP 2 mg.

Inactive Ingredients: Citric Acid, Flavors, Glycerin, Sodium Benzoate, Sorbitol, Water.

Indications: For temporary relief of runny nose, sneezing, itching of the nose or throat, and itchy, watery eyes due to hay fever or other upper respiratory allergies.

Warnings: Do not take this product, unless directed by a physician, if you have a breathing problem such as emphysema or chronic bronchitis, or if you have glaucoma or difficulty in urination due to enlargement of the prostate gland. May cause drowsiness; alcohol, sedatives and tranquilizers may increase the drowsiness effect. Avoid alcoholic beverages while taking this product. Do not take this product if you are taking sedatives or tranquilizers without first consulting your physician. Use caution when driving a motor vehicle or operating machinery. May cause excitability, especially in children.
As with any drug, if you are pregnant or nursing a baby, seek the advice of a health professional before using this product.
KEEP THIS AND ALL DRUGS OUT OF THE REACH OF CHILDREN. IN CASE OF ACCIDENTAL OVERDOSE, SEEK PROFESSIONAL ASSISTANCE OR CONTACT A POISON CONTROL CENTER IMMEDIATELY.

Directions: Adults and children 12 years of age and over: 2 teaspoonfuls every four to six hours, not to exceed 12 teaspoonfuls in 24 hours, or as directed by a physician; children 6 to under 12 years: 1 teaspoonful every four to six hours, not to exceed 6 teaspoonfuls in 24 hours, or as directed by a physician; children under 6 years: Consult a physician.
Store at Controlled Room Temperature, between 20°C and 25°C (68°F and 77°F). Not a USP Elixir.

How Supplied: 4 oz bottle. Dose cup provided.

DIMETAPP® Allergy Sinus
(Previously Cold & Flu)

Description: Nasal Decongestant, Antihistamine, Pain Reliever-Fever Reducer.

Active Ingredients: Each caplet contains Acetaminophen, USP 500 mg, Phenylpropanolamine Hydrochloride, USP 12.5 mg and Brompheniramine Maleate, USP 2 mg.

Inactive Ingredients: Corn Starch, Hydroxypropyl Cellulose, Hydroxypropyl Methylcellulose, Magnesium Stearate, Methylparaben, Microcrystalline Cellulose, Polysorbate 20, Povidone, Propylparaben, Propylene Glycol, Stearic Acid, Titanium Dioxide.

Indications: For the temporary relief of minor aches, pains, and headache; for the reduction of fever; for the relief of nasal congestion due to the common cold or associated with sinusitis; and for the relief of runny nose, sneezing, itching of the nose or throat and itchy and watery eyes due to hay fever (allergic rhinitis). Temporarily restores freer breathing through the nose.

Warnings: Do not take this product if you have a breathing problem such as emphysema or chronic bronchitis or if you have heart disease, high blood pressure, thyroid disease, diabetes, glaucoma, or difficulty in urination due to enlargement of the prostate gland, unless directed by a physican.

Alcohol Warning: Avoid alcoholic beverages while taking this product. If you generally consume 3 or more alcohol-

Continued on next page

Whitehall-Robins—Cont.

containing drinks per day, you should consult your physician for advice on when and how you should take ths product or any other acetaminophen-containing product.
May cause drowsiness; alcohol, sedatives and tranquilizers may increase the drowsiness effect. Do not take this product if you are taking sedatives or tranquilizers without first consulting your physician. Use caution when driving a motor vehicle or operating machinery. May cause excitability, especially in children.
Do not exceed recommended dosage. If nervousness, dizziness or sleeplessness occur, discontinue use and consult a physician. Do not take this product for more than 7 days or for fever for more than 3 days. If pain or fever persists or gets worse, if new symptoms occur, or if redness or swelling is present, consult a physician because these could be signs of a serious condition.
As with any drug, if you are pregnant or nursing a baby, seek the advice of a health professional before using this product.

Drug Interaction Precaution: Do not use this product if you are now taking a prescription monoamine oxidase inhibitor (MAOI) (certain drugs for depression, psychiatric or emotional conditions, or Parkinson's disease), or for 2 weeks after stopping the MAOI drug. If you are uncertain whether your prescription drug contains an MAOI, consult a health professional before taking this product.
KEEP THIS AND ALL DRUGS OUT OF THE REACH OF CHILDREN. IN CASE OF ACCIDENTAL OVERDOSE, SEEK PROFESSIONAL ASSISTANCE OR CONTACT A POISON CONTROL CENTER IMMEDIATELY. PROMPT MEDICAL ATTENTION IS CRITICAL FOR ADULTS AS WELL AS FOR CHILDREN EVEN IF YOU DO NOT NOTICE ANY SIGNS OR SYMPTOMS.

Directions: Adults (12 years and over): Two caplets every 6 hours. DO NOT EXCEED 8 CAPLETS IN A 24-HOUR PERIOD.
Children under 12: Consult a physican.
Store at Controlled Room Temperature, between 20°C and 25°C (68°F and 77°F).

How Supplied: Blister packs of 12 (NDC 0031-2284-46)
Bottles of 24

DIMETAPP® Cold & Allergy
[*di 'mĕ-tap*]
Chewable Tablets

Description: Each chewable tablet contains:
Brompheniramine Maleate, USP .... 1 mg
Phenylpropanolamine Hydrochloride, USP .... 6.25 mg

Inactive Ingredients: Aspartame, Citric Acid, Crospovidone, D&C Red 30 Lake, D&C Red 7 Lake, FD&C Blue 1 Lake, Flavor, Glycine, Magnesium Stearate, Mannitol, Microcrystalline Cellulose, Pregelatinized Starch, Silicon Dioxide, Sorbitol, Stearic Acid.

Indications: For temporary relief of nasal congestion due to the common cold, hay fever, or other upper respiratory allergies or associated with sinusitis. Temporarily relieves runny nose, sneezing, and itchy, watery eyes due to hay fever (allergic rhinitis). Temporarily restores freer breathing through the nose.

Warnings: Do not to give this product to children who have a breathing problem such as chronic bronchitis, or who have glaucoma, high blood pressure, heart disease, diabetes, or thyroid disease, without first consulting the child's physician. This product may cause drowsiness: sedatives and tranquilizers may increase the drowsiness effect. Do not give this product to children who are taking sedatives or tranquilizers without first consulting the child's physician. May cause excitability, especially in children.
Do not exceed recommended dosage. If nervousness, dizziness, or sleeplessness occur, discontinue use and consult a doctor. If symptoms do not improve within 7 days, or are accompanied by a fever, consult a physician. As with any drug, if you are pregnant or nursing a baby, seek the advice of a health professional before using this product.

Drug Interaction Precaution: Do not give this product to a child who is taking a prescription monoamine oxidase inhibitor (MAOI) (certain drugs for depression, psychiatric or emotional conditions) or for 2 weeks after stopping the MAOI drug. If you are uncertain whether your child's prescription drug contains an MAOI, consult a health professional before taking this product.
KEEP THIS AND ALL DRUGS OUT OF THE REACH OF CHILDREN. IN CASE OF ACCIDENTAL OVERDOSE, SEEK PROFESSIONAL ASSISTANCE OR CONTACT A POISON CONTROL CENTER IMMEDIATELY.
Phenylketonurics: contains phenylalanine, 8 mg per tablet.

Directions: Children 6 to under 12 years of age: 2 chewable tablets every 4 hours. Children under 6: Consult a physician. DO NOT EXCEED 6 DOSES IN A 24-HOUR PERIOD.

Professional Labeling: The suggested dosage for children age 2 to under 6 years, only when the child is under the care of a physician, is 1 tablet every 4 hours, not to exceed 6 doses in a 24-hour period.

How Supplied: Purple tablet scored on one side and engraved with AHR 2290 on the other in bottles of 24 tablets.
Store at Controlled Room Temperature, Between 20°C and 25°C (68°F and 77°F).

DIMETAPP COLD & ALLERGY
[*dī' mĕ-tap*]
Phenylpropanolamine Hydrochloride and Brompheniramine Maleate

Description: Dimetapp® Cold & Allergy Quick Dissolve tablet is a grape-flavored instantly dissolving tablet that contains phenylpropanolamine hydrochloride, USP 6.25 mg and brompheniramine maleate, USP 1 mg.

Inactive Ingredients: Aspartame, FD&C Blue 2, FD&C Red 40, Flavors, Gelatin, Glycine, Mannitol.

Indications: Dimetapp Cold & Allergy is indicated for the temporary relief of nasal congestion due to the common cold, hay fever or other respiratory allergies or associated with sinusitis. It temporarily restores freer breathing through the nose. It temporarily relieves runny nose, sneezing and itchy, watery eyes due to hay fever (allergic rhinitis).

Warnings: Do not give this product to children who have a breathing problem such as chronic bronchitis, or who have glaucoma, heart disease, high blood pressure, thyroid disease or diabetes, unless directed by a physician. May cause drowsiness. Sedatives and tranquilizers may increase the drowsiness effect. Do not give this product to children who are taking sedatives or tranquilizers without first consulting the child's physician. May cause excitability, especially in children. Do not exceed the recommended dosage. If nervousness, dizziness or sleeplessness occur, discontinue use and consult a physician. If symptoms do not improve within 7 days, or are accompanied by fever, consult a physician. As with any drug, if you are pregnant or nursing a baby, seek the advice of a health professional before using this product. Keep this and all drugs out of the reach of children. In case of accidental overdose, seek professional assistance or contact a poison control center immediately.

DRUG INTERACTION PRECAUTION: Do not give this product to a child who is taking a prescription monoamine oxidase inhibitor (MAOI) (certain drugs for depression, psychiatric or emotional conditions) or for 2 weeks after stopping the MAOI drug. If you are uncertain whether your child's prescription drug contains an MAOI, consult a health professional before giving this product.
Phenylketonurics: This product contains phenylalanine 2.10 mg per tablet.

Directions: Children 6 to under 12 years of age: 2 tablets every 4 hours. Children under 6: consult a physician. Do not exceed 6 doses in a 24–hour period.
Store at controlled room temperature, between 20°C and 25°C (68°F and 77°F).

How Supplied: 10 instantly dissolving tablets
Revised: 2/16/96

DIMETAPP® Cold & Cough Liqui-Gels® Maximum Strength

[*dī'mĕ-tap*]

Description: Nasal Decongestant, Antihistamine, Cough Suppressant Liqui-Gels®

Active Ingredients: Each softgel contains: Brompheniramine Maleate, USP 4 mg, Phenylpropanolamine Hydrochloride, USP 25 mg, and Dextromethorphan Hydrobromide, USP 20 mg.

Inactive Ingredients: FD&C Red 40, Gelatin, Glycerin, Mannitol, Pharmaceutical Glaze, Polyethylene Glycol, Povidone, Propylene Glycol, Sorbitan, Sorbitol, Titanium Dioxide, Water.

Indications: Temporarily relieves cough due to minor throat and bronchial irritation as may occur with a cold. For temporary relief of nasal congestion due to the common cold, hay fever or other upper respiratory allergies or associated with sinusitis; temporarily relieves runny nose, sneezing, itching of the nose or throat, and itchy, watery eyes due to hay fever (allergic rhinitis). Temporarily restores freer breathing through the nose.

Warnings: Do not take this product unless directed by a doctor, if you have a breathing problem such as emphysema or chronic bronchitis, or persistent or chronic cough such as occurs with smoking or asthma, or if cough is accompanied by excessive phlegm (mucus). Likewise, if you have heart disease, high blood pressure, thyroid disease, diabetes, glaucoma or difficulty in urination due to enlargement of the prostrate gland, do not take this product unless directed by a physician. May cause drowsiness; alcohol, sedatives and tranquilizers may increase the drowsiness effect. Avoid alcoholic beverages while taking this product. Do not take this product if you are taking sedatives or tranquilizers without first consulting your physician. Use caution when driving a motor vehicle or operating machinery. May cause excitability, especially in children.

Do not exceed recommended dosage. If nervousness, dizziness or sleeplessness occur, discontinue use and consult a physican. A persistent cough may be a sign of a serious condition. If cough or other symptoms persist, do not improve within 7 days, tend to recur, or are accompanied by fever, rash, or persistent headache, consult a physician. As with any drug, if you are pregnant or nursing a baby, seek the advice of a health professional before using this product.

Drug Interaction Precaution: Do not use this product if you are now taking a prescription monoamine oxidase inhibitor (MAOI) (certain drugs for depression, psychiatric or emotional conditions or Parkinson's disease), or for 2 weeks after stopping the MAOI drug. If you are uncertain whether your prescription drug contains an MAOI, consult a health professional before taking this product.

KEEP THIS AND ALL DRUGS OUT OF THE REACH OF CHILDREN. IN CASE OF ACCIDENTAL OVERDOSE, SEEK PROFESSIONAL ASSISTANCE OR CONTACT A POISON CONTROL CENTER IMMEDIATELY.

Directions: Adults and children 12 years of age and over: one softgel every 4 hours. Children under 12: Consult a physician. DO NOT EXCEED 6 SOFTGELS IN A 24-HOUR PERIOD.

Store at Controlled Room Temperature, between 20°C and 25°C (68°F and 77°F). Not a USP Elixir.

How Supplied: Blister packs of 12's. Blister packs of 24's.

Liqui-Gels is a registered trademark of R.P. Scherer International Corporation

---

DIMETAPP Cold and Fever Suspension

[*dī'mĕ-tap*]

Description: Nasal Decongestant, Antihistamine, Pain reliever-Fever reducer Alcohol Free

Active Ingredients: Each 5 mL (1 teaspoonful) contains: Acetaminophen, USP, 160 mg; Pseudoephedrine Hydrochloride, USP, 15 mg; Brompheniramine Maleate, USP, 1 mg.

Inactive Ingredients: Carboxymethylcellulose Sodium, Citric Acid, D&C Red 33, Disodium Edetate, FD&C Blue 1, Flavors, Glycerin, High Fructose Corn Syrup, Maltol, Methylparaben, Microcrystalline Cellulose, Polysorbate 80, Potassium Sorbate, Propylene Glycol, Propylparaben, Sorbitol, Sucrose, Water, Xanthan Gum.

Indications: For temporary relief of nasal congestion, minor aches, pains, headache and sore throat and to reduce fever associated with a cold or sinusitis. Temporarily relieves runny nose and sneezing, itching of the nose or throat and itchy, watery eyes due to hay fever or other upper respiratory allergies.

Warnings: Do not give this product to children who have a breathing problem such as chronic bronchitis, or who have high blood pressure, heart disease, diabetes, thyroid disease, or glaucoma unless directed by a physician. May cause drowsiness; sedatives and tranquilizers may increase the drowsiness effect. Do not give this product to children who are taking sedatives or tranquilizers without first consulting the child's physician. May cause excitability, especially in children.

Do not exceed recommended dosage. If nervousness, dizziness or sleeplessness occur, discontinue use and consult a doctor. If symptoms do not improve within 7 days or are accompanied by a fever, consult a doctor. If sore throat is severe, persists for more than 2 days, is accompanied or followed by fever, headache, rash, nausea or vomiting, consult a physician promptly. Do not give this product for pain for more than 5 days or for fever for more than 3 days unless directed by a doctor. If pain or fever persists, or gets worse, if new symptoms occur or if redness or swelling is present, consult a physician because these could be signs of a serious condition.

Drug Interaction Precaution: Do not give this product to a child who is taking a prescription monoamine oxidase inhibitor (MAOI) (certain drugs for depression, psychiatric or emotional conditions, or Parkinson's disease), or for 2 weeks after stopping the MAOI drug. If you are uncertain whether your child's prescription drug contains an MAOI, consult a health professional before giving this product.

Directions: Shake Well Before Using. Children 6 to under 12: two teaspoonfuls every 4 hours (or as directed by a physician). Do Not Exceed 4 Doses in a 24-hour Period. Children under 6 years: consult a physician.

KEEP THIS AND ALL DRUGS OUT OF THE REACH OF CHILDREN. IN CASE OF ACCIDENTAL OVERDOSE, SEEK PROFESSIONAL ASSISTANCE OR CONTACT A POISON CONTROL CENTER IMMEDIATELY, PROMPT MEDICAL ATTENTION IS CRITICAL FOR ADULTS AS WELL AS CHILDREN EVEN IF YOU DO NOT NOTICE ANY SIGNS OR SYMPTOMS.

Storage: Store at Controlled Room Temperature, Between 20°C and 25°C (68°F and 77°F).

How Supplied: 4 oz bottle with dosage cup.

DIMETAPP® Decongestant Pediatric Drops

[*dī'mĕ-tap*]

Description: Nasal Decongestant (Pseudoephedrine Hydrochloride)

Active Ingredients: Each 0.8 mL (1 dropperful) contains: 7.5 mg Pseudoephedrine Hydrochloride, USP.

Inactive Ingredients: Caramel, Citric Acid, FD&C Blue 1, D&C Red 33, Flavors, Glycerin, High Fructose Corn Syrup, Maltol, Menthol, Polyethylene Glycol, Propylene Glycol, Sodium Benzoate, Sorbitol, Sucrose, Water.

Indications: For temporary relief of nasal congestion due to the common cold, hay fever, other upper respiratory allergies or associated with sinusitis.

Warnings: Do not exceed recommended dosage. If nervousness, dizziness, or sleeplessness occur, discontinue use and consult a physician. If symptoms do not improve within 7 days or are accompanied by a fever, consult a physician. Do not give this product to a child who has heart disease, high blood pressure, thyroid disease, or diabetes, unless directed by a physician.

Continued on next page

Whitehall-Robins—Cont.

Drug Interaction Precaution: Do not give this product to a child who is taking a prescription monoamine oxidase inhibitor (MAOI) (certain drugs for depression, psychiatric or emotional conditions), or for 2 weeks after stopping the MAOI drug. If you are uncertain whether your child's prescription drug contains an MAOI, consult a health professional before giving this product.
KEEP THIS AND ALL DRUGS OUT OF THE REACH OF CHILDREN. IN CASE OF ACCIDENTAL OVERDOSE, SEEK PROFESSIONAL ASSISTANCE OR CONTACT A POISON CONTROL CENTER IMMEDIATELY.

Directions: Children 2 to 3 years: Two dropperfuls (1.6 mL) every 4–6 hours (or as directed by a physician). Children under 2: Consult a physician. DO NOT EXCEED 4 DOSES IN A 24-HOUR PERIOD. Take by mouth only. Not for nasal use.
Store at Controlled Room Temperature, between 20°C and 25°C (68°F and 77°F).

How Supplied: ½ oz (15 mL) bottle with dropper.

DIMETAPP® Elixir
[*dī' mĕ-tap*]

Description: Each 5 mL (1 teaspoonful) contains:
Brompheniramine
Maleate, USP ....2 mg
Phenylpropanolamine
Hydrochloride, USP ....12.5 mg

Inactive Ingredients: Citric Acid, FD&C Blue 1, FD&C Red 40, Flavors, Glycerin, Saccharin Sodium, Sodium Benzoate, Sorbitol, Water.

Indications: For temporary relief of nasal congestion due to the common cold, hay fever or other upper respiratory allergies or associated with sinusitis. Temporarily relieves runny nose, sneezing, itching of the nose or throat, and itchy and watery eyes due to hay fever (allergic rhinitis). Temporarily restores freer breathing through the nose.

Warnings: Do not take this product if you have a breathing problem such as emphysema or chronic bronchitis, high blood pressure, heart disease, diabetes, thyroid disease, glaucoma, or difficulty in urination due to enlargement of the prostate gland, unless directed by a physician. May cause drowsiness; alcohol, sedatives and tranquilizers may increase the drowsiness effect. Avoid alcoholic beverages while taking this product. Do not take this product if you are taking sedatives or tranquilizers without first consulting your physician. Use caution when driving a motor vehicle or operating machinery. May cause excitability, especially in children.
Do not exceed the recommended dosage. If nervousness, dizziness or sleeplessness occur, discontinue use and consult a doctor. If symptoms do not improve within 7 days, or are accompanied by fever, consult a doctor.
As with any drug, if you are pregnant or nursing a baby, seek the advice of a health professional before using this product.
KEEP THIS AND ALL DRUGS OUT OF THE REACH OF CHILDREN. IN CASE OF ACCIDENTAL OVERDOSE, SEEK PROFESSIONAL ASSISTANCE OR CONTACT A POISON CONTROL CENTER IMMEDIATELY.

Drug Interaction Precaution: Do not use this product if you are now taking a prescription monoamine oxidase inhibitor (MAOI) (certain drugs for depression, psychiatric or emotional conditions, or Parkinson's disease) or for 2 weeks after stopping the MAOI drug. If you are uncertain whether your prescription drug contains an MAOI, consult a health professional before taking this product.

Directions: Adults and children 12 years of age and over: 2 teaspoonfuls every 4 hours; children 6 to under 12 years: 1 teaspoonful every 4 hours; DO NOT EXCEED 6 DOSES IN A 24-HOUR PERIOD. Children under 6 years: consult a physician.

Professional Labeling: The suggested dosage for children age 2 to under 6 years, only when the child is under the care of a physician, is 1/2 teaspoonful every 4 hours, not to exceed 6 doses in a 24-hour period. The dosage for children under 2 years should be determined by the physician on the basis of the patient's weight, physical condition, or other appropriate consideration. Dimetapp Elixir is contraindicated in neonates (children under the age of one month).

How Supplied: Purple, grape-flavored liquid in bottles of 4 fl oz, 8 fl oz, 12 fl oz, pints, and gallons.
Store at Controlled Room Temperature, between 20°C and 25°C (68°F and 77°F).
Not a USP elixir.

DIMETAPP® DM ELIXIR
[*dī'mĕ-tap*]

Description: Each 5 mL (1 teaspoonful) contains:
Brompheniramine
Maleate, USP .... 2 mg
Phenylpropanolamine
Hydrochloride, USP .... 12.5 mg
Dextromethorphan
Hydrobromide, USP .... 10.0 mg

Inactive Ingredients: Citric Acid, FD&C Blue 1, FD&C Red 40, Flavors, Glycerin, Propylene Glycol, Saccharin Sodium, Sodium Benzoate, Sorbitol, Water.

Indications: Temporarily relieves cough due to minor throat and bronchial irritation as may occur with a cold. For temporary relief of nasal congestion due to the common cold, hay fever or other upper respiratory allergies or associated with sinusitis. Temporarily relieves runny nose, sneezing, itching of the nose or throat and itchy, watery eyes due to allergic rhinitis (hay fever). Temporarily restores freer breathing through the nose.

Warnings: Do not take this product if you have a breathing problem such as emphysema or chronic bronchitis or persistent or chronic cough such as occurs with smoking or asthma, or cough that is accompanied by excessive phlegm (mucus) unless directed by a physician. Likewise, if you have high blood pressure, heart disease, diabetes, thyroid disease, glaucoma, or difficulty in urination due to enlargement of the prostate gland, do not take this product unless directed by a physician.
May cause marked drowsiness; alcohol, sedatives and tranquilizers may increase the drowsiness effect. Avoid alcoholic beverages while taking this product. Do not take this product if you are taking sedatives or tranquilizers without first consulting your physician. Use caution when driving a motor vehicle or operating machinery. May cause excitability, especially in children.
Do not exceed the recommended dosage. If nervousness, dizziness or sleeplessness occur, discontinue use and consult a physician. A persistent cough may be a sign of a serious condition. If cough or other symptoms persist, do not improve within 7 days, tend to recur, or are accompanied by fever, rash or persistent headache, consult a physician. As with any drug, if you are pregnant or nursing a baby, seek the advice of a health professional before using this product.
KEEP THIS AND ALL DRUGS OUT OF THE REACH OF CHILDREN. IN CASE OF ACCIDENTAL OVERDOSE, SEEK PROFESSIONAL ASSISTANCE OR CONTACT A POISON CONTROL CENTER IMMEDIATELY.

Drug Interaction Precaution: Do not use this product if you are now taking a prescription monoamine oxidase inhibitor (MAOI) (certain drugs for depression, psychiatric or emotional conditions, or Parkinson's disease) or for 2 weeks after stopping the MAOI drug. If you are uncertain whether your prescription drug contains an MAOI, consult a health professional before taking this product.

Directions: Adults and children 12 years of age and over: Two teaspoonfuls every 4 hours; children 6 to under 12 years: one teaspoonful every 4 hours. DO NOT EXCEED 6 DOSES IN A 24-HOUR PERIOD. Children under 6 years: consult a physician.

Professional Labeling: The suggested dosage for children age 2 to under 6 years, only when the child is under the care of a physician, is ½ teaspoonful every 4 hours, not to exceed 6 doses in a 24-hour period. The dosage for children under 2 years should be determined by the physician on the basis of the patient's weight, physical condition, or other appropriate consideration. Dimetapp DM

Elixir is contraindicated in neonates (children under the age of one month).

How Supplied: Red, grape-flavored liquid in bottles of 4 fl oz, 8 fl oz, and 12 fl oz.
Store at Controlled Room Temperature, Between 20°C and 25°C (68°F and 77°F)
Not a USP elixir.

DIMETAPP® Extentabs®
[dī' mĕ-tap]

Description: Each **Dimetapp Extentabs®** Tablet contains:
Brompheniramine Maleate, USP .... 12 mg
Phenylpropanolamine Hydrochloride, USP .... 75 mg

Inactive Ingredients: Acacia, Acetylated Monoglycerides, Calcium Sulfate, Carnauba Wax, Citric Acid, Edible Ink, FD&C Blue 1, Gelatin, Hydrogenated Castor Oil, Magnesium Stearate, Magnesium Trisilicate, Pharmaceutical Glaze, Polysorbates, Povidone, Silicon Dioxide, Stearyl Alcohol, Sucrose, Titanium Dioxide, White Wax. May also contain Wheat Flour.

Indications: For temporary relief of nasal congestion due to the common cold, hay fever or other upper respiratory allergies or associated with sinusitis; temporarily relieves runny nose, sneezing, and itchy and watery eyes due to allergic rhinitis (hay fever). Temporarily restores freer breathing through the nose.

Warnings: Do not take this product, unless directed by a physician, if you have a breathing problem such as emphysema or chronic bronchitis, or if you have high blood pressure, heart disease, diabetes, thyroid disease, glaucoma, or difficulty in urination due to enlargement of the prostate gland.
This product may cause drowsiness; alcohol, sedatives and tranquilizers may increase the drowsiness effect. Avoid alcoholic beverages while taking this product. Do not take this product if you are taking sedatives or tranquilizers without first consulting your physician. Use caution when driving a motor vehicle or operating machinery. May cause excitability, especially in children.
Do not exceed recommended dosage. If nervousness, dizziness or sleeplessness occur, discontinue use and consult a physician. If symptoms do not improve within 7 days, or are accompanied by fever, consult a physician.
Do not give this product to children under 12 years, except under the advice and supervision of a physician. Do not take this product if you are hypersensitive to any of the ingredients. As with any drug, if you are pregnant or nursing a baby, seek the advice of a health professional before using this product.
KEEP THIS AND ALL DRUGS OUT OF THE REACH OF CHILDREN. IN CASE OF ACCIDENTAL OVERDOSE, SEEK PROFESSIONAL ASSISTANCE OR CONTACT A POISON CONTROL CENTER IMMEDIATELY.

Drug Interaction Precaution: Do not use this product if you are now taking a prescription monoamine oxidase inhibitor (MAOI) (certain drugs for depression, psychiatric or emotional conditions, or Parkinson's disease) or for 2 weeks after stopping the MAOI drug. If you are uncertain whether your prescription drug contains an MAOI, consult a health professional before taking this product.

Directions: Adults and children 12 years of age and over: one tablet every 12 hours. DO NOT EXCEED 1 TABLET EVERY 12 HOURS OR 2 TABLETS IN A 24-HOUR PERIOD.

How Supplied: Pale blue sugar-coated tablets monogrammed DIMETAPP AHR in bottles of 100, 500; Dis-Co® Unit Dose Packs of 100; and blister packs of 12 tablets, 24 tablets and 48 tablets.
Store at Controlled Room Temperature, between 20°C and 25°C (68°F and 77°F).
Dimetapp Extentabs® Tablets are the A. H. Robins Company's uniquely constructed extended action tablets.

DIMETAPP® Tablets and Liqui-Gels®
[dī' mĕ-tap]
Maximum Strength

Description: Each **Dimetapp** Tablet or Liquigel® contains:
Brompheniramine Maleate, USP .... 4 mg
Phenylpropanolamine Hydrochloride, USP .... 25 mg

Inactive Ingredients: Tablets: Corn Starch, FD&C Blue 1 Aluminum Lake, Magnesium Stearate, Microcrystalline Cellulose. Liqui-Gels: D&C Red 33, Gelatin, Glycerin, Mannitol, Pharmaceutical Glaze, Polyethylene Glycol, Povidone, Propylene Glycol, Sorbitan, Sorbitol, Titanium Dioxide, Water.

Indications: For temporary relief of nasal congestion due to the common cold, hay fever or other upper respiratory allergies or associated with sinusitis. Temporarily relieves runny nose, sneezing, and itchy, watery eyes due to allergic rhinitis (hay fever). Temporarily restores freer breathing through the nose.

Warnings: Do not take take this product, unless directed by a physician, if you have a breathing problem such as emphysema or chronic bronchitis, or if you have high blood pressure, heart disease, diabetes, thyroid disease, glaucoma, or difficulty in urination due to enlargement of the prostate gland. This product may cause drowsiness; alcohol, sedatives and tranquilizers may increase the drowsiness effect. Avoid alcoholic beverages while taking this product. Do not take this product if you are taking sedatives or tranquilizers without first consulting your physician. Use caution when driving a motor vehicle or operating machinery. May cause excitability, especially in children. **Do not exceed the recommended dosage.** If nervousness, dizziness or sleeplessness occur, discontinue use and consult a physician. If symptoms do not improve within 7 days or are accompanied by fever, consult a physician. As with any drug, if you are pregnant or nursing a baby, seek the advice of a health professional before using this product.
KEEP THIS AND ALL DRUGS OUT OF THE REACH OF CHILDREN. IN CASE OF ACCIDENTAL OVERDOSE, SEEK PROFESSIONAL ASSISTANCE OR CONTACT A POISON CONTROL CENTER IMMEDIATELY.

Drug Interaction Precaution: Do not use this product if you are now taking a prescription monoamine oxidase inhibitor (MAOI) (certain drugs for depression, psychiatric or emotional conditions, or Parkinson's disease) or for 2 weeks after stopping the MAOI drug. If you are uncertain whether your prescription drug contains an MAOI, consult a health professional before taking this product.

Directions: Tablets: Adults and children 12 years of age and over: one tablet every 4 hours. Children 6 to under 12 years: one-half tablet every 4 hours. DO NOT EXCEED 6 DOSES IN A 24-HOUR PERIOD. Liqui-Gels: Adults and children 12 years of age and over: one softgel every 4 hours. Children under 12 years: consult a physician. DO NOT EXCEED 6 SOFTGELS IN A 24-HOUR PERIOD.

How Supplied: Tablets: Blue, scored compressed tablets engraved AHR and 2254 in consumer packages of 24 (individually packaged).
Liqui-Gels: Purple Liquigel imprinted AHR and 2255 in consumer packages of 12 and 24 (individually packaged).
Tablets and Liqui-Gels: Store at Controlled Room Temperature, between 20°C and 25°C (68°F and 77°F).
Liqui-Gels is a registered trademark of R.P. Scherer International Corporation.

ORUDIS® KT™
[Orūdĭs]

Description: Pain Reliever/Fever Reducer.

Active Ingredients: Each tablet or caplet contains ketoprofen 12.5 mg.

Inactive Ingredients: Cellulose, D&C Yellow 10 Lake, FD&C Blue 1 Lake, Iron Oxide, Pharmaceutical Glaze, Povidone, Silica, Sodium Benzoate, Sodium Lauryl Sulfate, Starch, Stearic Acid, Sugar, Titanium Dioxide, Wax. Contains FD&C Yellow 5 Lake (Tartrazine) as a color additive.

Indications: Temporarily relieves minor aches and pains associated with the common cold, headache, toothache, muscular aches, backache, minor pain of arthritis and menstrual cramps. Temporarily reduces fever.

Continued on next page

Whitehall-Robins—Cont.

Warnings: Do not take this product if you have had asthma, hives or any other allergic reaction after taking any pain reliever/fever reducer. Ketoprofen could cause similar reactions in patients allergic to other pain relievers/fever reducers. As with any drug, if you are pregnant or nursing a baby, seek the advice of a health professional before using this product. **IT IS ESPECIALLY IMPORTANT NOT TO USE KETOPROFEN DURING THE LAST 3 MONTHS OF PREGNANCY UNLESS SPECIALLY DIRECTED TO DO SO BY A DOCTOR BECAUSE IT MAY CAUSE PROBLEMS IN THE UNBORN CHILD OR COMPLICATIONS DURING DELIVERY.**

If you generally consume 3 or more alcohol-containing drinks per day, you should talk to your doctor for advice on when and how you should take ORUDIS® KT™ or other pain relievers.

Do not use: with any other pain reliever/fever reducer, with any other product containing ketoprofen, for more than 3 days for fever or for more than 10 days for pain. **Ask a doctor before use if:** the painful area is red or swollen, you take other drugs on a regular basis, you are under a doctor's care for any continuing medical condition or you have had problems or side effects with any pain reliever/fever reducer. **Ask a doctor after use if:** symptoms continue or worsen, new or unexpected symptoms occur or stomach pain occurs with use of this product.

Keep this and all drugs out of the reach of children. In case of accidental overdose, seek professional assistance or contact a poison control center immediately.

Directions: Take with a full glass of **water** or other **liquid**. **Adults:** Take 1 tablet every 4–6 hours. If pain or fever does not get better in 1 hour, you may take 1 more tablet. With experience, some people may find they need 2 tablets for the first dose. The smallest effective dose should be used. **Do not take more than:** 2 tablets in any 4–6 hour period; 6 tablets in any 24 hour period. **Children:** Do not give to children under age 16 unless directed by a doctor.

Store at room temperature. Avoid excessive heat 98°F (37°C).

How Supplied: Coated tablets in bottles of 24, 50, 100

Coated caplets in bottles of 24, 50, 100

ORUDIS is a registered trademark of RHONE-POULENC. KT and the appearance of the green ORUDIS KT tablet are trademarks of WHITEHALL-ROBINS HEALTHCARE.

If you have questions or comments, please call 1-800-Orudis2.

PREPARATION H®

[*prep-e 'rā-shen-āch*]

Hemorrhoidal Ointment and Cream

PREPARATION H®

Hemorrhoidal Suppositories

Description: Preparation H is available in ointment, cream and suppository product forms. The **Ointment** contains Petrolatum 71.9%, Mineral Oil 14%, Shark Liver Oil 3% and Phenylephrine HCl 0.25%.

The **Cream** contains Petrolatum 18%, Glycerin 12%, Shark Liver Oil 3% and Phenylephrine HCl 0.25%.

The **Suppositories** contain Cocoa Butter 85.5%, Shark Liver Oil 3%, and Phenylephrine HCL 0.25%.

Indications: Preparation H Ointment, Suppositories and Cream, temporarily shrink hemorrhoidal tissue and give temporary relief of the itching, burning and discomfort associated with hemorrhoids.

Warnings: In case of bleeding, or if condition worsens or does not improve within 7 days, consult a doctor promptly. Do not exceed the recommended daily dosage unless directed by a doctor. Keep this and all drugs out of the reach of children. In case of accidental ingestion, seek professional assistance or contact a poison control center immediately. As with any drug, if you are pregnant or nursing a baby, seek the advice of a health professional before using this product.

Ointment/Cream/Suppository: Do not use this product if you have heart disease, high blood pressure, thyroid disease, diabetes, or difficulty in urination due to enlargement of the prostate gland unless directed by a doctor.

Ointment: Do not use this product with an applicator if the introduction of the applicator into the rectum causes additional pain. Consult a doctor promptly.

Cream: Do not put this product into the rectum by using fingers or any mechanical device or applicator.

Drug Interaction Precaution: Ointment/Cream/Suppository—Do not use this product if you are presently taking a prescription drug for high blood pressure or depression, without first consulting your doctor.

Dosage and Administration:
Ointment/Cream/Suppositories—
ADULTS—When practical, cleanse the affected area by patting or blotting with an appropriate cleansing tissue. Gently dry by patting or blotting with toilet tissue or a soft cloth before application of this product.

Children under 12 years of age: consult a doctor.

Ointment—Apply to the affected area up to 4 times daily, especially at night, in the morning or after each bowel movement. Regular application and lubrication with Preparation H Ointment provide continual therapy for relief of hemorrhoidal symptoms. FOR INTRARECTAL USE: Before applying, remove protective cover from applicator. Attach applicator to tube. Lubricate applicator well, then gently insert applicator into the rectum. Thoroughly cleanse applicator after each use and replace protective cover. Also apply ointment to external area.

Cream—Apply externally to the affected area up to 4 times daily, especially at night, in the morning, or after each bowel movement. Preparation H Cream is to be applied externally or in the lower portion of the anal canal only. The enclosed dispensing cap is designed to control dispersion of the cream to the affected area in the lower portion of the anal canal. Before applying, remove protective cover from dispensing cap. Attach cap to tube. Lubricate dispensing cap well, then gently insert dispensing cap part way into the anus. Thoroughly cleanse dispensing cap after each use and replace protective cover. Regular application and lubrication with Preparation H Cream provides continual therapy for relief of hemorrhoidal symptoms.

Suppositories—Detach one suppository from the strip. Remove foil wrapper before inserting into the rectum as follows: Hold suppository with rounded end up. Carefully separate foil by inserting tip of fingernail at end marked "peel down". Peel foil slowly and evenly down both sides, exposing suppository. Remove exposed suppository from wrapper. Insert one suppository into the rectum up to 4 times daily, especially at night, in the morning or after each bowel movement. Regular application and lubrication with Preparation H Suppositories provide continual therapy for relief of hemorrhoidal symptoms.

Inactive Ingredients: Ointment—Beeswax, Benzoic Acid, BHA, Corn Oil, Glycerin, Lanolin, Lanolin Alcohol, Methylparaben, Paraffin, Propylparaben, Thyme Oil, Tocopherol, Water.

Cream—BHA, Carboxymethylcellulose Sodium, Cetyl Alcohol, Citric Acid, Edetate Disodium, Glyceryl Oleate, Glyceryl Stearate, Lanolin, Methylparaben, Propyl Gallate, Propylene Glycol, Propylparaben, Simethicone, Sodium Benzoate, Sodium Lauryl Sulfate, Stearyl Alcohol, Tocopherol, Xanthan Gum, Water.

Suppositories—Methylparaben, Propylparaben, Starch.

How Supplied: Ointment: Net Wt. 1 oz and 2 oz **Cream:** Net wt. 0.9 oz and 1.8 oz **Suppositories:** 12's, 24's and 48's. Store at room temperature or in cool place but not over 80° F.

PREPARATION H® HYDROCORTISONE 1%

[*prep-e 'ra-shen-ach*]

Anti-Itch Cream

Description: Preparation H® Hydrocortisone 1% is an antipruritic cream containing 1% Hydrocortisone.

Indications: For the temporary relief of external anal itch and itching associated with minor skin irritations and rashes. Other uses of this product should be only under the advice and supervision of a doctor.

Warnings: For external use only. Avoid contact with the eyes. If condition worsens, or if symptoms persist for more than 7 days or clear up and occur again within a few days, stop use of this product and do not begin use of any other hydrocortisone product unless you have consulted a doctor. Do not exceed the recommended daily dosage unless directed by a doctor. In case of bleeding, consult a doctor promptly. Do not put this product into the rectum by using fingers or any mechanical device or applicator. Do not use for the treatment of diaper rash; consult a doctor. Keep this and all drugs out of the reach of children. In case of accidental ingestion, seek professional assistance or contact a Poison Control Center immediately.

Directions: Adults: When practical, cleanse the affected area by patting or blotting with an appropriate cleansing tissue. Gently dry by patting or blotting with toilet tissue or soft cloth before application of this product. Apply to affected area not more than 3 to 4 times daily.
Children under 12 years of age: consult a doctor.

Inactive Ingredients: BHA, Cellulose Gum, Cetyl Alcohol, Citric Acid, Disodium EDTA, Glycerin, Glyceryl Oleate, Glyceryl Stearate, Lanolin, Methylparaben, Petrolatum, Propyl Gallate, Propylene Glycol, Propylparaben, Simethicone, Sodium Benzoate, Sodium Lauryl Sulfate, Stearyl Alcohol, Water, Xanthan Gum.

How Supplied: Available in Net Wt. 0.9 oz tube. Store at room temperature or in cool place but not over 80°F. If cellophane tear strip is missing or if cellophane wrap is broken or missing when purchased, do not use.

PRIMATENE®
[prīm 'a-tēn]
Mist
(Epinephrine Inhalation Aerosol Bronchodilator)

Description: Primatene Mist contains Epinephrine 5.5 mg/mL.

FDA approved uses.

Indications: For temporary relief of shortness of breath, tightness of chest, and wheezing due to bronchial asthma. Eases breathing for asthma patients by reducing spasms of bronchial muscles.

Directions: Inhalation dosage for adults and children 12 years of age and over, and children 4 to under 12 years of age: Start with one inhalation, then wait at least 1 minute. If not relieved, use once more. Do not use again for at least 3 hours. The use of this product by children should be supervised by an adult. Children under 4 years of age: Consult a physician. Each inhalation delivers 0.22 mg of epinephrine.

Warnings: Do not use this product unless a diagnosis of asthma has been made by a physician. Do not use this product if you have heart disease, high blood pressure, thyroid disease, diabetes, or difficulty in urination due to enlargement of the prostate gland unless directed by a physician. As with any drug, if you are pregnant or nursing a baby, seek the advice of a health professional before using this product. Do not use this product if you have ever been hospitalized for asthma or if you are taking any prescription drug for asthma unless directed by a physician. Keep this and all drugs out of the reach of children. In case of accidental overdose, seek professional assistance or contact a poison control center immediately. **DO NOT CONTINUE TO USE THIS PRODUCT BUT SEEK MEDICAL ASSISTANCE IMMEDIATELY IF SYMPTOMS ARE NOT RELIEVED WITHIN 20 MINUTES OR BECOME WORSE. DO NOT USE THIS PRODUCT MORE FREQUENTLY OR AT HIGHER DOSES THAN RECOMMENDED UNLESS DIRECTED BY A PHYSICIAN.** EXCESSIVE USE MAY CAUSE NERVOUSNESS AND RAPID HEART BEAT AND, POSSIBLY, ADVERSE EFFECTS ON THE HEART.

Drug Interaction Precaution: Do not use this product if you are now taking a prescription monoamine oxidase inhibitor (MAOI) (certain drugs for depression, psychiatric or emotional conditions, or Parkinson's disease), or for 2 weeks after stopping the MAOI drug. If you are uncertain whether your prescription drug contains an MAOI, consult a health professional before taking this product.

Caution: Contents under pressure. Do not puncture or throw container into incinerator. Using or storing near open flame or heating above 120° F (49° C) may cause bursting. Store at room temperature 59° F to 86° F (15° C to 30° C).

Directions For Use of Mouthpiece:
The Primatene Mist mouthpiece, which is enclosed in the Primatene Mist 15 mL size (not the refill size), should be used for inhalation only with Primatene Mist.

1. Take plastic cap off mouthpiece. (For refills, use mouthpiece from previous purchase.)
2. Take plastic mouthpiece off bottle.
3. Place other end of mouthpiece on bottle.
4. Turn bottle upside down. Place thumb on bottom of mouthpiece over circular button and forefinger on top of vial. Empty the lungs as completely as possible by exhaling.
5. Place mouthpiece in mouth with lips closed around opening. Inhale deeply while squeezing mouthpiece and bottle together. Release immediately and remove unit from mouth. Complete taking the deep breath, drawing the medication into your lungs and holding breath as long as comfortable.
6. Exhale slowly keeping lips nearly closed. This helps distribute the medication in the lungs.
7. Replace plastic cap on mouthpiece.

Care of the Mouthpiece:
The Primatene Mist mouthpiece should be washed once daily with soap and hot water, and rinsed thoroughly. Then it should be dried with a clean, lint-free cloth.
If the unit becomes clogged and fails to spray, please send the clogged unit to:
Whitehall Laboratories
5 Giralda Farms
Madison, N.J. 07940

Inactive Ingredients: Alcohol 34%, Ascorbic Acid, Fluorocarbons (Propellant), Water. Contains No Sulfites.

Warning: Contains CFC 12, 114, substances which harm public health and environment by destroying ozone in the upper atmosphere.

How Supplied:
1/2 Fl oz (15 mL) With Mouthpiece.
1/2 Fl oz (15 mL) Refill
3/4 Fl oz (22.5 mL) Refill

PRIMATENE®
[prīm 'a-tēn]
Tablets

Description: Primatene Tablets contain Ephedrine Hydrochloride 12.5 mg, USP, Guaifenesin, USP 200 mg.

Indications: For temporary relief of shortness of breath, tightness of chest, and wheezing due to bronchial asthma. Eases breathing for asthma patients by reducing spasms of bronchial muscles and helps loosen phlegm (mucus) and thin bronchial secretions to rid bronchial passageways of bothersome mucus and make coughs more productive.

Warnings: Do not use this product unless a diagnosis of asthma has been made by a doctor. Do not use this product if you have heart disease, high blood pressure, thyroid disease, diabetes or difficulty in urination due to enlargement of the prostate gland unless directed by a doctor. Do not use this product if you have ever been hospitalized for asthma or if you are taking any prescription drug for asthma unless directed by a doctor. **DRUG INTERACTION PRECAUTION:** Do not use this product if you are now taking a prescription monoamine oxidase inhibitor (MAOI) (certain drugs for depression, psychiatric or emotional conditions or Parkinson's disease), or for 2 weeks after stopping the MAOI drug. If you are uncertain whether your prescription drug contains an MAOI, consult a health professional before taking this product. Do not continue to use this product but seek medical assistance immediately if symptoms are not relieved within 1 hour or become worse. Some users of this product may experience nervousness, tremor, sleeplessness, nausea, and loss of appetite. If these symptoms persist or become

Continued on next page

Whitehall-Robins—Cont.

worse, consult your doctor. Do not take this product for persistent or chronic cough such as occurs with smoking, asthma, chronic bronchitis, or emphysema, or where cough is accompanied by excessive phlegm (mucus) unless directed by a doctor. A persistent cough may be a sign of a serious condition. If cough persists for more than one week, tends to recur, or is accompanied by fever, rash, or persistent headache, consult a doctor. As with any drug, if you are pregnant or nursing a baby, seek the advice of a health professional before using this product. Keep this and all drugs out of the reach of children. In case of accidental overdose, seek professional assistance or contact a poison control center immediately. Intentional abuse of this product can be harmful or fatal.

Directions: Adults and children 12 years of age and over: 2 tablets initially then two every 4 hours, as needed, not to exceed 12 tablets in 24 hours. Do not exceed recommended dosage unless directed by a doctor. For children under 12 years of age, consult a doctor.

Inactive Ingredients:
Crospovidone, D&C Yellow 10 Lake, FD&C Yellow 6 Lake, Magnesium Stearate, Microcrystalline Cellulose, Povidone, Silicon Dioxide.

How Supplied: Available in 24 and 60 tablet thermoform blister cartons.
Store at room temperature, between 20°C and 25°C (68°F to 77°F).

ROBITUSSIN® COLD & COUGH LIQUI-GELS®

[ro"bĭ-tuss'ĭn]

Description: Each Softgel contains:

Guaifenesin, USP .... 200 mg
Pseudoephedrine Hydrochloride, USP .... 30 mg
Dextromethorphan Hydrobromide, USP .... 10 mg

Inactive Ingredients: FD&C Blue 1, FD&C Red 40, Gelatin, Glycerin, Mannitol, Pharmaceutical Glaze, Polyethylene Glycol, Povidone, Propylene Glycol, Sorbitan, Sorbitol, Titanium Dioxide, Water.

Indications: Temporarily relieves cough due to minor throat and bronchial irritation and nasal congestion due to the common cold, hay fever or other upper respiratory allergies, or associated with sinusitis. Helps loosen phlegm (mucus) and thin bronchial secretions to make coughs more productive.

Warnings: Do not take this product for persistent or chronic cough such as occurs with smoking, asthma, chronic bronchitis, emphysema, or if cough is accompanied by excessive phlegm (mucus), unless directed by a physician. Likewise, if you have heart disease, high blood pressure, thyroid disease, diabetes, or difficulty in urination due to enlargement of the prostate gland, do not take this product unless directed by a physician.
Do not exceed the recommended dosage. If nervousness, dizziness or sleeplessness occur, discontinue use and consult a physician. A persistent cough may be a sign of a serious condition. If cough or other symptoms persist, do not improve within 7 days, tend to recur, or are accompanied by fever, rash, or persistent headache, consult a physician.
As with any drug, if you are pregnant or nursing a baby, seek the advice of a health professional before using this product.
KEEP THIS AND ALL DRUGS OUT OF THE REACH OF CHILDREN. IN CASE OF ACCIDENTAL OVERDOSE, SEEK PROFESSIONAL ASSISTANCE OR CONTACT A POISON CONTROL CENTER IMMEDIATELY.

Drug Interaction Precaution: Do not use this product if you are now taking a prescription monoamine oxidase inhibitor (MAOI) (certain drugs for depression, psychiatric or emotional conditions, or Parkinson's disease) or for 2 weeks after stopping the MAOI drug. If you are uncertain whether your prescription drug contains an MAOI, consult a health professional before taking this product.

Directions: Follow dosage below: DO NOT EXCEED 4 DOSES IN A 24-HOUR PERIOD. Adults and children 12 years of age and over: swallow two Softgels every 4 hours. Children 6 to under 12 years: swallow one Softgel every 4 hours. Children under 6–consult your doctor.

How Supplied: Red Liquigel imprinted AHR and 8600 in consumer packages of 12 and 20 (individually packaged).
Store at Controlled Room Temperature, between 20°C and 25°C (68°F and 77°F)
Liqui-Gels and Liquigel are registered trademarks of R.P. Scherer International Corporation.

ROBITUSSIN® COLD, COUGH & FLU LIQUI-GELS®

[ro"bĭ-tuss'ĭn]

Description: Pain Reliever, Fever Reducer, Cough Suppressant, Nasal Decongestant, Expectorant.

Active Ingredients: Acetaminophen 250 mg, Guaifenesin 100 mg, Pseudoephedrine HCl 30 mg, Dextromethorphan HBr 10 mg

Inactive Ingredients: D&C Yellow #10, FD&C Red #40, Gelatin, Glycerin, Mannitol, Polyethylene Glycol, Povidone, Propylene Glycol, Sorbitan, Sorbitol, Water

Indications: For the temporary relief of minor aches and pains, headache, muscular aches and sore throat associated with cold or flu, and to reduce fever. Temporarily relieves cough due to minor throat and bronchial irritation and nasal congestion as may occur with a cold. Helps loosen phlegm (mucus) and thin bronchial secretions to make coughs more productive.

Warnings: Do not take this product for persistent or chronic cough such as occurs with smoking, asthma, chronic bronchitis, emphysema, or if cough is accompanied by excessive phlegm (mucus), unless directed by a doctor. Likewise, if you have heart disease, high blood pressure, thyroid disease, diabetes, or difficulty in urination due to enlargement of the prostate gland, do not take this product unless directed by a doctor.

Alcohol Warning: If you generally consume 3 or more alcohol-containing drinks per day you should consult your physician for advice on when and how you should take this product or any other acetaminophen-containing product.
Do not exceed recommended dosage.
If nervousness, dizziness, or sleeplessness occur, discontinue use and consult a doctor. Do not take this product for more than 7 days (adults) or 5 days (children under 12) or for fever for more than 3 days unless directed by a doctor.
If pain or fever persists or gets worse, if new symptoms occur, or if redness or swelling is present, consult a doctor because these could be signs of a serious condition. If sore throat is severe, persists for more than 2 days, is accompanied or followed by fever, headache, rash, nausea, or vomiting, consult a doctor promptly. A persistent cough may be a sign of a serious condition. If cough or other symptoms persist, do not improve within 7 days, tend to recur, or are accompanied by fever, rash, or persistent headache, consult a doctor.
As with any drug, if you are pregnant or nursing a baby, seek the advice of a health professional before using this product.

Drug Interaction Precaution: Do not use this product if you are now taking a prescription monoamine oxidase inhibitor (MAOI) (certain drugs for depression, psychiatric or emotional conditions, or Parkinson's disease), or for 2 weeks after stopping the MAOI drug. If you are uncertain whether your prescription drug contains an MAOI, consult a health professional before taking this product.

Directions: Follow dosage below: Do not exceed 4 doses in a 24-hour period.
Adult Dose (and children 12 yrs. and over): Swallow 2 Softgels every 4 hrs.
Child Dose: (6 yrs. to under 12 yrs.): Swallow 1 Softgel every 4 hrs.
Children under 6—Consult your doctor.
KEEP THIS AND ALL DRUGS OUT OF THE REACH OF CHILDREN. IN CASE OF ACCIDENTAL OVERDOSE, SEEK PROFESSIONAL ASSISTANCE OR CONTACT A POISON CONTROL CENTER IMMEDIATELY. PROMPT MEDICAL ATTENTION IS CRITICAL FOR ADULTS AS WELL AS CHILDREN EVEN IF YOU DO NOT NOTICE ANY SIGNS OR SYMPTOMS.

How Supplied: Blister Packs of 12's
Blister Packs of 20's

Storage: Store at Controlled Room Temperature, Between 20°C and 25°C (68°F and 77°F).

ROBITUSSIN® SEVERE CONGESTION LIQUI-GELS®

[ro "bĭ-tuss 'ĭn]

Description: Each Robitussin Severe Congestion Liquigel® contains:

Guaifenesin, USP .... 200 mg
Pseudoephedrine Hydrochloride, USP .... 30 mg

Inactive Ingredients: FD&C Green 3, Gelatin, Glycerin, Mannitol, Pharmaceutical Glaze, Polyethylene Glycol, Povidone, Propylene Glycol, Sorbitan, Sorbitol, Titanium Dioxide, Water.

Indications: For the temporary relief of nasal congestion due to the common cold, hay fever or other upper respiratory allergies, or associated with sinusitis. Helps loosen phlegm (mucus) and thin bronchial secretions to make coughs more productive.

Warnings: Do not take this product for persistent or chronic cough such as occurs with smoking, asthma, chronic bronchitis, emphysema, or if cough is accompanied by excessive phlegm (mucus), unless directed by a physician. Likewise, if you have heart disease, high blood pressure, thyroid disease, diabetes, or difficulty in urination due to enlargement of the prostate gland, do not take this product unless directed by a physician.

Do not exceed the recommended dosage. If nervousness, dizziness or sleeplessness occur, discontinue use and consult a physician. A persistent cough may be a sign of a serious condition. If cough or other symptoms persist, do not improve within 7 days, tend to recur, or are accompanied by fever, rash, or persistent headache, consult a physician.
As with any drug, if you are pregnant or nursing a baby, seek the advice of a health professional before using this product.
KEEP THIS AND ALL DRUGS OUT OF THE REACH OF CHILDREN. IN CASE OF ACCIDENTAL OVERDOSE, SEEK PROFESSIONAL ASSISTANCE OR CONTACT A POISON CONTROL CENTER IMMEDIATELY.

Drug Interaction Precaution: Do not use this product if you are now taking a prescription monoamine oxidase inhibitor (MAOI) (certain drugs for depression, psychiatric or emotional conditions or Parkinson's disease) or for 2 weeks after stopping the MAOI drug. If you are uncertain whether your prescription drug contains an MAOI, consult a health professional before taking this product.

Directions: Follow dosage below: DO NOT EXCEED 4 DOSES IN A 24-HOUR PERIOD. Adults and children 12 years of age and over: swallow two Softgels every 4 hours. Children 6 to under 12 years: swallow one Softgel every 4 hours. Children under 6, consult a physician.

How Supplied: Aqua Liquigel imprinted AHR and 8501 in consumer packages of 12 and 20 (individually packaged).
Store at Controlled Room Temperature, between 20°C and 25°C (68°F and 77°F).
Liqui-Gels and Liquigel are registered trademarks of R.P. Scherer International Corporation.

ROBITUSSIN®

[ro "bĭ-tuss 'ĭn]
(Guaifenesin Syrup, USP)

Active Ingredients: Each teaspoonful (5 mL) contains:
Guaifenesin, USP .... 100 mg
Alcohol-Free Cough Formula

Inactive Ingredients: Caramel, Citric Acid, FD&C Red 40, Flavors, Glucose, Glycerin, High Fructose Corn Syrup, Saccharin Sodium, Sodium Benzoate, Water.

Indications: Helps loosen phlegm (mucus) and thin bronchial secretions to make coughs more productive.

Professional Labeling: Helps loosen phlegm and thin bronchial secretions in patients with stable chronic bronchitis.

Warnings: Do not take this product for persistent or chronic cough such as occurs with smoking, asthma, chronic bronchitis, emphysema, or where cough is accompanied by excessive phlegm (mucus) unless directed by a physician.
A persistent cough may be a sign of a serious condition. If cough persists for more than one week, tends to recur, or is accompanied by a fever, rash, or persistent headache, consult a physician.
Do not take this product if you are hypersensitive to any of the ingredients. As with any drug, if you are pregnant or nursing a baby, seek the advice of a health professional before using this product.
KEEP THIS AND ALL DRUGS OUT OF THE REACH OF CHILDREN. IN CASE OF ACCIDENTAL OVERDOSE, SEEK PROFESSIONAL ASSISTANCE OR CONTACT A POISON CONTROL CENTER IMMEDIATELY.

Directions: Follow dosage below. Dosage cup provided. **Do Not Exceed Recommended Dosage**. Adults and children 12 years and over: 2–4 teaspoonfuls every 4 hours; children 6 years to under 12 years: 1–2 teaspoonfuls every 4 hours. Children 2 years to under 6 years: ½–1 teaspoonful every 4 hours. Children under 2 years—consult your doctor.

How Supplied: Robitussin (wine-colored) in bottles of 4 fl oz, 8 fl oz, pint.
Store at Controlled Room Temperature, between 20°C and 25°C (68°F and 77°F).

ROBITUSSIN®-CF

[ro "bĭ-tuss 'ĭn]

Active Ingredients: Each teaspoonful (5 mL) contains:
Guaifenesin, USP .... 100 mg
Phenylpropanolamine Hydrochloride, USP .... 12.5 mg
Dextromethorphan Hydrobromide, USP .... 10 mg

Inactive Ingredients: Citric Acid, FD&C Red 40, Flavors, Glycerin, Propylene Glycol, Saccharin Sodium, Sodium Benzoate, Sorbitol, Water.

Indications: Temporarily relieves cough due to minor throat and bronchial irritation and nasal congestion as may occur with a cold. Helps loosen phlegm (mucus) and thin bronchial secretions to make coughs more productive.

Warnings: Do not take this product for persistent or chronic cough such as occurs with smoking, asthma, chronic bronchitis, emphysema, or if cough is accompanied by excessive phlegm (mucus) unless directed by a physician. Likewise, if you have heart disease, high blood pressure, thyroid disease, diabetes, or difficulty in urination due to enlargement of the prostate gland, do not take this product unless directed by a physician.

Do not exceed the recommended dosage. If nervousness, dizziness, or sleeplessness occur, discontinue use and consult a doctor. A persistent cough may be a sign of a serious condition. If cough or other symptoms persist, do not improve within 7 days, tend to recur, or are accompanied by fever, rash, or persistent headache, consult a physician. As with any drug, if you are pregnant or nursing a baby, seek the advice of a health professional before using this product.
KEEP THIS AND ALL DRUGS OUT OF THE REACH OF CHILDREN. IN CASE OF ACCIDENTAL OVERDOSE, SEEK PROFESSIONAL ASSISTANCE OR CONTACT A POISON CONTROL CENTER IMMEDIATELY.

Drug Interaction Precaution: Do not use this product if you are now taking a prescription monoamine oxidase inhibitor (MAOI) (certain drugs for depression, psychiatric or emotional conditions, or Parkinson's disease) or for 2 weeks after stopping the MAOI drug. If you are uncertain whether your prescription drug contains an MAOI, consult a health professional before taking this product.

Directions: Follow dosage below: Dosage cup provided. DO NOT EXCEED 6 DOSES IN A 24-HOUR PERIOD. Adults and children 12 years and over: 2 teaspoonfuls every 4 hours; children 6 years to under 12 years, 1 teaspoonful every 4 hours; children 2 years to under 6 years, ½ teaspoonful every 4 hours; children under 2 years—consult your doctor.

Continued on next page

Whitehall-Robins—Cont.

How Supplied: Robitussin-CF (red-colored) in bottles of 4 fl oz, 8 fl oz, and 12 fl oz.
Store at Controlled Room Temperature, between 20°C and 25°C (68°F and 77°F).

ROBITUSSIN®-DM
[ro "bĭ-tuss 'ĭn]

Active Ingredients: Each teaspoonful (5 mL) contains:
Guaifenesin, USP .... 100 mg
Dextromethorphan Hydrobromide, USP .... 10 mg

Inactive Ingredients: Citric Acid, FD&C Red 40, Flavors, Glucose, Glycerin, High Fructose Corn Syrup, Saccharin Sodium, Sodium Benzoate, Water.

Indications: Temporarily relieves cough due to minor throat and bronchial irritation as may occur with a cold and helps loosen phlegm (mucus) and thin bronchial secretions to make coughs more productive.

Warnings: Do not take this product for persistent or chronic cough such as occurs with smoking, asthma, chronic bronchitis, emphysema, or if cough is accompanied by excessive phlegm (mucus) unless directed by a physician.
A persistent cough may be a sign of a serious condition. If cough persists for more than one week, tends to recur, or is accompanied by a fever, rash, or persistent headache, consult a physician.
Do not take this product if you are hypersensitive to any of the ingredients. As with any drug, if you are pregnant or nursing a baby, seek the advice of a health professional before using this product.
KEEP THIS AND ALL DRUGS OUT OF THE REACH OF CHILDREN. IN CASE OF ACCIDENTAL OVERDOSE, SEEK PROFESSIONAL ASSISTANCE OR CONTACT A POISON CONTROL CENTER IMMEDIATELY.

Drug Interaction Precaution: Do not use this product if you are now taking a prescription monoamine oxidase inhibitor (MAOI) (certain drugs for depression, psychiatric or emotional conditions, or Parkinson's disease) or for 2 weeks after stopping the MAOI drug. If you are uncertain whether your prescription drug contains an MAOI, consult a health professional before taking this product.

Directions: Follow dosage below or use as directed by a doctor. Dosage cup provided. DO NOT EXCEED 6 DOSES IN A 24-HOUR PERIOD. Adults and children 12 years and over: 2 teaspoonfuls every 4 hours; children 6 years to under 12 years, 1 teaspoonful every 4 hours; children 2 years to under 6 years, 1/2 teaspoonful every 4 hours; children under 2 years—consult your doctor.

How Supplied: Robitussin-DM (cherry-colored) in bottles of 4 fl oz, 8 fl oz, 12 fl oz, pint and single doses: 6 premeasured doses—1/3 fl oz each.
Store at Controlled Room Temperature, between 20°C and 25°C (68°F and 77°F).

ROBITUSSIN®-PE
[ro "bĭ-tuss 'ĭn]

Active Ingredients: Each teaspoonful (5 mL) contains:
Guaifenesin, USP .... 100 mg
Pseudoephedrine Hydrochloride, USP .... 30 mg

Inactive Ingredients: Citric Acid, FD&C Red 40, Flavors, Glucose, Glycerin, High Fructose Corn Syrup, Maltol, Propylene Glycol, Saccharin Sodium, Sodium Benzoate, Water.

Indications: Temporarily relieves nasal congestion due to a cold. Helps loosen phlegm (mucus) and thin bronchial secretions to make coughs more productive.

Warnings: Do not take this product for persistent or chronic cough such as occurs with smoking, asthma, chronic bronchitis, emphysema, or if cough is accompanied by excessive phlegm (mucus) unless directed by a physician. Likewise, if you have heart disease, high blood pressure, thyroid disease, diabetes, or difficulty in urination due to enlargement of the prostate gland, do not take this product unless directed by a physician.
Do not exceed the recommended dosage. If nervousness, dizziness, or sleeplessness occur, discontinue use and consult a doctor. A persistent cough may be a sign of a serious condition. If cough or other symptoms persist, do not improve within 7 days, tend to recur, or are accompanied by fever, rash, or persistent headache, consult a physician. As with any drug, if you are pregnant or nursing a baby, seek the advice of a health professional before using this product.
KEEP THIS AND ALL DRUGS OUT OF THE REACH OF CHILDREN. IN CASE OF ACCIDENTAL OVERDOSE, SEEK PROFESSIONAL ASSISTANCE OR CONTACT A POISON CONTROL CENTER IMMEDIATELY.

Drug Interaction Precaution: Do not use this product if you are now taking a prescription monoamine oxidase inhibitor (MAOI) (certain drugs for depression, psychiatric or emotional conditions, or Parkinson's disease) or for 2 weeks after stopping the MAOI drug. If you are uncertain whether your prescription drug contains an MAOI, consult a health professional before taking this product.

Directions: Follow dosage below. Dosage cup provided. DO NOT EXCEED 4 DOSES IN A 24-HOUR PERIOD. Adults and children 12 years and over: 2 teaspoonfuls every 4 hours; children 6 years to under 12 years, 1 teaspoonful every 4 hours; children 2 years to under 6 years, 1/2 teaspoonful every 4 hours; children under 2 years—consult your doctor.

How Supplied: Robitussin-PE (orange-red) in bottles of 4 fl oz, and 8 fl oz.
Store at Controlled Room Temperature, Between 20°C and 25°C (68°F and 77°F).

ROBITUSSIN® MAXIMUM STRENGTH COUGH SUPPRESSANT
[ro "bĭ-tuss 'ĭn]

Description: Each 5 mL (1 teaspoonful) contains:
Dextromethorphan Hydrobromide, USP .... 15 mg

Inactive Ingredients: Alcohol 1.4%, Citric Acid, FD&C Red 40, Flavors, Glycerin, Glucose, High Fructose Corn Syrup, Saccharin Sodium, Sodium Benzoate, Water.

Indications: Temporarily relieves cough due to minor throat and bronchial irritation as may occur with a cold.

Warnings: Do not take this product for persistent or chronic cough such as occurs with smoking, asthma, emphysema, or if cough is accompanied by excessive phlegm (mucus) unless directed by a physician.
A persistent cough may be a sign of a serious condition. If cough persists for more than one week, tends to recur, or is accompanied by fever, rash, or persistent headache, consult a physician.
As with any drug, if you are pregnant or nursing a baby, seek the advice of a health professional before using this product.
KEEP THIS AND ALL DRUGS OUT OF THE REACH OF CHILDREN. IN CASE OF ACCIDENTAL OVERDOSE, SEEK PROFESSIONAL ASSISTANCE OR CONTACT A POISON CONTROL CENTER IMMEDIATELY.

Drug Interaction Precaution: Do not use this product if you are now taking a prescription monoamine oxidase inhibitor (MAOI) (certain drugs for depression, psychiatric or emotional conditions, or Parkinson's disease) or for 2 weeks after stopping the MAOI drug. If you are uncertain whether your prescription drug contains an MAOI, consult a health professional before taking this product.

Directions: Follow dosage recommendations below or use as directed by a doctor. Repeat every 6–8 hours as needed. DO NOT EXCEED 4 DOSES IN A 24-HOUR PERIOD. Adults and children 12 years and over: 2 teaspoonfuls every 6–8 hours, in medicine cup. Children under 12 years: consult your doctor.

Professional Labeling: Children 6 years to under 12 years, 1 teaspoonful every 6–8 hours; children 2 years to under 6 years, 1/2 teaspoonful every 6–8 hours. Do not exceed 4 doses in a 24-hour period.
Tamper-Evident Bottle Cap. If Breakable Ring Is Separated, Do Not Use.

How Supplied: Robitussin Maximum Strength (dark red-colored) in bottles of 4 fl oz and 8 fl oz.
Store at Controlled Room Temperature, between 20°C and 25°C (68°F and 77°F).

ROBITUSSIN® MAXIMUM STRENGTH COUGH & COLD
[*ro "bĭ-tuss 'ĭn*]

Description: Each teaspoonful (5 mL) contains:
Dextromethorphan Hydrobromide, USP .... 15 mg
Pseudoephedrine Hydrochloride, USP .... 30 mg

Inactive Ingredients: Alcohol 1.4%, Citric Acid, FD&C Red 40, Flavors, Glycerin, Glucose, High Fructose Corn Syrup, Saccharin Sodium, Sodium Benzoate, Water.

Indications: Temporarily relieves cough due to minor throat and bronchial irritation and nasal congestion as may occur with a cold.

Warnings: Do not take this product for persistent or chronic cough such as occurs with smoking, asthma, emphysema, or if cough is accompanied by excessive phlegm (mucus) unless directed by a physician. Likewise, if you have heart disease, high blood pressure, thyroid disease, diabetes, or difficulty in urination due to enlargement of the prostate gland, do not take this product unless directed by a physician.
Do not exceed the recommended dosage. If nervousness, dizziness, or sleeplessness occur, discontinue use and consult a doctor. A persistent cough may be a sign of a serious condition. If cough or other symptoms persist, do not improve within 7 days, tend to recur, or are accompanied by fever, rash, or persistent headache, consult a physician.
As with any drug, if you are pregnant or nursing a baby, seek the advice of a health professional before using this product.
KEEP THIS AND ALL DRUGS OUT OF THE REACH OF CHILDREN. IN CASE OF ACCIDENTAL OVERDOSE, SEEK PROFESSIONAL ASSISTANCE OR CONTACT A POISON CONTROL CENTER IMMEDIATELY.

Drug Interaction Precaution: Do not use this product if you are now taking a prescription monoamine oxidase inhibitor (MAOI) (certain drugs for depression, psychiatric or emotional conditions, or Parkinson's disease) or for 2 weeks after stopping the MAOI drug. If you are uncertain whether your prescription drug contains an MAOI, consult a health professional before taking this product.

Directions: Follow dosage recommendations below or use as directed by a doctor. Repeat every 6 hours as needed. DO NOT EXCEED 4 DOSES IN A 24-HOUR PERIOD. Adults and children 12 years and over: 2 teaspoonfuls every 6 hours in medicine cup. Children under 12 years: consult your doctor.

How Supplied: Red syrup in bottles of 4 fl oz and 8 fl oz.
Store at Controlled Room Temperature, Between 20°C and 25°C (68°F and 77°F).

ROBITUSSIN® NIGHT-TIME COLD FORMULA
[*ro "bĭ-tuss 'ĭn*]

Description: Cough Suppressant, Nasal Decongestant, Antihistamine, Pain Reliever-Fever Reducer

Active Ingredients: Acetaminophen 325 mg, Pseudoephedrine HCl 30 mg, Dextromethorphan HBr 15 mg, Doxylamine Succinate 6.25 mg.

Inactive Ingredients: D&C Green 5, D&C Yellow 10, FD&C Green 3, FD&C Yellow 6, Gelatin, Glycerin, Mannitol, Pharmaceutical Glaze, Polyethylene Glycol, Povidone, Propylene Glycol, Sodium Acetate, Sorbitan, Sorbitol, Titanium Dioxide, Water

Indications: For the temporary relief of minor aches and pains, headache, muscular aches and sore throat associated with cold or flu, and to reduce fever. Temporarily relieves cough due to minor throat and bronchial irritation and nasal congestion as may occur with a cold. Temporarily relieves runny nose, and sneezing, itching of the nose or throat, and itchy, watery eyes due to hay fever or other upper respiratory allergies (allergic rhinitis).

Warnings: Do not take this product for persistent or chronic cough such as occurs with smoking, asthma, chronic bronchitis, emphysema, or if cough is accompanied by excessive phlegm (mucus), unless directed by a doctor. Likewise, if you have heart disease, high blood pressure, thyroid disease, diabetes, or difficulty in urination due to enlargement of the prostate gland, do not take this product unless directed by a doctor.

Alcohol Warning: Avoid alcoholic beverages while taking this product. If you generally consume 3 or more alcohol-containing drinks per day, you should consult your physician for advice on when and how you should take this product or any other acetaminophen-containing product.
May cause marked drowsiness; alcohol, sedatives, and tranquilizers may increase the drowsiness effect. Do not take this product if you are taking sedatives or tranquilizers, without first consulting your doctor. Use caution when driving a motor vehicle or operating machinery. May cause excitability especially in children.
Do not exceed recommended dosage. If nervousness, dizziness or sleeplessness occur, discontinue use and consult a doctor. Do not take this product for more than 7 days or for fever for more than 3 days unless directed by a doctor. If pain or fever persists or gets worse, if new symptoms occur, or if redness or swelling is present, consult a doctor because these could be signs of a serious condition. If sore throat is severe, persists for more than 2 days, is accompanied or followed by fever, headache, rash, nausea, or vomiting, consult a doctor promptly. A persistent cough may be a sign of a serious condition. If cough or other symptoms persist for more than one week without improvement, tend to recur, or are accompanied by fever, rash or persistent headache, consult a doctor.
As with any drug, if you are pregnant or nursing a baby, seek the advice of a health professional before using this product.

Drug Interaction Precaution: Do not use this product if you are now taking a prescription monoamine oxidase inhibitor (MAOI) (certain drugs for depression, psychiatric or emotional conditions, or Parkinson's disease), or for 2 weeks after stopping the MAOI drug. If you are uncertain whether your prescription drug contains an MAOI, consult a health professional before taking this product.

Directions: Follow dosage below: Do not exceed 4 doses in a 24-hour period. Adult Dose (and children 12 yrs. and over): Swallow 2 Softgels every 6 hrs.
Not recommended for children under 12 years of age
KEEP THIS AND ALL DRUGS OUT OF THE REACH OF CHILDREN. IN CASE OF ACCIDENTAL OVERDOSE, SEEK PROFESSIONAL ASSISTANCE OR CONTACT A POISON CONTROL CENTER IMMEDIATELY. PROMPT MEDICAL ATTENTION IS CRITICAL FOR ADULTS AS WELL AS CHILDREN EVEN IF YOU DO NOT NOTICE ANY SIGNS OR SYMPTOMS.

Storage: Store at Controlled Room Temperature, Between 20°C and 25°C (68°F and 77°F).

How Supplied: Blister Pack of 12's
Blister Pack of 20's

ROBITUSSIN® PEDIATRIC COUGH & COLD FORMULA
[*ro "bĭ-tuss 'ĭn*]

Description: Each 5 mL (1 teaspoonful) contains:
Dextromethorphan Hydrobromide, USP .... 7.5 mg
Pseudoephedrine Hydrochloride .... 15 mg

Inactive Ingredients: Citric Acid, FD&C Red 40, Flavors, Glycerin, Propylene Glycol, Saccharin Sodium, Sodium Benzoate, Sorbitol, Water.

Indications: Temporarily relieves cough due to minor throat and bronchial irritation and nasal congestion as may occur with a cold.

Warnings: Do not take this product for persistent or chronic cough such as oc-

Continued on next page

Whitehall-Robins—Cont.

Age	Weight	Dose
Under 2 yrs.	Under 24 lbs.	Consult doctor
2 to under 6 yrs.	24–47 lbs.	1 Teaspoonful
6 to under 12 yrs.	48–95 lbs.	2 Teaspoonfuls
12 yrs. and older	96 lbs. and over	4 Teaspoonfuls

curs with smoking, asthma, or emphysema, or if cough is accompanied by excessive phlegm (mucus) unless directed by a physician. Likewise if you have heart disease, high blood pressure, thyroid disease, diabetes, or difficulty in urination due to enlargement of the prostate gland, do not take this product unless directed by a physician.
Do not exceed the recommended dosage. If nervousness, dizziness, or sleeplessness occur, discontinue use and consult a doctor. A persistent cough may be a sign of a serious condition. If cough or other symptoms persist, do not improve within 7 days, tend to recur, or are accompanied by fever, rash, or persistent headache, consult a physician.
As with any drug, if you are pregnant or nursing a baby, seek the advice of a health professional before using this product.
KEEP THIS AND ALL DRUGS OUT OF THE REACH OF CHILDREN. IN CASE OF ACCIDENTAL OVERDOSE, SEEK PROFESSIONAL ASSISTANCE OR CONTACT A POISON CONTROL CENTER IMMEDIATELY.

Drug Interaction Precaution: Do not use this product if you are now taking a prescription monoamine oxidase inhibitor (MAOI) (certain drugs for depression, psychiatric or emotional conditions, or Parkinson's disease) or for 2 weeks after stopping the MAOI drug. If you are uncertain whether your prescription drug contains an MAOI, consult a health professional before taking this product.

Directions: Follow dosage recommendations below or use as directed by a physician. Repeat every 6 hours as needed. DO NOT EXCEED 4 DOSES IN A 24-HOUR PERIOD. Dosage: choose by weight, if known; if weight is not known, choose by age.
[See table above.]

How Supplied: Robitussin Pediatric Cough & Cold formula (bright red) in bottles of 4 fl oz and 8 fl oz.
Store at Controlled Room Temperature, Between 20°C and 25°C (68°F and 77°F).

ROBITUSSIN® PEDIATRIC COUGH SUPPRESSANT

[ro "bĭ-tuss 'ĭn]

Description: Each 5 mL (1 teaspoonful) contains:
Dextromethorphan
Hydrobromide, USP .... 7.5 mg

Inactive Ingredients: Citric Acid, FD&C Red 40, Flavors, Glycerin, Propylene Glycol, Saccharin Sodium, Sodium Benzoate, Sorbitol, Water.

Indications: Temporarily relieves cough due to minor throat and bronchial irritation as may occur with a cold.

Warnings: Do not take this product for persistent or chronic cough such as occurs with smoking, asthma, emphysema, or if cough is accompanied by excessive phlegm (mucus) unless directed by a physician.
A persistent cough may be a sign of a serious condition. If cough persists for more than one week, tends to recur, or is accompanied by fever, rash, or persistent headache, consult a physician.
Do not take this product if you are hypersensitive to any of the ingredients. As with any drug, if you are pregnant or nursing a baby, seek the advice of a health professional before using this product.
KEEP THIS AND ALL DRUGS OUT OF THE REACH OF CHILDREN. IN CASE OF ACCIDENTAL OVERDOSE, SEEK PROFESSIONAL ASSISTANCE OR CONTACT A POISON CONTROL CENTER IMMEDIATELY.

Drug Interaction Precaution: Do not use this product if you are now taking a prescription monoamine oxidase inhibitor (MAOI) (certain drugs for depression, psychiatric or emotional conditions, or Parkinson's disease) or for 2 weeks after stopping the MAOI drug. If you are uncertain whether your prescription drug contains an MAOI, consult a health professional before taking this product.

Directions: Follow dosage recommendations below or use as directed by a physician. Repeat every 6–8 hours. DO NOT EXCEED 4 DOSES IN A 24-HOUR PERIOD. Dosage: choose by weight, if known; if weight is not known, choose by age.
[See table below.]

Age	Weight	Dose
Under 2 yrs.	Under 24 lbs.	Consult doctor
2 to under 6 yrs.	24–47 lbs.	1 Teaspoonful
6 to under 12 yrs.	48–95 lbs.	2 Teaspoonfuls
12 yrs. and older	96 lbs. and over	4 Teaspoonfuls

How Supplied: Robitussin Pediatric (cherry-colored) in bottles of 4 fl oz
Store at Controlled Room Temperature, Between 20°C and 25°C (68°F and 77°F).

ROBITUSSIN PEDIATRIC DROPS

[ro "bĭ-tuss 'ĭn]

Description: Nasal Decongestant/Cough Suppressant/Expectorant

Active Ingredients: Each 2.5 mL contains Guaifenesin, USP 100 mg, Pseudoephedrine Hydrochloride, USP 15 mg, Dextromethorphan Hydrobromide, US 5 mg in a pleasant tasting berry flavore syrup.

Inactive Ingredients: Citric Aci FD&C Red 40, Flavors, Glycerin, Hig Fructose Corn Syrup, Menthol, Pol ethylene Glycol, Propylene Glycol, Sa charin Sodium, Sodium Benzoate, S dium Carboxymethylcellulose, Sorbito Water.

Indications: Temporarily relieves coug due to minor throat and bronchial irrita tion, and nasal congestion due to a col Helps loosen phlegm (mucus) and thi bronchial secretions to make cough more productive.

Warnings: Do not give this product fc persistent or chronic cough such as o curs with asthma, or where cough is a companied by excessive phlegm (mucu unless directed by a physician. Likewis do not give this product to a child wh has heart disease, high blood pressur thyroid disease, or diabetes, unless d rected by a physician.
Do not exceed recommended dosag If nervousness, dizziness or sleeplessne occur, discontinue use and consult a ph sician. A persistent cough may be a sig of a serious condition. If cough or othe symptoms persist, do not improve withi 7 days, tend to recur, or are accompanie by fever, rash, or persistent headach consult a physician

Drug Interaction Precaution: Do n give this product to a child who is takin a prescription monoamine oxidase inhil itor (MAOI) (certain drugs for depre sion, psychiatric or emotional cond tions), or for 2 weeks after stopping th MAOI drug. If you are uncertai whether your child's prescription dru contains an MAOI, consult a health pr fessional before giving this product.
KEEP THIS AND ALL DRUGS OUT O THE REACH OF CHILDREN. IN CAS OF ACCIDENTAL OVERDOSE, SEE PROFESSIONAL ASSISTANCE O CONTACT A POISON CONTROL CEN TER IMMEDIATELY.

Directions: Follow recommended do age below or use as directed by a docto Repeat every 4 hours. Do Not Exceed Doses in a 24-Hour Period.

Dosage: Choose by weight. (If weight not known, choose by age):

Age	Weight	Dose
Under 2 yrs.	Under 24 lbs.	Consul doctor
2–under 6 yrs.	24–47 lbs.	2.5 mL

Store at Controlled Room Temperatur between 20°C and 25°C (68°F and 77°F)

How Supplied: 1 oz bottle with dosing syringe.

J.B. Williams Company, Inc.

65 HARRISTOWN ROAD
GLEN ROCK, NJ 07452

Address Inquiries to:
Consumer Affairs: (800) 254-8656
(201) 251-8100
FAX: (201) 251-8097

For Medical Emergency Contact:
(800) 254-8656

CĒPACOL®/CĒPACOL MINT
[sē ′pə-cŏl]
Antiseptic Mouthwash/Gargle

Ingredients: Cēpacol Antiseptic Mouthwash: Ceepryn® (cetylpyridinium chloride) 0.05%. Also contains: Alcohol 14%, Edetate Disodium, FD&C Yellow No. 5 (tartrazine) as a color additive, Flavors, Glycerin, Polysorbate 80, Saccharin, Sodium Biphosphate, Sodium Phosphate, and Water.
Cēpacol Antiseptic Mint Mouthwash: Ceepryn® (cetylpyridinium chloride) 0.05%. Also contains: Alcohol 14.5%, D&C Yellow No. 10, FD&C Green No. 3, Flavor, Glucono Delta-Lactone, Glycerin, Poloxamer 407, Saccharin Sodium, Sodium Gluconate, and Water.

Actions: Cēpacol/Cēpacol Mint is an effective antiseptic mouthwash/gargle. It kills germs that cause bad breath for a fresher, cleaner mouth.
Cēpacol/Cēpacol Mint has a low surface tension, approximately ½ that of water. This property is the basis of the spreading action in the oral cavity as well as its foaming action. Cēpacol/Cēpacol Mint leaves the mouth feeling fresh and clean and helps provide soothing, temporary relief of dryness and minor mouth irritations.

Uses: Recommended as a mouthwash and gargle for daily oral care; as an aromatic mouth freshener to provide a clean feeling in the mouth; as a soothing, foaming rinse to freshen the mouth.
Used routinely before dental procedures, helps give patient confidence of not offending with mouth odor. Often employed as a foaming and refreshing rinse before, during, and after instrumentation and dental prophylaxis. Convenient as a mouth-freshening agent after taking dental impressions. Helpful in reducing the unpleasant taste and odor in the mouth following gingivectomy.
Used in hospitals as a mouthwash and gargle for daily oral care. Also used to refresh and soothe the mouth following emesis, inhalation therapy, and intubations, and for swabbing the mouths of patients incapable of personal care.

Warning: In case of accidental ingestion seek professional assistance or contact a poison control center immediately. Do not use in children under 6 years of age. Children over 6 should be supervised when using Cēpacol. Keep out of reach of children.

Directions: Rinse vigorously before or after brushing or any time to freshen the mouth. Cēpacol/Cēpacol Mint leaves the mouth feeling refreshingly clean.
Use full strength every two or three hours as a soothing, foaming gargle, or as directed by a physician or dentist. May also be mixed with warm water.
Product label directions are as follows: Rinse or gargle full strength before or after brushing or as directed by a physician or dentist.

How Supplied: Cēpacol/Cēpacol Mint Antiseptic Mouthwash: 12 oz, 24 oz, and 32 oz. 4 oz trial size.

Shown in Product Identification Guide, page 527

CĒPACOL® Maximum Strength Sore Throat Spray; Cherry and Cool Menthol Flavors.

Ingredients:
Cherry: Active Ingredient: Dyclonine Hydrochloride 0.1%. Also contains: Cetylpyridinium Chloride, D&C Red No. 33, Dibasic Sodium Phosphate, FD&C Yellow No. 6, Flavors, Glycerin, Phosphoric Acid, Poloxamer, Potassium Sorbate, Sorbitol, and Water.
Cool Menthol: Active Ingredient: Dyclonine Hydrochloride 0.1%. Also contains: Cetylpyridinium Chloride, Dibasic Sodium Phosphate, FD&C Blue No. 1, Flavors, Glycerin, Phosphoric Acid, Poloxamer, Potassium Sorbate, Polysorbate 20, Sodium Saccharin, Sorbitol and Water.

Indications: For temporary relief of occasional minor sore throat pain and sore mouth. Also, for temporary relief of pain due to canker sores, minor irritation or injury to the mouth and gums, minor dental procedures, dentures or orthodontic appliances.

Directions: Adults: Spray 4 times into throat or affected area (children 2 to 12 years of age: spray 2–3 times) and swallow. Repeat as needed up to 4 times daily or as directed by a physician or dentist. Children 2 to 12 years of age should be supervised in product use. Children under 2 years: Consult physician or dentist.

Warnings: If sore throat is severe, persists for more than 2 days, is accompanied or followed by fever, headache, rash, nausea, or vomiting, consult a physician promptly. If sore mouth symptoms do not improve in 7 days, or if irritation, pain, or redness persists or worsens, see your dentist or physician promptly. Do not exceed recommended dosage. Keep this and all drugs out of the reach of children. In case of accidental overdose, seek professional assistance or contact a Poison Control Center immediately. As with any drug, if you are pregnant or nursing a baby, seek the advice of a health professional before using this product.
Store at room temperature. Do not freeze.

How Supplied: Available in Cherry and Cool Menthol flavors in 4 fl. oz. (118 mL) plastic bottles with pump sprayer.

Shown in Product Identification Guide, page 527

CĒPACOL®
[sē ′pə-cŏl]
Sore Throat Lozenges
Regular Strength Original Mint,
Regular Strength Cherry,
Maximum Strength Mint,
Maximum Strength Cherry.
Oral Anesthetic

Ingredients: (per lozenge)

Regular Strength Original Mint: Active Ingredient: Menthol 2 mg. Also contains: Cetylpyridinium Chloride (Ceepryn®), D&C Yellow No. 10, FD&C Yellow No. 6, Flavor, Glucose, and Sucrose.

Regular Strength Cherry: Active Ingredient: Menthol 3.6 mg. Also contains: Cetylpyridinium Chloride (Ceepryn®), D&C Red No. 33, FD&C Red No. 40, Flavor, Glucose, and Sucrose.

Maximum Strength Mint: Active Ingredients: Benzocaine 10 mg., Menthol 2 mg. Also contains: Cetylpyridinium Chloride (Ceepryn®), D&C Yellow No. 10, FD&C Yellow No. 6, Flavor, Glucose, and Sucrose.

Maximum Strength Cherry: Active Ingredients: Benzocaine 10 mg., Menthol 3.6 mg. Also contains: Cetylpyridinium Chloride (Ceepryn®), D&C Red No. 33, FD&C Red No. 40, Flavor, Glucose, and Sucrose.

Actions: Menthol provides a mild anesthetic effect and cooling sensation for symptomatic relief of occasional minor sore throat pain and minor throat irritations. Benzocaine in the Maximum Strength lozenges provides an anesthetic effect for additional symptomatic relief of minor sore throat pain.

Indications: For temporary relief of occasional minor sore throat pain and dry, scratchy throat.

Warnings: If sore throat is severe, persists for more than 2 days, is accompanied or followed by fever, headache, rash, nausea, or vomiting, consult a physician promptly. Do not administer to children under 6 years of age unless directed by physician or dentist. Keep this and all drugs out of the reach of children. In case of accidental overdose, seek professional assistance or contact a Poison Control Center immediately. As with any drug, if you are pregnant or nursing a baby, seek the advice of a health professional before using this product.

Continued on next page

J.B. Williams—Cont.

Directions: Adults and children 6 years of age and older: Dissolve 1 lozenge in the mouth every 2 hours as needed or as directed by a physician or dentist. For children under 6 years, consult a physician or dentist.

How Supplied:

Trade package:
18 lozenges in 2 pocket packs of 9 each.

Institutional package: Regular Strength Original Mint and Maximum Strength Mint: 648 lozenges in 72 blisters of 9 each.
Store at room temperature, below 86°F (30°C). Protect contents from humidity.

Shown in Product Identification Guide, page 527

The Winning Combination

For product information, please see **AML Laboratories**

Wyeth-Ayerst Laboratories

Division of American Home Products Corporation
P.O. BOX 8299
PHILADELPHIA, PA 19101

Direct General Inquiries to:
(610) 688-4400

For Professional Services
(For example: Sales representative information, product pamphlets, educational materials):
800-395-9938

For Medical Product Information Contact:
Medical Affairs
Day: (800) 934-5556 (8:30 AM to 4:30 PM, Eastern Standard Time, Weekdays only)
Night: (610) 688-4400 (Emergencies only; non-emergencies should wait until the next day)

Wyeth-Ayerst Tamper-Resistant/Evident Packaging

Statements alerting consumers to the specific type of Tamper-Resistant/Evident Packaging appear on the bottle labels and cartons of all Wyeth-Ayerst over-the-counter products. This includes plastic cap seals on bottles, individually wrapped tablets or suppositories, and sealed cartons. This packaging has been developed to better protect the consumer.

AMPHOJEL®

[am 'fo-jel]
Antacid
(aluminum hydroxide gel)
ORAL SUSPENSION • TABLETS

Composition: *Suspension—Peppermint flavored* —Each teaspoonful (5 mL) contains 320 mg aluminum hydroxide [Al$(OH)_3$] as a gel, and not more than 0.10 mEq of sodium. The inactive ingredients present are calcium benzoate, glycerin, hydroxypropyl methylcellulose, menthol, peppermint oil, potassium butylparaben, potassium propylparaben, saccharin, simethicone, sorbitol solution, and water. *Suspension—Without flavor* —Each teaspoonful (5 mL) contains 320 mg of aluminum hydroxide [Al $(OH)_3$] as a gel. The inactive ingredients present are butylparaben, calcium benzoate, glycerin, hydroxypropyl methylcellulose, methylparaben, propylparaben, saccharin, simethicone, sorbitol solution, and water. *Tablets* are available in 0.3 and 0.6 g strengths. Each contains, respectively, the equivalent of 300 mg and 600 mg aluminum hydroxide as a dried gel. The inactive ingredients present are artificial and natural flavors, cellulose, hydrogenated vegetable oil, magnesium stearate, polacrilin potassium, saccharin, starch, and talc. The 0.3 g (5 grain) strength is equivalent to about 1 teaspoonful of the suspension and the 0.6 g (10 grain) strength is equivalent to about 2 teaspoonfuls. Each 0.3 g tablet contains 0.08 mEq of sodium and each 0.6 g tablet contains 0.13 mEq of sodium.

Indications: For temporary relief of heartburn, upset stomach, sour stomach, and/or acid indigestion.

Directions: *Suspension* —Two teaspoonfuls (10 ml) to be taken five or six times daily, between meals and on retiring or as directed by a physician. Medication may be followed by a sip of water if desired. *Tablets* —Two tablets of the 0.3 g strength, or one tablet of the 0.6 g strength, five or six times daily, between meals and on retiring or as directed by a physician. It is unnecessary to chew the 0.3 g tablet before swallowing with water. After chewing the 0.6 g tablet, sip about one-half glass of water.

Warnings: Do not take more than 12 teaspoonfuls (60 ml) of suspension, or more than twelve (12) 0.3 g tablets, or more than six (6) 0.6 g tablets in a 24-hour period or use this maximum dosage for more than two weeks except under the advice and supervision of a physician. May cause constipation. Prolonged use of aluminum-containing antacids in patients with renal failure may result in or worsen dialysis osteomalacia. Elevated tissue aluminum levels contribute to the development of dialysis encephalopathy and osteomalacia syndromes. Also, a number of cases of dialysis encephalopathy have been associated with elevated aluminum levels in the dialysate water. Small amounts of aluminum are absorbed from the gastrointestinal tract and renal excretion of aluminum is impaired in renal failure. Prolonged use of aluminum-containing antacids in such patients may contribute to increased plasma levels of aluminum. Aluminum is not well removed by dialysis because it is bound to albumin and transferrin, which do not cross dialysis membranes. As a result, aluminum is deposited in bone and dialysis osteomalacia may develop when large amounts of aluminum are ingested orally by patients with impaired renal function. As with any drug, if you are pregnant or nursing a baby, seek the advice of a health professional before using this product.

Drug Interaction Precaution: Antacids may interact with certain prescription drugs. Do not use this product if you are presently taking a prescription antibiotic containing any form of tetracycline. If you are presently taking a prescription drug, do not take this product without checking with your physician.
Keep tightly closed and store at room temperature, Approx. 77°F (25°C).
Suspension should be shaken well before use. Avoid freezing.
Keep this and all drugs out of the reach of children.

How Supplied: *Suspension* —Peppermint flavored; without flavor—bottles of 12 fluidounces. *Tablets* —a convenient auxiliary dosage form—0.3 g (5 grain) bottles of 100; 0.6 g (10 grain), boxes of 100.

Shown in Product Identification Guide, page 527

Professional Labeling: Consult *199[illegible] Physicians' Desk Reference.*

BASALJEL®

[bā 'sel-jel]
(basic aluminum carbonate gel)
ORAL SUSPENSION • CAPSULES • TABLETS

Composition: *Suspension* —each 5 ml teaspoonful contains basic aluminum carbonate gel equivalent to 400 mg aluminum hydroxide [$Al(OH)_3$]. The inactive ingredients present are artificial and natural flavors, butylparaben, calcium benzoate, glycerin, hydroxypropyl methylcellulose, methylparaben, mineral oil, propylparaben, saccharin, simethicone, sorbitol solution, and water. *Capsule* contains dried basic aluminum carbonate gel equivalent to 608 mg of dried aluminum hydroxide gel or 500 mg aluminum hydroxide [$Al(OH)_3$]. The inactive ingredients present are D&C Yellow 10, FD&C Blue 1, FD&C Red 40, FD&C Yellow 6, gelatin, polacrilin potassium, polyethylene glycol, talc, and titanium dioxide. *Tablet* contains dried basic aluminum carbonate gel equivalent to 608 mg of dried aluminum hydroxide gel or 500 mg aluminum hydroxide. The inactive ingredients present are cellulose, hydrogenated vegetable oil, magnesium stearate, polacrilin potassium, starch and talc.

Indications: For the symptomatic relief of hyperacidity, associated with the diagnosis of peptic ulcer, gastritis, peptic esophagitis, gastric hyperacidity, and hiatal hernia.

Warnings: Do not take more than 24 tablets/capsules/teaspoonsful of BASALJEL in a 24-hour period, or use this maximum dosage for more than two weeks except under the advice and supervision of a physician. Dosage should be carefully supervised since continued overdosage, in conjunction with restriction of dietary phosphorus and calcium, may produce a persistently lowered serum phosphate and a mildly elevated alkaline phosphatase. A usually transient hypercalciuria of mild degree may be associated with the early weeks of therapy. Prolonged use of aluminum-containing antacids in patients with renal failure may result in or worsen dialysis osteomalacia. Elevated tissue aluminum levels contribute to the development of dialysis encephalopathy and osteomalacia syndromes. Also, a number of cases of dialysis encephalopathy have been associated with elevated aluminum levels in the dialysate water. Small amounts of aluminum are absorbed from the gastrointestinal tract and renal excretion of aluminum is impaired in renal failure. Prolonged use of aluminum-containing antacids in such patients may contribute to increased plasma levels of aluminum. Aluminum is not well removed by dialysis because it is bound to albumin and transferrin, which do not cross dialysis membranes. As a result, aluminum is deposited in bone, and dialysis osteomalacia may develop when large amounts of aluminum are ingested orally by patients with impaired renal function. As with any drug, if you are pregnant or nursing a baby, seek the advice of a health professional before using this product.

Dosage and Administration: *Suspension* —two teaspoonsful (10 mL) in water or fruit juice taken as often as every two hours up to twelve times daily. Two teaspoonsful have the capacity to neutralize 23 mEq of acid. *Capsules* —two capsules as often as every two hours up to twelve times daily. Two capsules have the capacity to neutralize 24 mEq of acid. *Tablets* —two tablets as often as every two hours up to twelve times daily. Two tablets have the capacity to neutralize 25 mEq of acid. The sodium content of each dosage form is as follows: 0.13 mEq/5 mL for the suspension, 0.12 mEq per capsule, and 0.12 mEq per tablet.

Precautions: May cause constipation. Adequate fluid intake should be maintained in addition to the specific medical or surgical management indicated by the patient's condition.

Drug Interaction Precaution: Alumina-containing antacids should not be used concomitantly with any form of tetracycline therapy.

How Supplied: Suspension—bottles of 12 fluidounces.
Capsules—bottles of 100 and 500.
Tablets (scored)—bottles of 100.

Shown in Product Identification Guide, page 527

Professional Labeling: Consult *1997 Physicians' Desk Reference.*

CEROSE®DM

[se-ros 'DM]

Antihistamine/Nasal Decongestant/ Cough Suppressant

Description: Each teaspoonful (5 mL) contains 15 mg dextromethorphan hydrobromide, 4 mg chlorpheniramine maleate, and 10 mg phenylephrine hydrochloride. Alcohol 2.4%. The inactive ingredients present are artificial flavors, citric acid, edetate disodium, FD&C Yellow 6, glycerin, saccharin sodium, sodium benzoate, sodium citrate, sodium propionate, and water.

Indications: For the temporary relief of cough due to minor throat and bronchial irritation as may occur with the common cold or with inhaled irritants. Temporarily relieves nasal congestion, runny nose, and sneezing due to the common cold, hay fever, or other upper respiratory allergies.

Directions: Adults and children 12 years of age and over: One teaspoonful every four hours as needed. Children 6 to under 12 years of age: One-half teaspoonful every four hours as needed. Do not exceed six doses in a 24-hour period. Consult a physician for use in children under 6 years of age.

Warnings: May cause marked drowsiness; alcohol, sedatives, and tranquilizers may increase the drowsiness effect. Avoid alcoholic beverages while taking this product. Do not take this product if you are taking sedatives or tranquilizers, without first asking your doctor. Use caution when driving a motor vehicle or operating machinery. May cause excitability, especially in children. Do not take this product if you have heart disease, high blood pressure, thyroid disease, diabetes, a breathing problem such as emphysema or chronic bronchitis, glaucoma, or difficulty in urination due to enlargement of the prostate gland unless directed by a doctor. Do not take this product for persistent or chronic cough such as occurs with smoking, asthma, or emphysema, or if cough is accompanied by excessive phlegm (mucus) unless directed by a doctor. A persistent cough may be a sign of a serious condition. If cough or other symptoms persist for more than one week without improvement, tend to recur, or are accompanied by fever, rash, or persistent headache, consult a doctor. **Do not exceed recommended dosage.** If nervousness, dizziness, or sleeplessness occur, discontinue use and consult a doctor. As with any drug, if you are pregnant or nursing a baby, seek the advice of a health professional before using this product.
Keep this and all drugs out of the reach of children. In case of accidental overdose, seek professional assistance or contact a Poison Control Center immediately.

Drug Interaction Precaution: Do not use this product if you are now taking a prescription monoamine oxidase inhibitor (MAOI) (certain drugs for depression, psychiatric or emotional conditions, or Parkinson's disease), or for 2 weeks after stopping the MAOI drug. If you are uncertain whether your prescription drug contains an MAOI, consult a health professional before taking this product.

How Supplied: Cases of 12 bottles of 4 fl. oz.; bottles of 1 pint.
Keep tightly closed—Store at room temperature, below 77° F (25° C).

Shown in Product Identification Guide, page 527

DONNAGEL®

[don 'nă-jel]

Liquid and Chewable Tablets

Each tablespoon (15 mL) of **Donnagel Liquid** contains: 600 mg Attapulgite, Activated, USP.

Inactive Ingredients: Alcohol 1.4%, Benzyl Alcohol, Carboxymethylcellulose Sodium, Citric Acid, FD&C Blue 1, Flavors, Magnesium Aluminum Silicate, Methylparaben, Phosphoric Acid, Propylene Glycol, Propylparaben, Saccharin Sodium, Sorbitol, Titanium Dioxide, Water, Xanthan Gum.

Each **Donnagel Chewable** Tablet contains: 600 mg Attapulgite, Activated, USP.

Inactive Ingredients: D&C Yellow 10 Aluminum Lake, FD&C Blue 1 Aluminum Lake, Flavors, Magnesium Stearate, Mannitol, Saccharin Sodium, Sorbitol, Water.

Indications: Donnagel is indicated for the symptomatic relief of diarrhea. It reduces the number of bowel movements, improves consistency of loose, watery bowel movements and relieves cramping.

DONNAGEL®	Liquid	Chewable Tablets
Adults	2 Tablespoons	2 Tablets
Children		
12 years and over	2 Tablespoons	2 Tablets
6 to under 12 years	1 Tablespoon	1 Tablet
3 to under 6 years	½ Tablespoon	½ Tablet
Under 3 years	Consult Physician	

Liquid should be shaken well. Tablets should be chewed thoroughly and swallowed.

Continued on next page

Wyeth-Ayerst—Cont.

Warnings: Patients are told that diarrhea may be serious. They are warned not to use this product for more than 2 days, or in the presence of fever, or in children under 3 years of age unless directed by a doctor.
This product should not be taken by patients who are hypersensitive to any of the ingredients. As with any drug, women who are pregnant or nursing a baby should seek the advice of a health professional before using this product.
KEEP THIS AND ALL DRUGS OUT OF THE REACH OF CHILDREN. IN CASE OF ACCIDENTAL OVERDOSE, SEEK PROFESSIONAL ASSISTANCE OR CONTACT A POISON CONTROL CENTER IMMEDIATELY.

Dosage and Administration: Full recommended dose should be administered at the first sign of diarrhea and after each subsequent bowel movement, NOT TO EXCEED 7 DOSES IN A 24-HOUR PERIOD.
[See table on bottom of preceding page.]

How Supplied: Donnagel Liquid (green suspension) in 4 fl. oz. (NDC 0008-0888-02), and 8 fl. oz. (NDC 0008-0888-04).
Donnagel Chewable Tablets (light-green, flat-faced, beveled-edged, round tablets with darker green flecks; one side engraved "W", obverse engraved Donnagel) in consumer blister packages of 18 (NDC 0008-0889-02.)
Store at controlled room temperature, between 20°C and 25°C (68°F and 77°F).

Shown in Product Identification Guide, page 527

Zila Pharmaceuticals, Inc.

**5227 NORTH 7th STREET
PHOENIX, AZ 85014-2800**

Direct Inquiries to:
Jerry Kaster,
Director of Marketing:
(602) 266-6700
World Wide Web Address
www.zila.com

ZILACTIN® Medicated Gel
ZILACTIN®-L Liquid
ZILACTIN®-B Medicated Gel with Benzocaine

Description: **Zilactin** Medicated Gel stops pain and speeds healing of canker sores, fever blisters and cold sores. Zilactin forms a tenacious, occlusive film which holds the medication in place while controlling pain. Intra-orally, the film can last up to 6 hours, usually allowing pain-free eating and drinking. Extra-orally, the film will last much longer.

Zilactin-L is a non film-forming liquid that treats and relieves the pain, itching and burning of developing and existing cold sores and fever blisters. Zilactin-L is specially formulated to treat the initial signs of tingling, itching or burning that signal an oncoming cold sore or fever blister. Zilactin-L can often prevent developing cold sores or fever blisters from breaking out. If a lesion does occur, Zilactin-L will significantly reduce the size and the duration of the outbreak.

Zilactin-B is a medicated gel containing benzocaine that forms a smooth, flexible and occlusive film on the oral mucosa. It's specially formulated to control pain and shield the mouth sores, canker sores, cheek bites and gum sores that occur from dental appliances from the environment of the mouth. The film can last up to 6 hours.

Clinical studies on the effectiveness of Zila's products are available on request.

Active Ingredients: Zilactin—Benzyl Alcohol (10%); **Zilactin-L**—Lidocaine (2.5%); **Zilactin-B**—Benzocaine (10%);

Application: Zilactin: FOR USE IN THE MOUTH AND ON LIPS. Apply every four hours for the first three days and then as needed. Dry the affected area. Apply a thin coat of Zilactin and allow 60 seconds for the gel to dry into a film. Outside the mouth, Zilactin forms a transparent film. Inside the mouth, the film is white.

Zilactin-L: FOR USE ON THE LIPS AND AROUND THE MOUTH. Apply every 1-2 hours for the first three days and then as needed. For maximum effectiveness use at first signs of tingling or itching. Moisten a cotton swab with several drops of Zilactin-L. Apply on lip area where symptoms are noted or directly on existing cold sore or fever blister and allow to dry for 15 seconds.

Zilactin-B: FOR USE IN THE MOUTH. Apply every four hours for the first three days and then as needed. Dry the affected area. Apply a thin coat of Zilactin-B and allow 60 seconds for the gel to dry into a film.

Warning: A mild, temporary stinging sensation may be experienced when applying Zilactin, Zilactin-L or Zilactin-B to an open cut, sore or blister. This may be minimized by first applying ice for a minute before application of the medication. DO NOT USE IN OR NEAR EYES. In the event of accidental contact with the eye, flush with water immediately and continuously for ten minutes. Seek immediate medical attention if pain or irritation persists. For temporary relief only. As with all medications, keep out of the reach of children. Do not use Zilactin-L or Zilactin-B if you have a history of allergy to local anesthetics such as benzocaine, lidocaine or other "caine" anesthetics.

How Supplied: Zila products are nonprescription and carried by most drug wholesalers, retail chains and independent pharmacies. Each product is available to physicians and dentists directly from Zila in single use packages.
For further information call or write:

Zila Pharmaceuticals, Inc.
5227 N. 7th Street, Phoenix, AZ 85014-2800, (602) 266-6700

U.S. patent numbers 4,285,934; 4,381,296; and 5,081,158

Shown in Product Identification Guide, page 528

EDUCATIONAL MATERIAL

Samples and literature are available to medical professionals on request.

ZP Tech Inc.

**12803 SCHABARUM AVE.
IRWINDALE, CA 91706**

Direct Inquiries to:
(800) 636-6289
(818) 337-4700
FAX: (818) 338-7676

BIO-NOVA™ *Ginkgo*
Maximum Strength Ginkgo Biloba Extract (60 mg/tablet)
[*Gin-ko Bi-lo-ba*]

A Daily supplement for Best Mental Performance produced only from Premium Standardized Ginkgo Biloba Extract (50:1).
Recent medical studies indicate **BIO-NOVA™ *Ginkgo*** to be a safe and natural supplement which promotes optimum brain performance in the areas of memory, cognition and concentration. **BIO-NOVA™ *Ginkgo*** uses only the highest quality standard Ginkgo Biloba Extract in the world to guarantee these unique functions.

Active Ingredients: Each tablet contains 60 mg of concentrated (50:1) Ginkgo Biloba Extract, which is standardized to 24% Ginkgo flavonoid glycosides and 6% terpene lactones in their proven ratios.
Also Contains: Dicalcium phosphate, Cellulose, Stearic Acid, Croscarmelose Sodium, Magnesium Stearate, Riboflavin, Titanium Dioxide, Yellow #6, Blue #2, Hydroxypropyl Methylcellulose and Polyethylene Glycol.

Suggested Use: When taken as directed, **BIO-NOVA™ *Ginkgo*** provides a natural alternative to stimulate circulation and oxygen flow to the brain resulting in the inhibiting of memory loss, improving concentration and enhancing mental focus.
Recommended Adult Intake: Adults and children over 12 years of age should take one tablet twice daily, swallowed whole, with water at mealtimes. Take consistently for optimum benefits. Not recommended for children under 12 years of age.

Cautions: Please keep this product out of the reach of children. If you are taking prescription medication, or are pregnant or lactating, consult your physician before taking **BIO-NOVA™** ***Ginkgo.***

These statements have not been evaluated by the Food and Drug Administration. This product is not intended to diagnose, treat, cure or prevent any disease.

Store at room temperature; avoid high humidity and excessive heat above 40°C (104°F) to maintain optimum potency and freshness.

Shown in Product Identification Guide, page 528

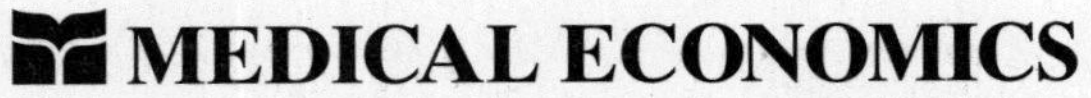

STATE BOARDS OF PHARMACY

Questions on local regulations governing prescription and over-the-counter drugs, controlled substances, and pharmacy licensure can often be answered by your local state board of pharmacy. For your convenience, a contact name, address, and phone number for each state board is listed in the directory that follows.

ALABAMA
Jerry Moore, R.Ph.
Executive Secretary
1 Perimeter Park S.
Suite 425 S
Birmingham, AL 35243
205-967-0130
Fax: 205-967-1009

ALASKA
Josephine Dawson
Licensing Examiner
Department of
Commerce and
Economic Development
Juneau, AK 99811
907-465-2589
Fax: 907-465-2974

ARIZONA
L.A. Lloyd, R.Ph.
Executive Director
5060 N. 19th Ave.
Suite 101
Phoenix, AZ 85015
602-255-5125
Fax: 602-255-5740

ARKANSAS
John T. Douglas, P.D.
Executive Director
101 E. Capitol Ave.
Suite 218
Little Rock, AR 72201
501-682-0190
Fax: 501-682-0195

CALIFORNIA
Patricia Harris
Executive Officer
400 "R" St., Suite 4070
Sacramento, CA 95814
916-445-5014
Fax: 916-327-6308

COLORADO
W. Kent Mount
Program Administrator
1560 Broadway
Suite 1310
Denver, CO 80202
303-894-7750—ext. 313
Fax: 303-894-7764

CONNECTICUT
Margherita R. Giuliano, R.Ph.
Board Administrator
State Office Building
Room 110
165 Capitol Avenue
Hartford, CT 06106
203-566-3290
Fax: 203-566-7630

DELAWARE
David W. Dryden, R.Ph., Esq.
Executive Secretary
P.O. Box 637
Dover, DE 19903
302-739-4798
Fax: 302-739-3071

DISTRICT OF COLUMBIA
Barbara Hagans
Contact Representative
614 "H" St., NW
Room 923
Washington, DC 20001
202-727-7832
Fax: 202-727-7662

FLORIDA
John D. Taylor, R.Ph.
Executive Director
Agency for Health Care Administration
Board of Pharmacy
1940 N. Monroe St.
Tallahassee, FL 32399
904-488-7546
Fax: 904-921-7865

GEORGIA
Gregg W. Schuder
Executive Director
166 Pryor St. SW
Atlanta, GA 30303
404-656-3912
Fax: 404-657-4220

HAWAII
Ruth Gushiken
Executive Officer
P.O. Box 3469
Honolulu, HI 96801
808-586-2698

IDAHO
R.K. Markuson, R.Ph.
Director
P.O. Box 83720
Boise, ID 83720-0067
208-334-2356
Fax: 208-334-3536

ILLINOIS
Ed Duffy, R.Ph.
Executive Administrator
Drug Compliance
Illinois Department of
Professional Regulation
100 W. Randolph
Suite 9-300
Chicago, IL 60601
312-814-4573
Fax: 312-814-3145

INDIANA
Frances L. Kelly
Director
402 W. Washington St.
Room 041
Indianapolis, IN 46204
317-232-2960
Fax: 317-233-4236

IOWA
Lloyd K. Jessen, R.Ph., J.D.
Exec. Sec./Director
1209 East Court Ave.
Executive Hills West
Des Moines, IA 50319
515-281-5944
Fax: 515-281-4609

KANSAS
Larry Froelich
Director
900 Jackson St.
Room 513
Topeka, KS 66612-1231
913-296-4056
Fax: 913-296-8420

KENTUCKY
Michael A. Moné, R.Ph., J.D.
Executive Director
1024 Capital Center Dr.
Suite 210
Frankfort, KY 40601
502-573-1580
Fax: 502-573-1582

LOUISIANA
Howard B. Bolton, R.Ph.
Executive Director
5615 Corporate Blvd., 8E
Baton Rouge, LA
70808-2537
504-925-6496
Fax: 504-925-6499

MAINE
Susan Greenlaw
Board Clerk
Department of
Professional and
Financial Regulation
35 State House Station
Augusta, ME 04333
207-624-8603
Fax: 207-624-8637

MARYLAND
Norene Pease
Executive Director
4201 Patterson Ave.
Baltimore, MD 21215
410-764-4755
Fax: 410-358-6207

MASSACHUSETTS
Lori Bassinger
Executive Director
100 Cambridge St.
Room 1514
Boston, MA 02202
617-727-0085
Fax: 617-727-2197

MICHIGAN
Sheldon Rich, R.Ph.
Chairman
611 W. Ottawa St.
P.O. Box 30018
Lansing, MI 48909
517-373-9102
Fax: 517-373-2179

MINNESOTA
David E. Holmstrom, R.Ph., J.D.
Executive Director
2829 University Ave. SE
Suite 530
Minneapolis, MN 55414
612-617-2201
Fax: 612-617-2212

MISSISSIPPI
William L. Stevens
Executive Director
P.O. Box 24507
C & F Plaza, Suite D
Jackson, MS 39225
601-354-6750
Fax: 601-354-6071

MISSOURI
Kevin E. Kinkade, R.Ph.
Executive Director
P.O. Box 625
Jefferson City, MO 65102
573-751-0093
Fax: 573-526-3464

MONTANA
Warren R. Amole, R.Ph.
Executive Director
111 N. Last Chance Gulch
Helena, MT 59620
406-444-1698
Fax: 406-444-1667

NEBRASKA
Katherine A. Brown
Executive Secretary
Board of Examiners in Pharmacy
P.O. Box 94986
Lincoln, NE 68509-4986
402-471-2118
Fax: 402-471-3577

NEVADA
Keith W. MacDonald, R.Ph.
Executive Secretary
1201 Terminal Way
Suite 212
Reno, NV 89502-3257
702-322-0691
Fax: 702-322-0895

NEW HAMPSHIRE
Paul G. Boisseau, R.Ph.
Executive Director
57 Regional Dr.
Concord, NH 03301
603-271-2350
Fax: 603-271-2856

NEW JERSEY
H. Lee Gladstein, R.Ph.
Executive Director
124 Halsey St., 6th Floor
Newark, NJ 07102
201-504-6450
Fax: 201-648-3355

NEW MEXICO
Richard W. Thompson
Executive Director
1650 University Blvd. NE
Suite 400-B
Albuquerque, NM 87102
505-841-9102
Fax: 505-841-9113

NEW YORK
Lawrence H. Mokhiber, R.Ph.
Executive Secretary
Cultural Education Center
Room 3035
Albany, NY 12230
518-474-3848
Fax: 518-473-6995

NORTH CAROLINA
David R. Work, R.Ph.
Executive Director
P.O. Box 459
Carrboro, NC 27510
919-942-4454
Fax: 919-967-5757

NORTH DAKOTA
William J. Grosz, Sc.D., R.Ph.
Executive Director
P.O. Box 1354
Bismarck, ND 58502
701-328-9535
Fax: 701-258-9312

OHIO
Franklin Z. Wickham, R.Ph.
Executive Director
77 S. High St., 17th Floor
Columbus, OH 43266
614-466-4143
Fax: 614-752-4836

OKLAHOMA
Bryan Potter, R.Ph.
Executive Director
4545 N. Lincoln Blvd.
Suite 112
Oklahoma City, OK 73105
405-521-3815
Fax: 405-521-3758

OREGON
Ruth Vandever, R.Ph.
Executive Director
State Office Bldg.
Suite 425
800 NE Oregon St., #9
Portland, OR 97232
503-731-4032
Fax: 503-731-4067

PENNSYLVANIA
W. Richard Marshman, R.Ph.
Executive Secretary
P.O. Box 2649
Harrisburg, PA 17105
717-783-7157
Fax: 717-787-7769

PUERTO RICO
Giselle Rivera, R.Ph., Pharm.D.
President
Call Box 10200
Santurce, PR 00908
809-725-8161
Fax: 809-725-7903

RHODE ISLAND
Mario Casinelli, Jr., R.Ph.
Chairman of the Board
Department of Health
Div. of Drug Control
Three Capitol Hill
Room 304
Providence, RI 02908
401-277-2837
Fax: 401-277-2499

SOUTH CAROLINA
Lynn J. Verzwyvelt, R.Ph.
Interim Administrator
P.O. Box 11927
Columbia, SC 29211
803-734-1010
Fax: 803-734-1552

SOUTH DAKOTA
Galen Jordre, R.Ph.
Secretary
P.O. Box 518
Pierre, SD 57501-0518
605-224-2338
Fax: 605-224-1280

TENNESSEE
Kendall M. Lynch
Director
500 James Robertson Pkwy.
Nashville, TN 37243
615-741-2718
Fax: 615-741-2722

TEXAS

Fred S. Brinkley, Jr., R.Ph.
Executive Director
333 Guadalupe
Suite 3-600, Box 21
Austin, TX 78701-3942
512-305-8001
Fax: 512-305-8075

UTAH

J. Craig Jackson
Director
Utah Department of Commerce
P.O. Box 146741
Salt Lake City, UT 84114
801-530-6628
Fax: 801-530-6511

VERMONT

Carla Preston
Staff Assistant
109 State St.
Montpelier, VT 05609
802-828-2875
Fax: 802-828-2496

VIRGINIA

Elizabeth Scott Russell, R.Ph.
Executive Director
6606 W. Broad St.
4th Floor
Richmond, VA 23230
804-662-9911
Fax: 804-662-9313

WASHINGTON

Donald H. Williams, R.Ph.
Executive Director
P.O. Box 47863
Olympia, WA 98504
360-753-6834
Fax: 360-586-4359

WEST VIRGINIA

Sam Kapourales, R.Ph.
President
236 Capitol St.
Charleston, WV 25301
304-558-0558
Fax: 304-558-0572

WISCONSIN

Patrick D. Braatz
Administrator
P.O. Box 8935
Madison, WI 53708
608-266-2811
Fax: 608-267-0644

WYOMING

Marilynn H. Mitchell, R.Ph.
Executive Director
1720 S. Poplar St., Suite 5
Casper, WY 82601
307-234-0294
Fax: 307-234-7226

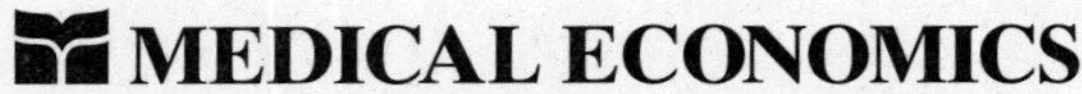
MEDICAL ECONOMICS

POISON CONTROL CENTERS

Many centers in this directory are certified members of the American Association of Poison Control Centers (AAPCC). Certified centers are marked by an asterisk after the name. They must meet certain criteria: for example, serve a large geographic area; be open 24 hours a day and provide direct dialing or toll-free access; be supervised by a medical director; and have registered pharmacists or nurses available to answer questions from healthcare professionals and the public.

Centers in each state are listed alphabetically by city. "TTY" numbers are reserved for the hearing impaired, and "TTD" numbers reach a telecommunication device for the deaf.

ALABAMA

BIRMINGHAM

Regional Poison Control Center Children's Hospital of Alabama (*)
1600 7th Ave. South
Birmingham, AL 35233-1711
Business: 205-939-9720
Emergency: 205-933-4050
205-939-9201
800-292-6678 (AL)
Fax: 205-939-9245

TUSCALOOSA

Alabama Poison Control Systems, Inc. (*)
408 A. Paul Bryant Dr. E.
Tuscaloosa, AL 35401
Business: 205-345-0600
Emergency: 205-345-0600
800-462-0800 (AL)
Fax: 205-759-7994

ALASKA

ANCHORAGE

Anchorage Poison Center Providence Hospital
P.O. Box 196604
3200 Providence Dr.
Anchorage, AK 99519-6604
Business: 907-562-2211 ext. 3633
Emergency: 907-261-3193
800-478-3193 (AK)
Fax: 907-261-3645

FAIRBANKS

Fairbanks Poison Control Center
1650 Cowles St.
Fairbanks, AK 99701
Business: 907-456-7182
Emergency: 907-456-7182
Fax: 907-458-5553

ARIZONA

PHOENIX

Samaritan Regional Poison Center (*) Good Samaritan Medical Center
1111 East McDowell Rd.
Phoenix, AZ 85006
Business: 602-495-4884
Emergency: 602-253-3334
Fax: 602-256-7579

TUCSON

Arizona Poison & Drug Information Center (*) University of Arizona Arizona Health Sciences Center
1501 North Campbell Ave. #1156
Tucson, AZ 85724
Emergency: 520-626-6016
800-362-0101 (AZ)
Fax: 520-626-2720

ARKANSAS

LITTLE ROCK

Arkansas Poison and Drug Information Center College of Pharmacy - UAMS
4301 West Markham St.
Slot 522-2
Little Rock, AR 72205
Business: 501-661-6161
Emergency: 800-376-4766 (AR)

CALIFORNIA

FRESNO

Central California Regional Poison Control Center (*) Valley Children's Hospital
3151 North Millbrook
Fresno, CA 93703
Business: 209-241-6040
Emergency: 209-445-1222
800-346-5922 (Central CA)
Fax: 209-241-6050

LOS ANGELES

Los Angeles County Regional Drug & Poison Information Center (*) LAC & USC Medical Center
1200 North State St.
Los Angeles, CA 90033
Business: 213-226-7741
Emergency: 213-222-3212
800-777-6476
Fax: 213-226-4194

SACRAMENTO

UC Davis Medical Center Regional Poison Control Center (*)
2315 Stockton Blvd.
Sacramento, CA 95817
Business: 916-734-3415
Emergency: 916-734-3692
800-342-9293 (N. CA only)
Fax: 916-734-7796

SAN DIEGO

San Diego Regional Poison Center (*) UCSD Medical Center
200 West Arbor Dr.
San Diego, CA 92103-8925
Business: 619-543-3666
Emergency: 619-543-6000
800-876-4766 (San Diego and Imperial counties only)
Fax: 619-692-1867

SAN FRANCISCO

San Francisco Bay Area Regional Poison Control Center (*) SF General Hospital
1001 Potrero Ave.
Bldg. 80
San Francisco, CA 94110
Business: 415-206-5524
Emergency: 800-523-2222
Fax: 415-821-8513

COLORADO

DENVER

Rocky Mountain Poison and Drug Center (*)
8802 East 9th Ave.
Bldg. 752
Denver, CO 80220
Business: 303-739-1100
Emergency: 303-629-1123
TTY: 303-739-1127
Fax: 303-739-1119

CONNECTICUT

FARMINGTON

Connecticut Poison Control Center (*)
University of Connecticut Health Center
263 Farmington Ave.
Farmington, CT 06032
Business: 203-679-3473
Emergency: 800-343-2722 (CT)
TTY: 203-679-4346
Fax: 203-679-1623

DISTRICT OF COLUMBIA

WASHINGTON, DC

National Capital Poison Center (*)
3201 New Mexico Ave., NW
Suite 310
Washington, DC 20016
Business: 202-362-3867
Emergency: 202-625-3333
TTY: 202-362-8563
Fax: 202-362-8377

FLORIDA

JACKSONVILLE

Florida Poison Information Center of Jacksonville
655 W. 8th St.
Jacksonville, FL 32209
Emergency: 904-549-4480
Fax: 904-549-4063

MIAMI

Florida Poison Information Center of Miami
P.O. Box 016960, R-131
Miami, FL 33101
Emergency: 305-585-5253
Fax: 305-242-9762

TAMPA

Florida Poison Information and Toxicology Resource Center (*)
Tampa General Hospital
P.O. Box 1289
Tampa, FL 33601
Emergency: 813-253-4444
800-282-3171 (FL)
Fax: 813-253-4443

GEORGIA

ATLANTA

Georgia Poison Center (*)
Grady Health System
80 Butler St. SE
P.O. Box 26066
Atlanta, GA 30335-3801
Emergency: 404-616-9000
800-282-5846 (GA)
Fax: 404-616-6657

MACON

Regional Poison Control Center
Medical Center of Central Georgia
777 Hemlock St.
Macon, GA 31201
Poison Ctr: 912-633-1427
Fax: 912-633-5082

ILLINOIS

CHICAGO

Chicago & NE Illinois Regional Poison Control Center
Rush-Presbyterian-St. Luke's Medical Center
1653 West Congress Pkwy.
Chicago, IL 60612
Business: 312-942-7064
Emergency: 312-942-5969
800-942-5969 (IL)
Fax: 312-942-4260

URBANA

ASPCA/National Animal Poison Control Center (*)
1717 Philo Rd., Suite 36
Urbana, IL 61801
Business: 217-333-2053
800-548-2423 (24-hour subscribers)
Fax: 217-244-1580

INDIANA

INDIANAPOLIS

Indiana Poison Center (*)
Methodist Hospital of Indiana
1701 North Senate Blvd.
P.O. Box 1367
Indianapolis, IN 46206-1367
Emergency: 317-929-2323
800-382-9097 (IN)
TTY: 317-929-2336
Fax: 317-929-2337

IOWA

DES MOINES

Variety Club Poison and Drug Information Center
Iowa Methodist Medical Center
1200 Pleasant St.
Des Moines, IA 50309
Business: 515-241-6254
Emergency: 800-362-2327 (IA)
Fax: 515-241-5085

IOWA CITY

Poison Control Center (*)
University of Iowa Hospitals and Clinics
200 Hawkins Dr.
Iowa City, IA 52242
Business: 319-356-2577
Emergency: 800-272-6477 (IA only)

KANSAS

KANSAS CITY

Mid-America Poison Control Center
University of Kansas Medical Center
3901 Rainbow Blvd.
Room B-400
Kansas City, KS 66160-7231
Business & Emergency: 913-588-6633
800-332-6633 (KS)
Fax: 913-588-2350

TOPEKA

Stormont-Vail Regional Medical Center
Emergency Department
1500 West 10th
Topeka, KS 66604
Business: 913-354-6000
Emergency: 913-354-6100
Fax: 913-354-5004

KENTUCKY

LOUISVILLE

Kentucky Regional Poison Center (*)
Kosair Children's Hospital
Medical Towers S.
Suite 572
P.O. Box 35070
Louisville, KY 40232-5070
Business: 502-629-7264
Emergency: 502-629-7275
502-589-8222
800-722-5725 (KY)
Fax: 502-629-7277

LOUISIANA

MONROE

Louisiana Drug and Poison Information Center (*)
Northeast Louisiana University School of Pharmacy
Monroe, LA 71209-6430
Business: 318-342-1710
Emergency: 800-256-9822 (LA)
Fax: 318-342-1744

MAINE

PORTLAND

Maine Poison Center (*)
Maine Medical Center
22 Bramhall St.
Portland, ME 04102
Business: 207-871-2950
Emergency: 800-442-6305 (ME)
Fax: 207-871-6226

MARYLAND

BALTIMORE

Maryland Poison Center (*)
University of Maryland School of Pharmacy
20 North Pine St.
Baltimore, MD 21201
Business: 410-706-7604
Emergency: 410-706-7701
800-492-2414 (MD only)
TTY: 410-706-1858
Fax: 410-706-7184

MASSACHUSETTS

BOSTON

Massachusetts Poison Control System (*)
300 Longwood Ave.
Boston, MA 02115
Emergency: 617-232-2120
800-682-9211
TTY: 617-355-6089
Fax: 617-738-0032

MICHIGAN

DETROIT

Poison Control Center (*) Children's Hospital of Michigan
Harper Professional Office Bldg., Suite 425
Detroit, MI 48201
Business: 313-745-5335
Emergency: 313-745-5711
Fax: 313-745-5493

GRAND RAPIDS

Blodgett Regional Poison Center (*) Blodgett Memorial Medical Center
1840 Wealthy St. SE
Grand Rapids, MI 49506
Business: 616-774-5329
Emergency: 800-764-7661 (MI)
Fax: 616-774-7204

MINNESOTA

MINNEAPOLIS

Hennepin Regional Poison Center (*) Hennepin County Medical Center
701 Park Ave.
Minneapolis, MN 55415
Business: 612-347-3144
Emergency: 612-347-3141
TTY: 612-904-4691
Fax: 612-904-4289

Minnesota Regional Poison Center (*)
8100 34th Ave. South
Box 1309
Minneapolis, MN 55440
Business: 612-851-8100
Emergency: 612-221-2113
Fax: 612-851-8166

MISSISSIPPI

HATTIESBURG

Poison Center
Forrest General Hospital
400 South 28th Ave.
Hattiesburg, MS 39401
Business: 601-288-4221
Emergency: 601-288-4235

JACKSON

Mississippi Regional Poison Control (*)
University of Mississippi Medical Center
2500 North State St.
Jackson, MS 39216
Business: 601-984-1675
Emergency: 601-354-7660
Fax: 601-984-1676

MISSOURI

KANSAS CITY

Poison Control Center (*)
Children's Mercy Hospital
2401 Gillham Rd.
Kansas City, MO 64108
Business: 816-234-3053
Emergency: 816-234-3430
Fax: 816-234-3421

ST. LOUIS

Cardinal Glennon Children's Hospital Regional Poison Center (*)
1465 South Grand Blvd.
St. Louis, MO 63104
Emergency: 314-772-5200
800-366-8888
Fax: 314-577-5355

MONTANA

DENVER, CO

Rocky Mountain Poison and Drug Center (*)
8802 E. 9th Ave.
Denver, CO 80220
Emergency: 303-629-1123
800-525-5042 (MT)
Fax: 303-739-1119

NEBRASKA

OMAHA

The Poison Center (*)
Children's Memorial Hospital
8301 Dodge St.
Omaha, NE 68114
Emergency: 402-390-5555 (Omaha)
800-955-9119 (NE, WY)
Fax: 404-354-3049

NEVADA

LAS VEGAS

Poison Center
Humana Medical Center
3186 Maryland Pkwy.
Las Vegas, NV 89109
Emergency: 800-446-6179 (NV)

RENO

Poison Center
Washoe Medical Center
77 Pringle Way
Reno, NV 89520
Business: 702-328-4129
Emergency: 702-328-4100
Fax: 702-328-5555

NEW HAMPSHIRE

LEBANON

New Hampshire Poison Information Center (*)
Dartmouth-Hitchcock Medical Center
1 Medical Center Dr.
Lebanon, NH 03756
Emergency: 603-650-5000 (ask for Poison Center)
800-562-8236 (NH only)
Fax: 603-650-8986

NEW JERSEY

NEWARK

New Jersey Poison Information and Education System
Newark Beth Israel Medical Center
201 Lyons Ave.
Newark, NJ 07112
Emergency: POISON-1 (800-764-7661)
TTY: POISON-1 (800-764-7661)
Fax: 201-705-8098

PHILLIPSBURG

Warren Hospital Poison Control Center
185 Roseberry St.
Phillipsburg, NJ 08865
Business: 908-859-6768
Emergency: 908-859-6767
800-962-1253 (NJ)
Fax: 908-859-6812

NEW MEXICO

ALBUQUERQUE

New Mexico Poison & Drug Information Center
University of New Mexico
Albuquerque, NM 87131-1076
Emergency: 505-843-2551
800-432-6866 (NM)
Fax: 505-277-5892

NEW YORK

BUFFALO

Western New York Regional Poison Control Center Children's Hospital of Buffalo
219 Bryant St.
Buffalo, NY 14222
Business: 716-878-7657
Emergency: 716-878-7654
800-888-7655 (NY & W. PA only)

MINEOLA

L.I. Regional Poison Control Center (*) Winthrop University Hospital
259 First St.
Mineola, NY 11501
Emergency: 516-542-2323
TTY: 516-747-3323
Fax: 516-739-2070

NEW YORK

New York City Poison Control Center (*) NYC Dept. of Health
455 First Ave., Room 123
New York, NY 10016
Business: 212-447-8154
Emergency: 212-340-4494
212-POISONS (212-764-7667)
TDD: 212-689-9014
Fax: 212-447-8223

NORTH TARRYTOWN

Hudson Valley Poison Center Phelps Memorial Hospital
701 N. Broadway
N. Tarrytown, NY 10591
Emergency: 914-353-1000
800-336-6997
Fax: 914-353-1050

ROCHESTER

Finger Lakes Regional Poison Control Center (*) University of Rochester Medical Center
601 Elmwood Ave.
Rochester, NY 14642
Business: 716-273-4155
Emergency: 716-275-3232
800-333-0542 (NY)
Fax: 716-244-1677

SYRACUSE

Central NY Poison Control Center SUNY Health Science Center
750 East Adams St.
Syracuse, NY 13210
Business: 315-464-7073
Emergency: 315-476-4766
800-252-5655 (NY)
Fax: 315-464-7077

NORTH CAROLINA

ASHEVILLE

Western North Carolina Poison Control Center (*) Memorial Mission Hospital
509 Biltmore Ave.
Asheville, NC 28801
Emergency: 704-255-4490
800-542-4225 (NC)
Fax: 704-255-4467

CHARLOTTE

Carolinas Poison Center (*)
P.O. Box 32861
Charlotte, NC 28232-2861
Business: 704-355-3054
Emergency: 704-355-4000 (Charlotte area)
800-848-6946

NORTH DAKOTA

FARGO

North Dakota Poison Information Center (*) Meritcare Medical Center
720 North 4th St.
Fargo, ND 58122
Business: 701-234-6062
Emergency: 701-234-5575
800-732-2200 (ND)
Fax: 701-234-5090

OHIO

AKRON

Akron Regional Poison Control Center Children's Hospital Medical Center
1 Perkins Square
Akron, OH 44308
Business: 330-258-3066
Emergency: 330-379-8562
800-362-9922 (OH)
TTY: 330-379-8446
Fax: 330-379-8447

CINCINNATI

Regional Poison Control System Cincinnati Drug and Poison Information Center (*) University of Cincinnati
College of Medicine
P.O. Box 670144
Cincinnati, OH 45267-0144
Emergency: 513-558-5111
800-872-5111 (OH)
Fax: 513-558-5301

CLEVELAND

Greater Cleveland Poison Control Center (*)
11100 Euclid Ave.
Cleveland, OH 44106
Emergency: 216-231-4455
888-231-4455
Fax: 216-844-3242

COLUMBUS

Central Ohio Poison Center (*)
700 Children's Dr.
Columbus, OH 43205-2696
Business: 614-722-2635
Emergency: 614-228-1323
800-682-7625
TTY: 614-228-2272
Fax: 614-221-2672

Greater Dayton Area Hospital Association (*) at Central Ohio Poison Center
700 Children's Dr.
Columbus, OH 43205
Business: 614-722-2635
Emergency: 513-222-2227
800-762-0727 (OH)

TOLEDO

Poison Information Center of NW Ohio (*) Medical College of Ohio Hospital
3000 Arlington Ave.
Toledo, OH 43614
Business: 419-381-3898
Emergency: 419-381-3897
800-589-3897 (OH)
Fax: 419-381-2818

ZANESVILLE

Drug Information/Poison Control Center (*)
Bethesda Hospital
2951 Maple Ave.
Zanesville, OH 43701
Business: 614-454-4246
Emergency: 614-454-4221
614-454-4000
800-686-4221 (OH)
Fax: 614-454-4059

OKLAHOMA

OKLAHOMA CITY

Oklahoma Poison Control Center (*) University of Oklahoma and Children's Hospital of Oklahoma
940 Northeast 13th St.
Oklahoma City, OK 73104
Emergency: 405-271-5454 (Bus.)
800-522-4611 (Bus.) (OK)
TDD: 405-271-1122
Fax: 405-271-1816

OREGON

PORTLAND

Oregon Poison Center (*)
Oregon Health Sciences University
3181 SW Sam Jackson Park Rd.
Portland, OR 97201
Emergency: 503-494-8968
800-452-7165 (OR)
Fax: 503-494-4980

PENNSYLVANIA

HERSHEY

Central Pennsylvania Poison Center (*)
University Hospital
Milton S. Hershey Medical Center
P.O. Box 850
Hershey, PA 17033
Emergency: 800-521-6110
Fax: 717-531-6932

LANCASTER

Poison Control Center (*)
St. Joseph Hospital and Health Care Center
250 College Ave.
Lancaster, PA 17604
Business: 717-299-4546
Emergency: 717-291-8111
Fax: 717-291-8346

PHILADELPHIA

The Poison Control Center (*)
3600 Market St.
Room 220
Philadelphia, PA 19104-2641
Business: 215-590-2003
Emergency: 215-386-2100
800-722-7112
Fax: 215-590-4419

PITTSBURGH

Pittsburgh Poison Center (*) Children's Hospital of Pittsburgh
3705 Fifth Ave.
Pittsburgh, PA 15213
Business: 412-692-5600
Emergency: 412-681-6669
Fax: 412-692-7497

RHODE ISLAND

PROVIDENCE

Rhode Island Poison Center (*)
Rhode Island Hospital
593 Eddy St.
Providence, RI 02903
Emergency: 401-444-5727
Fax: 401-444-8062

SOUTH CAROLINA

COLUMBIA

Palmetto Poison Center (*) College of Pharmacy
University of South Carolina
Columbia, SC 29208
Business: 803-777-7909
Emergency: 803-777-1117
800-922-1117 (SC)
Fax: 803-777-6127

SOUTH DAKOTA

ABERDEEN

Poison Control Center
St. Luke's Midland Regional Medical Center
305 South State St.
Aberdeen, SD 57401
Business: 605-622-5000
Emergency: 605-622-5100
800-592-1889 (SD, MN, ND, WY)

RAPID CITY

Rapid City Regional Poison Center
835 Fairmont Blvd.
P.O. Box 6000
Rapid City, SD 57709
Business & Emergency: 605-341-3333

SIOUX FALLS

McKennan Poison Center
McKennan Hospital
800 East 21st St.
P.O. Box 5045
Sioux Falls, SD 57117-5045
Business: 605-322-8305
Emergency: 605-322-3894
800-843-0505 (IA, MN, NE, ND)
800-952-0123 (SD)
Fax: 605-322-8378

TENNESSEE

MEMPHIS

Southern Poison Center (*)
847 Monroe Ave.
Suite 230
Memphis, TN 38163
Business: 901-448-6800
Emergency: 901-528-6048
800-288-9999 (TN only)
Fax: 901-448-5419

NASHVILLE

Middle Tennessee Poison Center (*)
501 Oxford House
1161 21st Ave. S.
Nashville, TN 37232
Business: 615-936-0760
Emergency: 615-936-2034
800-288-9999 (TN)
TDD: 615-936-2047
Fax: 615-936-2046

TEXAS

DALLAS

North Texas Poison Center
Texas Poison Center Network (*)
Parkland Memorial Hospital
5201 Harry Hines Blvd.
P.O. Box 35926
Dallas, TX 75235
Business: 214-590-6625
Emergency: 800-Poison-1 (800-764-7661)
Fax: 214-590-5008

EL PASO

West Texas Regional Poison Center (*)
4815 Alameda Ave.
El Paso, TX 79905
Business: 915-521-7661
Emergency: 800-764-7661 (800-POISON-1)
Fax: 915-521-7978

GALVESTON

Southeast Texas Poison Center (*)
University of Texas Medical Branch Trauma Center
Room 3-112
Galveston, TX 77555-1175
Emergency: 409-765-1420
800-764-7661 (TX only)
Fax: 409-772-3917

TEMPLE

Drug Information Center
Scott and White Memorial Hospital
2401 South 31st St.
Temple, TX 76508
Business: 817-724-4636
Fax: 817-724-1731

UTAH

SALT LAKE CITY

Utah Poison Control Center (*)
410 Chipeta Way
Suite 230
Salt Lake City, UT 84108
Emergency: 801-581-2151
800-456-7707 (UT)
Fax: 801-581-4199

VERMONT

BURLINGTON

Vermont Poison Center (*)
Fletcher Allen Health Care
111 Colchester Ave.
Burlington, VT 05401
Business: 802-656-2721
Emergency: 802-658-3456
Fax: 802-656-4802

VIRGINIA

CHARLOTTESVILLE

Blue Ridge Poison Center
Blue Ridge Hospital
P.O. Box 67
Charlottesville, VA 22901
Emergency: 804-924-5543
800-451-1428
Fax: 804-971-8657

RICHMOND

Virginia Poison Center
Virginia Commonwealth University
P.O. Box 980522
Richmond, VA 23298-0522
Emergency: 804-828-9123
Fax: 804-828-5291

WASHINGTON

SEATTLE

Washington Poison Center (*)
155 NE 100th St.
Suite 400
Seattle, WA 98125-8012
Business: 206-517-2351
Emergency: 206-526-2121
800-732-6985 (WA)
TTY: 206-517-2394
800-572-0638 (WA)
Fax: 206-526-8490

WEST VIRGINIA

CHARLESTON

West Virginia Poison Center (*) West Virginia University
3110 MacCorkle Ave. SE
Charleston, WV 25304
Business: 304-347-1212
Emergency: 304-348-4211
800-642-3625 (WV)
Fax: 304-348-9560

PARKERSBURG

Poison Center
St. Joseph's Hospital Center
19th St. and Murdoch Ave.
Parkersburg, WV 26101
Emergency: 304-424-4222
Fax: 304-424-4766

WISCONSIN

MADISON

Poison Control Center (*)
University of Wisconsin Hospital and Clinics
600 Highland Ave.
E5/238
Madison, WI 53792
Business: 608-262-7537
Emergency: 608-262-3702
800-815-8855 (WI)

MILWAUKEE

Children's Hospital Poison Center
Children's Hospital of Wisconsin
9000 W. Wisconsin Ave.
P.O. Box 1997
Milwaukee, WI 53201
Business: 414-266-2000
Emergency: 414-266-2222
800-815-8855 (WI)
Fax: 414-266-2820

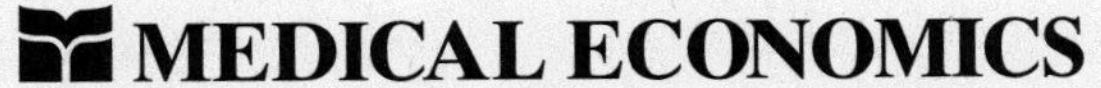
MEDICAL ECONOMICS

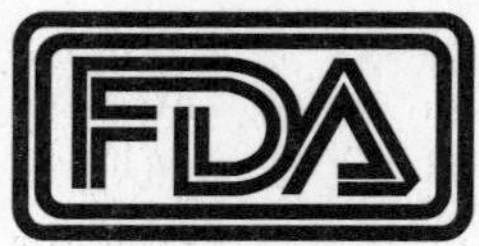

U.S. FOOD AND DRUG ADMINISTRATION

Professional and Consumer Information Numbers

Medical Product Reporting Programs

MedWatch (24 hour service) **800-332-1088**
Reporting of problems with drugs, devices, biologics (except vaccines), medical foods, dietary supplements.

Vaccine Adverse Event Reporting (24 hour service) **800-822-7967**
Reporting of vaccine-related problems.

Mandatory Medical Device Reporting **301-594-3886**
Reporting required from User facilities regarding device-related deaths and serious injuries.

Veterinary Adverse Drug Reaction Program (7:30 a.m. to 4:00 p.m., eastern time) **301-594-1751**
Reporting of adverse drug events in animals (collect calls accepted).

Medical Advertising Information (24 hour service) **800-238-7332**
Inquiries from health professionals regarding product promotion.

Information for Health Professionals

Drug Information Branch **301-827-4573**
Information on human drugs, including hormones.

Center for Devices and Radiological Health **301-443-4190**
Automated request for information on medical devices and radiation-emitting products.

Office of Health Affairs Medicine Staff **301-443-5470**
Information for health professionals on FDA activities.

General Information

General Consumer Inquiries **301-443-3170**
Consumer information on regulated products/issues.

Freedom of Information **301-443-6310**
Request for publicly available FDA documents.

Office of Public Affairs **301-443-1130**
Interviews/press inquiries on FDA activities.

Breast Implant Inquiries (24 hour service) **800-332-4440**
Prerecorded message/request information.

Seafood Hotline (24 hour service) **800-332-4010**
Prerecorded message/request information (English/Spanish).

All numbers accessible 8:00 a.m. to 4:30 p.m. eastern time, except where otherwise noted.

Appendix 1: Consumer Perceptions and OTC Use

Studies that have explored the ways consumers use and perceive nonprescription medicines shed light on the following issues:

- Americans' use of OTCs in comparison to other nationalities;
- OTCs as serious medicine;
- Safety and correctness of nonprescription drug use;
- Effect of age, sex, and economic status on self-medication habits;
- Product choice and availability;
- Impact of the rise of managed care and the national movement toward health care reform.

Important and far-reaching trends in these areas may be changing the way nonprescription—and prescription—drugs are used. In addition, the role that physicians and pharmacists play in the use of OTCs is paramount, and is discussed in a separate section.

Use Highest in the U.S.

Americans use more OTCs than people in other countries, according to a study comparing 14 national surveys on self-medication (see figure 1). The review ascribes this usage to the fact that the U.S. is the only country lacking a national health care program. It concludes: "Many U.S. citizens must pay for both doctor visits and prescription medicines; others [U.S. citizens] must pay a percentage of these costs. As a result, for common conditions, many Americans consider self-treatment with over-the-counter medicines a cost-saving alternative to doctor visits and prescription drugs."

Figure 1

Use of OTCs for Common Health Complaints: A Worldwide Comparison

Country	*Percent of Consumers Using OTCs*
United States	33%
Australia	28%
Germany	28%
Spain	24%
United Kingdom	24%
Sweden	24%
Switzerland	22%
Mexico	21%
Italy	20%
Japan	16%

Source: World Federation of Proprietary Medicine Manufacturers. "Health Care, Self-Care and Self-Medication" 1991.

Other consumer surveys bear out the importance of cost. In a national Gallup poll, nearly half of those surveyed cited low cost as the greatest advantage to using an OTC. Other important features are convenience (cited by 29 percent) and the fact that OTCs eliminate the need for a doctor's visit (23 percent).

Conditions for which OTCs are used are similar throughout the world. In all countries surveyed, the common cold is the most frequently reported ailment for which OTCs are used, followed by headache, digestive problems, and body aches and pains.

Satisfied Customers

OTCs can treat or cure about 400 different common health complaints. The average consumer reports suffering from about six of these every two weeks, ranging from headaches, which are treatable with an OTC according to more than three-quarters of consumers (76 percent), to dry skin and sinus problems (56 percent and 54 percent respectively) (see figure 2). By category, respiratory and feminine complaints are most likely to be treated with a nonprescription medication (see figure 3).

Figure 2

Top Ten Problems Most Likely to be Treated with OTCs

Complaint	*Percent Who Would Treat with OTCs*
Headache	76%
Athlete's foot	69%
Lip problems	68%
Common cold	63%
Chronic dandruff	59%
Pre-menstrual	58%
Menstrual	57%
Upset Stomach	57%
Painful/dry skin	56%
Sinus problems	54%

Source: Heller Research Group. "Self-Medication in the 90s: Practices and Perceptions." New York, 1992.

Figure 3

Major Categories for which OTCs are used

Condition	*Percent Treated with OTCs*
Respiratory	50%
Feminine	50%
Pain	46%
Digestive	44%
Eye/ear/mouth	41%
Skin	33%
General well being	8%

Source: Heller Research Group. "Self Medication in the 90s: Practices and perceptions." New York, 1992.

American consumers also say that OTCs are effective treatment for these conditions. Americans are, in fact, more satisfied with OTCs than consumers in other countries (see figure 4). Of all 14 countries surveyed, the U.S. had the highest level of satisfaction with nonprescription drugs.

Figure 4

Percentage of Consumers, by Country, who are Satisfied with OTCs.

Country	*%*
United States	92%
Mexico	90%
United Kingdom	83%
Canada	80%
Australia	75%

Source: World Federation of Proprietary Medicine Manufacturers. "Health Care, Self-Care and Self-Medication" 1991.

In a survey conducted in the U.S., 94 percent of those surveyed said they would retake OTCs they've used previously, and more than nine out of ten reported that they were satisfied with the products they had used. Indeed, nearly three-quarters of Americans say they believe OTCs are as effective as prescription medications.

Finally, studies have also probed the reasons consumers stop taking an OTC. Ninety percent of those surveyed said they discontinued use because the problem went away. Only 3 percent said they used a medicine that did not work.

The Safe Use of OTCs

No drug is completely safe, and consumers have shown that they appreciate the potential risk of taking any medication. In one survey, 94 percent of American consumers said that care must be used when taking medications, even those that are not prescription drugs. Ninety-five percent disagreed with the statement that "it is safe to take as many OTCs as you wish."

Over-medication with nonprescription drugs is rare among consumers. According to the Heller study, seven out of ten respondents prefer to fight symptoms without taking medications at all, and nine out of ten said they know all medications should only be used when absolutely necessary. In the same survey, 85 percent said it is nonetheless important to have nonprescription medications available to help relieve minor medical problems.

Americans rate second only to residents of the UK when it comes to reading the label before using an OTC, according to national surveys. Ninety-six percent of U.S. consumers said they read OTC labels, compared with 97 percent in the U.K. Many U.S. studies have confirmed this fact, reporting percentages ranging from 88 percent to 93 percent.

National surveys also show that:

- Americans generally take less than the maximum recommended daily dose when using OTC analgesics. (For colds, menstruation, and headache, the average number of tablets taken ranges from four to six; for arthritis, rheumatism, and backache, the average number taken each day of use is five);
- Nearly all OTCs are used for considerably less time than the standard ten-day limit-of-use warning;
- Consumer knowledge about OTCs is more accurate than consumer knowledge of many other areas, including banking, nutrition, and insurance. In comparative studies, consumers show a solid understanding, with scores of 75 percent or higher, for over half of the drug questions;
- Consumers read labels more carefully now than in the past.

Demographics of OTC Use

The way consumers approach self-medication with a nonprescription drug is affected by age, sex, and economic status, among other factors.

For example, the level of OTC use remains fairly constant with age, although younger consumers tend to use OTCs for acute conditions, whereas the elderly turn to them more often for chronic conditions.

The level of usage and conditions for which OTCs are used do differ with gender. Women not only buy more OTCs than men, they also use them more and use them to treat different types of conditions. Women take OTCs for anxiety, indigestion and stom-

Figure 5

Recent Additions to the OTC Market

Ingredient	*Category*	*Products*
Cimetidine	Heartburn relief	Tagamet HB
Clemastine fumarate	Antihistamine	Tavist-1
Clemastine fumarate with phenylpropanolamine HCl	Antihistamine/decongestant	Tavist -D
Famotidine	Acid controller	Pepcid AC
Hydrocortisone acetate	Antipruritic	Anusol, Caldecort
Ketoprofen	Internal analgesic	Orudis KT, Actron
Miconazole nitrate	Anticandidal	Monistat 7
Naphazoline HCl with pheniramine maleate	Antihistamine/decongestant eye drop	Opcon A
Naproxen	Internal analgesic/antipyretic	Aleve, Naprosyn

Source: Nonprescription Drug Manufacturers Association, 1995.

ach complaints, headaches, fatigue, sleep problems, arthritis, lip and skin conditions, and weight control. Among men, OTCs are used predominantly for aches and pains, cuts, and colds.

Economic status also affects how OTCs are used. Americans covered by Medicaid, for example, are less likely to take an OTC. They are more likely to seek a physician's care or use a prescription medication that is already in the home.

Increasing Product Choices

New categories and forms of OTCs in the market also affect consumer's self-medication choices. New drugs and whole new categories of products provide consumers with a growing number of effective alternatives for self-care. These new entities also increase the importance of physicians and pharmacists as OTC counselors.

Most of today's new nonprescription drugs contain ingredients that have recently been switched to OTC status. (Examples of these new OTCs are listed in figure 5.) And as noted above, consumer acceptance of switches is exceptionally high. For example, two feminine antifungal ingredients—clotrimazole and miconazole nitrate—became available over-the-counter in 1991. These products, which provide women with an entirely new class of over-the-counter remedies for treating vaginal infections, accounted for about 90 percent of Health and Beauty Care new-item sales volume in drugstores and other outlets in the year they appeared on the market.

The high use of switched products by consumers is also strongly demonstrated by a survey of top-selling OTCs. In 1992, 14 of the 15 best-selling OTCs introduced since 1975 were either switched brands or switch-related products, as shown in figure 6.

Figure 6

Consumer Preference for Switched Products

In 1992, 14 of the 15 best selling OTCs introduced since 1975 were either switched brands or switch-related products.

Product	*1992 Sales (in millions)*
Advil	$320
Monistat 7	114
Benadryl	92
Sudafed	92
Motrin IB*	87
Imodium AD	85
Dimetapp	77
Nuprin	67
Afrin	62
Gyne-Lotrimin	53
Oxy-line	52
Drixoral	49
Chlor-Trimeton	44
Actifed	44
Comtrex**	35

*Switch-related
**New proprietary product
Source: Sudler & Hennessy, New York, 1992.

Effects of Health Care Reform and Managed Care

Two trends that have affected every segment of health care delivery are health care reform and managed care. Since these trends are still evolving, their impact on the OTC market cannot yet be determined, but some outcomes can reasonably be projected.

Managed care probably has less of a direct effect on the use of OTCs than on other segments of health care since most third-party health care plans do not cover nonprescription drugs. By contrast, prescription drugs are often closely managed by the use of drug formularies; through financial incentives to members to use less expensive products, mail order pharmacies, and generics; and through drug utilization review. Nonetheless, because of the cost-effectiveness of OTCs, it is likely that their use will increase as health care costs rise and efforts to contain costs are exerted by payers and national reform programs. Self-medication will most likely be recognized as part of the solution to the problems of rising costs and limited access.

Managed care may also increase OTC use in another indirect way. Managed care typically uses capitated plans in which physicians and pharmacists are paid a flat rate per member by the managed care administrator, regardless of the amount of care provided. Plan members may also be given financial incentives to use fewer plan services. As a result, both providers and plan members often have an incentive to contain costs and use fewer of the medical services and products covered by the plan. Self-medication may therefore become more accepted and encouraged under this type of managed care reimbursement system.

By contrast, traditional fee-for-service health insurance plans provide reimbursement based on utilization rates. Under this system, self-care is, in effect, a form of competition for physicians and pharmacists since it decreases office visits and prescription drug use.

In addition, although most consumers are not reimbursed by health insurance companies for OTCs, nonprescription drugs nonetheless generally end up costing less than a prescription since the copay and/or deductible on an Rx drug usually exceeds the average price of an OTC.

Finally, health care reform, in an effort to make health care affordable and accessible, may also encourage the process of switching Rx products to over-the-counter status. In fact, experts predict that this trend may put a high number of new OTC products on the market in the near future.

Sources

World Federation of Proprietary Medicine Manufacturers. Health Care, Self-Care and Self Medication, 1991.

Market Research Corporation of America. Health care remedies usage study. February, 1990.

Consumer Federation of America. September, 1990.

Gallup Organization. *American Health,* March, 1989.

Gallup Organization. *American Health,* 1991.

Heller Research Group. Self-Medication in the '90s: Practices and perceptions. New York, 1992.

Holt G.A., Beck D., Williams M.M. Interview analysis regarding health status, health needs and health care utilization of ambulatory elderly. 40th Annual Conference of the National Council of Aging, Washington, DC, April, 1990.

Shanas E., Maddox G. Aging, health, and the organization of health resources. In: Binstock R., Shanas E., eds. *Handbook of Aging and the Social Sciences.* Van Nostrand Reinhold, New York, 1985.

Princeton Survey Research Associates. *Prevention,* 1992.

Gannon K. The Rx-to-OTC switch race: Drugstores setting the pace. *Drug Topics,* November 22, 1993.

Sudler & Hennessy. New York, 1992.

Rosendahl I. The private label story. *Drug Topics* June 13, 1994.

Appendix 2: Patient Counseling: A Critical Role for Physicians and Pharmacists

The Consumer's Self-Medication Bill of Rights, drafted by the Nonprescription Drug Manufacturers Association, states: "Next to safe and effective products, information is the most important commodity in self-care/self-medication." And as OTC use increases and the number of available products grows, consumers will require more information than ever to choose the right products and use them effectively and safely. For most consumers, that information comes from their health care providers. Physicians and pharmacists are in an ideal and unique position to provide patients with informed and up-to-date OTC advice. Through effective patient counseling on OTC use, physicians and phamacists can help improve medical outcomes and prevent costly incidents of drug misuse.

A Growing Need For Information

For most consumers, information on nonprescription drugs comes from product labels and advertising, but these can be confusing or incomplete. Consumers thus rely on the one-to-one relationship they possess with their doctors and pharmacists for additional information.

New products, line extensions, and OTC switches are just some of the factors that may overwhelm even the most well-informed patient. In 1993, for example, 97 percent of all pharmacists surveyed across the nation said that line extensions for adult cough/cold/flu preparations led to significant confusion among their customers. Switches for children's cough/cold preparations caused even more problems.

Such confusion, multiplied by the number of products on the market, can foster potential medical misadventures, including:

- use of an inappropriate medication;
- use of an inappropriate dosage;
- use of an OTC that is contraindicated;
- drug-drug interactions;
- inappropriate duration of OTC use;
- side effects.

In addition, although all consumers need counseling on OTCs, many have special needs. Groups requiring special attention include:

- patients with comprehension problems (20 percent of consumers are illiterate and nearly 10 percent say they are sometimes confused by OTC labels);
- blind and other visually impaired patients;
- deaf and other hearing-impaired patients;
- the elderly;
- children;
- patients with comprehension deficits;
- pregnant or nursing patients.

For these patients, self-medicating safely may pose difficulties, and counseling from a physician or pharmacist is particularly important.

All consumers have occasional questions about nonprescription medications. These range from requests for product recommendations to questions about cost. (Figure 1 lists the most commonly asked questions.) According to one national survey, almost two-thirds (65 percent) of consumers ask their physician for OTC advice and over half (54 percent) consult their pharmacist. (The total exceed 100 percent, since many consumers consult both physicians and pharmacists.) Consumers place a high value on the advice they receive. The same study revealed that 58 percent of patients are extremely satisfied with their doctor's advice, and 61 percent give the same high grade to pharmacists.

Figure 1

Commonly Asked Questions About OTCs

Question	*Percent of Pharmacists receiving the question*
Recommendations for the best OTC product for a specific ailment	94%
Side effects	54%
Dosage/duration of therapy	37%
Information on medical conditions	36%
Cost of OTC	35%

Source: Cardinale, V. "Pharmacists as OTC Counselors," *Drug Topics* (suppl.), 1994.

OTCs and Physicians

Nearly all (97 percent) physicians recommend OTCs to their patients, according to a recent survey by the international business consulting firm Kline & Co. They do so, in fact, for 27 percent of all their patients. As the professionals that consumers count on most, physicians and pharmacists play an important role in how OTCs are used. In turn, physician and pharmacy practices are also affected by the wide availability and effectiveness of these medications.

Americans take about one-tenth of their health problems to physicians. For the remainder of injuries and illnesses, they resort to no treatment or self-treatment; and 70 percent say they self-medicate regularly. For physicians, OTCs have a direct impact on the number of patients they see and the reasons for those office visits.

One study found that MD visits for the common cold dropped by 110,000 a year between 1976 and 1989. The study attributed the decrease to the high number of switched drugs available for treating cold symptoms. The number of visits for other ailments, including serious respiratory conditions, did not decrease in the same period. Another survey revealed that over half (54 percent) of Americans believe that new, switched OTCs saved them trips to the doctor.

Self-medication and seeking out a health care professional are not mutually exclusive. In fact, both approaches are increasing in frequency. Apparently, as their awareness grows, consumers place more reliance on physicians, as well as OTCs. For physicians, OTCs may often serve to screen out those patients with minor, self-treatable conditions, and free up valuable practice time for conditions that do require professional attention.

Some over-the-counter products actually encourage consumers to seek medical care. The greater availability of self-diagnostic and self-monitoring products, for example, serve to increase office visits by alerting patients to the need for a doctor's attention.

Finally, the impact of OTCs on physicians' practices in the future may be even greater under managed care programs. Capitated reimbursement systems, in which providers are reimbursed per enrollee, encourage practitioners to contain costs, reduce unnecessary services, and write fewer and less costly prescriptions. Under managed care, therefore, self-medication may be seen as an important component of cost-containment.

OTCs and Pharmacists

Year after year in national Gallup polls, consumers vote pharmacists the most trusted professional. It's not surprising that 98 percent of pharmacists say their customers generally or always follow their advice on OTCs and purchase the products they recommend.

Pharmacists are also the most accessible health care provider for consumers, and many prefer buying

Figure 2

Product Categories Causing Confusion Among Consumers

Product Category	*% of pharmacists asked for recommendation*	*Average number of recommendations per month*
Allergy relief products	99.5	28.0
Adult cough medications	99.5	31.2
Adult cold preparations	99.0	28.3
Antidiarrheals	98.5	14.5
Stool softeners/ other laxatives	98.5	13.6
Sinus remedies	98.1	25.4
Children's cough medications	98.1	24.5
Ibuprofens	98.0	22.5
Antacids	98.0	16.4
Vitamins, adult	97.0	15.8
Throat lozenges	94.6	15.6
Athlete's foot remedies	94.5	8.1
Children's cold preparations	94.4	22.9
Canker/cold sore remedies	91.1	7.7
Hemorrhoidal preparations	90.7	8.0
Topical anti-infectives	88.6	14.8
Acetaminophens	88.3	24.5
Naproxen sodium products	88.3	12.7
Eyedrops	88.0	9.4
Aspirins	88.0	14.0
Bulk laxatives	87.9	8.7
Flu remedies	87.0	15.8
Poison ivy treatments	86.4	10.6
Throat sprays	85.7	10.6
Blood glucose monitors	85.1	6.6
Jock itch remedies	84.3	4.6
Sleep aids	84.0	6.5
Wart removers	83.7	3.8
Vitamins, children's	83.5	9.8
Vaginal antifungals	83.1	7.8
Suntan/sunscreen products	78.5	8.7

Source: Rosendahl, I. "OTC Recommendations By Pharmacists Hit New High," *Drug Topics,* suppl., September, 1995.

their OTCs in a pharmacy because a pharmacist is on hand to provide counseling. There are, for instance, over three-quarters of a million OTC outlets, and only about 10 percent of these are pharmacies. Yet, about 45 percent of all the nation's OTCs are bought in drugstores. Consumers clearly go out of their way to purchase OTCs in a pharmacy.

Consumers often rely on their pharmacist to provide counseling on an OTC until they can make an appointment with a physician, and nearly all pharmacists report that patients occasionally or frequently come to them for OTC advice as an alternative to consulting their physician. In fact, patient counseling by pharmacists is a growing practice. In one recent study, pharmacists were shown to have made an average of 450 more OTC recommendations than they had in the previous year. In 1994, the number of OTC consultations per pharmacist reached 7,781—or almost 846 million per year nationwide—and the level is still rising. In 1995, over half (55 percent) of all pharmacists polled said that they were providing more OTC counseling. In addition, consumers ask pharmacists for help with every category of OTC product. Figure 2 ranks the percentage of pharmacists who were asked to make a product recommendation in that category. It also shows the average number of recommendations made per month.

OTCs are a crucial element in pharmacy practice. About 30 percent of pharmacy revenues come from OTC sales, and for chain drugstores the number is even higher. In addition, pharmacy owners who report expanding OTC sales cite pharmacist counseling as the number one reason for the increase.

With the rise of interest in pharmaceutical care, in which pharmacists are part of a health care team that plans, implements, and monitors patient care, some pharmacists today receive reimbursement for the time they spend counseling a patient. And many pharmacy plans provide financial incentives to pharmacists who encourage use of less expensive Rx or OTC medications. All of these factors may work to encourage OTC counseling by pharmacists in the near future, and may certainly change the way they dispense medications.

Figure 3

What Physicians Want to Know About OTCs

Physicians indicate that they often need more information about an OTC before making a recommendation to their patients. These categories were ranked as most important.

Type of Information	*% of Physicians*
Side effects, contraindications, symptoms and treatment of overdose	89
Clinical data from an independent source	77
Dosing, directions for use, how supplied	73
Direct comparison to similar products	50
Patient acceptance, compliance	41
Unique physical characteristics	41
Consumer pricing information	37
Reputation of company marketing the product	30
Unique packaging features	19
Clinical data from manufacturer	15
Differences in consumer and professional labeling	9
Type of consumer promotion and support	7
Market share data	2

Source: Griffie, K.G. "How Healthcare Providers Influence Drug Use," Kline & Co., Fairfield, NJ 1993.

Counseling Obstacles

Despite the increase in OTC use, and in patient counseling, studies show that consumers do not always receive the help they need from their health care providers. Physicians, constrained by time and the amount of other information that must be exchanged during a phone consultation or office visit, may neglect to discuss the OTCs their patients use.

Pharmacists also face busy schedules, and studies show that they cite time constraints as the main barrier to OTC counseling. Other obstacles for pharmacists include lack of reimbursement for counseling services, a need for more education on OTCs, and the absence of a physical area that provides privacy. Pharmacists report that insufficient staff and lack of management support are further disincentives for counseling.

Poor communication skills on the part of physicians and pharmacists may also impede effective patient counseling. The following elements of good communication can enhance the counseling process:

■ Listen to patients, ask them for details and clarification, and repeat their answers to confirm your understanding.
■ Assess the knowledge level of your patient. This process can often uncover special problems, such as a reading disability.
■ Use nontechnical terms with patients, and ask them to repeat the instructions you've given them.
■ Provide clearly-written instructions whenever possible. Oral instructions are often quickly forgotten.
■ Stay up-to-date on OTC products, and use current reference books, journals, product information from manufacturers, and other necessary sources, for the most recent and complete information. (Physicians and pharmacists both indicate that they would like to know more about the OTC products they recommend for their patients. Figure 3, for example, shows the percentage of doctors who seek more information on particular OTC topics.)

Finally, one useful aspect of patient counseling is often underused by pharmacists and physicians alike. This is the practice of recommending a companion OTC when a prescription is written or dispensed. Despite the benefits that companion OTCs can provide a patient, half of all pharmacists say they never recommend them. Many nonprescription drugs, however, can help control side effects and improve the efficacy of Rx drugs. Companion OTC recommendations also provide a useful service to patients, help build loyalty, encourage communication, and, for pharmacies, boost OTC sales. (Figure 4 shows which categories of OTC drugs can be helpful with which categories of Rx drugs.)

Figure 4

OTC Companions

OTCs are often overlooked for the relief they can bring from Rx drug side effects, or the added effectiveness they can bring to prescription drugs. Some examples are:

OTC Category	*Prescription Drug Category*
Antacids	Gastrointestinal drugs
Antacids	Glucocorticoids
Diabetes testing products and supplies	Antidiabetics
Anti-infective agents	Antifungals
Laxatives and vitamins	Cholesterol-lowering drugs
Antacids and analgesics	Rx analgesics
Analgesics	Cardiovascular drugs

Sources

IMS America. National Disease and Therapeutic Index, 1990.

Temin, P. Realized benefits from switching drugs. *J. Law Econ.* (25)2, 1992.

Gannon K. Pharmacists step up level of counseling on OTCs. *Drug Topics,* September 20, 1993.

Cardinale V. Pharmacists as OTC Counselors, *Drug Topics* (suppl.). 1994.

Gannon K. What do patient want to know about OTCs? *Drug Topics,* August 21, 1989

Epstein D. More counseling called for in medicating the illiterate. *Drug Topics,* November, 1988.

Rosendahl, I. OTC recommendations by pharmacists hit new high. *Drug Topics,* suppl., September, 1995.

Schering Laboratories. *What's Right with Pharmacy.* The Schering Report VII, Kenilworth, New Jersey.

Griffie K.G. *How Healthcare Providers Influence Drug Use.* Kline & Co., Fairfield, New Jersey, 1993.